Contraceptive Technology

Contraceptive Technology

Twenty-first Edition

Robert A. Hatcher, MD, MPH
Anita L. Nelson, MD
James Trussell, PhD
Carrie Cwiak, MD, MPH
Patty Cason, MS, FNP-BC
Michael S. Policar, MD, MPH
Alison B. Edelman, MD, MPH
Abigail R.A. Aiken, MD, MPH, PhD
Jeanne M. Marrazzo, MD, MPH, FACP, FIDSA
Deborah Kowal, MA, PA

Find us at www.contraceptivetechnology.com
Follow us on @ContraceptTech

AYER COMPANY PUBLISHERS, INC.
New York, NY
2018

Distributed by:
Managing Contraception LLC
Atlanta, GA

For all orders (including bulk purchase discounts) please visit the website contraceptivetechnology21st.com. You may also contact us by email info@contraceptivetechnology21st.com, by phone 404 875 5001, by fax 404 875 5030 and by mail:
Contraceptive Technology 21st
PO Box 79299 Atlanta, GA 30357.

Note to book sellers: All returns require written permission.

ISBN 978-1-7320556-0-5 (paperback)
ISBN 978-1-7320556-1-2 (hardback)
ISBN 978-1-7320556-2-9 (eBook)
ISBN 978-1-7320556-3-6 (bundle)

3 5 7 9 10 6 4 2

The paper used in this publication meets the minimum requirements of American National Standard for Information Sciences — Permanence of Paper for Printed Library Materials, ANSI Z39.48-1984. Printed in USA.

DISCLAIMER

The information contained herein is intended to be used by physicians and other qualified healthcare professionals. The information is not intended to be used for medical diagnosis or treatment by persons who are not qualified healthcare professionals. Such persons should not rely upon or use the information contained herein in place of a visit, call, or consultation with, or the advice of their personal physician or other qualified healthcare provider.

Physicians and other qualified healthcare professionals should recognize that this book is to be used only as a reference aid, and that this book is not intended to be a substitute for their exercise of professional judgment. Since medical science is always changing, physicians and other qualified healthcare professionals users are advised to confirm the information contained herein with an independent source. The authors and reviewers are not liable for errors and omissions.

Suggested full citation
Hatcher RA, Nelson AL, Trussell J, Cwiak C, Cason P, Policar MS, Edelman A, Aiken ARA, Marrazzo J, Kowal D, eds. Contraceptive technology. 21st ed. New York, NY: Ayer Company Publishers, Inc., 2018.

Dedication

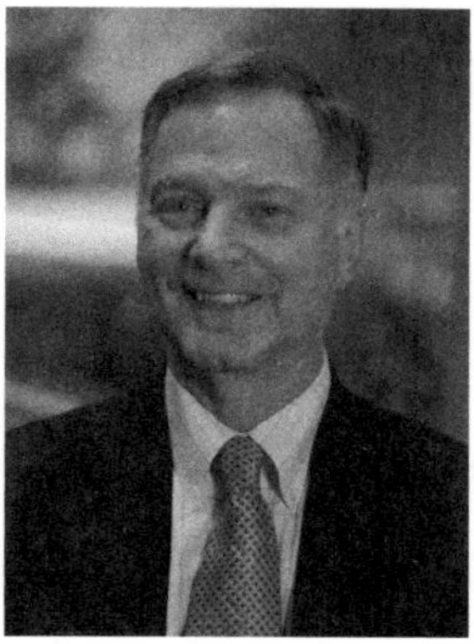

Willard (Ward) Cates, Jr.
1942–2016

Contraceptive Technology contributor since 1978 (9th edition)

We are deeply grateful for Ward's unending inspiration and his decades of mentoring us (his co-authors) and two generations of trainees in family planning and STD/HIV prevention.

"The world has lost one of its champions of public health and a pioneer researcher in the fields of HIV/AIDS and women's reproductive health."
— *The News & Observer / Raleigh, NC*

"Ward's energy, wisdom, love, and smiles encouraged us all. He was constantly looking for the best in people. His constructive, thoughtful cheerleading helped each person to be the best that he or she could be."
— Robert A. Hatcher, founding and lead author of *Contraceptive Technology*

"My first meeting with Ward Cates is cemented in my mind. I saw myself as a lowly research fellow, so I couldn't believe how excited he was to talk to me about my work. Later I realized he saw that value in all who cared about people's health and ways to improve it. He is irreplaceable."
— Jeanne Marrazzo, Ward's chosen successor as a *Contraceptive Technology* editor

"With his lifelong commitment to women's health and well-being, it is so fitting that Ward had two daughters—or "baby women," as he called them. He also crafted endearing nicknames for family and friends alike . . ."
—Ward's family, Joan (Bunsie), Deborah (Bootsie) and Sarah (Saysie)

Note to Readers:

Words Matter

Words we use have power, and their use can affect our thoughts and actions toward someone else. The authors of *Contraceptive Technology* endeavor to use words that encourage a collaborative and nonjudgmental partnership between provider and patient. Within the limitations of the English language and currently accepted grammar, we endeavor to use generic words that respect the patients we serve, equitably regardless of their gender identification, sexual orientation, ability, race, ethnicity, religion, or income. (Words that label gender or sexual preference, race/ethnicity, or other characteristics have been maintained when citing studies and documents.)

Preface

The true meaning of life is to plant trees under whose shade you do not expect to sit.
—Nelson Henderson

The seed that led to *Contraceptive Technology* was planted 50 years ago by Beech Conger, MD, when he said, "Hatcher, if you believe so much in birth control, why don't you have an outline to provide to medical students?" So in 1970, I gave Emory medical students mimeographed pages of that outline, and in 1971, I distributed the first bound edition of *Contraceptive Technology*, all twenty pages of it. From this sapling grew the 21 editions of *Contraceptive Technology*, now grown to a book of about 1,000 pages with 85 contributors performing the work of authoring, editing, and reviewing. It has been an exciting opportunity for me to watch the *Contraceptive Technology* tree grow from the small sapling I started more than 45 years ago.

Since 1970, *Contraceptive Technology* has told the remarkable story of reversible contraceptives, permanent contraception, the termination of unwanted pregnancies through safe legal abortions, the dramatic fall in teenage pregnancies, and the provision of emergency contraception pills or copper intrauterine devices following unprotected intercourse.

From the beginning, the book explored evidence on the safety and effectiveness of each of the available contraceptives. By the 16th edition (1998), we stopped using the word "contraindication," turning instead to a more accurate and nuanced approach to weighing the risks and benefits for any given contraceptive user. We now incorporate the Centers for Disease Control's *Medical Eligibility Criteria (MEC)* as the way to help clinicians, counselors, and clients understand the medical advisability of each of the contraceptive options for clients who may have any of the hundreds of medical conditions listed in the MEC.

In addition to bringing readers the improved process for helping clients select appropriate contraceptive methods, the authors of *Contraceptive Technology* describe different ways for effectively starting users on pills, injections, implants, and IUDs. This important task has evolved from complicated recommendations to just two words: *start today* or *quick start* method. Study after study has demonstrated that a delay in providing patients the method they want decreases the likelihood that they will ever initiate that method.

Contraceptive Technology has long addressed the problem of the 500,000 to 1 million pill users who become pregnant each year. It simply is not simple to take a pill every day, sometimes having to take it at the same time every day. Studies show that providing 13 cycles of pills makes pill use more effective. But for a number of reasons, providing 13 cycles at a time has not become the norm here in United States or worldwide. Further, the extended cycle pattern for taking pills is more effective than monthly cycling, but there has not been widespread provision of extended-cycle pills. Despite these and other strategies to improve pill use, the strategies simply have not been implemented often enough to lower failures. So the discouragingly high 5% to 10% typical-use failure rates of pills persist.

Because of the high typical-use failure rate of pills—and of patches, rings, and condoms—the authors of *Contraceptive Technology* encourage increasing access to long-acting reversible contraceptives (LARC methods). IUDs and implants are the most effective reversible contraceptives. Here are several conclusions that have evolved regarding LARC methods:

- They are very effective. More effective than permanent contraception in some studies.
- Generally, data have shown that LARC methods are effective for *more* years than they labeled to be effective.
- Long-acting reversible methods (IUDs and implants) may be used by almost everyone. There are very few conditions that strongly suggest that LARC methods be avoided.
- LARC methods lead to fewer serious complications than estrogenic contraceptives (pills, patches, or rings).
- Continuation rates of IUDs and implants are higher than continuation rates of other reversible methods.
- Patient satisfaction with LARC methods exceeds patient satisfaction with shorter-term contraceptives.

Among the important things providers of contraceptives have learned is that contraceptives offer so much more than just contraception. These "noncontraceptive benefits" include reducing dysmenorrhea and menstrual blood loss, offering first-line treatment for endometriosis, and preventing some types of cancer. Perhaps if we had started out calling oral contraceptive pills "the ovarian and endometrial cancer prevention pills," or if we had stressed that randomized controlled studies have demonstrated that the most effective outpatient approaches to both heavy menstrual bleeding and endometriosis is the levonorgestrel IUD, we would have had less opposition to our marvelous contraceptives.

Contraceptive Technology has focused on sensitive patient-centered communication. From Fifi Guest, an author of several editions, came an excellent counseling recommendation: Avoid using the word "should." We don't want our clients, she quipped, leaving the office saying to themselves: "Don't should all over me." Another outstanding piece of advice from Erica Monasterio, RN, MN, FNP: "If yours is the voice you hear most in your ear, it is not client-centered counseling."

Other "branches" to our *Contraceptive Technology* tree are our national conferences on the East Coast, West Coast, and in Atlanta, where our speakers present up-to-date evidence on reproductive health clinical practices. About 1,200 attendees conferences attend annually, as they have over the past 30 years. I hope the Contraceptive Technology conferences and book will long continue to grow and contribute to the process of informing providers on how to offer evidence-based and client-centered contraceptive services. Many of the superb clinicians who speak at our annual Contraceptive Technology conferences and author chapters of this book were trained in the family planning fellowship program[1] and the Ryan Program,[2] started by Phil Darney, MD, MSC, and Uta Landy, PhD. We would like to give a special thank you to them. They have trained hundreds of the field's leaders.

In addition, we authors of *Contraceptive Technology* thank each of you serving the reproductive health needs of people in our country and around the world. If it were not for you, the remarkable contraceptives and other reproductive health services described in this book would not be available today. Because of you, we can be certain that availability of high-quality voluntary contraceptive and abortion services will continue into the future. You are our "she-roes" and heroes. Thank you for your caring and your competence.

—Robert A. Hatcher, MD, MPH

[1]For more information, see www.familyplanningfellowship.org

[2]For more information, see http://bixbycenter.ucsf.edu/education-and-training

Table of Contents

List of Tables

List of Figures

List of Boxes

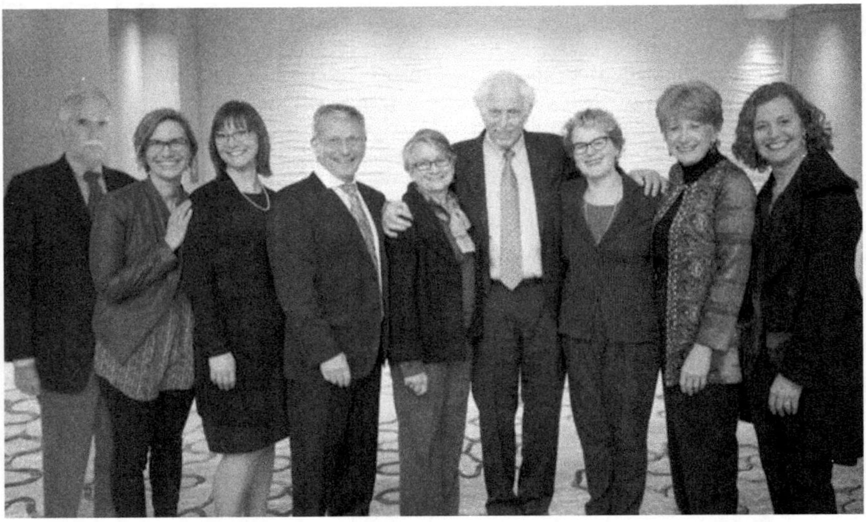

From left to right: James Trussell, Alison Edelman, Carrie Cwiak, Michael Policar, Deborah Kowal, Robert Hatcher, Jeanne Marrazzo, Anita Nelson, Patty Cason (not pictured, Abigail Aiken)

Editors

Robert A. Hatcher, MD, MPH
Professor Emeritus
Department of Gynecology and Obstetrics
Emory University School of Medicine
Atlanta, Georgia

Anita L. Nelson, MD
Professor Emeritus
Department of Obstetrics and Gynecology, David Geffen School of Medicine at UCLA
Clinical Professor, Obstetrics and Gynecology, University of Southern California
Professor and Chair, Obstetrics and Gynecology, Western University of Health Sciences
San Francisco, California

James Trussell, PhD
Office of Population Research
Charles and Marie Robertson Professor of Public and International Affairs, Emeritus
Princeton University
Princeton, New Jersey
Honorary Fellow
Edinburgh University
Edinburgh, Scotland

Carrie Cwiak, MD, MPH
Professor
Director, Division of Family Planning
Department of Gynecology and Obstetrics
Emory University School of Medicine
Atlanta, Georgia

Patty Cason, MS, FNP-BC
Assistant Clinical Professor
UCLA School of Nursing
Nurse Practitioner and Consultant
Envision SRH
Los Angeles, California

Michael S. Policar, MD, MPH
Professor Emeritus
Department of Obstetrics, Gynecology, and Reproductive Sciences
University of California San Francisco School of Medicine
San Francisco, California

Alison B. Edelman, MD, MPH
Professor
Director, Family Planning Fellowship
Department of Obstetrics and Gynecology
Oregon Health & Science University
Portland, Oregon

Abigail R.A. Aiken, MD, MPH, PhD
Assistant Professor
LBJ School of Public Affairs
Faculty Associate
Population Research Center
University of Texas, Austin
Austin, Texas

Jeanne M. Marrazzo, MD, MPH, FACP, FIDSA
Professor
Director, Division of Infectious Diseases
C. Glenn Cobbs, MD, Endowed Professor in Infectious Diseases
University of Alabama at Birmingham School of Medicine
Birmingham, Alabama

Deborah Kowal, MA, PA
CEO and President
Contraceptive Technology Communications, Inc.
Consultant, Maternal and Child Health Communications
Atlanta, Georgia

Authors

Abigail R.A. Aiken, MD, MPH, PhD
Assistant Professor
LBJ School of Public Affairs
Faculty Associate
Population Research Center
University of Texas, Austin

Rebecca H. Allen, MD, MPH
Associate Professor
Department of Obstetrics and Gynecology and Medical Science (Section of Medical Education)
The Warren Alpert Medical School of Brown University
Women & Infants Hospital of Rhode Island

Maureen K. Baldwin, MD, MPH
Assistant Professor
Department of Obstetrics and Gynecology, Family Planning Section
Oregon Health & Science University

Deborah Bartz, MD, MPH
Assistant Professor
Harvard Medical School
Associate Medical Director, Family Planning Clinic
Brigham and Women's Hospital

Amanda Black, MD, MPH
Professor
Department of Obstetrics and Gynecology, The Ottawa Hospital
Division of Pediatric and Adolescent Gynecology, Children's Hospital of Eastern Ontario
Medical Director, Shirley E. Greenberg Women's Health Centre
University of Ottawa

Anne E. Burke, MD, MPH
Associate Professor
Director, Division of Family Planning
Department of Gynecology and Obstetrics
Johns Hopkins University School of Medicine
Department of Population, Family, and Reproductive Health
Johns Hopkins Bloomberg School of Public Health

Patty Cason, MS, FNP-BC
Assistant Clinical Professor
UCLA School of Nursing
Nurse Practitioner and Consultant
Envision SRH

Kelly Cleland, MPA, MPH
Office of Population Research
Princeton University
Director, American Society for Emergency Contraception

Carrie Cwiak, MD, MPH
Professor
Director, Division of Family Planning
Department of Gynecology and Obstetrics
Emory University School of Medicine

Gillian Dean, MD, MPH
Senior Director, Medical Services
Planned Parenthood Federation of America

Alison B. Edelman, MD, MPH
Professor
Director, Family Planning Fellowship
Department of Obstetrics and Gynecology
Oregon Health & Science University

Crystal Goldsmith, MD, MSc
Director of Family Planning
Kaiser Permanente, East Bay, Oakland, CA

Jaclyn Grentzer, MD, MSCI
Associate Physician
Division of Family Planning
Women's Health Services
Kaiser Permanente Orange County

Stephanie Grilo, MA
Department of Sociomedical Sciences
Columbia University Mailman School of Public Health

Daniel Grossman, MD
Professor
Director, Advancing New Standards in Reproductive Health (ANSIRH)
Bixby Center for Global Reproductive Health
Department of Obstetrics, Gynecology and Reproductive Sciences
University of California, San Francisco

Kate A. Guthrie, FRCOG, FFSRH
Former Consultant and Clinical Director, Sexual and Reproductive Health
City Health Care Partnership CIC
Kingston Upon Hull, England

Kelli Stidham Hall, PhD, MS, FNP
Assistant Professor
Department of Behavioral Sciences & Health Education, Rollins School of Public Health
Department of Obstetrics & Gynecology, School of Medicine
Emory University

Leo Han, MD, MPH
Assistant Professor, Obstetrics and Gynecology
Oregon Health & Science University

Bryna Harwood, MD, MS
Director, Residency Program
Director, Division of Gynecologic Specialties
Department of Obstetrics and Gynecology
Cedars-Sinai Medical Center
Associate Professor,
David Geffen School of Medicine at UCLA

Jenny A. Higgins, PhD, MPH
Associate Professor
Department of Gender and Women's Studies
Department of Obstetrics and Gynecology
University of Wisconsin

Melody Y. Hou, MD, MPH, FACOG
Associate Professor
Division of Family Planning
Department of Obstetrics and Gynecology
University of California, Davis School of Medicine

Victoria H. Jennings, Ph.D.
Professor
Department of Obstetrics and Gynecology
Director, Institute for Reproductive Health
Georgetown University Medical Center

Rachel K. Jones, PhD
Principal Research Scientist
Guttmacher Institute

Kathy Irene Kennedy, DrPH, MA
Clinical Professor
Director, Maternal and Child Health
Colorado School of Public Health
University of Colorado Anschutz Medical Campus

Melissa Kottke, MD, MPH, MBA
Associate Professor
Director, Jane Fonda Center
Department of Gynecology and Obstetrics
Emory University School of Medicine

Jeanne M. Marrazzo, MD, MPH
Professor
Director, Division of Infectious Diseases
C. Glenn Cobbs, MD, Endowed Professor in Infectious Diseases
University of Alabama at Birmingham School of Medicine

Elizabeth Micks, MD, MPH
Assistant Professor
Department of Obstetrics and Gynecology
University of Washington

Kavita Nanda, MD, MHS
Director of Medical Research
Contraceptive Technology Innovation Department
Global Health, Population, and Nutrition
FHI360

Anita L. Nelson, MD
Professor Emeritus
Department of Obstetrics and Gynecology, David Geffen School of Medicine at UCLA
Clinical Professor, Obstetrics and Gynecology, University of Southern California
Professor and Chair, Obstetrics and Gynecology, Western University of Health Sciences

Brian Nguyen, MD, MSCP
Assistant Professor, Obstetrics & Gynecology
University of Southern California

Siripanth Nippita, MD, MS
Instructor
Department of Obstetrics, Gynecology, and Reproductive Biology
Harvard Medical School & Beth Israel Deaconess Medical Center

Ina U. Park, MD, MS
Associate Professor
Department of Family and Community Medicine
University of California San Francisco, School of Medicine
Medical Consultant,
Division of STD Prevention
Centers for Disease Control and Prevention

Maureen Paul, MD, MPH
Associate Professor
Department of Obstetrics,
Gynecology & Reproductive
Biology
Harvard Medical School
Director, Family Planning Division
Beth Israel Deaconess Medical
Center

Michael S. Policar, MD, MPH
Professsor Emeritus
Department of Obstetrics,
Gynecology, and Reproductive
Sciences
University of California San
Francisco School of Medicine

Chelsea B. Polis, PhD
Senior Research Scientist
Guttmacher Institute
Associate, Department of
Epidemiology
Johns Hopkins Bloomberg School
of Public Health

Elizabeth G. Raymond, MD, MPH
Senior Medical Associate
Gynuity Health Projects

Danielle Roncari, MD, MPH
Director of Family Planning, Tufts
Medical Center
Assistant Professor
Department of Obstetrics and
Gynecology
Tufts University School of
Medicine

John S. Santelli, MD, MPH
Professor
Departments of Population and
Family Health and Pediatrics
Columbia University

George F. Sawaya, MD
Professor
Department of Obstetrics,
Gynecology and Reproductive
Sciences
Epidemiology & Biostatistics.
University of California San
Francisco, School of Medicine

Eleanor Bimla Schwarz, MD, MS
Professor of Medicine
Division of General Internal
Medicine
University of California, Davis

Lee P. Shulman, MD
The Anna Ross Lapham Professor
Department of Obstetrics and
Gynecology
Chief, Division of Clinical Genetics
Feinberg School of Medicine of
Northwestern University
Chicago, Illinois

Diana Crabtree Sokol, MD
Clinical Instructor
Fellow, Family Planning
Department of Obstetrics and
Gynecology
University of Southern California

Julia R. Steinberg, PhD, MA
Assistant Professor
Department of Family Science
School of Public Health
University of Maryland,
College Park

Markus J. Steiner, PhD, MSPH
Senior Epidemiologist
Contraceptive Technology
Innovation Department
FHI 360

James Trussell, PhD
Office of Population Research
Charles and Marie Robertson Professor of Public and International Affairs, Emeritus
Princeton University
Princeton, New Jersey
Honorary Fellow
Edinburgh University
Edinburgh, Scotland

Lee Warner, PhD, MPH
Chief, Women's Health and Fertility Branch
Division of Reproductive Health
Centers for Disease Control and Prevention

Wan-Ju Wu, MD, MPH
Family Planning Fellow
Harvard Medical School

Reviewers

Pamela D. Berens, MD
Professor & Vice Chair of Clinical Affairs
Department of Obstetrics & Gynecology
University of Texas Health Science Center at Houston

Kelly Blanchard, MSc
President
Ibis Reproductive Health

Janet Bruno-Gaston, MD
Fellow in Reproductive Endocrinology and Infertility
Baylor College of Medicine
Department of Obstetrics and Gynecology

Maya Bunik, MD, MSPH
Professor
Department of Pediatrics
School of Medicine, University of Colorado Anschutz Medical Campus
Children's Hospital Colorado

Lisa Callegari, MD, MPH
Assistant Professor
Department of Obstetrics & Gynecology
University of Washington School of Medicine
Investigator, VA Health Services Research & Development

Angela Chen, MD, MPH
Associate Clinical Professor of Health Sciences
Fellowship Director, Division of Family Planning
David Geffen School of Medicine, UCLA

Melissa J. Chen, MD, MPH
Assistant Professor
Department of Obstetrics and Gynecology
University of California, Davis

Rebecca H. Cohen, MD
Assistant Professor
Division of Family Planning
Department of Obstetrics and Gynecology
University of Colorado Anschutz Medical Campus

Kaitlin Crawford, MPH
MD Candidate, 2019
University of California, Davis

Kelly R. Culwell, MD, MPH
Chief Medical Officer
WCG and Evofem Biosciences
Volunteer Clinical Faculty, Department of Reproductive Medicine
University of California, San Diego School of Medicine

Christine Dehlendorf, MD, MAS
Associate Professor
Director, Program in Woman-Centered Contraception
Department of Family & Community Medicine, UCSF

J. Dennis Fortenberry, MD, MS
Professor
Department of Pediatrics
Donald Orr MD Professor of Adolescent Medicine
Chief, Division of Adolescent Medicine
Indiana University School of Medicine

Liza Fuentes, DrPH
Senior Research Scientist
Research Division
Guttmacher Institute

Maria F. Gallo, PhD
Associate Professor
College of Public Health Division of Epidemiology
The Ohio State University

Aileen Gariepy, MD, MPH, FACOG
Assistant Professor
Department of Obstetrics, Gynecology, and Reproductive Sciences
Assistant Clinical Professor of Nursing

Laura Greenberg, MD
Reproductive Endocrinologist
Synergy Women's Healthcare

Sadia Haider, MD, MPH
Chief, Section of Family Planning and Contraceptive Research
Director, Fellowship in Family Planning
Associate Professor of Obstetrics and Gynecology
University of Chicago

Sarah Hardman, MBChB, MFSRH, DipGUM
Specialty Doctor, Sexual and Reproductive Health, Chalmers Centre, Edinburgh
Co-Director, Clinical Effectiveness Unit, Faculty of Sexual and Reproductive Healthcare

Nathalie Kapp, MD, MPH
Associate Medical Director
Ipas

Andrew M. Kaunitz, MD, FACOG, NCMP
University of Florida Research Foundation Professor and Associate Chairman
Department of Obstetrics and Gynecology
University of Florida College of Medicine-Jacksonville
Medical Director and Director of Menopause and Gynecologic Ultrasound Services
UF Women's Health Specialists-Emerson

Joan Kraft, PhD
Senior Health Scientist, Field Support Branch
Division of Reproductive Health
Centers for Disease Control and Prevention

Catherine M. Leclair, MD
Professor
Head, Division of General Obstetrics & Gynecology
Director, Program in Vulvar Health
Oregon Health & Science University

E. Steve Lichtenberg, MD, MPH
Professor
Department of Clinical Obstetrics and Gynecology
Northwestern University Feinberg School of Medicine
Medical Director, Family Planning Associates Medical Group, Limited

Sheila Marcus, MD
Clinical Professor
Section Chief, Child and Adolescent Psychiatry
Department of Psychiatry
University of Michigan

Isaac Maddow-Zimet, MS
Senior Research Associate
Research Division
Guttmacher Institute

Alan S. McNeilly, DSc, FRSB, FRSE
Honorary Professor
MRC Centre for Reproductive Health
Queen's Medical Research Institute
University of Edinburgh

Melissa Natavio, MD, MPH
Director, Family Planning Fellowship Program
Chief, Section of Family Planning
Assistant Professor
Department of Obstetrics and Gynecology
Keck School of Medicine of USC
University of Southern California

Robert Reid, MD, FRCSC
Professor
Department of Obstetrics and Gynecology
Head, Reproductive Endocrinology and Infertility
C.A.R.E. Fellowship Director
Queens University, Kingston, Canada

Maria I. Rodriguez, MD, MPH
Assistant Professor
Department of Obstetrics and Gynecology
Oregon Health & Science University

Jessica Sales, PhD
Associate Professor
Department of Behavioral Sciences and Health Education
Emory University

Jessica N. Sanders, PhD, MSPH
Family Planning Research Director
Division of Family Planning
Research Assistant Professor, Department of Obstetrics and Gynecology
University of Utah

Natasha Schimmoeller, MD, MPH, MA
Clinical Fellow, Family Planning
Department of Obstetrics and Gynecology
University of California, Davis

Salma Shabaik, MD
Medical Director & Clinical Assistant Professor
Physician Assistant Program
College of Science and Health
Charles R. Drew University of Medicine and Science

Katherine M. Stone, MD
Consultant
Tucson, AR

Phillip G. Stubblefield, MD
Emeritus Professor
Department of Obstetrics and Gynecology
Boston University School of Medicine

Hong-Thao Thieu, MD
Associate Professor
Department of Obstetrics and Gynecology
Assistant Fellowship Director, Pediatric and Adolescent Gynecology
Tufts University School of Medicine

David Turok, MD, MPH
Director, Division of Family Planning
Department of Obstetrics and Gynecology
University of Utah

Rachel Peragallo Urrutia, MD, MS
Clinical Assistant Professor
Department of Obstetrics and Gynecology
Division of General Obstetrics and Gynecology
University of North Carolina
Chapel Hill

Contraceptive Technology

Menstrual Cycle: Normal Patterns, Menstrual Disorders, and Menstrually-Related Problems

1

Anita L. Nelson, MD
Lee Shulman, MD

- The purpose of menstrual cycling is to achieve pregnancy.
- The menstrual cycle is the vital sign of a woman's* reproductive system.
- The normal menstrual cycle results from a complex orchestration of both stimulatory and inhibitory factors involving the hypothalamic-pituitary-ovarian axis and the uterus.
- The ovarian cycle is composed of three phases: the follicular phase, the LH surge, and the luteal phase.
- The endometrial cycle includes three phases: the proliferative phase, the secretory phase and menstrual sloughing.
- Abnormal uterine bleeding patterns include primary and secondary amenorrhea, infrequent bleeding, and heavy or prolonged bleeding as well as intermenstrual, postcoital and postmenopausal bleeding.
- Menstrually related problems, such as dysmenorrhea, premenstrual syndrome (PMS), premenstrual dysphoric disorder (PMDD), and catamenial exacerbations of medical problems, are quite common.

*It should be noted that in this chapter, the person who is experiencing menstrual cycling may be referred to as a "woman" and feminine pronouns may be used, in general and in reporting findings of studies that identify subjects as "women." The authors recognized that there are other people (such as transgender men) who might be cycling and may well need to be evaluated for menstrual abnormalities and for other problems described in this chapter. (See Chapter 22 on Sexuality & Contraception.) We beg the readers' indulgences for our shorthand and urge all involved in the care of our rich variety of patients to recognize the need to individualize the information provided here to the patient sitting in front of them.

The menstrual cycle results from a hormonal cascade coordinated among three separate organ systems: the brain, the ovaries, and the uterus. How the major roles of each of these organ systems were identified has been one of the more interesting detective stories in reproductive medicine, but many of the details are still being unraveled. This chapter outlines normal menstrual physiology, with a discussion of the individual contributions of each reproductive organ in establishing and maintaining normal menstrual cycling. Against the backdrop of normal cycling, the pathophysiology, diagnosis, and treatments for a wide range of abnormal menstrual patterns are reviewed. Finally, the chapter summarizes problems that are caused by or, at least, exacerbated by the hormonal changes that give rise to menstrual cycling.

ASSESSING THE MENSTRUAL CYCLE

The menstrual cycle is the vital sign of a woman's* reproductive health. As such, it should be assessed at every visit between menarche and menopause. The facts that are important to assess include the date of the last menses, the frequency of menses, cycle duration, and volume of blood lost. If possible, some estimate of cycle-to-cycle variability over 6 months can complete the description of the bleeding itself (See Table 1-1), but related issues such as dysmenorrhea and other menstrual problems should also be included in the history.

At the initial visit, information about age at menarche and obstetrical history provides a framework within which to evaluate reproductive health. Routine menstrual history is often absent from the medical records of non-gynecologic visits. Even when patients are being admitted to the hospital for profound anemia, clinicians often fail to inquire about menses.[2,3] This shortcut can easily result in lost opportunities for healthful interventions or, in other cases, can result in undiagnosed pregnancies.

When obtaining a menstrual history, avoid checkbox options. Ask very concrete questions. Self-characterizations of flow and cycling can be very misleading. A person who routinely bleeds for 10 to 12 days a month may check "normal" on the form because that pattern is all that she has ever known. Ask: When was the first day of your last period? The first day of the period before that? How many days do you usually flow? Do you ever have spotting or bleeding when you are not on your period? On your heaviest flow day, how many sanitary pads/internal protection products/etc. do you use? Do you ever have to change your protection or empty your menstrual cups more frequently than every two hours? Do you ever have staining or other accidents because you are not able to contain your flow? Box 1-1 provides information about frequently used reusable menstrual products. Also ask, what are your menstrual cramps like? Do you take any medication to control the pain? How much does

Table 1-1 Menstrual bleeding terminology and normal limits for menstrual parameters in mid-reproductive years

Category	Days (past 6 months)	Normal or Abnormal	✓
Frequency	Every □ □ □ days	Absent (no periods or bleeding) = amenorrhea Frequent (<24 days) Normal (24–38 Days) Infrequent (>38 days)	
Duration	Shortest: □ □ days Longest: □ □ days	Short (<4.5 days) Normal (4.5–8 days) Prolonged (>8 days)	
Regularity	Shortest: □ □ days Longest: □ □ days	Regular variation (shortest to longest ≤9 days) Irregular (shortest to longest 10+ days)	
Flow volume	As determined by the patient – based on her assessment of the impact on her quality of life	Heavy (>80 mL, if measured) Normal (5–79 mL, if measured) Light (<5 mL, if measured)	
Intermenstrual Bleeding (IMB) Bleeding Between Cyclically Regular Onset of Menses, without hormones	None Random Cyclic (Predictable)	Early Cycle Mid Cycle Late Cycle	
Unscheduled Bleeding on Hormone Medication (e.g., oral contraceptive pills, rings, or patches)	Not applicable (not on hormone medication) None (on hormone medication) Present		

Source: Modified from Munro MG, et al. (2017)[1]

it help you? What other problems do you have around the time of your period? It is also important to ask about contraceptive method use, which often can profoundly impact bleeding and risk for unintended pregnancy.[4] Encourage each reproductive-age woman to record menstrual cycles. Three top free menstrual cycle tracking apps were recently identified based on their accuracy and special features. Alphabetically they include: Clue, Glow, and Pink Pad Period Tracker Pro.[5] (For more information, see the Appendix on Digital Resources for Health and Medical Information.)

Compare the patient's bleeding patterns to normal values (5th-95th percentile) from the International Federation of Gynecology and Obstetrics (FIGO) displayed on Table 1-1. These FIGO values are generally accepted, with the exception that some authorities still define the normal cycle length to be 21 to 35 days.

Age has a strong influence on bleeding patterns. Recently menarcheal individuals (within 18 to 24 months of the first menses) and those who

Box 1-1 Re-useable Menstrual Products

Reusable Menstrual Cups
Many are concerned about the environmental impacts of used sanitary protection products, as well as their costs. New reusable products are now available.

DivaCup is one of the more popular brands and is available commercially. It is a conically shaped silicone cup that comes in two sizes (one for women <30 who have never delivered a pregnancy vaginally or have delivered only by Cesarean section and one for women ≥30 and those who have delivered a pregnancy). Some women complain that the DivaCup it is a little rigid, and blood may spill with removal. Women can learn more about this product by going to the website, www.divacup.com.

There are dozens of products with similar designs including Intimina lily cup, Ruby cup, Lunette cup, etc. Each has its own website.

Femmy Cycle is a softer silicone product that can be ordered online after the correct size has been determined. Those who are young, small, or who have never been pregnant should use the teen size. Most will use a regular size, especially if they have had Cesarean delivery. Those who have mild pelvic relaxation (a patient can touch her cervix after the second knuckle of the examining finger passes into the vagina) will use a low cervix model. Femmy Cycle is clear, easy to clean, and has a lip that helps prevent spillage when it is inverted during Placement, use and removal and also provides for easy emptying when it is everted after removal. The best website for information on this product is www.femmycycle.com.

Disposable Cups
There also are disposable menstrual cups that collect (not absorb) the menstrual flow. These are available in many commercial outlets alongside more standard absorbing products. Spillage with removal has been reported by users, but the advantage they report over products that absorb menstrual fluids is that users still have their own vaginal lubrication and do not have a detectable aroma. Users report that they use these cups to have intercourse during their menses.

are perimenopausal have the greatest variability in cycle-to-cycle length. Menstrual cycles are most predictable among those in their mid-to-late 30's. Most of the variability in ovulatory cycle length of occurs in the length of the follicular phase.

Abnormal bleeding patterns are discussed in more detail below, but first we will explore the elements that control menstrual cycling.

Overview of the Menstrual Cycle

The purpose of the menstrual cycle is to establish pregnancy. While much attention is paid to the ovaries and the uterus in describing the menstrual cycle, the control of that cycle actually rests in the brain. The hypothalamus and pituitary stimulate the ovaries to prepare a dominant follicle for ovulation, to enable release of that egg, and to produce the hormones needed at different times in the cycle to heal the lining of the uterus, to facilitate fertilization, to prepare the uterine lining for implantation, and to sustain the early pregnancy until it can become hormonally self-sufficient. If a pregnancy does not implant, the ovarian cycle ends, hormone levels fall, and menstrual sloughing occurs to clean up after the failed cycle. The body then prepares for the next cycle.

The ovaries are not passive, silent partners in this process. They are integrally linked in the hypothalamic-pituitary-ovarian (HPO) axis that controls hormonal production during the menstrual cycle. In response to the hypothalamic-pituitary stimulation, the ovaries make hormones and other proteins that are in turn closely monitored by the brain. This close monitoring allows the brain to adjust the signals it sends to the ovaries at different phases of the cycle to enable pregnancy. It is by hacking into this monitoring system that hormonal contraceptives can prevent ovulation. See Applications in Every Day Practice, below.

What are these signals? In brief, it can be said that—

- The hypothalamus uses gonadotropin releasing hormone (GnRH) to stimulate the pituitary.
- The pituitary uses two hormones to stimulate the ovaries in different ways at different times in the cycle:
  - — Follicle stimulating hormone (FSH) stimulates the final step in the production of estradiol (E_2) by the ovaries.
  - — Luteinizing hormone (LH) stimulates the ovary to produce both androgens and progesterone.
- Estradiol made by the follicles in the ovary causes the endometrial cells to proliferate (divide) before ovulation. It also thins cervical mucus at the time of the LH surge to facilitate sperm transport into the uterus and fallopian tubes.

Box 1-2 Highlights of Menstrual Cycle

- At the end of the previous cycle, the levels of estrogen, progesterone, and inhibins fell.
- The lack of negative feedback from the ovaries causes release of FSH and LH from the pituitary.
- A cohort of follicles, recruited in the ovaries, matures to produce estradiol and inhibin B.
- One dominant follicle emerges and, with the LH surge, extrudes its oocyte (ovulation), ready for fertilization.
- The residua of the dominant follicle collapses and transforms into a corpus luteum, which produces progesterone and estrogen to promote implantation and support the early pregnancy.
- If no implantation occurs, hormone levels fall, the endometrial lining sloughs, and a new menstrual cycle starts.

- Progesterone made by the corpus luteum formed in the ovary after ovulation causes the endometrial cells to hypertrophy (plump up) and prepare for implantation.

Principles of negative feedback

It is helpful to view the cycle from the perspective of each of the elements involved—the brain, the ovaries and the endometrium. But to understand how the HPO axis works, one must first understand the principle of negative feedback.

Negative feedback is the process involved in most endocrine systems to maintain normal circulating levels of hormones. When circulating levels of the hormone are low, the brain stimulates the end organ (thyroid, ovary, adrenal gland) to produce more of the needed hormone.

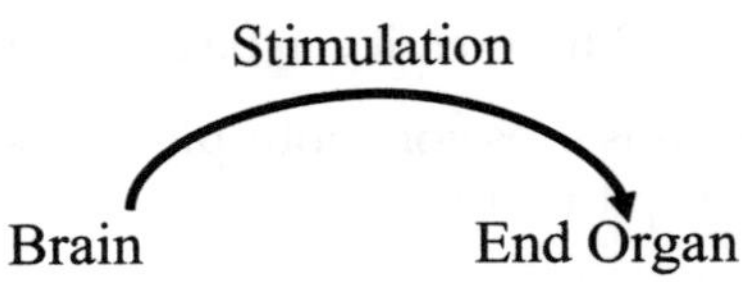

Figure 1-1 Stimulation phase of negative feedback

When the end organ responds, the hormone products made by the end organ are detected by the brain.

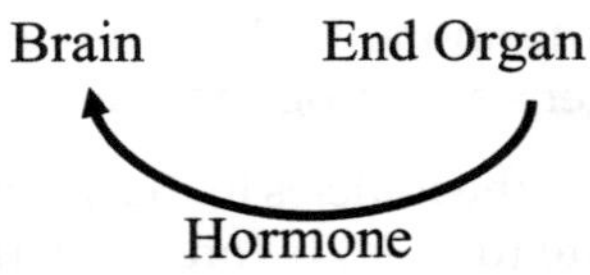

Figure 1-2 Braking phase of negative feedback

When hormone levels in circulation rise toward normal ranges, brain stimulation slows so less additional hormone is produced.

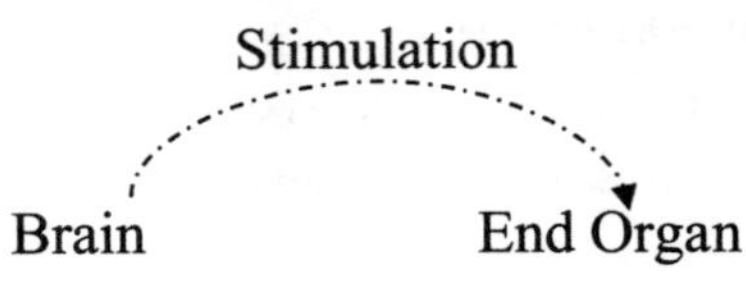

Figure 1-3 Reduced stimulation as result of negative feedback

When hormone levels are too high, all stimulation ceases. This process is called **negative feedback** because presence of the hormone controls future orders for its production. The lack of the hormone (the absence of negative feedback) induces increased stimulation from the brain to promote more production of the hormone by the end organ. This negative feedback system provides a way to administer synthetic hormones to interfere with cycling and to control fertility. (See Applications in Everyday Practice, below.)

The Menstrual Cycle in More Detail

Role of the Brain (Hypothalamus and Pituitary) in the Menstrual Cycle

The roles of each of the organs involved in the menstrual cycle are summarized diagrammatically in Figure 1-4 Regulation of the Menstrual Cycle.

The following sections will describe their actions in greater detail.

In the face of the extreme fluctuations in hormone levels throughout the cycle, questions arise. What are the target levels? What levels are too low and require greater stimulation? What levels are too high and require less stimulation? How does the pituitary know how much FSH and LH to release at any time?

The direct answer is that the hypothalamus controls how much FSH and LH the pituitary synthesizes and releases at every point in the cycle in response to the negative feedback it gets from the ovary. The hypothalamus releases GnRH in *pulses* that vary over the cycle in both frequency and amplitude. The response of the pituitary to these pulses of GnRH (how much FSH and LH it releases) depends not only on how often the GnRH signals come, but how strong they are and how much negative feedback the pituitary is getting from the ovary. For example, slow GnRH pulses increase FSH and decrease LH release when negative feedback is low. Rapid frequency, high amplitude GnRH pulses in the presence of high levels of estrogen cause high FSH and LH releases that enable both the LH surge and ovulation. This pulsatility provides another way to artificially interfere with the menstrual cycle to control fertility. (See Applications in Everyday Practice, below.)

The more complicated answer is that the hypothalamus itself is influenced not only by all of the hormones and proteins produced by the ovary, but also by neurotransmitters such as dopamine, endorphins, gamma-aminobutyric acid (GABA), and neuroendocrine factors. Other diverse factors such as leptin from peripheral fat cells and even sleep can affect GnRH release factors. Abnormalities in these factors are known to contribute to menstrual disorders and potentially to diminish fertility.

Ovarian Phases of the Menstrual Cycle

From the ovarian perspective, there are three major phases in the menstrual cycle: the follicular phase, the LH surge, and the luteal phase.

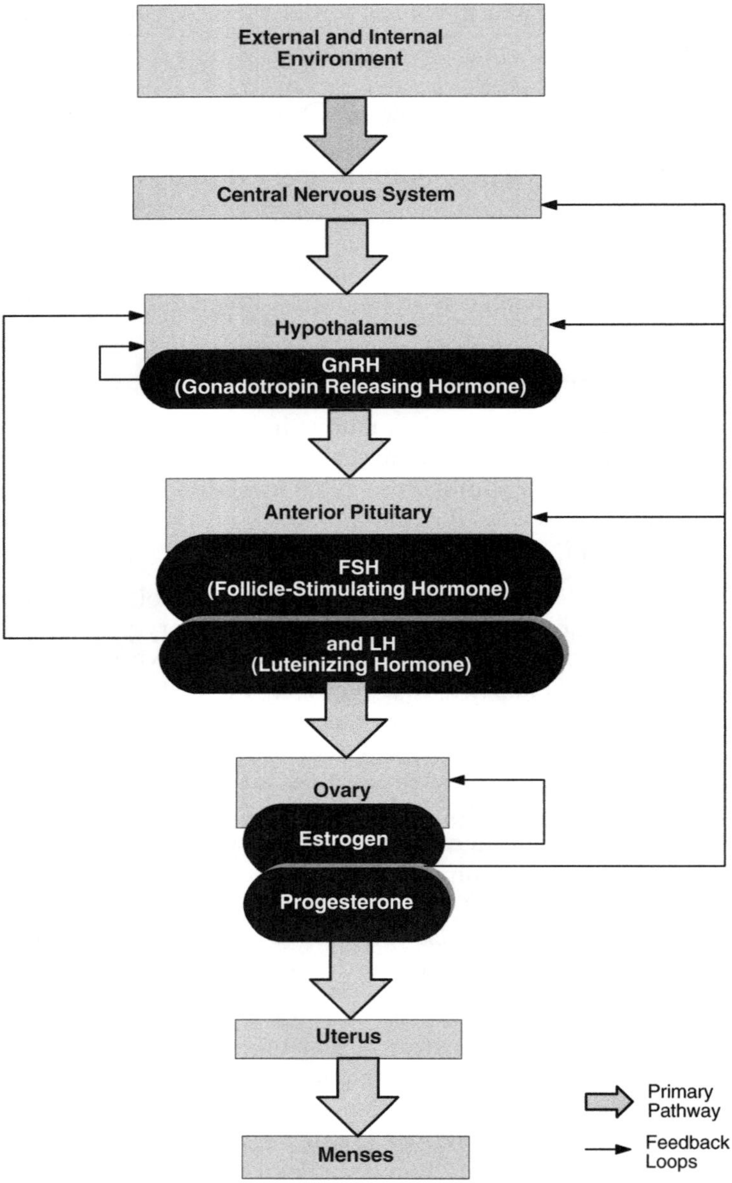

Primary hormone pathways (⇨) in the reproductive system are modulated by both negative and positive feedback loops (→). Prostaglandins, secreted by the ovary and by uterine endometrial cells, also play a role in ovulation, and may modulate hypothalamic function as well.

Figure 1-4 Regulation of the menstrual cycle

Table 1-2 GnRH pulse frequencies and amplitudes throughout the menstrual cycle

- Follicular phase: 90-100 minutes
- Mid-follicular: 60 minutes (amplitude attenuated)
- Late follicular: amplitude increases
- Midcycle: amplitude and frequency increase:
  - LH increases 10-fold
  - FSH increases 4-fold
- Luteal phase: amplitude higher, frequency decreases (Q4 hours)
- Premenstrually: frequency increases to 90 minutes
  - FSH levels rise

Follicular phase. The follicular phase starts on the first day of menses and ends around midcycle, on the day of the LH surge. Stimulation of the ovary starts with the involution of the corpus luteum in the prior cycle when estrogen and progesterone levels decline, which leads to menstruation. With the loss of negative feedback from the ovary, the pituitary increases its release of FSH and LH.

In the face of increasing FSH and LH levels, cohorts of small follicles measuring only millimeters in diameter are recruited in both ovaries. These tiny follicles are surrounded by two thin layers of cells with very limited numbers of receptors on them. The outer layer of cells are the theca cells. (See Figure 1-5.) In the follicular phase (see Figure 1-6), LH stimulates the theca cells to convert cholesterol into androgens. Some of these androgens escape into the general circulation, but many drift towards the inner circle of granulosa cells. When granulosa cells are stimulated by FSH, they aromatize those androgens into estradiol (E_2). FSH also stimulates the granulosa cells in the follicles to produce other important proteins such as inhibin B, activin, and folliculostatin. And importantly, FSH stimulates each granulosa cell to make more receptors on its surface for FSH.

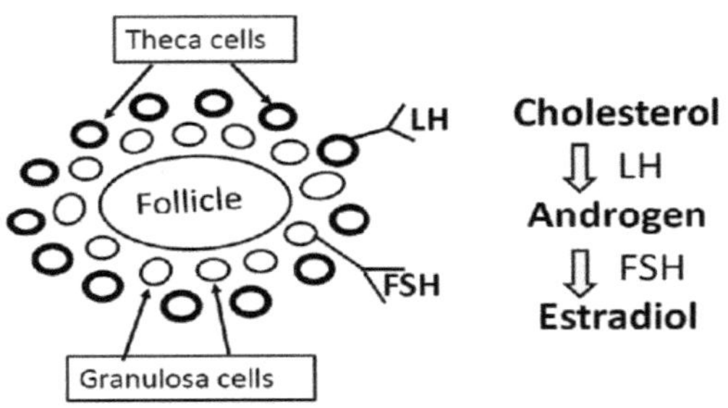

Figure 1-5 The two cell theory of ovarian steroid production

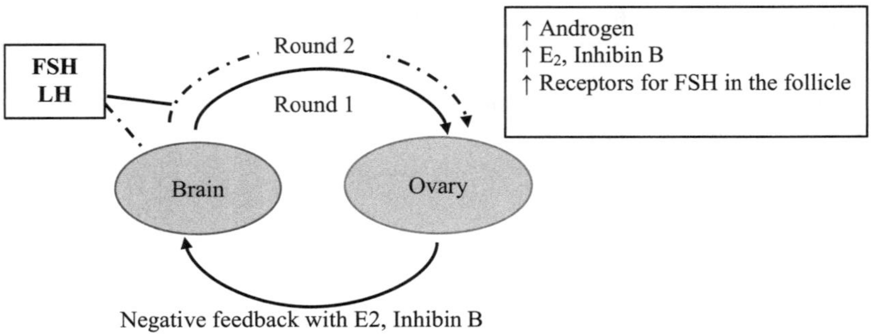

First	FSH stimulates ovarian production and release of E2 and inhibin B (Round 1).
Then	Some of the E2 and inhibin B is transported to the hypothalamus and pituitary, which respond by decreasing subsequent release of FSH (Round 2).

Figure 1-6 Negative feedback in the HPO axis during the *follicular phase*

The estradiol and inhibin B are released into the systemic circulation and are transported to the hypothalamus and pituitary as negative feedback, which determines the subsequent release of gonadotropins to stimulate further ovarian production of hormones.

How is it that only one of the follicles ovulates? What happens to all the other follicles that were recruited? Why is it that humans usually have singleton pregnancies and not litters of offspring? Again, the answer is negative feedback. Near the end of the follicular phase, there are dozens

Box 1-3 A Deeper Dive: Factors that Influence Ovarian Response to Pituitary Stimulation

- Some of the polypeptides from the granulosa cells contribute to the ovaries' negative feedback to the brain, while others modulate that feedback. As mentioned, estradiol and inhibin B provide the main negative feedback to the brain in the follicular phase. Progesterone and inhibin A perform a similar function in the luteal phase. On the other hand, activin stimulates FSH release from the anterior pituitary and increases the FSH activity in the ovaries. Follistatin mutes the effects of activin.
- Other peptide hormones and neuroendocrine factors also influence the hormonal production and the downstream effects of inhibin.
- Even systemic factors can influence the balance between androgen and estrogen production within the ovarian follicles. For example, insulin-like growth factor 1 (IGF-1) and insulin itself can amplify thecal cell response to LH. This results in overproduction of androgens and tips the androgen/estrogen balance within the follicle, creating androgen excess conditions, such as can be seen in some phenotypes of polycystic ovary syndrome (PCOS).

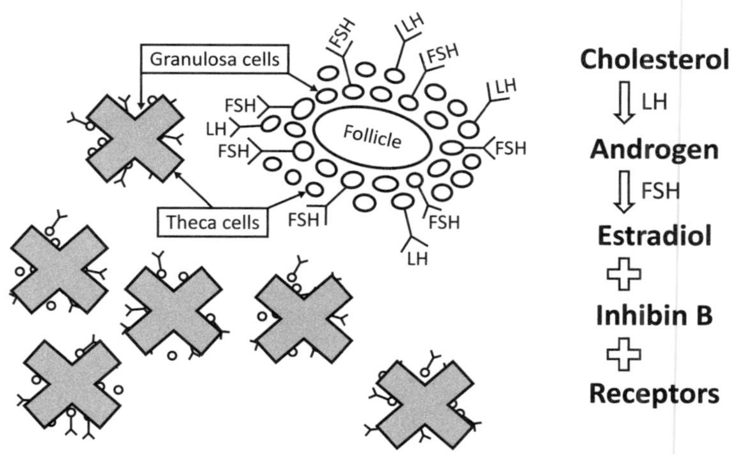

Figure 1-7 Emergence of the dominant follicle – atresia of all other follicles

of follicles in various stages of development with great differences in the numbers of receptors they possess for FSH. But every single follicle contributes to ever-increasing levels of circulating estradiol and inhibin B. As large amounts of E_2 and inhibin B enter into circulation, they provide very strong negative feedback to the hypothalamus and pituitary. The high levels of E_2 and inhibin force the pituitary to profoundly curtail LH and FSH release. With very little FSH and LH reaching the ovaries, only the follicle with the greatest number of receptors on its theca and granulosa cells is able to survive this gonadotropin drought. (See Figure 1-7.) All the other follicles undergo atrophy and stop producing estradiol and inhibin B.

The loss of all those smaller follicles causes a drop in E_2 and inhibin B, which is quickly detected by the brain. This drop in E_2 and inhibin B (the absence of negative feedback) induces the pituitary to release high levels of FSH and LH.

The sudden outpouring of FSH and LH triggers the *LH surge* by mechanisms that are not entirely delineated. One hypothesis is that the dominant follicle produces high levels of estrogen and low levels of progesterone in response to the rapid FSH rise. Once estradiol levels have been sustained at high levels (200pg/mL) for at least 50 hours, a *positive feedback* system is briefly established, replacing the negative feedback system. The LH surge starts, which marks the end of the follicular phase.

The LH surge at midcycle ends with ovulation in a successful cycle. To enable the final steps preparing the oocyte for ovulation, the hypothalamic-pituitary-ovarian axis switches, as noted, from a negative feedback system

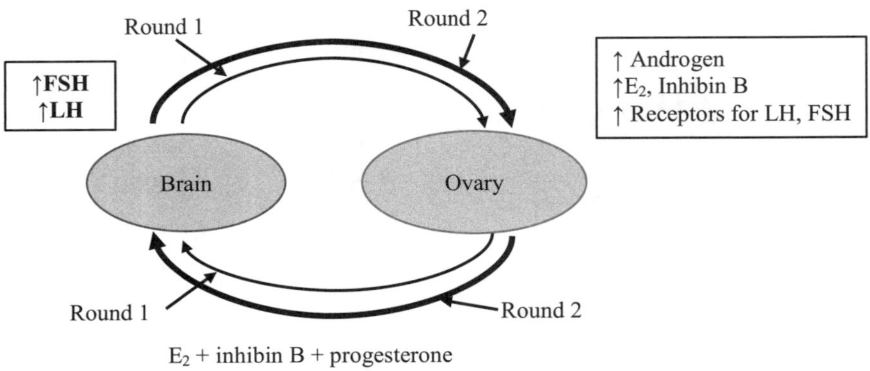

Figure 1-8 Positive feedback during the LH surge

to one based on positive feedback. This is a unusual system that could potentially spiral out of control. Estradiol and inhibin B from the ovaries prompt increased release of LH and FSH from the pituitary. In round after round, increasing levels of ovarian hormones trigger the pituitary to release even more LH to stimulate the ovary to produce even more hormones. (See Figure 1-8.)

The LH surge lasts for approximately 36 to 44 hours, after which negative feedback promptly takes over again. If local factors, such as prostaglandin activity, proteolytic enzymes, and contractile activity in the dominant follicle permit, then in about 10 to 12 hours after the LH peak, the follicle will rupture and the oocyte, covered by cumulus oophorous, will be extruded from the follicle (ovulation).

What has been going on inside the oocyte during this time? By the time of ovulation, the original oocyte has completed meiosis I. This means that it first created a large secondary oocyte, containing all the parent cell's cytoplasm and one full set of chromosomes. A smaller first polar body containing only the DNA from the second set of chromosomes was extruded. The large secondary oocyte then started into meiosis II. But that meiosis II was arrested in metaphase—at a time when the chromosomes were lined up and connected by spindle apparatus. If fertilization occurs in the next 12 to 24 hours, the oocyte will complete meiosis II and thereby create a haploid ovum that can be fertilized by a haploid sperm; a second small polar body with the DNA of the other haploid set of chromosomes will be extruded from the oocyte. If no fertilization occurs, the oocyte will degenerate, arrested in metaphase of meiosis II.

Luteal phase. A day after the LH surge, the ovaries enter the luteal phase. The remnant of the previous dominant follicle collapses and is converted into a corpus luteum. The corpus luteum is a temporary endocrine structure that produces relatively high levels of progesterone along with moderate levels of estrogen and inhibin A. Its yellow color derives from carotenoids in the diet. It grows to 2 to 5 cm in diameter. Within this corpus luteum, the former granulosa cells become *granulosa lutein cells* that produce estrogen, progesterone, and inhibin A. The former theca cells transform into *theca lutein cells* that make androgens and progesterone.

The corpus luteum will undergo apoptosis (programmed cell death) in 10 days and form a *corpus albicans* unless βhCG produced by cells in an implanted blastocyst are available to prolong its functional life. If no pregnancy occurs, then the corpus luteum undergoes that involution, and levels of estrogen, progesterone and inhibin A all plummet. This loss of hormones eliminates negative feedback from the ovaries to the hypothalamus and the pituitary and kick starts the next menstrual cycle.

Endometrial Phases of the Menstrual Cycle

The endometrium is the major target for hormones produced by the ovaries, but the myometrium and the endocervical cells also respond to those same hormonal signals and contribute to fertility. From the endometrial perspective, there are three phases of the menstrual cycle: the proliferative phase, the secretory phase and menstrual sloughing phase.

Proliferative phase. At the beginning of the proliferative phase, the endometrium is denuded. Many factors are involved in endometrial repair, including those that are classically involved in wound healing, such as macrophages and inflammatory agents. For complete functional healing, hormonal influences are particularly critical.[6,7] The endometrial cells in the basal layer (the cells close to the myometrium that were not shed in menses) rapidly proliferate under the influence of estradiol. Small glands form with narrow lumens. The stroma surrounding those glands proliferates and new vessels arise to perfuse this area, leading to thickening of the endometrial layer. Estrogen also stimulates the development of mitochondria, ribosomes, and other organelles within the glandular endometrial cells to provide energy. Estrogen also induces the formation of more receptors for estrogen and progesterone on the endometrial cells.

Secretory phase. Following ovulation and under the influence of progesterone, cellular proliferation in the endometrium ceases because progesterone down-regulates the estrogen receptors on the endometrial cells. The endometrial cells in the secretory phase undergo a series of distinctive changes that are so predictable that histologically, the endometrium can accurately be dated (which cycle day it is). First, each of the glandular cells hypertrophies (enlarges). The endometrium becomes even thicker. Glycogen vacuoles form within the glandular cells and are released into the endometrial cavity around cycle day 20 or 21, when the blastocyst would be expected to arrive into that cavity needing energy. A series of specific receptors develops on the endometrial cells, which help promote their receptivity to implantation. Progesterone quiets the myometrial cells so that they will not contract to expel the newly implanted blastocyst. The spiral arteries serving the endometrial cells increase greatly in number and caliber and become quite convoluted.

Menstrual phase. When the corpus luteum involutes, the endometrium undergoes its own *premenstrual involution*. The spiral arteries in the basal layer spasm shut, cutting off blood supply to the cells in the superficial functional layer of the endometrium. This induces ischemia distal to that vascular occlusion. Matrix metalloproteinase enzymes layered along the junction between the basal and functional layers of the endometrium are activated and start dissolving the connections between those two layers. Leukocytes infiltrate the area. The proximal portions of the spiral arteries relax and the blood that flows from them propels the necrotic material away from the uterine walls. The myometrium, which had been quieted by progesterone in the secretory phase, now contracts to help expel the waste products. This is what the individual sees as menstrual bleeding. To stop menstrual bleeding, blood flow from spiral arteries must be halted. Control over the spiral arteries is strongly influenced by local inflammatory factors, the ratio of local prostaglandins ($PGF_{2\alpha}$/PGE2) as well as the stability of the fibrin clots that form inside these vessels (see below). Once again, repair of the endometrium involves transforming growth factors and downstream intracellular transcription factors as well as estrogen-stimulated proliferation.[8]

Even before the menstrual bleeding starts, the follicular phase of ovarian function of the next cycle is already underway.

Applications in Everyday Practice

How does understanding the menstrual cycle help explain menstrual disorders or the mechanisms of action of hormonal contraceptive methods, or other therapies frequently used in women's health care? Here are some interesting ways that specific features of the menstrual cycle have been used therapeutically.

The pulsatility of GnRH stimulation of the pituitary can be masked by administering chronic high doses of a long-acting GnRH agonist, like Lupron, used to treat estrogen-dependent conditions such as endometriosis. Long-acting GnRH agonists flood the pituitary and make it impossible for it to detect the pulsatile messages from the hypothalamus. The pituitary ultimately stops responding; FSH and LH release is halted. Without FSH, the ovaries make no estrogen; the woman goes into pseudomenopause with hot flashes, dry vagina, and bone loss. But instead of the high FSH levels and low E_2 levels seen in natural menopause, treated women will have low FSH and low E_2 levels.

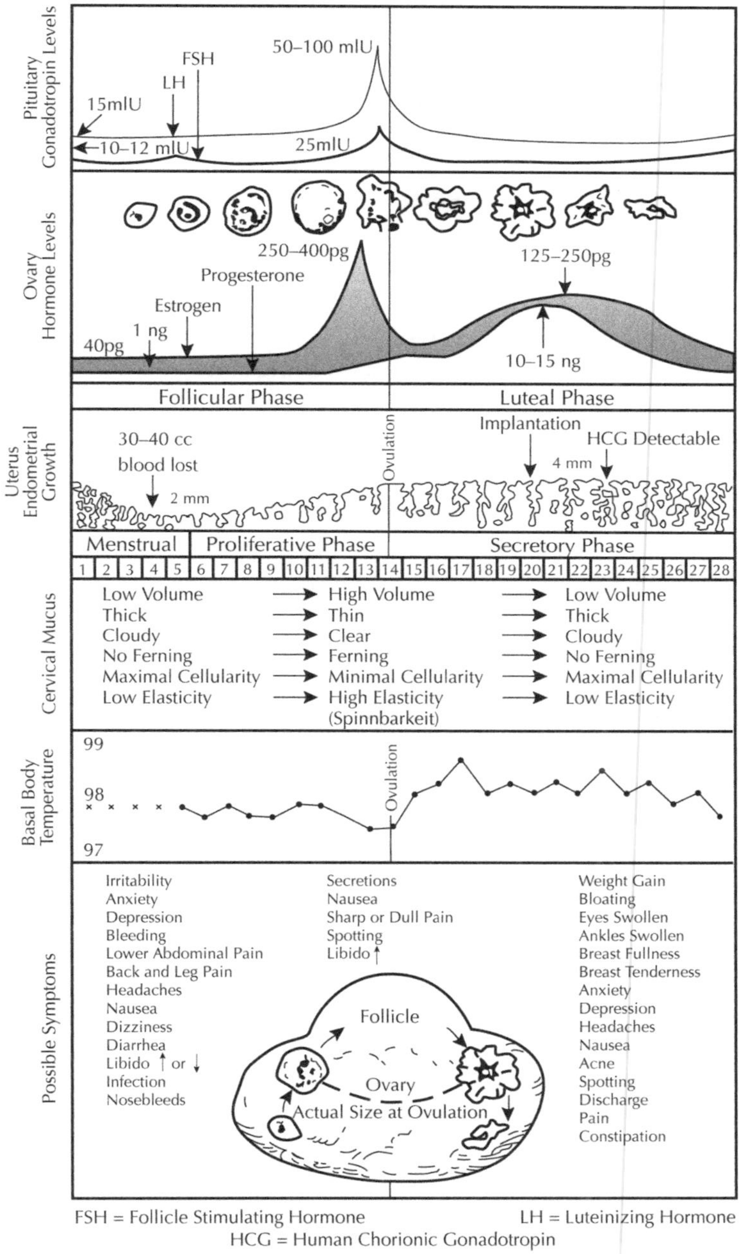

Figure 1-9 Comprehensive summary of menstrual cycle events

The negative feedback from the ovary to the hypothalamus and pituitary is key to how hormonal contraceptives block ovulation. The brain does not distinguish between estradiol and progesterone produced endogenously and synthetic estrogen and progestin derived from exogenous contraceptive agents. When pharmacologic doses of the synthetic hormones enter the circulation and reach the brain, the hypothalamus and pituitary detect their high levels and stop releasing FSH and LH. This halts ovarian follicular development and prevents the LH surge and ovulation.

The fact that the ovary uses two products – both estradiol and inhibin B – as messengers in the negative feedback loop to the brain means that in menopause we cannot rely on FSH levels to indicate that the dose of hormones we prescribed are adequate as we might rely on normalization of TSH levels to tell us levothyroxine doses were adequate. We have to rely on the patient's clinical response.

The fact that the hypothalamus is affected by an array of neurotransmitters and other factors described above can help explain why stress, obesity, and medications can disrupt ovulatory cycling.

The fact that the follicles within the ovary can be influenced by local imbalances between androgens and estrogens, or by high levels of insulin, can help explain the problems seen in many cases of PCOS.

The fact that progesterone down-regulates estrogen receptors on the endometrial cells can help explain the unscheduled spotting and amenorrhea that is often seen with progestin-only methods such as the levonorgestrel intrauterine device (LNG IUD) or depot medroxyprogesterone acetate (DMPA). The endometrial cells cannot detect the patient's estradiol, so no proliferation (healing) takes place and no endometrium builds up to be sloughed. The lack of high levels of estrogen at the time of ovulation also means that the cervical mucus never becomes thin and copious to trap the sperm and provide safe passage into the upper track. Instead the cervical mucus remains thick and impermeable to sperm penetration throughout the cycle.

As you read through the method chapters, try to relate the mechanisms of action of the methods back to what you know about the menstrual cycle. Also see if understanding these details can help you anticipate and explain the bleeding patterns observed with the different methods.

MENSTRUAL DISORDERS

TERMINOLOGY FOR ABNORMAL UTERINE BLEEDING

Many of the older terms used to describe menstrual irregularities were confusing and imprecise. For example, "menorrhagia" could mean heavy or prolonged bleeding or both. "Polymenorrhagia," and "oligomenorrhea" similarly had several possible interpretations, and the term "dysfunctional uterine bleeding" had no consistent definition at all.[9] The well-defined English terms listed in Table 1-1 have now replaced those imprecise, older terms. Some of the older terms that were sufficiently specific have been retained; these include "amenorrhea," "postcoital bleeding," "intermenstrual bleeding," and "postmenopausal bleeding." Together these terms are used to convey clearly the exact nature of each woman's menstrual experience. For example, if bleeding occurs every 40 days for 10 days and blood loss totals 60 mL of blood, we would describe it as infrequent, prolonged, with normal flow. While you are developing a differential diagnosis for abnormal bleeding and devising a plan to determine its underlying cause, use these terms in the assessment section of the initial visit note.

Once the etiology of abnormal bleeding has been identified, the assessment section in the record at the next visit would again list the pattern of abnormal uterine bleeding using the Table 1-1 terms. This entry would then be followed by short-hand documentation of the etiologies identified to explain nongestational abnormal uterine bleeding (AUB) using the FIGO PALM-COEIN classification system (see Figure 1-10).[4,10]

The PALM portion of the PALM-COEIN system refers to *structural or anatomical causes* of abnormal uterine bleeding, including **P**olyps, **A**denomyosis, **L**eiomyoma and **M**alignancy/hyperplasia. Leiomyoma are sub-classified by their position relative to the myometrium.[1] The COEIN portion of the rubric is used to describe *functional disorders* that may be causing abnormal uterine bleeding, including **C**oagulopathies, **O**vulatory dysfunctions, **E**ndometrial dysfunctions, **I**atrogenic causes and causes that are **N**ot otherwise classified. For example, if abnormal uterine bleeding is excessive because the patient's blood will not clot due to genetic factors or hematologic problems (von Willebrand disease), it would be categorized as AUB-C. If the bleeding is excessive because of anticoagulant use, it would be categorized as AUB-I. Abnormal bleeding due to obesity,

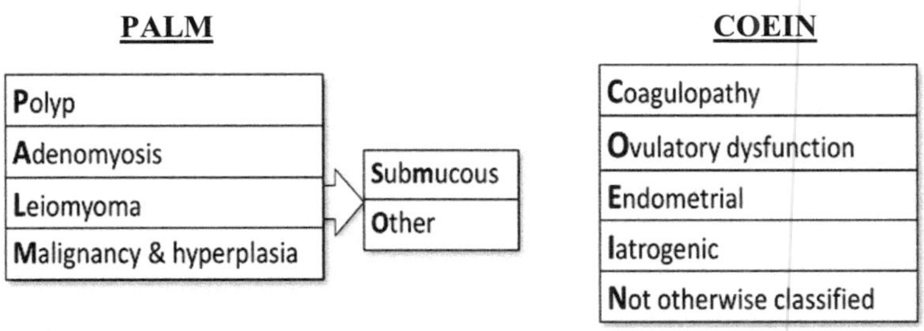

Source: Munro MG, et al. (2017),1 with permission

Figure 1-10 PALM-COEIN classification system for abnormal nongestational uterine bleeding

PCOS, or hypothyroidism interfering with ovulation would be charted as AUB-O. The category AUB-E is appropriate for many cases of lifelong idiopathic heavy menstrual bleeding due to endometrial prostaglandin imbalances described below.

Amenorrhea Overview

The most common causes of amenorrhea are pregnancy, lactation, menopause, and contraceptive use. However, for about 3% to 4% of those with amenorrhea, the cause is different. The majority of these patients have premature ovarian insufficiency or an extreme version of one of three other conditions: PCOS, hyperprolactinemia, or functional hypothalamic amenorrhea (FHA). Accounting for the remaining cases is an exhaustive list of uncommon genetic, anatomic, and enzymatic abnormalities.[11,12] See Table 1-3 for a summary of the major causes of amenorrhea—both primary and secondary.

Patients who never experience menstruation are more likely to have uncommon etiologies than are those who stop bleeding after menarche,

Table 1-3 Major causes of amenorrhea

Overflow tract	Pituitary	Hypothalamic	Other endocrine gland disorders
Congenital	Autoimmune disease	Eating disorder	Adrenal disease
Complete androgen resistance	Cocaine	Functional (overall energy deficit)	Adult-onset adrenal hyperplasia
Imperforate hymen	Cushing syndrome	Gonadotropin deficiency (e.g., Kallmann syndrome)	Androgen-secreting tumor
Müllerian agenesis	Empty sella syndrome	Infection (e.g., meningitis, tuberculosis syphilis),	Chronic disease
Transverse vaginal septum	Hyperprolactinemia	Malabsorption	Constitutional delay of puberty
Acquired	Infiltrative disease (e.g., sarcoidosis)	Rapid weight loss (any cause)	Cushing syndrome
Asherman syndrome (intrauterine synechiae)	Medications	Stress	Ovarian tumors (androgen producing)
Cervical stenosis	Antidepressants	Traumatic brain injury	Polycystic ovary syndrome (multifactorial)
	Antihistamines	Tumor	Thyroid disease
Primary ovarian insufficiency	Antihypertensives		
Congenital	Antipsychotics		**Physiologic**
Gonadal dysgenesis (other than Turner syndrome)	Opiates		Breastfeeding
Turner syndrome or variant	Other pituitary or central nervous system tumor		Contraception
Acquired	Prolactinoma		Exogenous androgens
Autoimmune destruction	Sheehan syndrome		Menopause
Chemotherapy or radiation			Pregnancy

Source: Klein DA, et al. (2013),[12] with permission

but the causes for both primary and secondary amenorrhea are often similar. Reproductive endocrinologists have persuasively argued that the distinction between primary amenorrhea (no menarche) or secondary amenorrhea (cessation of bleeding after menarche) should be eliminated. To evaluate women for any type of amenorrhea, the Endocrine Society recommends that a comprehensive set of hormonal laboratory tests be obtained initially, including β-human chorionic gonadotropin (β-hCG), free thyroxine (FT4), thyroid-stimulating hormone (TSH), prolactin (PRO), FSH, LH, E_2 and anti-Müllerian hormone (AMH).[13]

However, most family planning clinics and primary care providers have limited resources and may lack the expertise required to care for the more unusual causes associated with primary amenorrhea, while secondary amenorrhea is often comfortably within their scope of practice. Therefore, this chapter maintains a distinction between primary amenorrhea and secondary amenorrhea.

Primary Amenorrhea

The first manifestations of puberty are either thelarche (breast budding) or adrenarche (growth of sexual hair). The average age onset of puberty in the United States is 9.7 years, but normal age of onset ranges from 7 years to 13 years. Despite this great variability in the age of initiation of puberty, once puberty starts, it follows a very predictable pattern. The first menses generally follows thelarche within 2 years. This provides guidance about *when* the diagnosis of primary amenorrhea should be made and a diagnostic workup started:

- When there has been no adrenarche or thelarche by age 13.
- When there has been no menses by age 15.
- When adrenarche or thelarche started on time, but menses have not started within 5 years of that event.

The differential diagnosis for patients with primary amenorrhea (lack of menarche) includes anatomical, genetic, hormonal, enzymatic, and psychologic causes. Anatomical defects, such as an imperforate hymen or a transverse vaginal septum, may mask the actual onset of menses. In most such obstructive cases, surgical excision can allow normal outflow of menses along the reproductive tract. Most other cases of primary amenorrhea should be referred to reproductive endocrinologists, but generalists can often initiate the preliminary evaluation.

A comprehensive personal history, a physical exam, and a family history can suggest specific etiologies for primary amenorrhea. The work-up can be organized into four different categories based on the presence or absence on exam of breasts and a uterus.

Uterus, no breasts. Patients who have no breasts but have a uterus can be assumed to lack ovarian estrogen production. This ovarian insufficiency can be due to a wide variety of causes:

- Chromosomal abnormalities
  - — Turner syndrome, mosaicism, pure gonadal dysgenesis
- Ovarian enzyme deficiency
- Ovarian damage[14]
  - — Earlier radiation, chemotherapy
- Pituitary or hypothalamic dysfunction
  - — Congenital hypogonadotropic hypogonadism (e.g. Kallmann syndrome)

No breasts, no uterus. Patients who have neither breasts nor a uterus are extremely rare. Generally, affected patients have an enzyme deficiency (17,20 desmolase deficiency; 17 alpha-hydroxylase deficiencies in a 46,XY individual) or lack any gonads after birth (but in utero had testicular tissue to prevent the formation of a uterus).

Breasts, no uterus. For patients who have no uterus but have normal breast development demonstrating estrogen exposure, there are only a few major possible etiologies.

- *Androgen insensitivity syndrome*. Patients with this syndrome present with female secondary sexual characteristics, but possess a 46,XY chromosomal complement and bilateral testes (often appearing as inguinal masses). They have male levels of testosterone, to which they are unable to respond. However, they convert their testosterone peripherally, which explains in their high levels of circulating estrogens. Their testes need to be removed after puberty is complete, but before those organs undergo possible malignant transformation into gonadoblastoma. After diagnosis, patients with testosterone insensitivity should be allowed to retain their female sexual identity if they feel it is appropriate. If they desire children, they will need egg donation and surrogates to carry the pregnancy, or they can adopt.
- *Congenital absence of a uterus* (complete uterine Müllerian agenesis) is found in 10% of cases of primary amenorrhea. Müllerian agenesis is associated with other urogenital malformations, especially in the urinary tract (kidney and ureteral). Patients with congenital absence of the uterus, who desire their own children, must use surrogates to carry their pregnancies, but they can use their own eggs.

Breasts, uterus. Most patients with primary amenorrhea have both a uterus and normally developed breasts. As discussed above, congenital obstruction of menstrual flow (by vaginal septa, imperforate hymen, etc.) can be ruled out by examination or imaging studies. The remaining evaluations are virtually the same as the evaluations needed for secondary amenorrhea and are described in the following section.

Secondary Amenorrhea

When patients who have previously menstruated stop menstruating, do a pregnancy test. The only exception to this rule would be if the patient were asymptomatic and consistently used hormonal contraceptives that are known to reduce episodes of bleeding, such as the LNG IUD, DPMA, or extended cycle combined hormonal methods. It should be noted that with modern low-dose pills, it is no longer appropriate to attribute any significant delay in return of menses to "post-pill amenorrhea"; cyclic bleeding should not be delayed by more than 2 to 4 weeks after stopping any of the hormonal contraceptive methods except DMPA. If the onset of amenorrhea follows a uterine procedure (such as a dilation and curettage to treat a septic abortion or postpartum hemorrhage), evaluate the endometrial cavity for adhesions (Asherman syndrome). For amenorrhea following a cervical LEEP or cone biopsy, rule out cervical stenosis.

The question is: how *long* must a someone go without bleeding to be diagnosed as having secondary amenorrhea? Today the diagnosis is most appropriately made for those who had previously been *regularly cycling* after there has been no spotting or bleeding for 3 months. "Delayed menses" is used as the diagnosis before then. A patient with *infrequent menses* technically should not be diagnosed as having secondary amenorrhea until bleeding was missed for 2 times the expected normal menstrual cycle length. However, that patient would warrant earlier evaluation for infrequent menses (see below).

A lack of uterine bleeding can reflect one of two different endocrine states: a lack of *estrogen* to stimulate growth of the endometrium or a lack of *progesterone* to offset unopposed estrogen stimulation of the endometrium. Lack of estrogen carries with it the health risks experienced in menopause, such as osteoporosis, early cardiovascular disease, and genitourinary syndrome of menopause (GSM). On the other hand, exposure to estrogen without progesterone significantly increases the risk for endometrial hyperplasia and endometrial cancer. Rarely, in the presence of normal amounts of both estrogen and progesterone, other local factors can suppress the endometrium. For example, relatively high levels of testosterone (as seen with androgen-producing tumors or in transgender men) can block the ability of estrogen to stimulate endometrial cells. Of course, chronic endometrial suppression by progestins or estrogen-and-progestin combinations in hormonal contraception also results in amenorrhea, but this would not be of clinical concern.

Secondary amenorrhea in reproductive-aged patients not using hormonal contraception can signal either a problem confined to the reproductive system or a systemic medical problem. Even if someone with secondary amenorrhea does not desire fertility, amenorrhea must be evaluated because the medical problem underlying that lack of bleeding may require treatment.

History and physical examination. The evaluation of secondary amenorrhea begins with a thorough history and physical examination. Take a detailed menstrual history and inquire about vasomotor symptoms. Question the patient about recent changes in weight, acne, hair growth, and cold or heat tolerance. Ask about galactorrhea, recent pregnancy, recent breastfeeding, recent genital tract procedures or other surgeries (e.g. bariatric surgery), prior chemotherapy or irradiation, eating patterns (diet), stress, and exercise patterns. Medical problems, such as uncontrolled juvenile diabetes, end-stage renal disease, AIDS, malabsorption, hepatic failure, Cushing syndrome, sarcoidosis, acromegaly, and craniopharyngiomas can cause secondary amenorrhea. Also obtain a personal and family history of medical problems—especially endocrine problems—that might influence menstrual cycling.

Obtain a complete drug history, because all classes of medications (prescription, over-the-counter, and street recreational drugs) include some drugs that can induce amenorrhea or infrequent bleeding. Phenothiazine derivatives, phenothiazine-like compounds, haloperidol, selective serotonin reuptake inhibitors (SSRIs), reserpine derivatives, metoclopramide, sulpiride, promazine, cimetidine, verapamil, opiates, diazepams, tricyclic antidepressants, methyldopa, amphetamines and marijuana can cause amenorrhea, often by depleting dopamine levels or by blocking dopamine receptors. High levels of prolactin can cause amenorrhea; less dramatic elevations in prolactin are associated with infrequent menses (see below). Note that androgenic drugs, sometimes used to improve athletic performance or libido, may be compounded or obtained by patients in unconventional ways. Chemotherapeutic agents and radiation exposure after menarche can induce early ovarian insufficiency and present as secondary amenorrhea.[14]

On examination, pay close attention to signs of androgen excess (hirsutism, balding, acne, voice changes, and clitoromegaly), insulin resistance (acanthosis nigricans), hypoestrogenism (dry, flattened vaginal mucosa), prolactin excess (galactorrhea), thyroid dysfunction (skin, pulse, and reflex changes), or changes indicating other systemic diseases. Check the patient's index and middle fingers for any signs of calluses on the dorsal surfaces and look for yellow staining on the inner surfaces of teeth, which might suggest induced vomiting associated with eating disorders. Look for behaviors, such as excessive concern with weight or body image, as well as suggestive attitudes, such as perfectionism and stressors.

Laboratory tests. Order laboratory tests that are appropriate for the patient's history, physical exam, immediate fertility desires, and personal and family history. Once pregnancy is ruled out, the most common tests that are needed are TSH and prolactin, although total testosterone or FSH can also be very helpful in certain situations. However, not all tests are needed in every case, particularly in a resource-restricted clinical setting. For example:

- A 25-year-old with secondary amenorrhea who reports increasing weight and decreased energy may be best served by first testing TSH.
- A 23-year-old with secondary amenorrhea who complains of hot flashes and a dry vagina with a history of use of alkylating agents used to treat childhood cancer should have FSH tested first.[15]
- A 19-year-old amenorrheic patient with progressively worsening, severe hirsutism might need 17-α hydroxyprogesterone and total testosterone levels to rule out adult onset congenital adrenal hyperplasia and androgen-producing tumors.
- A 24-year-old nulliparous, hirsute patient with amenorrhea who desires pregnancy would most likely benefit from having all these tests done.

More extensive testing may be needed if the results of the first round of testing points toward a specific problem. For example, someone with elevated TSH needs additional testing to determine the cause of the thyroid deficiency. Someone with significantly elevated prolactin (prolactin >70 ng/dL) needs to have imaging studies (usually MRI) of the pituitary gland and adjacent areas to rule out pituitary prolactinoma, empty-sella syndrome, craniopharyngioma, and other obstructive lesions. The 23-year-old with no bleeding for 8 months, whose FSH is in the postmenopausal range, should have that diagnosis confirmed by repeat testing of FSH and testing of LH and estradiol levels. If both gonadotropins are elevated and estradiol is low, the patient has premature ovarian insufficiency (POI) and is menopausal. If there were not the history of childhood chemotherapy, additional tests would be needed. At age <30 years, with unexplained POI, an individual would need extensive testing to rule out chromosomal abnormalities.[16] If the patient were older (30 to 35 years), testing would be needed to rule out other autoimmune endocrinopathies, which could worsen with time.

Other than pregnancy, the two most common causes of secondary amenorrhea are PCOS and FHA. Each of those conditions presents clinically on a continuum from amenorrhea to subfertility. PCOS is discussed in greater detail in the section on infrequent menses below. FHA deserves more detailed discussion here due to the changes made in recommendations for therapies.[13]

Functional hypothalamic amenorrhea (FHA) The most common causes for FHA include weight loss, vigorous exercise, and stress. They often present together in different combinations, but they share the fact that the patient lacks estrogen. An *energy deficit* is the critical factor in both weight loss and exercise-induced forms of FHA, even if there have been no notable changes in weight with the latter. Low energy directly influences the HPO axis, inducing different clinical presentations in different people. FHA can occur as a result of abnormalities in GnRH receptors or dynamics induced by those problems.

An important subset of FHA is the *female athlete triad,* which is a medical condition found among those who are physically active, characterized by three components:[17]

1. Low energy availability, with or without disordered eating
2. Menstrual dysfunction (amenorrhea)
3. Low bone density

The female athlete triad can appear at any age, but it can have a more significant impact on the health of women in their adolescence who have not completed their bone mass accumulation.[18] Because the consequences of some of these conditions may not be completely reversible, ACOG points out that prevention, early diagnosis, and intervention are all critical and recommends that all active women should be assessed for components of the triad, and further investigation be performed if any of them is identified.[17]

Bone density, especially in young patients with FHA, can range from normal to low. Osteoporosis should be attributed to FHA only after excluding anatomic and organic pathology. In addition to the hormonal tests recommended above, the work-up of FHA also routinely includes CBC, electrolytes, liver and kidney function tests, and sedimentation rate or C-reactive protein tests. Magnetic resonance imaging is recommended in patients with presumed FHA as well as for other troubling signs or symptoms (e.g. headaches, vomiting, lateralizing neurological signs, etc.). For teens and adults with more than 6 months of amenorrhea due to FHA, a baseline bone mineral density measurement with DEXA is also recommended.

Treatments for Secondary Amenorrhea
Short-term therapies

While blood tests are being analyzed, it is quite reasonable to prescribe someone with secondary amenorrhea a short course of progestin therapy (medroxyprogesterone acetate [MPA]10 mg or norethindrone acetate

[NETA] 5 mg once daily for 10-12 days) to offset the possible adverse effects of unopposed estrogen on the endometrium. In the past, the result of this so-called *progestin challenge test* was used as part of the work-up of amenorrhea. Today the progestin is considered to be therapeutic, not diagnostic. This is because the results of the former "progestin challenge test" do not reliably support any diagnosis. The *presence* of withdrawal bleeding after progestin challenge does not necessarily demonstrate prior ovarian estradiol production. Peripheral aromatization of androgens can produce weaker estrogens that can stimulate the endometrium; some healthy postmenopausal women can even be induced to bleed following short-term treatment with progestin. On the other hand, the *absence* of bleeding after progestin therapy does not reliably verify the absence of ovarian estrogen production. High circulating levels of androgen can block the ability of estrogen to induce endometrial cells to proliferate.

Longer-term therapies

If a specific etiology is identified by the work-up, therapy should be targeted:

- Prolactinomas are generally treated medically with bromocriptine or cabergoline.
- Hypothyroidism can be treated with thyroxine replacement.
- Testosterone-producing tumors must be surgically removed.

The care of patients with functional hypothalamic amenorrhea is best provided by multidisciplinary teams involving, if possible, the patient, an obstetrician-gynecologist, nutritionist, parents, mental health care provider and, if indicated, coaches.[17] However, it is helpful for the initial clinician to counsel about the diagnosis and outline the care the patient can expect to receive. The most fundamental step in treating FHA is to correct the energy imbalance; this usually requires behavioral change and weight gain. Generally these goals can be achieved by any combination of increased caloric consumption, improved nutrition and/or decreased activity.[17] Cessation of self-induced vomiting is also important. Psychological support, such as cognitive behavioral therapy, can contribute greatly to the success of treatment. Combined oral contraceptives to induce menses or to protect bones are **not** recommended. In fact, a patient with FHA who does use combined hormonal contraception for birth control needs to know that those hormones may mask return of spontaneous menses and that even with COC use, bone loss may continue until the energy deficit is corrected. However, these same guidelines say that transdermal estradiol with cyclic oral progestin may be used if menses do not spontaneously resume after a trial of comprehensive therapy, but current evidence does not support the use of hormonal therapy for the sole purpose of improving bone mass in patients with FHA.[19,]

For reproductive-aged patients whose amenorrhea is caused by other cases of estrogen deficiency, such as premature ovarian insufficiency, ACOG recommends systemic hormone therapy with estrogen and progestin to treat the symptoms of hypoestrogenism and reduce the long-term health risks, as long as there are no contraindications to such therapy.[20] Combined hormonal contraceptives are usually first-line choices because they are considered to be age-appropriate and might protect patients with premature ovarian insufficiency from the infrequent (but real) risk of pregnancy. Therapy should be continued until age 50 or 51, unless contraindications develop.

Patients with persistent secondary amenorrhea due to chronic anovulation require a different approach. They need ongoing *progestin therapy* to mitigate the harmful effects that unopposed estrogen has on the endometrium. Progestin can be administered *cyclically*, following a variety of protocols. MPA or NETA can be given for the first 10 days of each month. Alternatively, patients may prefer to have some degree of *chronic* endometrial suppression using progestin-only methods, such as an LNG intrauterine contraceptive, the contraceptive implant, or progestin-only pills. Of course, anovulatory patients (except those with FHA) may be able to use combined hormonal contraceptive methods, either cyclically or continuously, if they do not have contraindications to estrogen.

Infrequent Menses

Infrequent menstruation is a common problem often caused by milder forms of conditions that cause secondary amenorrhea, such as hypothyroidism, androgen-excess conditions, and obesity. Once pregnancy is ruled out, most patients who have infrequent menses are found to have anovulation—i.e., estrogen production, but no progesterone. Occasionally, they may experience intermittent estrogen deficiency associated with episodic intermittent strenuous exercise, seasonal sports, periodic extreme stress, or severe depression.

The elements that should be included in the history and physical exam for people presenting with infrequent menses are almost identical to those outlined for secondary amenorrhea above, except that a more detailed history of recent menstrual trends is required. Ask about symptoms of ovulation (Mittelschmerz) and moliminal complaints (bloating, cramping, or breast tenderness symptoms that typically herald the onset of menses). Ask about bleeding patterns over time, and examine changes in these patterns in the context of events in the patient's life, activities, and changes in weight over time.

Polycystic Ovary Syndrome (PCOS)

Polycystic ovary syndrome (PCOS) is a common cause of infrequent bleeding and is the most common endocrinopathy of reproductive-aged patients. Depending upon the PCOS definition used, at least 7% to 10% of women meet all the criteria for PCOS, but up to 20% of reproductive-age women have some manifestation of androgen excess. With the increasing prevalence of obesity, prevalence estimates of PCOS may also increase substantially.[21]

One of the most significant new advances made in PCOS care has been the recognition that a diagnosis of "PCOS" may not be very informative. PCOS is a syndrome with a wide range of clinical presentations, different etiologies, and different long-term health implications. Each of the different subgroups needs targeted evaluations and therapies. Overall, the clinical manifestations of PCOS can include menstrual disorders, infertility, skin disorders (hirsutism, acne, androgenic alopecia), insulin resistance, metabolic syndrome, non-alcoholic fatty liver disease, sleep apnea, endometrial cancer risk factors, and mood disturbances and depression.[22] Pregnancy complications, including miscarriage, gestational diabetes, and premature delivery all have odds ratios well below 2.0, but their prevalence is statistically significantly higher than in controls.[23] Long-term hospitalization rates for women with PCOS are also substantially higher than for those without PCOS.[24]

The individual's clinical presentation and the clinical implications of PCOS certainly vary greatly by race and ethnicity as well as by the pathology underlying her PCOS.[25] To deal with this variety, efforts are underway to describe a series of *phenotypes* within PCOS so that both counseling and therapy may be better individualized to meet the specific needs of women who present with one or the other different subtypes of PCOS.[26-28] While we are awaiting a better understanding and definition for those phenotypes, the current generalized approach to PCOS is outlined in this section. However, in order to provide targeted evaluations and treatments where they are appropriate at certain junctions, we suggest individualization of care that may vary from existing comprehensive clinical guidelines. The recommendations outlined in this section may also not agree with observed community practice. Despite strong statements from professional societies, there are large knowledge gaps among clinicians about PCOS. In part, these gaps may be due to the clinical challenge of keeping up with a rapid growth in understanding and frequent changes in management recommendations for PCOS.[29]

The Rotterdam criteria are currently used to diagnose PCOS, although it is recognized that those criteria may over-diagnose PCOS and inflict unnecessary psychological harm.[30,31] The Rotterdam criteria state that, in the absence of other causes (e.g., congenital adrenal hyperplasia, androgen-secreting tumors, Cushing syndrome), adult women can be diagnosed with PCOS if they meet at least 2 of the 3 following criteria:[32]

1. Infrequent menses (<8 per year)
2. Hyperandrogenism or hyperandrogenemia
3. Polycystic appearing ovaries

As an aside, adolescents should not be evaluated for PCOS for at least 18 months following menarche and they should not be diagnosed with PCOS unless they meet *all 3 Rotterdam criteria.*

PCOS has traditionally been considered to be a condition of androgen excess or, more rarely, of androgen sensitivity.[26] Hyperandrogenemia (high normal or slightly elevated levels of circulating [free or total] testosterone or other androgens) or hyperandrogenism (hirsutism, acne, male-pattern balding) have traditionally been key elements in the clinical presentation. Hirsutism must be distinguished from virilization (e.g., irreversible androgen-induced changes, such as voice deepening, clitoromegaly). According to the Rotterdam criteria, in order to qualify as a polycystic appearing ovary (PAO), at least one ovary must have at least 12 preantral follicles, measuring 2 to 9 mm, in any one ultrasound image or have an ovarian volume of ≥10 mL. More recently studies have suggested that age-specific criteria are needed to reflect the decrease in volume and follicle number with increasing age.[33] For example, for women ≤24 years, the best sensitivity and specificity to define PCOS was achieved with a volume threshold of 12 mL and 13 follicles.[35] However, it is important to remember that PAO by itself does not make the diagnosis of PCOS, because any condition that causes chronic anovulation will induce polycystic-appearing ovaries.

PCOS is really a diagnosis of exclusion; other conditions that could explain the signs and symptoms must be excluded before a patient can be diagnosed with PCOS. First rule out pregnancy, thyroid dysfunction, prolactinoma, pituitary or hypothalamic suppression, and medication-induced infrequent menses. Your clinical evaluation should include questions, physical examination, and laboratory tests designed to rule out these other etiologies.[22]

The history should include a description of menstrual patterns over time in conjunction with contemporaneous estimates of weight, obstetrical history (including prior fertility challenges, gestational diabetes, excessive weight gain, macrosomia), and history of androgen-related symptoms and prior treatments. Hirsutism is a much more sensitive marker of PCOS than is either acne or alopecia. Family history of endocrine, reproductive, and metabolic disorders is important. On physical examination, take blood pressure, calculate body mass index (BMI), and measure waist circumference. Focus on signs that could either suggest another etiology, such as abnormal deep tendon reflexes (thyroid dysfunction), galactorrhea (prolactinoma), rapid excessive hair growth, decreased breast tissue or clitoromegaly (atypical congenital adrenal hyperplasia or androgen-producing tumors), and signs that could support the diagnosis of PCOS (acne, hirsutism, androgenic alopecia, acne, acanthosis nigricans, skin tags, or hidradenitis suppurativa).[26]

ACOG guidelines suggest that a panel of tests be performed to evaluate PCOS.[22] To establish biochemical hyperandrogenemia, those guidelines advise measuring either (1) total testosterone with sex hormone binding globulin (SHBG) or (2) bioavailable/free testosterone levels. To exclude other causes of PCOS symptoms, ACOG guidelines say to measure TSH, prolactin, 17-hydroxy-progesterone and to consider screening for Cushing disease or acromegaly. This list is certainly comprehensive and helpful in a workup for infertility or in a research setting for PCOS. However, in practice (particularly in less resource-rich areas), those tests may be prohibitively expensive. In the face of hyperandrogenism, the utility of ordering any tests for testosterone or DHEAS has been questioned.[34] This may be supported by new research implicating androstenedione or 11-oxygenated androgens rather than the classical testosterone as the root cause of PCOS hyperandrogenicity and metabolic risks.[35,36] Therefore, we may need to use each individual's history, physical findings, and immediate fertility desires to guide in selecting which are the more essential tests. The most common tests that are routinely needed in a family planning clinic would be TSH and perhaps a prolactin if galactorrhea were present. Other tests would be ordered only as indicated. For example, a young patient with progressive hirsutism would need a 17-hydroxy progesterone test. (See similar discussion in Secondary Amenorrhea.)

Other tests might be helpful in caring for those with PCOS. Many patients with PCOS have an increased risk of developing prediabetes and diabetes; they also tend to develop diabetes at a younger age.[37] Therefore, glucose tolerance testing may be very important to their health, even if it is not part of diagnosing PCOS. The best test is a 2-hour oral glucose tolerance test with a 75g glucose load. This test can clearly identify prediabetes (100-125 fasting blood glucose, or a 2-hour-glucose level between 140 to 200) as well as overt diabetes (>126 fasting blood glucose or a 2-hour glucose >200). Other tests, such as fasting glucose or hemoglobin A1C, can be used instead, but they are less sensitive in diagnosing diabetes and often miss the diagnosis of prediabetes. A substantial percent of women with PCOS (especially those with BMI >30 kg/m^2) also have metabolic syndrome, which may also put them at increased risk for future cardiovascular problems.[38] There are considerable racial and ethnic differences in the PCOS metabolic phenotype that will need to be addressed in the future.[39] But for now, when the diagnosis of PCOS is accompanied by hypertension or a BMI greater than 30 kg/m^2, a lipid profile may be important to include as part of well-person care. Also, carefully screen those with PCOS for depression.[40]

It is also important to know which tests are *not indicated* to diagnose PCOS. Routine testing for insulin resistance with fasting insulin levels is *not* indicated.[22] This is because there are no commercially available tests that can accurately diagnose insulin resistance and because knowing that a person has insulin resistance does *not* affect the choice of treatment. Older tests, such as the LH/FSH ratio, are also not relevant.[41] Finally, in the absence of a palpable pelvic mass, it is generally *not* necessary to order a pelvic ultrasound for adult patients who meet the other two criteria for PCOS.

Treatments for PCOS-related problems are discussed below with treatments for other causes of infrequent menses.

Other Causes of Infrequent Menses

Infrequent menses usually results from anovulation, as noted in the discussion of PCOS. Clinical symptoms such as fatigue, weight gain, constipation, and depressive moods can suggest hypothyroidism; an elevated TSH can confirm the diagnosis and distinguish it from depression. Prolactinomas more often cause infrequent menses than amenorrhea, especially when those pituitary tumors produce prolactin levels in the lower ranges of abnormal. Similarly, centrally acting medications, such as lithium and others that interfere with dopamine, modestly raise prolactin levels and commonly cause infrequent bleeding in their users.

An increasingly common cause of infrequent bleeding during reproductive years is obesity-related anovulation; patients with BMIs >30 kg/m^2 often have polycystic-appearing ovaries because of their chronic anovulation. Technically, criteria 1 and 3 of the Rotterdam definition would qualify them for the diagnosis of PCOS. However, since they have no androgen excess, some experts have objected to labeling these individuals as having PCOS. This issue should be clarified in subsequent refinements of the definition of PCOS, which will recognize different phenotypes within PCOS.

Treatments for Infrequent Menses (including PCOS)

Treatment of infrequent menses depends upon the underlying etiology, immediate fertility desires, and any other health challenges that are present. Patients with underlying medical problems, such as hyperprolactinemia and hypothyroidism, should receive targeted therapies for those issues, but they should also be provided progestin until their menses normalize. Contraception during this time is also important, because of episodic ovulation and unannounced return of fertility.

Lifestyle modification. The first-line intervention for those with excessive weight with or without PCOS focuses on *lifestyle changes*, with emphasis on weight loss and exercise.[22,42] It is important to stress to patients that a combination of long-term healthy eating, including a diet rich in fruits, vegetables, fiber, and lean proteins, *and* consistent engagement in physical activity, is key to losing excess weight and maintaining a healthy weight. While short-term studies may suggest superiority of one type of diet over another, there are no long-term studies demonstrating superior outcomes.[43] However, important genetic differences may make some people more resistant to weight loss with diets that may work for other people. Our goal is to encourage patients to find a safe diet they can follow over the long term.[22] To lose weight, women with PCOS must maintain low-calorie diets for prolonged periods of time. Reducing their intake to 500 to 600 kcal a day below subsistence level can mean that, without an exercise program, they are allowed to consume only 1000-1200 kilocalories a day.[44] In order to be successful on such stringent diets, they need significant support and understanding from their providers and from those around them. Behavioral therapy support will likely add to success.[45,46]

In a similar vein, providers should encourage patients to find a form of physical activity they enjoy and to make a lifetime commitment to engaging in exercise. Exercise is critically important to every weight loss program and to the maintenance of a healthy weight. To lose weight, calories consumed need to be lower than the calories being expended. Exercise helps consume calories, so overly restrictive caloric goals are not necessary. Aerobic exercise in women with PCOS results in reduction of fasting insulin and insulin resistance.[47] In addition, exercise promotes cardiovascular health, balance, and quality sleep. Sleep disorders associated with obesity or PCOS contribute to insulin resistance, which in turn, increases cardiovascular disease risk. Therefore, *sleep*, *diet*, and *exercise* comprise an interrelated triad of key health promotion messages for patients of all ages.

Therapeutic agents. Some medical agents have been shown to help patients with PCOS or obesity-related anovulation. One of the most successful agents to enhance weight loss is Orlistat, taken 60 mg orally before each meal. Orlistat works by blocking absorption of dietary fats from the intestine. When patients on Orlistat consume foods high in fat, they experience very unpleasant flatus and diarrhea. In a comparative clinical trial, the Orlistat-treated PCOS patients had over 4 times more weight loss than did those treated with Metformin.[48]

For patients with PCOS who are not seeking pregnancy, routine use of insulin-sensitizing agents is now discouraged by the ACOG, the American Society for Reproductive Medicine (ASRM), and the Endocrine Society.[22,41] Metformin may be appropriate in the treatment of PCOS in those who also have metabolic syndrome and prediabetes, but its use even in this context should still be individualized. Some experts have recommended dual therapies for subsets of high-risk patients. For example, it might be more effective to combine oral estrogen-progesterone therapy and metformin in treatment of those with factors indicating insulin resistance, such as metabolic syndrome, acanthosis nigricans, or a history of gestational diabetes.[49]

Patients with anovulatory cycling need special attention paid to their reproductive potential. Pregnancies should be planned and prepared for, because patients with PCOS, especially those with the hyperandrogenic phenotypes, have higher risks for developing gestational diabetes and requiring Cesarean delivery. Their infants are at risk for growth disorders, usually macrosomia.[50]

Because patients with high BMIs and PCOS do occasionally ovulate, they need *contraception* if they are sexually active. Progestin-only birth control methods such as LNG IUDs, DMPA, and progestin-only pills and extended cycle combined hormonal contraceptives provide both good pregnancy protection without inducing scheduled bleeding. Many with PCOS appreciate their freedom from bleeding and are excellent candidates for long-acting methods; however, some with PCOS or others with infrequent bleeding may desire monthly bleeding. Cyclic use of combined hormonal methods may be more appropriate for them, unless obesity would reduce efficacy (contraceptive patch) or would substantially increase the risk of thrombosis (as in older users) or other contraindications to estrogen exist.[51] (See Chapter 7 on the patch and ring and Chapter 8 on combined pills.)

Infertility treatment. The treatment of infertility due to PCOS has changed dramatically over the years. In patients with excessive weight, the first step has always been to encourage weight loss because a loss of only 10% to 15% of current weight can restore ovulation to a majority with elevated BMIs.[52] However, the utility of this approach has more recently been questioned.[52,53] If lifestyle interventions are not successful in inducing ovulation, ACOG recommends clomiphene citrate as first-line medical therapy for ovulation induction; insulin-sensitizing agents are not appropriate as sole therapy. More recently, the American Society for Reproductive Medicine (ASRM) has recommended either clomiphene citrate or letrozole alone as first-line therapies. Randomized comparative clinical trials have clearly demonstrated that both clomiphene citrate and letrozole as single therapies are superior to extended release metformin in producing higher rates of ovulation, pregnancy, and live births.[54] However, letrozole may be superior to clomiphene citrate, especially in PCOS with BMI >30 kg/m^2.[55] Second-line therapies recommended by ACOG for those who do not respond to clomiphene citrate include ovulation induction with menotropins, laparoscopic ovarian drilling and, perhaps, aromatase inhibitors. ACOG also recommends combining clomiphene citrate with metformin as a second-line option, although ASRM more recently has said that there is insufficient evidence that metformin increases live-birth rates either compared to placebo or when used in combination with other agents.[24,41] Progestin withdrawal prior to ovulation induction does not improve pregnancy rates.[56]

Long-term health promotion. Patients with annovulation-based infrequent menses need *long-term therapies* with a *progestin* to protect their endometrial linings from the long-term effects of unopposed estrogen: endometrial hyperplasia and endometrial carcinoma. Those who are at least 50 pounds overweight have a 10-fold increased risk of endometrial carcinoma. Patients with PCOS may be at higher risk for those endometrial problems because they have lower expression of both nuclear and membrane-bound progesterone receptors with their endometrial cells.[57] Progestin can be provided by contraceptive agents or by long-term cyclic progestin therapy.

Patients who have PCOS, especially those with obesity, tobacco use, dyslipidemia, hypertension, impaired glucose tolerance, or subclinical vascular disease need to be recognized as being at increased risk for cardiovascular disease. Hyperandrogenic PCOS and metabolic syndrome or Type 2 diabetes clearly raises the risk for developing cardiovascular disease (CVD) later in life.[38,58] Attention to these risks is part of a comprehensive well-person care. However, it is not clear that a history of PCOS during the reproductive years will increase the risk of CVD mortality after menopause.[59]

Attention to psychological health is also important since the prevalence of both depression and anxiety are higher in patients with PCOS. One good resource for patients with PCOS is the documentary "Scrambled: A journey through polycystic ovary syndrome (PCOS)" by Randi Cecchine; another is the PolyCysters website.

Intriguingly, early research has suggested that the fundamental dysfunction with POCS lies with faulty adipocytes and that statins may be very effective in normalizing many of the metabolic abnormalities with PCOS and in providing cardiovascular protection too.[60] Confirmation of these findings may fundamentally alter how some phenotypes of PCOS will be treated in the future.

Heavy or Prolonged Menstrual Bleeding

Heavy menstrual bleeding (HMB) is a common gynecologic problem affecting 9% to 14% of healthy women, although surveys have found that up to 30% of women consider their bleeding to be excessive.[61,59] HMB adversely impacts a variety of aspects of a woman's life.[62] Patients with HMB are 45% more likely to use health services and 27% less likely to work. If they do work outside the home, it has been estimated that annual income of those with heavy bleeding is nearly $2,000 less than those with normal menses.[63]

The prevalence of HMB depends upon how it is defined. The classic definition is the loss of greater than 80 mL of blood per cycle. However, in daily life, the amount of blood loss is very difficult to quantify. Pad counts are not a reliable measure because of differences in product absorbency and in patients' fastidiousness. Interpretation of hemoglobin levels can be complicated by variations in dietary intake of iron. Blood losses as great as 80 to 120 mL per cycle can occur without causing anemia in patients who consume iron-rich diets and iron supplements. However, by the time a patient does achieve anemia, a considerable amount of menstrual blood will have been lost.

A practical definition of HMB advances the idea that blood loss is excessive not only when it meets the classic objective measure of loss (>80 mL of blood loss per cycle), but also *when the patient says it is excessive*. This definition illustrates that a *key factor in making a diagnosis of HMB is not only the amount of blood being lost, but how much HMB disrupts one's life*. The NICE guidelines capture this by defining HMB as "excessive menstrual blood loss, which interferes with the woman's physical, social, emotional, and/or material quality of life, and which can occur along, or in combination with other symptoms."[64] For example, if total blood loss is only 60 mL/cycle, but the flow is so heavy for 2 hours each cycle that the person must remain sedentary, that bleeding is clearly excessive. On the other hand, blood loss so excessive that the patient becomes anemic must be evaluated even if the patient does not complain of heavy bleeding. Another important consideration is that menstrual flow includes much more fluid than just blood. Only about half of the menstrual fluid volume is blood; the rest of the flow is composed of cervical and uterine secretions.[65] When we estimate that blood loss is 150 mL/cycle, we need to recognize that the menstrual products need to contain over 300 mL of menstrual fluid each cycle, which can be a very challenging task, often resulting in staining episodes.

Etiologies of Heavy Menstrual Bleeding (HMB)

The differential diagnosis of heavy menstrual bleeding is extensive. Once pregnancy complications are ruled out, the PALM-COEIN classification system can guide the workup. As described above, structural/anatomic conditions that can cause HMB include endometrial and endocervical polyps, adenomyosis, uterine leiomyoma (fibroids), as well as endometrial hyperplasia, and cervical and endometrial malignancies. The functional causes of HMB include coagulation defects, ovulatory dysfunction, endometrial factors, iatrogenic and causes that are not otherwise classified.

Evaluation of Heavy Menstrual Bleeding

A variety of tools is available to assess the causes of abnormal bleeding in different situations. Cervical and endometrial biopsies are used to rule out endometrial hyperplasia and cervical or uterine carcinoma in reproductive-age patients with intermenstrual or postcoital bleeding and in high-risk patients with unexplained heavy or prolonged menstrual bleeding. Body mass index is more important than is age in deciding to do endometrial biopsy for those who are premenopausal.[66] A surgical dilation and curettage may be needed if the patient with acute excessive bleeding is hemodynamically unstable and if acute heavy bleeding does not respond to the recommended hormonal therapies. Ultrasound is the primary imaging tool used to evaluate anatomical abnormalities causing abnormal uterine bleeding.[67] Ultrasound studies can identify uterine leiomyoma that may contribute to heavy bleeding and can be used to evaluate the endometrial stripe of a patient with postmenopausal bleeding; 3–dimensional ultrasound can help identify adenomyosis. Saline infusion sonography or hysteroscopy can better visualize endometrial polyps and other intracavitary lesions. Saline infusion studies are better tolerated than traditional hysteroscopy, but the latter can provide direct visualization of focal areas of endometrial pathology.[68] Newer small office hysteroscopes are enabling endometrial imaging with less discomfort. Magnetic resonance imaging (MRI) is useful in determining the size, and location of individual leiomyoma. Computer tomographic (CT) scans can assess potential metastatic disease.

Although bleeding due to PALM (Figure 1-10) causes can be serious, even life-threatening, only about half of patients with HMB will be found to have any identifiable anatomical pathology even at the time of hysterectomy.[69] Patients with HMB more often have *functional* problems of the COEIN component (see Figure 1-10). For example, coagulopathy, excessive fibrinolysis, prostaglandin imbalances, vessel instability, prolonged or excessive matrix metalloproteinase activity and systemic causes can all induce HMB.

Coagulation defects, such as inherited and acquired disorders of hemostasis, are underdiagnosed.[70] In one study of women with unexplained HMB, 47% were found to have a hemostatic abnormality, such as von Willebrand disease, idiopathic thrombocytopenia purpura (ITP), aplastic anemia, or platelet disorders. The most common abnormality was a platelet aggregation defect.[71] Although classic teaching tells us that patients with coagulation defects generally have other symptoms, such as easy bruising or bleeding gums, HMB can be the only presenting symptom in a patient with a bleeding diathesis.[72] Bleeding patterns over time can suggest etiologies within this category. Patients with von Willebrand disease generally have lifelong histories of prolonged and HMB patterns.[73] In fact, 20% of adolescents with HMB are found to have a bleeding disorder.[74] On the other hand, patients with some acquired disorders, such as platelet aggregation disorders, are more likely to have histories of having experienced lighter menses earlier in their lives. All bleeding disorders in those with a family history, a personal history of lifelong heavy bleeding or a high bleeding score should be evaluated in collaboration with a hematologist. Baseline laboratory tests should include a CBC, activated partial thromboplastin time (aPTT), prothrombin time (PT), ristocetin cofactor activity, and antigen and factor VIII levels.[75]

Excessive blood loss can also result from systemic diseases or medication use. Hepatic cirrhosis and active hepatitis can disrupt production of clotting factors and vitamin K, resulting in HMB. HMB is also found with early renal failure, adrenal hyperplasia, and many hematologic cancers, as well as with thyroid dysfunction. Anticoagulants, some anticonvulsants (phenytoin, phenobarbital), digitalis, nonhormonal intrauterine contraceptives, and chronic use of aspirin or nonsteroidal anti-inflammatory drugs (NSAIDs) all increase menstrual blood loss.

Idiopathic bleeding is generally due to local endometrial factors, often involving increased local inflammation. In these cases of HMB, the menstrual fluid contains significantly elevated levels of cytokine TNF-α, which leads to increased prostaglandin signaling.[6] This in turn leads to an excess of prostaglandins that cause vasodilation (prostaglandin E_2) over those that cause the vasoconstriction (prostaglandin $F_{2\alpha}$) that is needed to halt bleeding.[76] Prostaglandin E_2 has been found in higher levels in the menstrual fluid of women with such HMB compared with controls. PGE_2 receptors are also found in higher concentrations in both the endometria and myometria of those with HMB.[77,78]

Treatments for Heavy Menstrual Bleeding

There are increasing numbers of treatments available for patients with HMB. Choice depends upon the age of the patient, the severity of symptoms, the presence of other pelvic pathology, and near-term plans for childbearing. Many of the therapies used are off-label applications, but they are based on substantial clinical experience. Treatments for acute excessive bleeding are generally different from those used for chronic heavy menstrual bleeding.

Acute excessive bleeding. Hormonal regimens form the bedrock of all therapies used to arrest acute HMB. However, only a few prospective studies involving limited numbers of women have ever been published addressing this problem. A classic treatment for acute excessive bleeding was intravenous estrogen therapy (conjugated equine estrogen 20 to 25 mg every 3 to 4 hours) for 24 hours or oral estrogen (conjugated equine estrogen 2.5 mg every 4-6 hours).[79] With either of these treatments, bleeding was expected to slow in 12 to 24 hours, at which time a progestin (MPA 5-10 mg daily) was added. The doses of the estrogen were reduced in 3 to 5 days and maintained for about 1 month, to allow the patient's hemoglobin to normalize with time. These regimens were generally replaced for outpatients by treatment with high-dose combined oral contraceptive (COC) pills, again with no published appropriate prospective trials. Initially, high dose oral contraceptives (50 mcg ethinyl estradiol [EE]/0.5 mg norgestrel) were given 4 times daily for 5 days to stop bleeding. The high doses of estrogen in all of these therapies caused considerable nausea and vomiting and increased the risk for venous thromboembolism. As a result, in regimens of COCs used, at least in the outpatient settings for hemodynamically stable patients, have significantly reduced the doses of estrogen used over time. First, the dose of estrogen-containing pills was reduced to 2 times daily for 5 days, then both the dose and duration of therapy were reduced. The most recent COC regimen recommended is substantially lower than any prior recommendation. It calls for any 1/35 EE/NETA pill 2 tabs, to be given orally; that initial dose should be followed by the rest of the EE/NETA pills taken 1 tab a day until the packet is empty.[80]

The latest development in the hormonal treatment of acute excessive uterine bleeding is that the hormones used have been changed. Estrogen has been removed entirely in the newer therapy. A regimen of high-dose progestin therapy (MPA 20 mg given 3 times daily for 7 days, followed by MPA 20 mg once daily for 21 days) was tested in the largest published randomized clinical trial in the English language. It was found to be as effective as high-dose COCs.[81] Because this progestin-only regimen is well-tolerated and does not expose patients to any estrogen-related adverse events (e.g. thrombosis), it should be considered first line treatment to arrest acute excessive bleeding, at least in the outpatient setting. Progestin-only therapies are effective outpatient treatment for acute heavy bleeding caused by a full range of endometrial pathologies, from endometrial atrophy to hyperplasia.[82] However, no studies have shown that progestin-only therapy is effective in arresting acute bleeding in patients who require hospitalization.

If progestin-only treatments fail, some clinicians have used estrogen therapies for second-line rescue regimens. Adjuvant therapy with high-dose NSAIDs can be used with any hormonal therapy. Antiemetics may be very helpful, especially in regimens that use high-dose estrogen or if the patient has a history of gastrointestinal complaints with prior

Box 1-4 Current first-line outpatient treatment for acute HMB

Progestin-only regimens are the recommended first-line treatment of acute excessive vaginal bleeding of individuals who are medically eligible for outpatient therapy:

Medroxyprogesterone acetate (MPA) 10 mg

1. 2 tabs by mouth 3 times daily for 7 days,
2. followed by 2 tabs by mouth once daily for the next 21 days.

(You may need to add a note to the pharmacist that you really do mean to prescribe these high doses.)

hormonal use. However, remember to counsel patients about the sedating effects of the antiemetic agents.

Surgical procedures, such as dilation and curettage, uterine packing, tamponade with a Foley balloon, uterine artery embolization or hysterectomy may be needed in the face of life-threatening hemorrhage or if medical therapies fail.[83]

Chronic heavy bleeding. Treatment for chronic HMB can be directed to correct the pathophysiology underlying HMB or it can simply attempt to suppress the endometrium, especially if there are only local causes for the HMB.

NSAIDS. NSAIDs exert their anti-inflammatory effect by inhibiting cyclooxygenase. High-dose NSAIDs also increase the ratio of prostaglandin $F_{2\alpha}$/prostaglandin E_2 to increase the ability of the spiral arteries to constrict. When taken from the onset of menses until the end of the heavy flow days, these NSAIDs can reduce total menstrual blood loss by 20% to 45% and offer the additional benefit of analgesia for pain associated with uterine cramping. See Table 1-4 for appropriate doses. A Cochrane Systematic Database Review demonstrated that blood loss reduction was not affected by the particular NSAID used, but found that low-dose NSAIDs were far less effective than high-dose regimens.[84] NSAIDs can also be used in conjunction with other therapies (such as hormonal therapies) to boost the efficacy of those treatments. Patients with peptic ulcers and those who have coagulation disorders should avoid NSAIDs or couple the therapy with proton-pump inhibitors (PPIs).

Antifibrinolytic agents. Some women with chronic heavy and prolonged bleeding have increased endometrial plasminogen activity that promotes fibrinolysis.[86] When normal blood clots form in the spiral arteries of these women at the end of menses, those clots are rapidly lysed, so their bleeding persists. The antifibrinolytic agent, tranexamic acid, has

Table 1-4 Oral NSAID regimens for treatment of chronic heavy menstrual bleeding

Mefenamic acid
- 500 mg TID first 4-5 days of menses
- 500 mg TID from 4-5 days prior to menses to cessation (rarely needed)
- 500 mg initially; 200 mg QID for 3-5 days

Naproxen
- 500 mg at onset and 3-5 hours later; 500 mg BID for 5 days
- 500 mg in AM and 250 in PM for 2 days; 250 mg BID for 7 days
- 500 mg; 250 mg QID for 4 days
- 550 mg; 275 mg QID for 5 days

Ibuprofen
- 600 mg daily or 1200 mg daily- not as effective
- 800 mg TID for 5 days (Norplant trial)[85]

been used in Europe for treatment of HMB for more than 3 decades and is available over-the-counter in some of those countries. A recent review reported that such antifibrinolytic therapy resulted in a 34% to 59% reduction in mean blood loss.[87] Tranexamic acid is now available by prescription in the United States (Lysteda). In clinical trials, women who used this tranexamic acid regimen (650 mg 2 tabs orally 3 times a day for up to the first 5 days of menses) experienced a 40% reduction in menstrual blood loss.[88] Reflecting previous theoretical concerns that drugs that block lysis of fibrin clots might create a hypercoagulable state, the FDA labeling for Lysteda advises caution in prescribing this product for women who use hormonal contraceptives (presumably only those with estrogen). These agents can also be helpful in women with von Willebrand disease especially in conjunction with hormonal treatments.[73]

Hormonal therapies are even more effective than nonhormonal medications in treating HMB.[89] Progestins form the basis of hormonal therapies to effectively control chronic excessive menstrual blood loss. Cyclic progestin (medroxyprogesterone acetate (MPA) 10 mg or norethindrone acetate (NETA) 5 mg) daily for 10 days a month is most useful for patients with chronic anovulation. Unexpectedly, these luteal phase therapies can increase blood loss in women who ovulate and have monthly cycling. Progestin-only pills, progestin injections, and progestin-containing intrauterine contraceptives offer variable control of bleeding as well as contraceptive protection. The progestin-only pill (POP) decreases estrogen-stimulated endometrial proliferation. DMPA initially increases unscheduled spotting and bleeding, but over the longer term, it usually results in cessation of spotting and bleeding.[90] DMPA is a first-line treatment for patients with underlying bleeding disorders. There is one oral combined contraceptive product (Natazia) that is approved by the FDA for treatment of heavy or prolonged menstrual bleeding. In clinical trials of this estradiol valerate (E2V)/dienogest multiphasic pill, the reduction in blood loss reduction was almost as great as that seen in the U.S. clinical trials of Mirena for treatment of HMB.[91] However, other COC formulations are routinely used off-label to reduce cyclic bleeding. Most of the studies demonstrating clinical efficacy of COCs in the treatment of HMB are based on higher dose formulations, but there is one clinical trial of a 20 mcg EE pill that reduced menstrual blood loss by 68%.[92] Cyclic use of the contraceptive vaginal ring (NuvaRing) has been found to be more effective than COCs in treating HMB because it offered better cycle control.[93] Use of extended-cycle COCs or vaginal rings also reduces total blood loss in patients with HMB by reducing the numbers of episodes of scheduled bleeding as well as the amount of blood lost per episode.[94,95]

The LNG intrauterine contraceptive is the most effective medical therapy for HMB.[96] The LNG-IUS 20 (Mirena) is approved for the treatment of HMB by the U.S. FDA and by regulatory authorities in over 100 other countries. In clinical trials of women with HMB documented by eluting hemoglobin from sanitary pads, women who randomized to this LNG intrauterine contraceptive had a median reduction in blood loss of 62% by 3 months and a 71% reduction by 6 months.[97] The LNG-IUS has been shown to be effective in controlling bleeding due to most of the PALM-COIEN causes.[98] It also is the most effective medical therapy for endometrial hyperplasia and it reduces HMB and pain due to adenomyosis.[99-101] It is also effective in women using oral anticoagulant therapy.[102] The LNG-IUS20 (Liletta) is approved for treatment of HMB in the European Union (Levosert) because its use led to an impressive reduction in blood loss.[103]

Other agents that are effective for short-term use include GnRH agonists, such as leuprolide acetate (Lupron), nafarelin acetate (Synarel) and goserelin acetate (Zoladex), or buserelin (Suprecur). Pseudomenopause is induced after about two weeks of use and amenorrhea rates approach 90%.[90] Because of concerns about osteoporosis and other hypoestrogenic conditions, the duration of GnRH agonists use is generally limited to 4 to 6 months unless an estrogen-progestin add-back is given.

Newer medical therapies to treat HMB related to leiomyoma may become available in the United States. Selective progesterone receptor modulation (SPRMs) exert partial progesterone antagonistic effects while maintaining estradiol levels, thus avoiding hypoestrogenism seen with many other hormonal therapies.[104] Characteristic histologic changes are seen in the endometrium called PAEC (progesterone receptor modulator associated endometrial changes) look like hyperplasia, but these changes apparently do not have the potential for malignancy. In particular, low-dose ulipristal acetate (UPA) has been found to be very effective in establishing amenorrhea in patients with fibroid-induced anemia to increase hemoglobin prior to myomectomy. Long-term use is being investigated.[105,106]

Procedural treatments

Outpatient endometrial ablation has been popular for the treatment of HMB. At their peak, ablations were almost as common as hysterectomies in the United States.[107] Patients who are treated with endometrial ablation must have finished their childbearing and be committed to using effective contraception until menopause. Pregnancies that occur after this partial destruction of the endometrium pose increased risk of spontaneous abortion and very serious problems with placentation, including placenta accreta and placenta percreta.[108] Clinical trials have shown that after 3 to 12 months, there is no difference in efficacy of endometrial ablation and LNG intrauterine therapy.[109-111] Compared with endometrial ablation, the high-dose LNG IUS has a better record of cost, safety, and reversibility, making it a first-line therapy.[112]

Several other procedures are approved for treatment of women with symptomatic fibroids, including myomectomy, uterine artery embolization of leiomyoma, cryotherapy, and ultrasonic destruction of leiomyoma, etc.

The ultimate therapy is hysterectomy, but studies have also demonstrated a comparable benefit of the high-dose LNG IUS compared to hysterectomy as first-line therapy for women with HMB who have no other pelvic pathology. One randomized 10-year study comparing LNG IUD use to hysterectomy found that 54% of women who randomized to the LNG IUD avoided surgery.[113] Reserving hysterectomy for use only in women with pelvic pathology and to those who do not respond to LNG IUD therapy would significantly reduce health care costs and risks associated with treatment of HMB.

Other Abnormal Bleeding Patterns in the Premenopause

Traumatic Bleeding

Postcoital bleeding or increased or renewed bleeding after removal of tampons may raise concerns about cervical or vaginal pathology. In younger individuals, the most common cause is chlamydia cervicitis. In older individuals, benign lesions such as cervical polyps and more serious problems, such as cervical carcinoma, classically present with this type of bleeding.

Intermenstrual Bleeding

Bleeding between menses is often associated with significant endometrial pathology, such as endometrial hyperplasia or carcinoma. Rarely, reproductive-aged individuals may have midcycle spotting associated with ovulation. Individuals who miss birth control pills have unscheduled spotting and bleeding, which could be labeled as "intermenstrual," but is not clinically concerning for pathology.

Menstrually Related Problems

Painful Menses (Dysmenorrhea)

Greek for painful menstruation, dysmenorrhea is classified as *primary dysmenorrhea* (intrinsic and usually of early onset) or *secondary dysmenorrhea* (due to some other physical cause and usually of later onset). Even though the word to describe this problem comes from ancient roots, dysmenorrhea has only recently been recognized as a medical problem. Before the 1970s, there were virtually no scientific articles studying any aspect of the condition. Dysmenorrhea is painfully prevalent among modern women who are limiting numbers of pregnancies and the time they spend breastfeeding. In a study of college students, 84% of those surveyed reported having experienced dysmenorrhea; only 9% missed exams due to dysmenorrhea, but 48.7% reported poor satisfaction with their academic performance because of menstrual pain.[114] Many patients with dysmenorrhea also experience nausea, vomiting, diarrhea, headaches, or lightheadedness. Symptoms often vary in severity from cycle to cycle but generally are present each month throughout the reproductive years. Younger patients lose days at school, and older patients are hampered at home and in the workplace.

Primary Dysmenorrhea

Primary dysmenorrhea has physiologic—not psychological—causes. While early investigators believed that dysmenorrhea occurred in "maladjusted women who were intensely rejecting their feminine role and who suffered from deep hostility,"[115] today we understand that the problem is not in the patient's head, but in the uterus. Measurements with intrauterine pressure catheters demonstrate that women with primary dysmenorrhea generate intrauterine pressures with menstrual contractions similar to intrauterine pressures seen during the second stage of labor.

Symptoms of primary dysmenorrhea usually do not begin until cycles are ovulatory and progesterone is present. Progesterone stimulates the production of prostaglandins, which are released as the functional layer is sloughed. Persons with primary dysmenorrhea produce excessive amounts of prostaglandin $F_{2\alpha}$.[116] Prostaglandin $F_{2\alpha}$ increases the force of uterine contractions. These strong uterine contractions reduce uterine blood flow to the myometrium, causing ischemia. This ischemia directly causes pain and sensitizes afferent nerve fibers in the uterus to other painful stimuli, which augments the patient's perception of pain. When uterine contractions inject these same prostaglandins into the general circulation, they can cause headache, nausea, vomiting, and diarrhea. Other etiologies of early onset dysmenorrhea, such as structural abnormalities of the uterus (blind horns), cervix (stenotic os), or vagina (transverse septa), can usually be ruled out by a careful pelvic examination and radiographic studies.

Regular exercise is likely to improve dysmenorrhea symptoms and should be recommended.[117] Prostaglandin synthetase inhibitors such as NSAIDs are first-line medical therapy for most women; approximately 80% of women with dysmenorrhea feel relief from cramping pain, backache, headaches, and blood loss with these agents. In some women, NSAIDS may cause gastrointestinal symptoms.[118] All currently available NSAIDs are of comparable efficacy and safety.[119] In contrast, aspirin is no more effective than placebo for dysmenorrhea and can increase menstrual blood loss. While COX-2 inhibitors also significantly reduce dysmenorrhea, they have been linked to cardiovascular risk and are more expensive, so they are generally not prescribed for this indication.

Suppression of ovulation is associated with decreased menstrual pain.[119] Hormonal contraceptives have been used extensively off-label to reduce menstrual cramping and have been shown to be effective in a placebo-controlled, double-blind clinical trial.[120] A review of studies using lower dose formulations (especially when they were used for extended periods of time) concluded that COCs were the preferred therapy for dysmenorrhea for women who wish to use contraception, because the additional benefit of such relief was not linked to any other risks and eliminated the risks of NSAID use.[121]

Amenorrhea induced by any medication is beneficial for treatment of primary dysmenorrhea.[119] Women can achieve profound relief from dysmenorrhea by using extended cycles of COCs or contraceptive vaginal rings.[122] DMPA is also helpful in treating dysmenorrhea.[123] After their third injections, nearly half of DMPA users become amenorrheic and avoid dysmenorrhea entirely. The high-dose LNG IUS is also an excellent choice for patients with dysmenorrhea, because menstrual blood loss and duration of bleeding are significantly reduced over time. By 12 months of use, 20% of users have amenorrhea. The contraceptive implant has been found to reduce dysmenorrhea symptoms in over 80% of users[124] Other therapies that have been studied as treatments for dysmenorrhea include vasopressin antagonists,[125] progesterone receptor modulators,[126] and dienogest.[127]

Alternative complementary therapies include dietary supplements, acupuncture, and high-frequency transcutaneous electrical nerve stimulation. A recent systematic review studied the effectiveness of a full range of dietary supplements in treating dysmenorrhea, including herbs or other botanicals, vitamins, minerals, enzymes, and amino acids; traditional Chinese medications were excluded. The bottom line was that there is no high-quality evidence to support the effectiveness or safety of any dietary supplement for dysmenorrhea.[128]

Trials with acupuncture compared to sham (placebo) procedures have not consistently demonstrated effectiveness.[129] However, many case reports and some placebo-controlled studies have shown that acupuncture reduced pain and related menstrual symptoms. A four-arm dose-finding study without a placebo arm showed that every acupuncture method studied at every intensity reduced menstrual pain intensity and duration.[130] A smart phone app-based self-acupressure therapy was recently found to reduce mean pain intensity more than did the usual cure in a randomized but not blinded study.[131]

Surgical approaches provide relief for patients who do not respond to medical therapies. Endometrial ablation can reduce dysmenorrhea when it occurs in conjunction with heavy or prolonged menstrual bleeding. Some evidence exists to support the effectiveness of laparoscopic nerve ablation in selected cases. Hysterectomy is the definitive, effective treatment for primary dysmenorrhea when other measures fail.

Secondary Dysmenorrhea

Patients with secondary dysmenorrhea also complain of painful uterine cramping with menses but may have other accompanying complaints, such as dyspareunia or non-menstrual pelvic pain. By definition, the pain that patients experience with secondary dysmenorrhea is due to uterine or other pathology.

The most common causes of secondary dysmenorrhea are adenomyosis, endometriosis, pelvic adhesions, and neoplasia. *Adenomyosis* is the presence of endometrial glands and stroma deep in the myometrium. With *endometriosis,* the endometrial glands and stoma implant outside the uterus on the serosa of the uterus, the fallopian tubes, the ovaries, the intestines, and other peritoneal surfaces. The endometrial cells within the endometriotic implants proliferate early in the cycle and are sloughed at the end of the cycle into the surrounding tissue; this induces intense, usually painful, local inflammation. Long-term, extensive adhesive disease, nodules, or ovarian endometriomas may develop.

The latest Canadian Society of Obstetrics and Gynecology guidelines report that both primary and secondary dysmenorrhea are likely to respond to the same medical therapies, so initiation of therapy should not depend on establishing a precise diagnosis.[119] However, the choice of therapy should reflect the desire for fertility. Ovulation suppression or, better yet, *menstrual suppression* is usually effective.[121] Progestin-only pills that suppress ovulation (desogestrel) have been found to be better than cyclic combined estrogen-progestin contraceptive pills.[132] In particular, Depo-subQ provera 104 is an FDA-approved therapy for the treatment of dysmenorrhea associated with endometriosis. The magnitude of pain reduction seen in the clinical trials with Depo-subQ provera 104 matched the pain score reductions seen with gonadotropin releasing hormone (GnRH) agonists with fewer adverse hypoestrogenic impacts.[123] In clinical trials, the high-dose LNG IUD has been effective in the treatment of dysmenorrhea caused by endometriosis, and also has shrunk the size of endometriotic implants, particularly those that are located near the uterus. In a comparative trial of extended cycle use of the vaginal contraceptive ring vs. oral contraceptives, mean pain score reductions were greater among ring users.[122] The contraceptive implant is as effective as DMPA in treating dysmenorrhea associated with endometriosis.[133]

Other medications are available to treat dysmenorrhea by inducing amenorrhea, but their use is limited by side effects and cost. GnRH agonists induce amenorrhea and, thereby, eliminate dysmenorrhea. However, GnRH use is limited to 4 to 6 months because it causes hypoestrogenic side effects such as vasomotor symptoms (hot flashes), vaginal dryness, and loss of bone mineralization. GnRH agonists have been combined with either progestin-only or combined estrogen/progestin add-back therapy for long-term treatment of endometriosis.[134] Danazol, an androgen that was used more frequently in the past to treat endometriosis, effectively induces amenorrhea but can be used for only 4 to 6 months due to androgenic side effects, such as acne, hirsutism, oily skin, clitoral enlargement, and voice deepening. Other therapies on the horizon, especially for endometriosis-related dysmenorrhea include selective progesterone (or estrogen) receptor modulators, aromatase inhibitors, immunomodulators and antiangiogenic agents.[135]

If medical therapies are not effective, or if the patient wants to become pregnant, more definitive surgical approaches may be needed. For example, secondary dysmenorrhea caused by pelvic scarring may benefit from surgical lysis of adhesions, although recurrence of such adhesions is very common. Hysterectomy is reserved for treatment of incapacitating dysmenorrhea unresponsive to more conservative measures and is appropriate only for patients who do not desire future childbearing.

Premenstrual Syndrome (PMS) and Premenstrual Dysphoric Disorder (PMDD)

Nearly 90% of cycling women experience some discomfort with their menses. With ovulation, problems with fluid retention, bloating, mood disorders, and breast tenderness are common. Caucasian women are more likely to experience PMS than are African American women. For many women, these symptoms are not significant, but in 20% to 30%, they affect a woman's activities,[136] and in 1.2% to 6.4% of women, the problem rises to the level that it qualifies as a psychiatrically defined disorder.[137] (See also Chapter 23 on Mental Health and Contraception.)

Premenstrual syndrome (PMS) is a heterogeneous collection of signs and symptoms that share one common characteristic: a temporal relationship to the menstrual cycle. PMS is the cyclic appearance of at least one symptom during the luteal phase, which abates as menstruation begins and is followed by an entirely symptom-free period.[138] There are many symptoms associated with PMS, including physical symptoms of abdominal bloating, breast tenderness, headaches, extremity edema, and emotional symptoms of anxiety, depression, confusion, social withdrawal, angry outbursts, and irritability.[139] Other commonly reported manifestations of PMS include fatigue, thirst, appetite changes, and crying spells. To be considered clinically significant, PMS symptoms must interfere with work, lifestyle, or interpersonal relationships. PMS can increase relationship strain, sexual dysfunction, social isolation, work absenteeism, and risk for suicide. Studies have demonstrated that PMS results in poorer self-reported mental and physical health, increased use of health services, and higher health care costs for sufferers.

Table 1-5 Criteria for premenstrual dysphoric disorder

Diagnostic and Statistical Manual of Mental Disorders, Fifth Edition Premenstrual Dysphoric Disorder

A. In most menstrual cycles, the following symptoms must be present in final week before onset of menses, start to improve within few days after onset of menses, and become minimal or absent in week post-menses—A least 1 symptom must be either (1), (2), (3) or (4) and individual must experience at least 5 total symptoms:

1. Marked affective lability (e.g., mood swings; feeling suddenly sad or tearful or increased sensitivity to rejection)
2. Marked irritability or anger or increased interpersonal conflicts
3. Marked depressed mood, feelings of hopelessness, or self-deprecating thoughts
4. Marked anxiety, tension, feelings of being "keyed up," or "on edge"
5. Decreased interest in usual activities (e.g., work, school, friends, hobbies)
6. Subjective difficulty in concentration
7. Lethargy, easy fatigability, or marked lack of energy
8. Marked change in appetite, overeating, or specific food cravings
9. Hypersomnia or insomnia
10. A sense of being overwhelmed or out of control
11. Physical symptoms such as breast tenderness or swelling, joint or muscle pain, sensation of "bloating," weight gain

B. Symptoms are associated with clinically significant distress or interference with work, school, usual social activities, or relationships.
C. Disturbance is not merely exacerbation of symptoms of another disorder.
D. Criteria on A should be confirmed by prospective daily ratings during at least 2 symptomatic cycles (diagnosis may be made provisionally prior to this confirmation).
E. Symptoms are not due to direct physiological effects of substance (e.g., drug of abuse, medication, or other treatment) or another medical condition (e.g., hyperthyroidism).

Premenstrual Dysphoric Disorder Work Group (2013)[140]

Premenstrual dysphoric disorder (PMDD) is a more severe form of PMS with a very specific definition. The American Psychiatric Association requires the manifestation of at least 5 symptoms during the final week before the onset of menses that start to improve after the onset of menses and become minimal or absent in the week following menses.[138] See Table 1-5. By definition, at least one of the five required symptoms must represent a change in mood that is severe enough to interfere with occupational or social functions for at least two consecutive cycles.

Etiologies

What causes PMS/PMDD? Multiple factors likely are involved. Early investigators suggested that PMS was due to a lack of progesterone,[141] but subsequent research failed to find a difference between PMS sufferers and controls in levels of progesterone or any other major hormones including estradiol, FSH, LH, prolactin, SHBG, or testosterone.[142,143] However, individuals with PMS may be more biologically vulnerable to normal fluctuations in hormone levels than are those without the syndrome.[144] Such sensitive individuals may have a pathological response to either withdrawal or exposure to allopregnanolone, the agonist to gamma-aminobutyric acid (GABA), and the neurotransmitter that reduces neuronal excitability. Blockage of allopregnanolone reduces premenstrual symptoms in these patients.

Another older hypothesis was that premenstrual disorders are due to a deficit in the function of the serotonin system, because a deficit in the tryptophan or exposure to serotonin receptor antagonist can elicit premenstrual symptoms.[138] Other investigators have hypothesized that PMS may be caused by low beta-endorphin levels, low adrenocorticotropic levels, abnormal prostaglandin production, or endogenous hormone allergies, but again research has not consistently supported any of these hypotheses. Studies of PMS sufferers have also failed to identify deficiencies of magnesium, zinc, vitamin A, vitamin E, thiamine, or vitamin B6.[145] An association between post-traumatic stress disorder (PTSD) or trauma and PMS/PMDD has also been suggested.[146]

Diagnosis

The differential diagnosis of PMS/PMDD includes other dysthymic and depressive disorders, generalized anxiety disorder, and hypothyroidism. Take a detailed history to begin differentiating among these conditions. Include a careful medical, gynecological, and psychiatric history. Also ask about diet and exercise. For many individuals, clinical depression and other serious problems worsen premenstrually but never completely abate; patients who do not experience a symptom-free interval do not have PMS or PMDD alone. As many as half of those with self-diagnosed PMS have other problems that require careful evaluation and may need therapies that may differ from those used to treat PMS.[147] Some patients may have PMDD symptoms as well as an underlying or concomitant psychiatric problem; in one study, 59% of women diagnosed with PMDD also had clinical depression or an anxiety disorder.[148]

Laboratory tests are generally not needed to diagnose PMS. In some cases, however, the clinician must rule out hypothyroidism, because a patient with low levels of thyroid hormone may present with fatigue, bloating, depression, and irritability. Laboratory testing to measure sex steroid hormone levels is completely unnecessary in the evaluation of PMS or PMDD.

The patient should chart her symptoms for at least 1 to 2 menstrual cycles. This is the best tool to use to diagnose PMS/PMDD. Two cycles of charting help control for cycle-to-cycle variability. Research studies have validated assessment tools for this purpose, including the Calendar of Premenstrual

Experiences (COPE), and the Daily Record of Severity of Problems (DRSP).[138] A patient generally can successfully document menstrually-related symptoms by taking notes on a regular calendar or in an app, noting the symptoms experienced each day, along with their severity, and recording the dates of menses. A patient who is overwhelmed by a large number of complaints can chart only the 3 to 5 complaints that are the most profoundly bothersome. Ideally, this chart should also include body weight and, if possible, a record of basal body temperature or home ovulation test results. Ask the patient to document any medications used during this time.

The patient should return to the office after collecting these data. Carefully study the pattern of symptoms. Symptoms do not need to recur with equal intensity in each cycle; different symptoms may occur during different cycles. Again, the key to diagnosing PMS/PMDD is the *timing* of symptoms—they must appear in the luteal phase and disappear soon after the onset of menses.

Treatment of Premenstrual Syndrome

PMS treatment is strongly influenced by a placebo effect. In a wide range of studies, researchers report that 40% to 94% of patients with PMS will improve in the short term regardless of the treatment used. This reinforces the need to rely on placebo-controlled studies rather than on case reports or personal testimonials to determine the true efficacy of a particular drug or treatment for PMS.

Treatment requires a comprehensive, individualized approach. However, all patients deserve reassurance, emotional support, and education. Both the patient and family may benefit from a discussion of the hormonal changes associated with PMS. Charting the symptoms not only validates the diagnosis, but it may also help the patient gain more insight into the problem and gain a greater sense of control. If therapy is initiated, the patient should continue charting to identify which interventions improve symptoms.

According to recent guidelines, first-line treatments for PMS include exercise, vitamin B-6, cognitive behavioral therapy (CBT), oral contraceptives, and intermittent or continuous selective serotonin reuptake inhibitors (SSRIs).[149] Cognitive behavioral therapy typically used for about 12 sessions is particularly helpful for patients who do not want medication. Smoking cessation, limits on alcohol intake, and regular sleep have all been found to be helpful.

If symptoms are mild, it may be reasonable to start with diet (complex carbohydrates in the late luteal phase), exercise, vitamin B6 (100 mg daily), and calcium (1,000 mg daily). For mild cases, also consider directing treatment toward specific symptoms. Breast tenderness can be eased with a fitted support or sports bra. Abdominal pain and backache respond well to the therapies outlined under the discussion of dysmenorrhea. Vigorous exercise may improve mood as well as reduce stress and physical complaints in PMS, but evidence is minimal.[150] Stronger evidence exists that a complex carbohydrate diet during the luteal phase may help women with PMS.[151,152] However, premenstrual chocolate craving may be a cultural phenomenon because such cravings are unusual elsewhere in the world. Stronger evidence also exists for the use of calcium supplementation in PMS. In the Nurses Health Study II, a large longitudinal cohort study, women who consumed the most vitamin D and calcium were the least likely to develop PMS during 10 years of follow-up.[153] In addition, randomized controlled trials have demonstrated a reduction of PMS symptoms among women taking 1,200 to 1,600 mg of calcium carbonate daily.[154,155] Even 500 mg per day of calcium supplements has been shown to significantly decrease in symptoms of moderate to severe PMS.[156] High doses of calcium should be avoided in women with histories of renal stones.

Herbal agents have grown in popularity in the United States and are used frequently by women to treat themselves for PMS. Chasteberry tree extract 20 to 40 mg/d (*Vitex agnus-castus* in Latin) is used commonly in Europe to treat PMS and cyclic breast pain; it is approved by the German Commission E for these indications. Meta-analysis shows a large pooled effect of *Vitex agnus-castus*, but because of poor quality of data, this result should be seen as exploratory; it overestimates the effects of this agent.[157] Evening primrose oil is also popularly used in Europe for PMS and breast tenderness (mastalgia), but randomized controlled studies have not validated the efficacy of this herb in the treatment of PMS. Ginkgo biloba and St. John Wort have shown some efficacy in small-scale trials.[158,159]

Trials of cognitive therapy, group therapy, and relaxation therapy have shown that these modalities may improve physical or psychological symptoms of PMS, although few studies have randomized patients.[160] Stress management, anger management, self-help, biofeedback, acupuncture, or light therapy may help some individuals.

Continuous transdermal low-dose estrogen with progestogen has been found to have a small to moderate beneficial effect based on low-quality evidence.[161] Progesterone supplementation, often with hormonal products marketed as natural or bio-identical, remains popular as a treatment for any degree of PMS, despite a recent comprehensive review failing to find evidence that progesterone as a treatment for PMS is either effective *or* ineffective.[162]

Ovulation suppressants or SSRI treatments are recommended for those who have moderate to severe symptoms that lead to the functional impairment and for those who do not respond to first-line therapies for milder symptoms.[138] Combined hormonal contraceptives given cyclically have been reported to slightly attenuate menstrual cycle symptom changes.[163]

However, for some COCs users, symptoms of depression, breast tenderness, and bloating worsen with pill use, especially during the placebo-pill days. Randomized, controlled trials of cyclic COC use for treatment of PMS have generated mixed results. One exception was the 35mcg EE/drospirenone (DSRP) oral contraceptive (Yasmin) that was found to reduce physical symptoms of PMS, especially bloating and mastalgia.[164] Extended-cycle dosing of COCs and vaginal contraceptive rings and use of DMPA may aid PMS sufferers not only by suppressing ovulation, but also by reducing the number of scheduled bleeding episodes (and episodes of associated symptoms) that users experience.

Treatment for Premenstrual Dysphoric Disorder (PMDD)

PMDD generally requires medication to deal with its severe symptoms and mood disorders, although some of the measures used for PMS may be added. There are two classes of medications approved by the FDA to treat the physical and emotional symptoms of PMDD. The first is SSRIs. The FDA has specifically approved three SSRIs for treatment of PMDD (fluoxetine, sertraline, and paroxetine). These agents can be given at low doses continuously (every day) or intermittently (only during the luteal phase) to reduce both the physical and psychological symptoms of PMDD.[165,166,167] Research has found that other agents related to SSRIs are equally effective, including citalopram and venlafaxine.[168] Patients who have severe physical symptoms usually respond better to daily treatment than they do to SSRI use only during the luteal phase.[169] SSRIs should be continued for at least 1 or (better) 2 months before declaring failure. If one agent is not successful, try another one before abandoning SSRIs as a class, because an individual's response may vary from drug to drug. Recommend that the patient use effective contraception while using SSRIs.

Most people tolerate SSRIs without incident, but these medications can cause side effects including nausea, decreased libido, and insomnia. The risk for side effects is related to dose; the use of low-dose SSRIs often suffices and may minimize side effects. In contrast to experience with SSRIs used for depression, rapid improvement of PMDD symptoms can be noted within a day or two of the dose even if it is given only during luteal phase.[170] Side effects can develop as rapidly. Clinicians should counsel patients about these potential side effects and inquire about them at follow-up visits.

The other FDA-approved therapy for the symptoms of PMDD is a monophasic oral contraceptive regimen with active pills containing 20 mcg EE and 3 mg drospirenone in a 24/4 formulation (Yaz). Randomized, prospective, placebo-controlled, double-blinded clinical prospective studies found that this COC reduced both mood disorders and physical complaints of PMDD by about 50%, which was significantly superior to the placebo effect.[171,172] This is about the same magnitude of response seen with SSRIs.

Second-line therapies include more profound suppression of monthly cycling with GnRH agonists with estrogen-progestin add-back started at 6 months.[138] Only after GnRH agonist therapies fail to relieve a patient's symptoms should surgical interventions be considered.

Clinical experience also supports off-label use of other medications to treat PMDD. For those who cannot tolerate SSRIs but who would benefit from psychotropic medication, buspirone, and anxiolytic medications provide alternatives.[172] Alprazolam has demonstrated efficacy in PMDD, but the most effective pattern of use for that drug has not been defined. Some studies have found therapeutic response with intermittent use of alprazolam (e.g., 4 to 5 days preceding menses), while other studies have found such protocols no better than placebo. To avoid withdrawal symptoms, taper the alprazolam each time it is discontinued. Be careful when prescribing anxiolytic medicines because they are habit-forming and have potential for abuse.[171] Patients with histories of alcoholism or other substance abuse are not appropriate candidates. Caution that the drug may induce drowsiness; the first dose should be taken at home, before bedtime, to gauge its sedating effect the next day.

The clinician must individualize therapy to symptoms and strongly consider referral to a mental health specialist for patients with a PMDD diagnosis meeting DSM-V criteria. Counseling may be very beneficial for patients with PMDD and their families. Stress management, anger management, self-help support groups, individual and couples therapy, cognitive behavioral therapy, and light therapy all have been reported to provide relief. Selection depends upon an individual patient's symptoms and ability to access resources.

MENSTRUAL EXACERBATION OF OTHER MEDICAL CONDITIONS

Medical conditions commonly worsen during the luteal phase and menses.[173] This may reflect the complex and often poorly understood interplay of hormones with other physiologic processes throughout the body. A classic example is *menstrual migraines*.[174] About 7% to 9% of women with migraine headaches have them only with menses. Another 35% to 40% of migraine sufferers experience worsening of headaches with menses.[175] Attacks of menstrual migraines are usually more debilitating, last longer, are more likely to recur, and are less responsive to medical therapies than non-menstrual migraine attacks.[176,177] One therapeutic approach to menstrual migraine headaches has been to treat prophylactically with standard migraine treatments during at-risk times. Some have recommended home fertility monitors to predict menses more accurately so therapy can be better timed.[178] However, because headaches have been definitely linked to a decline in estrogen levels,[179] another approach has been to suppress menses with extended cycle hormones or to provide estrogen supplementation during bleeding days. The use of estrogen is appropriate only for patients under 35 years of age who do not suffer neurologic auras preceding the onset of their migraines and do not suffer worsening of their headaches with estrogen exposure. The progestin-only pill with desogestrel (not available in the United States), which reliably suppresses ovulation, has been found to be equally effective as combination oral contraceptives, but is not contraindicated in migraineurs with aura.[180] DMPA, which suppresses ovulation and induces amenorrhea, would be preferred over LNG IUS, which does not control the hormonal cycling. Triptans have also been found to be effective for both acute treatment and for short-term prevention of menstrual migraine.[176]

Patients with *seizure disorders* frequently experience acute exacerbations of their convulsive activity with menstruation. More than one third of women with epilepsy are affected by catamenial (menses-related) epilepsy;[181,182] these seizures rarely respond to antiepileptic medications. Premenstrual increases in *asthma* attacks have been reported in up to 40% of women with asthma.[183] Virtually every woman knows that acne tends to blossom around the time of menses. Less common medical conditions that flare at menses include acute intermittent porphyria, diabetes, erythema multiforme, glaucoma, hereditary angioedema, rheumatoid arthritis, and multiple sclerosis.

Mental health problems tend to become more symptomatic with menses. Patients with anxiety disorders and pain disorders tend to experience more anxiety and panic attacks during menses. Symptoms of obsessive-compulsive disorders have been found to increase before menstruation, and patients with psychotic disorders also tend to suffer more intense symptoms during menses.[184] Worsening of schizophrenia symptoms during the luteal phase has been reported.[184] There is some evidence that women with bulimia may experience increased food cravings premenstrually.[185]

Suppressing ovulation alone (ENG implant) or eliminating menses by controlling the endometrium alone (LNG IUD) may not be sufficient therapy for patients whose medical conditions fluctuate in response to hormonal cycling. However, it is possible to prevent hormonal fluctuations with DMPA or extended cycle use of combined hormonal methods. Selection of the appropriate method depends upon underlying health, as well as personal preferences and specific symptom(s) presentation.

Author Disclosures: Nelson: Grants/Research—Agile Pharma, ContraMed, Estetra SPRL, Evofem Inc, FHI (MonaLisa), Merck. Speakers Bureau—Allergan, Bayer, Merck. Consultant/Advisory Board—Agile, Allergan, AMAG Pharma, Bayer, ContraMed, Merck, PharmaNest; Shulman: Speakers Bureau—AMAG Pharma, Allergan, Roche Labs. Consultant—Allergan, AMAG Pharma, Bayer, Lunada, Merck, NeoSeq Labs, Sera Prognostics.

References

1. Munro MG, Critchley H, Fraser IS. Research and clinical management for women with abnormal uterine bleeding in the reproductive years: More than PALM-COEIN. BJOG 2017;124:185–189.
2. Nelson AL, Ritchie JJ. Severe anemia from heavy menstrual bleeding requires heightened attention. Am J Obstet Gynecol 2015;213:97.e1–6.
3. Lam C, Anderson B, Lopes V, Schulkin J, Matteson K. Assessing abnormal uterine bleeding: Are physicians taking a meaningful clinical history? J Womens Health (Larchmt) 2017;26:762–767.
4. Mengesha B, Griffin L, Nagle A, Kiley J. Assessment of contraceptive needs in women undergoing bariatric surgery. Contraception 2016;94:74–7.
5. Chen KT. Top free menstrual cycle tracking apps for your patients. OBG Management 2017;29:44–46.
6. Smith OP, Jabbour HN, Critchley HO. Cyclooxygenase enzyme expression and E series prostaglandin receptor signalling are enhanced in heavy menstruation. Hum Reprod 2007;22:1450–6.
7. Maybin JA, Thiruchelvam U, Madhra M, Saunders PTK, Critchley HOD. Steroids regulate CXCL4 in the human endometrium during menstruation to enable efficient endometrial repair. J Clin Endocrinol Metab 2017;102:1851–1860.
8. Maybin JA, Boswell L, Young VJ, Duncan WC, Critchley HOD. Reduced transforming growth factor-β activity in the endometrium of women with heavy menstrual bleeding. J Clin Endocrinol Metab 2017;102:1299–1308.
9. Fraser IS, Critchley HO, Broder M, Munro MG. The FIGO recommendations on terminologies and definitions for normal and abnormal uterine bleeding. Semin Reprod Med 2011;29:383–90.
10. Munro MG. Practical aspects of the two FIGO systems for management of abnormal uterine bleeding in the reproductive years. Best Pract Res Clin Obstet Gynaecol 2017;40:3–22.
11. Deligeoroglou E, Athanasopoulos N, Tsimaris P, Dimopoulos KD, Vrachnis N, Creatsas G. Evaluation and management of adolescent amenorrhea. Ann N Y Acad Sci 2010;1205:23–32.
12. Klein DA, Poth MA. Amenorrhea: an approach to diagnosis and management. Am Fam Physician 2013;87:781–8. Table 1 ©2013 reprinted with permission, American Academy of Family Physicians. All rights reserved.
13. Gordon CM, Ackerman KE, Berga SL, et al. Functional hypothalamic amenorrhea: An Endocrine Society clinical practice guideline. J Clin Endocrinol Metab 2017;102:1413–1439.
14. Morgan S, Anderson RA, Gourley C, Wallace WH, Spears N. How do chemotherapeutic agents damage the ovary? Hum Reprod Update 2012;18:525–35.
15. Chemaitilly W, Li Z, Krasin MJ, et al. Premature ovarian insufficiency in childhood Cancer survivors: A report from the St. Jude Lifetime Cohort. J Clin Endocrinol Metab 2017;102:2242–2250.
16. Jiao X, Zhang H, Ke H, et al. Premature ovarian insufficiency: phenotypic characterization within different etiologies. J Clin Endocrinol Metab 2017;102:2281–2290.
17. ACOG Committee Opinion 702: Female athlete triad. Committee on Adolescent Health Care. Obstet Gynecol 2017;e160–e167.
18. Weiss Kelly AK, Hecht S; Council on Sports Medicine and Fitness. The female athlete triad. Pediatrics 2016;138:e20160922.
19. Altayar O, Nofal AA, Leon GC, et al. Treatments to prevent bone loss in functional hypothalamic amenorrhea: A systematic review and meta-analysis. J Endocrine Society. 2017;Epub ahead of print.
20. Committee on Gynecologic Practice. Committee Opinion No. 698: Hormone therapy in primary ovarian insufficiency. Obstet Gynecol 2017;129:e134–e141.
21. Yildiz BO, Knochenhauer ES, Azziz R. Impact of obesity on the risk for polycystic ovary syndrome. J Clin Endocrinol Metab 2008;93162–8.

22. ACOG Committee on Practice Bulletins—Gynecology. ACOG Practice Bulletin No. 108: Polycystic ovary syndrome. Obstet Gynecol 2009;114:936–49.
23. Rees DA, Jenkins-Jones S, Morgan CL. Contemporary reproductive outcomes for patients with polycystic ovary syndrome: A retrospective observational study. J Clin Endocrinol Metab 2016;101:1664–72.
24. Hart R, Doherty DA. The potential implications of a PCOS diagnosis on a woman's long-term health using data linkage. J Clin Endocrinol Metab 2015;100:911–9.
25. Chan JL, Kar S, Vanky E, et al. Racial and ethnic differences in the prevalence of metabolic syndrome and its components of metabolic syndrome in women with polycystic ovary syndrome: a regional cross-sectional study. Am J Obstet Gynecol 2017;217: 189.e1–189.e8.
26. Legro RS, Arslanian SA, Ehrmann DA, et al. Endocrine Society. Diagnosis and treatment of polycystic ovary syndrome: an Endocrine Society clinical practice guideline. J Clin Endocrinol Metab 2013;98:4565–92.
27. Azziz R. Polycystic ovary syndrome: what's in a name? J Clin Endocrinol Metab 2014;99:1142–5.
28. Dunaif A. Perspectives in polycystic ovary syndrome: From hair to eternity. J Clin Endocrinol Metab 2016;101:759–68.
29. Dokras A, Saini S, Gibson-Helm M, Schulkin J, Cooney L, Teede H. Gaps in knowledge among physicians regarding diagnostic criteria and management of polycystic ovary syndrome. Fertil Steril 2017;107:1380–1386.e1.
30. Fauser BC, Tarlatzis BC, Rebar RW, et al. Consensus on women's health aspects of polycystic ovary syndrome (PCOS): the Amsterdam ESHRE/ASRM-Sponsored 3rd PCOS Consensus Workshop Group. Fertil Steril 2012;97:28–38.e25.
31. Copp T, Jansen J, Doust J, Mol BW, Dokras A, McCaffery K. Are expanding disease definitions unnecessarily labelling women with polycystic ovary syndrome? BMJ 2017;358:j3694.
32. The Rotterdam ESHRE/ASRM Sponsored PCOS consensus Workshop Group. Human Reprod 2004;19:40–47.
33. Kim HJ, Adams JM, Gudmundsson JA, Arason G, Pau CT, Welt CK. Polycystic ovary morphology: age-based ultrasound criteria. Fertil Steril 2017;108:548–553.
34. Reid RL, Magee BA. A pragmatic approach to hormonal testing in the assessment of disorders of female reproduction. Intl J Womens Health Wellness 2016;2:022.
35. O'Reilly MW, Kempegowda P, Jenkinson C, et al. 11-Oxygenated C19 steroids sre the predominant androgens in polycystic ovary syndrome. J Clin Endocrinol Metab 2017;102:840–848.
36. O'Reilly MW, Taylor AE, Crabtree NJ, et al. Hyperandrogenemia predicts metabolic phenotype in polycystic ovary syndrome: the utility of serum androstenedione. J Clin Endocrinol Metab 2014;99:1027–36.
37. Wang ET, Calderon-Margalit R, Cedars MI, et al. Polycystic ovary syndrome and risk for long-term diabetes and dyslipidemia. Obstet Gynecol 2011;117:6–13.
38. Jovanovic VP, Carmina E, Lobo RA. Not all women diagnosed with PCOS share the same cardiovascular risk profiles. Fertil Steril 2010;94(3):826–32.
39. Engmann L, Jin S, Sun F, et al. Racial and ethnic differences in the polycystic ovary syndrome metabolic phenotype. Am J Obstet Gynecol 2017;216:493.e1–493.e13.
40. Kerchner A, Lester W, Stuart SP, Dokras A. Risk of depression and other mental health disorders in women with polycystic ovary syndrome: a longitudinal study. Fertil Steril 2009;91:207–12.
41. Practice Committee of the American Society for Reproductive Medicine. Role of metformin for ovulation induction in infertile patients with polycystic ovary syndrome (PCOS): a guideline. Fertil Steril 2017: S0015–0282:30485–5.
42. Domecq JP, Prutsky G, Mullan RJ, et al. Lifestyle modification programs in polycystic ovary syndrome: systematic review and meta-analysis. J Clin Endocrinol Metab 2013; 98:4655–63.

43. Gardner CD, Kiazand A, Alhassan S, et al. Comparison of the Atkins, Zone, Ornish, and LEARN diets for change in weight and related risk factors among overweight premenopausal women: the A TO Z Weight Loss Study: a randomized trial. JAMA 2007;297:969–77.
44. Heymsfield SB, Wadden TA. Mechanisms, pathophysiology, and management of obesity. N Engl J Med 2017;376:254–266
45. Lv N, Azar KMJ, Rosas LG, Wulfovich S, Xiao L, Ma J. Behavioral lifestyle interventions for moderate and severe obesity: A systematic review. Prev Med 2017;100:180–193.
46. Brennan L, Teede H, Skouteris H, Linardon J, Hill B, Moran L. Lifestyle and behavioral management of polycystic ovary syndrome. J Womens Health (Larchmt) 2017;26:836–848.
47. Redman LM, Elkind-Hirsch K, Ravussin E. Aerobic exercise in women with polycystic ovary syndrome improves ovarian morphology independent of changes in body composition. Fertil Steril 2011;95:2696–9.
48. Jayagopal V, Kilpatrick ES, Holding S, Jennings PE, Atkin SL. Orlistat is as beneficial as metformin in the treatment of polycystic ovarian syndrome. J Clin Endocrinol Metab 2005;90:729–33.
49. Barbieri RL. Treating polycystic ovary syndrome: start using dual medical therapy. OBG Mgmt 2017;4:9–13.
50. de Wilde MA, Lamain-de Ruiter M, Veltman-Verhulst SM, et al. Increased rates of complications in singleton pregnancies of women previously diagnosed with polycystic ovary syndrome predominantly in the hyperandrogenic phenotype. Fertil Steril 2017;108:333–340.
51. Yildiz BO. Approach to the patient: contraception in women with polycystic ovary syndrome. J Clin Endocrinol Metab 2015;100:794–802.
52. van Oers AM, Mutsaerts MAQ, Burggraaff JM, et al. Cost-effectiveness analysis of lifestyle intervention in obese infertile women. Hum Reprod 2017:1–9
53. Mutsaerts MA, van Oers AM, Groen H, et al. Randomized trial of a lifestyle program in obese infertile women. N Engl J Med 2016;374:1942–53.
54. Legro RS, Barnhart HX, Schlaff WD, et al. Cooperative Multicenter Reproductive Medicine Network. Clomiphene, metformin, or both for infertility in the polycystic ovary syndrome. N Engl J Med 2007;356:551–66.
55. Legro RS, Brzyski RG, Diamond MP, et al. Letrozole versus clomiphene for infertility in the polycystic ovary syndrome. N Engl J Med 2014;371:119–29.
56. Diamond MP, Kruger M, Santoro N, et al. Endometrial shedding effect on conception and live birth in women with polycystic ovary syndrome. Obstet Gynecol 2012;119:902–8.
57. Paulson M, Sahlin L, Hirschberg AL. Progesterone receptors and proliferation of the endometrium in obese women with polycystic ovary syndrome-a lifestyle intervention study. J Clin Endocrinol Metab 2017;102:1244–1253.
58. Wild RA, Carmina E, Diamanti-Kandarakis E, et al. Assessment of cardiovascular risk and prevention of cardiovascular disease in women with the polycystic ovary syndrome: a consensus statement by the Androgen Excess and Polycystic Ovary Syndrome (AE-PCOS) Society. J Clin Endocrinol Metab 2010;95:2038–49.
59. Merz CN, Shaw LJ, Azziz R, et al. Cardiovascular disease and 10-year mortality in postmenopausal women with clinical features of polycystic ovary syndrome. J Womens Health (Larchmt) 2016;25:875–81.
60. Banaszewska B, Pawelczyk L, Spaczynski RZ, Duleba AJ. Effects of simvastatin and metformin on polycystic ovary syndrome after six months of treatment. J Clin Endocrinol Metab 2011;96:3493–501.
61. Weisberg E, McGeehan K, Fraser IS. Effect of perceptions of menstrual blood loss and menstrual pain on women's quality of life. Eur J Contracept Reprod Health Care 2016;21:431–435.
62. Karlsson TS, Marions LB, Edlund MG. Heavy menstrual bleeding significantly affects quality of life. Acta Obstet Gynecol Scand 2014;93:52–7.
63. Côté I, Jacobs P, Cumming D. Work loss associated with increased menstrual loss in the United States. Obstet Gynecol 2002;100:683–7.

64. NICE Clinical Guidelines No. 44. Heavy menstrual bleeding : assessment and management. London: RCOG Press National Institute for health and Clinical Excellence, 2007. Available at www.nice.org.uk/guidance/cg44. Last accessed Sept. 19, 2017.
65. Fraser IS, McCarron G, Markham R, Resta T. Blood and total fluid content of menstrual discharge. Obstet Gynecol 1985;65:194–8.
66. Wise MR, Gill P, Lensen S, Thompson JM, Farquhar CM. Body mass index trumps age in decision for endometrial biopsy: cohort study of symptomatic premenopausal women. Am J Obstet Gynecol 2016;215:598.e1–598.e8.
67. ACOG Committee on Practice Bulletins-Gynecology. Practice Bulletin No. 128: diagnosis of abnormal uterine bleeding in reproductive-aged women. Obstet Gynecol 2012;120:197–206.
68. Widrich T, Bradley LD, Mitchinson AR, Collins RL. Comparison of saline infusion sonography with office hysteroscopy for the evaluation of the endometrium. Am J Obstet Gynecol 1996;174:1327–34.
69. Clarke A, Black N, Rowe P, Mott S, Howle K. Indications for and outcome of total abdominal hysterectomy for benign disease: a prospective cohort study. Br J Obstet Gynaecol 1995;102:611–20.
70. Munro MG, Lukes AS. Abnormal Uterine Bleeding and Underlying Hemostatic Disorders Consensus Group. Abnormal uterine bleeding and underlying hemostatic disorders: report of a consensus process. Fertil Steril 2005;84:1335–7.
71. Miller CH, Philipp CS, Stein SF, et al. The spectrum of haemostatic characteristics of women with unexplained menorrhagia. Haemophilia 2011;17:e223–9.
72. Byams VR, Kouides PA, Kulkarni R, et al. Surveillance of female patients with inherited bleeding disorders in United States Haemophilia Treatment Centres. Haemophilia 2011;17 Suppl 1:6–13.
73. Leebeek FW, Eikenboom JC. Von Willebrand's disease. N Engl J Med 2016;375:2067–2080.
74. James AH, Kouides PA, Abdul-Kadir R, et al. Evaluation and management of acute menorrhagia in women with and without underlying bleeding disorders: consensus from an international expert panel. Eur J Obstet Gynecol Reprod Biol 2011;158:124–34
75. Davies J, Kadir RA. Heavy menstrual bleeding: An update on management. Thromb Res 2017;151 Suppl 1:S70–S77.
76. Rees MC, Anderson AB, Demers LM, Turnbull AC. Prostaglandins in menstrual fluid in menorrhagia and dysmenorrhoea. Br J Obstet Gynaecol 1984;91:673–80.
77. Adelantado JM, López Bernal A, Turnbull AC. Topographical distribution of prostaglandin E receptors in human myometrium. Br J Obstet Gynaecol 1988;95:348–53.
78. Hagenfeldt K. The role of prostaglandins and allied substances in uterine haemostasis. Contraception 1987;36:23–35.
79. DeVore GR, Owens O, Kase N. Use of intravenous Premarin in the treatment of dysfunctional uterine bleeding—a double-blind randomized control study. Obstet Gynecol 1982;59:285–91.
80. Fritz MA. Clinical Gynecologic Endocrinology and Infertility. Lippincott Williams Wilkins. Philadelphia. 2011:591–620.
81. Munro MG, Mainor N, Basu R, Brisinger M, Barreda L. Oral medroxyprogesterone acetate and combination oral contraceptives for acute uterine bleeding: a randomized controlled trial. Obstet Gynecol 2006;108:924–9.
82. Ammerman SR, Nelson AL. A new progestogen-only medical therapy for outpatient management of acute, abnormal uterine bleeding: a pilot study. Am J Obstet Gynecol 2013;208:499.e1–5.
83. ACOG Committee Opinion No. 606: Options for prevention and management of heavy menstrual bleeding in adolescent patients undergoing cancer treatment. Obstet Gynecol 2014;124:397–402.
84. Lethaby A, Duckitt K, Farquhar C. Non-steroidal anti-inflammatory drugs for heavy menstrual bleeding. Cochrane Database Syst Rev 2013:CD000400.pub3
85. Díaz S, Croxatto HB, Pavez M, Belhadj H, Stern J, Sivin I. Clinical assessment of treatments for prolonged bleeding in users of Norplant implants. Contraception 1990;42: 97–109.

86. Gleeson N, Devitt M, Sheppard BL, Bonnar J. Endometrial fibrinolytic enzymes in women with normal menstruation and dysfunctional uterine bleeding. Br J Obstet Gynaecol 1993;100:768–71.
87. Lumsden MA, Wedisinghe L. Tranexamic acid therapy for heavy menstrual bleeding. Expert Opin Pharmacother 2011;12:2089–95.
88. Lukes AS, Moore KA, Muse KN, et al. Tranexamic acid treatment for heavy menstrual bleeding: a randomized controlled trial. Obstet Gynecol 2010;116:865–75.
89. Bradley LD, Gueye NA. The medical management of abnormal uterine bleeding in reproductive-aged women. Am J Obstet Gynecol 2016;214:31–44.
90. Maybin JA, Critchley HO. Medical management of heavy menstrual bleeding. Womens Health (Lond) 2016;12:27–34.
91. Bitzer J, Heikinheimo O, Nelson AL, Calaf-Alsina J, Fraser IS. Medical management of heavy menstrual bleeding: a comprehensive review of the literature. Obstet Gynecol Surv 2015;70:115–30.
92. Endrikat J, Shapiro H, Lukkari-Lax E, Kunz M, Schmidt W, Fortier M. A Canadian, multicentre study comparing the efficacy of a levonorgestrel-releasing intrauterine system to an oral contraceptive in women with idiopathic menorrhagia. J Obstet Gynaecol Can 2009;31:340–7.
93. Dahiya P, Dalal M, Yadav A, Dahiya K, Jain S, Silan V. Efficacy of combined hormonal vaginal ring in comparison to combined hormonal pills in heavy menstrual bleeding. Eur J Obstet Gynecol Reprod Biol 2016;203:147–51.
94. Anderson FD, Hait H. A multicenter, randomized study of an extended cycle oral contraceptive. Contraception 2003;68:89–96.
95 Miller L, Verhoeven CH, Hout J. Extended regimens of the contraceptive vaginal ring: a randomized trial. Obstet Gynecol 2005;106:473–82.
96. Lethaby A, Hussain M, Rishworth JR, Rees MC. Progesterone or progestogen-releasing intrauterine systems for heavy menstrual bleeding. Cochrane Database Syst Rev. 2015;(4):CD002126.pub3.
97. Kaunitz AM, Bissonnette F, Monteiro I, Lukkari-Lax E, Muysers C, Jensen JT. Levonorgestrel-releasing intrauterine system or medroxyprogesterone for heavy menstrual bleeding: a randomized controlled trial. Obstet Gynecol 2010;116:625–32.
98. ACOG Committee on Adolescent Health Care; Committee on Gynecologic Practice. Committee Opinion No.580: von Willebrand disease in women. Obstet Gynecol 2013;122:1368–73.
99. Abu Hashim H, Ghayaty E, El Rakhawy M. Levonorgestrel–releasing intrauterine system vs oral progestins for non-atypical endometrial hyperplasia: a systematic review and metaanalysis of randomized trials. Am J Obstet Gynecol 2015;213:469–78.
100. Zhang Q, Qi G, Kanis MJ, et al. Comparison among fertility-sparing therapies for well differentiated early-stage endometrial carcinoma and complex atypical hyperplasia. Oncotarget. 2017;8:57642–57653.
101. Li L, Leng JH, Zhang JJ, et al. Changes of menstruation patterns and adverse effects during the treatment of LNG-IUS for symptomatic adenomyosis. Zhonghua Fu Chan Ke Za Zhi 2016;51:657–662.
102. Braga GC, Brito MB, Ferriani RA, et al. Oral anticoagulant therapy does not modify the bleeding pattern associated with the levonorgestrel-releasing intrauterine system in women with thrombophilia and/or a history of thrombosis. Contraception 2014;89: 48–53.
103. Mawet M, Nollevaux F, Nizet D, et al. Impact of a new levonorgestrel intrauterine system, Levosert(®), on heavy menstrual bleeding: results of a one-year randomised controlled trial. Eur J Contracept Reprod Health Care 2014;19:169–79.
104. Donnez J, Donnez O, Matule D, et al. Long-term medical management of uterine fibroids with ulipristal acetate. Fertil Steril 2016;105:165–173.e4.
105. Safrai M, Chill HH, Reuveni Salzman A, Shushan A. Selective progesterone receptor modulators for the treatment of uterine leiomyomas. Obstet Gynecol. 2017;130:315–318.

106. Archer DF, Stewart EA, Jain RI, et al. Elagolix for the management of heavy menstrual bleeding associated with uterine fibroids: results from a phase 2a proof-of-concept study. Fertil Steril 2017;108:152–160.e4.
107. Farquhar CM, Naoom S, Steiner CA. The impact of endometrial ablation on hysterectomy rates in women with benign uterine conditions in the United States. Int J Technol Assess Health Care 2002;18:625–34.
108. Hare AA, Olah KS. Pregnancy following endometrial ablation: a review article. J Obstet Gynaecol 2005;25:108–14.
109. Marjoribanks J, Lethaby A, Farquhar C. Surgery versus medical therapy for heavy menstrual bleeding. Cochrane Database Syst Rev 2006:CD003855.pub
110. Kaunitz AM, Meredith S, Inki P, Kubba A, Sanchez-Ramos L. Levonorgestrel-releasing intrauterine system and endometrial ablation in heavy menstrual bleeding: a systematic review and meta-analysis. Obstet Gynecol 2009;113:1104–16.
111. de Souza SS, Camargos AF, de Rezende CP, Pereira FA, Araújo CA, Silva Filho AL. A randomized prospective trial comparing the levonorgestrel-releasing intrauterine system with thermal balloon ablation for the treatment of heavy menstrual bleeding. Contraception 2010;81:226–31.
112. Spencer JC, Louie M, Moulder JK, et al. Cost-effectiveness of treatments for heavy menstrual bleeding. Am J Obstet Gynecol 2017;217:574.e1–574.e9.
113. Heliövaara-Peippo S, Hurskainen R, Teperi J, et al. Quality of life and costs of levonorgestrel-releasing intrauterine system or hysterectomy in the treatment of menorrhagia: a 10-year randomized controlled trial. Am J Obstet Gynecol 2013;209:535.e1–535.e14.
114. Kamel DM, Tantawy SA, Abdelsamea GA. Experience of dysmenorrhea among a group of physical therapy students from Cairo University: an exploratory study. J Pain Res 2017;10:1079–1085.
115. Berry C, McGuire FL. Menstrual distress and acceptance of sexual role. Am J Obstet Gynecol 1972;114:83–7.
116. Sultan C, Gaspari L, Paris F. Adolescent dysmenorrhea. Endocr Dev 2012;22:171–80.
117. Geneen LJ, Moore RA, Clarke C, Martin D, Colvin LA, Smith BH. Physical activity and exercise for chronic pain in adults: an overview of Cochrane Reviews. Cochrane Database Syst Rev 2017;4:CD011279.pub3.
118. Zahradnik HP, Hanjalic-Beck A, Groth K. Nonsteroidal anti-inflammatory drugs and hormonal contraceptives for pain relief from dysmenorrhea: a review. Contraception 2010;81:185–96.
119. Burnett M, Lemyre M. No. 345-Primary dysmenorrhea consensus guideline. J Obstet Gynaecol Can 2017;39:585–595.
120. Harada T, Momoeda M. Evaluation of an ultra-low-dose oral contraceptive for dysmenorrhea: a placebo-controlled, double-blind, randomized trial. Fertil Steril 2016;106: 1807–1814.
121. Coffee AL, Sulak PJ, Kuehl TJ. Long-term assessment of symptomatology and satisfaction of an extended oral contraceptive regimen. Contraception 2007;75:444–9.
122. Priya K, Rajaram S, Goel N. Comparison of combined hormonal vaginal ring and low dose combined oral hormonal pill for the treatment of idiopathic chronic pelvic pain: a randomised trial. Eur J Obstet Gynecol Reprod Biol 2016;207:141–146.
123. Schlaff WD, Carson SA, Luciano A, Ross D, Bergqvist A. Subcutaneous injection of depot medroxyprogesterone acetate compared with leuprolide acetate in the treatment of endometriosis-associated pain. Fertil Steril 2006;85:314–25.
124. Funk S, Miller MM, Mishell DR Jr, et al. Safety and efficacy of Implanon, a single-rod implantable contraceptive containing etonogestrel. Contraception 2005;71:319–26.
125. Johnson PS, Ryckmans T, Bryans J, et al. Discovery of PF-184563, a potent and selective V1a antagonist for the treatment of dysmenorrhoea. The influence of compound flexibility on microsomal stability. Bioorg Med Chem Lett 2011;21:5684–7.
126. Fu J, Song H, Zhou M, et al. Progesterone receptor modulators for endometriosis. Cochrane Database Syst Rev 2017;7:CD009881.pub2.

127. Osuga Y, Watanabe M, Hagino A. Long-term use of dienogest in the treatment of painful symptoms in adenomyosis. J Obstet Gynaecol Res 2017;43:1441–48.
128. Pattanittum P, Kunyanone N, Brown J, et al. Dietary supplements for dysmenorrhoea. Cochrane Database Syst Rev 2016;3:CD002124.pub2.
129. Smith CA, Armour M, Zhu X, Li X, Lu ZY, Song J. Acupuncture for dysmenorrhoea. Cochrane Database Syst Rev 2016;4:CD007854.pub3.
130. Armour M, Dahlen HG, Zhu X, Farquhar C, Smith CA. The role of treatment timing and mode of stimulation in the treatment of primary dysmenorrhea with acupuncture: An exploratory randomised controlled trial. PLoS One 2017;12:e0180177.
131. Blödt S, Pach D, Eisenhart-Rothe SV, et al. Effectiveness of app-based self-acupressure for women with menstrual pain compared to usual care: A randomized pragmatic trial. Am J Obstet Gynecol 2017:Epub ahead of print.
132. Casper RF. Progestin-only pills may be a better first-line treatment for endometriosis than combined estrogen-progestin contraceptive pills. Fertil Steril 2017;107:533–536.
133. Walch K, Unfried G, Huber J, et al. Implanon versus medroxyprogesterone acetate: effects on pain scores in patients with symptomatic endometriosis—a pilot study. Contraception 2009;79:29–34.
134. Soliman AM, Bonafede M, Farr AM, Castelli-Haley J, Winkel C. Analysis of adherence, persistence, and surgery among endometriosis patients treated with leuprolide acetate plus norethindrone acetate add-back therapy. J Manag Care Spec Pharm 2016;22: 573–87.
135. Bedaiwy MA, Alfaraj S, Yong P, Casper R. New developments in the medical treatment of endometriosis. Fertil Steril 2017;107:555–565.
136. Arias RD. Premenstrual syndrome. In: Mishell DR Jr, Goodwin TM, Brener PF (eds). Management of common problems in obstetrics and gynecology, 4th ed. Boston: Blackwell Publishers, 2001.
137. Qiao M, Zhang H, Liu H, et al L. Prevalence of premenstrual syndrome and premenstrual dysphoric disorder in a population-based sample in China. Eur J Obstet Gynecol Reprod Biol 2012;162:83–6.
138. Yonkers KA, Simoni MK. Premenstrual disorders. Am J Obstet Gynecol 2017;S0002–9378. Epub ahead of print.
139. ACOG Premenstrual Syndrome. (PMS) ACOG FAQ057. May 2015. Available at: www.acog.org/Patients/FAQs/Premenstrual-Syndrome-PMS. Last accessed: 8/25/2017.
140. Premenstrual Dysphoric Disorder Work Group. Diagnostic and Statistical. Manual of diagnostic and statistical manual of mental disorders: DSM-V. 5th ed. American Psychiatric Association Arlington 2013.
141. Dalton K. The premenstrual syndrome and progesterone therapy, 2nd ed. Chicago: Mosby-Year Book Medical Publisher, 1984.
142. Rubinow DR, Hoban MC, Grover GN, et al. Changes in plasma hormones across the menstrual cycle in patients with menstrually related mood disorder and in control subjects. Am J Obstet Gynecol 1988;158:5–11.
143. Freeman EW, Rickels K, Sondheimer SJ, Polansky M. A double-blind trial of oral progesterone, alprazolam, and placebo in treatment of severe premenstrual syndrome. JAMA 1995;274:51–7.
144. Schmidt PJ, Nieman LK, Danaceau MA, Adams LF, Rubinow DR. Differential behavioral effects of gonadal steroids in women with and those without premenstrual syndrome. New Engl J Med 1998;338:209–16.
145. Mira M, Stewart PM, Abraham SF. Vitamin and trace element status in premenstrual syndrome. Am J Clin Nutr 1988;47:636–641.
146. Perkonigg A, Yonkers KA, Pfister H, Lieb R, Wittchen HU. Risk factors for premenstrual dysphoric disorder in a community sample of young women: the role of traumatic events and posttraumatic stress disorder. J Clin Psychiatry 2004;65:1314–22.
147. Harrison WM, Rabkin JG, Endicott J. Psychiatric evaluation of premenstrual changes. Psychosomatics 1985;26:789–92,795,798–9.

148. Fava M, Pedrazzi F, Guaraldi GP, Romano G, Genazzani AR, Facchinetti F. Comorbid anxiety and depression among patients with late luteal phase dysphoric disorder. J Anxiety Disorders 1992;6:325–35.
149. Green L, O'Brien P, Panay N, Craig, M. Royal College of Obstetricians and Gynecologists. Management of premenstrual symptoms. *BJOG* 2016;124:e73–e105.
150. Hartlage SA, Freels S, Gotman N, Yonkers K. Criteria for premenstrual dysphoric disorder: secondary analyses of relevant data sets. Arch Gen Psychiatry 2012;69:300–5.
151. Sayegh R, Schiff I, Wurtman J, Spiers P, McDermott J, Wurtman R. The effect of a carbohydrate-rich beverage on mood, appetite, and cognitive function in women with premenstrual syndrome. Obstet Gynecol 1995;86:520–8.
152. Miller ER, Pastor-Barriuso R, Dalal D, et al. Meta-analysis: high-dosage vitamin E supplementation may increase all-cause mortality. Ann Intern Med 2005;142:37–46.
153. Bertone-Johnson ER, Hankinson SE, Bendich A, et al. Calcium and vitamin D intake and risk of incident premenstrual syndrome. Arch Intern Med 2005;165:1246–52.
154. Thys-Jacobs S, Ceccarelli S, Bierman A, Weisman H, Cohen M, Alvir J. Calcium supplementation in premenstrual syndrome: a randomized crossover trial. J Gen Intern Med 1989;4:183–9.
155. Thys-Jacobs S, Starkey P, Bernstein D, Tian J. Calcium carbonate and the premenstrual syndrome: effects on premenstrual and menstrual symptoms. Premenstrual Syndrome Study Group. Am J Obstet Gynecol 1998;179:444–52.
156. Shobeiri F, Araste FE, Ebrahimi R, Jenabi E, Nazari M. Effect of calcium on premenstrual syndrome: a double-blind randomized clinical trial. Obstet Gynecol Sci 2017;60: 100–105.
157. Verkaik S, Kamperman AM, van Westrhenen R, Schulte PFJ. The treatment of premenstrual syndrome with preparations of Vitex agnus castus: a systematic review and meta-analysis. Am J Obstet Gynecol 2017;217:150–166.
158. Ozgoli G, Selselei EA, Mojab F, Majd HA. A randomized, placebo-controlled trial of Ginkgo biloba L. in treatment of premenstrual syndrome. J Altern Complement Med 2009;15:845–51.
159. Canning S, Waterman M, Orsi N, Ayres J, Simpson N, Dye L. The efficacy of Hypericum perforatum (St John's wort) for the treatment of premenstrual syndrome: a randomized, double-blind, placebo-controlled trial. CNS Drugs 2010;24:207–25.
160. Goodale IL, Domar AD, Benson H. Alleviation of premenstrual syndrome symptoms with the relaxation response. Obstet Gynecol 1990;75:649–55.
161. Naheed B, Kuiper JH, Uthman OA, O'Mahony F, O'Brien PM. Non-contraceptive oestrogen-containing preparations for controlling symptoms of premenstrual syndrome. Cochrane Database Syst Rev 2017;3:CD010503.pub2.
162. Ford O, Lethaby A, Roberts H, Mol BW. Progesterone for premenstrual syndrome. Cochrane Database Syst Rev 2012;14:CD003415.pub4.
163. Yonkers KA, Cameron B, Gueorguieva R, Altemus M, Kornstein SG. The influence of cyclic hormonal contraception on expression of premenstrual syndrome. J Womens Health (Larchmt) 2017;26:321–328.
164. Rapkin A. A review of treatment of premenstrual syndrome and premenstrual dysphoric disorder. Psychoneuroendocrinology 2003;28 Suppl 3:39–53.
165. Steiner M, Steinberg S, Stewart D, et al. Fluoxetine in the treatment of premenstrual dysphoria. N Engl J Med 1995; 332:1529–1534.
166. Yonkers KA, Halbreich U, Freeman E, et al. Symptomatic improvement of premenstrual dysphoric disorder with sertraline treatment. A randomized controlled trial. Sertraline Premenstrual Dysphoric Collaborative Study Group. JAMA 1997;278:983–8.
167. Steiner M, Hirschberg AL, Bergeron R, et al. Luteal phase dosing with paroxetine controlled release (CR) in the treatment of premenstrual dysphoric disorder. Am J Obstet Gynecol 2005;193:352–60.
168. Freeman EW, Rickels K, Yonkers KA, et al. Venlafaxine in the treatment of premenstrual dysphoric disorder. Obstet Gynecol 2001;98:737–44.

169. Marjoribanks J, Brown J, O'Brien PM, Wyatt K. Selective serotonin reuptake inhibitors for premenstrual syndrome. Cochrane Database Syst Rev 2013:CD001396.pub3.
170. Halbreich U, Smoller JW. Intermittent luteal phase sertraline treatment of dysphoric premenstrual syndrome. J Clin Psychiatry 1997;58:399–402.
171. Yonkers KA, Brown C, Pearlstein TB, Foegh M, Sampson-Landers C, Rapkin A. Efficacy of a new low-dose oral contraceptive with drospirenone in premenstrual dysphoric disorder. Obstet Gynecol 2005;106:492–501.
172. Rapkin AJ, Winer SA. The pharmacologic management of premenstrual dysphoric disorder. Expert Opin Pharmacother 2008;9:429–45.
173. Pinkerton JV, Guico-Pabia CJ, Taylor HS. Menstrual cycle-related exacerbation of disease. Am J Obstet Gynecol 2010;202:221–31.
174. Brandes JL. The influence of estrogen on migraine: a systematic review. JAMA 2006; 295:1824–30.
175. Granella F, Sances G, Allais G, et al. Characteristics of menstrual and nonmenstrual attacks in women with menstrually related migraine referred to headache centres. Cephalalgia 2004;24:707–16.
176. Nierenburg Hdel C, Ailani J, Malloy M, Siavoshi S, Hu NN, Yusuf N. Systematic review of preventive and acute treatment of menstrual migraine. Headache 2015;55:1052–71
177. Pavlović JM, Stewart WF, Bruce CA, et al. Burden of migraine related to menses: results from the AMPP study. J Headache Pain 2015;16:24.
178. MacGregor EA, Frith A, Ellis J, Aspinall L. Predicting menstrual migraine with a home-use fertility monitor. Neurology 2005;64:561–3.
179. Somerville BW. The role of estradiol withdrawal in the etiology of menstrual migraine. Neurology 1972;22:355–365.
180. Warhurst S, Rofe CJ, Brew BJ, et al. Effectiveness of the progestin-only pill for migraine treatment in women: A systematic review and meta-analysis. Cephalalgia 2017: 333102417710636. Epub ahead of print.
181. Khishfe BF. Catamenial epilepsy: The menstrual cycle as a clue to predict future refractory seizures. J Emerg Med 2017;52:235–237.
182. Foldvary-Schaefer N, Falcone T. Catamenial epilepsy: pathophysiology, diagnosis, and management. Neurology 2003;61:S2–15.
183. Tan KS. Premenstrual asthma: epidemiology, pathogenesis and treatment. Drugs 2001;61:2079–86.
184. Hsiao MC, Hsiao CC, Liu CY. Premenstrual symptoms and premenstrual exacerbation in patients with psychiatric disorders. Psychiatry Clin Neurosci 2004;58:186–90.
185. Gladis MM, Walsh BT. Premenstrual exacerbation of binge eating in bulimia. Am J Psychiatry 1987;144:1592–5.

2

Engaging With Unintended Pregnancy Through Patient-Centered Reproductive Goals and Contraceptive Counseling

Patty Cason, MS, FNP-BC
Abigail R.A. Aiken, MD, MPH, PhD

- Unintended pregnancy is a complex and nuanced concept.
- Sexuality and reproduction are core reflections of the way people choose to express their humanity and their decisions with regard to sexuality and reproduction are not inherently medical issues.
- Providers can help patients achieve their goals by engaging in patient centered reproductive goals counseling and, if appropriate, contraceptive counseling to clarify patients' values, preferences, and goals.
- Communication and counseling skills derived from active listening and adult learning principles can be applied to patient-centered reproductive goals and contraception counseling.
- Applying shared decision making to contraceptive counseling is an effective and patient-centered way to facilitate informed decision making.

What exactly is an unintended pregnancy? Can we safely assume that all unintended pregnancies are mistakes of timing destined to lead to negative life events? What implications do the answers to these questions have for how we counsel patients? And how do we measure the prevalence of unintended pregnancy in the population?

From a clinical perspective, our goal is to help people identify and fulfill their personal reproductive desires. From a public health surveillance perspective, we direct resources and shape policies based on the epidemiologic measures of the burden of unintended pregnancy in the population. In the following sections, we explore dimensions of pregnancy preferences and take a look at the evidence linking unintended pregnancies to both negative and positive health outcomes. We discuss how current estimates of unintended pregnancy in the United States are calculated, as well as how their methodological strengths and limitations determine the value we get from them. Armed with this knowledge, you can review the detailed strategies in this chapter for assessing pregnancy preferences with your patients and providing contraceptive counseling.

UNINTENDED PREGNANCY IN THE UNITED STATES

Many of our goals as clinicians, public health advocates, and researchers are motivated by the statistic that almost half of all pregnancies in the United States each year are unintended.[1,3] Having hovered at around 50% for the past decade,[2] the most recent data show a decline in the proportion of pregnancies that were unintended from 49% of all pregnancies in 2006[2] to 45% in 2011.[1]

But how often do you stop to think about where the figure "almost half of all pregnancies are unintended" comes from and what it represents? Estimates of unintended pregnancy in the United States come from the National Survey of Family Growth (NSFG), a large survey representative of the non-incarcerated, non-institutionalized U.S. population.[4] Current estimates rely upon asking women to report in retrospect on whether or not their last pregnancy occurred at the right time. Women who take part in the NSFG survey are asked, with respect to their last pregnancy, "Right before you became pregnant (with your (nth) pregnancy, which ended on (DATE)/this time), did you yourself want to have another baby at any time in the future?" If the answer is "no," then that pregnancy is classified as *unwanted*. If the answer is "yes," the person is asked a follow-up question: "So would you say you became pregnant too soon, at about the right time, or later than you wanted?" If the answer is "too soon," then that pregnancy is classified as *mistimed*.

The proportion of pregnancies that are "unintended" comprises both those that are "unwanted" and those that are "mistimed."[1] Due to the under-reporting of abortion in the NSFG, the proportion of pregnancies ending in abortion that are unintended is estimated using data from the nationally representative Abortion Patient Survey, which includes an NSFG-style question about pregnancy intentions.[1] The proportions of pregnancies ending in birth or miscarriage that are unintended are calculated using the NSFG data. These estimates are weighted to represent all pregnancies in the United States and then combined to determine the total number of unintended pregnancies.[1]

Because it is derived from a nationally representative sample, the NSFG estimate of unintended pregnancy has the major strength of being generalizable to the U.S. population. Estimates can also be calculated and compared across different demographic groups, revealing disparities by socioeconomic status, relationship status, and race/ethnicity. Rates of unintended pregnancy are highest among young women, women with incomes between 100% and 199% of the federal poverty level, women of color, those who do not have a high school education, and those who are in cohabiting relationships.[1,2] Between 2008 and 2011, disparities in the rates of unintended pregnancies across these groups narrowed but persisted.[1] Recent evidence suggests that sexual minority women (defined as those who are not exclusively in heterosexual relationships) also experience an elevated risk of unintended pregnancy.[5]

Limitations of Current Estimates

Despite our reliance on these estimates, they are not without limitations. First, the NSFG estimate is retrospective. Women are asked to think back to before they became pregnant and describe their intentions with respect to a pregnancy that has already occurred. This approach leaves women's responses vulnerable to recall bias, where intentions are inaccurately recalled, or retrospective bias, where the pregnancy becomes more positively viewed over time, particularly after birth.[6–10] For some, a process of adaption or changing circumstances may even mean that an unwanted pregnancy later becomes a wanted pregnancy.[11–13] There is also the potential for social desirability bias,[14] whereby women may be reluctant to say that their pregnancy was unwanted, especially if they feel they are attaching a negative label to an existing child.

A second limitation is that the NSFG measure is cross-sectional, meaning that it is measured at only a single time-point. But women's descriptions of their pregnancy intentions may vary, even over relatively short time periods.[15] It is possible that women's views about their pregnancy may change depending on their prevailing life circumstances, leading to a range of different answers if asked whether the pregnancy is wanted or unwanted at a number of different time points. Thus, our current measure provides only a snapshot of pregnancy intentions.

A third limitation is that the NSFG measure captures only a single dimension of women's attitudes towards their pregnancy: *timing-based intentions*. Despite being called a measure of "unintended pregnancy," the NSFG measure is actually based solely on *when* women said they *wanted* to become pregnant.[4] What is more important, however, is that these "wants" or "intentions" are timing-based (i.e., the pregnancy is classified as having been wanted then, later, or not at all). Yet when women actually describe the circumstances surrounding their pregnancies in conversation, most women don't describe them according to a strict timing-based "wanted" versus "unwanted" dichotomy. Instead, women's attitudes towards their pregnancies tend to fall along a spectrum, with many shades between wanted and unwanted (or intended and unintended).[16] By focusing on a single dimension of pregnancy preferences and constructing a binary intended versus unintended comparison, our current measure leaves little room for pregnancies that were viewed ambivalently, uncertainly, or indifferently.[17] It is also worth noting that attitudes towards pregnancy and attitudes towards childbearing may not be interchangeable. For example, a person may wish to test personal fertility or may find the idea of pregnancy with a partner exciting without feeling prepared to give birth to and raise a child.[18,19]

Unintended Pregnancy and the Question of Adverse Health Outcomes

Continuing to reduce unintended pregnancy is a national goal in the United States,[3] one that is underpinned by a conventional wisdom that unintended pregnancy leads to a host of adverse health outcomes. Is there thus an irreconcilable tension between individual reproductive autonomy and our public health goal of reducing poor health outcomes? In other words, are ambivalent attitudes towards pregnancy and "happy accidents" okay?

Despite the ubiquitous presence of the claim that unintended pregnancies lead to adverse outcomes in the biomedical and social science literature, there is surprisingly little high-quality evidence for a strong causal link between unintended pregnancy and a wide range of negative health effects, particularly in high-income countries like the United States.[20] Moreover, what we do know is limited by the challenges of accounting for multiple confounding influences that affect both the risk of unintended pregnancy and the likelihood of potential adverse outcomes, the selection bias created by pregnancies that end in abortion, and the complexities of defining and measuring unintended pregnancy. We briefly consider each in turn below.

Methodological Pitfalls

Examination of the health consequences of unintended pregnancy is mainly focused upon pregnancies that end in live births.[20] While this focus clearly makes sense from the point of view of examining health outcomes for neonates and children, it has two important drawbacks. First, it is likely to overlook health impacts for the person carrying the pregnancy and giving birth, which might differ depending on whether they continue or end an unwanted pregnancy. Second, the exclusion of pregnancies that end in abortion means that pregnancies that are viewed more positively may be over-represented and that the potential for abortion to result in positive health outcomes for individuals may be overlooked. The Turnaway Study, a longitudinal prospective cohort study comparing U.S. women who either received or were denied a wanted abortion provides important insight into the impacts of ending an unwanted pregnancy versus carrying it to term. Insights from the study suggest that women who continued unwanted pregnancies to term were more likely to remain in relationships with abusive partners.[21] Moreover, women who were denied wanted abortions initially had higher levels of stress, anxiety, and low self-esteem than did women who received abortions, although these differences appeared to converge over time.[22–24] The proportion of unwanted pregnancies that result in live births due to lack of access to or acceptability of abortion is likely to vary widely across geographical areas and demographic groups. Where abortion services are not readily accessible or acceptable, any potential health impacts of unwanted pregnancies that are continued may be more visible compared with populations where women have the option to end a pregnancy. In addition, unwanted pregnancies can clearly pose serious health risks in populations where abortion is restricted and individuals may resort to unsafe methods of ending their pregnancies.[25]

A second major challenge for these studies is the inability to control for the multiple confounding influences that are related to *both* the risk of unintended pregnancy and the risk of adverse pregnancy outcomes. Factors associated with a higher risk of unintended pregnancy—including socioeconomic disadvantage, living in a neighborhood with high rates of violence, lower education, lack of access to healthcare, and extremes of maternal age—may also be associated both with increased risk of negative health behaviors during pregnancy and with adverse maternal and neonatal health outcomes.[20] Any causal effects relating to the "unintendedness" of a pregnancy are therefore extremely difficult to disentangle. Studies vary in the extent to which they are able control for the myriad possible confounding factors. Rarely do different studies include the same set of controls, making comparisons across studies difficult. Moreover, apparent associations between unintended pregnancy and adverse health outcomes are often diluted or negated once potentially confounding socioeconomic influences are controlled for.[20] A further issue, particularly when investigating the relationships between intention status and longer-term health impacts, relates to the temporal separation between event and outcome. Variability in socioeconomic influences such as family relationships and resources over time makes the relative contribution of baseline pregnancy intentions very difficult to isolate and quantify.

The third methodological problem is that many studies examining the relationship between unintended pregnancy and adverse outcomes in the United States focus solely on binary (intended vs. unintended) and timing-based measures of intention.[20] There is evidence, however, that an individual's emotional response to a pregnancy may be more important than whether or not the pregnancy was planned or expected, as discussed below. Most studies also rely on retrospective reporting of intentions, which are subject to recall bias and do not account for adaptability and changing circumstances between the time the pregnancy was recognized and the time of reporting.[20]

Current Evidence

In light of these methodological limitations, it is perhaps not surprising that current evidence on the health impacts of unintended childbearing on women and infants is mixed and inconclusive. In economically more developed countries, including the United States, the rarity of infant mortality and maternal mortality makes it very difficult to study any association with unintended pregnancy.[20] Both mistimed and unwanted births, as well as undesired births, are more likely than intended or desired ones to be recognized later in pregnancy.[20,26] But although initiation of prenatal care is more likely to be delayed, the overall number of visits does not appear to be lower.[20,26] Current evidence does not suggest a strong or consistent association between pregnancies that are unintended and preterm birth.[20,26] There is some evidence to suggest that access to contraception, and to long-acting reversible methods in particular, is associated with a lower risk of preterm birth.[27] However, it is unclear whether this association is underpinned by a reduction in unintended pregnancy or a reduction in any pregnancy that might pose additional health risks, whether intended or not.

Some studies have suggested that maternal behavioral risk factors for adverse infant outcomes, including maternal smoking, depression and high alcohol consumption, were more strongly associated with being unhappy about pregnancy than with pregnancy intention.[28] Moreover, recent evidence suggests that positive maternal affect during pregnancy is associated with longer gestation and reduced risk of preterm delivery and that the risk of preterm birth was not increased among women experiencing pregnancies that were unintended but was increased in women with high stress levels during pregnancy.[29]

The lack of attention to feelings in the literature may explain some of the mixed results from various studies. For example, the best available evidence at present from higher-income countries suggests a consistent association between unintended births and an increased likelihood of low birthweight, as well as a reduced likelihood of breastfeeding.[20,26]

These associations do not appear to hold, however, when pregnancy desires (i.e., the extent to which one desires to achieve and to avoid pregnancy) are measured instead of pregnancy intentions and when the most desired births are compared to the least desired births.[26] A cohort from the Missouri Maternal and Infant Health Study demonstrated that, after adjustment for socioeconomic factors, low infant birthweight was not more likely among women whose pregnancies were unintended, but it was more likely among women who reported that they had felt unhappy about the pregnancy.[30]

These studies open up a line of inquiry suggesting that rather than focusing on pregnancies that are intended or unintended based upon timing, it might be more fruitful to distinguish between those pregnancies not specially intended or wanted at a certain time but nonetheless welcomed versus those viewed as a seriously negative life event. The inconsistency of current evidence highlights the fact that unintended pregnancies cannot be treated as a monolithic group. Future studies that develop more nuanced measures and assess their predictive outcomes will advance us toward a more definitive answer regarding which types of pregnancy result in negative health outcomes.[31] Another important goal of future research is to look beyond maternal behavioral outcomes and neonatal outcomes to examine obstetric outcomes (e.g., mode of delivery, birth experience, and postpartum mental health issues), health impacts during pregnancy including impacts on existing health conditions, and short-term and longer-term life impacts on individuals and families.

In the meantime, the lack of strong, conclusive evidence that unintended pregnancy will necessarily result in adverse health outcomes should not deter us from our work to help all people achieve their reproductive goals. Instead, what is needed is a shift in how we as health care and public health professionals approach this aspect of reproductive life. Rather than claiming an absolute public health imperative to reduce adverse outcomes, we can move forward with the goal of advancing reproductive rights, ensuring that all individuals have the freedom to decide the number, spacing, and timing their children.[32]

REPRODUCTIVE GOALS

COMPLEXITY OF PREGNANCY PREFERENCES

Eliciting prospective pregnancy preferences first requires that we become familiar with concepts beyond simply timing-based intentions. For some, timing-based intentions about *if or when* they are planning to get pregnant may simply not apply.[33] Some of your own patients no doubt hold beliefs or live in circumstances that make planning impossible or irrelevant. For example, while many people are aware of social norms that require waiting until financial, educational, and relationship circumstances are ideal before having a child, these circumstances may be unattainable in the near future or, in some cases, ever. Those who do not see their circumstances improving anytime soon may not want to delay having a child indefinitely. Indeed, for some, pregnancy may be a rational response to their circumstances given the status motherhood may confer in their community.[34] Moreover, for those who live in circumstances where cumulative psychosocial stresses including racism, discrimination, and socioeconomic disadvantage take a biological toll over the life course, there may be very real biological advantages to having children first and then concentrating on finishing education and investing time in building a career (the concept of allostatic load).[35,36] Others may not know anyone who has ever planned a pregnancy, or they believe that the number of children they will have is up to God.[33,37] Still others may feel there is no good method of contraception for them, or they may experience a lack of autonomy due to reproductive coercion from an intimate partner.[33] By contrast, others may simply not wish to plan and may find the idea of not knowing for sure whether or when a pregnancy will happen exciting or emotionally satisfying.[19]

For many, thinking about pregnancy or childbearing intentions in terms of long-term timing may be much more difficult than pin-pointing immediate desires to achieve or to avoid pregnancy. For example, you may have encountered some patients who hold ambivalent pregnancy desires (i.e. they simultaneously hold some degree of desire to get pregnant *and* some degree of desire to avoid pregnancy).[38] When asked about their pregnancy intentions or plans over the next year, these folks may often answer that they simply don't know. Similarly, those who are indifferent or "OK either way" (i.e. they don't have strong desires either to get pregnant or to avoid pregnancy)[38] may also struggle to translate this indifference into a plan or intention over the next year, 5 years, or 10 years. Even those who express strong desire to avoid or to get pregnant in the context of a single clinical encounter may experience fluctuation in these desires as health, relationships, financial situations, and life opportunities change over time.[15]

Some people may prefer to talk neither in terms of timing-based plans or intentions nor in terms of desires to achieve or avoid pregnancy. Instead, they may attach most meaning to their emotional orientations or feelings about pregnancy and childbearing—i.e., whether a pregnancy would be greeted with happiness or unhappiness. These feelings may reflect the anticipated impacts of a pregnancy on a person's life, including economic considerations, personal opportunity costs, social support, and the reactions of partners, families, and even communities.[39] Indeed, it is not uncommon for people to express emotional orientations towards pregnancy that appear to be at odds with their timing-based intentions.[40] A prime example of this is expressing happiness at the prospect of pregnancies they simultaneously acknowledge would be unintentional: so-called "happy accidents." For some, happiness may represent the idea that they and their partner would be able to "rise to the occasion" and take care of another child even if they were not specifically planning for one. For others, happiness may be a reflection of a deeply-felt joy in having and raising children even outside socially-sanctioned "ideal" circumstances.[39]

A Reproductive Rights Approach

Comprehensive sexual and reproductive health rests on the concept that all people have agency over their own sexual and reproductive life. Indeed, sexuality and reproduction are core reflections of the way people choose to express their humanity. Therefore, as health care providers, we do not consider people's decisions with regard to sexuality and reproduction to be medical issues. Our support of sexual and reproductive health can entail helping our patients prevent or manage risks associated with sex and reproduction such as sexually transmitted infections, sexual violence, unwanted pregnancy, or negative pregnancy or birth outcomes. But this should not distract us from the principle that a core part of free will is having control over sexual and reproductive choices. (See Chapter 22 on Sexuality & Contraception for more information.)

Patient-Centered Care

Health care providers can assist our patients with these choices[41] by starting with a clear understanding of our role, which we propose is to help our patients figure out what they want and then help them get it. We can accomplish this by applying principles of patient-centered care, which the Institute of Medicine defines as, "Providing care that is respectful of, and responsive to, individual patient preferences, needs, and values, and ensuring that patient values guide all clinical decisions." These principles include 1) highlighting that the patient's primary purpose for visiting the service site must be respected, 2) noting the high importance of confidential services and suggesting ways to provide them, 3) encouraging the availability of the comprehensive range of contraceptive methods so that patients can make a selection based on their individual needs and preferences, and 4) reinforcing the need to deliver services in a culturally competent manner so as to meet the needs of all patients, including adolescents, those with limited English proficiency, those with disabilities, and those who are lesbian, gay, bisexual, transgender, or questioning their sexual identity (LGBTQ). (See Chapter 22 on Sexuality & Contraception for more information.)

Reproductive Goals Counseling

The various dimensions of reproductive goals and pregnancy preferences described above—plans, intentions, desires, feelings, and the interactions between them—are no doubt complex and perhaps even seem daunting to clinicians and researchers alike. But acknowledging and valuing them is a vital component of patient-centered care. A good first step in family planning counseling conversations is to explore whether and when someone may want to reproduce. Beginning with efficient questions to elucidate reproductive goals is important because if the patient is currently interested in getting pregnant or causing pregnancy, conversations about contraception are less relevant than a discussion about preconception care. By the same token, if a person would like to prevent pregnancy, a discussion about contraception is relevant.

Reproductive goals counseling has several purposes:

- Help patients gain clarity about what they want in terms of reproduction.
- Identify patients with serious medical problems who would like to get pregnant or who are at risk of unintended pregnancy.
- Inform the provider about the direction of the visit (offering to discuss preconception care, fertility support, contraception).
- Guide the provider to avoid teratogens when prescribing medication for patients who desire pregnancy or who are at risk of unintended pregnancy.
- Help patients consider their future rather than just a current partner or sexual experience.
- Clarify their reproductive goals so they can make choices that are aligned with those goals.
- Demonstrate to the patients that your priority is helping them figure out what is important to them.
- Support a patient's reproductive autonomy and agency.
- Build rapport by letting them know you are listening.

The purpose of the reproductive goals counseling does NOT include any of the following:

- To give you as the provider information so you can decide which intervention or contraceptive is best for the patient

- To create a concrete "plan" that the patient should commit to
- To make the patient feel like they "should" have a "plan"

Three general strategies that providers use to elicit a person's reproductive goals have been described in the literature: Reproductive Life Plan,[51] One Key Question,[52] and the PATH[53] questions. There are studies in process, but at this time none of these approaches is evidence-based. Brief descriptions of Reproductive Life Plan and One Key Question are below. PATH questions are described in more detail because the strategy moves beyond timing-based intentions and allows a more effective open-ended approach.

Reproductive Life Plan

Family planning guidelines from the Centers for Disease Control and Prevention (CDC) recommend that all persons capable of having a child should have what is termed a "reproductive life plan."[60] CDC does not endorse a specific set of questions designed to clarify reproductive goals; however, the guidelines recommend that providers discuss a reproductive life plan with patients receiving contraceptive counseling, pregnancy testing and counseling, basic infertility services, sexually transmitted disease services, and preconception health services. The concept of a static "reproductive life plan" as described by CDC may not take into account the idea that many patients hold beliefs or live in circumstances that make planning impossible or irrelevant or for whom intentions about *if or when* they are planning to get pregnant may simply not apply.[20]

One Key Question[52]

"Would You Like to Become Pregnant in the Next Year?"

One Key Question was originally developed as a simple way for primary care providers to screen for pregnancy intention. Note that this approach is designed only for use with women of childbearing age. The following algorithm[54] uses the pronouns she and her; clinicians should use whatever pronoun the patient prefers.

IF YOUR PATIENT ANSWERS 'YES'

Preconception Care

- Screen for conditions that can affect pregnancy.
- Review medications.
- Recommend folic acid.

- Talk about the benefits of birth spacing recommended by One Key Question, depending on the patient's response.

IF YOUR PATIENT ANSWERS 'NO'

Contraceptive Services

- Ask if she is currently using a birth control method.
- Check on her satisfaction with current method.
- Offer more options, including long-acting reversible contraceptives (IUD, implant).
- Include information on emergency contraception.

IF YOUR PATIENT ANSWERS 'UNSURE' OR 'OK EITHER WAY'

- Offer a combination of contraception and preconception care.
- Discuss relevant issues.

Many women are unsure or ambivalent, especially if they have never been asked. You can start a conversation:

- "Is now the right time?"
- "Do you have the resources you need for another child (money, time, child care, space)?"
- "How would having another child impact family work plans, education plans, financial status?"

FOLLOW UP QUESTIONS

Use a 1-10 scale to gauge ambivalence or ask—

- "How important is it to you to prevent pregnancy?"
- "Why would you say you aren't a lower number?"
- "Why do you think your number might not be higher on the scale?"
- "I hear you have mixed feelings, but it's something you're thinking about. How can I help?"

FOLLOW UP RESPONSES

- "I would recommend you chose a contraceptive method to protect against pregnancy until you are sure."
- "I want you to know that in a year's time, 85 out of 100 women who have unprotected sex will become pregnant.
- "What would you like to do?"
- "How can I help you reach your goal?"

The PATH Questions

The PATH questions were developed for use with patients of any gender or sexual orientation. The PATH questions are designed to give patients an opportunity to verbalize their attitudes about reproduction and, if they would like to prevent pregnancy, to explore the degree to which they are motivated to prevent pregnancy. The PATH questions encourage a discussion about timeframe in a way that is relevant to the individual. This allows a provider to personalize the contraception counseling conversation and more effectively assist patients to achieve their goals. The **PATH** acronym can help you remember the questions:

Pregnancy / Parenthood Attitudes:

Do you think you might like to have (more) children at some point?

Timing:

When do you think that might be?

How important:

How important is it to you to prevent pregnancy (until then)?

1. Pregnancy/parenthood attitudes:

"Do you think you might like to have (more) children at some point?"

Including the word "might" in this question encourages patients to clarify their feelings and attitudes in addition to their thoughts about parenting. Note that this first question does not assume that all people want to be parents, so it is important not to skip over this and go straight to a timing question unless the patient has already mentioned a desire to have children. If you know the patient wants to have children now or sometime in the future because it has already been mentioned, you would not ask this first question.

If the person already has a child or children, ask "Do you think you might like to have *more* children at some point?" or "Do you think you might like to have *another* child at some point?

If the answer to the first question is NO, ***skip to question 3.*** There is no need to ask about timing if the patient has said no children are desired in the future. Skip to question 3 if your patient gives an answer similar to the following:

- "No, I really don't think so; I've really got my hands full with the three I've got!"
- "No, I know it sounds strange but I've never thought of myself as wanting to be a parent."

- "I seriously doubt it, I mean I love kids and all but I think it would be too much to deal with for me."

If the patient answers "Yes" to first question, proceed with question 2. However, listen carefully to the responses because patients often give an expanded answer that effectively answers the following two questions as well. For example—

> "Yes! I definitely want to be a mom someday. I am pretty traditional and family is one of the most important things in my life but I definitely want to be married first, which I don't see happening any time soon." In this example, this person seeks to prevent pregnancy at the current time and does not want to reproduce "any time soon." Therefore, you can proceed to ask, "How important is it to you to prevent pregnancy until you are married?"

2. *Timing:*

"When do you think that might be?"

If someone has indicated that they are considering future parenthood, a follow-up question assesses thoughts on timing in an open-ended manner recognizing that some people may not hold timing-based pregnancy intentions. Use of the words "think" and "might" is deliberate. These words allow for the possibility that the person has not given the matter a lot of thought, and they do not assume that any response is more correct than any other. The words do not to stigmatize.

If the patient answers "now" or "trying for a while," ***skip question 3***.

There is no need to press the patient for an exact answer about length of time. It is enough if they express clearly that there is no interest in becoming a parent "any time soon." The length of time until someone would like to parent is relevant when discussing preparation for pregnancy but not necessarily relevant when discussing prevention of pregnancy. Potential length of use is merely one of many features that may or may not be important to a patient requesting contraception. The "timing" question is not intended to inform contraceptive choice, because other than permanent contraception all of them are reversible and can be stopped at any time. The exception to this is if a person would like to conceive within the next couple of years, in which case a DMPA injection does not reliably provide immediate return to fertility. (See Chapter 6 on Injectable Contraceptives.)

3. *How important:*

"How important is it to you to prevent pregnancy (until then)?"

This question can provide context for preferences regarding the importance of contraceptive efficacy. If your patient has indicated a lack of interest in having children (or more children), you would have skipped question 2, but it is still important to ask question 3. If this is the case, leave off "until then." If they feel strongly about no future children, offer to discuss permanent contraception.

Considering what the impact might be if a pregnancy occurred before a patient is ready helps clarify priorities and helps determine if contraceptive effectiveness is a priority. Providers often assume that effectiveness is the most important attribute of a contraceptive method, but we cannot assume that our patients share this sentiment. Research shows that most people are seeking effectiveness in their method,[55,56] but some do not prioritize effectiveness.

Question 3 can flow into a conversation about the relative effectiveness of different contraceptive methods. Offer to discuss preconception care if the patient has indicated that the degree of effectiveness is not a priority in selecting a contraceptive method.

The PATH questions are not gender-specific.

PATH questions work exactly the same way for any gender or sexual orientation. Or if you prefer, you can change the third question as follows: How important is it to you not to *cause* a pregnancy until then?

CONTRACEPTIVE COUNSELING

There is consensus in the current medical literature that when patients are choosing among more than one reasonable option, such as when choosing a contraceptive method, providers should assist their patients in making these decisions by providing them with relevant information and helping them to identify their preferences in the context of their values. This shared decision-making approach[42] is an effective way to apply the principles of patient-centered care during contraception counseling.[43] Contraceptive counseling among family planning providers has undergone a transformation over the past decade. Below we describe the two general ways that providers historically have provided contraception counseling and then present a shared decision-making model which is the approach that we prefer.

Consumerist Counseling Or The "Menu" Approach

In what is known as an "informed choice" or consumerist counseling model,[44,45] providers function as information-givers who are neutral in the decision-making process. This can be thought of as a "menu" approach whereby the consumer (patient) is told about every available method in an effort to support patient autonomy. This approach places the decision in the hands of the patient, which is where most family planning providers believe the decision should rest. However, there is arguably too much information about contraception for an uninformed person to digest. The goal of patient-centered counseling should be for patients to have the information they need to make an informed choice given their individual needs and preferences, and not necessarily to be given all the information on all methods. In this model, the provider does not assist the patient in decision-making.

Directive Counseling

In contrast to the consumerist model are directive counseling approaches. Directive counseling is a more traditional model, in which a care provider prescribes the same treatment for most patients with similar diagnoses or conditions with little consideration of a patient's unique concerns, preferences, and values. When applying a directive counseling approach to contraception, providers form opinions about what they believe is best for the patient and counsel according to these opinions. This may mean that a provider offers information in a way that is designed to encourage patients to choose more effective methods.[46] An example of this is a tiered approach to counseling, which is an approach that promotes increased awareness of the most effective methods by presenting or describing them first, before presenting more user-dependent methods such as pills and condoms.[60]

Shared Decision-Making

A shared decision-making approach is associated with high levels of patient satisfaction in a wide variety of clinical settings[47] including contraceptive counseling.[48] Shared decision-making has been shown to increase a patient's engagement in self-care as well as improve patient outcomes and health status.[49] The quality of interpersonal care associated with shared decision-making approaches has been shown to influence contraceptive use[50] and, when applied to contraception counseling, it is also associated with increased satisfaction with method choice.

When practicing shared decision-making, providers do not communicate about and are not motivated by their own values or preferences. The contribution of the provider is to offer a framework that assists the patients in clarifying their preferences and goals and to facilitate the patients' informed decision-making. To achieve this, a health care provider asks the patient clarifying questions, listens to the responses, and explains the relevant science in a way that helps the patient understand and integrate the scientific information into their decision-making. Once a patient makes an informed decision that is consistent with personal preferences and goals, the health care provider's role is to perform services appropriate to the patient's objectives.

A FRAMEWORK FOR COUNSELING

Below, we present a detailed framework that providers can use to help clarify patients' goals and preferences. We then present information on a variety of patient-centered counseling and communication skills that encourage providers to listen purposefully to their patients and check their own biases continuously.

KEY PATIENT-CENTERED QUESTIONS

Open-Ended Or Yes/No Questions

"Yes" or "no" questions are appropriate for factual history taking. However when the conversation is geared toward helping patients clarify what is important to them or what their preferences are regarding contraception or any other sexual or reproductive health topic, open-ended questions will yield more nuanced information.

Health care providers often think that one potential downside of an open-ended approach is the time required to engage in meaningful discussions, particularly when people are not clear about their reproductive desires. However, counseling does not need to resolve ambiguity or address all issues that arise in one visit. Counseling can identify concrete steps to help people move toward their goals or create an agenda for future visits. A patient-centered counseling framework that prioritizes use of open-ended questions may also uncover social, economic, and relationship concerns related to reproductive hopes and goals, such as mental health, relationship violence, or unstable housing.

Clarifying Questions

A patient-centered approach entails full participation and engagement on the part of the patient. In order to encourage patients to be an equal partner in counseling conversations it is helpful to ask them questions. The PATH questions and the One Key Question are examples of clarifying questions designed to elicit and clarify preferences about reproduction and motivation about pregnancy prevention. In the next sections we describe the use of questions designed to elicit patients' specific preferences

Box 2-1 Characteristics of Contraceptives

- Effectiveness
- Hormones, whether or not and which
- Effect on the menstrual cycle
- Bleeding profile
- Partner preference
- Ability to use the method confidentially. This could mean—
  - — Avoiding methods that require "supplies"
  - — Needing to have a bleeding pattern that is unaffected/unchanged
- Length of (potential) use
- Control over removal
- A foreign object in the body
- Return to fertility
- Non-contraceptive benefits
- Side effects
- Risks
- Cost

about contraceptive characteristics and questions designed to help a patient integrate information that you have given.

Elicit contraceptive preferences. Contraceptive methods have characteristics associated with their use. (See Box 2-1 on Characteristics of Contraceptives.) Ask your patients about their preferences. Here are two options for how to ask:

- "Do you have a sense of what is important to you about your method?"[57]
- "Do you have a sense of what you are looking for in a contraceptive method?"

Patients can make informed choices that are consistent with their preferences when they understand which method(s) are most closely aligned with what they are seeking. Help them think about particular characteristics that they do or do not want in their method.

Note that these questions are not—

- "What are you looking for in a method?" Framed this way, the question could make someone feel as though they are expected to have a formulated answer. Adding the phrase "Do you have a sense . . ." allows for the likely possibility that no one has asked them that question before and they may need a moment to consider it.

Box 2-2 Follow-up questions to integrate information

- "How would it (or that) be for you?"
- "Knowing that, what do you think?"
- "Has that ever happened before?"
- "How did you manage it?"
- "How would you manage that?"

- "What is *most* important to you about your method?" Again, this could make someone feel pressured to have a formulated answer. More concerning is that in this example the person is expected to know what is "most" important to them before they have had an opportunity to consider the various wide range of things they may be seeking in a contraceptive method. Once a patient has clarified two or more characteristics that are important, it will become necessary to ask which is more important if there is not a method that fulfills all of the criteria.

Integrate information. Help a patient integrate information that you have given by asking a follow-up question like one of the examples in Box 2-2 immediately after you have given the information.

Because the follow-up questions in Box 2-2 are about the information just provided, include something about the topic in the question, for example—

"Knowing that, *how would it be for you* if you did not have periods?"

When you want to encourage the patient to ask for information, it is far preferable to ask, "What questions do you have?" rather than, "Do you have any questions?"

Patient-Centered Contraceptive Counseling Skills

As the practice of patient-centered care has matured, providers have used a variety of well-known communication and counseling skills that stem from active listening and adult learning principles.[58,59]

Active Listening communication techniques, first developed by Carl Rogers and Richard Evans Farson in 1957,[58] foreshadowed Shared Decision-Making by highlighting the role of the highly skilled yet non-directive listener (clinician) and the self-efficacy ascribed to the speaker (patient):

"It is called "active" because the listener has a very definite responsibility. He does not passively absorb the words which are spoken to him. He actively tries to grasp the facts and feelings in what he hears, and he tries, by his listening, to help the speaker work out his own problems."

Paraphrasing

A patient-centered way to respond to answers to clarifying questions and keep control of the time and focus of the visit is to paraphrase. This helpful counseling skill requires a bit of practice, so try it with friends or family before using it with patients. Paraphrasing can help in many ways:

- Build rapport.
- Demonstrate that you are listening and that you have heard what is important to them.
- Give patients the opportunity to hear their own priorities, preferences, and desires spoken out loud. Your paraphrasing can help them gain insight into what matters to them.
- Give patients the opportunity to correct, clarify, or confirm your paraphrasing.
- Allow you to be efficient and control the length and focus of the conversation.
- Allow you to summarize in order to move toward decision-making.

How to paraphrase. Pay close attention to what patients say about reproductive goals or contraception preferences. In addition to listening to the words, pay attention to tone of voice (happy, fearful, negative, concerned), body language (leaning forward, open stance or arms crossed indicating they are closed off), and facial expression. For example, does the person seem to be excited about the idea of being a parent someday (or having another child?) or do they seem put off by the idea?

Paraphrasing is not repeating what was said. Re-phrase what the person has said using different words to capture the essence of what was meant. You can be more succinct (or more detailed) than your patient was when you paraphrase. If you are not clear on a point, use paraphrasing to clarify. You can gather together bits of information your patient has mentioned throughout the conversation as well as things that you know about your patient when you use paraphrasing as a way to provide a summary.

Begin each paraphrase with an introduction like the following: "So I'm hearing you say . . ." and then after you have paraphrased say something like, "Did I get that right?" It helps to intermittently clarify, repeat, or summarize the attitudes and decisions that a patient has made during the counseling session.

Empathy

Central to patient-centered communication is the ability to exhibit empathy—verbally and non-verbally—by reflecting and validating a patient's feelings. Empathy means communicating that one cares about another person's feelings. You can demonstrate empathy by acknowledging feelings and communicating that someone's reaction to a situation is normal and common to others in similar situations. Avoid some of the common communications that actually create barriers to effectively expressing empathy:

- Underplaying (or overstating) the intensity of the emotion
- Saying "I know how you feel"
- Incorrectly "labeling" someone's feelings

Because each of us has different descriptions for each emotion, it is best not to "label" someone else's feelings. This is particularly true with negative emotions like anger or anxiety. For example, labeling an emotion by saying "I can see that you are angry" at a time when the patient would have used the word "annoyed" to describe the feeling has the potential to damage rapport. It is possible to be truly empathetic in a more general way (see Box 2-3).

Box 2-3 Phrases to demonstrate empathy without labeling

- "I can see that was really concerning you."
- "It seems like that was hard to deal with!"
- "I think anyone would find that situation very difficult to manage."
- "I can't even imagine how that must have been for you."

Positive Feedback

An excellent way to build rapport is to notice and point out your patient's health-supporting behaviors or health-related knowledge. (See Box 2-4.) This demonstrates to that you are paying attention to whom your patient is as a unique individual and that you are on the same side. Note that this is not complimenting patients for doing what a health care provider has told them to do. In contrast, you are noticing when their behavior supports their own sexual and reproductive health in a way that is aligned with their own values. By weaving positive feedback into the conversation, your patients hear that you respect their perspective. Examples of what you can say are below:

- "It's great that you were so strong in standing up for yourself (fill in a situation . . .)"
- "It's great you picked up on that . . ."
- "You've clearly thought about this a lot, what do you make of this situation?"

Box 2-4 Examples of health supporting behaviors or health related knowledge

Notice and point out:

- Insightful questions
- Condom use
- Adherence to a birth control method
- Exercise
- Diet improvement
- Smoking cessation
- Weight loss
- Ways in which someone is knowledgeable about health-related topics
- Whenever someone knows something about contraception, STDs or health
- If the person is in the field (an RN, MA, dental assistant . . .)
- If someone is studying biology or science

- "That is a great question."
- "Not many people (your age) act so responsibly about using a condom every time."
- "You are clearly interested in protecting yourself."

Patient Education

Patient education is not synonymous with counseling; however, it is part of counseling and shared decision-making because to make an informed choice, an individual needs to have the pertinent scientific information.

Patient-centered patient education. When providing patient education, individualize the information; prioritize the information most important to the patient, focusing on expressed concerns and demonstrated knowledge gaps. When patients are presented with too much information at once that is passively received, they may forget or remember incorrectly much of the information provided. Learning theory[59] tells us that in order for someone to be able to apply new information, they need to have not only heard or read the information but must also understand, remember, and integrate the information in order to be able to recall and use the relevant facts when making an informed decision. Most important, we also know from learning theory that we can facilitate the integration of new knowledge by having the "learner" interact with the information. For example, each time you share a digestible piece of information, ask the patient a clarifying question that pertains to the new information. (See Box 2-2 for examples.)

Language considerations for patient education.[60] As health care providers, we are comfortable with use of percentages, relative risk, and absolute risk. Our patients often have considerably less understanding of these concepts and may not be able to use the "data" to help inform their decisions if they don't have appropriate context or background. Applied to conversations with patients, this means that we should use natural frequencies (3 women out of 1,000) rather than using percentages (.3%). When comparing characteristics such as effectiveness or risk of a particular outcome, use common denominators:

- "If 100 women have unprotected sex for a year, 85 of them will get pregnant as compared with maybe 1 or none using an IUD."
- "If a person switches from the pill to an implant, the chance of unintended pregnancy is reduced from 7 in 100 to less than 1 in 100."

Teach Back. When you want to check to be sure patients have successfully integrated new information, an excellent strategy is to ask them to repeat back to you what they heard you say. This is called "teach back," and some providers complain that this can seem awkward or condescending. When implementing "teach back," an easy way to avoid awkwardness and not appear condescending is to take full responsibility for the communication. So rather than starting with, "Can you please repeat back to me what we just discussed" try saying, "I would like to be sure that I was as clear as I could be . . ." or "We have gone over quite a lot of information and I want to be sure I didn't forget to tell you something important . . ." or "I don't always explain things as clearly as I think I have . . ."

Find the "yes! . . . and" rather than "no" or "but".

When you find yourself feeling the need to correct your patient, or saying "that's wrong/incorrect," "no," or "but," consider instead the following strategy:

1. Find a kernel of truth in what they are saying (if there is one).
2. Acknowledge whatever correct information they have communicated.
3. Then build on it by adding the information you would like them to know.

Rather than creating a polarizing situation with a "no" or a correction, it is preferable to build rapport and self-efficacy by finding something in what they are saying to agree with and then adding clarifying information.

Example: How to discuss amenorrhea from using contraceptives containing hormones:

> *Provider*: Most people are very happy with their bleeding pattern when they use this method and many of them don't get their period. How would it be for you if you didn't get your period while you are using this method?

Patient: My mom said it's not healthy not to get my period. (Note: at this point you may feel like correcting your patient.)

Provider: Your mother is completely right. When you are not on contraceptive hormones it is important to get your period . . .

. . . It's so great that you know that if you miss your period when you are not on contraceptive hormones it could mean something's wrong!

. . . I wish all of my patients knew that if they are not on contraceptive hormones and they miss periods they need to come in to the clinic so we can see what's up.

Patient: Well, what about if I am using hormones? (Note: People are more likely to be receptive to information if they have asked the question that the information answers.)

Provider: So . . . interestingly, when someone is using contraceptive hormones it keeps the uterus very healthy and keeps the lining very thin. (Show a diagram of a uterus.) Knowing that, how would it be for you to not get periods?

The provider could add the following message:

Provider: Contraceptive hormones actually prevent cancer of the uterus. Knowing that, how would it be for you not to get your period while using this method?

Patients go online to find out about things they are interested in so your patient may have learned misinformation about contraception. Rather than correcting the misinformation, you can acknowledge that going online to seek information was proactive (i.e., point out the positive) and then share a good website like www.bedsider.org.

One of the most perplexing situations is when patients say that something bad happened to a friend or relative (or even to themselves) that you know is not possible scientifically. A strategy that has been shown to resonate with patients is to emphasize that "everyone is different."[61] This can readjust their frame of thinking to allow for the possibility that the (unscientific) "bad outcome" could be a chance occurrence.

A wonderful sentence to use in this situation might be as follows:

"That's too bad your friend had that experience. I haven't heard of that before, and I can tell you it definitely doesn't happen frequently."[57]

Language for Discussing an IUD or Implant. For the most part, people using the currently available implant and IUDs cannot remove the devices themselves. Therefore, contraceptive methods that require placement and removal by a health care provider require that patients give up control over their own fertility until a provider removes the device for them.[62] Providers may feel reluctant to remove a device in a timeframe they consider "early."[63] When patients are considering use of one of these methods, they are deciding if they can accept giving up control over their reproduction until the device is removed, whether or not they can trust the provider's procedural competence, whether there will be a provider willing and able to remove the device on demand, and whether they will have coverage for the cost of the removal. The following suggestions offer language designed to be patient-centered when discussing these methods.

1. Consider using this phrase when discussing an IUD or implant:

   "This [*IUD or implant*] is good for up to *X* years (*fill in information for the particular method*), but if you want to get pregnant before then or you would like it removed for any reason, come in, we will take it out,* and your ability to get pregnant will return to whatever is normal for you . . . immediately."

   This phrase:

   - Tells the patient that the method is effective *up to* a certain amount of time.
   - Emphasizes that they are not expected to use it for any particular length of time.
   - Stresses that the patient has control over removal.
   - Points out immediate return to fertility.
   - Avoids overly medicalized language; "Ability to get pregnant" rather than "return to fertility".
   - Does not promise fertility; "Goes back to whatever is normal for you" rather than "you can get pregnant right away."

2. Consider using the words "to place," "placing," or "placement" rather than "to insert," "inserting," or "insertion" when referring to an IUD or implant. This may feel less invasive.

3. Patients generally do not know what the term LARC (Long-Acting Reversible Contraception) means. Each LARC method is a separate method. Grouping them together does not help patients learn about the characteristics of the methods because, while each of the long-acting reversible methods is highly effective, each has other characteristics that are likely to differentiate them more than group them. These characteristics include hormonal vs. non-hormonal (copper IUD), a range of menstrual effects, and placement in the uterus or sub-dermally.

4. Using the words "long-acting" and emphasizing the length of use may cause patients having an IUD or implant placed to perceive

---

*If barriers exist in the practice setting where the patient receives care, this part of the statement would not be true.

that they are expected to use the method for the full length of time. This perception can result in the person feeling a loss of control. Because implants and IUDs are highly effective, they are excellent choices for the short-term, too, and the fact that an implant or an IUD is good for "up to" 3 to 20 years is an added advantage but not always relevant. The emphasis is better placed on the "up to" than the number of years because the amount of time is only relevant if the patient is seeking contraception for that length of time. Otherwise, other characteristics may be more important. When you ask, "Do you have a sense of what is important to you about your method?" and the patient says something like "a method that will last a long time," then it is appropriate to refer to these methods as "long-acting."

Misconceptions

Patients often have negative associations with contraception, such as unpleasant side effects and alarming complications. Less frequently, they are aware of non-contraceptive benefits associated with use of contraception. Asking probing questions about a patient's understanding and beliefs allows an opportunity to share accurate information and to frame the messaging positively when appropriate. Some common misconceptions include the following:

- Contraception adversely impacts fertility.
- Pregnancy is safer than contraception.
- All methods are equally effective.
- Patients believe they or their partner are subfertile or less susceptible to pregnancy than they really are.

Patients with Serious Medical Conditions Including Substance Abuse and Mental Illness

People with medical conditions are as likely as the general population to have unintended pregnancies. However, patients with serious medical conditions, including substance abuse and mental illness, have unique risks for adverse outcomes were they to become pregnant. Many medical conditions have a potential deleterious effect on pregnancy, or pregnancy may have a detrimental effect on the disease process. In many cases, outcomes are best when pregnancy occurs during a period of stability, when the disease is in remission.

Providing patient-centered care and engaging in shared decision-making are as equally important for patients with serious medical

BOX 2-5 Recommendations for counseling patients with medical conditions

- State your medical recommendation in a clear straightforward manner using plain language. Re-state your recommendation as needed with alternative language to help the patient integrate the information.
- Use the skills outlined in this chapter plus "on the one hand" (a form of paraphrasing).
- Ask your patients questions that address their emotional reactions to their medical condition and its potential impact on their reproductive health. Then communicate empathy once the patient responds.
- Focus on patient education about methods as well as how a method (and pregnancy) may affect the patient's disease state and vice versa.
- Use the follow-up questions in Box 2-2 frequently.
- Use visual aids and "teach back" (as described on page 85).
- Using non-judgmental language, describe the important information your patient needs in order to make an informed choice.

conditions as it is for others. And contraception counseling conversations have the potential to be more time consuming as patients often have misinformation, controversial evidence, cognitive or emotional challenges, and complicated drug interactions.

You may not know all of the facts about your patient's serious medical condition. If you are very knowledgeable, it can be tempting to make assumptions about your patients' emotional reactions to their medical conditions and the impact of those conditions on their reproductive health. Even if you know the important facts about the disease, each patient's reaction to the medical condition is unique. So in order to appreciate the important nuances, ask your patients about both the facts of their condition and their feelings.(See Chapters 18 and 23 for more information on the intersection between medical conditions and reproductive health.)

Patients struggling with adherence or whose behavior seems at odds with their stated goals can benefit from a type of paraphrasing—"on the one hand." If the clinician notes that the patient is having difficulty with an aspect of "self-care" such as adherence to medication or STI protection with condoms, the clinician can help the patient explore what the barrier or obstacle is by mentioning the goal "on one hand" and either the obstacle or the inconsistent behavior "on the other hand." An example of this might be, "So I am hearing you say that *on the one hand* it is really important to you not to get pregnant until your diabetes is controlled and *on the other hand* part of you would love to have another baby in your life right now. Do I have that right?"

"Quick Start" is Patient-Centered

Chapters on particular methods in this book recommend "Quick Start." This patient-centered approach encourages providers to offer timely access to

BOX 2-6 How to be reasonably certain that a woman is not pregnant

A health care provider can be reasonably certain that a woman is not pregnant if she has no symptoms or signs of pregnancy and meets any one of the following criteria:

- Is ≤7 days after the start of normal menses
- Has not had sexual intercourse since the start of last normal menses
- Has been correctly and consistently using a reliable method of contraception
- Is ≤7 days after spontaneous or induced abortion
- Is within 4 weeks postpartum
- Is fully or nearly fully breastfeeding (exclusively breastfeeding or the vast majority [≥85%] of feeds are breastfeeds), amenorrheic, and <6 months postpartum

Source: Curtis KM, Jatlaoui TC, Tepper NK, et al. (2016)[64]

patients' chosen method of contraception by starting them on the contraceptive method on the day they request it. Box 2-6 assists clinicians in providing contraception with a Quick-Start approach. If it is reasonably certain that a patient is not pregnant, offer a Quick Start of the chosen method that day.

SUMMARY

Pregnancy preferences can be complex, variable, and nuanced, and may not necessarily follow conventional norms. Accomplishing reproductive goals counseling within a patient-centered framework that safeguards reproductive rights helps individuals make the best reproductive choices for themselves. Shared decision-making is an excellent model for applying principles of patient-centered care that can lead to clarifying patients' goals about reproduction and contraception and to providing individualized services.

Author Disclosures—Cason: Advisory Board/Consultant for Teva, Merck, ContraMed, Cooper Surgical; Trainer/speaker for Merck, Medicines360, Teva, ContraMed. Aiken: Consultant for Agile Therapeutics.

REFERENCES

1. Finer LB, Zolna MR. Declines in unintended pregnancy in the United States, 2008–2011. New Engl J Med 2016;374:843–52.
2. Finer LB, Zolna MR. Shifts in intended and unintended pregnancies in the United States, 2001–2008. Am J Public Health 2014;104:S43–8.
3. U.S. Department of Health and Human Services. Healthy People 2020. Washington DC: Office of Disease Prevention and Health Promotion. www.healthypeople.gov/2020/topics-objectives/topic/family-planning/objectives. Accessed June 20, 2017.

4. Centers for Disease Control and Prevention (CDC) National Center for Health Statistics (NHCS) National Survey of Family Growth (NSFG). www.cdc.gov/nchs/nsfg/about_nsfg.htm. Accessed June 20, 2017.
5. Hartnett CS, Lindley LL, Walsemann KM. Congruence across sexual orientation dimensions and risk for unintended pregnancy among adult US Women. Women Health Iss 2017;27:145–51.
6. Koenig M, Acharya R, Singh S, Roy TK. Do current measurement approaches underestimate levels of unwanted childbearing? Evidence from rural India. Pop Stud-J Demog 2006;60:243–56.
7. Rosenzweig M, Wolpin K. Maternal expectations and ex post realizations. J Hum Resour 1993;28:205–27.
8. Joyce T, Kaestner R, Korenman S. On the validity of retrospective assessments of pregnancy intention. Demography 2002;39:199–213.
9. Miller W, Barber J. The effects of preconception desires and intentions on pregnancy wantedness. J Popul Res 2009;26:327–357.
10. Bankole A, Westoff CF. The consistency and validity of reproductive attitudes: evidence from Morocco. J Biosoc Sci 1998;30:439–55.
11. Hass PH. Wanted and Unwanted Pregnancies: A fertility decision-making model. J Soc Issues 1974;30:125–165.
12. Miller WB. Relationships between the intendedness of conception and the wantedness of pregnancy. J Nerv Ment Dis 1974;159:396–406.
13. Stanford JB, Hobbs R, Jameson P, DeWitt MJ, Fischer RC. Defining dimensions of pregnancy intendedness. Matern Child Health 2000;4:183–9.
14. Krosnick JA. Survey research. Annu RevPsychol 1999;50:537–567.
15. Jones RK, Tapales A, Lindberg LD, Frost J. Using longitudinal data to understand changes in consistent contraceptive use. Perspect Sex Reprod Health 2015;47:131–9.
16. Bachrach CA, Newcomer S. Intended pregnancies and unintended pregnancies: distinct categories or opposite ends of a continuum? Fam Plann Perspect 1999;31:251–2.
17. Santelli J, Rochat R, Hatfield-Timajchy K, et al. The measurement and meaning of unintended pregnancy. Perspect Sex Reprod Health 2003;35:94–101.
18. Polis CB, Zabin LS. Missed conceptions or misconceptions: perceived infertility among unmarried young adults in the United States. Perspect Sex Reprod Health 2012;44:30–8.
19. Higgins JA, Hirsch JS, Trussell J. Pleasure, prophylaxis and procreation: a qualitative analysis of intermittent contraceptive use and unintended pregnancy. Perspect Sex Reprod Health 2008;40:130–7.
20. Gipson JD, Koenig MA, Hindin MJ. The effects of unintended pregnancy on infant, child, and parental health: a review of the literature. Stud Fam Plann 2008;39:18–38.
21. Mauldon J, Foster DG, Roberts S. Effect of abortion vs. carrying to term on a woman's relationship with the man involved in the pregnancy. Perspect Sex Reprod Health 2015;47:11–8.
22. Harris LF, Roberts SC, Biggs MA, Rocca CH, Foster DG. Perceived stress and emotional social support among women who are denied or receive abortions in the United States: a prospective cohort study. BMC Women's Health 2014;14:76.
23. Biggs MA, Upadhyay UD, Steinberg JR, Foster DG. Does abortion reduce self-esteem and life satisfaction?. QualLife Res 2014;23:2505–13.
24. Biggs MA, Upadhyay UD, McCulloch CE, Foster DG. Women's mental health and well-being 5 years after receiving or being denied an abortion: a prospective, longitudinal cohort study. JAMA Psychiatry. 2017;74:169–78.
25. Grimes DA, Benson J, Singh S, et al. Unsafe abortion: the preventable pandemic. Lancet 2006;368:1908–19.
26. Kost K, Lindberg L. Pregnancy intentions, maternal behaviors, and infant health: investigating relationships with new measures and propensity score analysis. Demography 2015;52:83–111.
27. Goldthwaite LM, Duca L, Johnson RK, Ostendorf D, Sheeder J. Adverse birth outcomes in Colorado: assessing the impact of a statewide initiative to prevent unintended pregnancy. Am J Public Health 2015;105:e60–6.

28. Blake SM, Kiely M, Gard CC, El-Mohandes AA, El-Khorazaty MN. Pregnancy intentions and happiness among pregnant black women at high risk for adverse infant health outcomes. Perspect Sex Reprod Health. 2007;39:194–205.
29. Voellmin A, Entringer S, Moog N, Wadhwa PD, Buss C. Maternal positive affect over the course of pregnancy is associated with the length of gestation and reduced risk of preterm delivery. J Psychosom Res. 2013;75:336–40.
30. Sable MR, Washington CC, Schwartz LR, Jorgenson M. Social well-being in pregnant women: intended versus unintended pregnancies. J Psychosoc Nurs Ment Health Serv 2007;45:24–31.
31. Hall JA, Benton L, Copas A, Stephenson J. Pregnancy intention and pregnancy outcome: systematic review and meta-analysis. Matern Child Health 2017;21:1–35.
32. United Nations International Conference on Population and Development Programme of Action. www.unfpa.org/publications/international-conference-population-and-development-programme-action#sthash.0mEwqmmi.dpuf . Accessed June 20, 2017
33. Borrero S, Nikolajski C, Steinberg JR, et al. "It just happens": a qualitative study exploring low-income women's perspectives on pregnancy intention and planning. Contraception 2015;91:150–6.
34. Edin K, Kefalas M. Promises I can keep: why poor women put motherhood before marriage. Berkeley, CA:University of California Press; 2005.
35. Geronimus AT. Black/white differences in the relationship of maternal age to birthweight: a population-based test of the weathering hypothesis. Soc Sci Med 1996;42: 589–97.
36. Geronimus AT. Damned if you do: Culture, identity, privilege, and teenage childbearing in the United States. Soc Sci Med 2003;57:881–93.
37. Casterline JB, El-Zeini LO. The estimation of unwanted fertility. Demography 2007;44:729–45.
38. Miller WB, Barber JS, Gatny HH. The effects of ambivalent fertility desires on pregnancy risk in young women in the USA. Pop Stud-J Demog 2013;67:25–38.
39. Aiken AR, Dillaway C, Mevs-Korff N. A blessing I can't afford: factors underlying the paradox of happiness about unintended pregnancy. Soc Sci Med 2015;132:149–55.
40. Aiken AR, Potter JE. Are Latina women ambivalent about pregnancies they are trying to prevent? evidence from the border contraceptive access study. Perspect Sex Reprod Health 2013;45:196–203.
41. Dehlendorf C, Henderson JT, Vittinghoff E, et al. Association of the quality of interpersonal care during family planning counseling with contraceptive use. Am J Obstet Gynecol 2016;215: 78.e71–79.
42. Fried, TR. Shared decision making—finding the sweet spot. N Engl J Med 2016;374: 104–106.
43. Elwyn G, Dehlendorf C, Epstein RM, Marrin K, White J, Frosch DL. Shared decision making and motivational interviewing: achieving patient-centered care across the spectrum of health care problems. Ann Fam Med 2014;12: 270–275.
44. Dehlendorf C, Kimport K, Levy K, Steinauer J. A qualitative analysis of approaches to contraceptive counseling. Perspect Sex Reprod Health 2014;46:233–40.
45. Upadhyay U. Informed choice in family planning: helping people decide. Popul Reports 2001 Series J, No. 50.
46. Moskowitz E, Jennings B. Directive counseling on long-acting contraception. Am J Public Health, 1996;86:787–790.
47. Barry, MJ, Edgman-Levitan S. Shared decision making—pinnacle of patient-centered care. N Engl J Med, 2012;366:780–781.
48. Dehlendorf C, Grumbach, K, Schmittdiel JA, Steinauer J. Shared decision making in contraceptive counseling. Contraception 2017;95:452–455.
49. Shay LA, JE Lafata. Where is the evidence? A systematic review of shared decision making and patient outcomes. Med Decis Making 2015;35:114–131.

50. Dehlendorf C, Henderson JT, Vittinghoff E, Grumbach K, Levy K, et al. Association of the quality of interpersonal care during family planning counseling with contraceptive use. Am J Obstet Gynecol 2016;215:78.e71–79.
51. Recommendations to improve preconception health and health care—United States: a report of the CDC/ATSDR Preconception Care Work Group and the Select Panel on Preconception Care. MMWR 2006;55(No. RR-6).
52. www.thenationalcampaign.org/select360. Accessed September 17 2017.
53. Callegari LS, Aiken AR, Dehlendorf C, Cason P, Borrero S. Addressing potential pitfalls of reproductive life planning with patient-centered counseling. Am J Obstet Gynecol 2017;216:129–134.
54. Oregon Foundation for Reproductive Health. One Key Question. www.orpca.org/Symposia/OKQ_OPCA_4_2015_2.pdf. Accessed September 17, 2017.
55. Lessard, L. N., et al. Contraceptive features preferred by women at high risk of unintended pregnancy. Perspect Sex Reprod Health 2012;44:194–200.
56. Madden T, Secura GM, Nease RF, Politi MC, Peipert JF. The role of contraceptive attributes in women's contraceptive decision making. Am J Obstet Gynecol 2015;213: 46.e41–46.
57. Christine Dehlendorf, MD MAS. Personal communication July 29th 2017
58. Rogers CR, Farson RE. Active Listening. Connecticut: Martino Publishing; 2015.
59. Knowles, M., Holton, E., Swanson, R. The adult learner: The definitive classic in adult education and human resource development (6th ed.). London: Butterworth-Heinemann, 2005.
60. Gavin L, Pazol K. Update: providing quality family planning services—Recommendations from CDC and the U.S. Office of Population Affairs, 2015. MMWR 2016;65:231–234.
61. Anderson N, Steinauer J, Valente T, Koblentz J, Dehlendorf C. Women's social communication about IUDs: a qualitative analysis. Perspect Sex Reprod Health 2014;46:141–148.
62. Amico JR, Bennett AH, Karasz A, Gold M. "She just told me to leave it": Women's experiences discussing early elective IUD removal. Contraception 2016;94:357–61.
63. Amico JR, Bennett AH, Karasz A, Gold M. "I wish they could hold on a little longer": physicians' experiences with requests for early IUD removal. Contraception 2017;96:106–10.
64. Curtis KM, Jatlaoui TC, Tepper NK, et al. U.S. Selected Practice Recommendations for Contraceptive Use, 2016. MMWR Recomm Rep 2016;65(No. RR-4):1–66.

3

Efficacy, Safety, and Personal Considerations

James Trussell, PhD
Abigail RA Aiken, MD, MPH, PhD
Elizabeth Micks, MD, MPH
Katherine A. Guthrie, FRCOG, FFSRH

- Use of the top-tier reversible contraceptives—the intrauterine devices (IUDs) and the contraceptive implant—entails the lowest risk of pregnancy.
- Correct and consistent use of most contraceptive methods results in a low risk of pregnancy.
- The simultaneous use of methods dramatically lowers the risk of pregnancy.
- Emergency contraception provides a last chance to prevent pregnancy after unprotected intercourse or when the extent of contraceptive protection is unclear.
- Most contraceptives pose little risk to most users' health, although personal risk factors should influence personal choice.
- Nearly half (45%) of all pregnancies are unintended: 2.8 million each year; excluding spontaneous abortions more than 4 in 10 unintended pregnancies end in an induced abortion and nearly half (45%) of all unintended pregnancies result from contraceptive failure.

Choosing a method of contraception is an important decision. A method that is not effective for an individual can lead to an unintended pregnancy. A method that is not safe for the user can create significant negative medical and social consequences. A method that does not fit the individual's personal lifestyle is not likely to be used correctly or consistently. Individuals themselves must make the decision about the contraceptive method they use, and will often take into consideration the feelings and attitudes of their partners. The best method of contraception for an individual or couple is one that is safe and that will be used correctly and consistently.

Because most people will use a variety of contraceptive methods throughout their lives, they should be knowledgeable about various contraceptive methods. The patient's choice of a contraceptive method depends on several major factors: efficacy, safety, cost, non-contraceptive benefits, and personal considerations, including impacts on sexual pleasure and perceived or experienced side-effects.[1] Through counseling, you can help your patient choose the most suitable contraceptive method. You also can influence the user's motivation and ability to use the method correctly. Encourage clients to educate themselves about the various methods available. Direct clients toward available resources (see Chapter 2 on Engaging with Unintended Pregnancy through Patient-Centered Reproductive Goals and Contraceptive Counseling).

Information on levels and trends in contraceptive use in the United States is based on the National Surveys of Family Growth (NSFG), periodic surveys conducted by the National Center for Health Statistics in which women ages 15 to 44 are interviewed about topics related to childbearing, family planning, and maternal and child health. Among the 61.5 million women of reproductive age (ages 15 to 44) in 2013-15, about 61% (37.8 million) were using some method of contraception, according to the 2013–2015 NSFG. Among the 39% (23.7 million) who were not currently using a method, only about one-fifth were at risk of pregnancy. The remaining four-fifths were not at risk because they had been sterilized for noncontraceptive reasons, were sterile, were trying to become pregnant, were pregnant, were interviewed within 6 weeks after the completion of a pregnancy, or did not have intercourse during the 3 months prior to the survey.[2]

Almost 90% of the women at risk for an unintended pregnancy were using a contraceptive method, but 10.5% of all women at risk of unintended pregnancy were not using any contraceptive method. Today, the most popular contraceptive methods are oral contraceptive pills (9.5 million), tubal occlusion (8.2 million), male condoms (5.5 million), intrauterine devices (4.4 million), withdrawal (3.0 million), and vasectomy (2.5 million).[2] The diaphragm has virtually disappeared (diaphragm is not in Table 3-1, because the estimate does not meet the standard of precision). But while the original diaphragms that were fitted by clinicians are no longer available, a new over-the-counter single-size diaphragm was approved in September 2014. See Table 3-1 for information on contraceptive method use by age of women.

Use of the male condom and withdrawal is higher than indicated in Table 3-1, because some women use condoms and withdrawal in addition to another method. In the 2013-2015 NSFG, women were asked to

Table 3-1 Percentage and number of women at risk[1] and percentage at risk currently using various methods from the 2013-2015 National Survey of Family Growth

	Percent Using Among Women at Risk[1]						
Contraceptive method	**15-44**	**15-19**	**20-24**	**25-29**	**30-34**	**35-39**	**40-44**
Oral contraceptive pill	22.7	42.1	38.7	26.8	17.9	11.9	10.0
Tubal occlusion	5.8	0.0	*	1.1	4.7	10.4	14.4
Condom	13.0	16.6	14.5	15.7	14.4	10.4	8.5
No method	10.5	14.3	8.8	10.6	11.1	9.1	10.9
Intrauterine devices	10.5	3.1	11.7	13.0	13.6	12.5	5.8
Withdrawal	7.1	3.1	7.8	10.9	5.5	8.7	5.3
Vasectomy	5.8	0.0	*	1.1	4.7	10.4	14.4
Injectable	3.5	12.7	5.7	2.9	2.3	2.0	0.8
Ring or patch	2.3	*	2.9	2.7	2.7	2.7	*
Implant	3.5	12.7	5.7	2.9	2.3	2.0	0.8
Fertility awareness-based methods	1.9	0.0	1.0	3.3	1.9	2.2	2.5
Calendar rhythm	1.7	0.0	1.0	3.1	1.5	1.8	*
Other methods[2]	0.6	*	1.0	0.6	1.3	*	*
	Number of Women in Cohort, Percent and Number at Risk[1]						
Number (thousands) of Women	61,492	9,426	10,472	10,725	10,647	9,918	10,304
Percent at Risk[1]	68.6	38.5	71.9	69.9	75.0	76.7	77.3
Number (thousands) at Risk[1]	42,184	3,629	7,529	7,497	7,985	7,607	7,965

Source: Daniels and Abma (2017)

Notes:
Percentages may not add to 100 due to rounding
[1]At risk = those who *either* are current contraceptive users *or* are nonusers who have had sex in the past 3 months and are not trying to become pregnant, are not pregnant, or were not interviewed within 6 weeks after the completion of a pregnancy and are not sterile. Percentages may not add to 100 due to rounding.
[2]Other methods includes all other methods not shown separately
*Figure does not meet standard of reliability or precision

report all contraceptive methods used in the current month for any reason (for protection against either pregnancy or STIs). When more than one method was reported, only the most effective method is coded as the current method. When the data in Table 3-1 are recoded to capture all use of the male condom, the fraction using male condoms among all women at risk rises by 52%, from 13.0% to 19.7%. Increases are greatest among women ages 15 to 19 (an 81% increase, from 16.6% to 30.1%) and among women ages 20 to 24 (an 81% increase, from 14.5% to 26.3%). When the data in Table 3-1 are recoded to capture all use of withdrawal, the fraction using withdrawal among all women at risk rises by 106%, from 7.1% to 14.6%. Increases are greatest among women ages 15 to 19 (a 400% increase, from 3.1% to 15.6%) *and* among women ages 20 to 24 (a 179% increase, from 7.8% to 21.7%).[2]

The mix of methods shown in Table 3-1, including the 10.1% of women at risk who do not use any method, resulted in a staggering 2.8 million unintended pregnancies in 2011, the latest year for which data are available.[3] These represent nearly half (45%) of the 6.1 million pregnancies occurring each year.[3] Moreover, nearly half (45%) of unintended pregnancies result from contraceptive failure.[4] Every day in the United States, about 9.6 million couples at risk of unintended pregnancy have intercourse; among these, about 28 thousand experience a condom break or slip (assuming a 1.5% breakage/slippage rate), and about 1 million are not protected against pregnancy at all.[2,5] (See Table 3-1 and Chapter 26 on Contraceptive Efficacy.)

EFFICACY: "WILL IT WORK?"

"Is the condom really effective?"

"Which would be the most effective method for me?"

"Why did one magazine say condoms are 98% effective and another say they're 87% effective?"

"Can you still get pregnant if you take your pills every day on schedule?"

"Will it work?" is the question usually asked first and most frequently about any method of contraception.[1,6] Although this question cannot be answered with certainty for any particular couple, clinicians and counselors can help patients understand something of the difficulty of quantifying efficacy.

It is useful to distinguish between measures of contraceptive effectiveness and measures of the risk of pregnancy during contraceptive use. Many people, including clinicians and clients, prefer positive rather than negative statements; instead of the negative statement that 20% of women using a method become accidentally pregnant during their first year of use, they prefer the alternative positive statement that the method is 80% effective. However, it does not follow that the method is 80% effective, because it is not true that 100% of these women would have become pregnant if they had not been using contraception. Contraceptive effectiveness must always be expressed with respect to the risk of pregnancy in the same year if no method is used, which is never 100%. If 90% of these method users would have become pregnant had they used no method, then the use of the method reduced the number of accidental pregnancies from 90% to 20% (not 100% to 20%), a reduction of 78%. In this sense, the method could be said to be 78% effective at reducing pregnancy in the first year. But if only 60% of these women would have become pregnant if they did not use contraception, then the method would be only 67% effective. Because no study can ascertain the proportion of women who would have become pregnant had they not used the contraceptive method under investigation, it is simply not possible to measure effectiveness directly. Therefore, we focus attention entirely on pregnancy rates or probabilities of pregnancy during contraceptive use, which are directly measurable. However, we continue to use the term effectiveness in its loose everyday sense of how well a method works throughout this book, and we use the terms effectiveness and efficacy interchangeably. We also provide estimates of the proportion of women who would become pregnant if they did not use contraception, so that the reader may calculate rough effectiveness rates if they are needed.

The Risk of Pregnancy During Typical and Perfect Use

Four pieces of information about contraceptive efficacy would help individuals and couples to make an informed decision when choosing a contraceptive method:

1. Pregnancy rates during *typical use* show how effective the different methods are during actual, real-life use (including inconsistent *or* incorrect use).
2. Pregnancy rates during *perfect use* show how effective methods can be, where perfect use is defined as following the directions for use exactly and consistently.
3. Pregnancy rates during *imperfect use* show how ineffective methods will be if they are used incorrectly or inconsistently—rates can be computed separately for different categories of imperfect use to reveal which types of imperfect use are most risky.[7]
4. The percentage of *perfect users* or percentage of months during which a method is used perfectly reveals how hard it is to use a method correctly and consistently.

The difference between pregnancy rates during *imperfect use* and pregnancy rates during *perfect use* reveals how forgiving of *imperfect use* a method is. The difference between pregnancy rates during *typical use* and pregnancy rates during *perfect use* reveals the consequences of *imperfect use;* this difference depends both on how unforgiving of *imperfect use* a method is and on how hard it is to use that method perfectly. Only the first of these two pieces of information is currently available. Our current understanding of the literature on contraceptive efficacy is summarized in Table 3-2.

Typical Use

In the second column of Table 3-2, we provide estimates of the probabilities of pregnancy during the first year of typical use of each method in the United States. This information is shown graphically in

Table 3-2 Percentage of women experiencing an unintended pregnancy during the first year of typical use and the first year of perfect use of contraception and the percentage continuing use at the end of the first year. United States

Method	% of Women Experiencing an Unintended Pregnancy within the First Year of Use		% of Women Continuing Use at One Year[3]
	Typical Use[1]	Perfect Use[2]	
No method[4]	85	85	
Spermicides[5]	21	16	42
Female condom[6]	21	5	41
Withdrawal	20	4	46
Diaphragm[7]	17	16	57
Sponge	17	12	36
Parous Women	27	20	
Nulliparous Women	14	9	
Fertility awareness-based methods[8]	15		47
Ovulation method[8]	23	3	
TwoDay method[8]	14	4	
Standard Days method[8]	12	5	
Natural Cycles[8]	8	1	
Symptothermal method[8]	2	0.4	
Male condom[6]	13	2	43
Combined and progestin-only pills	7	0.3	67
Evra patch	7	0.3	67
NuvaRing	7	0.3	67
Depo-Provera	4	0.2	56
Intrauterine contraceptives			
ParaGard (copper T)	0.8	0.6	78
Skyla (13.5 mg LNG)	0.4	0.3	
Kyleena (19.5 mg LNG)	0.2	0.2	
Liletta (52 mg LNG)	0.1	0.1	
Mirena (52 mg LNG)	0.1	0.1	80
Nexplanon	0.1	0.1	89
Tubal occlusion	0.5	0.5	100
Vasectomy	0.15	0.1	100

Emergency Contraceptives: Use of emergency contraceptive pills or placement of a copper intrauterine contraceptive after unprotected intercourse substantially reduces the risk of pregnancy. (See Chapter 10.)

Lactational Amenorrhea Method: LAM is a highly effective, *temporary* method of contraception.[9] (See Chapter 17.)

Source: See Chapter 26.

(continued)

Table 3-2 Percentage of women experiencing an unintended pregnancy during the first year of typical use and the first year of perfect use of contraception and the percentage continuing use at the end of the first year. United States—*(continued)*

[1]Among *typical* couples who initiate use of a method (not necessarily for the first time), the percentage who experience an accidental pregnancy during the first year if they do not stop use for any reason other than pregnancy. Estimates of the probability of pregnancy during the first year of typical use for fertility awareness-based methods, withdrawal, the male condom, the pill, and Depo-Provera are taken from the 2006–2010 National Survey of Family Growth (NSFG) corrected for under-reporting of abortion. See the text for the derivation of estimates for the other methods.

[2]Among couples who initiate use of a method (not necessarily for the first time) and who use it *perfectly* (both consistently and correctly), the percentage who experience an accidental pregnancy during the first year if they do not stop use for any other reason. See the text for the derivation of the estimate for each method.

[3]Among couples attempting to avoid pregnancy, the percentage who continue to use a method for 1 year.

[4]This estimate represents the percentage who would become pregnant within 1 year among women now relying on reversible methods of contraception if they abandoned contraception altogether. See text.

[5]150 mg gel, 100 mg gel, 100 mg suppository, 100 mg film.

[6]Without spermicides.

[7]With spermicidal cream or jelly.

[8]About 80% of segments of FABM use in the 2006-2010 NSFG were reported as calendar rhythm. Specific FABM methods are too uncommonly used in the US to permit calculation of typical use failure rates for each using NSFG data; rates provided for individual methods are derived from clinical studies. The Ovulation and TwoDay methods are based on evaluation of cervical mucus. The Standard Days method avoids intercourse on cycle days 8 through 19. Natural Cycles is a fertility app that requires user input of basal body temperature (BBT) recordings and dates of menstruation and optional LH urinary test results. The Symptothermal method is a double-check method based on evaluation of cervical mucus to determine the first fertile day and evaluation of cervical mucus and temperature to determine the last fertile day.

[9]However, to maintain effective protection against pregnancy, another method of contraception must be used as soon as menstruation resumes, the frequency or duration of breastfeeds is reduced, bottle feeds are introduced, or the baby reaches 6 months of age.

Figure 3.1 in a way that clients may find more useful.[8-10] The four methods in the top section of that Figure are sometimes called "forgettable"[11] or "top-tier" methods. The two reversible methods in the top tier have been called highly effective reversible (HER) methods[12] (partly to distinguish them from long-acting reversible contraceptives (LARC), which also include Depo-Provera in some countries[13] and also to avoid the term LARC. The term "long-acting" can be misleading, as there is no minimum duration of use for these methods and clients may opt to use them even if they intend to become pregnant in the near future or are uncertain about future pregnancy plans. The recent reduction in unintended pregnancy in the United States is at least in part due to increased use of HER methods.[3]

For five methods, estimates of typical use failure rates were derived from the experience of women in the 2006–2010 NSFG, so that the information pertains to nationally representative samples of users.[14,15] For the other methods, we based the estimates on evidence from surveys and clinical investigations. See Chapter 26 on Contraceptive Efficacy for more complete explanations and for tables summarizing the efficacy literature for each method.

Pregnancy rates during typical use reflect how effective methods are for the average person who does not always use methods correctly or consistently. Typical use does not imply that a contraceptive method was

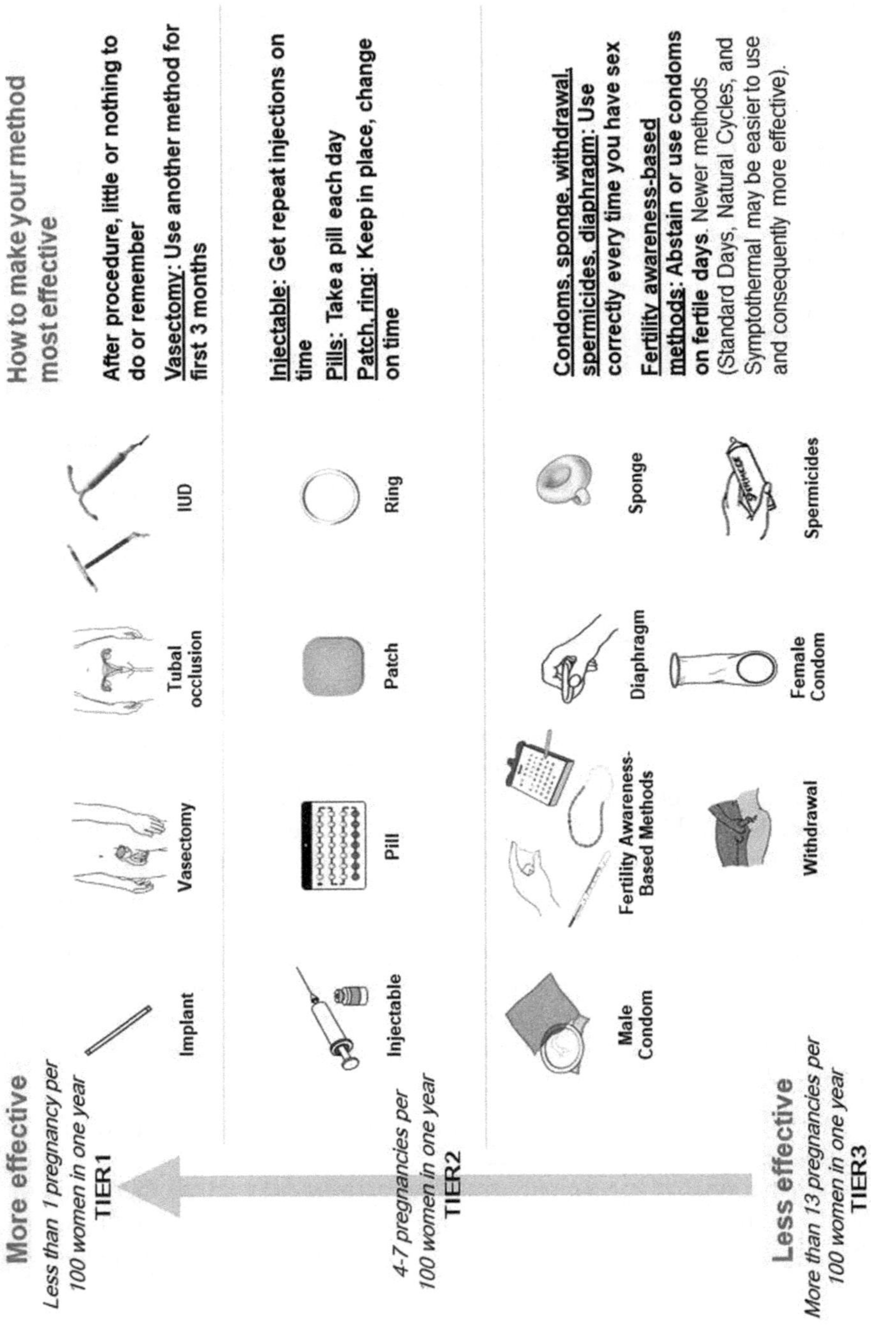

Figure 3-1 Comparing typical effectiveness of contraceptive methods

always used. In the NSFG and in most clinical trials, people are 'using' a contraceptive method if they consider themselves to be using that method. So typical use of the condom could include actually using a condom only occasionally, and a person could report that she is 'using' the pill even though the prescription ran out several months ago. In short, *use*—which is identical to *typical use*—is a very elastic concept that depends entirely on an individual's perception.

Perfect Use

In the third column, we provide our best guess of the probabilities of *method* failure (pregnancy) during the first year of perfect use. A method is used perfectly when it is used consistently according to a specified set of rules. For many methods in the third tier, perfect use requires use at every act of intercourse. Virtually all method failure rates reported in the literature have been calculated incorrectly and are too low (see the discussion of methodological pitfalls below). Hence, we cannot empirically justify our estimates except those for four fertility awareness-based methods,[7,16-18] the diaphragm,[19] the sponge,[20] the male condom,[21-23] the female condom,[24] spermicides,[25] and methods for which there are extensive clinical trials with very low pregnancy rates. (See Chapter 26 on Contraceptive Efficacy.) Even the estimates for the fertility awareness-based methods, female condom, diaphragm, spermicides, and sponge are based on only one or two studies. Our hope is that our understanding of efficacy during perfect use for these and other methods will be enhanced by additional studies.

Continuation

The fourth column displays the first-year probabilities of continuing use. They are based on the same sources used to derive the estimates in the second column (typical use). (See Chapter 26 on Contraceptive Efficacy.)

Comparison with Pregnancy Rates Among Women Using Isotretinoin (Accutane)

It is interesting to compare these estimates with pregnancy rates observed among women using isotretinoin, which is effective in treating severe acne but is also teratogenic. To minimize pregnancies among women undergoing treatment, the manufacturer and the U.S. Food and Drug Administration (FDA) implemented a pregnancy prevention program. Among 76,149 women who reported using contraception, 268 became pregnant, yielding a rate of 3.6 per 1,000 20-week courses of therapy;[26] this rate, if constant for a year, would be equivalent to an annual probability of pregnancy of 0.9%. The estimated annual probabilities of pregnancy were 0.8%, 2.1%, and 2.6% among women who reported using oral contraceptives, diaphragms, and condoms, respectively. Thus, women using diaphragms achieved lower rates of pregnancy than we estimate would occur during perfect use, and those using condoms and oral contraceptives experienced about the same pregnancy rates that would be expected during perfect use. Pregnancy rates for women using any of these three methods, however, were substantially below rates generally observed during typical use; this finding would appear to indicate that users' understanding of the teratogenic risks of isotretinoin substantially enhanced correct and consistent use. It is also possible that women in this study had lower than average fecundity, (because acne is a marker for excess androgen production associated with anovulation[27]), that they lowered their coital frequency during treatment, or that they under-reported their number of pregnancies (and abortions).

SIMULTANEOUS USE OF METHODS

Using two methods at once dramatically lowers the risk of unintended pregnancy, provided they are used consistently. If one of the methods is a condom or vaginal barrier, protection from disease transmission is an added benefit. For example, the probabilities of pregnancy during the first year of perfect use of male condoms and spermicides are estimated to be 2% and 16%, respectively, in Table 3-2. It is reasonable to assume that during perfect use the contraceptive mechanisms of condoms and spermicides operate independently, since lack of independence during typical use would most likely be due to imperfect use (either use both methods or not use either). The annual probability of pregnancy during simultaneous perfect use of condoms and spermicides would be 0.2%, about the same as that achieved by the combined pill (0.3%) and Depo-Provera (0.2%) during perfect use.[28]

EFFICACY OVER TIME

We confine attention to the first-year probabilities of pregnancy solely because probabilities for longer durations are generally not available. There are three main points to remember about the effectiveness of contraceptive methods over time.

- First, the risk of pregnancy during either perfect or typical use of a method should remain constant over time *for an individual* with a specific partner, providing that underlying fecundity and frequency of intercourse do not change. It is possible, however, that the risk of pregnancy could decline during typical use of certain methods because the individual learns to use the method correctly and consistently.
- Second, in contrast, the risk of pregnancy during typical use of a method will decline over time *for a group of users*, primarily

because those users prone to fail do so early, leaving a pool of more diligent contraceptive users or those who are relatively infertile or who have lower coital frequency or fecundity. This decline will be far less pronounced among users of those methods with little or no margin for imperfect use. By assuming that first-year probabilities of contraceptive failures would apply to probabilities in subsequent years of use, the *New York Times* greatly overstated the probabilities of failure over 10 years of use.[29] The risk of pregnancy during perfect use for a group of users should decline as well, but this decline will not be as pronounced as that during typical use, because only the relatively more fecund and those with higher coital frequency are selected out early. For these reasons, the probability of becoming pregnant during the second year of use of a contraceptive method will be lower than the probability of becoming pregnant during the first year of use.

- Third, probabilities of pregnancy cumulate over time. Suppose that 10%, 6%, and 4% of people using a method experience a contraceptive failure during years 1, 2, and 3, respectively. The probability of not becoming pregnant within 3 years is calculated by multiplying the probabilities of *not becoming pregnant* for each of the 3 years: 0.90 times 0.94 times 0.96, which equals 0.81. Thus, the percentage becoming pregnant within 3 years is 19% (= 100% − 81%).

The lesson here is that the differences among probabilities of pregnancy for various methods will increase over time. For example, suppose that each year the typical proportion of people becoming pregnant while taking the pill is 7% and while using the diaphragm is 17%. Within 5 years, 30% of pill users and 61% of diaphragm users will become pregnant.

Contraceptive Failures in a Lifetime

Data from the 1995 NSFG have been used to estimate age-specific contraceptive failure rates to produce a total lifetime contraceptive failure rate: the number of contraceptive failures that the typical woman would experience in a lifetime if she used reversible methods of contraception continuously (except for the time spent pregnant after a contraceptive failure) from exact age 15 to exact age 45. This estimate is based on the standard synthetic-cohort assumption: that the typical woman uses at each age the same mix of methods observed at each age in the NSFG and experiences the same rate of contraceptive failure observed at that age. The typical woman who uses reversible methods of contraception continuously from age 15 to age 45 would experience 1.8 contraceptive failures. If we consider both reversible methods and permanent contraception, the typical woman would experience only 1.3 contraceptive failures from age 15 to age 45.[30]

Factors That Influence Reported Efficacy

Our understanding of the efficacy of contraceptive methods is entirely dependent on results published in the literature and is influenced by three primary factors (1) the inherent efficacy of the method when used correctly and consistently (perfect use) and the technical attributes of the method that facilitate or interfere with proper use, (2) characteristics of the user, and (3) the quality of published evidence.

Inherent Method Efficacy

For some methods, such as permanent contraception, implants, and the levonorgestrel and the copper-T intrauterine devices (IUDs), the inherent efficacy is so high and correct and consistent use is so nearly guaranteed that extremely low pregnancy rates are found in all studies, and the range of reported pregnancy rates is quite narrow. For other methods such as the pill and injectable, inherent efficacy is high, but there is still the potential inconsistent or incorrect use (e.g., forgetting to take pills or failure to return on time for injections), so that the characteristics of the user can contribute to a wider range of reported probabilities of pregnancy. In general, the studies of permanent contraception, injectable, implant, pill, patch, ring, and IUD use have been competently executed and analyzed. Studies of fertility awareness-based methods, spermicides, and the barrier methods display a wide range of reported probabilities of pregnancy because the potential for misuse is high, the inherent efficacy is relatively low, and the quality of the evidence is mixed.

User Characteristics

Characteristics of the users can affect the pregnancy rate for any method under investigation, but the impact will be greatest for methods with the highest failure rates during typical use, either because the method has less inherent efficacy or because it is hard to use consistently or correctly.

Imperfect use. The most important user characteristic is imperfect use of the method. The importance of perfect use is demonstrated in the few studies where the requisite information on quality of use was collected. For example, in a World Health Organization (WHO) study of the ovulation method, the proportion of women becoming pregnant among those who used the method perfectly during the first year was 3.1%, whereas the corresponding proportion failing during a year of imperfect use was 86.4%.[7] In a large clinical trial of the cervical cap conducted in Los Angeles, among the 5% of the sample who used the method perfectly, the fraction failing during the first year was 6.1%. Among the remaining

95% of the sample who at least on one occasion used the cap imperfectly, the first-year probability of pregnancy was nearly twice as high (11.9%).[31,]

Frequency of intercourse. Among those who use a method consistently and correctly (perfect users), the most important user characteristic that determines the risk of pregnancy is frequency of intercourse. For example, in a study in which users were randomly assigned to either the diaphragm or the sponge, diaphragm users who had intercourse 4 or more times a week became pregnant in the first year twice as frequently as those who had intercourse fewer than 4 times a week.[32] In that clinical trial, among women who used the diaphragm at every act of intercourse, only 3.4% of those who had intercourse fewer than 3 times a week became pregnant in the first year, compared with 9.7% of those who had intercourse 3 or more times per week.[20]

Age. A female's biological capacity to conceive and bear a child declines with age. The decline in ovarian reserve is moderate until a woman reaches her late thirties.[33] Risk of tubal factor infertility also increases with age among women who are exposed to STIs such as gonorrhea and chlamydia. Although many investigators have found that contraceptive failure rates decline with age,[34-37] this effect almost surely overstates the pure age effect because age in many studies primarily captures the effect of coital frequency, which declines both with age and with marital duration.[38] User characteristics such as race and income seem to be less important determinants of contraceptive failure.

Regular cycles. Women with regular cycles were 7.2 times as likely as were women with irregular cycles (one or more cycles <17 days or >43 days) to become pregnant while using the Reality female condom.[39]

Quality of Published Evidence

When the published evidence is of poor quality, we cannot rely on it to help inform contraceptive decision-making. The reasons for poor quality data range from simple arithmetical mistakes to improper design or execution or analysis of studies to outright fraud.[40]

Fraud. One well-documented instance of fraud involved the Dalkon shield. In a two-page article published in the *American Journal of Obstetrics and Gynecology*, a first-year probability of pregnancy of 1.1% was presented and the claim made that "only the combined type of oral contraceptive offers slightly greater protection."[41] It was not revealed by the researcher that some women had been instructed to use spermicides as an adjunctive method to reduce the risk of pregnancy, nor that he was part-owner of the Dalkon Corporation. Furthermore, he never subsequently revealed (except to the A.H. Robins Company, which bought the shield from the Dalkon Corporation but did not reveal this information either) that as the original trial matured, the first-year probability of pregnancy more than doubled.[42]

What gets published. The incentives to conduct research on contraceptive failure vary widely from method to method. Many studies of the pill and IUD exist because companies wishing to market them must conduct clinical trials to demonstrate their efficacy. In contrast, few studies of withdrawal exist because there is no financial reward for investigating this method. Moreover, researchers face differing incentives to report unfavorable results. The vasectomy literature is filled with short articles by clinicians who have performed 500 or 1,000 or 1,500 vasectomies. When they report pregnancies (curiously, pregnancy is seldom mentioned in discussions of vasectomy "failures," which focus on the continued presence of sperm in the ejaculate), their pregnancy rates are invariably low. Surgeons with high pregnancy rates simply do not write articles calling attention to their poor surgical skills. Likewise, drug companies do not commonly publicize their failures. Even if investigators prepared reports describing failures, journal editors would not be likely to publish them.

Analytical pitfalls. Several analytical pitfalls can snare investigators. Three of the most common are (1) use of a misleading measure of contraceptive failure called the Pearl Index (2) the incorrect calculation of method failure rates, and (3) failure to follow up subjects in a trial. Other, more technical, errors that have biased reported results are discussed elsewhere.[40,43,44]

Pearl Index. The Pearl Index is obtained by dividing the number of unintended pregnancies by the number of years of exposure to the risk of unintended pregnancy contributed by all participants in the study. This measure can be misleading when one wishes to compare pregnancy rates obtained from studies with different average amounts of exposure. The likelihood of pregnancy declines over time because those most likely to become pregnant do so at earlier durations of contraceptive use and exit from observation. Those still using contraception after long durations are unlikely to become pregnant, so an investigator could (wittingly or unwittingly) drive the reported pregnancy rate toward zero by running the trial "forever." For example, two investigators using the NSFG could obtain Pearl-Index pregnancy rates of 7.5 and 4.4 per 100 woman-years of exposure for the condom.[45] One (who got 4.4) allowed each study subject to contribute a maximum of 5 years of exposure while the other (who got 7.5) allowed each study subject to contribute only 1 year. Which investigator is incorrect? Neither. The two rates are simply not comparable. Life-table measures of contraceptive failure are easy to interpret and control for the distorting effects of varying durations of use, but currently the FDA uses only the Pearl Index for primary effectiveness analysis.

Another problem occurs when deciding which pregnancies to count. Most studies count only the pregnancies observed and reported by the women. If, on the other hand, a pregnancy test were administered every month, the number of pregnancies (and hence the pregnancy rate) would increase because early pregnancy losses not observed by the woman would be added to the number of observed pregnancies. Such routine pregnancy testing in the more recent contraceptive trials has resulted in higher pregnancy rates than would otherwise have been obtained and makes the results not comparable to those from other trials.

Incorrect calculation of method failure rates. Unfortunately, nearly all investigators who have attempted to calculate "method" and "user" failure rates have done so incorrectly. Investigators routinely separate the unintended pregnancies into two groups. By convention, pregnancies that occur during a month in which a method was used improperly are classified as user failures (even though, logically, a pregnancy might be due to failure of the method, if it was used correctly on some occasions and incorrectly on others), and all other pregnancies are classified as method failures. But investigators do not separate the exposure (the denominator in the calculation of failure rates) into these two groups.

For example, suppose that 2 method failures and 8 user failures occur during 100 woman-years of exposure to the risk of pregnancy. Then the common calculation is that the user failure rate is 8% and the method failure rate is 2%; the sum of the two is the overall failure rate of 10%. By definition, however, method failures can occur only during perfect use and user failures cannot occur during perfect use. If there are 50 years of perfect use and 50 years of imperfect use in the total of 100 years of exposure, then the method failure rate would be 4% and the user failure rate would be 16%. The difference between the two rates (here 12%) provides a measure of how forgiving of imperfect use the method is. However, since investigators do not generally inquire about perfect use except when a pregnancy occurs, the proper calculations cannot be performed.

Loss to follow up. The standard assumption made at the time of analysis is that women who are lost-to-follow-up (LFU) experience unintended pregnancy at the same rate as those who are observed. This assumption is probably innocuous when the proportion LFU is small. But in many studies the proportion LFU may be 20% or higher, so that what really happens to these women could drastically affect the estimate of the proportion becoming pregnant. Our strong suspicion is that women LFU are more likely to experience a contraceptive failure than are those who remain in the trial. For example, one study found that the pregnancy rate for calendar rhythm rose from 9.4 to 14.4 per 100 woman-years of exposure as a result of resolution of cases LFU.[46]

GOALS FOR COMMUNICATING ABOUT EFFICACY

Keep these thoughts in mind when counseling about contraceptive efficacy:

1. **What matters most is correct and consistent use.** For example, the 7% probability of pregnancy during the first year for typical use of the pill will not protect the careless user. The 17% probability of pregnancy during the first year of typical diaphragm use need not overly discourage a person who is a careful and methodical method user and who has infrequent intercourse from using a diaphragm.
2. **Methods that protect a person for a long time and do not require daily or coital adherence** (permanent contraception, implants, and IUDs) **tend to be associated with lower pregnancy rates,** primarily because they allow little margin for user error.
3. **Abstinence is usually available as an option, as are "outercourse" and withdrawal.** Individuals do not always have a choice about sexual practices, but in most situations these methods are available if no other contraceptive method (or a less effective method) is available.
4. **Using two methods at once dramatically lowers the risk of unintended pregnancy,** provided they are used consistently. If one of the methods is a condom, protection from STI transmission is an added benefit.
5. **Emergency contraception provides a last chance to prevent pregnancy after unprotected intercourse.** Insertion of a copper IUD is the most effective option and provides up to 20 years of protection. Emergency contraceptive pills (ECPs) are an especially important second method for those relying on condoms, in cases of breakage or slippage, for those who do not actually use their ongoing method for whatever reason, and those who are forced to have unprotected intercourse.
6. **Make sure your staff provides consistent and correct information.** One study of the information provided by family planning staff indicated that providers tended to give the lowest reported probabilities of pregnancy for pills and IUDs, probabilities of pregnancy during typical use for diaphragms and spermicides, and higher-than-typical probabilities of pregnancy for condoms.[47] Thus, family planning providers may extensively bias their patient education in favor of methods they provide most frequently. Condoms and withdrawal get an undeserved low efficacy score within many family planning clinics and offices. You can avoid unintentional bias by deciding carefully what pregnancy rates your clinic or staff members are going to use and by using visual

aids, such as wall charts and handouts (reflecting information from Figure 3-1[10]).

7. **Technology fails people just as people fail technology.** Patients are sometimes told that unintended pregnancies are their own fault because they did not use their method correctly or carefully. Contraceptive methods are imperfect and can fail even the most diligent user.

SAFETY: "WILL IT HURT ME?"

"I smoke. Won't the pill give me a heart attack?"
"Could the IUD puncture my uterus?"
"Will I be able to get pregnant after stopping my method?"

In general, contraceptives pose few serious health risks to users. Moreover, the use of contraceptive methods is generally far safer than pregnancy. People in many developing countries will experience an even greater advantage in using contraceptive methods—in comparison with pregnancy-related mortality—than people in the developed world. Nonetheless, use of some contraceptive methods may entail potential risks.

- Use of the method may lead to side effects or, in rare cases, serious outcomes such as infection, hospitalization, surgery, loss of fertility, or even death.
- Contraceptive failure (pregnancy) is associated with risk: an individual must assess the likelihood of contraceptive failure and the dangers that a pregnancy would pose. Depending on where a person lives, she may face risks associated with delayed or unsafe abortion, or risks associated with pregnancy continuation and childbirth. These risks are all affected by an individual's health and sociocultural circumstances.

MAJOR HEALTH RISKS

When it comes to the most serious outcome of all—death—the absolute level of risk is extraordinarily low for most people. Table 3-3 puts into perspective some of the mortality risks of everyday life in the United States.[48-62] Other major health risks from contraceptive use are uncommon, and they are most likely to occur in individuals who have underlying medical conditions. (See Chapter 18 on Contraception for Women with Medical Conditions.)

Cardiovascular Disease

Use of combined hormonal contraceptive methods (CHCs), including combined oral contraceptives (COCs), the patch, and vaginal ring, are

Table 3-3 Voluntary risks in perspective

Activity	Risk of Death	Source
Risk per year		
While skydiving	0.5 in 100,000 skydives	U.S. Parachuting Association (2015)[48]
From an unintentional injury	42.7 in 100,000	CDC (2014)[49]
From an automobile accident	9.2 in 100,000	NHTSA (2015)[50]
From accidentally falling	10.0 in 100,000	CDC (2014)[49]
From accidental poisoning	13.2 in 100,000	CDC (2014)[49]
From homicide	5.0 in 100,000	CDC (2014)[51]
From a fire	1.1 in 100,000[50]	U.S. Fire Administration (2014)[52]
In an airplane crash	0.007 in 100,000	International Air Transport Association (2016)[53]
From being struck by lightning	0.1 in 100,000	National Weather Service (2015)[54]
From being a pedestrian hit by a car	1.7 in 100,000	NHTSA (2015)[50]
Risk per year for women preventing pregnancy		
Using combined oral contraceptives (and presumably the patch and ring as well)		Schwingl et al. (1999)[55]
Nonsmoker		
Aged 15–34	0.06 in 100,000	
Aged 35–44	3.0 in 100,000	
Smoker		
Aged 15–34	1.7 in 100,000	
Aged 35–44	19.2 in 100,000	
Undergoing tubal occlusion	1.5 in 100,000	Escobedo et al. (1989)[56]
Risk per year from using tampons	0.02 in 100,000	Hajjeh et al. (1999);[57] U.S Census Bureau (2003)[58]
Risk from live birth	10.4 in 100,000	Raymond and Grimes (2012)[59]
Risk from spontaneous abortion	0.7 in 100,000	Saraiya et al. (1999)[60]
Risk from legal induced abortion	0.6 in 100,000	Raymond and Grimes (2012)[59]
Mifepristone/misoprostol	0.5 in 100,000	Karnovsky (2017)[61]
Surgical		Zane (2015)[62]
≤8 weeks	0.3 in 100,000	
9–13 weeks	0.5 in 100,000	
14–17 weeks	2.5 in 100,000	
≥18 weeks	6.7 in 100,000	

associated with an increased risk of arterial and venous thromboembolism (VTE).[63] The most serious thrombotic events, myocardial infarction (MI) and stroke, are extremely rare and much less common than deep venous thrombosis (DVT). Smoking significantly increases the risk of MI, especially in users over age 35. However, studies have not consistently shown an increased risk of MI among nonsmoking, normotensive, nondiabetic women of any age who use CHCs.[64-66] The risk of stroke in nonsmoking women under age 35 may not be increased by use of CHCs,[67] except potentially in women with certain medical conditions such as migraines with aura.[68,69] The risk of VTE is increased by CHC use, but the absolute risk is quite low, ranging from 2 events per 10,000 woman-years among those aged 15 to 19, to 7 events per 10,000 woman-years among those aged 45 to 49.[70,71]

Cancer

Use of COCs (and presumably the patch and ring as well) protects users against cancers of the endometrium and ovary.[67] A comprehensive review concluded that use of COCs is associated with an increased risk of cancer of the cervix and liver, an increased risk of breast cancer in young women, and a decreased risk of colorectal cancer.[67] The risk of death is lower among ever-users of COCs than never-users for colorectal,[72,73] uterine,[72,74] ovarian,[72,74] and lymphatic and hematopoietic [73] cancer. The net effect of COC use on cancer is negligible,[67,72-74] and ever-users of COCs have a significantly lower death rate from all cancers than do never-users.[72]

Analysis of pooled data from 54 epidemiologic studies conducted in 25 countries found that women face a slightly increased risk (about 25% higher) for having breast cancer diagnosed while they are using COCs. Cancers diagnosed in these women were less advanced clinically than those diagnosed in women of the same age who had never used COCs.[75] A study of 1.8 million women in Denmark followed over an average of 10 years similarly found that COC use was associated with an elevated risk of breast cancer (about 20% higher), and that the risk increased slightly with duration of use.[76] However, the absolute increase in risk was very small, only 13 per 100,000 women. The elevated risk was observed in women using pills with 20 to 40 mcg of ethinyl estradiol, and appeared unrelated to estrogen dose or specific formulation. The risk decreased to baseline after cessation of use for most women, but persisted for at least 5 years after discontinuation among women with greater than 5 years of use. In general, the patterns of increased breast cancer risk are not typical for a carcinogenic agent but would be consistent with promotion of already existing tumors or with earlier diagnosis of breast cancer in women who have used COCs. This is an expected effect given that most breast cancers are positive for estrogen and/or progesterone receptors. However, studies in the United States and United Kingdom found that current or former COC use is not associated with an increased risk of diagnosis of breast cancer (with one exception, where current but not former users had a marginally significant higher risk[77]).[68,78] Moreover, COC use has neither a harmful nor a beneficial effect on breast cancer *mortality*.[72,74,79]

Few studies have evaluated cancer risk among users of progestin-only methods of contraception (including the progestin-only pill, injectables, implants, and levonorgestrel IUD). Use of injectable contraception substantially reduces the risk of endometrial cancer, but does not affect ovarian cancer risk.[80] A 2016 systematic review concluded that progestin-only methods of contraception do not appear to increase the risk of breast cancer,[81] however the large study from Denmark found that the levonorgestrel IUD, but not the implant or injectable, was associated with an increased risk of breast cancer.[76] In this study, levonorgestrel IUD users had a 20% higher risk of breast cancer, similar to women using COCs. Studies specifically evaluating an association between the levonorgestrel IUD and cancer have been inconsistent, with some showing an increase in breast cancer risk, but a decrease in endometrial, ovarian, pancreatic, and lung cancer.[82,83,84] The levonorgestrel IUD is commonly used to prevent and, in some cases, treat endometrial cancer.[85,86] It is unlikely that this method significantly affects the risk of non-gynecologic cancers given the low strength of association and methodological flaws of the studies, as well as lack of biological plausibility.

Persistent infection with certain types of human papillomavirus (HPV) is the etiologic agent responsible for cervical cancer (see Chapter 20 on Reproductive Tract Infections). The incidence of cervical cancer is increased in women using COCs, particularly long-term users, among women who test positive for HPV; this risk increases as duration of use increases.[87] Results from limited data also suggest a slight increase in the risk of cervical cancer among women who use injectable contraceptives for 5 years or longer. Results from one large cohort study in the UK found that ever users of COCs had a significantly higher risk of death from cervical cancer than did never users.[88] However, oral contraceptive use had neither a harmful nor a beneficial effect on cervical cancer mortality in an even larger UK cohort study.[72] There are several important sources of confounding among studies evaluating an association between contraceptive use and cervical cancer. First, women using hormonal contraception are less likely to use barrier methods, and may be more likely to acquire HPV. In addition, they are more likely to be screened for cervical cancer. Smoking status and the number of previous sexual partners also differ among women using hormonal versus barrier contraception, and affect cervical cancer risk. No studies have adjusted for all confounding factors simultaneously. A pooled analysis of 26 epidemiologic studies concluded that IUD use is associated with a decreased risk of cervical cancer.[89] However a more recent large prospective cohort study found no association between IUD use and HPV acquisition or clearance.[90] Neither study was able to provide data on IUD type. One retrospective study found increased clearance of HPV among users of the copper versus levonorgestrel IUD,[91] but no difference in cervical dysplasia. The authors hypothesized that the inflammatory changes induced by the copper IUD would promote faster clearance of HPV.

Side Effects

Often, the possibility of minor side effects of contraceptive methods, in addition to the more serious complications, influences whether an individual selects a certain method. "What physical changes will I undergo?" "Will it be messy when I use this method or will I have spotting, or cramping?" Do not dismiss the important role that side effects play when an individual must repeatedly assess whether to continue using a method or whether to use it consistently.

Side effects can be hormonally, chemically, or mechanically induced. Headaches, nausea, mood disturbances, dizziness and breast tenderness can be side effects of hormonal methods. Menstrual changes such as spotting and decreased or increased bleeding can be caused by hormonal methods and IUDs and are a major cause of method discontinuation. The vaginal ring and IUDs can lead to increased vaginal discharge, and all methods may lead to perceived changes in discharge amount or odor, or changes in the frequency of vaginal infections. Some individuals report weight gain with hormonal methods. Physical sensations such as decreased penile sensitivity, pressure on vaginal walls, or uterine cramping may be caused by mechanical methods. Other chemically-induced side effects include allergic reactions to latex and to copper.

For many reported side effects, it is unknown whether there is a true causal association with contraceptive use. The vast majority of contraceptive studies are not placebo-controlled, and many do not have an appropriate comparison group for rates of various side effects. Placebo-controlled studies of COCs have shown no significant difference in the frequency of most nonspecific side effects, yet side effects are the most common cause for discontinuation.[92] Patients may report symptoms that are temporally related to initiation of a method but not plausibly caused by the method. For some reported side effects, it may be helpful for a clinician to discuss with the patient whether the symptoms are possibly or likely caused by the method, or whether there might be another explanation. However, it is not useful to talk patients out of their symptoms or convince them to continue a method with which they are not satisfied (see Chapter 2 on Engaging with Unintended Pregnancy through Patient-Centered Reproductive Goals and Contraceptive Counseling).

With the great majority of side effects, instruction and patient education can help users understand and accept what is happening. The appearance of side effects that are not serious is not a medical reason to preclude use of a method. However, people who wish to discontinue using a method due to perceived or experienced side effects must be supported in doing so, even if the clinician does not believe that the side effect is harmful or related to the method. Similarly, a person's decision to discontinue a method must be respected even if pregnancy would pose substantial health risks. Clinicians have an important role to play in helping clients to feel listened to and to choose another method, if desired, but patient autonomy must always be respected.

Goals for Communicating About Safety

1. **Try to educate the patient about misconceptions.** Many patients hold false beliefs about contraceptive methods—that the pill is very dangerous even to healthy, nonsmoking young women or that injectables lead to permanent sterility (see Chapter 2 on Engaging with Unintended Pregnancy through Patient-Centered Reproductive Goals and Contraceptive Counseling). If you see that you are getting nowhere, stop. Help each client select a method that can be used correctly and consistently without fear, and support the patient in his or her own choice.
2. **Make sure that you and your staff know all about the major risks and side effects** of contraceptive methods and can communicate these clearly, such as the association between pill use and blood clots or reproductive cancers.
3. **Tell patients what they need to know** even if they do not ask. Patients do not always ask the questions they need answered. Usually, they do not know what they don't know.
4. **Compare risks of using contraception with pregnancy risks.** In general, the risks of pregnancy, abortion, and delivery are far greater than those for using a contraceptive method.
5. **Start with a sexual health assessment so you can help patients make a contraceptive method choice that will protect them from both STIs and pregnancy.** Safety concerns often overlap with worries about infections. With the exception of abstinence, currently available methods (male and female condoms) that protect against infection are not those that provide greatest protection against pregnancy. Conversely, the most highly effective methods of contraception provide *no* protection against infection. Therefore, highly effective protection against both risks requires use of two methods. Ask patients about specific sexual behaviors,

as even couples practicing "abstinence" may be engaging in oral and anal intercourse, which can result in STI transmission.

6. **Teach patients the danger signals** of the method they select. If a danger signal does appear, the informed user can quickly seek help.
7. **Use language that is appropriate for the patient.**

NONCONTRACEPTIVE BENEFITS

Noncontraceptive benefits are often a major determinant for an individual selecting a contraceptive method. (See Table 3-4.) Adolescents may opt for combined hormonal contraceptives (CHCs) to help improve their acne or reduce dysmenorrhea, and an increasing proportion of people opt for a levonorgestrel IUD to reduce or eliminate menstrual blood loss. In many cases, noncontraceptive benefits can help patients decide between two or more suitable methods. (See Table 3-4.) Awareness that a method of contraception has noncontraceptive benefits (cancer prevention, protection of future fertility or diminished menstrual cycle symptoms) may also increase the likelihood of continuing to use that method. Make it a practice to tell your patients about the noncontraceptive benefits of the various methods. If patients have additional reasons for using the contraceptive method, their motivation to use the method correctly and consistently will probably be improved.

Reducing the user's risk of STIs may weigh as heavily as preventing pregnancy. Any sexually active person who may be at risk of acquiring STIs should consider condoms (see Chapter 14 on Male Condoms and Chapter 20 on Reproductive Tract Infections), either alone or, preferably, with another method more effective in preventing pregnancy. Because condoms reduce the risk of STIs that cause PID and thus lead to infertility, they protect future fertility.[93]

Fertility awareness methods educate users about their menstrual physiology. This knowledge can also help couples achieve a planned pregnancy.

Most hormonal methods of contraception lead to reduced menstrual blood loss, particularly the levonorgestrel IUD, and can be used to manage heavy menstrual bleeding.[94] They also decrease dysmenorrhea and are first-line treatment for endometriosis.[95,96] Hormonal methods all contain a progestin and so can be used to protect the endometrium for individuals who are anovulatory or on hormone therapy.[97]

COCs, and presumably the patch and vaginal ring, can improve acne and PMDD/PMS. These CHC methods protect against ovarian, endometrial, and colorectal cancer and may improve bone health in women with low estrogen levels related to premature ovarian failure. In the case of a

Table 3-4 Major methods of contraception and some related safety concerns, side effects, and noncontraceptive benefits

Method	Dangers[1]	Side Effects	Noncontraceptive Benefits
Combined hormonal contraception (pill, patch, and vaginal ring)	Cardiovascular complications (stroke, heart attack, blood clots, high blood pressure), hepatic adenomas, increased risk of breast, cervical and liver cancer diagnosis	Nausea, headaches, dizziness, irregular bleeding or spotting, weight gain, breast tenderness, chloasma	Decreases dysmenorrhea, heavy menstrual bleeding, anemia and cyclic mood problems (PMS or PMDD); reduces acne, reduces risk of ectopic pregnancy, and symptomatic PID, and protects against ovarian, endometrial, and colorectal cancer
Progestin-only pill	None known	Acne and irregular bleeding or spotting	
Intrauterine devices	Infection post placement, uterine perforation, expulsion (and subsequent risk of pregnancy), anemia (with copper IUD). If pregnancy occurs, higher risk of ectopic	Irregular bleeding or spotting, increased bleeding or menstrual cramping with copper IUD; amenorrhea with levonorgestrel IUD	Levonorgestrel IUD reduces menstrual blood loss and dysmenorrhea, can be used to treat endometriosis, adenomyosis, and heavy bleeding, and can provide progestin for hormone therapy. Reduced risk of endometrial cancer, Lactation not disturbed. Copper IUD is the only method in the top two tiers without hormones
Male condom	Anaphylactic reaction to latex	Decreased sensation, allergy to latex	Protects against STIs, including HIV; delays premature ejaculation
Female condom	None known	Aesthetically unappealing and awkward to use for some	Protects against STIs
Progestin implant	Rare migration, rare infection at implant site; problems with removal, especially if inserted too deeply	Menstrual changes (increased or decreased bleeding and spotting, amenorrhea), acne, adverse effect on mood	Lactation not disturbed; decreases dysmenorrhea, usually reduces menstrual bleeding

Injectable	Allergic reactions, pathologic weight gain, decreased bone mineral density	Menstrual changes, amenorrhea, weight gain, adverse effects on lipids	Lactation not disturbed; reduces risk of catamenial seizures; may protect against ovarian and endometrial cancers
Permanent contraception	Anesthetic or surgical complications; if pregnancy occurs after tubal occlusion, high risk that it will be ectopic. With hysteroscopic occlusion risk of pain, tubal perforation, malpositioned inserts.	Pain at surgical site, psychological reactions, subsequent regret that the procedure was performed	Tubal occlusion reduces risk of ovarian cancer and may protect against PID
Abstinence	None known		Prevents STIs, including HIV, if anal and oral intercourse are avoided as well
Diaphragm, Sponge	Vaginal and urinary tract infections, toxic shock syndrome; possible increase in susceptibility to HIV/AIDS acquisition if exposed to positive partner	Vaginal discomfort, vaginal irritation, vaginal discharge if left in too long, allergy to spermicides or latex	None known
Spermicides	Vaginal and urinary tract infections; possible increase in susceptibility to HIV/AIDS acquisition if exposed to positive partner	Vaginal irritation, allergy	None known
Lactational Amenorrhea Method (LAM)	None known	None known	Breastfeeding provides excellent nutrition for infants
Withdrawal	None known	None known	None known

Note:
[1]Among healthy women with no concurrent medical conditions

method failure, the pregnancy is less likely to be ectopic if the woman is using a CHC because the thickening of the cervical mucus caused by hormonal methods potentially confers a slight benefit in regard to development of symptomatic pelvic inflammatory disease (PID). Higher-dose pills (those with 30 mcg ethinyl estradiol or higher) may protect against functional ovarian cysts and benign breast disease (see Chapter 8 on Combined Oral Contraceptives).

PERSONAL CONSIDERATIONS

The best method of contraception for patients is one that will be in harmony with their wishes, preferences, and lifestyle and takes their fears and other concerns into consideration: a method that will be used correctly.

A typical woman in the United States spends about 39 years—almost half of her lifespan of 81 years—at potential biological risk of pregnancy, during the time from menarche (at about age 12) to natural menopause (at about age 51).[98,99] Individuals have different priorities for their ideal contraceptive method. Some prioritize efficacy, while others might give greater importance to their ability to easily stop and start the method. Many people use contraception because they strongly wish to avoid pregnancy, but others may feel more ambivalent, or would welcome an unintended pregnancy.[100] What matters most to an individual when considering a contraceptive method often changes over the course of a reproductive lifespan. It is critical to discuss each client's reproductive goals, using a patient-centered approach (see Chapter 2 on Engaging with Unintended Pregnancy through Patient-Centered Reproductive Goals and Contraceptive Counseling). Different reproductive stages are associated with distinct fertility goals and sexual behaviors.[101] For individuals and couples who plan to have children, from menarche to first birth, the primary fertility goal is to postpone pregnancy and birth. Between the first birth and the time when a person intends to have no more children, the primary goal is to space pregnancies. Between the time when a person intends to have no more children and menopause, the goal is to cease childbearing altogether. For many people, their goal may be to avoid pregnancy throughout their reproductive lifespan and maintenance of fertility is not a concern.

Reproductive Goals. Individuals and couples often choose their contraceptive method based on the number of children they desire and the timing of those births. For example, people who plan on having a few children or having children early in their reproductive life cycle may have more flexible requirements about the spacing before and between pregnancies and may be more willing to risk a mistimed, but not unwanted, pregnancy. Such flexibility may mean that contraceptive method choices would not be limited to those with highest efficacy. Moreover, many people's desires to achieve or to avoid pregnancy are situated along a spectrum, which can include ambivalence or even indifference towards avoiding pregnancy. Rather than seeing this situation as a problem to be solved, providers should help individuals choose a method that best suits their needs, and when appropriate offer a conversation about preconception care if they would like to be prepared for the possibility of pregnancy, with interventions such as quitting smoking and initiating a prenatal vitamin with folic acid.

Pattern of sexual activity. In choosing their contraceptive method, individuals should consider their risk of acquiring an STI.

The number of partners affects the risk of exposure to STIs. People may have more than one partner at any given time, their partners may have other partners or they may have only one partner at a time but the relationships are short term. The practitioner recommending the use of male or female condoms must be prepared to take the time required to discuss risks of STIs, encourage safer sexual behaviors, and teach how to correctly use condoms.

The frequency of intercourse may have an influence a person's contraceptive method choice. For example, the woman who has infrequent intercourse may not wish to use a method that requires daily medication. On the other hand, infrequent intercourse may also indicate that a client has intercourse at unpredictable times. These clients may need skills in "expecting the unexpected." In general, if someone has said that preventing pregnancy is very important, efficacy will take precedence regardless of coital frequency.

Access to medical care. Many people in the United States have difficulty gaining access to health care: they lack health care coverage, find the system difficult to navigate, or find that the system shuns them. Others may find their access hampered by difficulties getting to a clinic, requirements for repeat visits, or too long a wait once they get there. Studies in other nations have shown that access has great bearing on contraceptive method adherence and choice.[102] The degree of access can also influence people in the United States. Individuals may decline a highly effective method such as the implant or IUD if there is no assurance that they will have access to timely removal. Conversely, people may opt for a longer-acting method if they anticipate losing insurance coverage or access to care. Access and adherence are improved by providing a full year's supply of contraceptives. While many clinicians provide 13 cycles of pills, for example, most do not offer sufficient quantities of condoms.

Intimate partner violence. It is important to routinely screen clients for intimate partner violence and provide appropriate resources if necessary. Reproductive coercion is a form of intimate partner violence in which a partner attempts to maintain control over reproductive health in the relationship. Coercive behaviors can include attempts to have unprotected intercourse, interfere with proper use of a contraceptive method and cause an unwanted pregnancy, or control the outcome of a pregnancy (such as obstructing pregnancy termination).[103] In such situations, these individuals may not be able to rely on their partners to use abstinence, withdrawal, or a condom; a non-coitally dependent or a female-controlled coital method should be offered. Many people may also require a method that is not visible to their partner and affords complete privacy, such as the IUD, implant, or injectable (see Chapter 2 on Engaging with Unintended Pregnancy through Patient-Centered Reproductive Goals and Contraceptive Counseling).

Goals for Communicating About Personal Considerations

Key concepts for discussing and teaching about contraceptive method choice and personal considerations include the following:

1. **The patient decides which personal considerations matter**. Only the potential user can weigh all the elements for personal choice, and the clinician will not be able to predict what matters. Privacy? Lubrication? Light periods? What her older sister uses? Do not make assumptions; ask using open-ended questions.
2. **It is a long way from the exam room to the bedroom**. We offer methods as medicines in a clinical setting, and then our patients go home and use them in a sexual setting, be it a bedroom, motel room, car seat, or tent. Remember to help your patient think through the sexual aspects of contraception (see Chapter 22 on Sexuality).
3. **Support patients in making a second (or third) contraceptive method choice**. They may not like the first method at all and will need to know that they are welcome to come back and try something else. Besides, it is always good to know how to use several methods.
4. **Encourage your patients to talk about contraceptive issues with their partners**. While the user of the method is the only one who can decide which method seems the best choice, partners can play a helpful and supportive role. Help your clients think about and practice discussing contraception with their partners if this is new territory for them. For example, discuss strategies for negotiating condom use.
5. **Personal considerations change over time**. Teenagers and 35-year-olds often use different criteria as they evaluate their contraceptive method choices. Encourage patients to think through their contraceptive method needs as their reproductive goals, sexual lives, and bodies change over time.

6. **Do not make assumptions about sexual preferences or sexual practices.** All individuals have a range of sexual preferences and practices, which may or may not put them at risk for pregnancy or STIs. These preferences and practices can change over time, too. Ask open-ended questions about sexuality and reproductive goals that are nonjudgmental and do not assume the sexual orientation or gender of their partners.

Suggested Reading

Brown SS, Eisenberg L. The best intentions: unintended pregnancy and the well-being of children and families. Washington DC: National Academy Press, 1995.

Harrison PF, Rosenfield A. Contraceptive research and development: looking to the future. Washington DC: National Academy Press, 1996.

Foreman M, Spieler J. Contraceptive evidence: questions and answers. Washington DC: Population Reference Bureau, 2013. Available at www.prb.org/pdf13/contraceptive-evidence-2013.pdf.

Author Disclosures: Trussell: Merck, Evofem, Agile; Aiken: Agile; Micks: Nexplanon trainer (Merck); Guthrie: none.

Acknowledgments: Joyce Abma and Kim Daniels (special tabulations of NSFG data)

References

1. Lessard LN, Karasek D, Ma S, et al. Contraceptive features preferred by women at high risk of unintended pregnancy. Perspect Sex Reprod Health 2012;44:194–200.
2. Daniels K, Abma J. Personal communication to James Trussell dated April 3, 2017.
3. Finer LB, Zolna MR. Declines in Unintended Pregnancy in the United States, 2008–2011. N Engl J Med 1016;374:843–52.
4. Personal communication from Mia Zolna and Larry Finer, September 15, 2017.
5. Smith, TW. (National Opinion Research Center, Chicago, IL). Conversation with: James Trussell (Office of Population Research, Princeton University, Princeton, NJ). 1993 Dec 13.
6. Madden T, Secura GM, Nease RF, Politi MC, Peipert JF. The role of contraceptive attributes in women's contraceptive decision making. Am J Obstet Gynecol 2015;213:46.e1–6.
7. Trussell J, Grummer-Strawn L. Contraceptive failure of the ovulation method of periodic abstinence. Fam Plann Perspect 1990;22:65–75.
8. Steiner MJ, Trussell J, Mehta N, Condon S, Subramaniam S, Bourne D. Communicating contraceptive effectiveness: a randomized controlled trial to inform a World Health Organization family planning handbook. Am J Obstet Gynecol 2006;195:85–91.
9. Steiner MJ, Trussell J, Johnson S. Communicating contraceptive effectiveness: an updated counseling chart. Am J Obstet Gynecol 2007;197:118.
10. Trussell J, Guthrie K. Lessons from the contraceptive CHOICE project: the Hull long-acting reversible contraception (LARC) initiative. J Fam Plann Reprod Health Care 2015;41:60–3.
11. Grimes DA. Forgettable contraception. Contraception 2009;80:497–9.
12. Trussell J, Schwarz EB, Guthrie K. Research priorities for preventing unintended pregnancy: moving beyond emergency contraceptive pills. Perspect Sex Reprod Health 2010;42:8–9.

13. National Collaborating Centre for Women's and Children's Health. Long-acting reversible contraception: the effective and appropriate use of long-acting reversible contraception. London: RCOG Press; 2005; [cited 2010 Jun 7]. Available from: http://www.nice.org.uk/CG030.
14. Sundaram A, Vaughan B, Kost K, Bankole A, Finer L, Singh S, Trussell J. Contraceptive failure in the United States: estimates from the 2006–2010 National Survey of Family Growth. Perspect Sexual Reprod Health 2017;49:7–16.
15. Personal communication from Aparna Sundaram and Barbara Vaughan, October 6, 2016.
16. Arévalo M, Jennings V, Sinai I. Efficacy of a new method of family planning: the Standard Days Method. Contraception 2002;65:333–8.
17. Arévalo M, Jennings V, Nikula M, Sinai I. Efficacy of the new TwoDay Method of family planning. Fertil Steril 2004;82:885–92.
18. Frank-Herrmann P, Heil J, Gnoth C, et al. The effectiveness of a fertility awareness based method to avoid pregnancy in relation to a couple's sexual behaviour during the fertile time: a prospective longitudinal study. Hum Reprod 2007;22:1310–9.
19. Schwartz JL, Weiner DH, Lai JJ, et al. Contraceptive efficacy, safety, fit, and acceptability of a single-size diaphragm developed with end-user input. Obstet Gynecol 2015;125:895–903.
20. Trussell J, Strickler J, Vaughan B. Contraceptive efficacy of the diaphragm, the sponge and the cervical cap. Fam Plann Perspect 1993;25:100–5, 135.
21. Frezieres RG, Walsh TL, Nelson AL, Clark VA, Coulson AH. Evaluation of the efficacy of a polyurethane condom: results from a randomized controlled clinical trial. Fam Plann Perspect 1999;31:81–7.
22. Walsh TL, Frezieres RG, Peacock K, Nelson AL, Clark VA, Bernstein L. Evaluation of the efficacy of a nonlatex condom: results from a randomized, controlled clinical trial. Perspect Sex Reprod Health 2003;35:79–86.
23. Steiner MJ, Dominik R, Rountree RW, Nanda K, Dorflinger LJ. Contraceptive effectiveness of a polyurethane condom and a latex condom: a randomized controlled trial. Obstet Gynecol 2003;101:539–47.
24. Farr G, Gabelnick H, Sturgen K, Dorflinger L. Contraceptive efficacy and acceptability of the female condom. Am J Public Health 1994;84:1960–4.
25. Raymond EG, Chen PL, Luoto J. Contraceptive effectiveness and safety of five nonoxynol-9 spermicides: a randomized trial. Obstet Gynecol 2004;103:430–9.
26. Mitchell AA, Van Bennekom CM, Louik C. A pregnancy-prevention program in women of childbearing age receiving isotretinoin. N Engl J Med 1995;333:101–6.
27. Speroff L, Glass RH, Kase NG. Clinical gynecologic endocrinology and infertility. 6th ed. Baltimore (MD): Williams & Wilkins; 1999.
28. Kestelman P, Trussell J. Efficacy of the simultaneous use of condoms and spermicides. Fam Plann Perspect 1991;23:226–7, 232.
29. Aisch G, Marsh B. How likely is it that birth control could let you down? New York Times, September 13, 2014.
30. Trussell J, Vaughan B. Contraceptive failure, method-related discontinuation and resumption of use: results from the 1995 National Survey of Family Growth. Fam Plann Perspect 1999;31:64–72, 93.
31. Richwald GA, Greenland S, Gerber MM, Potik R, Kersey L, Comas MA. Effectiveness of the cavity-rim cervical cap: results of a large clinical study. Obstet Gynecol 1989;74:143–8.
32. McIntyre SL, Higgins JE. Parity and use-effectiveness with the contraceptive sponge. Am J Obstet Gynecol 1986;155:796–801.
33. Menken J, Trussell J, Larsen U. Age and infertility. Science 1986;233:1389–94.
34. Grady WR, Hayward MD, Yagi J. Contraceptive failure in the United States: estimates from the 1982 National Survey of Family Growth. Fam Plann Perspect 1986;18:200–9.

35. Schirm AL, Trussell J, Menken J, Grady WR. Contraceptive failure in the United States: the impact of social, economic, and demographic factors. Fam Plann Perspect 1982;14:68–75.
36. Sivin I, Schmidt F. Effectiveness of IUDs: a review. Contraception 1987;36:55–84.
37. Vessey M, Lawless M, Yeates D. Efficacy of different contraceptive methods. Lancet 1982;1:841–2.
38. Trussell J, Westoff CF. Contraceptive practice and trends in coital frequency. Fam Plann Perspect 1980;12:246–9.
39. Steiner MJ, Hertz-Picciotto I, Raymond E, Trussell J, Wheeless A, Schoenbach V. Influence of cycle variability and coital frequency on the risk of pregnancy. Contraception 1999;60:137–43.
40. Trussell J, Kost K. Contraceptive failure in the United States: a critical review of the literature. Stud Fam Plann 1987;18:237–83.
41. Davis HJ. The shield intrauterine device: a superior modern contraceptive. Am J Obstet Gynecol 1970;106:455–6.
42. Mintz M. At any cost: corporate greed, women, and the Dalkon shield. New York: Pantheon Books; 1985.
43. Trussell J. Methodological pitfalls in the analysis of contraceptive failure. Stat Med 1991;10:201–20.
44. Trussell J, Hatcher RA, Cates W, Stewart FH, Kost K. A guide to interpreting contraceptive efficacy studies. Obstet Gynecol 1990;76:558–67.
45. Trussell J, Menken J. Life table analysis of contraceptive failure. In: Hermalin AI, Entwisle B, (eds). The role of surveys in the analysis of family planning programs. Liege (Belgium): Ordina Editions; 1982. p. 537–71.
46. Tietze C, Poliakoff SR, Rock J. The clinical effectiveness of the rhythm method of contraception. Fertil Steril 1951;2:444–50.
47. Trussell TJ, Faden R, Hatcher RA. Efficacy information in contraceptive counseling: those little white lies. Am J Public Health 1976;66:761–7.
48. United States Parachute Association. Safety Information. http://.test.uspa.org/facts-faqs/safety. Accessed March 29, 2017.
49. Centers for Disease Control and Prevention. National Center for Health Statistics. Accidents or Unintentional Injuries 2014. http://www.cdc.gov/nchs/fastats/accidental-injury.htm. Accessed March 29, 2017.
50. National Highway Traffic Safety Administration. Traffic Safety Facts 2015. http://.crashstats.nhtsa.dot.gov/Api/Public/ViewPublication/812375. Accessed March 29, 2017.
51. Centers for Disease Control and Prevention. National Center for Health Statistics. Assault or Homicide 2014. http://www.cdc.gov/nchs/fastats/homicide.htm. Accessed March 29, 2017.
52. United States Fire Administration. Fire Death Rates and Risk 2014. http://www.usfa.fema.gov/data/statistics/fire_death_rates.html. Accessed March 29, 2017.
53. International Air Transport Association. Airline Safety Performance 2016. http://www.iata.org/pressroom/pr/Pages/2017-03-10-01.aspx. Accessed March 29, 2017.
54. National Weather Service. National Oceanic and Atmospheric Administration. Odds of Becoming a Lightning Victim 2006–2015. http://www.lightningsafety.noaa.gov/odds.shtml. Accessed March 29, 2017.
55. Schwingl PJ, Ory HW, Visness CM. Estimates of the risk of cardiovascular death attributable to low-dose oral contraceptives in the United States. Am J Obstet Gynecol 1999;180:241–9.
56. Escobedo LG, Peterson HB, Grubb GS, Franks AL. Case-fatality rates for tubal sterilization in U.S. hospitals, 1979–1980. Am J Obstet Gynecol 1989;160:147–50.
57. Hajjeh RA, Reingold A, Weil A, Shutt K, Schuhat A, Perkins BA. Toxic shock syndrome in the United States, 1979–1996. Emerg Infect Dis 1999;5:807–10.
58. US Bureau of the Census. Statistical abstract of the United States: 2003. Washington (DC): Government Printing Office; 2003. Table 11, Resident population by age and sex: 1980–2002. p. 13.

59. Raymond EG, Grimes DA. The comparative safety of legal induced abortion and childbirth in the United States. Obstet Gynecol 2012;119:215–9.
60. Saraiya M, Green CA, Berg CJ, Hopkins FW, Koonin LM, Atrash HK. Spontaneous abortion-related deaths among women in the United States—1981–1991. Obstet Gynecol 1999;94:172–6.
61. Karnovsky, R. (Danco Laboratories, New York, NY). Email to: James Trussell (Office of Population Research, Princeton University, Princeton, NJ). 2017 Mar 28.
62. Zane S, Creanga AA, Berg CJ, Pazol K, Suchdev DB, Jamieson DJ, Callaghan WM. Abortion-related mortality in the United States: 1998–2010. Obstet Gynecol 2015;126:258–65.
63. Tepper NK, Dragoman MV, Gaffield ME, Curtis KM. Nonoral combined hormonal contraceptives and thromboembolism: a systematic review. Contraception 2017;95:130–139.
64. Horton LG, Simmons KB, Curtis KM. Combined hormonal contraceptive use among obese women and risk for cardiovascular events: a systematic review. Contraception 2016;94:590–604.
65. Lidegaard Ø, Løkkegaard E, Jensen A, Skovlund CW, Keiding N. Thrombotic stroke and myocardial infarction with hormonal contraception. N Engl J Med 2012;366:2257–66
66. Tanis BC, van den Bosch MA, Kemmeren JM, Cats VM, Helmerhorst FM, Algra A, van der Graaf Y, Rosendaal FR. Oral contraceptives and the risk of myocardial infarction. N Engl J Med 2001;345:1787–93.
67. Burkman R, Schlesselman JJ, Zieman M. Safety concerns and health benefits associated with oral contraception. Am J Obstet Gynecol 2004;190 Suppl 4:S5–22.
68. Ischaemic stroke and combined oral contraceptives: results of an international, multicentre, case-control study. WHO Collaborative Study of Cardiovascular Disease and Steroid Hormone Contraception. Lancet 1996;348:498–505.
69. Horton LG, Simmons KB, Curtis KM. Combined hormonal contraceptive use among obese women and risk for cardiovascular events: A systematic review. Contraception 2016;94:590–604.
70. Lidegaard Ø, Løkkegaard E, Svendsen AL, Agger C. Hormonal contraception and risk of venous thromboembolism: national follow-up study BMJ 2009;339:b2890.
71. Heinemann LA, Dinger JC. Range of published estimates of venous thromboembolism incidence in young women. Contraception 2007;75:328–36.
72. Hannaford PC, Iversen L, Macfarlane TV, Elliott AM, Angus V, Lee AJ. Mortality among contraceptive pill users: cohort evidence from Royal College of General Practitioners' oral contraception study. BMJ 2010;340:c927.
73. Iversen L, Sivasubramaniam S, Lee AJ, Fielding S, Hannaford PC. Lifetime cancer risk and combined oral contraceptives: the Royal College of General Practitioners' Oral Contraception Study. Am J Obstet Gynecol 2017;216:580.e1–580.e9.
74. Vessey M, Yeates D, Flynn S. Factors affecting mortality in a large cohort study with special reference to oral contraceptive use. Contraception 2010;82:221–9.
75. Collaborative Group on Hormonal Factors in Breast Cancer. Breast cancer and hormonal contraceptives: collaborative reanalysis of individual data on 53,297 women with breast cancer and 100,239 women without breast cancer from 54 epidemiological studies. Lancet 1996;347:1713–27.
76. Mørch LS, Skovlund CW, Hannaford PC, Iversen L, Fielding S, Lidegaard Ø. Contemporary hormonal contraception and the risk of breast cancer. N Engl J Med 2017;377:2228–39.
77. Hunter DJ, Colditz GA, Hankinson SE, Malspeis S, Spiegelman D, Chen W, Stampfer MJ, Willett WC. Oral contraceptive use and breast cancer: a prospective study of young women. Cancer Epidemiol Biomarkers Prev 2010;19:2496–502.
78. Hannaford PC, Selvaraj S, Elliott AM, Angus V, Iversen L, Lee AJ. Cancer risk among users of oral contraceptives: cohort data from the Royal College of General Practitioner's oral contraception study. BMJ 2007;335:651.
79. Wingo PA, Austin H, Marchbanks PA, Whiteman MK, Hsia J, Mandel MG, Peterson HB, Ory HW. Oral contraceptives and the risk of death from breast cancer. Obstet Gynecol 2007;110:793–800.

80. Kaunitz AM. Depot medroxyprogesterone acetate contraception and the risk of breast and gynecologic cancer. J Reprod Med 1996;41:419–27.
81. Samson M, Porter N, Orekoya O, Hebert JR, Adams SA, Bennett CL, Steck SE. Progestin and breast cancer risk: a systematic review. Breast Cancer Res Treat 2016;155:3–12.
82. Soini T, Hurskainen R, Grénman S, Mäenpää J, Paavonen J, Pukkala E. Cancer risk in women using the levonorgestrel-releasing intrauterine system in Finland. Obstet Gynecol 2014;124:292–9.
83. Soini T, Hurskainen R, Grénman S, Mäenpää J, Paavonen J, Pukkala E. Impact of levonorgestrel-releasing intrauterine system use on the cancer risk of the ovary and fallopian tube. Acta Oncol 2016;55:1281–1284.
84. Soini T, Hurskainen R, Grénman S, et al. Levonorgestrel-releasing intrauterine system and the risk of breast cancer: A nationwide cohort study. Acta Oncol 2016;55:188–92.
85. Wan YL, Holland C. The efficacy of levonorgestrel intrauterine systems for endometrial protection: a systematic review. Climacteric 2011;14:622–32.
86. Kim MK, Seong SJ, Kim YS, Song T, Kim ML, Yoon BS, Jun HS, Lee YH. Combined medroxyprogesterone acetate/levonorgestrel-intrauterine system treatment in young women with early-stage endometrial cancer. Am J Obstet Gynecol 2013;209:358.e1–4.
87. Smith JS, Green J, Berrington de Gonzalez A, Appleby P, Peto J, Plummer M, Franceschi S, Beral V. Cervical cancer and use of hormonal contraceptives: a systematic review. Lancet 2003;361:1159–67.
88. Vessey M, Yeates D, Flynn S. Factors affecting mortality in a large cohort study with special reference to oral contraceptive use. Contraception 2010;82:221–9.
89. Castellsagué X, Díaz M, Vaccarella S, de Sanjosé S, Muñoz N, Herrero R, Franceschi S, Meijer CJ, Bosch FX. Intrauterine device use, cervical infection with human papillomavirus, and risk of cervical cancer: a pooled analysis of 26 epidemiological studies. Lancet Oncol 2011;12:1023–31.
90. Averbach SH, Ma Y, Smith-McCune K, Shiboski S, Moscicki AB. The effect of intrauterine devices on acquisition and clearance of human papillomavirus. Am J Obstet Gynecol 2017;216:386.e381–386.e385.
91. Lekovich JP, Amrane S, Pangasa M, Pereira N, Frey MK, Varrey A, Holcomb K. Comparison of human papillomavirus infection and cervical cytology in women using copper-containing and levonorgestrel-containing intrauterine devices. Obstet Gynecol 2015;125:1101–5.
92. Grimes DA, Schulz KF. Nonspecific side effects of oral contraceptives: nocebo or noise? Contraception 2011;83:5–9.
93. Ness RB, Randall H, Richter HE, et al.; Pelvic Inflammatory Disease Evaluation and Clinical Health Study Investigators. Condom use and the risk of recurrent pelvic inflammatory disease, chronic pelvic pain, or infertility following an episode of pelvic inflammatory disease. Am J Public Health 2004;94:1327–9.
94. Lethaby A, Hussain M, Rishworth JR, Rees MC. Progesterone or progestogen-releasing intrauterine systems for heavy menstrual bleeding. Cochrane Database Syst Rev 2015 Apr 30;(4).
95. Imai A, Matsunami K, Takagi H, Ichigo S. Levonorgestrel-releasing intrauterine device used for dysmenorrhea: five-year literature review. Clin Exp Obstet Gynecol 2014;41:495–8.
96. Brown J, Farquhar C. An overview of treatments for endometriosis. JAMA 2015;313: 296-7.
97. Bahamondes L, Valeria Bahamondes M, Shulman LP. Non-contraceptive benefits of hormonal and intrauterine reversible contraceptive methods. Hum Reprod Update 2015;21:640–51.
98. Kochanek KD, Murphy SL, Xu J, Tejada-Vera B. Deaths: final data for 2014. Natl Vital Stat Rep 2016;65:1–122.
99. Finer LB, Philbin JM. Trends in ages at key reproductive transitions in the United States, 1951-2010. Women Health Iss 2014;24:e271–9.

100. Callegari LS, Aiken AR, Dehlendorf C, Cason P, Borrero S. Addressing potential pitfalls of reproductive life planning with patient-centered counseling. Am J Obstet Gynecol 2017;216:129–134
101. Forrest JD. Timing of reproductive life stages. Obstet Gynecol 1993;82:105–10.
102. Tsui AO, Ochoa LH. Service proximity as a determinant of contraceptive behaviour: evidence from cross-national studies of survey data. In: Philips JF, Ross JA, (eds). Family planning programmes and fertility. Oxford (England): Clarendon Press; 1992. p. 222–56.
103. American College of Obstetricians and Gynecologists. ACOG Committee opinion no. 554: reproductive and sexual coercion. Obstet Gynecol 2013;121:411–5.

Contraceptive Implant

4

Anita L. Nelson, MD
Diana Crabtree Sokol, MD
Jaclyn Grentzer, MD, MSCI

- The U.S. implant (Nexplanon) provides pregnancy protection that is at least as effective as permanent contraception and is not reduced by the user's weight or BMI.
- Mechanisms of action:
  - Profound ovulation suppression, thickened cervical mucus
  - No post-fertilization impacts have been documented
- Bleeding patterns are not predictable prior to placement. Counseling improves acceptance of abnormal bleeding patterns. It may also help to provide NSAIDS in advance of need for treatment of prolonged or heavy bleeding that may occur.
- Both placement and removal of the implant can be accomplished quickly. Same day placement is very feasible, even in busy practices.

Contraceptive implants are safe and convenient contraceptives that can be used by virtually every person. They provide reversible pregnancy protection that is at least as effective as permanent contraception. Nexplanon is the only contraceptive implant currently available in the United States.

Implanon was the system that preceded Nexplanon and is still used in many other countries. It differs from Nexplanon only in that it has no barium sulfate and can be imaged only by ultrasound and MRI, not by x-ray or x-ray computer tomography (CT). With the change from Implanon to Nexplanon, a new one-hand introducer was developed to decrease the risk of deep or nonpalpable implant placement that had been occasionally reported with Implanon's trocar applicator.[1,2] Although placement with the new applicator system is rapid and straightforward, formal training is still required by the Food and Drug Administration (FDA).

Nexplanon is a single rod system measuring 4 cm in length and 2 mm in diameter. The firm, semi-flexible white rod is made of an ethylene vinyl acetate core that contains 68 mg of etonogestrel (ENG), 15 mg of barium sulfate and 0.1 mg of magnesium stearate. ENG is an active metabolite of the third-generation progestin desogestrel, which is found in commonly used combined oral contraceptives (COC), such as Mircette and Ortho-Cept, as well as in the vaginal contraceptive NuvaRing. Barium sulfate renders the implant radiopaque to help with its localization using x-ray.[3]

Because many patients from other countries may seek care in the United States, clinicians should be aware that globally there are also two other implant systems—the 3-year single-rod etonogestrel-releasing implant (Implanon) and the 5-year two-rod levonorgestrel-releasing systems (Sino II and Jadelle II).

MECHANISM OF ACTION

The etonogestrel implant was designed by the Population Council to provide adequate hormone levels to guarantee ovulation suppression in 100% of users for 2 years. This was done specifically to address the concerns of couples who might be opposed to any post-fertilization activity and want reassurance that it was purely contraceptive. Calculations determined that etonogestrel levels of at least 90 pg/mL would achieve that goal. Those levels of etonogestrel also thickened cervical mucus to prevent sperm penetration into the upper genital tract. One study of 244 ultrasound scans of the implant users found 1 episode of ovulation at 16 months, but other investigators have not shown any evidence of any early ovulation.[4] Following the initial clinical trial, subsequent experience and studies demonstrated low failure rates with the single implant for up to 3 years. Later a pharmacokinetic and pharmacodynamic study showed that mean serum progesterone levels remained sub-ovulatory for more than 3 years.[5] This raised the question of how long ovulation suppression could be guaranteed. To determine how long ovulation was reliably suppressed, investigators studied follicular development, endometrial thickness and serum concentrations of 17 β-estradiol and progesterone twice weekly for 3 years. They found that this ENG implant universally suppressed ovulation for 30 months. Between 30 to 36 months, 3% of users showed some evidence of ovulation, but no pregnancies occurred because the thickened cervical mucus prevented sperm entry into the upper genital tract.[6]

EFFECTIVENESS

Implants are in the top tier of contraceptive efficacy. In the international clinical trials and in the U.S. studies, no pregnancies were reported when the implant was in place. In the trials done in the United States,

6 pregnancies were reported in over 20,000 cycles of use, but each of those conceptions most likely occurred during the required 14-day study follow-up period after the implant had been removed. Including those pregnancies, the Pearl Index for the implant was 0.38%.

After the product was introduced into practice, higher failure rates were noted, but analysis found that this was due primarily to two problems: either pregnancy started prior to implant placement or the patient never actually received the implant. To deal with the first problem, the manufacturer lists optimal times to place the implant but also provides for same day placement if the clinician is reasonably confident that the patient is not pregnant.[7] To address the second issue, clinicians are taught to double check the applicator to ensure that the implant has been released from it and to palpate the arm immediately after placement to verify its presence. In the CHOICE study (based in St. Louis, MO, USA), implant users had a pregnancy rate of 0.2 per 100 user-years.[8] Among teen users in the CHOICE study, there were no reported pregnancies in 633.3 teen-years.[9]

Efficacy in Users with Body Mass Index (BMI) ≥30 kg/m²

In U.S. clinical trials, only subjects whose weights were less than 30% above their ideal body weights were enrolled. As a result, product labeling states that it is not known if those with higher BMI's would have higher failure rates. Since those original clinical trials, many studies have investigated the pharmacokinetics and efficacy of the implant in users with BMI ≥30 kg/m^2; the conclusion from each of those studies has been that the implant may be offered as a first-line contraceptive method to candidates of all BMIs. Current evidence on this issue is summarized in the following paragraphs.[10,11]

The CHOICE study has provided robust data about the efficacy, safety and continuation rates of users of all ages and of all body mass indices. In that study, there was no significant difference in failure rates in users with different BMI categories. Normal and overweight users had failure rates of 0.000/100 user-years compared with a rate of 0.231/100 user-years in those who were obese.[10] However, that marginally higher Pearl Index in obese women occurred because there was 1 pregnancy in a study participant with a BMI ≥30 kg/m^2 who was transitioning from COC use to implant. The investigators commented that they could not be certain that the participant had taken the prior oral contraceptives correctly and concluded that a luteal phase pregnancy was the most logical explanation for the 1 observed pregnancy in the study.

Early work showed that ENG levels at 6 months were lower in those with BMI >30 kg/m^2, but at 1 year the levels were comparable within a wide range of BMIs.[12,13] At the end of 3 years of use, subjects with BMI ≥30 kg/m^2

had median etonogestrel levels of 188.2 pg/mL (range 75.9, 520.9). These levels were not any different from median level of those with normal weights, which was 193.7 pg/mL (range 118.3, 802.3). However, a few subjects with BMI $\geq$30 kg/m^2 fell below the target 90 pg/mL level for guaranteed ovulation suppression.[14] A second study confirmed that ENG levels are independent of BMI through 3 years of use.[13] A review also concluded that the failure rates in users with BMI's greater than 30 kg/m^2 were as low as in those with normal BMI's.[15]

Cumulatively, evidence supports the conclusion that once the implant is in place, it provides convenient, "forgettable," ongoing pregnancy protection that is not affected by BMI.[12,15]

Drugs that Impact Efficacy

Implants rely for efficacy on adequate systemic levels of ENG, which makes them susceptible to drug-drug interactions. The most significant threat comes from drugs that increase activity of the hepatic cytochrome P-450 enzyme system that promotes metabolic clearance of etonogestrel. (See "Medication Interactions and the Impact on COC Effectiveness" in Chapter 8.) Table 4-1 contrasts two listings of the drugs and herbal products that reduce ENG levels: one listing is from the implant product labeling and the other is from the U.S. Medical Eligibility Criteria for Contraceptive Use (MEC). Clinicians should note that the U.S. MEC categorizes the listed agents as no worse than category 2. It is important that clinicians be familiar with FDA labeling so they can counsel women who might be told by others that they are not candidates.

Table 4-1 Potential adverse drug-drug interactions: Nexplanon product labeling vs. U.S. MEC

Drugs and Herbal Products Listed on Product Labeling[20]	Drugs and Herbal Products Listed in U.S. MEC*
Barbiturates	Barbiturates
Bosentan	
Carbamazepine	Carbamazepine
Felbamate	
Griseofulvin	
Oxcarbazepine	Oxcarbazepine
Phenytoin	Phenytoin
Rifampin	Rifampin or rifabutin
St. John's Wort	St. John's Wort
Topiramate	Topiramate
Ritonavir-boosted protease inhibitors	Fosamprenavir
	Primidone

All of the listed drugs are Category 2 or 2 for either initiation or continuation on the U.S. MEC 2016.

Several drugs are on both lists. Anticonvulsants are important because they are used for a broad array of clinical indications, including treatment of several non-epileptic neurologic and psychiatric conditions.[16] For up to 30 days after the user has taken the last dose of St. John's Wort, hepatic enzyme activity can remain increased. Studies of St. John's Wort with implants are not directly available, but St. John's Wort showed a pattern of small to moderate induction of metabolism of contraceptive steroids, including progestin when given with COCs.[17] Ritonavir-boosted protease inhibitors can suppress circulating ENG after 2 years of implant use, so implant replacement at that time might be prudent to avoid an ENG drop below therapeutic levels. Case reports of pregnancies in HIV-infected people using efavirenz have raised issues about this antiretroviral agent as well.[18] However, in combination with lopinavir, neither ritonavir nor efavirenz impaired the efficacy of the implant. Discuss medications—both prescription and nonprescription—and supplements with patients considering Nexplanon, and remind them of the potential for deleterious drug-drug interactions while they have the implant.[19]

DURATION OF USE

Product labeling states that the ENG implant is to be used for no more than 3 years. If a longer period of time of use is desired, labeling recommends that this implant be removed and replaced by a new unit.[20] However, in a follow-up of the CHOICE study, no pregnancies occurred during 2 years of extended use. The researchers followed 291 subjects who wanted to use their implants for longer periods of time and who provided 444 user-years of extended use. The median circulating ENG level at the end of the fifth year was 153.0 pg/mL (range 72.1–538.8 pg/mL). Interestingly, higher levels of ENG were found in overweight users compared with those in other BMI groups.[21] In an earlier 7-country study, 390 users consented to keep the implant beyond 3 years. Over 200 of them used the implant for at least 5 years. Again, no pregnancies occurred in the additional 2 years of follow-up.[22] Based on these findings, ACOG Practice Bulletin 186 published November 2017 stated, "the etonogestrel implant is effective for at least 4 years."[94]

On the other hand, users may request early removal. Occasionally those requests may seem almost frivolous or for complaints that could be easily managed, but these cases remind us that we must consistently respect patient requests, especially when method discontinuation requires action by a clinician. We need to remember that all users must be in control of their contraception at all times.[23,24] If the patient wants the implant removed, counseling or reassurance may be appropriate at first, but if the patient's desires do not change, promptly remove the implant. (See Chapter 2 on Engaging in Unintended Pregnancy Through Patient-Centered Reproductive Goals and Contraceptive Counseling.)

CANDIDATES FOR IMPLANT USE

The U.S. MEC lists only one category 4 condition contraindicating initiation of the ENG implant: current or recent (<5 years) breast cancer. More conditions are rated as category 3, including the following: systemic lupus erythematosus (SLE) with positive or unknown antiphospholipid antibodies, unexplained abnormal vaginal bleeding, past breast cancer, hepatocellular adenoma, and hepatoma. (See the U.S. MEC summary chart insert in this book.) Most common medical conditions, such as hypertension, diabetes and migraine headaches are *not* contraindications to implant use. Product labeling includes many more contraindications to implant use than does the U.S. MEC (see Table 4-2). Again, these on-label contraindications are displayed here to remind providers to counsel candidates with these conditions as to why they may still be able to use implants according to the more modern evidence presented by the U.S. MEC. We do not want anyone to worry that a mistake has been made. There have been isolated reports of allergy to the barium sulfate, which would be covered by the recommendation to avoid use in those with allergies to any product compounds.[25,26]

Table 4-2 Contraindications to use of ENG implant listed in product labeling vs. U.S. MEC 2016

Product-Labeling Contraindications[20]	U.S. MEC Category
Known or suspected pregnancy	2
Current or past history of thrombosis or thromboembolic disease	2
Liver tumor	
Benign	2
Malignant	3
Active liver disease	1
Undiagnosed abnormal genital bleeding	3
Known or suspected breast cancer	
In last 5 years	4
>5 years ago	3
Family history of breast cancer	1
Other progestin-sensitive cancer now or in the past	Not listed
Allergic reaction to any of the compounds of Nexplanon	Assumed 4

REQUIREMENTS FOR IMPLANT PROVIDERS

All clinicians who wish to provide the ENG contraceptive implant must attend an FDA-approved, company-sponsored training program and have their competency in placement and removal of implants in artificial models certified by the course faculty.[27] Completing this training enables clinicians to order implants from the distributors. Technically, formal training may not be required for implant removal, but it is very helpful (see tips on placement and removal below). Of course, providers should be familiar with the anatomy of the arm for both placement and removal.

Because the implant has so very few contraindications and the placement procedure is rapid and straightforward, the implant is an ideal method for busy primary care clinicians to offer and supply. This is especially important for those patients with medical problems, which could seriously complicate pregnancy.

ADVANTAGES

1. **Safety.** Virtually every person seeking contraception (even those with serious medical conditions) is eligible for use of the ENG implant based on the US MEC.[28] Because the implant has no estrogen, users face no increased risk of venous thromboembolism, according to recent systematic review, despite the fact that the etonogestrel used is an active metabolite of the third generation desogestrel.[29] (See Chapter 8 on COCs.) This same review found that there were no increased odds of stroke or acute myocardial infarction with implant use.[29] Metabolic safety studies suggest that the implant induces changes consistent with a *lower risk* of insulin resistance and dyslipidemia.[30,31] In a prospective cohort sub-study within the CHOICE study, implant users experienced the same changes in body weight and composition after 6 and 12 months as did copper IUD users, who had no exposure to hormones.[32] There are minimal risks associated with the implant placement and removal procedures and allergic reaction are rare (see below in the Disadvantages section).

2. **Highest efficacy.** Implants offer pregnancy protection that is superior to the protection provided by any IUD or even by permanent contraception.[33] In typical use, the implant is essentially as effective as it is with correct and consistent use, because there are few things that can reduce its efficacy. U.S. labeling quotes a first-year failure rate of 0.38% but also notes that all six of the observed

pregnancies were most likely conceived after implants had been removed, during the 14-day follow-up period.[34]

3. **Convenience.** Once the implant has become active (≤7 days) after placement, there is nothing else that needs to be done to achieve pregnancy protection. This convenience makes the implant a particularly attractive option for busy patients as well as those who may have difficulty remembering daily, weekly, or monthly methods. The implant can be placed postpartum before discharge home, even if the patient will be breastfeeding.[35,36] The implant can also be started directly after abortion. There are only a few drugs that diminish the implant's efficacy. The only *inconvenience* a user may experience would result from having to deal with side effects, most notably bleeding disturbances. (See Disadvantages below.)

4. **Discreet.** The implant is palpable, but it should not be visibly detected except for the small telltale skin puncture scar near the base of the implant. The method does not require that supplies be concealed or periodically purchased. Unlike the IUD or barrier methods, the implant cannot be detected during intercourse.

5. **High rates of continuation.** Numerous clinical trials have shown high continuation rates with the implant. There are two types of "discontinuation" that potentially can affect the efficacy of any method. The classic discontinuation rate answers the question: what percentage of users prematurely stops using the method entirely before its useful life is over? The second question asks: what percentage of users has temporary interruption in their use of the method? This latter may represent incorrect use (missed pills) or inconsistent use (not refilling pill packs, not using condoms with each act of intercourse, or returning late for DMPA injection). Implants are not subject to either incorrect or inconsistent use; they provide user-independent pregnancy protection at all times. Even if the patient is somewhat late returning for removal of the implant, studies show that the implant provides prolonged protection beyond the FDA-approved duration of use.

   Estimates of early discontinuation of the implant vary greatly. In the clinical trials in the United States, the 3-year discontinuation rates for adverse events were low. Fewer than 20% of study subjects requested early removal due to adverse events (side effects) that they attributed to the implant. Despite popular professional beliefs, only 11.1% of study participants requested implant removal due to complaints about abnormal bleeding during the 3-year trial.[20] For other adverse events, the rates for early removal ranged from 1.0 to 2.38% (see Side Effects, below).

Continuation rates have been studied in many different settings and have been very reassuring, even among high-risk groups. In a clinical 12-month trial comparing the LNG-IUS 8 (Skyla, Jaydess) and Nexplanon, discontinuation rates were 7.2% lower with LNG-IUS 8 (19.6% vs. 26.8%); LNG-IUS users were more likely to be very or somewhat satisfied with their bleeding patterns.[37] That pattern of early higher discontinuation among the implant was also seen in the CHOICE study. However, over the longer term, more implant users continued use of their method. The overall first-year continuation rate with the implant in the CHOICE study was 83%.[38] Teens aged 14 to 18 years in that study also had high continuation rates (82%).[39] In an Australian study, teen mothers given the implant used it for an average of 18.7 months and demonstrated a longer mean time to repeat pregnancy than patients given COCs or depo-medroxyprogesterone acetate (DMPA).[40] In a mixed-payer setting, a retrospective study reported that 2-year continuation rates were similar for each of the long-acting methods: LNG-IUS 20 (77.8%), copper IUD (73.1%) and implant (75.9%).[41] In an outpatient pediatric clinic, 89.7% of 750 patients continued the ENG implant at 12 months. Older age, history of prior pregnancy and ≥1 visit for implant concerns were predictive of early discontinuation.[42]

6. **Decreased dysmenorrhea.** Clinical evidence suggests that dysmenorrhea may be improved with use of the ENG implant. Among U.S. users with baseline dysmenorrhea, 81% showed improvement with implant use.[43] International studies found similar results; 82% with baseline dysmenorrhea reported improvement in symptoms at the end of the study.[44] The implant is as effective as DMPA in relieving pain scores with endometriosis.[45] Implants can be combined with the LNG-IUS to treat severe pain from endometriosis, especially when the endometriotic implants are deep in the pelvic ligaments or at a distance from the uterus.[46]

7. **Rapid return of fertility.** As shown by the 6 pregnancies that occurred within 14 days of implant removal in the U.S. clinical studies, return to fertility is rapid. In another study, which followed return to fertility among those desiring pregnancy, 13.8% became pregnant within 90 days of removal of the implant.[47] A later study concluded that pregnancy rates (76% to 100%) seen 1 year after implant removal are usually no different from pregnancy rates following cessation of other contraceptive methods. Of note, they reported that there is no increase in the risk of ectopic implantation, fetal malformation, or impaired infant health in pregnancies conceived during implant use or after implant removal.[48]

8. **Ectopic pregnancy prevention**. Because ovulation is suppressed, pregnancy is rare, making ectopic pregnancy extremely rare (0% in clinical trials). (For more discussion, see #4 in Disadvantages.)

9. **Other noncontraceptive benefits.** The only FDA-approved indication for the ENG-implant is prevention of pregnancy, but other menstrual-related benefits have been reported. Because ovulation is reliably suppressed, users will not form hemorrhagic corpus luteal cysts, which can represent surgical emergencies. The lack of ovulation also means that anticoagulated users face less risk of hemoperitoneum.

10. **Highly cost-effective.** Intermediate to long-term use (12 to 24 months) of the implant is cost effective.[49]

DISADVANTAGES

1. **Procedure-related risks.** Implant placement does require a minor office-based procedure and another such procedure is needed for removal. The placement procedure carries risks of erythema (3.3%), hematoma (3.0%), bruising (2.0%), pain (1.0%), and swelling (0.7%). Infection occurred in less than 1% of cases. More rarely, other complications have occurred, such as pain or paresthesia from neural compression or damage, or superficial venous thrombosis from vascular compression.[1] In trials with the new applicator, hematomas were reported in 2.7% of cases and implant site erythema was seen in 2.0%; no infections were reported in the 301 placements.[2] Intramuscular placements complicate removal and may cause discomfort with muscle contraction. Implants that are placed too close to the skin puncture site are more likely to be expelled.

   Removal of the implant is generally quite straightforward, but risks similar to those seen with placement are possible. In clinical trials, mean time required for removal was 119 seconds and the median time was 78 (range 8–730) seconds. Removal time exceeded 10 minutes in 4 out of 296 of cases. No complications were reported in 94.6% of removals, but the rest were complicated by fibrosis.[2] In the pooled data from 11 international trials of Implanon that had been placed with the original introducer system, 1.7% had complications with removal, including breaking the implant, inability to palpate the implant before removal, removal difficulty due to deep placement, implant fixed by fibrous tissue, implant too flexible for easy removal, implant adherent to underlying tissue, and difficulty locating the implant.[50] Those deeply placed or nonpalpable implants present special challenges that are discussed below.

2. **Migration of implants.** Distant migration of contraceptive implants is a rare complication. Usually migration is limited, but migration of several centimeters has been reported; such as into the ipsilateral axilla.[51] There are now reports of some (albeit very few) implants having been placed intravascularly and migrating to the thoracic cavity in the pulmonary artery.[52,53] These reports prompted the change in instructions for implant placement; *clinicians are now advised to avoid placement in the biceps groove, no matter how superficial that placement might be.*

3. **Unpredictable bleeding.** With the suppression of ovulation and the progestin's effects on the endometrium, implant users do not usually have predictable bleeding. While it is not possible to anticipate what the bleeding patterns will be for any one user, reanalysis of clinical study results has revealed some overall patterns among users as a group. In the first 3 months of use, about one third of implant users will experience what they characterize as "satisfactory" bleeding patterns; these patterns tended to predict future patterns for those patients. In the second 3 months, another third of users develops satisfactory patterns. But even after 6 months of use, a third still experiences bleeding patterns that are not satisfactory to them.

In general, prolonged or frequent bleeding or spotting occurs more frequently in the early months of implant use. Patients switching from combined hormonal contraception are less likely to have heavy or prolonged bleeding during the early transitional months.[55] Some work suggests that unfavorable bleeding patterns may be more common among users with lower BMIs.[55] It is important to recognize that counseling patients about these potential changes can be influential. It also helps to see what actions users take when faced with bleeding they experienced with the implant. In the U.S. trials, only 11.1–14% of users asked for early implant removal because of bleeding complaints. Reassure patients that there are no long-lasting impacts on menses: normal menses almost always return within 3 months after removal of the implants.[54] In addition to providing explicit counseling and reassurance about this issue, it also may be important to provide patients with tools to deal with the prolonged or heavy bleeding episodes (see below).

Several other analyses about bleeding patterns can be helpful when counseling interested candidates. In 75% of 90-day reference periods, the number of bleeding-spotting days reported by users was less than or the same as they had experienced with their normal cycles, but those bleeding-spotting days occurred at unpredictable intervals.[55] Tables 4-3 and 4-4 show data from

Table 4-3 Percent of implant users with bleeding patterns by 90-day reference periods[55]

90-Day Reference Period	Amenorrhea No B/S* Episodes	Infrequent <3 B/S* Episodes	Normal 3–5 B/S* Episodes	Frequent >5 B/S* Episodes	Prolonged >14 B/S* Uninterrupted
1	10%	39%	39%	12%	31%
2	19%	34%	39%	8%	21%
4	23%	32%	39%	6%	17%
6	21%	33%	41%	6%	15%
8	17%	33%	47%	4%	15%
10	17%	35%	44%	4%	17%
12	12%	34%	52%	2%	17%

*Bleeding and/or spotting

different studies and display slightly different aspects to help counsel those considering the implant about their possible bleeding patterns. Table 4-3 displays the numbers of days of bleeding per 90-day reference period. Table 4-4 shows the numbers of episodes of bleeding by 90-day reference period.

4. **Other hormonally-related potential side effects.** A systematic review of several clinical studies reported that the most commonly reported complaints over a 3-year period of implant use were headache (15.5%), weight increase (11.8%), acne (12%), breast pain (10.2%), emotional lability (5.8%), and abdominal pain (5.2%).[43,50] Interestingly, in a comparative trial, once adjustment had been made for confounding variables, implant users gained no more weight than copper IUD users.[56] And body composition of ENG implant users did not differ that from copper IUD users.[32] The ability of postpartum users with BMI >30 kg / m^2 to lose weight by 6 months was not statistically different from postpartum patients who did not get the implant.[50]

Table 4-4 Percent of implant users reporting abnormal bleeding patterns over time in 90-day reference periods

Total Days of Spotting or Bleeding in 90-Day Reference Period	Percentage of Patients		
	Treatment Days 91–180 (N = 566)	Treatment Days 271–360 (N = 657)	Treatment Days 631–720 (N = 547)
0 days	19%	24%	17%
1–7 days	15%	13%	12%
8 to 21 days	30%	30%	37%
>21 days	35%	33%	35%

Nexplanon Product Information: www.accessdata.fda.gov/drugsatfda_docs/label/2015/021529s011lbl.pdfslide

Acne deserves special mention. Whereas 16% of users in the U.S. clinical trial reported development of acne while using the implant, 60% who had acne when they had the implant placed reported improvement of that problem while using the system.[43]

As a progestin, etonogestrel can induce angioedema at almost any time after exposure. Pseudotumor cerebri has been rarely associated with progestin use, but with the implant, it has been suggested that rapid weight gain may have been the trigger for the development of the rare cases of angioedema that have been reported in implant users.[57] There have also been cases reported of delayed-type hypersensitivity reaction against Nexplanon.[26]

5. **Pregnancy issues.** Theoretically, should a pregnancy occur, ectopic pregnancy risk would be increased because progestins slow ciliary motion within the fallopian tube. In a systemic review of 42 studies, reports of ectopic pregnancy were extremely uncommon. Only one study with insufficient information reported any pregnancies at all.[58] However, localization of the pregnancy is always important in implant users. With widespread use, there have been case reports of ectopic pregnancies with an implant in place that have caused serious complications.[59] (For more discussion, see #8 in Advantages.)

   Generally, it is advisable to remove the implant when pregnancy is diagnosed because it provides no benefits in pregnancy. If a pregnancy is terminated, and the user wishes to continue to use the implant, it would be prudent to determine why the implant failed in the first place. If a cause can be identified and corrected (such as use of a drug that diminished the implant's effectiveness), then continued reliance on the implant for contraception may be reasonable.

6. **Decreased interest in sex.** In the CHOICE study, implant users were 60% more likely to report lack of interest in sex compared to copper IUD users when surveyed 6 months after method initiation, even when controlling for age.[60] However, in a prospective study specifically designed to measure sexual function, more users reported sexual function improvement; negative sexual changes were largely attributed to increased vaginal bleeding.[61]

7. **Lower use of male condoms.** Early analysis of adolescent users of IUDs or implants shows that they were about 60% less likely to use condoms than were teens using pills. However, this may be true because pill users had to use male condoms for back-up methods when they skipped pills, but it may show less concern for STD risk.[62]

PROVIDING THE METHOD

COUNSELING AND INFORMED CONSENT

Provide counseling not only about the risks associated with placement and removal procedures but also about the hormone-related side effects that may be experienced with implant use. The FDA specifies that in order to give informed consent, those considering the implant should read the product information provided within the product labeling. The manufacturer also provides an informed consent form in the product packaging. Ask the patient to sign this form, which indicates that the patient has read the FDA material, had all the questions answered, and desires to use this implant. That consent form should be incorporated into the patient's medical record.

People tend to form negative impressions from the stories they hear from others about the implant.[63] In part that may be because they do not know much about either implants or IUDs.[64] Focus groups have revealed that teens do not know the difference between IUDs and implants, but teens have bunched those methods together as what they call "invasive methods." College students reported not wanting a foreign object in their body, not knowing enough about the method, and preferring a "controllable method" as top reasons for not wanting an implant or IUD. Studies have shown that how we deliver the counseling—in groups, one-on-one, intensity, etc.—makes little impact on discontinuation. However, the words we use seem to be very important. Instead of saying we will be "inserting" the implant into the arm, consider using less threatening terms. For example, you could say that you will be "placing" an implant or "sliding" it just beneath the skin. Some people have said they reject implants because they do not want to have pressure or throbbing pain in their arms for three years. This misconception may have come from our promise that the user would always be able to feel the implant. To avoid this problem, we might want to say that they will not even know the implant is in their arm, but they can "feel" it with their fingertips whenever they want to check it.

TIMING OF INITIATION

In order to ensure that the patient is not pregnant prior to placement of the implant, product labeling recommends that the procedure be performed when the patient is on menses or when switching methods. However, labeling also states that if the implant is placed at any other time in the cycle, the clinician should insure that the candidate is not pregnant and will use a backup method (including abstinence) for at least 7 days. History is the best way to rule out pregnancy, using the questions posed by the U.S. Selected

Practice Recommendations for Contraceptives, 2016.[7] (See Box 2-6 on "How to be reasonably certain that a woman is not pregnant" in Chapter 2.) Pregnancy testing is appropriate only if the history is not convincing. The incidence of luteal phase pregnancy is $<1\%$.[65] If switching from an effective method, such as an IUD, it may be reasonable to let the two methods overlap. Place the implant, wait at least 7 days, and then remove the IUD.

The importance of same day implant placement was highlighted in the CHOICE study. In those who had delayed initiation of the implant or the IUD they had selected as their method, the risk of unintended pregnancy was increased by 60% over those who got same-day placement. Delays for implant placement in that study were as long as 16 weeks.[8]

Immediate postabortal placement of implants is associated with high continuation rates among young users and reduces the incidence of births and abortions for at least 2 years.[66–68] Postpartum placement is also associated with excellent protection with no adverse impacts on duration of lochia or on overall breastfeeding success and no increase in the risk of expulsion, such as seen with immediate postpartum IUD placement.[69–74] Please see Chapter 17 for more information.

Implant Placement Principles

Average time for placement after preparation and administration of anesthesia is 27 to 29 seconds.[2] Please note, the new instructions for insertion state that the implant should **not** be placed in the biceps groove, as had been previously advised, but over the triceps muscle starting 8 to 10 cm above the epicondyle.[34]

Practical tips on implant placement and removal

Implant placement

Formal training, which is required prior to being able to order and use the implant, stresses the following points:

1. Make certain the patient is not pregnant prior to placement.
2. Select a site for the implant in the inner aspect of the non-dominant upper arm, just below the skin in the subcutaneous tissue overlying a muscle mass (preferably the triceps) and avoiding the biceps grove.
3. Placement using all the steps should be performed under direct visualization.

   Sit directly facing the inner surface of the patient's arm to place the implant under direct visualization. Introduce the applicator through the skin starting at the distal (elbow) end of desired placement site, then while tenting the skin, advance the introducer just beneath the skin toward the shoulder. Be sure to stretch the skin before puncturing it with the trocar tip.

BUT

This will not work when the patient and the clinician have mismatches in their handedness. For example, if a right-handed clinician is trying to put an implant into the right arm of a left-handed patient these instructions are not possible to follow. In that case, the clinician should ***stand*** over the shoulder of the patient and lean over the patient's arm to watch the advancement of the implant from above.

OR

Stand at the patient's elbow and lean over laterally to observe each step carefully.

Implant removal

Palpable Rods

- To visualize the implant, the labelling says to mark skin over each end of the implant.
- **BUT** this can create tattoos if the marked skin is punctured.
- **SO** it is much easier to clean the entire area with betadine and while the betadine is still wet, drag the wooden part of a sterile Q-tip along the skin from the upper to the lower edge of the area along the axis of the arm. This will scrape the betadine off the skin overlying the implant and reveal its presence on the skin like the negative of a photo. (See Figure 4-1.)

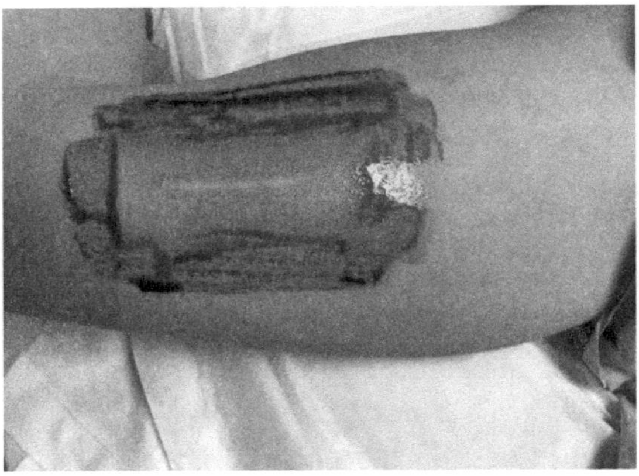

Figure 4-1 "Betadine stripping" technique to visualize implant for removal

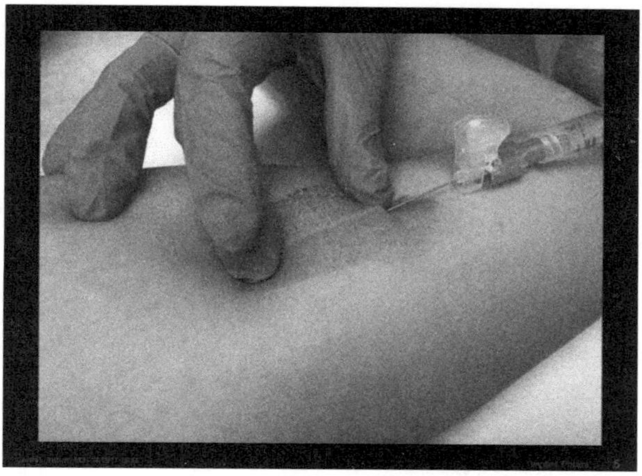

Figure 4-2 Maintain pressure on implant during anesthetic infusion below implant

- Place the anesthesia at the distal tip of the implant and just underneath it. (See Figure 4-2.)
- *Always* keep the implant stabilized under pressure with the distal tip of the implant pressing up against the skin when you are removing the implant. (See Figure 4-3.) To get the implant positioned for removal, follow these steps.
  - — Press with the ring finger of your non-dominant hand down on the proximal tip of the implant. Press down to the floor and towards the elbow.
  - — Drag the skin overlying the implant from the top of the implant along its length to tighten it. Pull the skin laterally toward yourself and trap it below the thumb of your non-dominant hand; this will expose the distal tip of the implant under tension.
  - — Do not move your fingers holding the implant in place until the implant is completely out of the arm.
  - — Hold the scalpel in your dominant hand like a pencil, and stabilize your hand against the arm. Incise the skin **longitudinally** about 2–3 mm starting just over tip of the implant cutting thru the fibrous sheath to expose the distal end of the implant. (See Figure 4-3.) **Do not make a transverse incision.**
  - — Put your scalpel down.
  - — Remove the implant: slide the nail of your thumb or index finger of your dominant hand beneath the exposed tip of the implant and it will jump out.

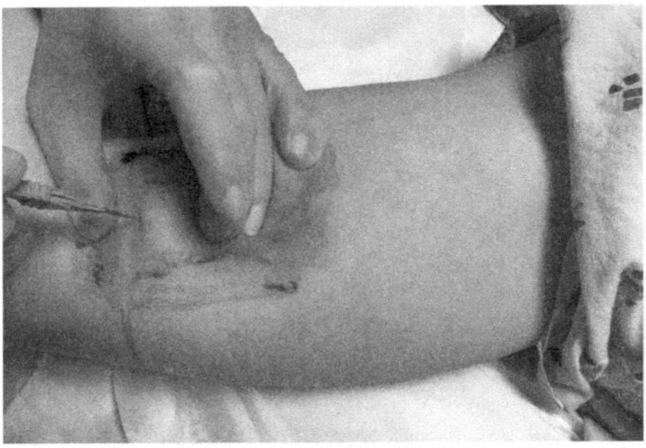

Figure 4-3 Maintain pressure to stabilize implant during vertical incision for removal

— Grasp the implant with your thumb and index finger or with forceps to remove it from the fibrous sheath. (See Figure 4-4.)

- This should take less than 30 seconds!

Difficult Removals

Nonpalpable Implants

Localization of Deeply Placed or Nonpalpable Implants

Always know exactly where the implant is before you try to remove it.[75]

If you have *any* trouble palpating the full length of the implant, **STOP**. Apply lubricant (KY jelly) and repeat the exam. Rock the proximal and distal ends like a teeter-totter to identify the tips of the implant. If you cannot

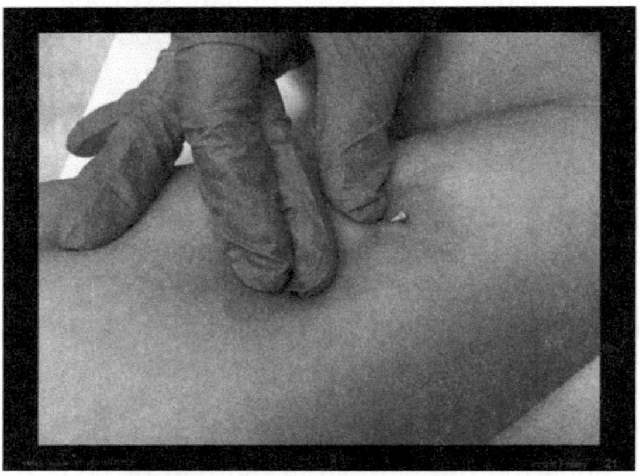

Figure 4-4 Maintain pressure on implant to enable it to pop out once fibrous tissue is incised

palpate the implant, perform imaging to localize it. Ultrasound is usually the most effective imaging tool. A CT or an MRI can help define in which tissue the implant is located, though not as effectively. An X-ray may help identify that the Nexplanon implant is present in the arm, but is not helpful in localization for removal. If you cannot localize the implant or do not wish to perform the removal, refer the patient for removal to centers able to do so.

- Tip: If the implant moves with muscle contraction, it is likely within the muscle.[76]

> Throughout the country, there are many Centers of Experience with the ability to accept referrals of patients with nonpalpable implants as well as those in whom the removal may be challenging, whether or not the user has insurance coverage. For general advice and support for nonpalpable implants visit www.merckconnect.com/nexplanon/overview.html.

To localize the implant with ultrasound, use a linear array transducer with at least 10 megahertz (15 or 18 megahertz is preferred)[77]

— Place the transducer at right angles to the implant.

— Find the echogenic shadow cast by the implant (the "eclipse sign").

— The implant will be at the top of that shadow.

— Rotate the transducer along the length of the implant to see where it is closest to the skin.

— Turn on the Doppler flow to see if there are any adjacent vessels (and nerves) near the implant. It is important to avoid these to prevent hemorrhage and nerve damage.

Removal Techniques Available for Deeply Placed or Nonpalpable Implants

Deeply placed implants can be removed as outpatient procedures by those with additional training and imaging tools. Here are some of the options:

— Removal under real-time ultrasound guidance has been shown to be quite effective.[79–82] The best approach to the implant is identified by ultrasound. Under real-time guidance (if needed), anesthesia can be placed through the overlying skin and along the track from the skin to the implant and beneath the implant. Make a longitudinal incision in the overlying skin and a track through the subcutaneous tissue and (if needed) through the fascia down to the implant. The implant and its fibrous sheath are grasped with a Norgrasp or no-vasectomy clamp and elevated out of the incision. The fibrous sheath is incised, and the implant is maneuvered out.

— A hook wire can be placed beneath implant under ultrasound guidance to guide the dissection to the implant.[81]

— Fluoroscopy can be combined with ultrasound to localize the implant and guide removal.[82]

— The implant can be localized with ultrasound and the skin is marked just prior to surgical removal.[83]

Tips on placing a new implant after removal of prior one

— Infuse anesthesia along the tract in which the new implant will be placed.

— While holding the introducer *parallel* to floor, slide the tip into top of the incision that you used to remove the prior implant.

- Do *not* approach the skin at the 20 to 30° angle. Come in flat to avoid deep placement of the new implant.

MANAGING PROBLEMS AND FOLLOW-UP

Follow-up visits after implant placement are not routinely needed, but always reassure users that if they have any problems or questions, you will see them promptly. Some higher-risk patients, such as those who are anxious or young, may be offered follow-up appointments in 2 to 3 weeks to ensure they are doing well. Do suggest that users record their bleeding patterns; apps on cell phones are particularly useful to help identify bleeding pattern trends (see Chapter 1 on the Menstrual Cycle). At each subsequent office visit, document how satisfied the patient is with the implant and what bleeding patterns the user has been experiencing.

MANAGING ABNORMAL BLEEDING

Once pregnancy and other gynecological problems have been ruled out as causes of abnormal bleeding, reassurance can be helpful, especially for infrequent bleeding or amenorrhea. Review the patient's bleeding patterns (phone apps) to see if there has been improvement over time. If a patient with heavy or prolonged bleeding has not already tried NSAIDs, offer that as first-line therapy. Treatment options that have been tested for abnormal bleeding with progestin-only methods are listed below. Because the circulating levels of ENG are so low, the addition of combined hormonal contraceptives to control bothersome heavy or prolonged bleeding or spotting is generally well tolerated. Monophasic combined oral contraceptives can be given cyclically or continuously (using only active pills).

Box 4-1 Practice tips: how to control excessive or prolonged bleeding with progestin-only implant

Pre-placement counseling and reassurance during use is important.

- Advise users to keep menstrual calendars (apps helpful). All treatments stop current episodes only. Recurrence is common.[84]
- Provide a prescription of NSAIDs (in advance of need) after implant placement, if there are no medical contraindications to NSAID use.
  - — Tell them to use Ibuprofen 800mg 3 times a day for up to 5 days or naproxen 500mg 2 times a day for up to 5 days to stop bleeding that is too heavy or prolonged.[85–87] Treatment can be repeated if problem bleeding returns.
- Advise return for consultation if NSAIDs do not provide enough help. At that time, you can recommend other nonhormonal therapy or hormonal therapies.
  - — Other nonhormonal therapies—
    - ○ Tranexamic acid 650 mg three times a day for up to 5 days.[88]
  - — Hormonal therapies—
    - ○ Any combination pill.
      - – Short term—daily for 14 days.[89]
      - – Longer term—cyclic or extended use.[90]
    - ○ NuvaRing—1 ring for up to 35 days. Repeat as needed.
    - ○ Estrogen only (conjugated equine estrogen 1.25 mg or estradiol 2 mg) daily for 1–2 weeks.[84]
    - ○ Tamoxifen 10 mg twice daily for 7–190 days.[91,92]
  - — Future therapies under consideration: ulipristal acetate (UPA), mifepristone, doxycycline with ethinyl estradiol.[93]

The vaginal ring is especially useful in treating such abnormal bleeding, because it provides continuous steady levels of hormonal support. Most patients usually only need 2 to 3 months of treatment to give them some relief, but others may benefit from more lengthy use of the combination therapy—implant for contraception, pill or vaginal ring for bleeding control. However, some may prefer implant removal if short-term interventions do not provide them adequate relief.

Managing Other Problems

Local superficial venous thrombosis following placement can usually be managed with warm compresses and NSAIDs after neurological involvement has been ruled out. Rapid removal is recommended whenever neural compression is suspected. Involve neurologists if any neurological deficits are suspected. If the implant is thought to be in the thoracic cavity, consult with pulmonary specialists.

USER INSTRUCTIONS*

Before you decide to use the Nexplanon implant, be sure to read the FDA-approved product information so you can sign the informed consent. Your clinician or websites such as Bedsider.org can provide you up-to-date information and answer your questions (see the Appendix on Digital Resources for Health and Medical Information).

The contraceptive implant provides the most effective pregnancy protection of any method—including tubal ligation.

1. The implant is placed just under your skin on the inside of your arm. Your clinician will pick a site on your arm, cleanse your skin, and give you numbing medicine. Once that takes effect, your clinician will place the implant in a procedure that takes about 30 seconds.

   Because you have a nick in your skin, there is a small chance that you may have several days of bruising or even a collection of blood under your skin (hematoma). You could get an infection, and there is a very small chance the implant could press against a blood vessel and give you a blood clot in your vein or do nerve damage. In very rare cases, the implant may migrate. You can always touch your arm to make sure it is in place. There are similar risks at the time of removal. If the implant is deeply placed, you may need extra tests and a referral to specialists to get it taken out.
2. With the implant, your periods will change. They generally become lighter with time, but users can have all kinds of different bleeding patterns at the beginning, even heavier or prolonged bleeding. There is a good chance you will have spotting or bleeding on days of the month that you do not generally bleed. Ask your clinician what you can use to try to control the extra bleeding in case you get that problem.
3. The convenience and efficacy of the implant are unsurpassed. Only a few drugs can diminish how well it protects against pregnancy. Its ease of placement and removal make it possible for many different clinicians to offer the implant to patients. If you want to get pregnant, the implant must be removed by a clinician, but once it is taken out there will be virtually no delay in your return of fertility.
4. Individuals who are at risk of STI's should use condoms in addition to their Implant.

Author Disclosures—Nelson: Research grants, honoraria for speaker's bureau and advisory board for Merck. Crabtree: none. Grentzer: none.

Acknowledgement: The authors thank Erica Chang, MD, for providing the photos used in this chapter.

*These instructions are intended to guide providers in educating patients in how to use their method.

References

1. Brown M, Britton J. Neuropathy associated with etonogestrel implant insertion. Contraception 2012;86:591–3.
2. Mommers E, Blum GF, Gent TG, Peters KP, Sørdal TS, Marintcheva-Petrova M. Nexplanon, a radiopaque etonogestrel implant in combination with a next-generation applicator: 3-year results of a noncomparative multicenter trial. Am J Obstet Gynecol 2012;207:388.e1–6.
3. Schnabel P, Merki-Feld GS, Malvy A, Duijkers I, Mommers E, van den Heuvel MW. Bioequivalence and x-ray visibility of a radiopaque etonogestrel implant versus a non-radiopaque implant: a 3-year, randomized, double-blind study. Clin Drug Investig 2012;32:413–22.
4. Van den Bosch T, Donders GG, Riphagen I, et al. Ultrasonographic features of the endometrium and the ovaries in women on etonogestrel implant. Ultrasound Obstet Gynecol 2002;20:377–80.
5. Bennink HJ. The pharmacokinetics and pharmacodynamics of Implanon, a single-rod etonogestrel contraceptive implant. Eur J Contracept Reprod Health Care 2000; 5 Suppl 2:12–20.
6. Mäkäräinen L, van Beek A, Tuomivaara L, Asplund B, Coelingh Bennink H. Ovarian function during the use of a single contraceptive implant: Implanon compared with Norplant. Fertil Steril 1998;69:714–21.
7. Curtis KM, Jatlaoui TC, Tepper NK, et al. U.S. Selected practice recommendations for contraceptive use (US SPR) for Contraceptive Use, 2016. MMWr Recomm Rep 2016;65;RR-#3. At www.cdc.gov/reproductivehealth/contraception/mmwr/spr/summary.html. Accessed June 16, 2017.
8. Reeves MF, Zhao Q, Secura GM, Peipert JF. Risk of unintended pregnancy based on intended compared to actual contraceptive use. Am J Obstet Gynecol 2016;215:71.e1–6.
9. Secura GM, Madden T, McNicholas C, et al. Provision of no-cost, long-acting contraception and teenage pregnancy. N Engl J Med 2014;371:1316–23.
10. Xu H, Wade JA, Peipert JF, Zhao Q, Madden T, Secura GM. Contraceptive failure rates of etonogestrel subdermal implants in overweight and obese women. Obstet Gynecol 2012;120:21–6.
11. Lopez LM, Bernholc A, Chen M, et al. Hormonal contraceptives for contraception in overweight or obese women. Cochrane DB Syst Rev 2016:CD008452.
12. Mornar S, Chan LN, Mistretta S, Neustadt A, Martins S, Gilliam M. Pharmacokinetics of the etonogestrel contraceptive implant in obese women. Am J Obstet Gynecol 2012;207:110.e1–6.
13. Morrell KM, Cremers S, Westhoff CL, Davis AR. Relationship between etonogestrel level and BMI in women using the contraceptive implant for more than 1 year. Contraception 2016;93:263–5.
14. McNicholas C, Maddipati R, Zhao Q, Swor E, Peipert JF. Use of the etonogestrel implant and levonorgestrel intrauterine device beyond the U.S. Food and Drug Administration-approved duration. Obstet Gynecol 2015;125:599–604.
15. Robinson JA, Burke AE. Obesity and hormonal contraceptive efficacy. Womens Health (Lond) 2013;9:453–66.
16. Lazorwitz A, Davis A, Swartz M, Guiahi M. The effect of carbamazepine on etonogestrel concentrations in contraceptive implant users. Contraception 2017;05:571–577.
17. Berry-Bibee EN, Kim MJ, Tepper NK, Riley HE, Curtis KM. Co-administration of St. John's Wort and hormonal contraceptives: a systematic review. Contraception 2016;94:668–677.
18. Leticee N, Viard JP, Yamgnane A, Karmochkine M, Benachi A. Contraceptive failure of etonogestrel implant in patients treated with antiretrovirals including efavirenz. Contraception 2012;85:425–7.
19. Vieira CS, Bahamondes MV, de Souza RM, et al. Effect of antiretroviral therapy including lopinavir/ritonavir or efavirenz on etonogestrel-releasing implant pharmacokinetics in HIV-positive women. J Acquir Immune Defic Syndr 2014;66:378–85.

20. Product Labeling etonogestrel implant. At www.accessdata.fda.gov/drugsatfda_docs/label/2009/021529s004lbl.pdf. Accessed June 16, 2017.
21. McNicholas C, Swor E, Wan L, Peipert JF. Prolonged use of the etonogestrel implant and levonorgestrel intrauterine device: 2 years beyond Food and Drug Administration-approved duration. Am J Obstet Gynecol 2017;216:586 e1–586.
22. Ali M, Akin A, Bahamondes L, et al. WHO study group on subdermal contraceptive implants for women—Extended use up to 5 years of the etonogestrel-releasing subdermal contraceptive implant: comparison to levonorgestrel-releasing subdermal implant. Hum Reprod 2016;31:2491–2498.
23. Amico JR, Bennett AH, Karasz A, Gold M. "She just told me to leave it": Women's experiences discussing early elective IUD removal. Contraception 2016;94:357–61.
24. Amico JR, Bennett AH, Karasz A, Gold M. "I wish they could hold on a little longer": physicians' experiences with requests for early IUD removal. Contraception 2017;96:106–110.
25. Pedroso C, Martins I, Palma F, Machado AI. Implant site Nexplanon reaction? BMJ Case Rep 2015.
26. Serati M, Bogani G, Kumar S, Cromi A, Ghezzi F. Delayed-type hypersensitivity reaction against Nexplanon®. Contraception 2015;91:91–2.
27. Creinin MD, Kaunitz AM, Darney PD, et al. The US etonogestrel implant mandatory clinical training and active monitoring programs: 6-year experience. Contraception 2017;95:205–210.
28. Curtis KM, Peipert JF. Long-acting reversible contraception. N Engl J Med 2017;376: 461–468.
29. Tepper NK, Whiteman MK, Marchbanks PA, James AH, Curtis KM. Progestin-only contraception and thromboembolism: A systematic review. Contraception 2016;94:678–700.
30. Villas-Boas J, Vilodre LC, Malerba H, Pontremoli Salcedo M, Foresti Jiménez M, El Beitune P. Metabolic safety of the etonogestrel contraceptive implant in healthy women over a 3-year period. Eur J Obstet Gynecol Reprod Biol 2016;202:51–4.
31. Oderich CL, Wender MC, Lubianca JN, Santos LM, de Mello GC. Impact of etonogestrel-releasing implant and copper intrauterine device on carbohydrate metabolism: a comparative study. Contraception 2012;85:173–6.
32. Silva Dos Santos PN, Madden T, Omvig K, Peipert JF. Changes in body composition in women using long-acting reversible contraception. Contraception 2017;95:382–389.
33. Bahamondes L, Brache V, Meirik O, Ali M, Habib N, Landoulsi S; WHO Study Group on Contraceptive Implants for Women. A 3-year multicentre randomized controlled trial of etonogestrel- and levonorgestrel-releasing contraceptive implants, with non-randomized matched copper-intrauterine device controls. Hum Reprod 2015;30:2527–38.
34. Stoddard A, McNicholas C, Peipert JF. Efficacy and safety of long-acting reversible contraception. Drugs 2011;71:969–80.
35. Bryant AG, Bauer AE, Stuart GS, et al. Etonogestrel-releasing contraceptive implant for postpartum adolescents: a randomized controlled trial. J Pediatr Adolesc Gynecol 2017;30:389–394.
36. Braga GC, Ferriolli E, Quintana SM, Ferriani RA, Pfrimer K, Vieira CS. Immediate postpartum initiation of etonogestrel-releasing implant: A randomized controlled trial on breastfeeding impact. Contraception 2015;92:536–42.
37. Apter D, Briggs P, Tuppurainen M, et al. A 12-month multicenter, randomized study comparing the levonorgestrel intrauterine system with the etonogestrel subdermal implant. Fertil Steril 2016;106:151–157.e5.
38. Peipert JF, Zhao Q, Allsworth JE, et al. Continuation and satisfaction of reversible contraception. Obstet Gynecol 2011;117:1105–13.
39. Rosenstock JR, Peipert JF, Madden T, Zhao Q, Secura GM. Continuation of reversible contraception in teenagers and young women. Obstet Gynecol 2012;120:1298–305.
40. Lewis LN, Doherty DA, Hickey M, Skinner SR. Implanon as a contraceptive choice for teenage mothers: a comparison of contraceptive choices, acceptability and repeat pregnancy. Contraception 2010;81:421–6.

41. Sanders N, Turok DK, Gawron LM, Law A, Wen L, Lynen R. Two-year continuation of intrauterine devices and contraceptive implants in a mixed-payer setting: a retrospective review. Am J Obstet Gynecol 2017;216:590.e1–590.e8.
42. Berlan E, Mizraji K, Bonny AE. Twelve-month discontinuation of etonogestrel implant in an outpatient pediatric setting. Contraception 2016;94:81–6.
43. Funk S, Miller MM, Mishell DR Jr, et al. Implanon US Study Group. Safety and efficacy of Implanon, a single-rod implantable contraceptive containing etonogestrel. Contraception 2005;71:319–26.
44. Croxatto HB. Mechanisms that explain the contraceptive action of progestin implants for women. Contraception 2002;65:21–7.
45. Walch K, Unfried G, Huber J, et al. Implanon versus medroxyprogesterone acetate: effects on pain scores in patients with symptomatic endometriosis—a pilot study. Contraception 2009;79:29–34.
46. Al-Jefout M, Palmer J, Fraser IS. Simultaneous use of a levonorgestrel intrauterine system and an etonogestrel subdermal implant for debilitating adolescent endometriosis. Aust N Z J Obstet Gynaecol 2007;47:247–9.
47. Croxatto HB, Urbancsek J, Massai R, Coelingh Bennink H, van Beek A. A multicentre efficacy and safety study of the single contraceptive implant Implanon. Implanon Study Group. Hum Reprod 1999;14:976–81.
48. Glasier A. Implantable contraceptives for women: effectiveness, discontinuation rates, return of fertility, and outcome of pregnancies. Contraception 2002;65:29–37.
49. Committee on Gynecologic Practice Long-Acting Reversible Contraception Working Group. Committee Opinion No. 642: Increasing access to contraceptive implants and intrauterine devices to reduce unintended pregnancy. Obstet Gynecol 2015;126:e44–8.
50. Darney P, Patel A, Rosen K, Shapiro LS, Kaunitz AM. Safety and efficacy of a single-rod etonogestrel implant (Implanon): results from 11 international clinical trials. Fertil Steril 2009;91:1646–53.
51. Diego D, Tappy E, Carugno J. Axillary migration of Nexplanon®: Case report. Contraception 2017;95:218–220.
52. Gallon A, Fontarensky M, Chauffour C, Boyer L, Chabrot P. Looking for a lost subdermal contraceptive implant? Think about the pulmonary artery. Contraception 2017;95:215–217.
53. Choi JH, Kim HY, Lee SS, Cho S. Migration of a contraceptive subdermal device into the lung. Obstet Gynecol Sci 2017;60:314–317.
54. Zheng SR, Zheng HM, Qian SZ, Sang GW, Kaper RF. A randomized multicenter study comparing the efficacy and bleeding pattern of a single-rod (Implanon) and a six-capsule (Norplant) hormonal contraceptive implant. Contraception 1999;60:1–8.
55. Mansour D, Korver T, Marintcheva-Petrova M, Fraser IS. The effects of Implanon on menstrual bleeding patterns. Eur J Contracept Reprod Health Care 2008;13 Suppl 1:13–28.
56. Vickery Z, Madden T, Zhao Q, Secura GM, Allsworth JE, Peipert JF. Weight change at 12 months in users of three progestin-only contraceptive methods. Contraception 2013;88:503–8.
57. Kassen N, Wells CL, Moodley A. Pseudotumor cerebri and Implanon: Is rapid weight gain the trigger? Euroophthalmology 2015;39:281–284.
58. Callahan R, Yacobson I, Halpern V, Nanda K. Ectopic pregnancy with use of progestin-only injectables and contraceptive implants: a systematic review. Contraception 2015; 92:514–22.
59. Bouquier J, Fulda V, Bats AS, Lécuru F, Huchon C. A life-threatening ectopic pregnancy with etonogestrel implant. Contraception 2012;85:215–7.
60. Boozalis A, Tutlam NT, Chrisman Robbins C, Peipert JF. Sexual desire and hormonal contraception. Obstet Gynecol 2016;127:563–72.
61. Higgins JA, Sanders JN, Palta M, Turok DK. Women's sexual function, satisfaction, and perceptions after starting long-acting reversible contraceptives. Obstet Gynecol 2016;128:1143–1151.

62. Steiner RJ, Liddon N, Swartzendruber AL, Rasberry CN, Sales JM. Long-acting reversible contraception and condom use among female U.S. high school students: Implications for sexually transmitted infection prevention. JAMA Pediatr 2016;170:428–34.
63. Inoue K, Kelly M, Barratt A, et al. Australian women's attitudes towards and understandings of the subdermal contraceptive implant: a qualitative study of never-users. J Fam Plann Reprod Health Care 2017;43:128–134.
64. Hall KS, Ela E, Zochowski MK, et al. "I don't know enough to feel comfortable using them." Women's knowledge of and perceived barriers to long-acting reversible contraceptives on a college campus. Contraception 2016;93:556–64.
65. Richards M, Teal SB, Sheeder J. Risk of luteal phase pregnancy with any-cycle-day initiation of subdermal contraceptive implants. Contraception 2017;95:364–370.
66. Cohen R, Sheeder J, Arango N, Teal SB, Tocce K. Twelve-month contraceptive continuation and repeat pregnancy among young mothers choosing postdelivery contraceptive implants or postplacental intrauterine devices. Contraception 2016;93:178–83.
67. Rose SB, Garrett SM. Postabortion initiation of long-acting reversible contraception by adolescent and nulliparous women in New Zealand. J Adolesc Health 2016;58:160–6.
68. Madden T, Eisenberg DL, Zhao Q, Buckel C, Secura GM, Peipert JF. Continuation of the etonogestrel implant in women undergoing immediate postabortion placement. Obstet Gynecol 2012;120:1053–9.
69. Eggebroten JL, Sanders JN, Turok DK. Immediate postpartum intrauterine device and implant program outcomes: a prospective analysis. Am J Obstet Gynecol 2017;217:51.e1–51.e7.
70. Wilson S, Tennant C, Sammel MD, Schreiber C. Immediate postpartum etonogestrel implant: a contraception option with long-term continuation. Contraception 2014;90:259–64.
71. Bahamondes L, Bahamondes MV, Modesto W, et al. Effect of hormonal contraceptives during breastfeeding on infant's milk ingestion and growth. Fertil Steril 2013;100:445–50.
72. Carmo LSMP, Braga GC, Ferriani RA, Quintana SM, Vieira CS. Timing of etonogestrel-releasing implants and growth of breastfed infants: a randomized controlled Trial. Obstet Gynecol 2017;130:100–107.
73. Iltemir Duvan C, Onaran Y, Aktepe Keskin E, et al. Effects of the etonogestrel contraceptive implant (Implanon(®)) on bone metabolism during lactation: a prospective study. J Fam Plann Reprod Health Care 2017;43:113–117.
74. Dobromilsky KC, Allen PL, Raymond SH, Maindiratta B. A prospective cohort study of early postpartum etonogestrel implant (Implanon®) use and its effect on duration of lochia. J Fam Plann Reprod Health Care 2016;42:187–93.
75. Pearson S, Stewart M, Bateson D. Implanon NXT: Expert tips for best-practice insertion and removal. Aust Fam Physician 2017;46:104–108.
76. Biskamp C, Kauffman RP. Arm flexion during ultrasound assists localization of an intramuscular etonogestrel contraceptive implant. Contraception 2016;93:273–5.
77. Persaud T, Walling M, Geoghegan T, Buckley O, Stunell H, Torreggiani WC. Ultrasound-guided removal of Implanon devices. Eur Radiol 2008;18:2582–5.
78. Nelson AL, Sinow RM. Real-time ultrasonographically guided removal of nonpalpable and intramuscular Norplant capsules. Am J Obstet Gynecol 1998;178:1185–93.
79. Chen MJ, Creinin MD. Removal of a nonpalpable etonogestrel implant with preprocedure ultrasonography and modified vasectomy clamp. Obstet Gynecol 2015;126:935–8.
80. Mansour D, Walling M, Glenn D, et al. Removal of nonpalpable etonogestrel implants. J Fam Plann Reprod Health Care 2008;34:89–91.
81. Nouri K, Pinker-Domenig K, Ott J, Fraser I, Egarter C. Removal of nonpalpable Implanon® with the aid of a hook-wire marker. Contraception 2013;88:577–80.
82. Guiahi M, Tocce K, Teal S, Green T, Rochon P. Removal of a Nexplanon implant located in the biceps muscle using a combination of ultrasound and fluoroscopy guidance. Contraception 2014;90:606–8.

83. Vollans SR, Grainger A, O'Connor P, Limb D. Hormone-releasing contraceptive implants: our experience of complex removals using preoperative ultrasound. Contraception 2015;92:81–3.
84. Zigler RE, McNicholas C. Unscheduled vaginal bleeding with progestin-only contraceptive use. Am J Obstet Gynecol 2017;216:443–450.
85. Phaliwong P, Taneepanichskul S. The effect of mefenamic acid on controlling irregular uterine bleeding second to Implanon use. J Med Assoc Thai 2004;87 Suppl 3:S64–8.
86. Díaz S, Croxatto HB, Pavez M, Belhadj H, Stern J, Sivin I. Clinical assessment of treatments for prolonged bleeding in users of Norplant implants. Contraception 1990; 42:97–109.
87. Abdel-Aleem H, d'Arcangues C, Vogelsong KM, Gaffield ML, Gülmezoglu AM. Treatment of vaginal bleeding irregularities induced by progestin only contraceptives. Cochrane Database Syst Rev 2013;10:CD003449.pub5.
88. Phupong V, Sophonsritsuk A, Taneepanichskul S. The effect of tranexamic acid for treatment of irregular uterine bleeding secondary to Norplant use. Contraception 2006;73:253–6.
89. Guiahi M, McBride M, Sheeder J, Teal S. Short-term treatment of bothersome bleeding for etonogestrel implant users using a 14-day oral contraceptive pill regimen: A randomized controlled trial. Obstet Gynecol 2015;126:508–13.
90. Hou MY, McNicholas C, Creinin MD. combined oral contraceptive treatment for bleeding complaints with the etonogestrel contraceptive implant: a randomized controlled trial. Eur J Contracept Reprod Health Care 2016;21:361–6.
91. Simmons KB, Edelman AB, Fu R, Jensen JT. Tamoxifen for the treatment of breakthrough bleeding with the etonogestrel implant: a randomized controlled trial. Contraception 2017;95:198–204.
92. Abdel-Aleem H, Shaaban OM, Amin AF, Abdel-Aleem AM. Tamoxifen treatment of bleeding irregularities associated with Norplant use. Contraception 2005;72:432–7.
93. Weisberg E, Hickey M, Palmer D, et al. A randomized controlled trial of treatment options for troublesome uterine bleeding in Implanon users. Hum Reprod 2009;24: 1852–61.
94. ACOG Practice Bulletin number 186. Long-acting reversible contraception: implants and intrauterine devices. Obstet Gynecol 2017;130:e251–e269.

Intrauterine Devices (IUDs) 5

Gillian Dean, MD, MPH
Eleanor Bimla Schwarz, MD, MS

- IUDs are among the safest, most convenient, and well-liked methods of contraception.
- IUDs are the most commonly used reversible contraceptives in the world.
- IUDs are over twenty times more effective than pills and as effective as surgical sterilization.
- IUDs are among the most cost-effective contraceptives available.
- IUDs are safe for adolescents and nulliparous individuals.
- IUDs are promptly reversible and pose no risk to future fertility.
- Levonorgestrel IUDs reduce dysmenorrhea, anemia and risk of endometrial cancer.
- The Copper T 380A IUD is the most effective form of emergency contraception.

Intrauterine devices (IUDs) are among the most effective, safest, and most well-liked methods of contraception available. The term intrauterine contraceptive (IUC) is a commonly used synonym. IUDs containing levonorgestrel (LNG) are also sometimes referred to as intrauterine systems (IUS). Worldwide, the IUD is the most commonly-used reversible method of contraception.[1] In China, Korea, and Vietnam, IUDs are used by over 40% of married women of reproductive age; in Europe, 6% to 16% of such women use IUDs.[1] The United States (U.S.) has been slower to adopt intrauterine contraception, and in 2002, only 2% of U.S. contraceptive users chose an IUD.[2] However, by 2013 this number had grown to 10.3%.[3,4] It is estimated that 40% of U.S. family planning clinicians use an IUD for their personal contraceptive needs.[5]

Widespread use of IUDs in the United States was historically limited by a history of negative publicity, misinformation about the risks of ectopic pregnancy, infection, and subsequent infertility, misconceptions about the mechanism of action, lack of clinician training, and fears of litigation.[6] In the 1970s, only 10% of U.S. contraceptive users chose IUDs.[7] Research from this period associated IUDs, particularly the Dalkon Shield, with increased risk of pelvic inflammatory disease (PID)[8] and septic abortion, and use of IUDs subsequently fell until the first part of the 21st century.[4] In addition, in the 1970s, it was not yet possible to test for asymptomatic chlamydia. As such, early studies of the associations between IUDs and PID suffered from methodological flaws; data on modern IUDs show no increase in PID with IUD use.[9]

The IUDs available in the 1970s differed from modern IUDs in design and efficacy. Early IUDs were inert (plastic only) and had 1st year failure rates of 2%[10] to 9%,[11,12] while modern IUDs have copper or LNG added to a polyethylene frame; these additions improve contraceptive efficacy by an order of magnitude.[11] Modern IUDs have monofilament threads which have not been associated with infections[13] or other adverse outcomes.[14] In recent years, a number of new IUDs have been introduced to the U.S. and international markets. All available IUDs are safer and more effective than oral contraceptives. When cost is an issue, Liletta is noteworthy as a low-cost option. Otherwise, the primary difference among currently available IUDs is their effect on menstrual bleeding patterns and potential duration of use.

IUD Options in the United States

As of 2018, there are five IUDs available in the United States. See Table 5–1. All of these are made of polyethylene with barium sulfate added to create x-ray visibility, and can be safely imaged using MRI.[15] The copper IUD is highly echogenic on ultrasound and thus relatively easy to locate within the uterus. LNG IUDs produce an echolucent (dark) sonographic shadow and can be more difficult to identify with ultrasound, although two of the newer IUDs contain a silver ring on the stem to aid in identification. The Progestasert IUD, which contained progesterone[12] and was only effective for one year, was sold in the US from 1986-1988[16] and is no longer on the market.

Copper T 380A (ParaGard) IUD

The copper T 380A (TCu380A) was introduced in the United States in 1988. It is now available in most countries around the world and has been used by tens of millions of people. The copper T 380A is the only highly effective, reversible contraceptive method that is hormone-free. Fine copper wire is wound around the vertical stem of the T, and each of the two horizontal arms holds a sleeve of copper. The combined

Table 5-1 Characteristics of IUDs available in the United States in 2018

	ParaGard	Mirena	Liletta*	Kyleena	Skyla**
Contains	380 mm^2 copper	52 mg LNG	52 mg LNG	19.5 mg LNG	13.5 mg LNG
LNG release/day (1st year)	0 mcg	20 mcg	20 mcg	12 mcg	8 mcg
Evidence-based use	**12–20 years**[17,18]	**7 years**[19]	**7 years**[19]	**5 years**[20]	**3 years**[20]
FDA-labeled use	10 years	5 years	3 years	5 years	3 years
FDA approval year	1984	2000	2015	2016	2013
LNG serum concentration over 3 years of use[21]	0 ng/L	218 ng/L	218 ng/L	114 ng/L	74.3 ng/L
Placement tube diameter	4.01 mm	4.40 mm	4.80 mm	3.80 mm	3.80 mm
Size of frame (mm)	32×36	32×32	32×32	28×30	28×30
Silver ring on T	No	No	No	Yes	Yes
Thread color	White	Brown	Blue	Blue	Brown
Ovulatory cycles (%)	All	45% at 1 yr 75% at 4 yrs[22]	45% at 1 yr 75% at 4 yrs[22]	Almost all	Almost all
Amenorrhea at 1 year	0%	15%[23] to 24%[19]	15%[23] to 24%[19]	13%[19]	6%[24]
Amenorrhea at 2 years	0%	10%[19] to 26%[25]	10%[19] to 26%[25]	20%[26]	10%[24]
1st year Pearl Index (95% CI)	0.7[27]	0.19[28]	0.15 (0.02–0.55)[29]	0.16 (0.02–0.58)[30]	0.48 (0.13–1.23)[24]
Lifetime Pearl Index (95% CI)	0.52 (0.42–0.64)[31]	0.06 (0.04–0.09)[31]	0.06 (0.04–0.09)[31]	0.29 (0.16–0.50)[30]	0.9 (0.4–1.9)[24]
Need for back up contraception[32] after placement***	None	7 days	7 days	7 days	7 days

*Marketed as Levosert in the UK

**Marketed as Jaydess in Asia

***Unless placed post-abortion, post-partum, or within 7 days of beginning last menstrual period copper surface area of the stem and sleeves is 380 ± 23 mm^2. The device is latex-free and clinically-relevant allergy to copper is extremely rare.[33] Serum copper levels are higher in TCu380A users compared with non-users and may be above the normal blood copper level range;[34] however, adverse clinical effects of this elevated blood copper level have not been noted among the millions of women who have used TCu380A IUDs worldwide. The TCu380A is labeled for 10 years of use, although data indicate high effectiveness for 12 years,[17] and no pregnancies were reported among the few who retained the TCu380A for 20 years.[18] Cumulative pregnancy rates for the TCu380A are 0.5% to 0.8% (first year),[35,36] 1.4% to 2.5% (7 years),[33,37,38] and 2.2% (12 years).[17] Inert IUDs and copper IUDs with less than 380 mm^2 of copper are less effective than those containing 380 mm^2 or more of copper and are no longer available in the United States.[39,40] In 2005, the U.S. Food and Drug Administration (FDA) clarified package labeling for the TCu380A, removing any proscription against use by nulliparous individuals or individuals with more than one sexual partner. TCu380A labeling now also supports placement immediately after an abortion or delivery.

Levonorgestrel IUDs

There are currently four LNG IUDs available in the United States. All have T-shaped frames with a reservoir containing levonorgestrel dispersed in polydimethylsiloxane molded around the vertical stem. The reservoirs are covered with a silicone membrane that regulates the release of the hormone. The stems have monofilament polyethylene threads attached to the base to assist with removal. Mirena and Liletta have identical frame sizes and contain 52 mg of LNG. Kyleena and Skyla have slightly smaller frames and lower doses of LNG (19.5 mg and 13.5 mg, respectively). Small amounts of levonorgestrel are systemically absorbed and some systemic side effects can occur. However, the daily systemic dose of levonorgestrel with use of a 52 mg LNG IUD[41–43] is about 10% that of an oral contraceptive containing 150 mcg LNG,[44] and the systemic dose of lower-dose LNG IUDs is even lower.

52 mg LNG IUDs (Mirena, Liletta) Millions of women in 120 countries around the world[1] have used a 52 mg LNG IUD. The first 52 mg LNG IUD (Mirena) was approved for use in Europe in the early 1990s and in the United States in 2000; it was first sold in the United States in 2001. In 2015, the FDA approved the lower-cost Liletta IUD,[45] which has an identical frame size (32 mm in both height and width), levonorgestrel content, and performance characteristics, although a different inserter. These IUDs release LNG into the endometrial cavity at an initial rate of 19 to 20 mcg per day,[25] declining to 10 mcg per day after five years.[22,43] Cumulative pregnancy rates for the 52 mg LNG IUD are 0.1% to 0.2% (first year),[46,47] 0.5% to 1.1% (5 years),[48,49] and 0.5% (7 years).[19,37,41,50–53]

19.5 mg LNG IUD (Kyleena) FDA-approved in 2016, the newest IUD available in the United States contains 19.5 mg of LNG at initial placement, with an average daily release rate of 9.8 mcg after 1 year and 7.4 at 5 years.[26] This IUD is labeled by the FDA for 5 years of use, and its cumulative 5-year pregnancy rate is 1.1% ±0.5%.[48] Extended use of this IUD beyond 5 years may be reasonable given the studies of IUDs containing lower doses of LNG,[23,54] described below.

13.5 mg LNG IUD (Skyla) FDA-approved in 2013, this IUD contains 13.5 mg of LNG at initial placement, and has an average daily release rate of 8 mcg in the first year,[54] declining to approximately 5 mcg at 3 years. This IUD is labeled by the FDA for 3 years of use; it has a first year Pearl Index of 0.48 and a lifetime Pearl Index of 0.9.[23]

MECHANISM OF ACTION

IUDs work primarily by preventing sperm from fertilizing ova.[55] Pregnancy is prevented by a combination of the "foreign body effect" of the plastic frame and the specific action of the active ingredient (copper or levonorgestrel) that is released. Exposure to a foreign body causes changes in the intrauterine environment that are toxic to sperm and ova and may impair implantation.[56,57] The production of cytotoxic peptides and activation of enzymes lead to inhibition of sperm motility, reduced sperm capacitation and survival, and increased phagocytosis of sperm.[58,59] Copper ions released by the TCu380A cause an increase in enzymes, prostaglandins, and white blood cells (macrophages) in uterine and tubal fluids; these impair sperm function and prevent fertilization. The progestin in LNG IUDs thickens cervical mucus, suppresses the endometrium by reducing uterine artery blood flow,[60] and impairs sperm function by changing the uterine immune microenvironment.[61,62] In addition, ovulation may be impaired as a result of systemic absorption of levonorgestrel.[51] Ovulation suppression is greatest in the initial year of use and with higher LNG levels. According to package inserts, among women using a 52 mg LNG IUD for 1 year, 45% of cycles were ovulatory, and at 4 years, 75% were ovulatory, while with the 19.5 mg and 13.5 mg LNG IUDs, almost all cycles are ovulatory.

Three lines of evidence indicate that IUDs primarily work early in the reproductive process to prevent fertilization, rather than implantation.[35] First, human chorionic gonadotropin assays for early pregnancy do not reveal "chemical pregnancies" in women using IUDs.[63–65] Second, studies in women undergoing tubal sterilization at mid-cycle, in which the fallopian tubes were flushed and the fluid examined with a microscope to identify fertilized eggs, show markedly fewer fertilized, normally-dividing eggs were recovered from IUD users than women using no contraception.[66] Third, IUD users have a significantly decreased risk of ectopic pregnancy compared to women using no contraception,[31,67] which implies that IUDs inhibit fertilization.

EFFECTIVENESS

All IUDs available in the United States rank in the top tier of contraceptive effectiveness. IUDs are typically over twenty times as effective as oral contraceptives.[68] (See Figure 3-1 in Chapter 3.) IUDs with 52 mg LNG are the most effective IUDs,[31,67] with a cumulative 7-year pregnancy rate of 0.5%, compared with 2.5% for the TCu380A.[19] The effectiveness of the TCu380A is comparable to tubal sterilization (which has pregnancy rates of 1.3% at 5 years and 1.9% at 10 years[69]). The only contraceptive option more effective than the 52 mg LNG IUD is the subdermal contraceptive implant.[70] As an IUD's LNG dose decreases, the efficacy of the IUD decreases; however, the 13.5 mg LNG IUD appears to be at least as effective as the TCu380A.[71] The effectiveness of the TCu380A remains high over long-term use; at 12 years the cumulative pregnancy rate is only 2.2%.[17]

Cost-effectiveness

One office visit for IUD placement can provide years of highly effective contraception at a low daily cost. Although the initial cost of an IUD can be high, the overall cost decreases with each year of use,[72] and the costs of undesired pregnancy are considerably higher.[73] For obese individuals, a levonorgestrel IUD is also a potentially cost-effective strategy for prevention of deaths from endometrial cancer.[74]

ADVANTAGES

- High effectiveness
- Impressive safety
- Few contraindications to use; no estrogen
- Convenient and private
- High user satisfaction
- Long-term protection
- Rapid reversibility

- Reduce endometrial cancer risk (particularly important for women facing obesity, or taking tamoxifen or postmenopausal estrogen)
- Reduce dysmenorrhea and menstrual blood loss (LNG IUDs)
- Nearly 100% effective as emergency contraception (TCu380A)
- Immediate placement after end of pregnancy (post abortion, miscarriage, or delivery)
- The possibility of self-removal

The possibility of self-removal by the user is an important difference between IUDs and the other highly effective reversible contraceptive, the subdermal implant. Thread length affects ability to self-remove an IUD, as was demonstrated in one study, in which only 20% of patients who attempted self-removal were successful; therefore, clinicians should clarify patients' preferences before trimming IUD threads.[75] For individuals facing reproductive coercion, IUDs can be made undetectable (except by clinical imaging) by completely removing the threads.

User Satisfaction and Continuation Rates

Several studies have demonstrated the effectiveness of the TCu380A and 52 mg LNG IUDs beyond the duration of use noted on product labels. As IUD replacement often causes some discomfort and carries a small risk of uterine perforation or ascending infection, continued use is often advantageous. Satisfaction and continuation rates for IUDs are higher than for all other reversible contraceptives at 1 year (ranging from 78%, as shown in Table 27-1, to 90%[50,76–79]). Although satisfaction and continuation rates are a bit higher for the 52 mg LNG than TCu380A IUD users at one year (84% versus 88%),[79] continuation rates for both IUDs are 77% to 79% at 2 years,[80] 70% at 3 years,[81] greater than 60% at 4 years, and 50% at 5 years.[82]

Ectopic Pregnancy Prevention

Individuals with a history of ectopic pregnancy can safely use either a copper or LNG IUD.[83] In fact, people using no contraception are 10 times more likely than IUD users to develop an ectopic pregnancy.[84]

Protection from pelvic inflammatory disease (PID)

Individuals with multiple partners, a history of sexually transmitted infection (STI), or PID can safely use an IUD. LNG IUDs, like all progestin-containing contraceptives, decrease risk of PID by thickening cervical mucus, which acts as a barrier to ascending infection.[85,86]

All individuals at risk of STI should be encouraged to consistently use condoms. Screening asymptomatic patients for STI may be done at the time of IUD placement; those found to be carrying an asymptomatic STI can be treated with the IUD in place.[87]

Cancer Protection

Copper IUD use has been associated with lower rates of cervical cancer,[88,89] even after controlling for rates of screening for cervical cancer. Both copper and LNG IUDs have been associated with a reduction in the risk of endometrial cancer. Although the specific mechanism of action by which the copper IUD protects against endometrial cancer is unknown, it may relate to alterations in the endometrium.[90,91] Similarly, progestin-releasing intrauterine contraception has also been shown to protect against endometrial cancer[92] by decreasing endometrial proliferation, as do contraceptives that deliver a progestin systemically.[93] LNG IUDs suppress the endometrium by reducing uterine artery blood flow.[60] The 52 mg LNG IUD has been used to prevent development of endometrial hyperplasia in women using perimenopausal estrogen therapy[94–96] or tamoxifen;[92,97,98] other LNG IUDs may also provide this endometrial protection but have not been studied. The 52 mg LNG IUD has also been used for the treatment of nonatypical endometrial hyperplasia, atypical hyperplasia and grade 1 stage I endometrial cancer.[99–102] LNG IUD use has also been associated with lower rates of ovarian cancer,[103,104] pancreatic cancer, and lung cancer.[104,105]

Emergency Contraception

The TCu380A is the most effective method of emergency contraception (EC) and is highly effective for up to 7 days from unprotected intercourse; limited data support its use through 10 days from unprotected sex.[106] Although most guidelines recommend placing a copper IUD for EC within 5 days of unprotected sex, some evidence suggests that a copper IUD is highly effective if placed at any time in the menstrual cycle.[185] In 42 studies conducted in 6 countries between 1979 and 2011 that included a total of 7,034 participants, the pregnancy rate was 0.09%.[106] No published data support the use of LNG IUDs for EC; however, when an LNG IUD is placed at the time LNG EC pills are taken, pregnancy rates within 2 weeks are less than 1%.[107] (See Chapter 10 on Emergency Contraception.)

Noncontraceptive Benefits of LNG IUDs

Overall, LNG IUD use is associated with a reduction in menstrual blood loss compared with women using no contraception and women using copper IUDs.[50] LNG IUDs reduce dysmenorrhea and menstrual blood loss by inducing endometrial decidualization and atrophy,[108] and the proportion of LNG IUD users with amenorrhea increases with duration of use.[109,36,50] Rates of amenorrhea among IUD users differ markedly by LNG dose (Table 5-1),[110,111] and lower-dose LNG IUDs have not been as well-studied for the management of menorrhagia. With use of a 52 mg LNG IUD, overall blood loss drops about 90%; this translates into clinically important increases in hemoglobin and iron stores.[36,50] The reduction in menstrual blood loss occurs both for patients with normal coagulation parameters and those with bleeding diatheses or using anticoagulant therapy.[112–114] Some evidence supports using a 52 mg LNG IUD to treat heavy bleeding associated with adenomyosis[115] and leiomyomas.[116] Trials have compared this approach to medical treatments with an oral progestin, a nonsteroidal anti-inflammatory drug, or mefenamic acid (which is not available in the United States)[113] and found 52 mg LNG IUDs superior to the other alternatives. In addition, the 52 mg LNG IUD is an acceptable and cost-effective alternative to endometrial ablation or hysterectomy.[117–120]

DISADVANTAGES AND CAUTIONS

Common but benign side effects

- Changes in menstrual patterns
- Cramping
- Expulsion of the IUD
- Concern of weight gain
- Actinomyces-like organisms seen on Papanicolaou smear

Rare but concerning health risks

- Pelvic infection
- Uterine perforation
- Pregnancy complications, in the unlikely event that pregnancy occurs with IUD use

CHANGES IN MENSTRUAL PATTERNS

Changes in menstrual patterns are the most common side effects of intrauterine contraception. Irregular bleeding and spotting are common in the early months of use and the most frequent cause of discontinuation. Thus, anticipatory counseling about expected menstrual changes is very important.

TCu380A

Copper IUD users may find that their menses become heavier, longer, or more uncomfortable, particularly in the first several cycles of TCu380A use. Heavy menses and dysmenorrhea are the most frequent reasons for copper IUD removal in the first year of use.[121] Although these side effects may decrease over time,[122] approximately 2 of every 100 users discontinue use in subsequent years due to bleeding and pain.[50,78] Average monthly menstrual blood loss may be increased by up to 55% throughout the duration of copper IUD use, although this rarely leads to anemia.[123]

LNG IUDs

Irregular but light bleeding or spotting is the norm in the early months of using an LNG IUD, with considerable improvement after the first 3 months. Overall, LNG IUDs are associated with a reduction in menstrual blood loss and may result in amenorrhea. The majority of LNG IUD users have ovulatory cycles and may continue to experience other cyclic symptoms (e.g. acne or mood changes) while amenorrheic.[50,109,124] The lower the LNG dose, the more likely the individual is to ovulate and have ovulatory symptoms. Side effects that may lead to early discontinuation of an LNG IUD include hormonal side effects, such as breast tenderness, mood changes, hair loss, and acne,[50,76,86] although systemic levels of levonorgestrel are far lower than with other hormonal methods.[41,125] Over time, plasma levels of levonorgestrel gradually decline[41] and cyclic symptoms may increase.

Cramping and Pain

Most people experience discomfort at the time of IUD placement. Use of intravaginal lidocaine gel or cream may reduce discomfort due to tenaculum placement.[126,127] Immediately following IUD placement, some patients experience 10 to 30 minutes of uterine cramping accompanied by nausea or feeling faint. Some clinicians offer oral non-steroidal anti-inflammatory drugs prior to placement, a paracervical block, or both, although most patients do not require either. Despite hopes that misoprostol might facilitate IUD placement, multiple randomized trials have not found misoprostol to reduce cramping or increase ease of IUD placement in most cases.[128] However, misoprostol may facilitate IUD placement after a previous failed attempt at IUD placement[129] or for those with multiple prior Cesarean sections.[130] Approximately a third of nulliparous patients report requiring pain medication for at least 3 days after IUD placement.[127] Along with unscheduled bleeding, dysmenorrhea is one of the primary reasons for discontinuation of use of a TCu380A IUD[121,122] and may also affect LNG IUD users.[110] When pelvic pain develops weeks after IUD placement, consider whether the IUD may be partially expelled or dislodged into the cervix and evaluate for infection or pregnancy.

IUD Expulsion

IUD expulsions can be complete (i.e., the IUD is completely outside of uterine cavity and cervical canal) or partial (i.e., all or part of the IUD is in the cervix). Expulsions can be symptomatic (producing cramping, bleeding, pain, dyspareunia, change in thread length, or a palpable IUD at cervix) or asymptomatic. The risk of IUD expulsion is greatest in the first year of use,[131] when expulsion occurs in 3% to 10% of TCu380A users and 3% to 6% of LNG IUD users. The risk of expulsion is higher for individuals who are nulliparous, younger than 20, have menorrhagia or severe dysmenorrhea, or have an IUD placed immediately postpartum or after a second trimester abortion;[121,132,133] however, IUDs can be successfully used in all of these clinical scenarios. Placement immediately after first trimester abortion does not increase expulsion risk.[186] An individual who has expelled one IUD is more likely to experience a repeat expulsion; limited data on repeat expulsion place the risk between 14% and 31% within a year of replacement.[133] Because some IUD expulsions are asymptomatic, some clinicians encourage IUD users to routinely check their IUD threads, especially during the first 6 months of use, when risk of IUD expulsion is greatest.

Concern of Weight Gain

Although up to 10% of women will report concerns that their weight has increased after placement of an LNG IUD,[110] mean weight change at 1 year for LNG IUD users is 1 kg, which is less than seen with use of subdermal or injectable contraception.[134]

Pelvic Infection

Flaws in early research led to exaggerations in estimates of the risk of upper-genital-tract infection associated with use of IUDs.[9] Rigorous studies[135,136] and reviews of the literature[137] have now established that the risk of infection and infertility among users of modern IUDs is very low. Both epidemiological[138] and bacteriological evidence[139] indicates that the insertion process, and not the device or its thread, poses a small transient risk of infection. No procedure that requires traversing the cervical canal can be devoid of all pathogenic organisms. Although sterile technique should be used, endocervical bacteria are routinely introduced to the endometrial cavity regardless of technique.[139] However, antibiotic prophylaxis should not be routinely used before IUD placement.[140] A large randomized controlled trial that evaluated the potential benefit of prophylactic azithromycin given before IUD placement[135] found no benefit. More importantly, this study found that salpingitis was rare with or without prophylaxis: only one women out of about a thousand in each group developed salpingitis in the early months of IUD use. International experience with IUDs has been similarly favorable. In large trials sponsored by the World Health Organization (WHO), the elevated risk of upper-genital-tract infection was limited to the first 20 days after insertion.[136] Afterwards, the risk returned to a low level and remained there for years. More recent studies have found similarly low risk of PID (0.2–0.5%) and no initial increase in infection following IUD placement.[87,141] LNG IUDs appear to protect users from pelvic inflammatory disease (PID) because progestins thicken cervical mucus reducing bacterial infiltration of the upper genital tract.[85,86]

Early assessments of the risk of tubal infertility among IUD users exaggerated risks as well.[142,143] IUD users have no significant differences in return to fertility, whether the IUD was removed because of a desire for pregnancy or because of problems with the IUD.[144,145] Indeed, in a Mexican case-control study,[146] prior use of a copper IUD was not significantly related to tubal pathology, whereas the presence of Chlamydia antibodies was, underscoring that sexually transmitted infections (STI), not IUDs, cause salpingitis. IUD placement does not increase risk of PID compared with no IUD placement among women with asymptomatic cervical infection or high risk of STI.[147,148] IUDs can be safely used by people with human immunodeficiency virus (HIV)[149] and those requiring treatment with immunosuppressant medications.[150]

Perforation

Perforation of the uterus can occur at the time of IUD placement; no evidence supports the theory that IUDs can migrate outside the uterus thereafter. The most important determinant of the risk of perforation is the skill of the person placing the IUD. In experienced hands, the risk of perforation is 1 per 1,000 insertions or fewer.[35] Particular care is required when placing IUDs for women who are breastfeeding as perforation is more likely.[14] However, in a large cohort study, no uterine perforations led to serious illness or to injury of intra-abdominal or pelvic structures.[14] The terms "embedment" and "translocation" refer to the position of the IUD relative to the body of the uterus. Bimanual examination of the uterus (to determine size and position) is recommended before attempting to place an IUD in order to guide correct placement in the endometrial cavity.

Pregnancy Complications

Pregnancy is very rare with an IUD in place. However, when an individual does conceive with an IUD in place, there is an increased risk that the pregnancy is ectopic compared with women using no contraception.

It is estimated that among women using no contraception, 2% of pregnancies are ectopic; among women using an IUD, 6% to 50% of pregnancies are ectopic.[151,152] Nonetheless, a person is much less likely to develop an ectopic pregnancy while using an IUD than while using less-effective or no contraception.

PROVIDING THE IUD

Most women, including teens, are good candidates for intrauterine contraception. IUDs can be used safely by individuals who are nulliparous, have multiple partners, have history of ectopic pregnancies, or those with a history of PID as long as they have no symptomatic cervical infection at the time of IUD placement. All IUDs can also be used by people with contraindications to estrogen. IUDs can be removed whenever desired, and may be appropriate for women who desire pregnancy in the next year or two.

CHOOSING WHICH IUD

Most patients can safely use either a copper or LNG IUD. When counseling a patient about choice of IUD, it is helpful to know her menstrual history, her medical history, her desire for lighter or less painful menses, and her feelings about amenorrhea, unscheduled bleeding or spotting, and hormonal contraception. A current history of anemia, menorrhagia, or dysmenorrhea may be compounded by use of the TCu380A IUD. When choosing among the LNG IUDs, the patient's feelings about amenorrhea and spotting are more important than her anticipated duration of IUD use. (See Chapter 2 for more complete discussion of patient-centered contraception counseling.)

CONTRAINDICATIONS TO IUD USE

Few absolute contraindications exist to IUD placement or continued use. The Medical Eligibility Criteria for Contraceptive Use published by the WHO and U.S. Centers for Disease Control and Prevention (CDC)[153] offer clinicians guidelines for determining safe candidates for IUD use. (See the U.S. MEC summary chart in this book.). The vast majority of women worldwide are good candidates for an IUD. However, intrauterine contraception is contraindicated in people with active pelvic infection, including PID, endometritis, mucopurulent cervicitis and pelvic tuberculosis, because the presence of a foreign body may impede resolution of the infection. Do not place an IUD for women with known or suspected pregnancy. An IUD should not be newly inserted in individuals awaiting treatment for cervical or endometrial cancer, but may be continued in previously treated patients, and may be placed for those with a history of abnormal Pap tests. Evaluate abnormal uterine bleeding before placing an IUD, so the abnormal bleeding will not be erroneously attributed to the IUD rather than to the preexisting pathology. Placement of an IUD may be difficult with severe cervical stenosis. IUD placement may not be possible with severe uterine distortion from anatomic abnormalities such as bicornuate uteri or fibroids severely distorting the uterine cavity. However, nondistorting fibroids are not a contraindication to intrauterine contraception. IUDs should not be placed for patients with gestational trophoblastic neoplasia who have persistently elevated beta hCG levels or malignant disease with evidence or suspicion of intrauterine disease, although continued use of a previously placed IUD may be acceptable. The TCu380A should not be used by individuals with Wilson's disease or copper allergy.[153]

Special Issues

Adolescents and Nulliparous Individuals

Adolescent and nulliparous individuals are excellent candidates for IUD use; the American Academy of Pediatrics recommends IUDs and subdermal implants as preferred contraceptive options for sexually active adolescents.[154] Future fertility is not affected by IUD use[146] and return to fertility after IUD removal is prompt. Younger age, which is associated with nulliparity, is associated with IUD expulsion; however, rates of IUD expulsion remain relatively low.[155] Although nulliparity increases the likelihood of discomfort with IUD placement, IUD placement is well tolerated by most teens and nulliparous individuals[156] without requiring use of a smaller-framed IUD. When necessary, cervical dilation with a 13 to 15 Fr Pratt dilator can be performed at the time of the insertion. Prophylaxis with an oral nonsteroidal anti-inflammatory drug and paracervical anesthesia[157,158] may help as well. However, multiple trials have found that most nonsteroidal anti-inflammatory drugs are not effective for reducing pain during IUD placement, although naproxen (300 mg to 550 mg) had some effect.[159] Spraying the cervix with lidocaine 10% also improves comfort.[160] Topical lidocaine gel may reduce need for dilation with IUD placement but does not significantly reduce discomfort.[126,127] Misoprostol does not reduce pain or facilitate IUD placement for nulliparous women.[159]

Women Who are Breastfeeding

IUDs can be placed immediately after delivery of the placenta. Be careful when placing an IUD for a breastfeeding mother as uterine perforation is six times more common than for those who are not breastfeeding.[161]

However, the absolute risk of perforation remains rare,[14] and breastfeeding is not a contraindication to IUD placement. Women who are concerned that they may experience difficulties initiating breastfeeding may choose to delay initiation of hormonal contraception until they are confident in their breastfeeding abilities.[162]

Individuals Who are Immunocompromised

IUD use appears safe and effective for people who are immunosuppressed due to organ transplantation,[163] autoimmune disease,[164] or HIV infection.[165] For all of these individuals, the benefits of IUD use generally outweigh the potential or known risks, including the risks associated with potential pregnancy. Risk of complications, including infection, when IUDs are used by HIV-infected individuals appear to be equivalent to IUD users without HIV.[166,167] Moreover, a randomized controlled trial found that clinical HIV disease progression was slower among CuT380A users than among those using hormonal contraception and that HIV-positive patients assigned to intrauterine contraception were half as likely to become pregnant as those assigned to hormonal contraception. [168]

Individuals with Heart Valve Abnormalities or Shunts

Intrauterine contraception may be used safely by individuals with cardiac disease and structural abnormalities.[153] The risk of infectious complications, such as bacterial endocarditis, following IUD placement or removal is negligible, even among those with heart valve abnormalities or shunts. No evidence suggests that antibiotic prophylaxis is warranted. Whether bacteremia may result from removal of an infected IUD is controversial; prophylaxis (with an antibiotic active against enterococci administered 1 hour before removal of the infected IUD) may therefore be reasonable for those with prosthetic heart valves or a history of cardiac transplantation.[169]

Individuals with Diabetes Mellitus

Intrauterine contraception has significant benefits for individuals with diabetes mellitus who are at increased risk of vascular disease and adverse birth outcomes if they conceive while glycemic control is poor.[153] Good evidence supports IUD use by individuals with either Type 1 or Type 2 diabetes.[170–173] A rigorous trial of 52 mg LNG IUD use by patients with Type 1 diabetes confirmed no adverse effect on glucose metabolism or insulin requirements.[174] Vascular complications are less common among patients with diabetes who use IUDs than injectable contraception or progestin-only pills.[175]

Individuals with a History of Breast Cancer

The CuT380A IUD is generally the preferred contraceptive option for patients with a history of breast cancer who desire future fertility or whose male partners are not interested in vasectomy. However, the LNG IUD may be preferable for patients being treated with tamoxifen, because tamoxifen induces endometrial hyperplasia which LNG reduces.[98,176] Individuals with a history of breast cancer who are considering using an LNG IUD should be counseled that one study reported that patients using an LNG IUD at the time they were diagnosed with breast cancer who did not have their IUD removed had an increased risk of recurrence compared to those who never used an IUD[177] (although this arguably is not the relevant comparison group[178] and many oncologists consider this an acceptable option for breast cancer patients).[179] However, more research is needed on any potential effects of an LNG IUD on breast cancer treatment and risk of recurrence.

In the general population, data on whether LNG IUD use is associated with breast cancer diagnosis is mixed. A Danish study found an age-adjusted risk difference of 16 additional breast cancer diagnoses per 100,000 woman-years of use of a LNG IUD compared to women who had never used hormonal contraception.[180] Similarly, a Finnish study found a slightly increased standardized incidence ratio for breast cancer among LNG IUD users.[104] However, a case-control study conducted in Germany and Finland found no association between LNG IUD use and breast cancer diagnosis.[105] Importantly, there is no data to suggest that LNG IUD use increases breast cancer mortality.[181]

Individuals at Risk of Sexually Transmitted Infections

Individuals who are at risk of acquiring STIs should be advised to use condoms but are generally still good candidates for IUD use.[153]

Individuals with a History of Venous Thromboembolism

All IUDs may be used safely by patients with a history of deep venous thrombosis and pulmonary embolism.[153] The 52 mg LNG IUD is preferred for individuals currently on chronic anticoagulation therapy to treat or prevent menorrhagia.[112–114] LNG IUDs, unlike hormonal contraception containing estrogen, are not associated with an increased risk of venous thrombosis,[182] even when used by patients with other vascular risk factors.[175]

Individuals with Prior Cesarean Delivery

Patients may safely use an IUD after cesarean section. IUDs can be placed easily at the time of cesarean delivery.[183] Misoprostol may facilitate

IUD placement for some patients previously delivered only by cesarean section,[130] but may cause side-effects.

Transgender and Gender Nonconforming Individuals

Transgender and gender nonconforming individuals may benefit from either a copper or LNG IUD for contraception; testosterone, which causes menstrual suppression, is teratogenic.[184] LNG IUDs, which reduce menstrual bleeding, may be preferred by transgender or gender nonconforming individuals who are not on testosterone and wish to suppress menses.

Counseling About IUDs

Let people handle and examine sample IUDs; many are surprised at how small and flexible IUDs are. Discussing the option of IUD self-removal may increase interest in IUD use among individuals with concerns that their clinicians may not respect their reproductive autonomy or that they may have poor access to health care in the future.[75] Be aware of common myths and misconceptions about IUDs (e.g., that the IUD can "float off" and lodge in distant parts of the body, such as heart and brain). Address these sensitively but directly. Use a checklist to remember to share important information with each of your patients, and ask patients to repeat important information back to you to confirm understanding. Give each new IUD user an identification card with the type of IUD placed, date of placement, and date replacement is recommended if continued use is desired.

Table 5-2 Myths and misconceptions about the IUD

Myth	Fact
IUDs must be used for years.	IUDs can be removed whenever the user desires and have been self-removed by many users.
IUDs are abortifacients.	IUDs prevent fertilization.
IUDs increase the risk of ectopic pregnancy.	IUDs significantly reduce the risk of an ectopic pregnancy compared with the risk if not using contraception or using a less effective contraceptive.
IUDs increase the risk of PID.	The risk of PID with IUD placement is very small and prophylactic antibiotics are not warranted.
IUDs should not be used by people who have not had a child.	IUDs can be easily placed for nulliparas, who have a rapid return of fertility after IUD removal.
IUDs increase the risk of sexually transmitted infections.	People who are at risk of acquiring STIs should be advised to use condoms but are generally still good IUD candidates.

Clinician Training

With appropriate training, IUDs can safely be placed by physicians, nurse practitioners, midwives, and physician assistants. Because IUD packaging and loading techniques vary, clinicians should receive training for each type of IUD they wish to offer patients. IUD placement should first be practiced with a model and then an adequate number of IUDs should be placed under supervision to demonstrate proficiency. Rather than an absolute number of insertions, credentialing should be based on a level of proficiency in different uterine positions and clinical situations.

Timing of IUD Placement

The copper IUD may be placed at any time during the menstrual cycle, provided a urine pregnancy test is negative.[185] An LNG IUD may be placed at any time during the menstrual cycle, provided reasonable assurance exists that the patient is not pregnant.[32] The U.S. CDC Selected Practice Recommendations state that a clinician can be reasonably sure a patient is not pregnant if she has no signs or symptoms of pregnancy and meets any of the following criteria[32]:

- Is ≤7 days from the first day of her last normal menses
- Has not had intercourse since her last normal menses
- Is using a reliable method of contraception correctly and consistently
- Is ≤7 days from induced or spontaneous abortion
- Is ≤4weeks post-partum
- Is ≤6 months post-partum, amenorrheic, and exclusively breast feeding

Testing for chlamydia, gonorrhea, and any other STI that may be indicated can be performed at the time of the IUD placement visit but is not required. Clients who wish to use an IUD should not have to make two clinic visits.[186] In the past, IUD placement during menstrual bleeding was suggested,[35,187] but this approach has no benefits and constrained clients' access to IUDs. Copper IUDs are immediately effective. A "backup" contraceptive should be used for 1 week after initiating use of an LNG IUD placed more than 7 days after the first day of the last menstrual period. No backup contraception is needed when an LNG IUD is placed immediately after abortion, miscarriage, delivery, or for a patient who had consistently been using another hormonal contraceptive. No published data support the necessity of waiting to resume normal activities such as exercise, sexual activity, tampon use, bathing and swimming.

Extensive clinical experience has shown the safety and feasibility of IUD placement immediately after abortion or delivery. A systematic review of randomized controlled trials of immediate post-abortion insertion showed low rates of perforation and pelvic inflammatory disease.[188] Immediate placement after first-trimester abortion is not associated with an increased rate of expulsion; however, continuation rates of IUDs at 6 months are significantly higher among patients who had immediate post-abortion placement compared with patients who delayed (94% vs. 83%) placement.[189] Insertion of IUDs after second-trimester abortion was associated with a slightly higher expulsion rate (7%); however, 54% of patients scheduled to return for delayed insertion after a second-trimester abortion did not return,[190] making provision of post-abortion IUDs an effective way to reduce rates of repeat induced abortion.[191,192]

Insertion of IUDs immediately after delivery is popular in many countries, and is offered in a growing number of U.S. maternity hospitals, as it is a highly cost-effective approach[193] to optimizing inter-pregnancy intervals. Expulsion rates are lowest when the IUD is placed within 10 minutes of the expulsion of the placenta, often referred to as postplacental insertion,[194] although expulsions appear to be higher with postpartum placement than with interval insertions (24% versus 4%), whether IUD placement was done by hand or with instruments. Expulsion of an IUD placed immediately postpartum appears more likely when the IUD contains LNG than copper (17% vs. 4%).[195]

Placement Technique

Review the IUD placement procedure with each patient. In general, a uterine cavity length of 6 cm to 10 cm leads to successful IUD use. IUDs may be placed in larger uterine cavities; however, less is known about the risks of IUD expulsion for these patients. Always place the IUD slowly and gently. Read and follow the manufacturer's instructions on placement (available online).

General Preparation

1. Perform a careful bimanual examination to identify the position and size of the uterus.
2. Many clinicians wash the cervix with an antiseptic, such as providone-iodine or chlorhexidine. However, no evidence supports this practice and its effect on bacterial colony counts in the endocervix is minimal.[196]
3. Although many people do not need anesthesia for IUD placement, lidocaine applied to the cervix (as a spray, gel, or injection)

may increase comfort during tenaculum placement.[159] A paracervical block is generally not indicated; however, it may be useful for those with a history of difficult or painful attempts at IUD placement or who require cervical dilation to facilitate insertion.

4. Gently place a tenaculum on the cervix. Apply traction to the tenaculum to stabilize the cervix and straighten the axis of the uterus.
5. Sound the uterus prior to placing the IUD. Advance the sound using the muscles in your fingers and wrist, not your elbow or shoulder.
6. Place the IUD at the fundus, remove the insertion tube and trim the threads so they extend 3 to 4 cm from the os and are long enough to curl up in the fornix.

CAUTION

Instrumentation of the cervical os may result in vasovagal reactions, including fainting. If a patient feels dizzy, nauseated, ringing in her ears, vision changes, or like she may faint, have her isometrically contract the muscles in her arms and hands to push blood back to the center of her body. Also consider wafting an alcohol swab under her nose, cooling the patient by removing extra blankets or placing a cool cloth on her forehead. Have the patient remain supine after IUD placement until she feels comfortable sitting up.

IUD REMOVAL

When removing an IUD, apply gentle, steady traction to the IUD threads using gloved hands. If this proves difficult, place a speculum and grasp the threads with a ring forceps. Most IUDs can be easily removed this way; if you cannot remove the IUD with gentle traction, a paracervical block may make the removal less painful. After placing the block, use a tenaculum to steady the cervix and straighten the anteversion or retroversion of the uterus and try again. If this technique does not work, dilate the cervix a small amount, and try again. If this is not successful, experienced clinicians may attempt removal with an alligator forceps or packing forceps: with transabdominal ultrasound guidance, grasp the IUD, twist and push gently upwards to dislodge the IUD and then attempt removal.

If the IUD threads are not visible or palpable, confirm the IUD is in the uterus with ultrasound. If it is, then try using an endocervical brush or small cotton swab to tease the threads out of the endocervical canal. If this is not successful, use of alligator forceps, packing forceps, or a manual vacuum aspirator with a size 6 cannula can help remove the IUD or bring the threads through the external cervical os. Administering a paracervical block before cervical manipulation can decrease pain before attempting to remove a "stringless IUD". If this is insufficient to control pain, consider placing an osmotic dilator overnight or using 400 mcg of misoprostol to dilate the cervix.

Rarely, on removal, an IUD is found not to be intact. When this happens, consider uterine manual vacuum aspiration with a size 6 cannula to remove the retained fragment.[197] Alternatively, obtain an abdominal x-ray to confirm that the fragment is retained; dislodged fragments may be spontaneously expelled.

People who desire pregnancy may attempt to conceive immediately after IUD removal.

Timing of IUD Removal for Perimenopausal Patients

Copper IUDs can be removed one year after the last menstrual period. Because LNG IUDs can cause amenorrhea, it can be difficult to identify when a patient has entered menopause. As the average age of menopause in the US is 51, consider removing an LNG IUD for those over 51 years of age. However, LNG IUDs may be safely left in place after menopause and provide protection from endometrial proliferation for patients using estrogen for menopausal symptoms.[198]

MANAGING PROBLEMS AND FOLLOW-UP

Routine follow-up examination after IUD placement is not required; however, some clinicians offer a follow-up visit approximately 1 month after IUD placement to check that the IUD is in place and that no signs of infection are evident. Further routine visits are not required,[199,200] but encourage IUD users to return at any time that they have problems, questions, or concerns. In particular, counsel IUD users to visit when they cannot feel IUD threads that were previously palpable, the threads seem too long, or the IUD (and not just the thread) is palpable in the cervix. Counseling about the expected changes in bleeding patterns before IUD placement may enhance tolerance of the IUD and anticipated side effects. Unexpected changes in bleeding patterns or changes that are not tolerable to the patient should be evaluated.

INTERMENSTRUAL BLEEDING, SPOTTING, OR EXCESSIVE MENSTRUAL FLOW

Copper IUD users should be counseled to expect some changes in their menstrual bleeding patterns; initial difficulties with bleeding and pain improve for many people after their first 2 months of use of a copper IUD.[122] Use of nonsteroidal anti-inflammatory drugs (NSAIDs), such as naproxen taken twice daily, can reduce excessive menstrual flow as well as dysmenorrhea.[201] Trials have not demonstrated the superiority of one NSAID product over another. Because local prostaglandin production is involved with excessive bleeding, any prostaglandin synthetase inhibitor should help; in contrast, aspirin and acetaminophen do not. If hemoglobin levels drop, consider oral iron supplementation. Patients with persistent heavy menses and dysmenorrhea may consider replacing their copper IUD with an LNG IUD.

Individuals initiating use of an LNG IUD should also be counseled to expect changes in their menses. For most users, the number of bleeding and spotting days decreases considerably after the first 3 months of use. When this bleeding is problematic, use of naproxen (500 mg twice daily for the first 5 days of each month) can be helpful.[202] Other therapies that have been used to manage irregular bleeding induced by progestin-only contraceptives include estrogen (or a combined hormonal contraceptive), tamoxifen, tranexamic acid, mifepristone combined with an estrogen, and doxycycline.[203]

New onset of postcoital, unscheduled or heavy bleeding in an IUD user may indicate IUD expulsion or pregnancy (intrauterine or ectopic), and so should be promptly evaluated. Persistent abnormal bleeding also requires clinical evaluation because not all nuisance bleeding can be attributed to the IUD. Other gynecologic disorders, such as cervicitis, cervical cancer, or endometrial polyps, may be responsible. In addition, bleeding may accompany endometritis. If there is concern of endometrial hyperplasia with use of a TCu380A, biopsy the endometrium using a pipelle with the TCu380A left in place.

Chlamydia or Gonorrhea Infection Among IUD Users

If an IUD user acquires chlamydia or gonorrhea infection, standard treatment for her and her partner(s) is indicated with the IUD in place. No evidence suggests that an IUD should be removed in this setting,[204] although concomitant condom use should be encouraged.

Pelvic Inflammatory Disease (PID)

Upper genital tract infections need prompt treatment. The CDC has published standard criteria for diagnosing PID, as well as treatment recommendations,[205] and recommends treating PID without IUD removal.[32] (See www.cdc.gov/std/treatment.) However, data on the management of PID with an IUD in place are limited.[206] If no clinical improvement is seen within 48–72 hours of antibiotic treatment, consider removal of the

IUD and sending the IUD for culture to assess for possible antibiotic resistant organisms. Individuals who wish to have their IUD removed after being diagnosed with PID should initiate antibiotics prior to removal to decrease the possibility of bacteremia. Those who wish to have an IUD replaced after treatment of PID should wait until complete resolution of the infection.

Abnormal Cervical Cytology

IUD users do not have an increased risk of abnormal cervical cytology. If a patient with an IUD requires treatment of a cervical abnormality, the IUD may be left in place. To preserve the IUD threads, loop electrosurgical excision procedures (LEEP) may be performed in two segments, or LEEP may be performed after pushing the threads into the cervical canal (and later bringing the threads back down with a cytobrush).

Actinomyces-Like Organisms Seen on Papanicolaou Smear

An asymptomatic IUD user who has "Actinomyces-like organisms" reported on Papanicolaou smear should be informed that this is a common finding of limited clinical significance. If she is asymptomatic, nothing more need be done; the IUD may be left safely in place, and subsequent Papanicolaou smears can follow standard timelines. Actinomyces-like organisms on Papanicolaou smear do not predict clinical illness. Actinomyces species are normal inhabitants of the female genital tract; vaginal culture is not helpful in diagnosing actinomycosis.[207]

If the IUD user is symptomatic (pelvic pain, discharge, or fever), the device should be removed after initiating antibiotics and the IUD should be sent for culture. The reason for recommending IUD removal when individuals are symptomatic is that, unlike usual gynecological pathogens, this genus of bacterium preferentially grows on foreign bodies. Pelvic actinomycosis is a very rare, serious, and poorly understood infection. Actinomyces species are sensitive to a variety of antibiotics, including penicillin.

Thread Problems

Missing threads may signal an unsuspected perforation or spontaneous expulsion; alternatively, some threads ascend into the endometrial cavity and descend without known explanation. Ultrasound examination can quickly confirm the presence of the IUD within the endometrial cavity.

An IUD that is in the endometrial cavity may be left in place even if the threads are not palpable or visible; no additional surveillance or follow-up is required. However, the patient should be informed that, when removal is desired, this should be done by a clinician experienced in "stringless IUD" removal. If the IUD is not visible in the uterus with ultrasound, perform an abdominal X-ray to determine whether the IUD has been expelled or perforated into the peritoneal cavity. When considering potential causes of missing threads, remember the possibility of (a) expulsion, (b) an intrauterine pregnancy, (c) an IUD in the uterus with coiled or short threads, (d) IUD embedment in the uterine wall, and (e) IUD perforation.

If the male partner complains of penile discomfort from the thread, one option is to cut the threads shorter to the level of the endocervical canal. This may eliminate the barb-like sensation and obviate the need to replace the IUD. Avoid trimming the threads too short with IUD placement to prevent this. If the threads are too long, simply trim them.

Expulsion

Some IUD expulsions are asymptomatic. Users with previous amenorrhea on an LNG IUD who experience return to normal menstrual cycles should be evaluated for asymptomatic IUD expulsion. At other times, expulsions present with symptoms. IUD users complaining of cramping, vaginal discharge, intermenstrual or postcoital bleeding or spotting, male or female dyspareunia, or lengthened or newly absent strings should be evaluated for partial or complete expulsion. The diagnosis of complete expulsion is confirmed by an ultrasound showing that the IUD is not in the uterus, followed by x-ray demonstrating that the IUD is not in the abdomen or pelvis. Individuals who have expelled an IUD should be offered emergency contraception if needed. A new IUD can be placed at the time expulsion is diagnosed.

Malpositioned IUDs

On occasion, an ultrasound done for unrelated purposes will diagnose a displaced or malpositioned IUD. An IUD is considered well-positioned if the top of the device is in the uterine fundus. An IUD is considered malpositioned if any part extends into the cervical canal, if it is positioned within the lower uterine segment, or if it is rotated. Approximately 10% of IUDs are incidentally found to be malpositioned.[208] When a malpositioned IUD is identified on ultrasound, assess for symptoms such as cramping, heavy menstrual bleeding, or new intermenstrual bleeding or spotting. If the patient is asymptomatic and the IUD is in the lower uterus (not the cervix), removal is not necessary.

PERFORATION

If a copper IUD is found outside the endometrial cavity, it should be removed promptly, because copper in the peritoneal cavity induces adhesion formation, which may involve the adnexa, omentum, and bowel. Laparoscopy is the preferred approach for removal. In contrast, nonmedicated and progestin-bearing devices do not evoke similar intraperitoneal adhesions. No clear medical indication exists for removal of IUDs that do not contain copper,[209] although this is commonly done.

PREGNANCY WITH AN IUD IN PLACE

If an individual becomes pregnant with an IUD in place, confirm the pregnancy location (intrauterine or ectopic) as soon as possible. If she wishes to continue the pregnancy, she should be advised that she has an increased risk of adverse pregnancy outcomes, including spontaneous miscarriage or preterm delivery, septic abortion and chorioamnionitis, even after removal of the IUD.[210] Regardless of her plans for the pregnancy, early removal reduces the risk of these adverse outcomes.[35,211] Delaying IUD removal may increase the difficulty of removal as the uterus grows and the threads are drawn upwards.

If the IUD threads are not visible in the first trimester, removal can be attempted under ultrasound guidance using alligator or packing forceps or hysteroscopy;[212] consider antibiotic prophylaxis against infection with this approach. If the threads are not visible in the early second trimester, depending on the IUD location relative to the pregnancy, consider attempting removal with forceps under ultrasound guidance or simply leaving the IUD in place.[213] The IUD may be removed at the time of surgical abortion. Removal is required before mifepristone administration for medication abortion. An IUD left in place during pregnancy carries no known risk of teratogenesis, although data are insufficient regarding the risk of fetal levonorgestrel exposure.[210]

USER INSTRUCTIONS FOR INTRAUTERINE CONTRACEPTION†

- Many people have cramps for a few days after IUD placement. This is normal. If you want to take something for pain, products that contain ibuprofen or naproxen are best.

†These instructions are intended to guide providers in educating patients in how to use their method.

- Expect some spotting in the first few weeks after IUD placement. This is normal. You can use pads or tampons.
- When you feel ready, you can start having sex. Use condoms for protection from STIs as your IUD will not protect you from these infections. You can also return to other activities, such as exercising, taking baths, swimming, and using tampons, as soon as you feel ready.
- If you want, you can check to make sure that you can feel your IUD threads about once a month and whenever you have had a heavy period. Contact your clinician if you cannot feel IUD threads that you were previously able to feel, and be sure to use another method of birth control until you have a clinician check whether your IUD is still in your uterus.
- Call your clinician right away if you
  — Can feel part of the IUD, and not just the threads
  — Have pain or bleeding with sex
  — Have unusually heavy bleeding from your vagina
  — Think you are pregnant
  — Have been, or might have been, exposed to an STI
  — Have unusual pelvic pain, cramping, or soreness in your abdomen
  — Have unexplained fever or chills
- If you are not happy with your IUD, talk to your clinician about ways to reduce your symptoms. There are lots of contraceptive options and your clinician can help you find the one that best meets your current needs.

Copper IUD (ParaGard)

- Works as soon as it is placed; no backup method is needed.
- During the first 1 to 3 months that you use ParaGard, you may have some irregular bleeding or spotting and your next few menstrual periods may be longer, heavier, and you may have more cramping than usual. Consider using ibuprofen or naproxen to reduce this cramping.
- Call your health care provider right away if your period is late and you think you might be pregnant.
- Discuss with your healthcare provider the pros and cons of replacing your ParaGard after 12 years.

LNG IUDs

- Use condoms or another contraceptive method (i.e., a "backup method") for 7 days after your LNG IUD is placed. If the day your LNG IUD is placed is less than one week since the first day of your last menstrual period, a backup method is not needed.
- You may have some irregular bleeding or spotting in addition to your monthly period while you use an LNG IUD, especially during the first 3 to 6 months. If you find this bothersome, talk to your clinician about ways to decrease your bleeding.
- Some people stop having periods right after the IUD is placed, while others notice that their periods get lighter with time. Many people eventually stop having their period—this is perfectly safe. It doesn't mean that you are pregnant.
- Side effects are most common during the first 3 months of IUD use and usually subside over time. You may experience any or none of the following: menstrual changes, lower abdominal pain, back pain, breast tenderness, headache, mood changes, nausea, acne.
- Discuss with your healthcare provider the suggested timing for replacing your LNG IUD.

Author Disclosures—Dean: none. Schwarz: none.

References

1. Buhling KJ, Zite NB, Lotke P, Black K, Group IW. Worldwide use of intrauterine contraception: a review. Contraception 2014;89:162–73.
2. Mosher WD, Martinez GM, Chandra A, Abma JC, Willson SJ. Use of contraception and use of family planning services in the United States: 1982–2002. Advance data 2004:1–36.
3. Kavanaugh ML, Jerman J, Finer LB. Changes in Use of Long-Acting Reversible Contraceptive Methods Among U.S. Women, 2009-2012. Obstet Gynecol 2015;126:917–27.
4. Branum AM, Jones J. Trends in long-acting reversible contraception use among U.S. women aged 15–44. NCHS Data Brief 2015:1–8.
5. Stern LF, Simons HR, Kohn JE, Debevec EJ, Morfesis JM, Patel AA. Differences in contraceptive use between family planning providers and the U.S. population: results of a nationwide survey. Contraception 2015;91:464–9.
6. Stanwood NL, Garrett JM, Konrad TR. Obstetrician-gynecologists and the intrauterine device: a survey of attitudes and practice. Obstet Gynecol 2002;99:275–80.
7. Hubacher D, Cheng D. Intrauterine devices and reproductive health: American women in feast and famine. Contraception 2004;69:437–46.
8. Sivin I. Another look at the Dalkon Shield: meta-analysis underscores its problems. Contraception 1993;48:1–12.
9. Hubacher D, Grimes DA, Gemzell-Danielsson K. Pitfalls of research linking the intrauterine device to pelvic inflammatory disease. Obstet Gynecol 2013;121:1091–8.
10. Farr G, Amatya R, Acosta M, Ekwempu C, Kisninci H. Clinical performance of the TCu 380A and Lippes Loop IUDs in three developing countries. Contraception 1995;52:17–22.

11. Randic L, Haller H, Perovic M, Farr G. The effect of adding copper onto Lippes Loop IUDs: results from a ten-year study in Yugoslavia. Contraception 1991;43:229–39.
12. Newton J, Szontagh F, Lebech P, Rowe P. A collaborative study of the progesterone intrauterine device (Progestasert). The World Health Organization Task Force on Methods for the Regulation of Implantation. Contraception 1979;19:575–89.
13. Jatlaoui TC, Riley HE, Curtis KM. The safety of intrauterine devices among young women: a systematic review. Contraception 2017;95:17–39.
14. Heinemann K, Reed S, Moehner S, Minh TD. Risk of uterine perforation with levonorgestrel-releasing and copper intrauterine devices in the European Active Surveillance Study on Intrauterine Devices. Contraception 2015;91:274–9.
15. Ciet P, Litmanovich DE. MR safety issues particular to women. Magn Reson Imaging C 2015;23:59–67.
16. Soderstrom RM. Progestasert intrauterine progesterone contraceptive system. In: Proceedings from the Fourth International Conference on IUDs; Editors: Bardin CW and Mishell DR. 1994; Boston, Massachusetts: Butterworth-Heinemann. p. 319–27.
17. Long-term reversible contraception. Twelve years of experience with the TCu380A and TCu220C. Contraception 1997;56:341–52.
18. Sivin I. Utility and drawbacks of continuous use of a copper T IUD for 20 years. Contraception 2007;75:S70-5.
19. Rowe P, Farley T, Peregoudov A, et al. Safety and efficacy in parous women of a 52-mg levonorgestrel-medicated intrauterine device: a 7-year randomized comparative study with the TCu380A. Contraception 2016;93:498–506.
20. Gemzell-Danielsson K, Apter D, Dermout S, et al. Evaluation of a new, low-dose levonorgestrel intrauterine contraceptive system over 5 years of use. Eur J of Obstet Gyn R B 2016;210:22–8.
21. Apter D, Gemzell-Danielsson K, Hauck B, Rosen K, Zurth C. Pharmacokinetics of two low-dose levonorgestrel-releasing intrauterine systems and effects on ovulation rate and cervical function: pooled analyses of phase II and III studies. Fertil Steril 2014;101:1656–62 e1–4.
22. Mirena package insert. 2016 December 21. (Accessed March 10, 2017, at www.labeling.bayerhealthcare.com/html/products/pi/Mirena_PI.pdf.)
23. Mejia M, McNicholas C, Madden T, Peipert JF. Association of baseline bleeding pattern on amenorrhea with levonorgestrel intrauterine system use. Contraception 2016;94:556–60.
24. Fan G, Kang S, Ren M, et al. A single-arm phase III study exploring the efficacy and safety of LNG-IUS 8, a low-dose levonorgestrel intrauterine contraceptive system (total content 13.5 mg), in an Asia-Pacific population. Contraception 2017;95:371–7.
25. Liletta Package insert. 2015 February. Accessed March 10, 2017, at www.pi.actavis.com/data_stream.asp?product_group=1960&p=pi&language=E.
26. Kyleena Levonorgestrel-releasing intrauterine system (19.5mg). 2016. Available at www.omr.bayer.ca/omr/online/kyleena-pm-en.pdf.
27. Sivin I GF, Schmidt F, Waldman SN. The Copper T 380 intrauterine device : a summary of scientific data New York: The Population Council; 1992.
28. Application Number 21–225: Medical review of Mirena. Center for Drug Research and Evaluation; 2000.
29. Eisenberg DL, Schreiber CA, Turok DK, et al. Three-year efficacy and safety of a new 52-mg levonorgestrel-releasing intrauterine system. Contraception 2015;92:10–6.
30. Gemzell-Danielsson K, Apter D, Dermout S, et al. Evaluation of a new, low-dose levonorgestrel intrauterine contraceptive system over 5 years of use. Eur J Obstet Gyn R B 2017;210:22–8.
31. Heinemann K, Reed S, Moehner S, Minh TD. Comparative contraceptive effectiveness of levonorgestrel-releasing and copper intrauterine devices: the European Active Surveillance Study for Intrauterine Devices. Contraception 2015;91:280–3.
32. Curtis KM, Jatlaoui TC, Tepper NK, et al. U.S. selected practice recommendations for contraceptive use, 2016. MMWR Recomm Rep 2016;65:1–66.

33. Fage SW, Faurschou A, Thyssen JP. Copper hypersensitivity. Contact Dermatitis 2014;71:191–201.
34. De la Cruz D, Cruz A, Arteaga M, Castillo L, Tovalin H. Blood copper levels in Mexican users of the T380A IUD. Contraception 2005;72:122–5.
35. World Health Organization. Mechanism of action, safety and efficacy of intrauterine devices: technical report series 753. Geneva: World Health Organization; 1987.
36. Sivin I, Schmidt F. Effectiveness of IUDs: a review. Contraception 1987;36:55–84.
37. Sivin I, Stern J, Coutinho E, et al. Prolonged intrauterine contraception: a seven-year randomized study of the levonorgestrel 20 mcg/day (LNg 20) and the Copper T380 Ag IUDS. Contraception 1991;44:473–80.
38. The TCu380A, TCu220C, multiload 250 and Nova T IUDS at 3,5 and 7 years of use—results from three randomized multicentre trials. World Health Organization. Special Programme of Research, Development and Research Training in Human Reproduction: Task Force on the Safety and Efficacy of Fertility Regulating Methods. Contraception 1990;42:141–58.
39. O'Brien PA, Kulier R, Helmerhorst FM, Usher-Patel M, d'Arcangues C. Copper-containing, framed intrauterine devices for contraception: a systematic review of randomized controlled trials. Contraception 2008;77:318–27.
40. French R, Cowan F, Mansour D, et al. Hormonally impregnated intrauterine systems (IUSs), versus other forms of reversible contraceptives as effective methods of preventing pregnancy. Cochrane Database Syst Rev 2001:CD001776.
41. Nilsson CG, Lahteenmaki PL, Luukkainen T, Robertson DN. Sustained intrauterine release of levonorgestrel over five years. Fertil Steril 1986;45:805–7.
42. Liletta NDA Number: 206229 Clinical Pharmacology Review. US FDA, 2014. Available at www.fda.gov/downloads/Drugs/DevelopmentApprovalProcess/DevelopmentResources/UCM446653.pdf.
43. Creinin MD, Jansen R, Starr RM, Gobburu J, Gopalakrishnan M, Olariu A. Levonorgestrel release rates over 5 years with the Liletta(R) 52-mg intrauterine system. Contraception 2016;94:353–6.
44. Basaraba CN, Westhoff CL, Pike MC, Nandakumar R, Cremers S. Estimating systemic exposure to levonorgestrel from an oral contraceptive. Contraception 2017;95:398–404
45. Shreffler KM, McQuillan J, Greil AL, Johnson DR. Surgical sterilization, regret, and race: contemporary patterns. Soc Sci Res 2015;50:31–45.
46. Luukkainen T, Allonen H, Haukkamaa M, et al. Effective contraception with the levonorgestrel-releasing intrauterine device: 12-month report of a European multicenter study. Contraception 1987;36:169–79.
47. Sivin I, Stern J, Diaz J, et al. Two years of intrauterine contraception with levonorgestrel and with copper: a randomized comparison of the TCu 380Ag and levonorgestrel 20 mcg/day devices. Contraception 1987;35:245–55.
48. Sivin I, el Mahgoub S, McCarthy T, et al. Long-term contraception with the levonorgestrel 20 mcg/day (LNg 20) and the copper T 380Ag intrauterine devices: a five-year randomized study. Contraception 1990;42:361–78.
49. Andersson K, Odlind V, Rybo G. Levonorgestrel-releasing and copper-releasing (Nova T) IUDs during five years of use: a randomized comparative trial. Contraception 1994;49:56–72.
50. Sivin I, Stern J. Health during prolonged use of levonorgestrel 20 micrograms/d and the copper TCu 380Ag intrauterine contraceptive devices: a multicenter study. International Committee for Contraception Research (ICCR). Fertil Steril 1994;61:70–7.
51. Barbosa I, Olsson SE, Odlind V, Goncalves T, Coutinho E. Ovarian function after seven years' use of a levonorgestrel IUD. Adv Contracept 1995;11:85–95.
52. Xiao B, Zeng T, Wu S, Sun H, Xiao N. Effect of levonorgestrel-releasing intrauterine device on hormonal profile and menstrual pattern after long-term use. Contraception 1995;51:359–65.
53. Hidalgo MM, Hidalgo-Regina C, Bahamondes MV, Monteiro I, Petta CA, Bahamondes L. Serum levonorgestrel levels and endometrial thickness during extended use of the levonorgestrel-releasing intrauterine system. Contraception 2009;80:84–9.

54. Gemzell-Danielsson K, Apter D, Hauck B, et al. The effect of age, parity and body mass index on the efficacy, safety, placement and user satisfaction associated with two low-dose levonorgestrel intrauterine contraceptive systems: subgroup analyses of data from a phase III trial. PloS one 2015;10:e0135309.
55. Rivera R, Yacobson I, Grimes D. The mechanism of action of hormonal contraceptives and intrauterine contraceptive devices. Am J Obstet Gynecol 1999;181:1263–9.
56. El-Habashi M, El-Sahwi S, Gawish S, Osman M. Effect of Lippes loop on sperm recovery from human fallopian tubes. Contraception 1980;22:549–55.
57. Ortiz ME, Croxatto HB, Bardin CW. Mechanisms of action of intrauterine devices. Obstet Gynecol Surv 1996;51:S42–51.
58. Sagiroglu N. Phagocytosis of spermatozoa in the uterine cavity of woman using intrauterine device. Int J Fertil 1971;16:1–14.
59. Ammala M, Nyman T, Strengell L, Rutanen EM. Effect of intrauterine contraceptive devices on cytokine messenger ribonucleic acid expression in the human endometrium. Fertil Steril 1995;63:773–8.
60. Haliloglu B, Celik A, Ilter E, Bozkurt S, Ozekici U. Comparison of uterine artery blood flow with levonorgestrel intrauterine system and copper intrauterine device. Contraception 2011;83:578–81.
61. Shanmugasundaram U, Hilton JF, Critchfield JW, et al. Effects of the levonorgestrel-releasing intrauterine device on the immune microenvironment of the human cervix and endometrium. Am J Reprod Immunol 2016;76:137–48.
62. Achilles SL, Creinin MD, Stoner KA, Chen BA, Meyn L, Hillier SL. Changes in genital tract immune cell populations after initiation of intrauterine contraception. Am J Obstet Gynecol 2014;211:489 e1–9.
63. Segal SJ, Alvarez-Sanchez F, Adejuwon CA, Brache de Mejia V, Leon P, Faundes A. Absence of chorionic gonadotropin in sera of women who use intrauterine devices. Fertil Steril 1985;44:214–8.
64. Wilcox AJ, Weinberg CR, Armstrong EG, Canfield RE. Urinary human chorionic gonadotropin among intrauterine device users: detection with a highly specific and sensitive assay. Fertil Steril 1987;47:265–9.
65. Videla-Rivero L, Etchepareborda JJ, Kesseru E. Early chorionic activity in women bearing inert IUD, copper IUD and levonorgestrel-releasing IUD. Contraception 1987;36:217–26.
66. Alvarez F, Brache V, Fernandez E, et al. New insights on the mode of action of intrauterine contraceptive devices in women. Fertil Steril 1988;49:768–73.
67. Ganacharya S, Bhattoa HP, Batar I. Ectopic pregnancy among non-medicated and copper-containing intrauterine device users: a 10-year follow-up. Eur J Obstet Gyn R B 2003;111:78–82.
68. Winner B, Peipert JF, Zhao Q, et al. Effectiveness of long-acting reversible contraception. N Engl J Med 2012;366:1998–2007.
69. Peterson HB, Xia Z, Hughes JM, Wilcox LS, Tylor LR, Trussell J. The risk of pregnancy after tubal sterilization: findings from the U.S. Collaborative Review of Sterilization. Am J Obstet Gynecol 1996;174:1161–8; discussion 8–70.
70. Tocce K, Sheeder J, Python J, Teal SB. Long acting reversible contraception in postpartum adolescents: early initiation of etonogestrel implant is superior to IUDs in the outpatient setting. Journal of pediatric and adolescent gynecology 2012;25:59–63.
71. Nelson A, Apter D, Hauck B, et al. Two low-dose levonorgestrel intrauterine contraceptive systems: a randomized controlled trial. Obstet Gynecol 2013;122:1205–13.
72. Foster DG, Rostovtseva DP, Brindis CD, Biggs MA, Hulett D, Darney PD. Cost savings from the provision of specific methods of contraception in a publicly funded program. Am J Public Health 2009;99:446–51.
73. Crespi S, Kerrigan M, Sood V. Budget impact analysis of 8 hormonal contraceptive options. Am J Manag Care 2013;19:e249–55.
74. Dottino JA, Hasselblad V, Secord AA, Myers ER, Chino J, Havrilesky LJ. Levonorgestrel intrauterine device as an endometrial cancer prevention strategy in obese women: a cost-effectiveness analysis. Obstet Gynecol 2016;128:747–53.

75. Foster DG, Grossman D, Turok DK, et al. Interest in and experience with IUD self-removal. Contraception 2014;90:54–9.
76. Backman T, Huhtala S, Blom T, Luoto R, Rauramo I, Koskenvuo M. Length of use and symptoms associated with premature removal of the levonorgestrel intrauterine system: a nation-wide study of 17,360 users. BJOG 2000;107:335–9.
77. Jensen JT, Nelson AL, Costales AC. Subject and clinician experience with the levonorgestrel-releasing intrauterine system. Contraception 2008;77:22–9.
78. Hubacher D, Reyes V, Lillo S, et al. Preventing copper intrauterine device removals due to side effects among first-time users: randomized trial to study the effect of prophylactic ibuprofen. Hum Reprod 2006;21:1467–72.
79. Peipert JF, Zhao Q, Allsworth JE, et al. Continuation and satisfaction of reversible contraception. Obstet Gynecol 2011;117:1105–13.
80. O'Neil-Callahan M, Peipert JF, Zhao Q, Madden T, Secura G. Twenty-four-month continuation of reversible contraception. Obstet Gynecol 2013;122:1083–91.
81. Diedrich JT, Zhao Q, Madden T, Secura GM, Peipert JF. Three-year continuation of reversible contraception. Am J Obstet Gynecol 2015;213:662 e1–8.
82. Diedrich JT, Madden T, Zhao Q, Peipert JF. Long-term utilization and continuation of intrauterine devices. Am J Obstet Gynecol 2015;213:822 e1–6.
83. Ory HW. Ectopic pregnancy and intrauterine contraceptive devices: new perspectives. The Women's Health Study. Obstet Gynecol 1981;57:137–44.
84. Sivin I. Dose- and age-dependent ectopic pregnancy risks with intrauterine contraception. Obstet Gynecol 1991;78:291–8.
85. Toivonen J. Intrauterine contraceptive device and pelvic inflammatory disease. Ann Med 1993;25:171–3.
86. Toivonen J, Luukkainen T, Allonen H. Protective effect of intrauterine release of levonorgestrel on pelvic infection: three years' comparative experience of levonorgestrel- and copper-releasing intrauterine devices. Obstet Gynecol 1991;77:261–4.
87. Turok DK, Eisenberg DL, Teal SB, Keder LM, Creinin MD. A prospective assessment of pelvic infection risk following same-day sexually transmitted infection testing and levonorgestrel intrauterine system placement. Am J Obstet Gynecol 2016;215:599 e1–e6.
88. Roura E, Travier N, Waterboer T, et al. The influence of hormonal factors on the risk of developing cervical cancer and pre-cancer: results from the EPIC Cohort. PloS one 2016;11:e0147029.
89. Castellsague X, Diaz M, Vaccarella S, et al. Intrauterine device use, cervical infection with human papillomavirus, and risk of cervical cancer: a pooled analysis of 26 epidemiological studies. Lancet Oncol 2011;12:1023–31.
90. Guleria K, Agarwal N, Mishra K, Gulati R, Mehendiratta A. Evaluation of endometrial steroid receptors and cell mitotic activity in women using copper intrauterine device: Can Cu-T prevent endometrial cancer? J Obstet Gynaecol Res 2004;30:181–7.
91. Curtis KM, Marchbanks PA, Peterson HB. Neoplasia with use of intrauterine devices. Contraception 2007;75:S60–9.
92. Gardner FJ, Konje JC, Bell SC, et al. Prevention of tamoxifen induced endometrial polyps using a levonorgestrel releasing intrauterine system long-term follow-up of a randomised control trial. Gynecol Oncol 2009;114:452–6.
93. Depot-medroxyprogesterone acetate (DMPA) and risk of endometrial cancer. The WHO Collaborative Study of Neoplasia and Steroid Contraceptives. Int J Cancer 1991;49: 186–90.
94. Suvanto-Luukkonen E, Kauppila A. The levonorgestrel intrauterine system in menopausal hormone replacement therapy: five-year experience. Fertil Steril 1999;72:161–3.
95. Suhonen S, Holmstrom T, Lahteenmaki P. Three-year follow-up of the use of a levonorgestrel-releasing intrauterine system in hormone replacement therapy. Acta Obstet Gynecol Scand 1997;76:145–50.
96. Varila E, Wahlstrom T, Rauramo I. A 5-year follow-up study on the use of a levonorgestrel intrauterine system in women receiving hormone replacement therapy. Fertil Steril 2001;76:969–73.

97. Gardner FJ, Konje JC, Abrams KR, et al. Endometrial protection from tamoxifen-stimulated changes by a levonorgestrel-releasing intrauterine system: a randomised controlled trial. Lancet 2000;356:1711–7.
98. Schwarz EB, Hess R, Trussell J. Contraception for cancer survivors. J Gen Intern Med 2009;24 Suppl 2:S401–6.
99. Buttini MJ, Jordan SJ, Webb PM. The effect of the levonorgestrel releasing intrauterine system on endometrial hyperplasia: an Australian study and systematic review. Aust N Z J Obstet Gynaecol 2009;49:316–22.
100. Dhar KK, NeedhiRajan T, Koslowski M, Woolas RP. Is levonorgestrel intrauterine system effective for treatment of early endometrial cancer? Report of four cases and review of the literature. Gynecol Oncol 2005;97:924–7.
101. Varma R, Soneja H, Bhatia K, et al. The effectiveness of a levonorgestrel-releasing intrauterine system (LNG-IUS) in the treatment of endometrial hyperplasia—A long-term follow-up study. Eur J Obstet Gyn R B 2008;139:169–75.
102. Bahamondes L, Ribeiro-Huguet P, de Andrade KC, Leon-Martins O, Petta CA. Levonorgestrel-releasing intrauterine system (Mirena) as a therapy for endometrial hyperplasia and carcinoma. Acta Obstet Gynecol Scand 2003;82:580–2.
103. Soini T, Hurskainen R, Grenman S, Maenpaa J, Paavonen J, Pukkala E. Impact of levonorgestrel-releasing intrauterine system use on the cancer risk of the ovary and fallopian tube. Acta Oncologica 2016;55:1281–4.
104. Soini T, Hurskainen R, Grenman S, Maenpaa J, Paavonen J, Pukkala E. Cancer risk in women using the levonorgestrel-releasing intrauterine system in Finland. Obstet Gynecol 2014;124:292–9.
105. Dinger J, Bardenheuer K, Minh TD. Levonorgestrel-releasing and copper intrauterine devices and the risk of breast cancer. Contraception 2011;83:211–7.
106. Cleland K, Zhu H, Goldstuck N, Cheng L, Trussell J. The efficacy of intrauterine devices for emergency contraception: a systematic review of 35 years of experience. Hum Reprod 2012;27:1994–2000.
107. Turok DK, Sanders JN, Thompson IS, Royer PA, Eggebroten J, Gawron LM. Preference for and efficacy of oral levonorgestrel for emergency contraception with concomitant placement of a levonorgestrel IUD: a prospective cohort study. Contraception 2016;93:526–32.
108. ACOG committee opinion. No. 337: Noncontraceptive uses of the levonorgestrel intrauterine system. Obstet Gynecol 2006;107:1479–82.
109. Ronnerdag M, Odlind V. Health effects of long-term use of the intrauterine levonorgestrel-releasing system. A follow-up study over 12 years of continuous use. Acta Obstet Gynecol Scand 1999;78:716–21.
110. Gemzell-Danielsson K, Schellschmidt I, Apter D. A randomized, phase II study describing the efficacy, bleeding profile, and safety of two low-dose levonorgestrel-releasing intrauterine contraceptive systems and Mirena. Fertil Steril 2012;97: 616–22 e1–3.
111. Hidalgo M, Bahamondes L, Perrotti M, Diaz J, Dantas-Monteiro C, Petta C. Bleeding patterns and clinical performance of the levonorgestrel-releasing intrauterine system (Mirena) up to two years. Contraception 2002;65:129–32.
112. Kadir RA, Chi C. Levonorgestrel intrauterine system: bleeding disorders and anticoagulant therapy. Contraception 2007;75:S123–9.
113. Kilic S, Yuksel B, Doganay M, et al. The effect of levonorgestrel-releasing intrauterine device on menorrhagia in women taking anticoagulant medication after cardiac valve replacement. Contraception 2009;80:152–7.
114. Lukes AS, Reardon B, Arepally G. Use of the levonorgestrel-releasing intrauterine system in women with hemostatic disorders. Fertil Steril 2008;90:673–7.
115. Fedele L, Bianchi S, Raffaelli R, Portuese A, Dorta M. Treatment of adenomyosis-associated menorrhagia with a levonorgestrel-releasing intrauterine device. Fertil Steril 1997;68:426–9.

116. Grigorieva V, Chen-Mok M, Tarasova M, Mikhailov A. Use of a levonorgestrel-releasing intrauterine system to treat bleeding related to uterine leiomyomas. Fertil Steril 2003;79:1194–8.
117. Brown P, Farquhar C, Lethaby A, Sadler L, Johnson N. Cost-effectiveness analysis of levonorgestrel intrauterine system and thermal balloon ablation for heavy menstrual bleeding. BJOG 2006;113:797–803.
118. Shaw RW, Symonds IM, Tamizian O, Chaplain J, Mukhopadhyay S. Randomised comparative trial of thermal balloon ablation and levonorgestrel intrauterine system in patients with idiopathic menorrhagia. Aust N Z J Obstet Gynaecol 2007;47:335–40.
119. Hurskainen R, Teperi J, Rissanen P, et al. Clinical outcomes and costs with the levonorgestrel-releasing intrauterine system or hysterectomy for treatment of menorrhagia: randomized trial 5-year follow-up. JAMA 2004;291:1456–63.
120. Busfield RA, Farquhar CM, Sowter MC, et al. A randomized trial comparing the levonorgestrel intrauterine system and thermal balloon ablation for heavy menstrual bleeding. Obstet Gynecol Surv 2006;61:444–5.
121. Rivera R, Chen-Mok M, McMullen S. Analysis of client characteristics that may affect early discontinuation of the TCu-380A IUD. Contraception 1999;60:155–60.
122. Hubacher D, Chen PL, Park S. Side effects from the copper IUD: do they decrease over time? Contraception 2009;79:356–62.
123. Milsom I, Andersson K, Jonasson K, Lindstedt G, Rybo G. The influence of the Gyne-T 380S IUD on menstrual blood loss and iron status. Contraception 1995;52:175–9.
124. Nilsson CG, Lahteenmaki PL, Luukkainen T. Ovarian function in amenorrheic and menstruating users of a levonorgestrel-releasing intrauterine device. Fertil Steril 1984;41:52–5.
125. Xiao BL, Zhou LY, Zhang XL, Jia MC, Luukkainen T, Allonen H. Pharmacokinetic and pharmacodynamic studies of levonorgestrel-releasing intrauterine device. Contraception 1990;41:353–62.
126. Abbas AM, Abdellah MS, Khalaf M, et al. Effect of cervical lidocaine-prilocaine cream on pain perception during copper T380A intrauterine device insertion among parous women: A randomized double-blind controlled trial. Contraception 2017;95:251–6.
127. Rapkin RB, Achilles SL, Schwarz EB, et al. Self-administered lidocaine gel for intrauterine device insertion in nulliparous women: a randomized controlled trial. Obstet Gynecol 2016;128:621–8.
128. Zapata LB, Jatlaoui TC, Marchbanks PA, Curtis KM. Medications to ease intrauterine device insertion: a systematic review. Contraception 2016;94:739–59.
129. Bahamondes MV, Espejo-Arce X, Bahamondes L. Effect of vaginal administration of misoprostol before intrauterine contraceptive insertion following previous insertion failure: a double blind RCT. Hum Reprod 2015;30:1861–6.
130. Abdellah MS, Abbas AM, Hegazy AM, El-Nashar IM. Vaginal misoprostol prior to intrauterine device insertion in women delivered only by elective cesarean section: a randomized double-blind clinical trial. Contraception 2017;95:538–43.
131. Aoun J, Dines VA, Stovall DW, Mete M, Nelson CB, Gomez-Lobo V. Effects of age, parity, and device type on complications and discontinuation of intrauterine devices. Obstet Gynecol 2014;123:585–92.
132. Zhang J, Feldblum PJ, Chi IC, Farr MG. Risk factors for copper T IUD expulsion: an epidemiologic analysis. Contraception 1992;46:427–33.
133. Bahamondes L, Diaz J, Marchi NM, Petta CA, Cristofoletti ML, Gomez G. Performance of copper intrauterine devices when inserted after an expulsion. Hum Reprod 1995;10:2917–8.
134. Vickery Z, Madden T, Zhao Q, Secura GM, Allsworth JE, Peipert JF. Weight change at 12 months in users of three progestin-only contraceptive methods. Contraception 2013;88:503–8.
135. Walsh T, Grimes D, Frezieres R, et al. Randomised controlled trial of prophylactic antibiotics before insertion of intrauterine devices. IUD Study Group. Lancet 1998;351:1005–8.

136. Farley TM, Rosenberg MJ, Rowe PJ, Chen JH, Meirik O. Intrauterine devices and pelvic inflammatory disease: an international perspective. Lancet 1992;339:785–8.
137. Grimes DA. Intrauterine device and upper-genital-tract infection. Lancet 2000;356:1013–9.
138. Lee NC, Rubin GL, Ory HW, Burkman RT. Type of intrauterine device and the risk of pelvic inflammatory disease. Obstet Gynecol 1983;62:1–6.
139. Mishell DR, Jr., Bell JH, Good RG, Moyer DL. The intrauterine device: a bacteriologic study of the endometrial cavity. Am J Obstet Gynecol 1966;96:119–26.
140. Grimes DA, Schulz KF. Prophylactic antibiotics for intrauterine device insertion: a metaanalysis of the randomized controlled trials. Contraception 1999;60:57–63.
141. Sufrin CB, Postlethwaite D, Armstrong MA, Merchant M, Wendt JM, Steinauer JE. Neisseria gonorrhea and Chlamydia trachomatis screening at intrauterine device insertion and pelvic inflammatory disease. Obstet Gynecol 2012;120:1314–21.
142. Daling JR, Weiss NS, Metch BJ, et al. Primary tubal infertility in relation to the use of an intrauterine device. N Engl J Med 1985;312:937–41.
143. Cramer DW, Schiff I, Schoenbaum SC, et al. Tubal infertility and the intrauterine device. N Engl J Med 1985;312:941–7.
144. Wilson JC. A prospective New Zealand study of fertility after removal of copper intrauterine contraceptive devices for conception and because of complications: a four-year study. Am J Obstet Gynecol 1989;160:391–6.
145. Skjeldestad F, Bratt H. Fertility after complicated and non-complicated use of IUDs. A controlled prospective study. Adv Contracept 1988;4:179–84.
146. Hubacher D, Lara-Ricalde R, Taylor DJ, Guerra-Infante F, Guzman-Rodriguez R. Use of copper intrauterine devices and the risk of tubal infertility among nulligravid women. N Engl J Med 2001;345:561–7.
147. Jatlaoui TC, Simmons KB, Curtis KM. The safety of intrauterine contraception initiation among women with current asymptomatic cervical infections or at increased risk of sexually transmitted infections. Contraception 2016;94:701–12.
148. Birgisson NE, Zhao Q, Secura GM, Madden T, Peipert JF. Positive Testing for Neisseria gonorrhoeae and Chlamydia trachomatis and the Risk of Pelvic Inflammatory Disease in IUD Users. J Womens Health 2015;24:354–9.
149. Tepper NK, Curtis KM, Nanda K, Jamieson DJ. Safety of intrauterine devices among women with HIV: a systematic review. Contraception 2016;94:713–24.
150. Kim CR, Martinez-Maza O, Magpantay L, et al. Immunologic evaluation of the endometrium with a levonorgestrel intrauterine device in solid organ transplant women and healthy controls. Contraception 2016;94:534–40.
151. Furlong LA. Ectopic pregnancy risk when contraception fails. A review. J Reprod Med 2002;47:881–5.
152. Backman T, Rauramo I, Huhtala S, Koskenvuo M. Pregnancy during the use of levonorgestrel intrauterine system. Am J Obstet Gynecol 2004;190:50–4.
153. Curtis KM, Tepper NK, Jatlaoui TC, et al. U.S. Medical Eligibility Criteria for Contraceptive Use, 2016. MMWR Recomm Rep 2016;65:1–103.
154. Ott MA, Sucato GS, Committee on A. Contraception for adolescents. Pediatrics 2014;134:e1257–81.
155. Deans EI, Grimes DA. Intrauterine devices for adolescents: a systematic review. Contraception 2009;79:418–23.
156. Brockmeyer A, Kishen M, Webb A. Experience of IUD/IUS insertions and clinical performance in nulliparous women—a pilot study. Eur J Contracept Reprod Health Care 2008;13:248–54.
157. Thiery M. Pain relief at insertion and removal of an IUD: a simplified technique for paracervical block. Adv Contracept 1985;1:167–70.
158. Penney G, Brechin S, de Souza A, et al. FFPRHC Guidance (January 2004). The copper intrauterine device as long-term contraception. J Fam Plan Reprod Health 2004;30:29–41.
159. Lopez LM, Bernholc A, Zeng Y, et al. Interventions for pain with intrauterine device insertion. Cochrane Database Syst Rev 2015:CD007373.

160. Aksoy H, Aksoy U, Ozyurt S, Acmaz G, Babayigit M. Lidocaine 10% spray to the cervix reduces pain during intrauterine device insertion: a double-blind randomised controlled trial. J Fam Plann Reprod H 2016;42:83–7.
161. Andersson K, Ryde-Blomqvist E, Lindell K, Odlind V, Milsom I. Perforations with intrauterine devices. Report from a Swedish survey. Contraception 1998;57:251–5.
162. Chen B, Creinin M, Reeves M, Schwarz E. Breastfeeding continuation among women using the levonorgestrel-releasing intrauterine device after vaginal delivery. Contraception;80:204–5.
163. Browne H, Manipalviratn S, Armstrong A. Using an intrauterine device in immunocompromised women. Obstet Gynecol 2008;112:667–9.
164. Culwell KR, Curtis KM, del Carmen Cravioto M. Safety of contraceptive method use among women with systemic lupus erythematosus: a systematic review. Obstet Gynecol 2009;114:341–53.
165. Curtis KM, Nanda K, Kapp N. Safety of hormonal and intrauterine methods of contraception for women with HIV / AIDS: a systematic review. AIDS 2009;23 Suppl 1:S55–67.
166. Sinei SK, Morrison CS, Sekadde-Kigondu C, Allen M, Kokonya D. Complications of use of intrauterine devices among HIV-1-infected women. Lancet 1998;351:1238–41.
167. Morrison CS, Sekadde-Kigondu C, Sinei SK, Weiner DH, Kwok C, Kokonya D. Is the intrauterine device appropriate contraception for HIV-1-infected women? BJOG 2001;108:784–90.
168. Stringer EM, Kaseba C, Levy J, et al. A randomized trial of the intrauterine contraceptive device vs hormonal contraception in women who are infected with the human immunodeficiency virus. Am J Obstet Gynecol 2007;197:144 e1–8.
169. Wilson W, Taubert KA, Gewitz M, et al. Prevention of infective endocarditis: guidelines from the American Heart Association: a guideline from the American Heart Association Rheumatic Fever, Endocarditis, and Kawasaki Disease Committee, Council on Cardiovascular Disease in the Young, and the Council on Clinical Cardiology, Council on Cardiovascular Surgery and Anesthesia, and the Quality of Care and Outcomes Research Interdisciplinary Working Group. Circulation 2007;116:1736–54.
170. Kjos SL, Ballagh SA, La Cour M, Xiang A, Mishell DR, Jr. The copper T380A intrauterine device in women with type II diabetes mellitus. Obstet Gynecol 1994;84:1006–9.
171. Skouby SO, Molsted-Pedersen L, Petersen KR. Contraception for women with diabetes: an update. Baillieres Clin Obstet Gynaecol 1991;5:493–503.
172. Kimmerle R, Heinemann L, Berger M. Intrauterine devices are safe and effective contraceptives for type I diabetic women. Diabetes Care 1995;18:1506–7.
173. Petersen KR, Skouby SO, Jespersen J. Contraception guidance in women with pre-existing disturbances in carbohydrate metabolism. Eur J Contracept Reprod Health Care 1996;1:53–9.
174. Rogovskaya S, Rivera R, Grimes DA, et al. Effect of a levonorgestrel intrauterine system on women with type 1 diabetes: a randomized trial. Obstet Gynecol 2005;105:811–5.
175. O'Brien SH, Koch T, Vesely SK, Schwarz EB. Hormonal contraception and risk of thromboembolism in women with diabetes. Diabetes Care 2017;40:233–8.
176. World Health Organization. Medical eligibility criteria for contraceptive use 5th ed. Geneva: World Health Organization; 2015.
177. Trinh XB, Tjalma WA, Makar AP, Buytaert G, Weyler J, van Dam PA. Use of the levonorgestrel-releasing intrauterine system in breast cancer patients. Fertil Steril 2008;90:17–22.
178. Neven P, Amant F, Poppe W, Van den Broecke R. Levonorgestrel-releasing intra-uterine systems (LNG-IUS) and breast cancer. Fertil Steril 2009;91:e5; author reply e6.
179. Fu Y, Zhuang Z. Long-term effects of levonorgestrel-releasing intrauterine system on tamoxifen-treated breast cancer patients: a meta-analysis. Int J Clin Exp Patho 2014;7:6419–29.
180. Morch LS, Skovlund CW, Hannaford PC, Iversen L, Fielding S, Lidegaard O. Contemporary hormonal contraception and the risk of breast cancer. New Engl J of Med 2017;377:2228–39.

181. Dominick S, Hickey M, Chin J, Su HI. Levonorgestrel intrauterine system for endometrial protection in women with breast cancer on adjuvant tamoxifen. Cochrane Database Syst Rev 2015:CD007245.
182. Lidegaard O, Lokkegaard E, Svendsen AL, Agger C. Hormonal contraception and risk of venous thromboembolism: national follow-up study. BMJ 2009;339:b2890.
183. Levi EE, Stuart GS, Zerden ML, Garrett JM, Bryant AG. Intrauterine device placement during cesarean delivery and continued use 6 months postpartum: a randomized controlled trial. Obstet Gynecol 2015;126:5–11.
184. Cipres D, Seidman D, Cloniger C, 3rd, Nova C, O'Shea A, Obedin-Maliver J. Contraceptive use and pregnancy intentions among transgender men presenting to a clinic for sex workers and their families in San Francisco. Contraception 2017;95:186–9.
185. Turok DK, Godfrey EM, Wojdyla D, Dermish A, Torres L, Wu SC. Copper T380 intrauterine device for emergency contraception: highly effective at any time in the menstrual cycle. Hum Reprod 2013;28:2672–6.
186. American College of O, Gynecologists Committee on Gynecologic P, Long-Acting Reversible Contraception Working G. ACOG Committee Opinion no. 450: Increasing use of contraceptive implants and intrauterine devices to reduce unintended pregnancy. Obstet Gynecol 2009;114:1434–8.
187. White MK, Ory HW, Rooks JB, Rochat RW. Intrauterine device termination rates and the menstrual cycle day of insertion. Obstet Gynecol 1980;55:220–4.
188. Grimes D, Schulz K, Stanwood N. Immediate postabortal insertion of intrauterine devices. Cochrane Database Syst Rev 2002:CD001777.
189. Bednarek PA, Creinin MD, Reeves MF, et al. Immediate versus delayed IUD insertion after uterine aspiration. N Engl J Med 2011;364:2208–17.
190. Hohmann HL, Reeves MF, Chen BA, Perriera L, Hayes JL, Creinin MD. Immediate versus delayed insertion of the levonorgestrel-releasing intrauterine device following dilation and evacuation: a randomized controlled trial. Contraception 2012;85:240–5.
191. Goodman S, Hendlish SK, Reeves MF, Foster-Rosales A. Impact of immediate postabortal insertion of intrauterine contraception on repeat abortion. Contraception 2008;78:143–8.
192. Reeves MF, Smith KJ, Creinin MD. Contraceptive effectiveness of immediate compared with delayed insertion of intrauterine devices after abortion: a decision analysis. Obstet Gynecol 2007;109:1286–94.
193. Washington CI, Jamshidi R, Thung SF, Nayeri UA, Caughey AB, Werner EF. Timing of postpartum intrauterine device placement: a cost-effectiveness analysis. Fertil Steril 2015;103:131–7.
194. Eroglu K, Akkuzu G, Vural G, et al. Comparison of efficacy and complications of IUD insertion in immediate postplacental/early postpartum period with interval period: 1 year follow-up. Contraception 2006;74:376–81.
195. Eggebroten JL, Sanders JN, Turok DK. Immediate postpartum intrauterine device and implant program outcomes: a prospective analysis. Am J Obstet Gynecol 2017.
196. Osborne NG, Wright RC. Effect of preoperative scrub on the bacterial flora of the endocervix and vagina. Obstet Gynecol 1977;50:148–51.
197. Wilson S, Tan G, Baylson M, Schreiber C. Controversies in family planning: how to manage a fractured IUD. Contraception 2013;88:599–603.
198. Wildemeersch D. Safety and comfort of long-term continuous combined transdermal estrogen and intrauterine levonorgestrel administration for postmenopausal hormone substitution—a review. Gynecol Endocrinol 2016;32:598–601.
199. Hubacher D, Fortney J. Follow-up visits after IUD insertion. Are more better? J Reprod Med 1999;44:801–6.
200. Janowitz B, Hubacher D, Petrick T, Dighe N. Should the recommended number of IUD revisits be reduced? Stud Fam Plann 1994;25:362–7.
201. Ylikorkala O. Prostaglandin synthesis inhibitors in menorrhagia, intrauterine contraceptive device-induced side effects and endometriosis. Pharmacol Toxicol 1994; 75 Suppl 2:86–8.

202. Madden T, Proehl S, Allsworth JE, Secura GM, Peipert JF. Naproxen or estradiol for bleeding and spotting with the levonorgestrel intrauterine system: a randomized controlled trial. Am J Obstet Gynecol 2012;206:129.e1–8.
203. Abdel-Aleem H, d'Arcangues C, Vogelsong KM, Gaffield ML, Gulmezoglu AM. Treatment of vaginal bleeding irregularities induced by progestin only contraceptives. Cochrane Database Syst Rev 2013:CD003449.
204. Soderberg G, Lindgren S. Influence of an intrauterine device on the course of an acute salpingitis. Contraception 1981;24:137–43.
205. Workowski KA, Bolan GA, Centers for Disease Control and Prevention. Sexually transmitted diseases treatment guidelines, 2015. MMWR Recomm Rep 2015;64:1–137.
206. Tepper NK, Steenland MW, Gaffield ME, Marchbanks PA, Curtis KM. Retention of intrauterine devices in women who acquire pelvic inflammatory disease: a systematic review. Contraception 2013;87:655–60.
207. Lippes J. Pelvic actinomycosis: a review and preliminary look at prevalence. Am J Obstet Gynecol 1999;180:265-9.
208. Braaten KP, Benson CB, Maurer R, Goldberg AB. Malpositioned intrauterine contraceptive devices: risk factors, outcomes, and future pregnancies. Obstet Gynecol 2011;118:1014–20.
209. Adoni A, Ben Chetrit A. The management of intrauterine devices following uterine perforation. Contraception 1991;43:77–81.
210. Brahmi D, Steenland MW, Renner RM, Gaffield ME, Curtis KM. Pregnancy outcomes with an IUD in situ: a systematic review. Contraception 2012;85:131–9.
211. Foreman H, Stadel BV, Schlesselman S. Intrauterine device usage and fetal loss. Obstet Gynecol 1981;58:669–77.
212. Owen C, Sober S, Schreiber CA. Controversies in family planning: desired pregnancy, IUD in situ and no strings visible. Contraception 2013;88:330–3.
213. Schiesser M, Lapaire O, Tercanli S, Holzgreve W. Lost intrauterine devices during pregnancy: maternal and fetal outcome after ultrasound-guided extraction. An analysis of 82 cases. Ultrasound Obst Gyn 2004;23:486–9.

Injectable Contraceptives

6

Wan-Ju Wu, MD, MPH
Deborah Bartz, MD, MPH

- Contraceptive injections are an effective, convenient method of birth control and an important option for many patients who cannot use estrogen.
- The high progestin dose in injectable contraceptives allows use in overweight and obese patients without concern for decreased efficacy, though it often results in local and systemic side effects. Counseling patients about the menstrual cycle changes associated with injectable contraceptives can substantially lower discontinuation rates.
- Patients who gain more than 5% of their baseline body weight with early DMPA use may be at risk of continued weight gain.
- Progestin-only injectable contraceptives, while producing a transient decrease in bone mineral density, have not been associated with increased fracture risk; therefore, concerns about skeletal health should not limit use in most patients.
- A causal association between injectable contraceptives and increased HIV acquisition has not been clearly established. However, the data remain inconclusive and given the importance of DMPA for preventing pregnancy, use should not be restricted because the benefits outweigh the theoretical risk.

***Depo-Provera** (DMPA-IM) 150 mg/1 ml.* The most commonly used injectable contraceptive is depot medroxyprogesterone acetate (DMPA), marketed as Depo-Provera, given in a deep intramuscular (IM) injection of 150 milligrams (mg) every 13 weeks. DMPA is extremely effective, in part because it is forgiving for patients who return up to 2 weeks late for an injection.[1]

***Depo-subQ Provera** 104 (DMPA-SC) 104 mg/0.65 ml.* This branded formulation of DMPA has been dose-adjusted and reformulated to be given subcutaneously every 3 months (13 weeks). Its efficacy and side effect profile are similar to that of DMPA-IM.[2,3] There are no safety concerns specific to DMPA-SC in comparison with DMPA-IM. Patients who are eligible for progestin injectables can choose either formulation.[4]

Short-term injectable contraceptives. Although not available in the United States, these short-term injectables are popular methods in China, Eastern Asia, and Latin America; they are not discussed further in this chapter.

1. Medroxyprogesterone acetate 25 mg and estradiol cypionate 5 mg (Lunelle or Cyclofem). This highly effective combined IM monthly injectable is associated with less irregular bleeding and amenorrhea than progestin-only injectables.[5]
2. Norethindrone ethanate 50 mg and estradiol valerate 5 mg (Mesigyna). This IM monthly injectable has even less irregular bleeding and amenorrhea than Lunelle and faster return to fertility after discontinuation than DMPA.[6]
3. Dihydroxyprogesterone acetophenide 150 mg and estradiol enanthate 10 mg. This monthly IM injectable has bleeding patterns similar to Lunelle.[6]
4. Norethindrone ethanate 200 mg (NET-EN, Noristerat, and Syngestal). This bimonthly IM injectable has the same mechanism of action and similar advantages and disadvantages as DMPA.[6]

MECHANISM OF ACTION

DMPA prevents pregnancy primarily by inhibiting ovulation.[7] The dose of DMPA provided in each injection suppresses levels of follicle stimulating hormone (FSH) and luteinizing hormone (LH) and eliminates the LH surge. The pituitary gland remains responsive to gonadotropin-releasing hormone (GnRH), which suggests that the site of action of DMPA is the hypothalamus and the primary mechanism of action is inhibition of GnRH pulsatility.[8] After a patient discontinues DMPA, there is a great deal of variability in when ovulation resumes after an injection, with most patients resuming ovulation 15 to 49 weeks from the last injection.[9] Secondarily, DMPA prevents pregnancy by thickening and decreasing cervical mucus, an anti-estrogenic effect that prevents sperm penetration.[10,11] Furthermore, DMPA alters the endometrium, making it atrophic; however, given the effectiveness of DMPA at inhibiting ovulation and thickening the cervical mucus, it is unclear if this endometrial atrophy significantly contributes to the contraceptive effect of DMPA.[11,12]

EFFECTIVENESS

DMPA-IM (150 mg)

DMPA-IM is highly effective (see Figure 3-1 in Chapter 3 on Efficacy, Safety, and Personal Considerations). With correct and consistent use, the probability of pregnancy is only 0.2%. With typical use, the failure rate in the first year of use is 4% (see Chapter 26 on Contraceptive Efficacy). These estimates apply to injections of 11 to 13 week intervals, with each injection providing 150 mg of DMPA per 1 cc. (For a comparative view of first-year contraceptive failure rates, see Table 26-1.) Efficacy is not compromised by greater body weight. Furthermore, because DMPA avoids first-pass metabolism, its efficacy is unaffected by a patient's use of most other medications that may increase hepatic enzyme activation.[2]

DMPA-SC (104 mg)

In two large, open-label, phase 3 studies of DMPA-SC, there were no reported pregnancies in a total of 16,023 woman-cycles of use.[3] In a recent large randomized study, the cumulative pregnancy rate over the 2-year study period was 0% in DMPA-SC users compared with 0.8% in the DMPA-IM group.[13]

DISCONTINUATION RATES

The St. Louis Contraceptive CHOICE Project reported discontinuation rates of 42.5% at 1 year and 62% at 2 years.[14] Data from the 2011–2013 National Survey of Family Growth (NSFG) indicate that among ever-users of DMPA, 45.6% reported stopping due to dissatisfaction. Seventy percent of the patients reported side effects as being the primary reason for method discontinuation.[15] Improved provider education and patient counseling regarding the expected hormonal effects on users' bleeding profiles can improve DMPA continuation rates.[16–18] In rural Mexico, 175 patients received detailed, structured counseling about the hormonal effects of DMPA at the pre-treatment visit and at each injection visit, while 175 received routine counseling and information. Over 12 months, only 8% of patients who received structured counseling discontinued use due to amenorrhea or irregular or heavy bleeding, compared with 32% of patients who received routine counseling. The cumulative life-table discontinuation rate was 17% among patients receiving structured counseling versus 43% among patients receiving routine counseling.[16] Simply encouraging patients to come in for a visit if they are having a problem with DMPA can also improve continuation rates.[17] It is likely that a combination of structured counseling, multiple provider contacts, and reminders are needed to improve hormonal contraceptive adherence and acceptability.[19] (See Chapter 2 for more complete discussion of patient-centered contraception counseling.)

In the past decade, concern about DMPA's effect on skeletal health has also become a reason for patients to discontinue the method or for clinicians to suggest discontinuation. (See section on Bone Density in Special Issues.) Upon discontinuing DMPA, many patients do not switch to another effective contraceptive method; two studies reported unintended pregnancy rates of 20% to 22% within 9 months of stopping DMPA.[20,21]

While not FDA-approved for at-home administration, self-administered DMPA-SC could potentially lead to improved continuation rates due to greater convenience. In one survey study of 176 patients who were currently using DMPA, 67% expressed an interest in self-administration of their DMPA at home.[22] In a follow-up survey of 313 users of other contraceptive methods, 64% reported they would like fewer clinic visits relating to contraceptive needs, while 26% of never-DMPA users and 40% of ex-DMPA users reported they would consider using DMPA if self-administration were possible.[22] Several studies, including those conducted with adolescents, have consistently affirmed patients' willingness and ability to self-administer subcutaneous DMPA.[23,24] One randomized clinical trial comparing clinic versus self-administration of DMPA-SC demonstrated that 90 of 91 patients randomized to the self-administration group were able to do so correctly. The study showed similar continuation rates between the two groups at 1 year—71% for the self-administration group and 63% for the clinic group.[24]

ADVANTAGES

1. **No estrogen.** DMPA does not contain estrogen and can be safely used for patients with contraindications to estrogen, including endometrial hyperplasia, migraine with aura, and smoking over the age of 35.[25] Studies thus far have not shown that serious cardiovascular effects are associated with use of progestin-only contraceptives.[12,26,27]

2. **Reversibility.** DMPA does not cause long-term loss of fertility. While return to fertility may be delayed, DMPA's contraceptive mechanism is reversed once the effect of the last injection wears off.

3. **Effective contraception, even for obese (BMI >30) users.** DMPA provides 3 months of highly effective contraception per injection. There is no decrease in the efficacy of DMPA among overweight or obese patients.[3,28]

4. **Infrequent dosing.** Because the efficacy of DMPA does not require frequent dosing or partner cooperation, this method is ideal for populations that may have contraceptive adherence difficulties, such as adolescents. Compared with adolescent users of oral contraceptive pills, teenagers using DMPA have higher continuation rates over time and lower repeat pregnancy rates.[29–31] DMPA is a discreet contraceptive method that can be used by patients at risk for reproductive coercion and birth control sabotage.[32] Other high-risk populations may benefit from the ease of adherence with DMPA.

5. **Reduced risk of ectopic pregnancy.** Compared with patients using no contraceptive at all, patients who use DMPA have an overall decreased pregnancy risk and therefore a reduced risk for having an ectopic pregnancy.[33] One study showed that 1.5% of patients who got pregnant on DMPA had an ectopic pregnancy, the same ectopic rate as patients who conceived while not using contraception.[34]

6. **Absence of menstrual bleeding.** Following the endometrial stabilization that occurs with the first one to three doses, DMPA typically results in very light or absent bleeding. During the first year of DMPA use, approximately 10% to 30% of patients have amenorrhea after one injection and 40% to 50% have amenorrhea after four injections.[35,36] By the end of the fifth year of use, approximately 80% of patients have amenorrhea. In a study of teenagers, nearly two thirds of DMPA users reported amenorrhea at 6 months.[37] Similar amenorrhea rates are reported with DMPA-SC.[38] If patients have been fully informed about the likelihood of this bleeding pattern change, it is considered by many to be advantageous.

7. **Improvement of cyclic menstrual symptoms.** Given its mechanism of action that shuts down the hypothalamic-pituitary-ovarian axis, DMPA is associated with a decrease in ovulation pain and symptoms that often accompany menses, such as cramps, mood changes, headaches, breast tenderness, and nausea.[39]

8. **Minimal drug interactions.** There has been no demonstrated interaction between DMPA and antibiotics, antiretrovirals, or enzyme-inducing drugs.[40,41] The only drug that decreases the effectiveness of DMPA is aminoglutethimide, an aromatase inhibitor that blocks the conversion of cholesterol to pregnenolone. It is used to suppress adrenal function in some patients with Cushing's disease. Aminoglutethimide increases the metabolism of progestins.[42]

9. **Fewer seizures.** In small studies, DMPA use has been potentially associated with decrease in frequency of grand mal seizures.[43,44]

While the biologic mechanism is poorly understood, improvement in seizure control is thought to be mediated, in part, by the inhibitory effects of progestin metabolites on gamma-aminobutyric acid (GABA) receptors in the hippocampus.[45] Taking anti-seizure medications has no impact on the contraceptive efficacy of DMPA.[46]

10. **Fewer sickle cell crises.** DMPA may stabilize the membrane of red blood cells, making cells less prone to sickling, and reduce the frequency of resultant pain crises. In a randomized trial, DMPA use was associated with a greater reduction in the frequency of sickle cell crises than were combined oral contraceptive use or no intervention. After 1 year of DMPA use, 70% of patients with sickle cell disease were pain-free (compared with 50% of patients not using hormones), and of the patients who had continuing crises, only 16% reported the ongoing pain as intense.[47] Additional evidence is needed to support the use of DMPA above other contraceptive options for patients with sickle cell disease.

11. **Less pain from endometriosis.** DMPA has been shown to reduce pain associated with endometriosis.[48,49] A randomized, blinded trial compared DMPA-SC to leuprolide acetate, a GnRH agonist, for management of the pain associated with endometriosis. This trial found equivalent pain reduction with both treatment options and less bone mineral density loss with DMPA-SC.[50] There is some evidence that DMPA-SC reduces the symptoms of endometriosis during use and for months following discontinuation.[4] In 2005, the FDA approved use of DMPA-SC for this indication. As DMPA-IM has the same mechanism of action as DMPA-SC, it likely has similar effect on endometriosis-related symptoms.[13]

12. **Benefits for patients with myomas.** While there are no randomized trials that have studied the effect of DMPA on myomas,[51] DMPA has been shown in open label trials to decrease the bleeding associated with myomas and improve hemoglobin levels.[52,53] DMPA use may also shrink myomas[53]; however, the evidence on this is conflicting.[52] One case-control study showed that DMPA use was associated with a lower risk of recurrent myomas after myomectomy.[54]

13. **Decreased risk of pelvic inflammatory disease.** As with other progestin hormonal methods, the thickened cervical mucus produced with DMPA use may prevent ascent of cervical pathogens to the upper genital tract.[55]

14. **Decreased risk of endometrial and ovarian cancer.** A large case-control study showed that DMPA use was associated with as much as an 80% reduction in risk of endometrial cancer; DMPA use had a greater protective effective against endometrial cancer

than oral contraceptive use.[56] Another multi-centered case control study found DMPA use was associated with an overall 39% reduction in risk of epithelial ovarian cancer and a significant risk reduction of 83% when DMPA use was greater than 3 years.[57]

Potential Additional Advantages of DMPA-SC

1. Subcutaneous injections may be less painful than IM injections.
2. Although not FDA-approved, self-administration of DMPA-SC may be acceptable to many patients.[22] Self-injection may improve adherence with the method by eliminating the need for patients to periodically return to a health care provider for injections.[23,58]

DISADVANTAGES AND CAUTIONS

1. **Menstrual cycle disturbances.** Bleeding patterns with DMPA use are unpredictable during the first few months of use.[35] The overall incidence of irregular bleeding is 70% in the first year, with a decrease in irregular bleeding with each reinjection, and rates as low as 10% after the first year.[59] Amenorrhea becomes more common over time among DMPA users. Approximately 40% to 50% of users experience amenorrhea after 1 year of use and 80% after 5 years of use.[35,36] Similar patterns have been observed with DMPA-SC use, with 55% of patients developing amenorrhea after 1 year of use.[3,38] Patients using DMPA rarely experience an increased number of days of heavy bleeding.

   Episodes of unpredictable bleeding, particularly in the first few months as the endometrium becomes more atrophic, is the most common reason for discontinuation of DMPA. Approximately 20% to 25% of patients will discontinue DMPA within the first year because of menstrual disturbances.[37,60–62] In one study, of the patients who discontinued for menstrual disturbances, 35% discontinued because of undesired amenorrhea and 30% discontinued due to prolonged bleeding.[63] The irregular bleeding associated with progestin-only contraception has been associated with an increased fragility of endometrial capillaries as a result of endometrial atrophy.[64]

2. **Weight changes.** Weight gain is common in many people with age; the manner in which DMPA may affect this weight gain is not well understood, largely because it does not appear to have a consistent effect on all users. In one study of 206 Brazilian patients, those using DMPA gained an average of 9 pounds over

5 years, significantly more than the 5 pounds gained by IUD users over the same time interval.[65] However, in another large study of 1,994 Chinese patients, DMPA use was associated with no weight gain over 1 year of use.[66] Among patients who gain weight while on DMPA, the weight gain has been demonstrated to be due to increases in fat deposition, not fluid retention.[67,68] Weight gain is commonly cited as a reason for discontinuation of DMPA, with 12% to 19% discontinuing for this reason.[60–62]

The only randomized trial to address the association of weight gain in DMPA users assigned 20 patients to DMPA versus placebo and then measured food intake, energy expenditure, and weight gain over 3 months. All patients in this trial were of normal weight at baseline. No significant difference in weight gain, food intake, or resting metabolism was observed between the groups when comparing the pre- with post-injection intervals. As compared to baseline weight, the mean body weight was 0.1 kg (0.22 lbs) lower 3 months post-injection in the DMPA group and 0.7 kg (1.54 lbs) higher 3 months post-injection in the placebo group.[69]

It is possible that, while on average, overall weight does not change significantly in a population, there may be subsets of that patients are more likely to experience significant weight gain with DMPA.[70] One study of adult patients suggests that the subset of patients who gained more than 5% of their body weight (early weight gainers) in the first 3 to 6 months of DMPA use were more likely to continue to gain weight with ongoing use; the weight differences became more pronounced at 36 months as compared to 12 and 24 months. This study showed that the early weight gainers, which comprised of 26% of the study population, gained an average of 7.03 kg (15.5 lbs) more than regular weight gainers over 36 months. At 36 months the mean weight gain of the regular weight gainers was 2.49 kg (5.5 lbs) as compared to 11.08 kg (24.4 lbs) for the early weight gainers. Baseline BMI <30, multiparity, and self-reported increased appetite were associated with early weight gain.[71]

Similar to studies in adults, one study showed that adolescents who gained >5% of their baseline weight at 6 months of DMPA use were more likely to continue to gain weight with continued DMPA. Twenty-one percent of the adolescents had early weight gain. The early gainers had a mean increase in BMI of 7.6 kg/m^2 over 18 months as compared to an increase in BMI of only 2.3 kg/m^2 in non-early weight gainers over the same time period. Early weight gain consistently predicted later weight gain, regardless of baseline characteristics such as age at menarche, BMI, race, ethnicity, parity, or reported physical activity.[72] Baseline obesity appears to be a second, less powerful predictor of weight gain among adolescent

DMPA users. One observational study found that at 18 months mean weight gain for obese adolescent DMPA users was 9.5kg as compared to 4kg for nonobese adolescents. This study, however did not account for early weight gain in its analyses.[73] Use of DMPA by obese adolescents is rated category 2 by the U.S. CDC Medical Eligibility Criteria for Contraceptive Use (MEC), while use by obese adult patients is considered category 1.[25]

These data suggest that in both adult and adolescent DMPA-users, there may be a subset of patients who can be identified by rapid weight gain in the first 6 months of DMPA use who are at greatest risk for continued weight gain. Weight monitoring is reasonable for patients who are concerned about potential weight gain associated with DMPA use.

3. **Depression.** Depression is a common, chronic and recurrent condition for patients. Data on the impact of DMPA on mood are limited and conflicting. One study of 183 subjects found an association between DMPA use and depressive symptoms, but the study was not designed to establish a causal relationship.[74] Other studies have shown no association, including a prospective cohort study that enrolled 495 patients who were interviewed regarding depressive symptoms at baseline and again after 12 months of use.[75–77] The U.S. MEC rates DMPA use in patients with depression as category 1.[25,78] A history of depression should not be a contraindication to DMPA use. Patients on DMPA who experience symptoms suggestive of depression or have worsening of depressive symptoms should be screened. DMPA discontinuation should be considered on a case-by-case basis after discussion between patients and providers.

   Data on the association of DMPA and postpartum depression are also limited. One retrospective study did not show an increased likelihood of developing postpartum depression among DMPA users.[79] Given the limited data, the decision to initiate DMPA in patients with a history of severe postpartum depression should be made by providers and their patients after careful discussion of the risks and benefits.

4. **Bone density decrease.** Long-term DMPA users may develop temporary and usually reversible decreased bone density. (See section on Bone Density in Special Issues.)

5. **Allergic reactions.** Although rare, severe allergic reactions may occur following any type of injection.[80] For this reason it is recommended that patients remain in the vicinity of the clinic for 20 minutes after their first injection. There have been rare case reports of anaphylaxis after DMPA-IM injection.[81]

6. **Glucose and lipoprotein effects.** A multicenter clinical trial by the World Health Organization (WHO) did find an increase in total cholesterol and low-density lipoprotein cholesterol accompanied by a brief decrease in high-density lipoprotein cholesterol in the first weeks following injection when serum hormone levels were the highest.[82] A second study demonstrated similar results and showed that the adverse lipoprotein changes were temporary and improved over time even if DMPA was continued.[83] Lastly, data from one recent experimental study suggested that DMPA may have negative effects on glucose regulation in obese patients,[84] however there are no conclusive data that DMPA affects carbohydrate metabolism. The clinical significance of these findings is unclear.

7. **Venous thromboembolism event (VTE) risk.** The data on increased risk of VTE with DMPA use are controversial. One systematic review of 26 studies on progestin-only contraception and thromboembolism identified two case-control studies that showed statistically increased odds of VTE risk among DMPA users.[85] The first study found a 3.6-fold increased odds of VTE among DMPA users as compared with patients not using hormonal contraceptives.[86] A second case control study found a 2.2-fold increased odds of VTE among DMPA users. In this study, patients who were carriers of Factor V Leiden had five-fold increased odds of VTE as compared to noncarriers who were not using progestin contraceptives.[86] The evidence included in the systematic review generally found no statistically significant increased VTE risk among people in the general population using progesterone-only pills, implants, or LNG-IUD.[85] The biologic mechanism for theoretic increased VTE risk remains unclear. Studies have generally shown no negative impact of DMPA on coagulation or inflammation markers.[87,88]

   Based on the available data it appears that any increased risk is likely small and represents only a slight increase in the absolute numbers of VTE events at the population level.[85] Among the general population the benefits of DMPA in preventing pregnancy and pregnancy-associated VTE risks likely outweigh the theoretical, small increased risk of VTE. The U.S. MEC guidelines classify DMPA use as category 2 for patients with acute or history of VTE. Providers should be aware that the potential risk of VTE might be compounded in patients with baseline medical conditions that already place them at increased VTE risk.

8. **Other adverse effects.** In one of the largest studies of DMPA users, 17% of the 3,875 patients complained of headaches, 11% of nervousness, 5% of decreased libido, and 3% of breast discomfort at some point during the 5 year trial.[36] The attribution of these symptoms to DMPA is unclear.

9. **Not possible to discontinue immediately.** Possible negative side effects related to DMPA use, such as weight gain, depression, breast tenderness, and menstrual irregularities may continue until DMPA is cleared from a patient's body, which may take as long as 6 to 8 months after the last injection for total clearance. Approximately half of patients who discontinue DMPA will have resumption of normal menses within 6 months after the last injection, while 25% will wait a year before a normal bleeding pattern returns.[59]

10. **Delay in return of fertility.** After discontinuing DMPA, the median time to conception is 9 to 10 months, which is longer than with other hormonal contraceptive methods.[1,36] A systematic review demonstrated a wide range in resumption of ovulation, ranging from 15 to 49 weeks after the last injection, making fertility prediction difficult following DMPA discontinuation. While duration of use did not predict return of fertility, patients' body weights did have an association. Patients with higher body weights took longer to conceive after DMPA discontinuation. This is likely due to storage of biologically active metabolites of DMPA in adipose tissue.[89] Because of the delay in return to fertility in DMPA users, providers may consider recommending patients discontinue DMPA use 12–18 months prior to when they desire a pregnancy.

11. **Return visits required every 3 months.** For some patients, clinic visits for repeated injections of DMPA are unacceptable. Approximately 20% to 50% of patients continue to use DMPA at 1 year, and many who discontinue do so because of the difficulty in returning for injections.[17,61,62,90] Convenient access to DMPA injections through flexible and expanded clinic hours or pharmacist-administered injections may improve continuation rates.[91,92] With DMPA-SC, self-injection may be possible, which would decrease the need for return visits.

PRECAUTIONS

Two documents—the 2016 U.S. MEC and the 2015 World Health Organization (WHO) MEC—guide health care providers in determining who can safely use various contraceptive methods. Compared with estrogen-containing methods, DMPA has only one absolute contraindication (category 4): current breast cancer within the last 5 years.[25,78] There are several conditions listed as category 3 (risks usually outweigh benefits). Generally these conditions include evidence of current cardiovascular disease, abnormal liver function or liver tumors, a remote history of breast cancer, and unexplained vaginal bleeding prior to evaluation.

Providing DMPA in these circumstances requires careful clinical judgment that often includes multidisciplinary teams, access to clinical follow-up, and consideration of alternative available options. [25,78] (See the U.S. MEC summary chart in this book.)

Special Issues

Breastfeeding Patients

There used to be concerns that progestin-only methods may thwart lactation if they are initiated before the post-delivery withdrawal of progesterone that triggers milk synthesis.[93–95] However, clinical experience has not substantiated that hypothesis.[96] Despite this clinical experience and because of theoretical concerns over early neonatal exposure to exogenous steroids, several international organizations have urged that progestin-only methods not be initiated until at least 6 weeks postpartum. [78,97–99] Studies of DMPA initiated within 1 to 3 days postpartum,[96] 7 days postpartum,[100] or within 6 weeks postpartum[101] have found no adverse effects on neonatal outcomes. There are insufficient data to suggest early breastfeeding cessation or decreased breast milk quality with DMPA use.[95,102] In the U.S MEC, family planning experts have endorsed the safety of administering DMPA immediately postpartum in patients, classifying DMPA as category 2 immediately postpartum regardless of breastfeeding status.[74,103,104] Because prothrombic concerns for DMPA are inconclusive, it may be initiated immediately after delivery with likely minimal increase in risk of thromboembolism. (See Chapter 17 Contraception after Pregnancy.)

Cancer Risk and DMPA

Breast cancer. Overall, it appears that there is no increase in the risk of breast cancer with DMPA use. In a pooled international study including 1,768 patients with breast cancer and more than 13,000 controls, the overall relative risk associated with the use of DMPA was statistically insignificant (RR 1.1, 95% CI=0.97–1.4). When subjects were stratified by duration of DMPA use, there was also no increased risk with longer use of DMPA. However, patients who had used DMPA within the past 5 years had an increased risk of breast cancer (RR=2.0; 95%CI=1.5–2.8).[105] If this is a true effect, the increased risk may reflect either increased detection of breast cancer in DMPA users due to increased surveillance or accelerated growth of preexisting tumors. However, two more recent studies have shown no association between DMPA use and breast cancer in subjects with recent or current use.[106,107] Based on the available data, we would not recommend restricting use of DMPA due to concerns for increased breast cancer risk, but providers should inform patients that in rare cases of an existing occult tumor, DMPA may accelerate its growth.[105]

Reproductive tract cancers. There does not appear to be any association between invasive cervical cancer and DMPA use. A WHO Collaborative Study of 2,009 patients with invasive cervical cancer and more than 9,000 controls failed to demonstrate a significantly increased risk (RR=1.1; 95% CI=1.0–1.3). There was no association between adenocarcinoma or squamous carcinoma of the cervix and DMPA use. [108,109] Two other large case-control studies have similarly demonstrated that DMPA use is not associated with an overall increase in ovarian cancer, and the data suggest that, similar to combined oral contraceptive pills, DMPA may actually be protective against epithelial ovarian cancer, especially when the duration of use is >3 years.[56,57] Furthermore, like OCPs, DMPA is associated with a significantly decreased risk of endometrial cancer (RR 0.2; 95% CI=0.1, 0.8).[56]

Bone Density and DMPA

DMPA suppresses ovarian production of estradiol.[110] Estrogen deficiency is associated with deceases in bone mineral density or bone mass. This has led to concern that DMPA may put patients at risk of osteoporosis and, subsequently, bone fractures. Because minimal-trauma bone fractures occur infrequently in reproductive-age patients, bone mineral density (BMD) has instead been examined in many populations of current and previous DMPA users. DMPA is associated with a decrease in BMD[111–115] that is generally temporary and reversible.[116–118] This loss in BMD occurs within the first 2 years of use, but after 2 years further loss of BMD slows and even plateaus.[117–119] Although patients have a decrease in BMD while using DMPA, studies have consistently demonstrated that BMD is regained back to baseline levels equivalent to that seen in non-DMPA users when DMPA is discontinued.[116–118] For patients over age 21 years, BMD values among patients who had previously used DMPA return to similar values to those of never-users by 30 months post-discontinuation. [117] Other studies comparing past users of DMPA to never users have similarly shown no difference in BMD.[120] The recovery in BMD was seen as soon as 24 weeks after discontinuation of DMPA.[121] Similar effects on BMD have been found with DMPA-SC.[13]

It is debatable whether BMD is the best surrogate marker of skeletal health, as ultimately, the most important question is whether DMPA use increases the risk of fracture, the clinically relevant outcome of interest. Our literature review identified only one case report of a low-trauma fracture in a long-term DMPA user.[122] A study of female military recruits found increased stress fracture risk in white study participants, but this increased risk was no longer significant when adjusted for other factors.[123] Another study, a cross-sectional study of developmentally delayed patients, suggests an increased risk of fractures in previous users of DMPA, a result that again may not be generalizable.[124] One retrospective cohort study demonstrated increased fracture risk with DMPA use, but DMPA users in this study had higher fracture risk than nonusers prior to DMPA initiation. This study did not show a causal relationship between DMPA use and fracture, but instead suggests that there are possibly unmeasured baseline differences in behavior, lifestyle, or unreported medical history, between patients who choose to use DMPA and patients who choose other methods that could explain the different fracture risks.[125] A recent systematic Cochrane review of 14 studies including 2 high quality studies on progestin-only contraceptives found insubstantial evidence to implicate DMPA and other hormonal contraceptives as a risk factor for elevated fracture risk.[126] A similar pattern of the decline in BMD followed by recovery that is seen in DMPA use is also observed with the low estrogen state that occurs with pregnancy and lactation.[127,128] Similar to the evidence on DMPA use, epidemiological evidence of BMD declines following pregnancy and lactation has not demonstrated any negative effect on fracture risk.[129]

The decreasing adolescent pregnancy rate in the United States has been paralleled by increased DMPA use in teenagers.[130,131] While this decreasing pregnancy rate has multiple contributing factors, the convenience of DMPA dosing for adolescents has likely played a role. Since the effects of contraceptives on bone mass may be particularly important for adolescents who have not yet reached peak bone mass, it is important to know if teenagers who have used DMPA regain bone mass after discontinuing DMPA.[132] Studies suggest they do regain bone mass, and they regain it more quickly than older populations. A study of 170 adolescents (80 DMPA users and 90 controls) ages 14 to 18 years who underwent BMD testing every 6 months for 24 to 36 months, even after discontinuation of DMPA, found that use was associated with significant declines in BMD, but upon discontinuation, former users had a rapid and significant gain in BMD beyond the bone gain observed in control patients.[118] Another study found that BMD in adolescents declined in the first 2 to 3 years of DMPA use, but it substantially or fully recovered to baseline following discontinuation.[133] This is reassuring and suggests that the bone loss associated with DMPA use is transient. Whether adolescents who use DMPA ultimately reach the same peak bone mass as they would have had they not used DMPA remains unknown. Similarly, we do not know the impact of prolonged DMPA use during adolescence on the risk of fracture later in life.

A separate, important question is whether prolonged DMPA use during the premenopausal years is associated with an increased risk of fracture after menopause. Limited data address this question. One study from New Zealand assessing bone density in post-menopausal previous

DMPA users, did not demonstrate an association between prior DMPA use and postmenopausal fractures, although the study had limited statistical power to detect differences in fracture risk.[134] Another small study found similar BMD levels among patients entering natural menopause without exogenous hormone administration as compared to patients with a history of prolonged DMPA use who continued this use until they became menopausal. Those entering menopause naturally had a rapid decline in BMD as compared to those on DMPA who had little additional loss with the transition to menopause, resulting in equivalent post-menopausal BMD levels between arms. This suggests that peri-menopausal DMPA users had already "lost the estrogen-sensitive component of bone" but suffered no further bone loss secondary to menopause[135] (see Chapter 19, Contraception in the Later Reproductive Years).

In November 2004 the FDA added a black box warning to the label of DMPA: Patients "who use Depo-Provera Contraceptive Injection may lose significant bone mineral density. Bone loss is greater with increasing duration of use and may not be completely reversible. It is unknown if use of Depo-Provera Contraceptive Injection during adolescence or early adulthood, a critical period of bone accretion, will reduce peak bone mass and increase the risk for osteoporotic fracture in later life. Depo-Provera Contraceptive Injection should be used as a long-term birth control method (e.g., longer than 2 years) only if other birth control methods are inadequate."[136]

In June 2005, the World Health Organization reviewed the evidence on this subject. They concluded, "there should be no restriction on the use of DMPA, including no restriction on duration of use, among patients aged 18 to 45 who are otherwise eligible to use the method." They further recommended that, "Among adolescents (menarche to < 18) and patients over 45, the advantages of using DMPA usually outweigh the theoretical safety concerns regarding fracture risk. Since data are insufficient to determine if this is the case with long-term use among these age groups, the overall risks and benefits for continuing use of the method should be reconsidered over time with the individual user."[137,138] The Society for Adolescent Medicine advocates for continued use of DMPA in teenage girls: "Continue prescribing DMPA to adolescent girls needing contraception with adequate explanation of benefits and potential risks" and recommends adequate calcium and vitamin D intake, along with weight-bearing exercise for all adolescents on DMPA.[139] The American College of Obstetricians and Gynecologists states: "skeletal health concerns should not restrict use of DMPA in adult patients. In adolescents, the advantages of DMPA likely outweigh the theoretical safety concerns regarding bone mineral density and factures. However, in the absence of long-term data in this population, consideration of long-term use should be individualized."[140,141]

Clinical management should be dictated by evidence that measures outcomes of interest (such as fracture risk), not by surrogate markers of unclear clinical significance (such as BMD in healthy premenopausal patients).[142] According to the WHO, "since the effect of DMPA on bone mineral density is largely reversible, any lifetime increase in fracture risk is likely to be small."[137] Despite product labeling, BMD testing should play no role in the routine management of healthy DMPA users, because in premenopausal patients there is no good correlation between bone densitometry results and fracture risk.[140,143,144] Similarly, using amenorrhea or serum estradiol levels to guide management is not helpful, because these factors have not consistently been associated with lower BMD or higher fracture risk among DMPA users.[115,119,145]

Based on the available evidence, we recommend providers counsel adult and adolescent patients on the risks and benefits of DMPA including the "black box" warning. In most situations the benefits of DMPA use will outweigh the theoretical fracture risks. However, patients with conditions that place them at high risk for osteoporosis and fracture, such as chronic corticosteroid use, disorders of bone metabolism, a strong family history of osteoporosis (that may represent a genetic mutation associated with fracture), or anorexia nervosa—may not be well suited for long-term DMPA use. Additional, individualized counseling is warranted for these subgroups.

Risk of Sexually Transmitted Infections and DMPA

DMPA provides no protection against acquisition of sexually transmitted infections (STIs), including HIV. DMPA use has been inconsistently associated with acquisition of gonorrhea and chlamydia.[55,146–148] It has been proposed that DMPA might increase the risk of chlamydia because progestins may enhance the growth of chlamydia or influence host immune factors that enable growth, but no randomized controlled trial has addressed this question. Any relationship may be due to bias inherent in observational studies.[55,147] In one observational study, patients who chose DMPA had a higher chlamydia infection rate at baseline as compared to oral contraceptive users (8.9 v 3.1%).[149] Despite the potential weak association between DMPA use and cervical chlamydia acquisition, DMPA use is associated with a decreased risk of pelvic inflammatory disease (PID).[55,147] One proposed mechanism is that progestins thicken cervical mucus and inhibits ascent of bacteria. Based on the available data, we would not recommend restrictions in use of DMPA among patients who may be at increased risk for STI infection.

The association between DMPA and HIV acquisition remains controversial. The evidence has not established a clear causal association. Plausible biologic mechanisms to explain the increased risk of HIV transmission with hormonal contraception include disruption of epithelial barriers, alterations in genital tract immune cell populations due to hormonal influence, and local mucosal inflammatory responses.[150–154] Studies have used inconsistent approaches that often fail to account for differences in study population characteristics. The existing observational data are difficult to interpret due to inability to account for different hormones used, varying dosages, contraceptive adherence, and rate of method discontinuation.[153,155]

Earlier studies in high-risk populations, including sex workers in Kenya and Thailand, demonstrated an association between DMPA and HIV acquisition,[156–158] while studies in the general population have been mixed.[146,159,160] A recent meta-analysis of the available epidemiologic evidence on the risk of HIV acquisition while using DMPA concludes that if the association is causal, the magnitude of effect is likely small, with only a 1.5-fold (or less) of increased risk of HIV acquisition.[152] There are no data to support that use of NET-EN (a long-acting progestin-only injectable) affects the risks of HIV acquisition[152] (see Chapter 20 on Reproductive Tract Infections).

Though the data remain inconclusive, the WHO recently released a report stating that the data continue to show a possible increased risk of HIV infection among progestin-only injectable users, but it is unclear whether this is due to a causal relationship or methodological limitations of available research. The WHO has changed the guidance on use of progestin-only injectable contraceptives among patients at high risk of HIV infection from "use without restriction" to "benefits outweigh theoretical or proven risks."[161] This change is qualified by the WHO statement: "In many settings, unintended pregnancies and/or pregnancy related morbidity and mortality are common, and progestogen-only injectables are among the few types of methods widely available. Women should not be denied the use of progestogen-only injectables because of concerns about the possible increased risk [of HIV infection]. Women considering progestogen-only injectables should be advised about these concerns, about the uncertainty over whether there is a causal relationship, and about how to minimize their risk of acquiring HIV." [161]

The statement reaffirms that all individuals at high risk of HIV or other STI infection need access to prevention strategies such as condoms and, when appropriate, pre-exposure prophylaxis.[161] The U.S. MEC guidelines have not been changed in regard to their recommendations for DMPA use and is classified as category 1 for the listed STI conditions.[25]

PROVIDING DMPA

DMPA-IM is provided in either 1 cc vials or prefilled syringes containing 150 mg/mL. The vial and the syringe should be vigorously shaken. The label states a 2-year shelf-life. Using a sterile needle and syringe, inject the

DMPA deeply into the deltoid or the gluteal muscle. The 21- to 23-gauge needle should be 2.5 to 4 cm long.[40] For obese patients, a spinal needle may be needed to allow injection deep enough to be in the muscle. Immediately after injection do not massage the area over the injection, because it could lower the effectiveness of DMPA. DMPA-SC is available in prefilled, single-use syringes. Subcutaneous DMPA injections can be given in the anterior thigh or abdominal wall.

If a DMPA injection is given within 5 to 7 days of a normal last menstrual period or when switching from another effective contraceptive method, onset of contraceptive efficacy is within 24 hours and no back-up contraception is needed.[7] DMPA can be given at any time in a menstrual cycle if the patient can be reasonably certain that she is not pregnant. If DMPA is given later than day 7 in the menstrual cycle, it is important that patients use back-up contraception for 7 days and receive a follow-up pregnancy test several weeks later to diagnose pregnancy in a timely fashion. A recent study of immediate initiation of DMPA among 149 patients who presented on cycle day 8 or later found that 47% of patients continued to a second dose of DMPA, 92% returned for their follow-up pregnancy test (half required many reminders), and 3 patients were pregnant (2%).[162] Other studies have shown that this *Quick Start* (or *Depo Now*) method, administering DMPA at any time that the patient presents to clinic provided she and the provider are reasonably sure she is not pregnant, is safe, improves adherence, and results in fewer unwanted pregnancies in long-term follow-up.[163–165] (See Figure 6-1.)

Schedule DMPA injections for every 13 weeks. After a single IM or SC DMPA injection, ovulation does not occur for at least 14 weeks (98 days).[2,166] One systematic review found no pregnancies in the 2-week interval following reinjection date as well as extremely low pregnancy rates (0.4 per 100) for the 4-week interval following reinjection. However, the data were limited and one study included many breastfeeding patients.[9,167] The CDC expert group did not consider the data to be generalizable to the U.S. population and therefore continues to recommend a grace period of no more than 2 weeks beyond 13-week dosing interval. There are no time limitations on early injections.[168] For patients who return more than 15 weeks after a previous injection, exclude pregnancy before re-injection, offer emergency contraception (except ulipristal acetate) if they have had unprotected intercourse in the last 5 days, and recommend back-up contraception for 7 days after resuming DMPA (see Figure 6-1).

Giving DMPA injections in early pregnancy should be avoided if possible, because exposure has been associated with low-birthweight infants.[169] There is no increased risk of birth defects from pregnancies exposed to DMPA.[170,171]

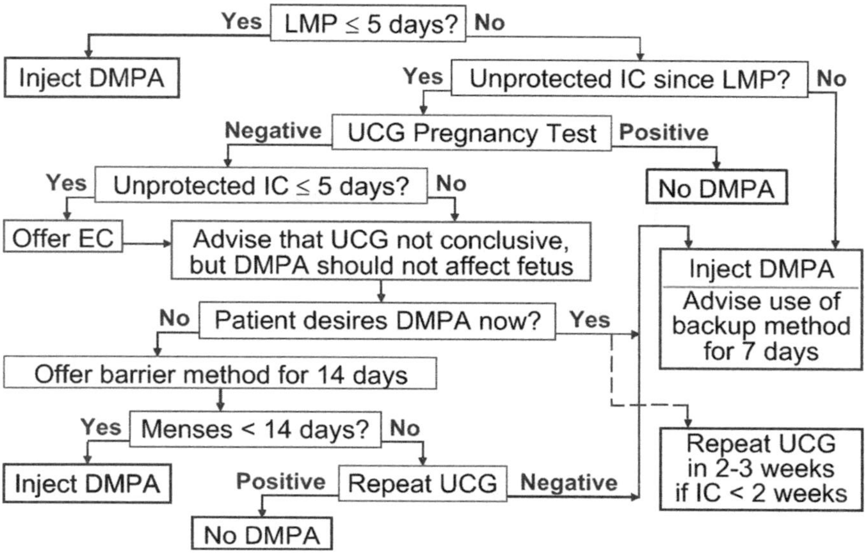

Source: Nelson AL, Katz T (2007),[164] with permission.

Figure 6-1 Flow sheet of Same Day Start DMPA protocol. EC, emergency contraception; IC, intercourse; UCG, sensitive urine pregnancy test

At each re-injection visit, ask about any problems or concerns, the date of the last menstrual period, and any need for change in contraceptive or STI prevention. Consider monitoring weight changes if the patient is concerned about potential weight gain associated with contraceptive use. If the patient is not having any unacceptable symptoms or problems, the patient may continue getting DMPA injections. Advise your patient that after 2 years of continuous use you will have to 1) discuss the impact of DMPA on BMD and the question of fracture risk, 2) reassess any underlying risk factors for bone fragility or fractures, and 3) re-evaluate whether DMPA continues to be the best contraceptive option for the patient. If DMPA remains the patient's best contraceptive option, the patient may continue to get injections.

MANAGING DMPA PROBLEMS AND FOLLOW-UP

Menstrual changes. Inform patients in advance that changes will occur in their menstrual cycles. Do not dismiss the impact of bleeding changes: they are the major reason that patients discontinue this method. If bleeding occurs shortly after beginning DMPA, counsel patients that irregular bleeding decreases over time with use of DMPA. Unscheduled bleeding and spotting observed in prolonged use of DMPA may be managed initially by a 5 to 7 day course of non-steroidal anti-inflammatory drugs.[172,173] If this does not adequately control symptoms, other options include one or more cycles of combined oral contraceptives or exogenous estrogen.[174] Each of these interventions has been shown to decrease bleeding in the short term; however, when these interventions are discontinued, irregular bleeding patterns resume.[173,174] Patient may be educated to repeat these interventions as needed when symptoms recur.

A Cochrane review concluded that, while some patients may benefit to a degree from these interventions, there is not enough evidence to recommend routine use of any one regimen to treat menstrual irregularities with DMPA, especially in the long term.[175] Other agents that show promising data for management of irregular bleeding include antiprogestins such as mifepristone[176] and antifibrinolytics such as tranexamic acid,[177] but additional larger, well-controlled studies are needed.[175] Matrix metalloproteinase inhibitors such as doxycycline, have not been found to be effective in improving irregular bleeding with DMPA.[178]

Counseling helps continuation rates (see Discontinuation, in the Effectiveness section). Patients should be informed that the irregular bleeding might return but that over time the likelihood of amenorrhea will increase; in the context of DMPA use, amenorrhea is not harmful and does not require treatment.

Allergic reactions. Fortunately, severe anaphylactic reactions are rare. However, because DMPA is irreversible once injected, have on hand emergency supportive measures such as epinephrine and diphenhydramine. Encourage patients to stay in the clinic/office area for 20 minutes following their first injection. Those considering self-injection of DMPA-SC should receive their first one or two injections in a clinical setting, both to monitor for an allergic reaction and to learn safe self-injection technique.

USER INSTRUCTIONS FOR DMPA*

DMPA injections are very effective if you return on time for a repeat injection. Of 1,000 patients who consistently get repeat injections on time, only 2 will become pregnant over a year's time. DMPA works mainly by preventing ovulation and thickening the cervical mucus.

1. DMPA injections have many *noncontraceptive benefits*. DMPA injections may decrease—
   - Menstrual blood flow
   - Menstrual cramping

*These instructions are intended to guide providers in educating patients in how to use their method.

- Risk of anemia (low blood count)
- Risk of fibroids and bleeding from fibroids
- Risk of endometrial cancer
- Risk of ovarian cancer
- Risk of pelvic infection
- Risk of ectopic pregnancy (a pregnancy outside of the uterus)
- Risk of a sickle cell crisis
- Frequency of grand mal seizures

2. **To use DMPA, you must be willing to accept unpredictable, frequent, or absent menstrual bleeding.** About 40% to 50% of patients using DMPA will stop having any menstrual bleeding or spotting after a year of injections. This is to be expected and is not harmful to you.
3. **Have on hand a back-up contraceptive method** such as male or female condoms, contraceptive sponge, spermicidal foam, tablets, or suppositories. Depending on the timing of the injection, you may need to use your back-up method for 1 week after your first injection. This precaution may not be necessary if the first shot is given during the first 7 days after the beginning of your normal menstrual period. Ask your clinician to give you a package of or a prescription for the levonorgestrel emergency contraceptive pill, such as Plan B One-Step or Take Action, as a backup in case you have unprotected sex in the first week after your injection or if you are late for your next injection.
4. **Have condoms ready if you—**
    - Are late for your injection
    - May be at risk for a sexually transmitted infection, including infection with HIV, the virus that causes AIDS
5. Because of the rare possibility of an *allergic reaction*, you may be asked to remain in the vicinity of the clinic for 20 minutes after having your first DMPA injection.
6. **Make a return appointment. Before you leave the office**, schedule an appointment for your next injection. Mark your calendar for your next DMPA shot to be sure you will be on time.
7. Depression and premenstrual symptoms may improve or become worse.
8. DMPA can decrease estrogen levels, which can cause a decrease in the density of your bones. There is no evidence that DMPA use in reproductive-age patients increase the risk of fractures later

in life. However, given the theoretical risk of fractures, let your clinician know if you frequently take corticosteroids or heparin, if you have fractured bones with minimal trauma, if you have a bone metabolism disease, if you have a strong family history of osteoporosis and fractures, or if you have (or had) anorexia nervosa. Also, discuss bone health with your clinician if you plan to use DMPA for more than 2 years and are less than 18 years old or over 45 years old.[137]

9. Some DMPA users may gain weight. Be sure to eat a healthy balanced diet and exercise regularly. If you continue to gain weight excessively despite diet and exercise, discuss this with your clinician.

Late for Injection

1. **If you are more than 15 weeks (>2 weeks late) from your last injection** use a back-up method or abstain from intercourse as soon as you realize that you are going to be late. If you have had unprotected intercourse use emergency contraception right away. If you do not have emergency contraception on hand, you can get emergency contraception from your pharmacy without a prescription, but you will have to pay out of pocket. You should use a progestin-only emergency contraceptive (such as *Plan B One-Step* or *Take Action*). The generic medications cost on average $40. Anyone can buy emergency contraception without showing ID and regardless of age or gender. Visit your clinician as soon as possible for your injection. You will need to continue using a back-up method until you get your injection and for a week after that injection. Many clinicians will perform a pregnancy test to make sure you are not pregnant.
2. If you are afraid you will forget your appointment for your next injection, there are mobile apps available that can help you set reminders. Visit www.bedsider.org/reminders_app for directions to download one of these apps. Your clinician's office or clinic may also be able to call you or email you with reminders.

DMPA and Your Periods

1. DMPA will usually make your bleeding less regular and predictable. Eventually most patients on DMPA stop bleeding completely. This is not harmful. Do *not* choose DMPA if you do not desire changes to your periods.
2. If your pattern of bleeding concerns you, contact your clinician. Your clinician may recommend that you return to the clinic for

an evaluation to rule out the possibility of pregnancy or infection. If your bleeding is frequent or heavy, your clinician may want to rule out anemia. Your clinician may recommend medications that you can use to decrease your bleeding.

3. If you stop using DMPA, it may be a number of months before your periods return to normal after the last injection. However, there are medications, such as birth control pills, that can give you monthly bleeding after you stop using DMPA.

Discontinuing DMPA

1. If you do not wish to return for your next DMPA injection and do not want to become pregnant, start using a new contraceptive within 14 weeks after your last shot. This ensures that you will not be pregnant at the time you start the new contraceptive method. You may start birth control pills, have a contraceptive implant or intrauterine contraceptive placed, or use another contraceptive *before* the time you would have been due for your next injection.
2. If you stop DMPA because you want to become pregnant, remember that the contraceptive effect may take a number of months to go away. Start taking prenatal vitamins as soon as you decide to attempt pregnancy. Be patient.

DMPA and Pregnancy

1. DMPA injections may keep you from getting pregnant for 15 weeks after your last shot. Fifty percent of patients who stop DMPA to get pregnant will become pregnant within 10 months of the last injection. DMPA does not decrease your fertility in the long run.
2. If you are over age 35 and want to become pregnant in the near future, you may want to use an alternative contraceptive that has minimal or no delay in return of fertility after you stop using that method.
3. If you get pregnant while using DMPA, there is no increased risk of birth defects.[170,171]

DMPA Warning Signals

Serious health problems are very rare with DMPA use. Although DMPA is a highly effective contraceptive method, pregnancies do occur. If you feel pregnant, or think you might be pregnant, check with a pregnancy test. See your clinician if you develop any of the following warning signals or if any other symptoms concern you. Many of these symptoms are not due to DMPA use but may represent serious health problems:

- Heavy bleeding
- Depression
- Severe, lower abdominal pain (may be a sign of pregnancy)
- Pus, prolonged pain, redness, itching or bleeding at injection site (may be a sign of infection).

Author Disclosures—Wu: none. Bartz: none.

References

1. Mishell DR, Jr. Pharmacokinetics of depot medroxyprogesterone acetate contraception. J Reprod Med 1996;41:381–90.
2. Jain J, Dutton C, Nicosia A, Wajszczuk C, Bode F, Mishell D. Pharmacokinetics, ovulation suppression and return to ovulation follwoing a lower dose subcutaneous formulation of Depo-Provera. Contraception 2004;70:11–8.
3. Jain J, Jakimiuk A, Bode F, Ross D, Kaunitz A. Contraceptive efficacy and safety of DMPA-SC. Contraception 2004;70:269–75.
4. Dragoman MV, Gaffield ME. The safety of subcutaneously administered depot medroxyprogesterone acetate (104mg/0.65mL): A systematic review. Contraception 2016;94:202–15.
5. Gallo MF, Grimes DA, Lopez LM, Schulz KF, d'Arcangues C. Combination injectable contraceptives for contraception. Cochrane Database Syst Rev 2008:CD004568.
6. Haider S, Darney PD. Injectable contraception. Clin Obstet Gynecol 2007;50:898–906.
7. Petta CA, Faundes A, Dunson TR, et al. Timing of onset of contraceptive effectiveness in Depo-Provera users. II. Effects on ovarian function. Fertil Steril 1998;70:817–20.
8. Ismail AA, el-Faras A, Rocca M, el-Sibai FA, Toppozada M. Pituitary response to LHRH in long-term users of injectable contraceptives. Contraception 1987;35:487–95.
9. Paulen ME, Curtis KM. When can a woman have repeat progestogen-only injectables—depot medroxyprogesterone acetate or norethisterone enantate? Contraception 2009; 80:391–408.
10. Petta CA, Faundes A, Dunson TR, et al. Timing of onset of contraceptive effectiveness in Depo-Provera users: Part I. Changes in cervical mucus. Fertil Steril 1998;69:252–7.
11. Croxatto HB. Mechanisms that explain the contraceptive action of progestin implants for women. Contraception 2002;65:21–7.
12. Mishell DR, Jr. Long-acting contraceptive steroids. Postcoital contraceptives and antiprogestins. In: Mishell DR, Jr., Davajan V, Lobo R, eds. Infertility, contraception and reproductive endocrinology. Cambridge: Blackwell Scientific Publications; 1991.
13. Kaunitz AM, Darney PD, Ross D, Wolter KD, Speroff L. Subcutaneous DMPA vs. intramuscular DMPA: a 2-year randomized study of contraceptive efficacy and bone mineral density. Contraception 2009;80:7–17.
14. O'Neil-Callahan M, Peipert JF, Zhao Q, Madden T, Secura G. Twenty-four-month continuation of reversible contraception. Obstet Gynecol 2013;122:1083–91.
15. Daniels K, Daugherty J, Jones J. Current contraceptive status among women aged 15–44: United States, 2011–2013. NCHS Data Brief 2014:1–8.
16. Canto De Cetina TE, Canto P, Ordonez Luna M. Effect of counseling to improve compliance in Mexican women receiving depot-medroxyprogesterone acetate. Contraception 2001;63:143–6.

17. Hubacher D, Goco N, Gonzalez B, Taylor D. Factors affecting continuation rates of DMPA. Contraception 1999;60:345–51.
18. Moreau C, Cleland K, Trussell J. Contraceptive discontinuation attributed to method dissatisfaction in the United States. Contraception 2007;76:267–72.
19. Halpern V, Lopez LM, Grimes DA, Stockton LL, Gallo MF. Strategies to improve adherence and acceptability of hormonal methods of contraception. Cochrane Database Syst Rev 2013:CD004317.
20. Davidson AR, Kalmuss D, Cushman LF, Romero D, Heartwell S, Rulin M. Injectable contraceptive discontinuation and subsequent unintended pregnancy among low-income women. Am J Public Health 1997;87:1532–4.
21. Goldberg AB, Cardenas LH, Hubbard AE, Darney PD. Post-abortion depot medroxyprogesterone acetate continuation rates: a randomized trial of cyclic estradiol. Contraception 2002;66:215–20.
22. Lakha F, Henderson C, Glasier A. The acceptability of self-administration of subcutaneous Depo-Provera. Contraception 2005;72:14–8.
23. Williams RL, Hensel DJ, Fortenberry JD. Self-administration of subcutaneous depot medroxyprogesterone acetate by adolescent women. Contraception 2013;88:401–7.
24. Beasley A, White KO, Cremers S, Westhoff C. Randomized clinical trial of self versus clinical administration of subcutaneous depot medroxyprogesterone acetate. Contraception 2014;89:352–6.
25. Curtis KM, Tepper NK, Jatlaoui TC, et al. U.S. Medical Eligibility Criteria for Contraceptive Use, 2016. MMWR Recomm Rep 2016;65:1–103.
26. McCann MF, Potter LS. Progestin-only oral contraception: a comprehensive review. Contraception 1994;50:S1–195.
27. Speroff L, Darney PD. A clinical guide for contraception. Third ed. Philadelphia: Lippincott Williams & Wilkins; 2001.
28. Lopez LM, Bernholc A, Chen M, et al. Hormonal contraceptives for contraception in overweight or obese women. Cochrane Database Syst Rev 2016:CD008452.
29. Fu H, Darroch JE, Haas T, Ranjit N. Contraceptive failure rates: new estimates from the 1995 National Survey of Family Growth. Fam Plann Perspect 1999;31:56–63.
30. Stevens-Simon C, Kelly L, Kulick R. A village would be nice but . . . it takes a long-acting contraceptive to prevent repeat adolescent pregnancies. Am J Prev Med 2001;21:60–5.
31. Diedrich JT, Zhao Q, Madden T, Secura GM, Peipert JF. Three-year continuation of reversible contraception. Am J Obstet Gynecol 2015;213:662 e1–8.
32. Steinauer JE, Upadhyay UD, Sokoloff A, Harper CC, Diedrich JT, Drey EA. Choice of the levonorgestrel intrauterine device, etonogestrel implant or depot medroxyprogesterone acetate for contraception after aspiration abortion. Contraception 2015;92:553–9.
33. Callahan R, Yacobson I, Halpern V, Nanda K. Ectopic pregnancy with use of progestin-only injectables and contraceptive implants: a systematic review. Contraception 2015;92:514–22.
34. Borgatta L, Murthy A, Chuang C, Beardsley L, Burnhill MS. Pregnancies diagnosed during Depo-Provera use. Contraception 2002;66:169–72.
35. Belsey EM. Vaginal bleeding patterns among women using one natural and eight hormonal methods of contraception. Contraception 1988;38:181–206.
36. Schwallie PC, Assenzo JR. Contraceptive use—efficacy study utilizing medroxyprogesterone acetate administered as an intramuscular injection once every 90 days. Fertil Steril 1973;24:331–9.
37. Cromer BA, Smith RD, Blair JM, Dwyer J, Brown RT. A prospective study of adolescents who choose among levonorgestrel implant (Norplant), medroxyprogesterone acetate (Depo-Provera), or the combined oral contraceptive pill as contraception. Pediatrics 1994;94:687–94.
38. Arias RD, Jain JK, Brucker C, Ross D, Ray A. Changes in bleeding patterns with depot medroxyprogesterone acetate subcutaneous injection 104 mg. Contraception 2006;74:234–8.

39. Kaunitz AM. Injectable depot medroxyprogesterone acetate contraception: an update for U.S. clinicians. Int J Fertil Womens Med 1998;43:73–83.
40. Injectable contraceptives: their role in family planning. Geneva: World Health Organization; 1990.
41. Nanda K, Amaral E, Hays M, Viscola MA, Mehta N, Bahamondes L. Pharmacokinetic interactions between depot medroxyprogesterone acetate and combination antiretroviral therapy. Fertil Steril 2008;90:965–71.
42. Hatcher RA, Schnare S. Ask the experts: progestin-only contraceptives. Contracept Technol Update 1993;14:114–5.
43. Mattson RH, Cramer JA, Darney PD, Naftolin F. Use of oral contraceptives by women with epilepsy. JAMA 1986;256:238–40.
44. Mattson RH, Rebar RW. Contraceptive methods for women with neurologic disorders. Am J Obstet Gynecol 1993;168:2027–32.
45. Rhodes ME, Frye CA. Actions at GABA(A) receptors in the hippocampus may mediate some antiseizure effects of progestins. Epilepsy Behav 2005;6:320–7.
46. Hoopes AJ, Simmons KB, Godfrey EM, Sucato G. 2016 Updates to US Medical Eligibility Criteria for Contraceptive Use and Selected Practice Recommendations for Contraceptive Use: Highlights for adolescent patients. J Pediatr Adolesc Gynecol 2017.
47. de Abood M, de Castillo Z, Guerrero F, Espino M, Austin KL. Effect of Depo-Provera or Microgynon on the painful crises of sickle cell anemia patients. Contraception 1997;56:313–6.
48. Surrey ES. The role of progestins in treating the pain of endometriosis. J Minim Invasive Gynecol 2006;13:528–34.
49. Walch K, Unfried G, Huber J, et al. Implanon versus medroxyprogesterone acetate: effects on pain scores in patients with symptomatic endometriosis—a pilot study. Contraception 2009;79:29–34.
50. Crosignani PG, Luciano A, Ray A, Bergqvist A. Subcutaneous depot medroxyprogesterone acetate versus leuprolide acetate in the treatment of endometriosis-associated pain. Hum Reprod 2005.
51. Sangkomkamhang US, Lumbiganon P, Laopaiboon M, Mol BW. Progestogens or progestogen-releasing intrauterine systems for uterine fibroids. Cochrane Database Syst Rev 2013:CD008994.
52. Johnson N, Fletcher H, Reid M. Depo medroxyprogesterone acetate (DMPA) therapy for uterine myomata prior to surgery. Int J Gynaecol Obstet 2004;85:174–6.
53. Venkatachalam S, Bagratee JS, Moodley J. Medical management of uterine fibroids with medroxyprogesterone acetate (Depo Provera): a pilot study. J Obstet Gynaecol 2004;24:798–800.
54. Lumbiganon P, Rugpao S, Phandhu-fung S, Laopaiboon M, Vudhikamraksa N, Werawatakul Y. Protective effect of depot-medroxyprogesterone acetate on surgically treated uterine leiomyomas: a multicentre case—control study. Br J Obstet Gynaecol 1996;103:909–14.
55. Baeten J, Nyange P, Richardson B, et al. Hormonal contraception and risk of sexually transmitted disease acquisition: results from a prospective study. Am J Obstet Gynecol 2001;185:380–5.
56. Depot-medroxyprogesterone acetate (DMPA) and risk of endometrial cancer. The WHO Collaborative Study of Neoplasia and Steroid Contraceptives. Int J Cancer 1991;49: 186–90.
57. Wilailak S, Vipupinyo C, Suraseranivong V, et al. Depot medroxyprogesterone acetate and epithelial ovarian cancer: a multicentre case-control study. BJOG 2012;119:672–7.
58. Prabhakaran S. Self-administration of injectable contraceptives. Contraception 2008;77:315–7.
59. Gardner JM, Mishell DR, Jr. Analysis of bleeding patterns and resumption of fertility following discontinuation of a long acting injectable contraceptive. Fertil Steril 1970;21:286–91.

60. Paul C, Skegg DC, Williams S. Depot medroxyprogesterone acetate. Patterns of use and reasons for discontinuation. Contraception 1997;56:209–14.
61. Polaneczky M, Liblanc M. Long-term depot medroxyprogesterone acetate (Depo-Provera) use in inner-city adolescents. J Adolesc Health 1998;23:81–8.
62. Potter LS, Dalberth BT, Canamar R, Betz M. Depot medroxyprogesterone acetate pioneers. A retrospective study at a North Carolina Health Department. Contraception 1997;56:305–12.
63. Gray RH, Parker RA, Diethelm P. Vaginal bleeding disturbances associated with the discontinuation of long-acting injectable contraceptives. From the World Health Organization Special Programme for Research, Development, and Research Training in Human Reproduction; Task Force on Long-acting Systemic Agents for the Regulation of Fertility. Br J Obstet Gynaecol 1981;88:317–21.
64. Hickey M, Dwarte D, Fraser IS. Superficial endometrial vascular fragility in Norplant users and in women with ovulatory dysfunctional uterine bleeding. Hum Reprod 2000;15:1509–14.
65. Bahamondes L, Del Castillo S, Tabares G, Arce XE, Perrotti M, Petta C. Comparison of weight increase in users of depot medroxyprogesterone acetate and copper IUD up to 5 years. Contraception 2001;64:223–5.
66. Danli S, Qingxiang S, Guowei S. A multicentered clinical trial of the long-acting injectable contraceptive Depo Provera in Chinese women. Contraception 2000;62:15–8.
67. Amatayakul K, Sivasomboon B, Thanangkul O. A study of the mechanism of weight gain in medroxyprogesterone acetate users. Contraception 1980;22:605–22.
68. Bonny A, Britto M, Huang B, Succop P, Slap G. Weight gain, adiposity, and eating behaviors among adolescent females on depot medroxyprogesterone acetate (DMPA). J Pediatr Adolesc Gynecol 2004;17:109–15.
69. Pelkman CL, Chow M, Heinbach RA, Rolls BJ. Short-term effects of a progestational contraceptive drug on food intake, resting energy expenditure, and body weight in young women. Am J Clin Nutr 2001;73:19–26.
70. Steenland MW, Zapata LB, Brahmi D, Marchbanks PA, Curtis KM. Appropriate follow up to detect potential adverse events after initiation of select contraceptive methods: a systematic review. Contraception 2013;87:611–24.
71. Le YC, Rahman M, Berenson AB. Early weight gain predicting later weight gain among depot medroxyprogesterone acetate users. Obstet Gynecol 2009;114:279–84.
72. Bonny AE, Secic M, Cromer B. Early weight gain related to later weight gain in adolescents on depot medroxyprogesterone acetate. Obstet Gynecol 2011;117:793–7.
73. Bonny AE, Ziegler J, Harvey R, Debanne SM, Secic M, Cromer BA. Weight gain in obese and nonobese adolescent girls initiating depot medroxyprogesterone, oral contraceptive pills, or no hormonal contraceptive method. Arch Pediatr Adolesc Med 2006;160:40–5.
74. Civic D, Scholes D, Ichikawa L, et al. Depressive symptoms in users and non-users of depot medroxyprogesterone acetate. Contraception 2000;61:385–90.
75. Westhoff C, Truman C, Kalmuss D, et al. Depressive symptoms and Depo-Provera. Contraception 1998;57:237–40.
76. Berenson AB, Odom SD, Breitkopf CR, Rahman M. Physiologic and psychologic symptoms associated with use of injectable contraception and 20 microg oral contraceptive pills. Am J Obstet Gynecol 2008;199:351 e1–12.
77. Gupta N, O'Brien R, Jacobsen LJ, et al. Mood changes in adolescents using depot-medroxyprogesterone acetate for contraception: a prospective study. J Pediatr Adolesc Gynecol 2001;14:71–6.
78. World Health Organization. Medical Eligibility Criteria for Contraceptive Use. 5th ed. Geneva 2015.
79. Tsai R, Schaffir J. Effect of depot medroxyprogesterone acetate on postpartum depression. Contraception 2010;82:174–7.
80. Selo-Ojeme DO, Tillisi A, Welch CC. Anaphylaxis from medroxyprogesterone acetate. Obstet Gynecol 2004;103:1045–6.

81. Lestishock L, Pariseau C, Rooholamini S, Ammerman S. Anaphylaxis from depot medroxyprogesterone acetate in an adolescent girl. Obstet Gynecol 2011;118:443–5.
82. Kongsayreepong R, Chutivongse S, George P, et al. A multicentre comparative study of serum lipids and apolipoproteins in long-term users of DMPA and a control group of IUD users. World Health Organization. Task Force on Long-Acting Systemic Agents for Fertility Regulation Special Programme of Research, Development and Research Training in Human Reproduction. Contraception 1993;47:177–91.
83. Berenson AB, Rahman M, Wilkinson G. Effect of injectable and oral contraceptives on serum lipids. Obstet Gynecol 2009;114:786–94.
84. Segall-Gutierrez P, Xiang AH, Watanabe RM, et al. Deterioration in cardiometabolic risk markers in obese women during depot medroxyprogesterone acetate use. Contraception 2012;85:36–41.
85. Tepper NK, Whiteman MK, Marchbanks PA, James AH, Curtis KM. Progestin-only contraception and thromboembolism: A systematic review. Contraception 2016;94:678–700.
86. van Hylckama Vlieg A, Helmerhorst FM, Rosendaal FR. The risk of deep venous thrombosis associated with injectable depot-medroxyprogesterone acetate contraceptives or a levonorgestrel intrauterine device. Arterioscler Thromb Vasc Biol 2010;30:2297–300.
87. Whigham KA, Howie PW, Mack A, Prentice CR. The effect of an injectable progestogen contraceptive on blood coagulation and fibrinolysis. Br J Obstet Gynaecol 1979;86: 806–9.
88. Goldstein J, Cushman M, Badger GJ, Johnson JV. Effect of depomedroxyprogesterone acetate on coagulation parameter: a pilot study. Fertil Steril 2007;87:1267–70.
89. Schwallie PC, Assenzo JR. The effect of depo-medroxyprogesterone acetate on pituitary and ovarian function, and the return of fertility following its discontinuation: a review. Contraception 1974;10:181–202.
90. Nelson AL, Westhoff C, Schnare SM. Real-world patterns of prescription refills for branded hormonal contraceptives: a reflection of contraceptive discontinuation. Obstet Gynecol 2008;112:782–7.
91. Picardo C. Pharmacist-administered depot medroxyprogesterone acetate. Contraception 2006;73:559–61.
92. Picardo C, Ferreri S. Pharmacist-administered subcutaneous depot medroxyprogesterone acetate: a pilot randomized controlled trial. Contraception 2010;82:160–7.
93. Kennedy KI, Short RV, Tully MR. Premature introduction of progestin-only contraceptive methods during lactation. Contraception 1997;55:347–50.
94. Truitt ST, Fraser AB, Grimes DA, Gallo MF, Schulz KF. Combined hormonal versus nonhormonal versus progestin-only contraception in lactation. Cochrane Database Syst Rev 2003:CD003988.
95. Lopez LM, Grey TW, Stuebe AM, Chen M, Truitt ST, Gallo MF. Combined hormonal versus nonhormonal versus progestin-only contraception in lactation. Cochrane Database Syst Rev 2015:CD003988.
96. Halderman LD, Nelson AL. Impact of early postpartum administration of progestin-only hormonal contraceptives compared with nonhormonal contraceptives on short-term breast-feeding patterns. Am J Obstet Gynecol 2002;186:1250–6; discussion 6–8.
97. International Planned Parenthood Federation. IMAP statement on breast feeding, fertility and postpartum contraception. IPPF Med Bull 1996;30:1–3.
98. Medical eligibility criteria for contraceptive use, fourth edition. Geneva: World Health Organization; 2009.
99. Brownell E, Howard CR, Lawrence RA, Dozier AM. Delayed onset lactogenesis II predicts the cessation of any or exclusive breastfeeding. J Pediatr 2012;161:608–14.
100. McCann MF, Liskin LS, Piotrow PT, Rinehart W, Fox G. Breast-feeding, fertility, and family planning. Popul Rep J 1981:J525–75.
101. Effects of hormonal contraceptives on breast milk composition and infant growth. World Health Organization (WHO) Task Force on Oral Contraceptives. Stud Fam Plann 1988;19:361–9.

102. Brownell EA, Fernandez ID, Fisher SG, et al. The effect of immediate postpartum depot medroxyprogesterone on early breastfeeding cessation. Contraception 2013;87:836–43.
103. Rodriguez MI, Kaunitz AM. An evidence-based approach to postpartum use of depot medroxyprogesterone acetate in breastfeeding women. Contraception 2009;80:4–6.
104. Speroff L, Mishell DR, Jr. The postpartum visit: it's time for a change in order to optimally initiate contraception. Contraception 2008;78:90–8.
105. Skegg DC, Noonan EA, Paul C, Spears GF, Meirik O, Thomas DB. Depot medroxyprogesterone acetate and breast cancer. A pooled analysis of the World Health Organization and New Zealand studies. JAMA 1995;273:799–804.
106. Shapiro S, Rosenberg L, Hoffman M, et al. Risk of breast cancer in relation to the use of injectable progestogen contraceptives and combined estrogen/progestogen contraceptives. Am J Epidemiol 2000;151:396–403.
107. Strom BL, Berlin JA, Weber AL, et al. Absence of an effect of injectable and implantable progestin-only contraceptives on subsequent risk of breast cancer. Contraception 2004;69:353–60.
108. Depot-medroxyprogesterone acetate (DMPA) and risk of invasive squamous cell cervical cancer. The WHO Collaborative Study of Neoplasia and Steroid Contraceptives. Contraception 1992;45:299–312.
109. Thomas DB, Ray RM. Depot-medroxyprogesterone acetate (DMPA) and risk of invasive adenocarcinomas and adenosquamous carcinomas of the uterine cervix. WHO Collaborative Study of Neoplasia and Steroid Contraceptives. Contraception 1995;52:307–12.
110. Clark MK, Sowers M, Levy BT, Tenhundfeld P. Magnitude and variability of sequential estradiol and progesterone concentrations in women using depot medroxyprogesterone acetate for contraception. Fertil Steril 2001;75:871–7.
111. Berenson A, Breitkopf C, Grady J, Rickert V, Thomas A. Effects of hormonal contraception use on bone mineral density after 24 months of use. Obstetrics and Gynecology 2004;103:899–906.
112. Clark MK, Sowers M, Levy B, Nichols S. Bone mineral density loss and recovery during 48 months in first-time users of depot medroxyprogesterone acetate. Fertil Steril 2006;86:1466–74.
113. Cromer B, Stager M, Bonny A, et al. Depot medroxyprogesterone acetate, oral contraceptives and bone mineral density in a cohort of adolescent girls. J Adolescent Health 2004;35:434–41.
114. Cundy T, Cornish J, Roberts H, Elder H, Reid I. Spinal bone density in women using depot medroxyprogesterone contraception. Obstetrics and Gynecology 1998;92:569–73.
115. Paiva L, Pinto-Neto A, Faundes A. Bone density among long-term users of medroxyprogesterone acetate as a contraceptive. Contraception 1998;58:351–5.
116. Cundy T, Cornish J, Evans MC, Roberts H, Reid IR. Recovery of bone density in women who stop using medroxyprogesterone acetate. BMJ 1994;308:247–8.
117. Scholes D, Lacroix A, Ichikawa L, Barlow W, Ott S. Injectable hormone contraception and bone density: results from a prospective study. Epidemiology 2002;13:581–7.
118. Scholes D, Lacroix A, Ichikawa L, Barlow W, Ott S. Change in bone mineral density among adolescent women using and discontinuing depot medroxyprogesterone acetate contraception. Archives of Pediatric and Adolescent Medicine 2005;159:139–44.
119. Clark M, Sowers M, Nichols S, Levy B. Bone mineral density changes over two years in first-time users of depot medroxyprogesterone acetate. Fertil Steril 2004;82:1580–6.
120. Petitti DB, Piaggio G, Mehta S, Cravioto MC, Meirik O. Steroid hormone contraception and bone mineral density: a cross-sectional study in an international population. The WHO Study of Hormonal Contraception and Bone Health. Obstet Gynecol 2000;95: 736–44.
121. Kaunitz AM, Arias R, McClung M. Bone density recovery after depot medroxyprogesterone acetate injectable contraception use. Contraception 2008;77:67–76.

122. Harkins GJ, Davis GD, Dettori J, Hibbert ML, Hoyt RA. Decline in bone mineral density with stress fractures in a woman on depot medroxyprogesterone acetate. A case report. J Reprod Med 1999;44:309–12.
123. Lappe JM, Stegman MR, Recker RR. The impact of lifestyle factors on stress fractures in female Army recruits. Osteoporos Int 2001;12:35–42.
124. Watson KC, Lentz MJ, Cain KC. Associations between fracture incidence and use of depot medroxyprogesterone acetate and anti-epileptic drugs in women with developmental disabilities. Womens Health Issues 2006;16:346–52.
125. Lanza LL, McQuay LJ, Rothman KJ, et al. Use of depot medroxyprogesterone acetate contraception and incidence of bone fracture. Obstet Gynecol 2013;121:593–600.
126. Lopez LM, Grimes DA, Schulz KF, Curtis KM, Chen M. Steroidal contraceptives: effect on bone fractures in women. Cochrane Database Syst Rev 2014:CD006033.
127. Chantry CJ, Auinger P, Byrd RS. Lactation among adolescent mothers and subsequent bone mineral density. Arch Pediatr Adolesc Med 2004;158:650–6.
128. Sowers M, Corton G, Shapiro B, et al. Changes in bone density with lactation. JAMA 1993;269:3130–5.
129. Karlsson MK, Ahlborg HG, Karlsson C. Maternity and bone mineral density. Acta Orthop 2005;76:2–13.
130. Santelli JS, Abma J, Ventura S, et al. Can changes in sexual behaviors among high school students explain the decline in teen pregnancy rates in the 1990s? J Adolesc Health 2004;35:80–90.
131. Santelli JS, Lindberg LD, Finer LB, Singh S. Explaining recent declines in adolescent pregnancy in the United States: the contribution of abstinence and improved contraceptive use. Am J Public Health 2007;97:150–6.
132. Curtis KM, Chrisman CE, Peterson HB. Contraception for women in selected circumstances. Obstet Gynecol 2002;99:1100–12.
133. Harel Z, Johnson CC, Gold MA, et al. Recovery of bone mineral density in adolescents following the use of depot medroxyprogesterone acetate contraceptive injections. Contraception 2010;81:281–91.
134. Orr-Walker BJ, Evans MC, Ames RW, Clearwater JM, Cundy T, Reid IR. The effect of past use of the injectable contraceptive depot medroxyprogesterone acetate on bone mineral density in normal post-menopausal women. Clin Endocrinol (Oxf) 1998;49:615–8.
135. Cundy T, Cornish J, Roberts H, Reid I. Menopausal bone loss in long-term users of depot medroxyprogesterone acetate contraception. Am J Obstet Gynecol 2002;186:978–83.
136. Depo-Provera label. Pharmacia & Upjohn, 2004. At www.accessdata.fda.gov/drugsatfda_docs/label/2004/20246s025lbl.pdf. Accessed April 8, 2010.
137. WHO statement on hormonal contraception and bone health. Wkly Epidemiol Rec 2005;80:302–4.
138. World Health Organization. Technical consultation on the effects of hormonal contraception on bone health. Geneva, Switzerland: World Health Organization 2007.
139. Cromer BA, Scholes D, Berenson A, Cundy T, Clark MK, Kaunitz AM. Depot medroxyprogesterone acetate and bone mineral density in adolescents—the Black Box Warning: a Position Paper of the Society for Adolescent Medicine. J Adolesc Health 2006;39:296–301.
140. ACOG Committee Opinion No. 415: Depot medroxyprogesterone acetate and bone effects. Obstet Gynecol 2008;112:727–30.
141. Committee Opinion No. 602: Depot medroxyprogesterone acetate and bone effects. Obstet Gynecol 2014;123:1398–402.
142. Grimes DA, Schulz KF. Surrogate end points in clinical research: hazardous to your health. Obstet Gynecol 2005;105:1114–8.
143. Diagnosis of osteoporosis in men, premenopausal women, and children. J Clin Densitom 2004;7:17–26.
144. Lewiecki EM. Premenopausal bone health assessment. Curr Rheumatol Rep 2005;7:46–52.

145. Gbolade B, Ellis S, Murby B, Randall S, Kirkman R. Bone density in long term users of depot medroxyprogesterone acetate. British Journal of Obstetrics and Gynaecology 1998;105:790–4.
146. Morrison CS, Turner AN, Jones LB. Highly effective contraception and acquisition of HIV and other sexually transmitted infections. Best Pract Res Clin Obstet Gynaecol 2009;23:263–84.
147. Morrison C, Bright P, Wong E, et al. Hormonal contraceptive use, cervical ectopy, and the acquisition of cervical infections. Sexually Transmitted Diseases 2004;31:561–7.
148. Jacobson DL, Peralta L, Farmer M, Graham NM, Gaydos C, Zenilman J. Relationship of hormonal contraception and cervical ectopy as measured by computerized planimetry to chlamydial infection in adolescents. Sex Transm Dis 2000;27:313–9.
149. Dayan L, Donovan B. Chlamydia, gonorrhoea, and injectable progesterone. Lancet 2004;364:1387–8.
150. Hickey M, Marino JL, Tachedjian G. Critical review: mechanisms of HIV transmission in Depo-Provera users: the likely role of hypoestrogenism. J Acquir Immune Defic Syndr 2016;71:1–7.
151. Haddad LB, Polis CB, Sheth AN, et al. Contraceptive methods and risk of HIV acquisition or female-to-male transmission. Curr HIV / AIDS Rep 2014;11:447–58.
152. Polis CB, Curtis KM, Hannaford PC, et al. An updated systematic review of epidemiological evidence on hormonal contraceptive methods and HIV acquisition in women. AIDS 2016;30:2665–83.
153. Hel Z, Stringer E, Mestecky J. Sex steroid hormones, hormonal contraception, and the immunobiology of human immunodeficiency virus-1 infection. Endocr Rev 2010;31: 79–97.
154. Murphy K, Irvin SC, Herold BC. Research gaps in defining the biological link between HIV risk and hormonal contraception. Am J Reprod Immunol 2014;72:228–35.
155. Polis CB, Westreich D, Balkus JE, Heffron R, Participants of the HCHIVOAM. Assessing the effect of hormonal contraception on HIV acquisition in observational data: challenges and recommended analytic approaches. AIDS 2013;27 Suppl 1:S35–43.
156. Baeten JM, Benki S, Chohan V, et al. Hormonal contraceptive use, herpes simplex virus infection, and risk of HIV-1 acquisition among Kenyan women. AIDS 2007;21:1771–7.
157. Martin HL, Jr., Nyange PM, Richardson BA, et al. Hormonal contraception, sexually transmitted diseases, and risk of heterosexual transmission of human immunodeficiency virus type 1. J Infect Dis 1998;178:1053–9.
158. Ungchusak K, Rehle T, Thammapornpilap P, Spiegelman D, Brinkmann U, Siraprapasiri T. Determinants of HIV infection among female commercial sex workers in northeastern Thailand: results from a longitudinal study. J Acquir Immune Defic Syndr Hum Retrovirol 1996;12:500–7.
159. Bulterys M, Chao A, Habimana P, Dushimimana A, Nawrocki P, Saah A. Incident HIV-1 infection in a cohort of young women in Butare, Rwanda. AIDS 1994;8:1585–91.
160. Morrison CS, Richardson BA, Mmiro F, et al. Hormonal contraception and the risk of HIV acquisition. AIDS 2007;21:85–95.
161. Gaffield ME, Rodriguez MI. Hormonal contraceptive eligibility for women at high risk of HIV, Guidance Statement. Geneva, Switzerland: World Health Organization; 2017.
162. Sneed R, Westhoff C, Morroni C, Tiezzi L. A prospective study of immediate initiation of depo medroxyprogesterone acetate contraceptive injection. Contraception 2005;71: 99–103.
163. Lopez LM, Newmann SJ, Grimes DA, Nanda K, Schulz KF. Immediate start of hormonal contraceptives for contraception. Cochrane Database Syst Rev 2008:CD006260.
164. Nelson AL, Katz T. Initiation and continuation rates seen in 2-year experience with Same Day injections of DMPA. Contraception 2007;75:84–7.
165. Rickert VI, Tiezzi L, Lipshutz J, Leon J, Vaughan RD, Westhoff C. Depo Now: preventing unintended pregnancies among adolescents and young adults. J Adolesc Health 2007;40:22–8.

166. Kaunitz AM. Long-acting injectable contraception with depot medroxyprogesterone acetate. Am J Obstet Gynecol 1994;170:1543–9.
167. Steiner MJ, Kwok C, Stanback J, et al. Injectable contraception: what should the longest interval be for reinjections? Contraception 2008;77:410–4.
168. Curtis KM, Jatlaoui TC, Tepper NK, et al. U.S. Selected Practice Recommendations for Contraceptive Use, 2016. MMWR Recomm Rep 2016;65:1–66.
169. Pardthaisong T, Gray RH. In utero exposure to steroid contraceptives and outcome of pregnancy. Am J Epidemiol 1991;134:795–803.
170. Dahlberg K. Some effects of depo-medroxyprogesterone acetate (DMPA): observations in the nursing infant and in the long-term user. Int J Gynaecol Obstet 1982;20:43–8.
171. Katz Z, Lancet M, Skornik J, Chemke J, Mogilner BM, Klinberg M. Teratogenicity of progestogens given during the first trimester of pregnancy. Obstet Gynecol 1985;65:775–80.
172. Nathirojanakun P, Taneepanichskul S, Sappakitkumjorn N. Efficacy of a selective COX-2 inhibitor for controlling irregular uterine bleeding in DMPA users. Contraception 2006;73:584–7.
173. Tantiwattanakul P, Taneepanichskul S. Effect of mefenamic acid on controlling irregular uterine bleeding in DMPA users. Contraception 2004;70:277–9.
174. Said S, Sadek W, Rocca M, et al. Clinical evaluation of the therapeutic effectiveness of ethinyl oestradiol and oestrone sulphate on prolonged bleeding in women using depot medroxyprogesterone acetate for contraception. World Health Organization, Special Programme of Research, Development and Research Training in Human Reproduction, Task Force on Long-acting Systemic Agents for Fertility Regulation. Hum Reprod 1996;11 Suppl 2:1–13.
175. Abdel-Aleem H, d'Arcangues C, Vogelsong KM, Gaffield ML, Gulmezoglu AM. Treatment of vaginal bleeding irregularities induced by progestin only contraceptives. Cochrane Database Syst Rev 2013:CD003449.
176. Jain JK, Nicosia AF, Nucatola DL, Lu JJ, Kuo J, Felix JC. Mifepristone for the prevention of breakthrough bleeding in new starters of depo-medroxyprogesterone acetate. Steroids 2003;68:1115–9.
177. Senthong AJ, Taneepanichskul S. The effect of tranexamic acid for treatment irregular uterine bleeding secondary to DMPA use. J Med Assoc Thai 2009;92:461–5.
178. Abdel-Aleem H, Shaaban OM, Abdel-Aleem MA, Fetih GN. Doxycycline in the treatment of bleeding with DMPA: a double-blinded randomized controlled trial. Contraception 2012;86:224–30.

Contraceptive Patch and Vaginal Contraceptive Ring

7

Kavita Nanda, MD, MHS
Anne Burke, MD, MPH

- Both the weekly contraceptive patch and the monthly vaginal contraceptive ring are highly effective in clinical trials, with pregnancy rates less than 1 per 100. However, of 100 typical patch or ring users, approximately 7 will become pregnant within a year (see Chapter 26).
- Neither the contraceptive patch nor the vaginal contraceptive ring requires daily use—which could facilitate consistent and correct use for some users—as compared with combined oral contraceptives (COCs).
- Serum estrogen levels with the patch are higher than with COCs, while levels with the vaginal ring are the lowest of the three. It is unclear whether the difference in levels leads to clinically significant differences in adverse outcomes.
- Reported side effects associated with use of the contraceptive patch and ring are similar to those associated with COC use, except for skin reactions and more frequent and pronounced breast tenderness associated with patch use and vaginal symptoms associated with ring use.

CONTRACEPTIVE PATCH

A transdermal contraceptive patch (Ortho Evra) was approved by the Food and Drug Administration (FDA) in 2002. Ortho Evra is no longer marketed in the United States, but a generic version of the Ortho Evra patch (Xulane) was found to be bioequivalent and was approved by the FDA in 2014. It is a thin, flexible patch with three layers: a beige outer protective polyester layer; a middle medicated adhesive layer; and a clear liner. The Ortho Evra patch contained 6 mg of norelgestromin (the primary active metabolite of norgestimate) and 0.75 mg of ethinyl estradiol (EE) in each 20 cm^2 patch, while Xulane contains 4.86 mg of norelgestromin and 0.53 mg of EE in each 14 cm^2 patch. Both patches release 150 micrograms (mcg) of norelgestromin and 20 mcg of EE daily. The patch can be applied to the buttocks, upper arm, lower abdomen, or upper torso (excluding the breasts). The dosing schedule is designed to mimic the 28-day dosing schedule of combined oral contraceptives (COCs), with 21 days of active hormones. Each patch provides contraceptive protection for 7 days. Users apply a new 7-day patch for each of 3 weeks, and then they have a 7-day patch-free interval. Several other formulations are under investigation, or used in other countries. These will be briefly discussed at the end of this chapter.

MECHANISM OF ACTION

The patch, like other combined hormonal contraceptives, works mainly by suppressing gonadotropins and preventing ovulation.[1] Other likely mechanisms of action include thickening of the cervical mucus to prevent sperm penetration and endometrial changes that could affect implantation.

EFFECTIVENESS AND SUCCESSFUL USE

In clinical trials and as reported in a Cochrane Review,[2] failure rates for patches were similar to those with COCs. Pearl Indices for the patch range from 0.71 to 1.24 per 100 person-years with overall use in trials, to 0.59 to 0.99 with perfect use.[3,4] In a pooled analysis of the three pivotal clinical trials, 15 pregnancies occurred in 22,160 treatment cycles, with an overall life-table failure rate of 0.8% (95% CI, 0.3%–1.3%) and overall Pearl Index of 0.88 (95% CI, 0.44–1.33).[5] In this analysis, the contraceptive patch was less effective in obese women (see Special Populations).

Although clinical trials showed higher correct and consistent use with the patch than with COCs,[4,6] pregnancy rates are similar to or higher than those with COCs.[2] In observational studies of typical use, patch users in the United Kingdom's General Practice Database had slightly higher pregnancy rates (0.34 per 100 person-years, 95% CI 0.13–0.69) compared with users of second- and third-generation COCs (0.16, 95% CI 0.14–0.17 and 0.12, 95% CI 0.10–0.15, respectively); however, women using the patch were younger than women using COCs.[7] In another observational study of new hormonal contraceptive users at high risk of unintended pregnancy, the Pearl Index was 3.62 for COCs and 14.84 for the patch in a total of 3,206 cycles.[8] Patch users in this study were less educated, had more prior pregnancies and abortions, and were more likely to be lost to follow-up immediately after receiving a prescription.

Continuation: Discontinuation is a challenge to the effectiveness of short-acting contraceptive methods: users who discontinue a short-acting method without replacement are at almost immediate risk of unintended pregnancy. Despite its convenience, the contraceptive patch does not have higher continuation rates or lower failure rates than COCs.[7–9] In comparative studies, continuation rates with the patch in typical use populations were lower than with the vaginal ring (88% vs. 95% over 3 cycles, $p = 0.03$)[10] or with COCs (67% vs. 89% over 3 cycles, $p < .001$; and 57% vs. 76% at 1 year, $p = .004$).[8] Another large cohort of young women showed very low continuation rates for the patch; the 12-month continuation rate was 10.9 per 100 person-years compared with 32.7 per 100 person-years for COCs; reported side effects were the most common reasons for discontinuation.[11] In contrast, the contraceptive CHOICE study found continuation rates for the patch were low, but similar to those with COCs and rings, with 1-, 2-, and 3-year patch continuation rates of 49%, 40%, and 28%.[12–14]

SPECIAL POPULATIONS

Patients with higher body weight: Body weight is associated with lower serum levels of EE and norelgestromin in contraceptive patch users.[5] Furthermore, limited evidence suggests that persons weighing more than 90 kg (198 lbs) may be at higher risk of pregnancy when using the contraceptive patch, but evidence is inconsistent. In a pooled analysis of the three pivotal trials, 5 of the 15 pregnancies that occurred in patch users were in women weighing more than 90 kg, though such women comprised only 3% of the study population.[5] In contrast, another recent observational study found no increased risk of contraceptive failure among overweight, obese, and morbidly obese contraceptive patch users, though data were combined with pill and ring user data.[15]

Adolescents: In one observational study of teen mothers during the first year postpartum, repeat pregnancy rates were similar for patch users (32%) and COC users (30%) and higher than those of DMPA users (14%).[9] In another cohort study of women aged 15 to 24, self-reported pregnancy rates were of 30.1 per 100 person-years among patch users, compared with 15.6 per 100 person-years among COC users.[11] However, in the contraceptive CHOICE study, failure rates in participants using COCs, patch, or ring were similar and were combined: 4.8%, 7.8%, and 9.4% in years 1, 2, and 3.[16]

Although continuation rates among adolescent patch users in one study were higher at 3 months than for COCs (71% vs. 51%), approximately half of both patch and COC users stopped the method by 1 year.[9] Another observational study found that only 38% of adolescent patch users (compared with 60% of COC users) were still using their method after nine cycles, even though no differences were noted in reported side effects or quality of life.[17] In the study of young women reported above, 1-year continuation rates were lowest for patch and depot medroxyprogesterone acetate initiators, 10.9 and 12.1 per 100 person-years, compared with 29.4 and 32.7 per 100 person-years for ring and pill users.[11]

DOSING REGIMENS

Conventional use of the patch follows a 28-day cycle. A user applies a new patch weekly for 3 weeks, leaves the patch off for a week to allow withdrawal bleeding, and then applies a new patch. Extended use of combined hormonal contraceptives has been studied in healthy women who wish to avoid estrogen-withdrawal side effects during the hormone-free week or to avoid withdrawal bleeding.[18] Likewise, extended (84 days) use of the patch resulted in fewer days of bleeding and episodes of bleeding or spotting when compared with cyclic use.[19] Women in both groups reported more headache days during the patch-off weeks compared with patch-on weeks, but women in the extended group also reported more headache days per week while wearing the patch. Both regimens led to decreased headache frequency over time, and women in both groups were highly satisfied.[19] In one new study of 12 weeks of extended patch use, slow accumulation of EE levels was noted over time.[20] No published data evaluate long-term risks of extended patch use; the safety of this practice is unproven.

ADVANTAGES

CONTRACEPTIVE BENEFITS

1. **Convenience.** Some users find the weekly patch regimen more convenient than a daily pill regimen. In study populations, the weekly regimen appears to enhance consistent and correct use when compared with daily COC use, particularly among younger women.[3,4,6,21] Adolescents using the contraceptive patch are more likely to use them consistently and correctly than those using COCs, making the patch a method particularly appropriate for teens.[6,21] Ease of use, the lack of need for daily adherence, and the ease of concealment are among the reported advantages.

However, adolescents are more likely than older users to experience problems with adherence and use.[21,22]

2. **Forgiving.** Hormone levels remain therapeutic for at least 9 days after application of the second patch, suggesting that ovulation inhibition would be maintained even if a scheduled patch change was missed for as long as 2 days.[23] Additionally, missed patches (either forgetting to start a new patch or forgetting to change a patch) are less likely to lead to follicular growth or ovulation than are missed COCs.[1] Hormone levels and ovulation are surrogate markers, however, and no studies have evaluated pregnancy rates with missed patches.

3. **Adheres well under a variety of conditions.** In clinical trials, very few patches (< 5%) needed replacement because of complete or partial detachment. Heat, humidity, and exercise do not affect patch adhesion or pharmacokinetics.[23,24] In typical use, however, patch adhesion may be lower. In one 3-cycle study, almost half of the women reported that the patch fell off at least once.[10] Adolescents are more likely to experience problems with application site reactions and patch detachment, so they should receive anticipatory counseling.[21,22]

4. **Verifiable.** The user can easily verify the presence of the patch. This reassurance about continued protection may reduce the anxiety some individuals report with COCs—questioning whether they remembered to take their daily pill and worrying that they might forget to take it.

5. **Rapidly reversible.** Fertility returns rapidly when users discontinue the patch; FSH and LH levels return to nearly baseline levels, and 86% of women ovulate in the month following patch discontinuation.[1]

Menstrual Benefits

Cycle control comparable to COCs. Although patch users may experience more breakthrough bleeding and spotting in the first 2 cycles, subsequent cycle control is comparable to that seen with COCs.[3,4] In a randomized cross-over trial comparing patch use to vaginal ring use, however, women switching to the patch were more likely than women switching to the ring to experience longer periods (38% compared with 9%) and increased dysmenorrhea (29%compared with 16%).[10]

Noncontraceptive Benefits

Because the hormone levels and mechanisms of action are similar to those of COCs, the contraceptive patch may provide many of the same advantages and noncontraceptive health benefits (see Chapter 8 on

Combined Oral Contraceptives). Data about long-term health benefits are not yet available.

1. **No significant weight gain.** In a randomized placebo-controlled trial, the contraceptive patch was not associated with weight gain. In a pooled analysis of the clinical trials, the mean change in body weight from baseline to the end of treatment was an increase of 0.3 kg, and 79% of participants remained within 5% of their baseline weight.[25]

2. **No clinically significant metabolic effects.** Although the patch has not been studied in individuals with cardiovascular or other diseases, studies in healthy women have shown no clinically meaningful changes in hematology, blood chemistry, or bone turnover.[26–29] However, the impact of the patch on surrogate markers, such as cholesterol or coagulation tests, may not reflect the impact on outcomes of clinical interest such as myocardial infarction or stroke.[30]

3. **No need for oral administration.** Patches can be used by individuals who cannot take a pill orally or who have abnormal intestinal drug absorption.

4. **No effect on sexual function.** In one recent study, women switching from COCs to the patch had slightly higher sexual functioning scores.[31]

DISADVANTAGES AND CAUTIONS

POTENTIALLY SERIOUS HEALTH EFFECTS

1. **Risk of venous thromboembolism (VTE) or arterial thromboembolism (ATE).** Serum ethinyl estradiol levels of patch users appear to be higher than those of women using a COC containing 35 mcg EE.[32] However, pharmacokinetic measures are surrogate markers and do not necessarily correlate with the magnitude of risk of rare estrogen-related complications such as VTE, stroke, or myocardial infarction, and epidemiologic data are inconsistent. Several studies have been published, with some studies finding risks similar to those associated with COC use while others noting higher risks with patch.[33–41] The FDA conducted its own review of several databases and found an increased risk of VTE with the contraceptive patch compared with certain COCs, leading to a change in the warning label. In contrast, the CDC MEC does not distinguish between the different combined hormonal methods (patch, ring, COC) when categorizing conditions associated with risk of VTE.[42] In any event, any risk of VTE with patch use is still far below the risk of VTE during pregnancy and the postpartum period.

In the Cochrane review, the risk of VTE with patch use was estimated to be 53 per 100,000 women (95% CI 1 to 294).[2]

The risk of ATE does not appear increased among women using the patch compared with those using COCs.[41] One retrospective cohort study found a tripling of thrombotic stroke risk among patch users compared with women *not* using hormonal contraceptives.[43]

2. **Other health complications.** In pivotal studies, other serious adverse events reported with patch use included migraine, cholecystitis, paresthesia at the patch site, cervical adenocarcinoma in situ, and menorrhagia.[25] Although data are scarce, the contraceptive patch may also be associated with some of the rare but serious health complications associated with COCs, such as cholestatic jaundice, hepatic adenomas, or other conditions.

Reported Side Effects

1. **Skin reactions.** One unique side effect, experienced by up to half of patch users, is a transient skin reaction, such as irritation, redness, pigment changes, or rash at the site of patch application. These reactions lead to patch discontinuation less than 3% of the time, however. Most application-site reactions are mild to moderate, and the reactions do not appear more frequently over time.[25,44]

2. **Breast symptoms.** In a pooled analysis of the three pivotal clinical trials, 22% of patch users reported breast discomfort, engorgement, or pain, mainly in cycles 1 and 2. Breast symptoms were generally mild or moderate, decreased with continued use, and rarely led to patch discontinuation.[25] Compared with women using COCs and the vaginal ring, women using the patch are more likely to experience breast symptoms.[10,25]

3. **Headache.** In one study, 22% of women using either the patch or COCs reported headaches. Headaches led to discontinuation in 1.1% of patch users—a higher rate than in COC users.[25] Whether these symptoms are actually caused by the patch is unknown.

4. **Nausea.** Nausea is another frequent complaint, reported by approximately one fifth of both patch and COC users in a pooled study.[25] In the clinical trials, nausea led to patch discontinuation in 1.5% of women.[4] In the cross-over trial of patch vs. ring use, women switching to the patch were more likely than women switching to the ring to report frequent nausea (8% compared with 1%).[10]

See section on Providing the Contraceptive Patch and Vaginal Ring, Managing Problems, and User Instructions.

VAGINAL CONTRACEPTIVE RING

A vaginal contraceptive ring (NuvaRing) was approved by the FDA in 2001. NuvaRing is a soft, transparent, flexible ring of ethylene vinyl acetate copolymer, with an outer diameter of 54 mm and a cross-sectional diameter of 4 mm. The ring releases 120 mcg of etonogestrel (3-keto desogestrel) (ENG), the major metabolite of desogestrel, and 15 mcg of ethinyl estradiol (EE) daily.

The vaginal contraceptive ring is considered a combined hormonal contraceptive, along with the contraceptive patch and oral contraceptives. About 6% of American women have ever used the ring.[45] Of those currently using a contraceptive method, 2.6% report using the ring.[46]

While the ENG/EE vaginal contraceptive ring is currently the only one available in the United States, there are several other formulations under investigation or in use in other countries. These will be briefly discussed at the end of this chapter. Most of this chapter will focus on the ENG/EE ring (NuvaRing).

MECHANISM OF ACTION

The contraceptive mechanism of action of the combined vaginal ring is primarily ovulation suppression. Other likely mechanisms include effects on cervical mucus viscosity and endometrial thinning.[47]

EFFECTIVENESS AND SUCCESSFUL USE

Failure rates with the vaginal contraceptive ring in clinical trials are low and similar to the patch and COCs.[48] Pearl Indices range from 0.25 to 0.96 per 100 person-years with perfect use, to 0.65 to 1.23 overall.[48,49] In one study, more pregnancies occurred in North American sites than in European sites; the overall Pearl Index was 1.75 in North America and 0.65 in Europe. Reasons for this difference are unclear but likely reflect differences in participant characteristics among different study settings.[50,51] Typical-use pregnancy rates among those using the ring are about 7% in the first year. (See Chapter 26).

Theoretically, improved ease of adherence to ring regimens could lead to typical-use pregnancy rates lower than those with COCs, which require daily attention. However, this has not been conclusively demonstrated. One recent systematic review noted that, among 8 clinical trials, pregnancy rates were similar between the vaginal ring and oral contraceptives.[2] Another systematic review found a trend toward lower pregnancy rates with the ring compared to COCs, though the trend did not meet statistical significance (OR 0.52, 95%CI 0.26-1.04).[52]

Findings about whether adherence is improved with the ring compared with the pill are mixed. Although a non-comparative trial showed a high rate of correct and consistent ring use (91%),[53] randomized comparative trials generally have demonstrated similar adherence rates for both methods.[2,48,49] Recently, a systematic review found that the number of study participants able to adhere correctly to ring and pill regimens was similar (63.4% vs. 61.2%), but the number of "compliant cycles" was slightly higher for the ring than COCs (88.3% vs. 86.4%).[52] In trials, 86% to 91% of ring users report perfect adherence,[49,50,53–56] although clinical trial settings likely represent a best-case scenario. Studies of typical use find lower adherence rates than seen in clinical efficacy trials.[57]

Continuation: A randomized crossover study found higher 3-month continuation rates with the ring (94.6%) compared with the patch (88.2%) among women switching from COC,[10] but this short-term study may not reflect real-world experience for those choosing the ring. Twelve-month continuation rates of the ring are in the range of 40% to 55%, generally similar to those of the pill.[14,56,57]

Special Populations

Patients with higher body weight: Generally, there are few appropriately designed studies for any contraceptive method that explore the relationship between contraceptive efficacy and obesity. No published trials compare efficacy of the ring between non-obese and obese contraceptive users.[58] One study found similar etonogestrel levels and similar suppression of ovarian follicular development between obese and non-obese women using the ring. Effects persisted for up to 6 weeks of continuous use.[59,60]

Adolescents: The vaginal contraceptive ring is appropriate for adolescents, because it offers both privacy and the convenience of monthly dosing. Improved consistent and correct use could ultimately lead to improved typical-use effectiveness. Some adolescents may feel uncomfortable with a vaginal device. In one study of women aged 18 to 41, there was a trend toward increased sexual comfort with ring use with increasing age, for both the woman and her partner.[61] While adolescents who desire combined hormonal contraception may be excellent candidates for the ring, they may lack familiarity with the method or have concerns about a vaginal insert: one study reported that only 17% of adolescents reported willingness to use a vaginal ring, while 39% were undecided.[62] Concerns based on lack of familiarity or comfort level can be addressed through patient-centered counseling.

DOSING REGIMENS

Each ring is designed to be placed vaginally once every 28 days. Labeling advises that the ring be kept in place for 21 days and removed for a 7-day ring-free period to allow a withdrawal bleed. While monthly cycling is the conventional use regimen, data support use of the ring continuously or in extended cycles. Extended use of combined hormonal contraceptives has been used to avoid estrogen-withdrawal side effects during the hormone-free week, to avoid bleeding in individuals who prefer amenorrhea, and to allow them to control the timing and frequency of bleeding.

Extended or continuous ring cycles are safe and practical for many. Individuals can choose the duration of extended use that they prefer; regimens of 84 or 91 days of consecutive use are best studied, but options ranging from 49 to 364 days (changing the ring every 21 or 28 days) are well-tolerated and acceptable. Extended use is associated with fewer episodes of scheduled bleeding but may be associated with more unscheduled bleeding. Unscheduled bleeding tends to be more common in the first months and then decreases significantly over the first year of use.[63–65]

Those who experience persistent or prolonged breakthrough bleeding/spotting with extended ring cycling may benefit from a 4-day hormone-free interval.[66] One recommendation is to follow a flexible "bleeding-signaled" regimen. That is, individuals use the ring continuously until they experience 4 or more days of consecutive bleeding or spotting, at which point they remove ring for 4 days, and then insert a new ring on the fifth day. A recent study demonstrated that this approached stopped the bleeding episode within 4 days in about 50% of ring users, and within 7 days in over 90%.[65]

ADVANTAGES

CONTRACEPTIVE BENEFITS

1. **Convenience.** Participants in clinical trials report that the ring is easy to insert, comfortable to use, and easy to remove.[50,53,56] Users may easily verify that the device is in place. The ring's effectiveness does not depend on its position, because hormonal absorption occurs through the vaginal walls. The ring rests against the vaginal wall, near or around the cervix;[56] walking and usual movement do not lead to expulsion.[67] Although ring users and their partners report feeling the ring during intercourse, this did not affect acceptability or continuation for most individuals in clinical trials.[53,54] Because the ring doesn't require daily action and

is not coitally dependent, it may be more convenient than other methods such as the diaphragm or COCs.

2. **Forgiving.** Hormone levels remain therapeutic for at least 35 days after application of the vaginal ring. This suggests that ovulation inhibition would be maintained even if a person forgets to remove the ring for up to 2 weeks beyond schedule. A recent study demonstrated that contraceptive hormone levels are sustained for up to 6 weeks of use of the same ring, although the incidence of breakthrough bleeding began to increase after 21 days.[5] Ring use for as few as 3 days has been shown to suppress ovarian follicular growth (compared with 7 days for COCs).[68] Removal after 3 days is not recommended, however, and follicular size and ovulation are only surrogate markers; no studies have evaluated the risk of pregnancy due to dosing errors in ring use.

3. **Vaginal hormone delivery.** The vaginal route of delivery increases the bioavailability of hormones, thus enabling the use of a lower total hormone dose. The ring can be used by individuals who cannot swallow a pill and by individuals with abnormal intestinal absorption. The steady release of hormones via vaginal route also has the potential to decrease side effects that may be associated with oral dosing.

4. **Rapidly effective and rapidly reversible.** Hormone levels needed to suppress ovulation are achieved within the first day of vaginal ring use,[69] and as few as 3 consecutive days of vaginal ring use interfere with follicular growth. Return to ovulation after ring removal is rapid, occurring in a median of 17 to 19 days.[70] Return to fertility can be extrapolated from what we know about COC discontinuation, for which the median time to pregnancy is 3 cycles, with 74% to 95% of those seeking fertility becoming pregnant within a year of discontinuation.[71]

5. **No adverse effects on cervico-vaginal epithelium.** Ring use does not appear to have adverse effects on the cervico-vaginal epithelium or on cervical cytology.[50,72]

6. **No adverse endometrial effects.** Ring use for up to 2 years did not lead to endometrial hyperplasia or other adverse effects on endometrial histology.[73]

7. **Can be used concurrently with tampons.** Occasionally, a user may need to insert a ring while still having withdrawal bleeding. A pharmacokinetic study showed that tampons can be used concurrently with the ring without any effects on hormone absorption.[74] Ring users need to ensure that the ring is not inadvertently withdrawn at the time of tampon removal.

8. **Can be removed for up to 3 hours without compromising effectiveness.** Although most individuals and their partners do not report discomfort due to the ring during vaginal intercourse, the ring can be removed or left out for up to 3 hours in any 24-hour period without requiring a backup method. The same ring can then be reinserted.[75] Caution should be exercised in making this recommendation, as insertion within the narrow 3-hour window may not always occur. Those who choose to remove and reinsert the ring for this reason should make sure to reinsert within the 3 hours, or it is possible that ring effectiveness could be compromised.

Menstrual Benefits

Excellent cycle control. Compared with COCs, the ring may be less likely to produce irregular bleeding, especially in the first few cycles.[52] Most vaginal ring users experience withdrawal bleeding on schedule.[50,76–78] Extended or continuous use may be associated with an increase in unscheduled bleeding, as can prolonged (>21 day) use of a single ring.[59,65,66] The frequency and duration of unscheduled bleeding episodes tend to be highest in the first few months of use and decrease over time.

Noncontraceptive Benefits

Because the hormonal levels and mechanisms of action are similar, the vaginal contraceptive ring may provide many of the same advantages and non-contraceptive health benefits that COCs do, although data about long-term health benefits are not yet available. Such benefits include control of menstrually related symptoms, such as headaches, pelvic pain, and dyspareunia. Extended regimens may offer further improvement in menstrually related and premenstrual symptoms.

1. **Does not cause weight gain.** In clinical studies, women are as likely to lose weight as to gain it when using the ring for a year.[48,79] A recent randomized review noted no large effect on weight among ring users, though the authors noted that available data were limited.[80]

2. **Safe in individuals with latex allergies.** Because the ring is made from vinyl acetate, individuals with latex allergies can use it safely.

3. **No clinically significant metabolic effects.** In healthy individuals, the vaginal ring has had no clinically important adverse effects on surrogate markers of disease such as heart rate, blood pressure, blood chemistries, lipids, adrenal and thyroid function, carbohydrate metabolism, or hematology.[50,53,81,82] In a study

of women with type 1 diabetes, ring use did not adversely affect glycemic control or other metabolic measures.[83] These surrogate markers may not reflect the actual risk of adverse outcome, and no studies have examined long-term metabolic outcomes.

4. **Does not affect bone density.** In one study, bone mineral density showed no change from baseline after as long as 24 months of contraceptive ring use.[84] The study did not include adolescents or perimenopausal individuals. One study of adolescents and young women found no decrease in bone density at the spine after 12 months of use.[29] No study has looked at risk of fractures.

DISADVANTAGES AND CAUTIONS

POTENTIAL SERIOUS HEALTH RISKS

1. **Risk of venous thromboembolism (VTE) or arterial thromboembolism (ATE).** Several cases of VTE have been reported with vaginal ring use.[85,86] The exploration of differential thrombotic risk among different progestins in combined hormonal contraceptives formulations continues to draw attention.[87] Etonogestrel, the progestin component of the ring, is a metabolite of desogestrel. Some studies have found that women using desogestrel-containing COCs are at increased risk of VTE compared with women using COCs containing other progestins, but study findings are not consistent in this regard.

   Although ring users have progestin levels similar to those of COC users, their EE levels are 2-fold lower than in individuals taking COCs with 35 mg EE and 3-fold lower than in individuals wearing the patch.[32] Pharmacokinetic measures are surrogate endpoints, however, and may not necessarily reflect a decreased risk of estrogen-related side effects or long-term risks. Studies of the ring based on analyses of large databases have also reported somewhat inconsistent results, with some showing a small increased risk of thrombosis among ring users compared with users of levonorgestrel (LNG)-containing oral contraceptives, and others showing no increase in risk.[39–41] In a Cochrane review of several randomized studies, the risk of VTE with ring use was estimated to be 149 per 100,000 women (95% CI: 18–538).[2]

   The risk of myocardial infarction (MI) does not appear to be significantly increased among ring users of the ring, compared either with COC users or non-users of combined hormonal contraception; the risk of thrombotic stroke may be about double that of women using no hormonal contraception.[43] ATE (stroke or MI) is even more rare than VTE among reproductive-aged women.

2. **Other health complications.** Although ring-specific data are scarce, the vaginal ring may be associated with other rare but serious health complications associated with COCs, such as cholestatic jaundice, gallbladder disease, hepatic adenomas, or other conditions.

3. **Toxic shock syndrome (TSS).** Very rare cases of TSS have been reported by ring users; some of these users were also using tampons.[75] Although causation has not been determined, any ring user with signs or symptoms of TSS should remove the ring and seek immediate medical evaluation and treatment.

Reported Side-Effects

1. **Headache.** Headache is the most common reported hormonal side-effect of the ring, reported by 6% of users.[50,53]

2. **Vaginal symptoms.** In the clinical trials that led to FDA approval of the ring, common reasons for ring discontinuation included vaginal symptoms such as foreign body sensation or coital problems; 1% to 2.6% of ring users discontinued because of these symptoms or because of ring expulsion.[88] Other self-reported vaginal symptoms include vaginitis, leukorrhea, and vaginal discomfort. In a randomized comparative trial with COCs, the only vaginal symptom significantly associated with ring use was vaginal wetness; 63% of ring users reported vaginal wetness compared with 43% of COC users. Microbiological evaluation showed that ring use was associated with an increase in hydrogen peroxide-producing Lactobacillus, the predominant species in the healthy human vagina, but not in other types of bacteria.[89]

3. **Irregular bleeding.** As discussed above, irregular bleeding may be a side effect of ring use. This can occur with monthly cycling regimens, particularly in the first few months of use. Irregular bleeding may be more common in those who choose continuous or extended cycling and tends to decrease in frequency and severity over time. In comparison to COCs, continuous ring use seems to be associated both with more episodes of prolonged amenorrhea, and more episodes of prolonged bleeding or spotting.[65] Irregular bleeding is frequently cited as a reason for discontinuation.[52]

4. **Other side effects.** Other reported side effects include decreased libido, nausea, and breast tenderness.[31,50,53,76] The incidence of nausea seems to be a little lower with rings than COCs (4% vs. 6%),[52] which is consistent with the fact that hormones released from

ring bypass the digestive tract. One study found that, in the first 3 months of use, fewer ring users called their providers about side effects than did patch or COC users.[90]

PROVIDING THE CONTRACEPTIVE PATCH AND VAGINAL RING

MEDICAL ELIGIBILITY CRITERIA (MEC)

Most healthy reproductive-age individuals at risk of pregnancy will be able to use the patch and ring safely. Those with certain health conditions, however, may face increased risks from estrogen-containing methods. Several of these health conditions are associated with increased risk of vascular events, such as hypertension and vascular complications from diabetes (Table 7-1). Neither age nor parity is an independent contraindication for the patch or ring.[42]

In most cases, U.S. MEC recommendations for the ring and patch are the same as for oral contraceptives. However, because these are non-oral regimens, they are still appropriate in some conditions for which COC may not be recommended, such as gastric bypass surgery.[42] (For more on the U.S. MEC, see Chapter 18 on Contraception for Women with Medical Conditions.)

Postpartum and postabortion use: The first 3 weeks postpartum, especially, are characterized by an elevated risk of venous thromboembolism (VTE), which generally returns to baseline by 6 weeks postpartum. Additionally, evidence conflicts as to whether combined hormonal contraceptives affect breastfeeding supply or continuation. There are few data specific to the patch or ring, and recommendations have largely been extrapolated from oral contraceptives.

The contraceptive vaginal ring and patch can be safely used immediately after first or second trimester abortion (U.S. MEC category 1).

Individuals who are obese. Data are limited regarding safety of the ring or patch in obese individuals. While the trials leading to patch or ring approval in the United States did not explicitly exclude obese individuals, they did not report differential safety outcomes based on weight. The U.S. MEC advises that, in the absence of other comorbidities, women who are obese can safely use the patch or ring (U.S. MEC category 2).[42] For the ring, the relatively lower EE exposure and the steady delivery system may pose advantages, though obese women may be more likely

Table 7-1. U.S. MEC (2016) Category 3 and 4 Conditions for use of the contraceptive patch and ring.[42]

Organ System	Health Condition	MEC Category	Rationale/notes
Cardiovascular	**Hypertension**		Among women with hypertension, CHC use increases risk of stroke, myocardial infarction, and arterial disease. Adequate control of blood pressure may decrease these risks.
	• Blood pressure adequately controlled or <160/100	**3**	
	• BP 160/100 or higher	**4**	
	• Evidence of vascular disease/other cardiovascular risk factors	**4**	
	Venous thromboembolism (VTE) (DVT/PE)		Estrogen in CHC formulations increases risk of VTE. The magnitude of this risk is higher among those who have a history of DVT/PE, particularly if they have **risk factors** for recurrence.
	• Acute DVT/PE	**4**	
	• History, with risk factors for recurrence (whether or not on anticoagulant therapy)	**4**	**Risk factors:** pregnancy-related, estrogen-related, or idiopathic DVT/PE; known thrombophilias; active cancer; history of recurrent DVT/PE.
	• Low risk of recurrence/no risk factors (whether or not on anticoagulant therapy)	**3**	
	• Major surgery with prolonged immobilization	**4**	
	Superficial venous thrombosis	**3**	This may be associated with increased VTE risk.
	Known thrombogenic mutations (e.g. Factor V Leiden, protein S or C deficiencies)	**4**	Such mutations significantly increase the risk of thrombosis with CHC use. Routine screening is not recommended, however.
	Ischemic heart disease (current or history)	**4**	CHC use increases risk of these events.
	Stroke	**4**	
	Peripartum cardiomyopathy		Evidence specific to CHC use in individuals with cardiomyopathy is lacking. CHC may induce fluid retention in some users, which could worsen heart failure. CHC-induced cardiac arrhythmias may also be more likely in those with cardiomyopathy.
	• Occurred <6 months ago or has moderate/severe impairment of cardiac function	**4**	
	• Occurred >6 months ago with normal function or only mild impairment	**3**	
Rheumatologic	**Systemic lupus erythematosus (SLE) with positive/unknown antiphospholipid antibodies**	**4**	SLE increases risk of stroke, heart disease, and VTE. Antiphospholipid antibodies are associated with increased thrombotic risk.
Neurologic	**Migraines *with aura*, at any age**	**4**	Migraine with aura and CHC use both increase the risk of ischemic stroke.
	Multiple sclerosis (MS) *with prolonged immobility*	**3**	Persons with MS are at higher risk of VTE, and prolonged immobility further increases this risk.

(continued)

Table 7-1. U.S. MEC (2016) Category 3 and 4 Conditions for use of the contraceptive patch and ring.[42]—*(continued)*

Organ System	Health Condition	MEC Category	Rationale/notes
Breast disease	**Breast cancer**		Breast cancer is hormonally sensitive. CHC use may worsen the prognosis for progression or recurrence in persons with breast cancer.
	• Current disease	4	
	• Past, and disease free for 5 years or more	3	
Endocrine	**Diabetes**		CHC use may increase the risk of vascular complications in persons who have vascular involvement from diabetes.
	• With nephropathy, neuropathy, retinopathy, or other vascular disease	3/4*	
	• Diabetes of >20 years' duration	3/4*	
Gastrointestinal	**Inflammatory bowel disease (IBD), *with risk factors for VTE***	3	Data for CHC use in IBD are lacking. Persons with IBD are at higher risk than unaffected women for VTE. The presence of additional **risk factors for VTE** (see above) further increases this risk.
	Gallbladder disease		CHC use may worsen gallbladder disease.
	Symptomatic, current and/or medically treated	3	
	Liver disease		Recommendations are based on the following: • Prior cholestasis with CHC use predicts recurrence. • There is limited evidence for CHC use in cases of active hepatitis. • Certain hepatic tumors may be hormone-sensitive, and severe liver disease may impair hormone metabolism.
	• History of cholestasis related to CHC use	3	
	• Viral hepatitis, acute or flare	3/4*§	
	• Cirrhosis, severe/ decompensated	4	
	• Hepatocellular adenoma	4	
	• Malignant hepatoma	4	
Solid organ transplant	Complicated: graft failure (acute or chronic), rejection, cardiac allograft vasculopathy	4	One study reported discontinuations of COC among transplant recipients as a result of serious medical complications.

CHC = combined hormonal contraceptives, DVT = deep venous thrombosis, PE = pulmonary embolism

*Determination of Category 3 vs. 4 should be based on clinical judgment of disease severity.

§For Initiation. Continuation if using patch/ring at time of diagnosis is Category 2.

(Postpartum recommendations (Table 7-2) and clinically relevant drug interactions (Box 7-1) are presented elsewhere in this chapter.)

For additional detail, the reference below can be accessed in its entirety at www.cdc.gov/mmwr/volumes/65/rr/rr6503a1.htm?s_cid=rr6503a1_w

Table 7-2 Medical Eligibility Criteria for use of the contraceptive patch/vaginal ring in the postpartum period[42]

	Breastfeeding	Not Breastfeeding
<21 days postpartum	4	4
21 – <30 days postpartum		
With additional risk factors for VTE*	3	3
With no additional VTE risk factors	3	2
30–42 days postpartum		
With additional risk factors for VTE*	3	3
With no additional VTE risk factors	2	2
>42 days postpartum	2	1

*VTE = venous thromboembolism; Additional risk factors for VTE include: age ≥35 years, previous VTE, thrombophilia, immobility, transfusion at delivery, peripartum cardiomyopathy, obesity, postpartum hemorrhage, cesarean delivery, preeclampsia, smoking

to experience breakthrough bleeding, possibly due to the lower estrogen levels.[60]

DRUG INTERACTIONS

Although data are limited, drugs that affect hepatic metabolism could reduce effectiveness of the patch or ring, just as they reduce the effectiveness of COCs (Box 7-1). In one pharmacokinetic study, a short course of oral tetracycline in patch users did not significantly affect the pharmacokinetics of norelgestromin or EE.[23] In a pharmacokinetic study of ring users, co-administration of three antimycotic formulations led to slight increases in etonogestrel and EE levels, with vaginal suppositories having the greatest effect.[9] In another study, a single-dose of 100 mg nonoxynol-9 gel did not affect the serum concentrations of etonogestrel or EE in ring users.[92] Serum concentrations of etonogestrel and EE in ring users were also not affected by concomitant administration of 10 days of oral amoxicillin or doxycycline in standard dosages.[23]

HOW TO PRESCRIBE THE CONTRACEPTIVE PATCH OR VAGINAL RING

Explore the potential user's medical, reproductive, and social history to ensure that there are no contraindications to use. Generally, those in need of contraception who have medical or other contraindications to COC use (except for those related to intestinal absorption, such as gastric bypass

Box 7-1 Medications that may interact with contraceptive patch and ring, leading to Category 3 Recommendations in the 2016 U.S. MEC[42]

Medication Category	Medication name	Rationale/ Notes
Antiretroviral therapy:	Fosamprenavir (FPV)	Interactions between FPV and hormonal contraceptives may lead to decreased FPV levels, which might diminish effectiveness
Anticonvulsant/ anti-epileptic therapy:	Phenytoin Carbamazepine Barbiturates Primidone Topiramate Oxcarbazepine	Certain anticonvulsants may interact with CHCs. This is not harmful, but may reduce the effectiveness of CHCs. Consider use of other contraceptives instead.
	Lamotrigine	Interactions between CHC and lamotrigine may significantly decrease lamotrigine levels, which can result in increased seizure activity. [This appears to be true when lamotrigine is used as monotherapy, not when it is combined with non-enzyme inducing anti-epileptic medications.]
Antimicrobial therapy	Rifampin/ Rifabutin	Interactions may reduce effectiveness of CHC. Consider use of other contraceptives instead.

Many medications and medication categories do *not* appear on this list, indicating that there is no concern for clinically significant drug-drug interaction with concomitant use of the contraceptive patch or ring. These include:

- **Most broad-spectrum antibiotics**
- **Antifungals**
- **Selective serotonin reuptake inhibitors (SSRI)**
- **Many antiretrovirals**

More detail on these recommendations can be found at www.cdc.gov/mmwr/volumes/65/rr/rr6503a1.htm?s_cid=rr6503a1_w

surgery) also have contraindications to the initiation and continuation of patch or ring use.

Although not absolute contraindications, generalized skin conditions such as psoriasis, eczema, or sunburn, may prevent successful patch use. Additionally, individuals may not be suitable candidates for the vaginal ring if they have significant pelvic relaxation, vaginal stenosis or obstruction (if it prevents placement or retention of the ring), conditions that make the vagina more susceptible to irritation or ulceration, or an inability or unwillingness to touch their genitalia.

Measure the person's blood pressure, if possible. No other screening tests are needed routinely before starting the contraceptive patch or vaginal ring unless the history or blood pressure measurement reveal a contraindication or a need for further assessment.[93]

Counseling

Advise potential patch or ring users of the advantages, potential risks, and side effects. Quality of counseling influences satisfaction with some contraceptive methods.[94] Individuals who have heard media reports about VTE-related deaths associated with the patch may express concerns. Counsel them that the overall risk of death with patch use is extremely low and that to determine the exact risk will require many more years of use by many users.[95] Remind them that pregnancy carries higher risks of death due to thromboembolic complications than do hormonal contraceptive methods.

Advise potential patch users weighing more than 90 kg (198 lbs) that they may want to consider using a backup method of contraception or another more effective method, particularly if they think they may forget to change patches on time. Any potential decrease in effectiveness does not preclude use of the patch by obese individuals, who may be at risk for adverse outcomes from unplanned pregnancies. Similar advice is not needed for heavier individuals who wish to use the ring.

Advise potential patch users to confirm periodically that the patch is firmly adherent, and to avoid using any creams, lotions, or oils near or at the patch site.

When Can a Person Start Using the Contraceptive Patch or Vaginal Ring?

Use of the patch and ring can be initiated at any time of the menstrual cycle, as long as pregnancy can be ruled out with reasonable certainty. (See Box 2-3 "How to be reasonably certain a woman is not pregnant" in Chapter 2.) Time initiation of the patch or ring to minimize the possibility that a person is already pregnant or might become pregnant between initiation and onset of effectiveness. The U.S. Selected Practice Recommendations for Contraceptive Use provides guidance.[96] In patch users, serum levels of norelgestromin reach therapeutic range in 24 to 48 hours.[1,97] A small randomized trial showed that immediate start of Ortho Evra on any cycle day was acceptable, although it did not lead to greater compliance or continuation rates compared with starting with menses.[98] Similarly, the ring inhibits ovulation even when it is started on cycle day 5, and 3 days of ring use inhibited ovulation even with a follicle of up to 13 millimeters size.[68]

Timing

- The contraceptive patch or vaginal ring can be initiated at any time if it is reasonably certain that the person is not pregnant[96] (see Box 2-3 in Chapter 2).

Need for Back-Up Contraception

- If combined hormonal contraceptives are started within the first 5 days since menstrual bleeding started, no additional contraceptive protection is needed.
- If contraceptive patches or rings are started >5 days since menstrual bleeding started, the person needs to abstain from sexual intercourse or use additional contraceptive protection for the next 7 days.

SPECIAL CONSIDERATIONS

Amenorrhea (Not Postpartum)

- **Timing:** Contraceptive patches or rings can be started at any time if it is reasonably certain that the person is not pregnant.
- **Need for back-up contraception:** The person needs to abstain from sexual intercourse or use additional contraceptive protection for the next 7 days.

Postpartum (Breastfeeding)

- **Timing:** Contraceptive patches or rings can be started when the person is medically eligible to use the method and if pregnancy has been reasonably excluded.

  Postpartum individuals who are breastfeeding should not use contraceptive patches or rings during the first 3 weeks after delivery (U.S. MEC category 4) because of concerns about increased risk for venous thromboembolism and generally should not use contraceptive patches or rings during the fourth week postpartum (U.S. MEC category 3) because of concerns about potential effects on breastfeeding. Postpartum breastfeeding individuals with other risk factors for venous thromboembolism generally should not use contraceptive patches or rings 4 to 6 weeks after delivery (U.S. MEC category 3).[42] (See Chapter 17 on Contraception After Pregnancy.)

- **Need for back-up contraception:** If the person is <6 months postpartum, amenorrheic, and fully or nearly fully breastfeeding (exclusively breastfeeding or the vast majority [≥85%] of feeds are breastfeeds)[96] no additional contraceptive protection is needed. (Please also refer to Chapter 17 on Contraceptive Use After Pregnancy.) Otherwise, a person who is ≥21 days postpartum and has not experienced return of menstrual cycles needs to abstain from sexual intercourse or use additional contraceptive protection for the next 7 days. If menstrual cycles have returned and it has been >5 days since menstrual bleeding started, the individual should abstain from sexual intercourse or use additional contraceptive protection for the next 7 days.

Postpartum (Not Breastfeeding)

- **Timing:** Contraceptive patches or rings can be started when the person is medically eligible to use the method and if pregnancy has been reasonably excluded.

  Postpartum individuals should not use contraceptive patches/rings during the first 3 weeks after delivery (U.S. MEC category 4) because of concerns about increased risk for venous thromboembolism. Those with other risk factors for venous thromboembolism generally should not use contraceptive patches or rings within 3 to 6 weeks after delivery (U.S. MEC category 3).

- **Need for back-up contraception:** If a person is <21 days postpartum, no additional contraceptive protection is needed. A person who is ≥21 days postpartum and whose menstrual cycles have not returned needs to abstain from sexual intercourse or use additional contraceptive protection for the next 7 days. If menstrual cycles have returned and it has been >5 days since menstrual bleeding started, the person should abstain from sexual intercourse or use additional contraceptive protection for the next 7 days.

Postabortion (Spontaneous or Induced)

- **Timing:** Contraceptive patches or rings can be started within the first 7 days following first-trimester or second-trimester abortion, including immediately postabortion (U.S. MEC category 1).
- **Need for back-up contraception:** The person needs to abstain from sexual intercourse or use additional contraceptive protection for the next 7 days unless contraceptive patches or rings are started at the time of a surgical abortion.

Switching from Another Contraceptive Method

- **Timing:** Contraceptive patches or rings can be started immediately if it is reasonably certain that the person is not pregnant. Delaying initiation until the next menstrual cycle is unnecessary and not recommended.
- **Need for back-up contraception:** If it has been >5 days since menstrual bleeding started, the person should abstain from sexual intercourse or use additional contraceptive protection for the next 7 days.
- **Switching from an IUD:** If the person has had sexual intercourse since the start of a current menstrual cycle and it has been >5 days since menstrual bleeding started, residual sperm theoretically might be in the genital tract, which could lead to fertilization if ovulation occurs. A health care provider may consider any of the following options:
  - — Advise the person to retain the IUD for at least 7 days after contraceptive patches or rings are initiated and return for IUD removal.
  - — Advise the person to abstain from sexual intercourse or use barrier contraception for 7 days before removing the IUD and switching to the new method.
  - — If the person cannot return for IUD removal and has not abstained from sexual intercourse or used barrier contraception for 7 days, advise the person to use emergency contraceptive pills (ECPs) at the time of IUD removal. Contraceptive patches or rings can be started immediately after use of ECPs (except for ulipristal acetate, UPA). Contraceptive patches or rings can be started no sooner than 5 days after use of UPA.

Note: If the provider is uncertain whether a woman may be pregnant, the benefits of starting combined contraception likely exceed the risk. The patch or ring can be initiated, with a follow-up pregnancy test in 2 to 4 weeks.[96]

MANAGING PROBLEMS OF CONTRACEPTIVE PATCH AND VAGINAL RING USERS

CONTRACEPTIVE PATCHES

Dislodged or detached patches: If the patch is partially or completely detached for less than 24 hours, instruct the user to try to reapply it firmly, applying pressure for 10 seconds, and confirm that the edges are sticking well. If it does not stick well, tell the user to remove the patch and apply a replacement. A user should not use other adhesives or wraps to hold the patch in place. No additional contraception is needed, and the patch change day will be the same. If the edges stick well, the user can continue to use the patch for the full 7 days.

If the patch has been partially or completely detached for more than 24 hours or if the user does not know how long it has been unstuck, instruct the person to start a new patch cycle immediately and use additional contraceptive protection for 7 days. The user will now have a new patch-change day; if unprotected intercourse has occurred, emergency contraception may be needed.

Missed or forgotten patches: Missed or forgotten patches may mean that a user has forgotten to place a patch at all in the first week of the cycle, or forgotten to remove and replace a patch during the 2nd or 3rd weeks. Management of forgotten patches depends upon which patch is missed and for how long (Table 7–3).

Application-site reactions: To decrease the risk of skin irritation, instruct users to rotate application sites when new patches are applied and not to apply the patch to areas of skin that are irritated or cut. If users experience skin reactions at patch application sites, they can remove the patch and apply a new patch in a different location.

Other side effects: If users experience breast symptoms, mild headaches, nausea, or breakthrough bleeding or spotting, advise them that these symptoms usually decrease over time; counsel them to try to continue using the patch.

VAGINAL RING

Expelled or removed ring: A user may accidentally remove or expel the ring while removing a tampon, engaging in intercourse, having a bowel movement, or engaging in strenuous physical activity such as marathon running. Instruct the user to rinse the ring with

Table 7-3 Management of missed or forgotten patches

When Patch Forgotten/Missed	Management
1st week	• If a patch is forgotten or is applied late during the first week, and the user has had unprotected intercourse, provide emergency contraception. • Ask the user to place a patch immediately. • The user should use an additional contraceptive method or abstain for 7 days. • Remind the user to change the patch each week, from now on, on the day of the week the new patch was applied.
2nd—3rd week	• 1–2 days late: If a user forgets to remove and replace a patch, advise to remove the old patch and replace it with a new patch immediately. The user needs no additional contraceptive method or emergency contraception, and the patch change day does not change. • *More than 2 days late*: Have the user remove the old patch and place a new one immediately. Provide emergency contraception if unprotected intercourse has occurred (especially if the user is 4 or more days late in applying the patch). Advise additional contraception or abstinence for 7 days; the next patch is applied 7 days later on the same day of the week that the new patch was applied.
4th week	• If a user forgets to remove the third patch, ask the person to remove the patch. • The user needs no additional contraceptive method or emergency contraception; a new patch is placed on the usual change day.

lukewarm water (for comfort) and reinsert it as soon as possible. If ring is lost, the user should insert a new ring and continue the regimen without alteration.

- If the ring has been *out for more than 3 hours, but less than 48 hours,* reinsert it as soon as possible, and continue wearing it until the scheduled removal day.[96] No additional contraceptive is needed. Consider emergency contraception with LNG if unprotected intercourse occurred in the first week of a cycle.
- If the ring has been *out for more than 48 hours*, instructions may vary depending on week of the cycle.
  - — Generally, reinsert the ring as soon as possible, and continue it until the scheduled removal day.
  - — Use additional contraception or avoid intercourse until the ring has been in for 7 days.

- If the prolonged ring removal occurs in the *third week of the cycle or later*:
    - ○ Omit the hormone-free week by finishing the third week of ring use and starting a new ring immediately.
    - ○ If unable to start a new ring immediately, use back-up contraception (e.g., condoms) or avoid sexual intercourse until a new ring has been worn for 7 consecutive days.

Forgotten or late ring: If a person reports that the ring was left in the vagina for more than 3 weeks (but less than 5 weeks), advise that it is still effective in preventing pregnancy. Counsel to remove the ring and insert a new one after a 1-week interval if following a monthly regimen, or immediately if extended or continuous use is preferred. If the ring was left in place for more than 5 weeks, contraceptive effectiveness could be compromised. A recent study is reassuring that serum ENG levels persist up to 6 weeks, but more data are needed to confirm contraceptive effectiveness. Consider pregnancy testing. Advise the woman to consider emergency contraception if indicated and to use an additional contraceptive method until a new ring has been in place for at least 7 days.

Disconnected (broken) ring: If users call to report that the contraceptive ring has disconnected or broken, counsel them to discard the ring and replace it with a new ring. They do not need additional contraception as long as they can insert a new ring quickly.

Vaginal symptoms: Advise individuals that they may perceive more vaginal discharge or wetness while using the ring, but that this does not signify infection. Counsel them that there is no increased risk of vaginal infection with ring use. However, if an individual complains of vulvovaginal itching or a foul odor, evaluation and any needed treatment are indicated. Even if there is no documented infection, if a person using the ring is bothered by increased vaginal discharge and wishes to change methods, this choice should be respected.

Other side effects: If a ring user experiences headache, nausea, or breast tenderness upon initiation, advise that these symptoms usually decrease over time. If they persist or become more severe, ring discontinuation and a switch to another method may be indicated.

Warning Signs with Patch or Ring Use

Severe new-onset headache, chest pain, or shortness of breath require immediate medical attention. They may be signs of rare but serious vascular complications, and these should be ruled out. Warning signs for patch and ring are the same as those for the combined pill.

(Please refer to Figure 8-3, ACHES handout, in Chapter 8 on Combined Oral Contraceptives.)

Dispensing Patches/Rings

It is recommended to prescribe a full year's prescription or supply of patches and rings at the first visit. Advise patch users to store patches at room temperature (25°C or 77°F) in their protective pouches.

Advise ring users to refrigerate the rings at 2° to 8°C (36–46°F) to extend the shelf-life beyond 4 months. Rings may be stored for up to 4 months at room temperature, 25°C (77°F).

User Instructions for the Contraceptive Patch*

Store patches at room temperature (25°C or 77°F) in their protective pouches, and do not put them in the refrigerator or freezer. Use 1 patch for 7 days. Apply a new patch once a week on the same day for 3 weeks in a row. During the fourth week, do not wear a patch. At the end of the week, start another cycle of patches.

Ask your clinician to provide you with a package of or a prescription for levonorgestrel emergency contraceptive pills. If you forget, you may also get these pills over-the-counter. You can use these pills if you have had sex that was not properly protected by the patch or by another contraceptive method (for example, you forget to place a patch during the first week of the cycle, or you are more than 2 days late replacing a patch in the second or third week of the cycle).

1. Each patch is packaged in an individual foil packet. Open the pouch by tearing along the top edge and one side edge. Peel the foil pouch apart and open it. Using a fingernail to peel the unit off the foil pouch, lift out the patch along with its clear plastic cover—take care not to remove the clear liner as you remove the patch.
2. Fold the patch open. While holding onto one half, peel the plastic off the other half. Avoid touching the adhesive surface after you remove the liner.
3. Apply the sticky side of the opened patch to your skin, and then remove the other half of the clear liner. You can put the patch on your buttocks, abdomen, upper torso (except the breasts), or on the outer upper arm. Avoid placing patches in areas of friction,

*These instructions are intended to guide providers in educating patients in how to use their method.

such as under bra straps or thongs. Only apply the patch to clean, dry skin, and never put it over skin that is irritated, sunburned, red, or infected. Make sure there are no creams, oils, powder, sunscreen, or sweat on the skin, as these prevent the patch from sticking properly. Press firmly on the patch for 10 seconds. Run your finger around the patch to make sure that all parts of the patch are sticking and to smooth out wrinkles.

4. Keep the patch in place for 7 days, and then remove it. Check the patch every day to make sure it is fully adherent. You can wear the patch while bathing, showering, swimming, and exercising.
5. To remove the patch, grasp it by an edge and pull it off. Fold it closed on itself on the adhesive side to seal in the medication.
6. Discard the patch in the garbage; do not flush it into the toilet.
7. If any stickiness or adhesive remains on your skin, remove it by using baby oil or lotions.
8. At the beginning of the second week, remove the first patch and apply a new patch in a different spot on your body. Every new patch should be applied on the same day of the week, called the "patch change day." Because the hormone levels remain protective for up to 9 days, you do not need to apply a new patch at the same time of the day. Wear the new patch for 7 days. Repeat the procedure for a third week.
9. During the fourth week, do not wear a patch. You will begin your menstrual period.
10. After a week without wearing a patch, apply a new "first week" patch on the same day of the week you applied your other patches.

USER INSTRUCTIONS FOR THE VAGINAL RING*

If multiple rings are given, refrigerate the rings at 2° to 8°C (36–46°F) to extend the shelf-life beyond 4 months. Rings may be stored for up to 4 months at room temperature, 25°C (77°F).

Ask your clinician to provide you with a package of or a prescription for emergency contraceptive pills. If you forget you may also get these pills over-the-counter. You can use these pills if you have had sex that was not properly protected by the ring or by another contraceptive method.

1. Each ring comes in a resealable foil pouch. After washing and drying your hands, remove the ring and keep the foil pouch for ring disposal.

*These instructions are intended to guide providers in educating patients in how to use their method.

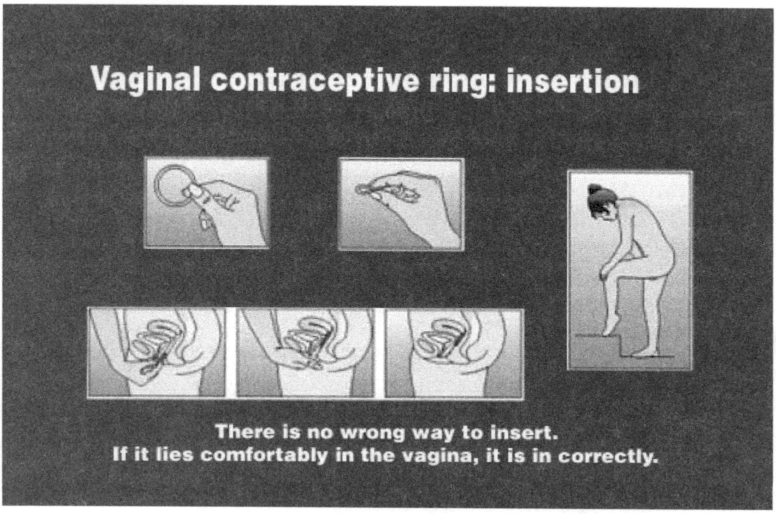

Source: Ballagh SA (2002), with permission courtesy of Organon USA.

Figure 7-1 Inserting the NuvaRing

2. To insert the ring into your vagina, use any position you find most comfortable: standing with one leg up, squatting, or lying down. Hold the ring between your thumb and index finger and press the sides of the ring together so that it makes a long loop. Insert the folded ring into your vagina and gently push it further up into vagina using your index finger until it is comfortable; the muscles of your vagina should keep it in place. The exact position of the ring is not critical for its function.

3. Leave the ring in place for 3 weeks. You do not need to remove the ring for intercourse. If you do remove the ring for intercourse, do not leave it out of the vagina for more than 3 hours in any 24-hour period.

4. After 3 weeks of use, remove the ring for 7 days. During this break, you will experience withdrawal bleeding. If using the ring continuously, have a new ring ready to insert when you remove the old one.

5. Before removing the ring, wash and dry your hands. Insert your index finger into your vagina until you feel the rim of the ring. Remove the ring by hooking your index finger under the forward rim or by grasping the rim between your index and middle finger and pulling it out. Place the used ring in the foil pouch and throw it away in a trash container out of the reach of children and pets (do not flush it down the toilet).

6. For cyclic (monthly) ring use, after the 7-day break, insert a new vaginal ring to begin the cycle again. Insert the new ring on the

same day of the week you inserted the previous ring, even if you have not finished your period. If you are using the ring continuously, insert the new ring right after you remove the old one. Do not take a break.

7. If the ring is out of your vagina for more than 3 hours during the 21-day period, re-insert it and use additional contraception for the next 7 days. If you have had unprotected intercourse, consider using emergency contraception.

NEW PATCHES AND RINGS IN DEVELOPMENT

Newer contraceptive vaginal patches and rings are in various phases of development. Another version of the combined EE/norelgestromin patch, called Evra, is available in Canada and Europe. This patch contains 6.0 mg of norelgestromin but only 0.6 mg of EE.

Two other combined contraceptive patches have currently completed clinical trials, but are not yet approved by the FDA. One is Twirla, also known as AG200-15, a weekly patch containing EE and levonorgestrel. In an earlier Phase III clinical trial that included obese women, pregnancy rates were higher than expected and compliance was low.[99] Results from a second trial have been submitted to the FDA.

Another smaller patch (Apleek) contains EE and gestodene. Approved in Europe, this patch is worn for 3 weeks and then removed for a week. One week after the last patch is removed, a new 4-week cycle is started by applying a new patch.

A new combined hormonal contraceptive vaginal ring, releasing 150 mcg of the progestin nestorone and 15 mcg EE daily, has been developed by the Population Council, and the New Drug Application (NDA) is planned for submission to the FDA.[100] This ring is designed to be effective for 1 year; users keep the ring in place for 3 weeks, and then remove it for 1 week, reinserting the same ring a week later. A 3-month progesterone-only ring, available in 8 countries in Latin America, is designed for use by breastfeeding women.[100]

Another ring formulation under study contains nestorone and estradiol (E2). Even earlier in the product development pathway is a ring containing etonogestrel and E2. The use of E2 is postulated to improve the safety profile compared to EE, which is a more potent estrogen.[101] Vaginal rings containing ulipristal, a progesterone receptor modulator, and intended to be effective for 3 months, are also under investigation.[102]

Author Disclosures—Nanda: none. Burke: research funding from Bayer and the National Institute of Child Health and Human Development (NICHD).

REFERENCES

1. Pierson RA, Archer DF, Moreau M, Shangold GA, Fisher AC, Creasy GW. Ortho Evra/Evra versus oral contraceptives: follicular development and ovulation in normal cycles and after an intentional dosing error. Fertil Steril 2003;80:34–42.
2. Lopez LM, Grimes DA, Gallo MF, Schulz KF, Stockton LL, Schulz KF. Skin patch and vaginal ring versus combined oral contraceptives for contraception. Cochrane Database Syst Rev 2013;(4):Cd003552.
3. Audet MC, Moreau M, Koltun WD, et al. Evaluation of contraceptive efficacy and cycle control of a transdermal contraceptive patch vs an oral contraceptive: a randomized controlled trial. JAMA 2001;285:2347–54.
4. Urdl W, Apter D, Alperstein A, et al. Contraceptive efficacy, compliance and beyond: factors related to satisfaction with once-weekly transdermal compared with oral contraception. Eur J Obs Gynecol Reprod Biol 2005;121:202–10.
5. Zieman M, Guillebaud J, Weisberg E, Shangold GA, Fisher AC, Creasy GW. Contraceptive efficacy and cycle control with the Ortho Evra/Evra transdermal system: the analysis of pooled data. Fertil Steril 2002;77(2 Suppl 2):S13-8.
6. Archer DF, Bigrigg A, Smallwood GH, Shangold GA, Creasy GW, Fisher AC. Assessment of compliance with a weekly contraceptive patch (Ortho Evra/Evra) among North American women. Fertil Steril 2002;77(2 Suppl 2):S27-31.
7. Jick SS, Hagberg KW, Kaye JA, Jick H. The risk of unintended pregnancies in users of the contraceptive patch compared to users of oral contraceptives in the UK General Practice Research Database. Contraception 2009;80:142–51.
8. Bakhru A, Stanwood N. Performance of contraceptive patch compared with oral contraceptive pill in a high-risk population. Obs Gynecol 2006;108:378–86.
9. Thurman AR, Hammond N, Brown HE, Roddy ME. Preventing repeat teen pregnancy: postpartum depot medroxyprogesterone acetate, oral contraceptive pills, or the patch? J Pediatr Adolesc Gynecol 2007;20:61–5.
10. Creinin MD, Meyn LA, Borgatta L, et al. Multicenter comparison of the contraceptive ring and patch: a randomized controlled trial. Obs Gynecol 2008;111:267–77.
11. Raine TR, Foster-Rosales A, Upadhyay UD, et al. One-year contraceptive continuation and pregnancy in adolescent girls and women initiating hormonal contraceptives. Obstet Gynecol 2011;117:363–71.
12. Peipert JF, Zhao Q, Allsworth JE, et al. Continuation and satisfaction of reversible contraception. Obstet Gynecol 2011;117:1105–13.
13. O'neil-Callahan M, Peipert JF, Zhao Q, Madden T, Secura G. Twenty-four-month continuation of reversible contraception. Obstet Gynecol 2013;122:1083–91.
14. Diedrich JT, Zhao Q, Madden T, Secura GM, Peipert JF. Three-year continuation of reversible contraception. Am J Obstet Gynecol 2015;213:662.e1–8.
15. McNicholas C, Zhao Q, Secura G, Allsworth JE, Madden T, Peipert JF. Contraceptive failures in overweight and obese combined hormonal contraceptive users. Obstet Gynecol 2013;121:585–92.
16. Winner B, Peipert JF, Zhao Q, et al. Effectiveness of long-acting reversible contraception. N Engl J Med 2012;366:1998–2007.
17. Sucato GS, Land SR, Murray PJ, Cecchini R, Gold MA. Adolescents' experiences using the contraceptive patch versus pills. J Pediatr Adolesc Gynecol 2011;24:197–203.
18. Miller L, Hughes JP. Continuous combination oral contraceptive pills to eliminate withdrawal bleeding: a randomized trial. Obs Gynecol 2003;101:653–61.
19. Stewart FH, Kaunitz AM, Laguardia KD, Karvois DL, Fisher AC, Friedman AJ. Extended use of transdermal norelgestromin/ethinyl estradiol: a randomized trial. Obs Gynecol 2005;105:1389–96.
20. Lavelanet AF, Rybin D, White KO. The pharmacokinetics of 12-week continuous contraceptive patch use. Contraception 2017;95:578–85.

21. Rubinstein ML, Halpern-Felsher BL, Irwin CE. An evaluation of the use of the transdermal contraceptive patch in adolescents. J Adolesc Heal 2004;34:395–401.
22. Bodner K, Bodner-Adler B, Grünberger W. Evaluation of the contraceptive efficacy, compliance, and satisfaction with the transdermal contraceptive patch system Evra: A comparison between adolescent and adult users. Arch Gynecol Obstet 2011;283:525–30.
23. Abrams LS, Skee D, Natarajan J, Wong FA. Pharmacokinetic overview of Ortho Evra/Evra. Fertil Steril 2002;77:S3-12.
24. Zacur HA, Hedon B, Mansour D, Shangold GA, Fisher AC, Creasy GW. Integrated summary of Ortho Evra/Evra contraceptive patch adhesion in varied climates and conditions. Fertil Steril 2002;77:S32-5.
25. Sibai BM, Odlind V, Meador ML, Shangold GA, Fisher AC, Creasy GW. A comparative and pooled analysis of the safety and tolerability of the contraceptive patch (Ortho Evra/Evra). Fertil Steril 2002;77:S19-26.
26. Creasy GW, Fisher AC, Hall N, Shangold GA. Transdermal contraceptive patch delivering norelgestromin and ethinyl estradiol. Effects on the lipid profile. J Reprod Med 2003;48:179–86.
27. Graziottin A. A review of transdermal hormonal contraception: focus on the ethinylestradiol/norelgestromin contraceptive patch. Treat Endocrinol 2006;5:359–65.
28. Kiriwat O, Petyim S. The effects of transdermal contraception on lipid profiles, carbohydrate metabolism and coagulogram in Thai women. Gynecol Endocrinol 26:361–5.
29. Massaro M, Di Carlo C, Gargano V, Formisano C, Bifulco G, Nappi C. Effects of the contraceptive patch and the vaginal ring on bone metabolism and bone mineral density: a prospective, controlled, randomized study. Contraception 81:209–14.
30. Grimes DA, Schulz KF. Surrogate end points in clinical research: hazardous to your health. Obs Gynecol 2005;105:1114–8.
31. Gracia CR, Sammel MD, Charlesworth S, Lin H, Barnhart KT, Creinin MD. Sexual function in first-time contraceptive ring and contraceptive patch users. Fertil Steril 93:21–8.
32. van den Heuvel MW, van Bragt AJ, Alnabawy AK, Kaptein MC. Comparison of ethinylestradiol pharmacokinetics in three hormonal contraceptive formulations: the vaginal ring, the transdermal patch and an oral contraceptive. Contraception 2005;72:168–74.
33. Jick SS, Kaye JA, Russmann S, Jick H. Risk of nonfatal venous thromboembolism in women using a contraceptive transdermal patch and oral contraceptives containing norgestimate and 35 microg of ethinyl estradiol. Contraception 2006;73:223–8.
34. Jick S, Kaye JA, Li L, Jick H. Further results on the risk of nonfatal venous thromboembolism in users of the contraceptive transdermal patch compared to users of oral contraceptives containing norgestimate and 35 microg of ethinyl estradiol. Contraception 2007;76:4–7.
35. Jick SS, Hagberg KW, Kaye JA. ORTHO EVRA and venous thromboembolism: an update. Contraception 81:452–3.
36. Cole JA, Norman H, Doherty M, Walker AM. Venous thromboembolism, myocardial infarction, and stroke among transdermal contraceptive system users. Obs Gynecol 2007;109:339–46.
37. Dore DD, Norman H, Loughlin J, Seeger JD. Extended case-control study results on thromboembolic outcomes among transdermal contraceptive users. Contraception 81:408–13.
38. Jick SS, Hagberg KW, Hernandez RK, Kaye JA. Postmarketing study of ORTHO EVRA and levonorgestrel oral contraceptives containing hormonal contraceptives with 30 mcg of ethinyl estradiol in relation to nonfatal venous thromboembolism. Contraception 81:16–21.
39. Lidegaard O, Nielsen LH, Skovlund CW, Lokkegaard E. Venous thrombosis in users of non-oral hormonal contraception: follow-up study, Denmark 2001–10. BMJ 2012;344:e2990.
40. Sidney S, Cheetham TC, Connell FA, et al. Recent combined hormonal contraceptives (CHCs) and the risk of thromboembolism and other cardiovascular events in new users. Contraception 2013;87:93–100.

41. Tepper NK, Dragoman M V, Gaffield ME, Curtis KM. Nonoral combined hormonal contraceptives and thromboembolism: a systematic review. Contraception 2017;95:130–9.
42. Curtis KM, Tepper NK, Jatlaoui TC, et al. U.S. Medical Eligibility Criteria for Contraceptive Use, 2016. MMWR Recomm reports Morb Mortal Wkly report Recomm reports 2016;65:1–103.
43. Lidegaard O, Lokkegaard E, Jensen A, Skovlund CW, Keiding N. Thrombotic stroke and myocardial infarction with hormonal contraception. N Engl J Med 2012;366:2257–66.
44. Weisberg F, Bouchard C, Moreau M, et al. Preference for and satisfaction of Canadian women with the transdermal contraceptive patch versus previous contraceptive method: an open-label, multicentre study. J Obs Gynaecol Can 2005;27:350–9.
45. Benson LS, Micks EA. Why Stop Now? Extended and continuous regimens of combined hormonal contraceptive methods. Obs Gynecol Clin North Am 2015;42:669–81.
46. Daniels K, Daugherty J, Jones J, Mosher W. Current contraceptive use and variation by selected characteristics among women aged 15-44: United States, 2011–2013. Natl Heal Stat Rep 2015;86:1–14.
47. Duijkers IJ, Klipping C, Verhoeven CH, Dieben TO. Ovarian function with the contraceptive vaginal ring or an oral contraceptive: a randomized study. Hum Reprod 2004;19:2668–73.
48. Oddsson K, Leifels-Fischer B, de Melo NR, et al. Efficacy and safety of a contraceptive vaginal ring (NuvaRing) compared with a combined oral contraceptive: a 1-year randomized trial. Contraception 2005;71:176–82.
49. Ahrendt HJ, Nisand I, Bastianelli C, et al. Efficacy, acceptability and tolerability of the combined contraceptive ring, NuvaRing, compared with an oral contraceptive containing 30 microg of ethinyl estradiol and 3 mg of drospirenone. Contraception 2006;74:451–7.
50. Dieben TO, Roumen FJ, Apter D. Efficacy, cycle control, and user acceptability of a novel combined contraceptive vaginal ring. Obs Gynecol 2002;100:585–93.
51. Gerlinger C, Trussell J, Mellinger U, et al. Different Pearl Indices in studies of hormonal contraceptives in the United States: impact of study population. Contraception 2014;90:142–6.
52. Lopez-Picado A, Lapuente O, Lete I. Efficacy and side-effects profile of the ethinylestradiol and etonogestrel contraceptive vaginal ring: a systematic review and meta-analysis. Eur J Contracept Reprod Heal Care 2017;22:131–46.
53. Roumen F. Contraceptive efficacy and tolerability with a novel combined contraceptive vaginal ring, NuvaRing. Eur J Contracept Reprod Heal Care 2002;7 Suppl 2:19.
54. Roumen FJ, op ten Berg MM, Hoomans EH. The combined contraceptive vaginal ring (NuvaRing): first experience in daily clinical practice in The Netherlands. Eur J Contracept Reprod Heal Care 2006;11:14–22.
55. Merki-Feld GS, Hund M. Clinical experience with the combined contraceptive vaginal ring in Switzerland, including a subgroup analysis of previous hormonal contraceptive use. Eur J Contracept Reprod Heal Care 2010;15:413–22.
56. Roumen FJ, Mishell Jr. DR. The contraceptive vaginal ring, NuvaRing((R)), a decade after its introduction. Eur J Contracept Reprod Heal Care 2012;17:415–27.
57. Lete I, Doval JL, Perez-Campos E, et al. Self-described impact of noncompliance among users of a combined hormonal contraceptive method. Contraception 2008;77:276–82.
58. Dragoman M V, Simmons KB, Paulen ME, Curtis KM. Combined hormonal contraceptive (CHC) use among obese women and contraceptive effectiveness: a systematic review. Contraception 2017;95:117–29.
59. Dragoman M, Petrie K, Torgal A, Thomas T, Cremers S, Westhoff CL. Contraceptive vaginal ring effectiveness is maintained during 6 weeks of use: a prospective study of normal BMI and obese women. Contraception 2013;87:432–6.
60. Westhoff CL, Torgal AH, Mayeda ER, et al. Pharmacokinetics and ovarian suppression during use of a contraceptive vaginal ring in normal-weight and obese women. Am J Obs Gynecol 2012;207:39.e1–6.

61. Novak A, de la Loge C, Abetz L, van der Meulen EA. The combined contraceptive vaginal ring, NuvaRing: an international study of user acceptability. Contraception 2003;67:187–94.
62. Maheux-Lacroix S, Leboeuf M, Dufresne A, Dodin S. Adolescents' willingness to use the contraceptive vaginal ring. J Obs Gynaecol Can 2011;33:353–60.
63. Miller L, Verhoeven CH, Hout J. Extended regimens of the contraceptive vaginal ring: a randomized trial. Obs Gynecol 2005;106:473–82.
64. Guazzelli CA, Barreiros FA, Barbosa R, de Araujo FF, Moron AF. Extended regimens of the vaginal contraceptive ring: cycle control. Contraception 2009;80:430–5.
65. Weisberg E, Merki-Feld GS, McGeechan K, Fraser IS. Randomized comparison of bleeding patterns in women using a combined contraceptive vaginal ring or a low-dose combined oral contraceptive on a menstrually signaled regimen. Contraception 2015;91:121–6.
66. Sulak PJ, Smith V, Coffee A, Witt I, Kuehl AL, Kuehl TJ. Frequency and management of breakthrough bleeding with continuous use of the transvaginal contraceptive ring: a randomized controlled trial. Obs Gynecol 2008;112:563–71.
67. Barnhart KT, Timbers K, Pretorius ES, Lin K, Shaunik A. In vivo assessment of NuvaRing(R) placement. Contraception 2005;72:196–9.
68. Killick S. Complete and robust ovulation inhibition with NuvaRing. Eur J Contracept Reprod Heal Care 2002;7 Suppl 2:13–9.
69. Timmer CJ, Mulders TM. Pharmacokinetics of etonogestrel and ethinylestradiol released from a combined contraceptive vaginal ring. Clin Pharmacokinet 2000;39:233–42.
70. Mulders TM, Dieben TO, Bennink HJ. Ovarian function with a novel combined contraceptive vaginal ring. Hum Reprod 2002;17:2594–9.
71. Mansour D, Gemzell-Danielsson K, Inki P, Jensen JT. Fertility after discontinuation of contraception: a comprehensive review of the literature. Contraception 2011;84:465–77.
72. Roumen FJ, Boon ME, van Velzen D, Dieben TO, Coelingh Bennink HJ. The cervico-vaginal epithelium during 20 cycles' use of a combined contraceptive vaginal ring. Hum Reprod 1996;11:2443–8.
73. Bulten J, Grefte J, Siebers B, Dieben T. The combined contraceptive vaginal ring (NuvaRing) and endometrial histology. Contraception 2005;72:362–5.
74. Verhoeven CH, Dieben TO. The combined contraceptive vaginal ring, NuvaRing, and tampon co-usage. Contraception 2004;69:197–9.
75. Merck & Dohme, Inc, Whitehouse Station, NJ 08889 USA S. Nuvaring (R) Prescribing Information. 2017;Available from: https://www.nuvaring.com/prescribing-information
76. Bjarnadottir RI, Tuppurainen M, Killick SR. Comparison of cycle control with a combined contraceptive vaginal ring and oral levonorgestrel/ethinyl estradiol. Am J Obs Gynecol 2002;186:389–95.
77. Oddsson K, Leifels-Fischer B, Wiel-Masson D, et al. Superior cycle control with a contraceptive vaginal ring compared with an oral contraceptive containing 30 microg ethinylestradiol and 150 microg levonorgestrel: a randomized trial. Hum Reprod 2005;20:557–62.
78. Milsom I, Lete I, Bjertnaes A, et al. Effects on cycle control and bodyweight of the combined contraceptive ring, NuvaRing, versus an oral contraceptive containing 30 microg ethinyl estradiol and 3 mg drospirenone. Hum Reprod 2006;21:2304–11.
79. O'connell KJ, Osborne LM, Westhoff C. Measured and reported weight change for women using a vaginal contraceptive ring vs. a low-dose oral contraceptive. Contraception 2005;72:323–7.
80. Gallo MF, Lopez LM, Grimes DA, Carayon F, Schulz KF, Helmerhorst FM. Combination contraceptives: effects on weight. Cochrane Database Syst Rev 2014;1:Cd003987.
81. Tuppurainen M, Klimscheffskij R, Venhola M, Dieben TO. The combined contraceptive vaginal ring (NuvaRing) and lipid metabolism: a comparative study. Contraception 2004;69:389–94.

82. Barreiros FA, Guazzelli CA, Barbosa R, de Assis F, de Araujo FF. Extended regimens of the contraceptive vaginal ring: evaluation of clinical aspects. Contraception 2010;81:223–5.
83. Grigoryan OR, Grodnitskaya EE, Andreeva EN, Chebotnikova T V, Melnichenko GA. Use of the NuvaRing hormone-releasing system in late reproductive-age women with type 1 diabetes mellitus. Gynecol Endocrinol 2008;24:99–104.
84. Massai R, Makarainen L, Kuukankorpi A, Klipping C, Duijkers I, Dieben T. The combined contraceptive vaginal ring and bone mineral density in healthy pre-menopausal women. Hum Reprod 2005.
85. Shum MK, Rajagopalan K, Lachant NA. Venous thromboembolic events in women using the NuvaRing(R). ASH Annu Meet Abstr 2007;110:3994.
86. Kolacki C, Rocco V. The combined vaginal contraceptive ring, nuvaring, and cerebral venous sinus thrombosis: a case report and review of the literature. J Emerg Med 2012;42:413–6.
87. Han L, Jensen JT. Does the progestogen used in combined hormonal contraception affect venous thrombosis risk? Obs Gynecol Clin North Am 2015;42:683–98.
88. Roumen FJ, Apter D, Mulders TM, Dieben TO. Efficacy, tolerability and acceptability of a novel contraceptive vaginal ring releasing etonogestrel and ethinyl oestradiol. Hum Reprod 2001;16:469–75.
89. Veres S, Miller L, Burington B. A comparison between the vaginal ring and oral contraceptives. Obs Gynecol 2004;104:555–63.
90. Victor I, Fink RA. Comparing patient telephone callback rates for different hormonal birth control delivery systems. Am J Ther 2006;13:507–12.
91. Verhoeven CH, van den Heuvel MW, Mulders TM, Dieben TO. The contraceptive vaginal ring, NuvaRing, and antimycotic co-medication. Contraception 2004;69:129–32.
92. Haring T, Mulders TM. The combined contraceptive ring NuvaRing and spermicide co-medication. Contraception 2003;67:271–2.
93. Stewart FH, Harper CC, Ellertson CE, Grimes DA, Sawaya GF, Trussell J. Clinical breast and pelvic examination requirements for hormonal contraception: Current practice vs evidence. JAMA 2001;285:2232–9.
94. Canto De Cetina TE, Canto P, Ordonez Luna M. Effect of counseling to improve compliance in Mexican women receiving depot-medroxyprogesterone acetate. Contraception 2001;63:143–6.
95. Grimes DA, Mishell DR. Assessing rare event reports: a numerator in search of a denominator. Dialogues Contracept 2004;8:7.
96. Curtis KM, Jatlaoui TC, Tepper NK, et al. U.S. Selected Practice Recommendations for Contraceptive Use, 2016. MMWR 2016;65:1–66.
97. Abrams LS, Skee DM, Natarajan J, Wong FA, Anderson GD. Pharmacokinetics of a contraceptive patch (Evra/Ortho Evra) containing norelgestromin and ethinyloestradiol at four application sites. Br J Clin Pharmacol 2002;53:141–6.
98. Murthy AS, Creinin MD, Harwood B, Schreiber CA. Same-day initiation of the transdermal hormonal delivery system (contraceptive patch) versus traditional initiation methods. Contraception 2005;72:333–6.
99. Kaunitz AM, Portman D, Westhoff CL, Archer DF, Mishell DRJ, Foegh M. Self-reported and verified compliance in a phase 3 clinical trial of a novel low-dose contraceptive patch and pill. Contraception 2015;91:204–10.
100. Sitruk-Ware R, A. N. Applying emerging science to contraception research: implications for the clinic. Expert Rev Endocrinol Metab 2015;10:115–26.
101. Stanczyk FZ, Archer DF, Bhavnani BR. Ethinyl estradiol and 17beta-estradiol in combined oral contraceptives: pharmacokinetics, pharmacodynamics and risk assessment. Contraception 2013;87:706–27.
102. Huang Y, Jensen JT, Brache V, et al. A randomized study on pharmacodynamic effects of vaginal rings delivering the progesterone receptor modulator ulipristal acetate: research for a novel estrogen-free, method of contraception. Contraception 2014;90:565–74.

8

Combined Oral Contraceptives (COCs)

Carrie Cwiak, MD, MPH
Alison Edelman, MD, MPH

- Combined oral contraceptives (COCs) are the most commonly used reversible contraceptive method in the United States.
- Not only are COCs safe and effective, but they also offer many non-contraceptive health benefits.
- Adherence to a daily method like COCs can be challenging; studies demonstrate that most patients miss several pills each month.[1]
- Decreasing barriers to COC use such as 'Quick Start' initiation or providing a year's worth of COCs may help improve adherence.[2,3]

Combined oral contraceptives (COCs) have been almost synonymous with contraception in the United States for over half a century. The creation of the "pill," coupled with the social and legal changes of the 1960s, was a critical step for women in the ongoing struggle for gender equity. Individuals (and couples) could plan and prepare for or prevent pregnancy, thus enabling women to take advantage of educational or professional opportunities. Additionally, by unlinking sexual intercourse and child-bearing, the pill enabled women to enjoy sexual activity without the fear of pregnancy.

The first COC approved by the United States Food and Drug Administration (FDA) in May 1960 was Enovid-10. Enovid-10 was a monophasic pill with 21 active pills (9.85 mg norethynodrel and 150 mcg mestranol) and 7 placebo pills. The amount of hormones contained in Enovid-10 was significantly higher than today's COCs. Over the years, the doses of the hormones in COCs have dramatically decreased and new synthetic hormones and formulations have since been developed. Initial studies of these higher-dose COCs should be interpreted in this context; health concerns about high-dose pills may not be clinically relevant to current low-dose COCs (i.e., formulations containing <50 mcg ethinyl estradiol).

Clinical Impact

Although the widespread public perception is that COCs are hazardous,[4] recent data about short- and long-term safety of COC use are very reassuring. Short-term safety is achieved by careful patient selection, and clinicians have better tools now to identify eligible COC users, as will be explained in this chapter. Long-term safety data about COCs are also reassuring. The Royal College of General Practitioners (RCGP) observed 46,112 women for up to 39 years, accumulating over 378,000 woman-years of observational data among never-users of COCs and 819,175 woman-years of experience among ever-users.[5] Ever-users of COCs had a significant 12% *lower* rate of death from any cause than did never-users. The estimated absolute reduction in all causes of mortality for ever-users of COCs from that study was 52 per 100,000 women-years. For example, COCs reduce the risk of ectopic pregnancy by 90%, a leading cause of maternal mortality in early pregnancy, because they substantially reduce the risk of pregnancy.[6,7] Other health benefits from COCs, besides contraception, have also been discovered and will be reviewed in this chapter. The pill's contributions to women's health have been so enormous that the Centers for Disease Control and Prevention (CDC) recognized family planning (with oral contraceptives and condoms, in particular) as one of the 10 greatest public health achievements of the 20th century, on par with the vaccination and control of infectious disease.[8]

Even with advancements made in other methods of contraception, COCs remain the most commonly used reversible contraceptive method in the United States: 26% of current contraceptors, or 9.7 million women, use COCs.[9] In the most recent National Survey for Family Growth, 82% of U.S. women who have ever been sexually active reported using COCs at some point in their lives.[10] COCs continue to be an ideal option for those who desire an effective, short-term, rapidly reversible method that allows for the option of a monthly bleeding pattern or the option for other non-contraceptive benefits, ranging from the treatment of menstruation-related issues to cancer prevention.

Readers of this chapter will become more effective COC advocates and providers by understanding how COCs work, their advantages and disadvantages, and how to manage bleeding changes and side effects. We will review several ways to overcome barriers to using COCs correctly and consistently—many of these barriers have been historically and arbitrarily created by us as providers and by our healthcare system. Finally, by providing clinically relevant information, we hope to make patient counseling messages more patient-centered and, hopefully, more effective.

MECHANISM OF ACTION

COCs prevent fertilization. There is no evidence that they work after fertilization. COCs are, therefore, contraceptive and not contragestive (which refers to agents that prevent or interrupt implantation in the uterus). The progestin component provides the main contraceptive effect through ovulation suppression. The estrogen component, typically ethinyl estradiol (EE), makes a small contribution to ovulation suppression but primarily helps with cycle control. Ovulation suppression occurs through a series of positive and negative feedback loops resulting in pituitary suppression thus suppressing the LH surge (progestin effect) and release of FSH (estrogen effect). (See Chapter 1 on the Menstrual Cycle for further explanation.) Ovulation suppression provided by low-dose COC formulations is profound: they suppress 99% to 100% of cyclic ovulations as reported in clinical trials that detected ovulation through measurement of progesterone, 17B-estradiol, FSH, and LH concentrations[11]

EE and progestins have other effects on the reproductive system, but it has not been well substantiated that any of these effects contributes significantly to COC effectiveness:

- Slowing of tubal motility (disruption of ova transport may interfere with fertilization)
- Thickening of cervical mucus (barrier to sperm transport). Blockage of sperm transport has been demonstrated with a levonorgestrel-releasing intrauterine system but has not been well studied in terms of COCs.[12,13]
- Endometrial atrophy, changes in function of endometrial vessels, and alterations in the matrix metalloproteinase content in the endometrium (These are progestin effects that might impede sperm motility and viability or, theoretically, could inhibit implantation.)
- Localized edema of the endometrium (an estrogen effect that might affect implantation)

COC HORMONAL COMPONENTS

COCs contain both an estrogen and a progestin. In today's COCs, the estrogen component is mostly EE, whereas there are many different types of progestins used in COCs (see below, Progestin Generations).

Estrogen

Estrogen was added to birth control pills to provide better cycle control. Estradiol, the estrogen produced by the ovary, was not used initially in COCs because it has low bioavailability (estradiol is extensively metabolized in the liver) and thus does not produce good cycle control.[14] Instead, the early COCs used mestranol, an estrogen contaminant in the first COC, Enovid. Mestranol is a prodrug that converts into EE. Over time, the doses of mestranol were reduced from 150 mcg eventually down to 50 mcg; today, the majority of COCs contain EE with doses as low as 10 mcg. Estradiol and estradiol esters, instead of EE, are also now being developed for use in COCs; for example, a COC containing estradiol valerate with dienogest is now commercially available in the US.[15]

Progestins

Because the progestin component provides the main contraceptive effect, therapeutic levels must be maintained for at least 24 hours, with an adequate margin to allow for individual variation in drug absorption and metabolism as well as some allowance for user adherence variability.[16] Natural progesterone is poorly absorbed from the gastrointestinal tract and is rapidly metabolized, thus it is not a good choice for contraceptive development. Synthetic progestins vary in their properties of bioavailability (percentage of drug eventually in the bloodstream), half-life (the time necessary for the blood level to fall to 50% of its maximum), and clearance. Thus, the progestin dose needed to suppress ovulation varies from type to type.[16]

Progestin Generations

The first progestins were structurally related to testosterone, which possibly leads to the androgenic side effects such as acne and unwanted hair growth. The classification system most commonly used for synthetic progestins recapitulates the history of pill development in the United States by categorizing them into so-called "generations"; for example, first generation = norethisterone, second generation = levonorgestrel, third generation = desogestrel. Fourth generation includes newer progestins, like drospirenone (see Box 8-1). Third and fourth generations are considered the least androgenic. All progestins contained in currently approved

Box 8-1 Drospirenone and potassium levels

- Drospirenone has antimineralocorticoid activity, and initially there was concern that it might increase potassium levels.
- The EURAS multinational study noted no increase in arrhythmias in users of drospirenone-containing COCs as compared with other COC formulations.[113]
- Routine testing of potassium levels is not necessary for healthy users of COCs containing drospirenone.

COCs appear to be well-tolerated, but progestin development has been ongoing in an attempt to solve issues such as unscheduled bleeding and to improve upon the possible androgen-related side effects. However, the latter issue may not be an issue at all given that EE-containing COCs increase sex-hormone binding globulin (sHBG), which likely offsets any androgen-related progestin activity.[17] The ongoing controversy regarding progestins is that they may or may not differentially modulate the risk of deep venous thrombosis (DVT) associated with the use of EE.[18]

COC Formulations

Over the decades, COC formulations have changed and the number available has increased. Clinicians and patients now have many options to choose from, which help to meet individual needs and desires, or insurance coverage. COC formulations are either monophasic or multiphasic. Monophasic formulations have the same combination of estrogen and progestin in each active pill. Multiphasic formulations have active pills with differing doses of estrogen and progestin; the pill doses increase as the cycle progresses. Typically, biphasic formulations have two different dose combinations of estrogen and progestin in the active pills, and triphasic formulations have three different dose combinations. COC formulations offering multiphasic combinations of hormones were introduced in an effort to minimize hormonal exposure—although the need for this improvement in regard to safety has not been substantiated given that the doses of modern day pills are so much lower (less than 50mcg EE).

Cycling Patterns

The original COC formulations included hormone-free days to induce a monthly scheduled bleed that patients would interpret as normal menstruation. This scheduled monthly bleeding was needed for initial acceptance of the pill. Today, it is recognized that this scheduled bleeding is not biologically necessary while using COCs and that it is safe to suppress menstruation.[19] Due to the atrophy caused by the progestin-dominant effect on the endometrial lining, the avoidance of a withdrawal bleed with COC use is safe. The withdrawal bleeding of menses is due to withdrawal of the hormones and not due to the need to shed a thickened endometrial lining. Thus, COC users can choose whether and at what intervals they may want to experience a scheduled bleed.

21/7 Formulations. The 21/7-day COC combination came from experience with the early high-dose COCs. Many formulations today still use a 21/7-day schedule. In order to prevent breakthrough ovulation in patients using these 21/7 formulations, it is very important that they do not delay in starting their next COC pack following the 7 placebo days.

Shortened hormone-free interval. Many of the newer COC formulations have increased the number of active pills and decreased the number of placebo pills. Shortening the hormone-free interval appears to improve COC efficacy—likely in its ability to prevent breakthrough ovulation and/or provides more room for error with the shorter hormone-free interval.[20] The hormone-free interval can be shortened with any monophasic COC formulation if a 24/4 formulation cannot be obtained or covered by insurance, or if a patient likes her current formulation. A patient can be instructed to adjust the hormone-free interval to be shorter than 7 days, but should be warned not to extend longer than 7 days because that could increase her risk of pregnancy.

Extended-cycle use. Many patients are afflicted with menstruation-related symptoms that can significantly impact their lives even if on 21/7 formulations,[21] and menstrual suppression through COC use is highly effective in alleviating these symptoms.[22]Additionally, most women would prefer to bleed less frequently than once a month.[23] COC users do not need a medical reason to extend the duration of time between scheduled bleeds. The downside of extended-cycling is that some users will experience more unscheduled bleeding in the first 3 to 6 months of use, but the bleeding will decrease over time in most users and is not harmful. Timely ingestion and good adherence likely decrease the amount of unscheduled bleeding. An occasional 3 to 4 day break [24] (no more frequently than every 30 days) or a pill containing norethindrone acetate[25] may result in more days of amenorrhea.

For some patients, menstrual bleeding reassures them that they are not pregnant. No evidence exists that missing a withdrawal bleed with COC use is indicative of a failure—in fact, many patients experience no bleeding routinely during the hormone-free interval.

EFFECTIVENESS

COCs are considered a second-tier contraceptive method in terms of effectiveness—moderately, but not highly, effective. Their first-year failure rate with *typical use* is 9% (see Figure 3-1 in Chapter 3 on Efficacy, Safety, and Personal Considerations). However, the first-year *perfect-use* failure rate of most COCs is less than 1%. The failure rates reported in clinical trials (i.e., "perfect use") should not be confused with the typical-use failure rate, because subjects in clinical trials are highly motivated, monitored closely, and compensated for their time. Typical-use failure rates, derived from real-world use in which some individuals use COCs correctly and others do not, are a better guide for patient counseling. Adolescents and young adults experience even higher typical-use failure rates than adults when using short-acting methods like COC, the ring, and the patch—almost twice as high.[26]

Barriers to successful COC use. The gap that exists between *perfect-use* failure rates and *typical-use* failure rates is due to human behavior and systems issues that negatively affect users' adherence. Substantial barriers may prevent a patient from gaining timely access to contraceptive supplies or to consistent use of those methods. A study demonstrated that by 1 month, only 72% of COC users returned to the pharmacy on a timely basis for refill.[27] Dispensing a 1-year supply as compared with only 1 to 3 pill packs was associated with a 30% reduction in the odds of an unintended pregnancy. Requiring patients to return each month for refills constitutes a major barrier to successful COC use, plus other routine medications are allowed a 90-day supply.[2]

Possession of the COC pack does not guarantee correct daily use. One study, in which a computer chip was placed in the COC pack to record the date and time a pill was removed from the pack, found that although most COC users thought that they took the pills on a daily basis, but during the third cycle 54% of users actually missed 3 or more pills.[1,28] Taking a daily pill for an asymptomatic condition is challenging. Plus, many patients are ambivalent about pregnancy desires.[29,30] Unfortunately, using a smart phone app, signing up for a text messaging service, or setting the alarm on cell phones to remind the patient does not appear to make adherence better, though it did not make it worse.[31] As mentioned earlier, using formulations with fewer placebo pills (24/4) has demonstrated lower pregnancy rates,[20] and it is expected that extended-use will have lower pregnancy rates as well.

COC users should be notified that fertility returns quickly with discontinuation[32] so if pregnancy is not desired, another method should be started immediately. Studies show that 11% of COC users discontinue their COCs in the first month of use, and 19% of those who discontinue fail to adopt a new method.[28]

Impact of Body Weight on COC Effectiveness

Given the growing number of reproductive-age women who are obese, the impact that weight might have on COC efficacy is important for public health as well as for personal health. Although it does appear that obesity adversely affects contraceptive steroid hormone pharmacokinetics (e.g. drug levels and how drugs are metabolized),[33,34] the literature has been conflicting regarding the impact on COC effectiveness.[35] The majority of studies are not large enough to investigate the main outcome of interest: pregnancy. However, a study of 10,000 women demonstrated that there may be a slight increased risk of pregnancy[36] as did a meta-analysis performed by the U.S. FDA of individual study participant data.[37] Likely, obesity plays a small role in decreasing effectiveness, but the small impact is masked by the overwhelming issues of adherence.

Both extended-cycle use of a 20 mcg EE COC and 21/7 use of a 35 mcg EE COC provided better suppression of ovarian activity than 21/7 use of a 20 mcg EE COC.[22] For healthy obese individuals, COCs are a CDC Medical Eligibility Criteria (MEC) category 2[38] and thus safe to use, but as most providers would likely prefer to use a lower-dose formulation to minimize VTE, an extended cycle with a 20 mcg EE COC may be more acceptable. For patients of any weight or BMI, COCs are still considered second-tier in terms of effectiveness, so if a highly effective or first-tier method is desired, then a long-acting reversible or permanent method should be recommended.

Bariatric Surgery and the Impact on COC effectiveness

After bariatric surgery, effective contraceptive use is very important initially because fertility and ovulation rates increase, and the CDC advises against pregnancy in the first 2 years post-surgery as pregnancy outcomes are worse.[39] No clinical trials have assessed the effectiveness of COCs used after bariatric surgery. A case series noted 2 COC failures in patients after surgery for malabsorption syndromes (biliopancreatic diversion, Roux-en-Y bypass). Nutritional deficiencies have been noted in patients after these surgeries, suggesting that COCs may also have contributed to their decreased gastrointestinal absorption. These patients can use COCs with caution if no other method is available or acceptable (category 3), and then use of a back-up method of contraception is also recommended. These patients can still use other hormonal methods including transdermal patch or the transvaginal ring. Patients who have restrictive procedures (banding, gastrectomy) may use COCs (category 1).

Medication Interactions and the Impact on COC Effectiveness

One medication can alter the effectiveness of another medication in many ways. The most important way a medication can interact with COCs is through the liver's cytochrome P-450 enzyme activation.[14,16] Induction of P-450 will cause more rapid clearance of medications, including oral contraceptives, that are metabolized by this pathway. Medication development is ongoing, thus the knowledge regarding whether a new medication interacts with a COC often lags. However, most medication labeling will contain information on its metabolism pathway—if it is a P450 inducer, then it is possible that it could decrease COC effectiveness.

The major class of medications to be aware of that often decrease COCs' effectiveness is anticonvulsants such as carbamazepine, phenytoin, topiramate. Lamotrigine (Lamictal) is a special case as the COC is not affected but the lamotrigine level is. Lamotrigine levels drop almost by half when COCs are started[40] because increases in cytochrome P-450 start rapidly after COC initiation, and they are slow to normalize after COC cessation. Involving the provider who prescribes lamotrigine in the decision about COC use is critical. *For the most up-to-date list, please refer to the CDC MEC.*[38]

Antiretrovirals (ARV) and COCs appear to have either no impact on each other, the COCs may impact the ARV, or the ARV may impact the COC. Medication development and treatment regimens for HIV is rapidly changing thus *for the most up to date list of potential interactions, please refer to the CDC MEC.*[38]

The majority of antibiotics have no impact on the effectiveness of COCs. A systematic review of nearly 200 articles found that only rifampin impaired the effectiveness of COCs.[41] Specific studies of tetracycline, doxycycline, ampicillin, metronidazole, and quinolones demonstrated no impact on medication levels.[42–46]

St. John's Wort is an over-the-counter herbal product that is used to treat mild depression; evidence is limited but it may decrease the effectiveness of COCs.[47] Other psychotropic medications do not appear to be of concern.[48]

ADVANTAGES

COCs provide patients with safe, effective, and rapidly reversible control of their fertility; patients can plan and prepare for any pregnancies they may desire. In addition, COCs solve many menstruation-related problems, not only by reducing menstrual blood loss but also by suppressing ovulation. COCs also provide other non-contraceptive health benefits.

Contraceptive Benefits

1. **Rapid reversibility.** A comprehensive review of the literature concluded that the return to fertility in patients who stop COCs in order to conceive occurs within the first few months after cessation and is comparable to that observed following discontinuation of other contraceptive methods, even with extended use of COCs.[32] Baseline cycling resumes within the first few months. With long-term use, up to 10 years or more, there is similarly no clinically significant delay in return to fertility.[49]

2. **Regulation of bleeding.** Taken cyclically, COCs produce predictable scheduled bleeding. In a randomized controlled trial of patients with abnormal uterine bleeding (AUB), use of COCs was associated with an 80% improvement in bleeding pattern compared with less than 50% with placebo.[50] This includes AUB related to anovulation, which is commonly associated with adolescence, perimenopause, obesity, or polycystic ovarian syndrome (PCOS). Predictability in bleeding episodes allows patients to plan their scheduled bleeding to fit their lives, rather than scheduling their lives to fit their bleeding. Patients who use extended-cycle COCs similarly gain control over their scheduled bleeding and, with time, over unscheduled bleeding.[22] Scheduling bleeding can be done merely for personal preference or convenience. In particular, developmentally or physically disabled adolescents and adults whose menstrual bleeding presents a hygiene challenge to them and their caregivers can benefit.

3. **Decreased menstruation. Decreased menstrual blood loss.** COCs decrease the number of days of bleeding and the amount of blood loss with each menstruation. In a randomized trial of 45 women with heavy menstrual bleeding (HMB), use of a 30 mcg EE COC was associated with a 43% decrease in menstrual blood loss.[51] Observational studies have shown that use of COCs can reduce menstrual blood loss and increase hemoglobin levels, and this use is supported in clinical practice guidelines.[52,53] Patients who use extended-cycle regimens similarly reduce their numbers of scheduled bleeding episodes compared with patients who use COCs cyclically. The resulting total blood loss is decreased, though the total number of days of bleeding or spotting is the same.[22] This benefit is particularly important for patients with pre-existing anemia from idiopathic heavy menstrual bleeding, adenomyosis, iron-deficiency anemia, or coagulation defects. COCs may also be effective medical therapy for heavy menstrual bleeding due to uterine leiomyomas, especially for patients who wish to preserve their fertility.[52]

   - **Decreased dysmenorrhea.** COCs significantly decrease menstruation-related cramping. In a randomized clinical trial of treatment for dysmenorrhea, low-dose COC users reported significantly lower pain scores, fewer absences from school and work, and less need for analgesics than did placebo users.[54] A recent review of the existing literature concluded that for women who wish to use contraception, low-dose COCs are the preferred therapy for pain relief from dysmenorrhea; because there are risks associated with taking NSAIDs, COC use is a more suitable long-term option.[55] Extended-cycle

COC use, which eliminates scheduled bleeding episodes, may provide even more relief from dysmenorrhea. (See Chapter 1 on the Menstrual Cycle.)

- **Decreased symptoms of endometriosis.** Current COC use is associated with a 50% lower incidence of symptomatic endometriosis among parous patients.[56] The risk of developing endometriomas has been found to be significantly lower in current and past COC users over the age of 25.[57] In addition, long-term cyclic or extended use of COCs following laparoscopic excision of ovarian endometriomas has been found to significantly reduce or delay their recurrence.[58] In addition, COCs decrease menstrual pain with endometriosis.[59] This benefit is enhanced by use of extended-cycle COCs, which reduce the number of painful scheduled bleeding episodes. Also, with extended use of COCs, the progestins induce pseudodecidualization of the endometriotic implants, which makes them inactive and less likely to induce painful inflammation reactions during menstruation.[60] However, such treatment is not curative; the endometriotic implants undergo atrophy during treatment but remain ready for reactivation whenever COCs are stopped.[61]

- **Decreased menstruation-related migraines.** Menstrual migraines are caused by estrogen withdrawal before menstruation, prostaglandin release during menstruation, or both. It is unclear whether use of COCs is associated with increased frequency of migraine or other headaches as most studies did not control for baseline frequency of headaches or compare COCs with placebo.[62] On the other hand, menstrual migraines can be prevented with the use of extended cycle regimens.[63,64] (See the section on Headaches, in Managing Side Effects.)

- **Decreased endometrial cancer risk.** COC use for at least 12 months reduces the risk of developing endometrial cancer by approximately 40%.[65] A meta-analysis found that longer durations of use were associated with greater decreases in risk, up to a 72% decrease in patients who used COCs for at least 12 years compared with non-users, and the protection against endometrial cancer endures for up to 20 years after COC discontinuation.[66] Studies suggest that the protection against endometrial cancer is conferred with low-dose COCs as well.[52] For patients who currently have endometrial hyperplasia (a precursor to endometrial carcinoma), COCs can be used as a treatment to prevent endometrial carcinoma.[38]

4. **Suppression of ovulation.**

- **Decreased premenstrual symptoms.** There is limited evidence that cyclic use of COCs containing older progestins decrease the symptoms of premenstrual syndrome (PMS) such as breast pain, bloating, and negative affect compared with placebo. In a non-placebo controlled trial, drospirenone-containing COCs reduced PMS symptoms more than did levonorgestrel-containing COCs.[67] A comparative trial of extended versus cyclic use of a low-dose drospirenone-containing COC noted that extended use was associated with a significant decrease in premenstrual symptoms, including negative mood. The greatest improvement was noted after 6 months of use.[68] A greater clinical benefit may be seen for premenstrual dysphoric disorder (PMDD). As many as 18% of women of reproductive age may have PMDD, which by definition means that their symptoms are severe enough to cause distress.[69] A Cochrane review of randomized clinical trials concluded that use of low-dose drospirenone-containing COCs reduced the severity of symptoms of PMDD. Subjects' ability to function and to interact socially during menses also improved.[70] Based on these studies, drospirenone-containing COCs gained approval from the FDA as treatment for the symptoms of PMDD. Extended use of levonorgestrel-containing COCs may also be effective treatment for PMS or PMDD, though studies are not consistent in this finding.[71] (See Chapter 23 on Mental Health and Contraception.)

- **Decreased functional ovarian cysts.** The use of low-dose COCs is associated with a reduced prevalence of functional (i.e., post-ovulatory or luteal) cysts.[72,73,74] The clinical significance of this benefit is unclear, as most functional cysts regress without needing therapy, although hemorrhagic corpus luteal cysts can rarely pose a surgical emergency. Low-dose COCs taken cyclically (21/7) do not protect as well against ovarian follicle formation, because they do not sufficiently suppress FSH levels.[75–78] Extended cycle use of low-dose COCs more effectively reduces ovarian follicle formation. COCs are not a treatment for existing ovarian cysts because their use does not accelerate regression of cysts,[79] but COCs may prevent the formation of a new cyst, which might be mistaken for the original cyst on repeat exam. And COCs may eliminate mittelschmerz, the midcycle pain associated with ovarian follicle extrusion.

- **Decreased ovarian cancer risk.** A collaborative reanalysis of data from 45 studies showed that ever-users of COCs had a 27% reduced risk of ovarian cancer that persisted for 30 years.[80] The longer the duration of use, the greater the protection: the relative risk decreased by 20% for every 5 years of COC use. Low-dose COC formulations were associated with a similar decrease in risk as provided by older, high-dose formulations containing 50 mcg or more of EE.[81] The Royal College of General Practitioners (RCGP) observational study with up to 39 years of follow-up found that ever-users were 47% less likely to die from ovarian cancer than were nonusers (RR 0.53 (0.38–0.72)).[5] A meta-analysis of three observational studies found a similar protective effect among women with BRCA1 and BRCA2 mutations who are at higher risk of developing ovarian and breast cancer. Again, the longer the duration of use, the greater the effect. A compelling argument can be made that COCs should be offered to otherwise healthy patients who are at high risk for developing ovarian cancer, even if they do not need contraception.[82]

- **Decreased risk of benign breast conditions.** COC users are less likely to develop fibrocystic breast changes, cysts, or fibroadenoma, especially with longer durations of COC use.[83,84] In one case-control study with over 500 women, the risk of benign breast conditions was lower in the COC users, regardless of dose of EE, and markedly lower in subjects who started COC use before their first full-term pregnancy.[85] COC use does not reduce nor does it elevate the risk of developing ductal hyperplasia with atypia.[84]

5. **Benefits related to the estrogen component.**

- **Improvement of acne.** Three brand name COC formulations have received formal FDA approval for treatment of mild to moderate acne, but all COC formulations are effective.[86,87] A recent Cochrane review concluded that in nine randomized clinical trials, all COCs were significantly more effective than placebo in reducing the number, severity, and self-assessment of facial acne lesions. In comparative trials of COCs containing progestins of differing generations, few differences were found in effectiveness against acne.[88] COCs reduce acne by suppressing ovarian production of androgens and by inducing hepatic production of sex hormone binding globulin (SHBG). SHBG binds circulating testosterone and, thereby, reduces serum concentrations of free (biologically active) testosterone by up to 50%. In addition, conversion of testosterone to dihydrotestosterone in skin and hair follicles is decreased. Extended-cycle regimens suppress endogenous androgen production more than 21/7 regimens.[89] COCs do not have an immediate impact on acne; patients need to be advised that maximal effect may not be seen for up to 6 months.[90,91] SHBG levels may remain elevated for several months after discontinuation of COCs.[92]

- **Improvement of hirsutism.** Just as estrogen in COCs helps reduce androgen levels and activation of sebum production, it also helps reduce androgenic stimulation of hair growth. With COC use, patients with hirsutism have a reduction in the hair shaft diameter.[93,94] It generally takes 6 months to see the beneficial effect of COCs on hirsutism, and continued use of COCs is necessary to prevent recurrence. In patients with significant androgenic symptoms, as often seen with PCOS, drospirenone-containing COCs may be more effective than other COC formulations in decreasing testosterone levels and symptomatology.[95,96] In addition, extended-cycle regimens suppress androgen production more than do cyclic 21/7 regimens.[89]
- **Treatment for hot flashes and other perimenopausal symptoms.** One 3-year observational study found that 90% of perimenopausal women with vasomotor symptoms had relief with COC therapy compared with 40% with placebo.[97] Extended use of COCs may be more effective as users would not experience a drop in EE during the placebo week. (See Chapter 19 on Contraception in the Later Reproductive Years.)
- **Favorable impact on bone for high-risk patients.** Patients who have hypothalamic amenorrhea have low levels of circulating estrogens and are at higher at risk for osteoporosis and, later in life, for fractures. COC use increases bone mineral density (BMD) in adolescents with hypothalamic amenorrhea.[98] COC use by patients with osteopenia due to anorexia nervosa is not sufficient to completely protect bone, but when added to anabolic agents such as insulin growth factor, COC use significantly improved that agent's effectiveness. [99] A systematic review concluded there is a possible benefit of COC use in preserving BMD in perimenopausal patients.[100] For patients with normal estrogen levels, the effect of low-dose COCs on BMD is less clear. A review of all observational studies found use of low-dose COCs in healthy women had no effect on bone health overall or fracture risk.[101]

DISADVANTAGES AND CAUTIONS

Before patients decide to use COCs, they should consider if they would be able to use them correctly and consistently. They should also balance the benefits they would get with COC use against the possible risks they pose in the context of their individual medical status.

Contraceptive Disadvantages

1. **Daily administration.** Inconsistent use of COCs reduces the effectiveness of protection from pregnancy and increases the incidence of some side effects, especially unscheduled bleeding and spotting. Studies demonstrate that most patients miss several pills each month.[1]

2. **Expense and access challenges.** If insurance companies do not provide contraceptive coverage as a benefit, many patients, whether insured or uninsured, must pay out of pocket for their contraception.[102] So for short-term methods like COCs, out-of-pocket costs may be required every 1 to 3 months. The cost of branded COCs may easily exceed $80 per pack. Generic formulations are typically less expensive but often cost $30 or more per month. Pharmacies that have generic prescription programs (such as Wal-Mart or Target) sell a limited number of generic COC formulations for $9 a pack. For systems that do provide contraceptive coverage, there may be a high copayment, especially for the more expensive formulations. Find out about patients' coverage and their financial constraints when you help them choose COCs. *Often, the number of packs dispensed at pharmacies is severely restricted, so patients are required to return to pharmacies each month to purchase another pack.* The mismatch between calendar months with 30 to 31 days and COC packs with only 28 pills can present additional challenges in COC use. Patients who desire to use extended cycles of pills are faced with even more difficulties in obtaining adequate pill supplies.

3. **Need for privacy as well as ready access.** Adolescents and adults whose parents or partners do not want them to use contraception may not have a secure place to store their COC packs. Practitioners may need to guide them to more private contraceptive methods, if needed.

Health Risks

1. **Venous thromboembolism (VTE).** The best evidence suggests the increased risk of **VTE in COC users is from the estrogen component dependent on dose and duration**, and independent of the progestin used.[103] Higher doses of estrogen are associated with a greater risk of VTE. VTE risk with 50 mcg EE formulations is higher than that with 35 mcg EE formulations, which is one reason why use of 50 mcg EE COCs is discouraged. Clinically significant VTE occurs when there is an imbalance between two sets of factors that control blood clot formation. Estrogen increases hepatic production of elements that promote clot formation by the extrinsic clotting system (Factor VII, Factor VIII, Factor X) and

decreases the production of elements that promote clot lysis (tissue plasminogen activator, antiplasmin). COC users also develop an increased resistance to anticoagulant effect of activated protein C. The net result is a prothrombotic effect.

Progestins alone have virtually no impact on the clotting system, but when combined with estrogen, some progestins can modulate the strength of estrogen's production of extrinsic clotting factors, antithrombin,[104] fibrinolytics, and other steps in blood clot formation. In the mid-1990s, international studies indicated that COCs containing the third-generation progestins, desogestrel and gestodene (not available in the US), were associated with higher rates of thrombosis (up to a 2-fold increase) compared with formulations containing the second-generation progestins, levonorgestrel and norgestrel.[105–107] Because third-generation progestins were designed to reduce the androgenicity of progestin to allow fuller expression of the COC's estrogen component, such concerns were biologically plausible. Re-analyses of those early studies showed no increase in VTE risk with third-generation progestins once corrections were made for biases related to duration of COC use and patient selection.[108] Although more recent observational studies also found as much as a 2-fold increased risk of VTE associated with third-generation progestins, the overall incidence of VTEs was expectedly rare (i.e., 6.3 per 10,000).[109,110] Furthermore, for drospirenone-containing COCs, two large cohort studies found no increased VTE risk associated with their use compared with other COC formulations.[111,112] Overall, there is no strong evidence to suggest clinicians need to change their prescribing patterns of COCs containing newer generation progestins. Discussing the potential benefits vs. risks of these newer COCs formulations with patients who may be good candidates for them is key to patient informed consent before use.

Though the *relative risk* of thrombosis is increased with COC use, most COC users face a low *absolute risk* of thrombosis because VTE is a rare event in the healthy young user. A systematic review of the literature estimated the incidence of VTE in reproductive-aged women to be 5 to 10 per 10,000 women-years, which is higher than previous estimates.[113] The most recent meta-analysis concluded that the risk of VTE was increased 3 to 4 times in COC users compared with nonusers, and peaks in the first 12 months of use before declining with future use.[114] A population-based cohort found the VTE risk during pregnancy is increased at least 4 times, and during the postpartum period at least 20 times.[115]

The risk of VTE increases with age, with nearly a 5-fold increase from age 25 to age 50.[116] Another risk factor for VTE is obesity: obese COC users have as much as a 3-fold increased risk of VTE when compared with COC users of normal weight.[112] The American College of Obstetricians and Gynecologists (ACOG) recommends caution in prescribing estrogen-containing contraception to patients over age 35 with a BMI >30,[117] although the U.S. MEC rates obesity as a category 2 condition. Tobacco use also increases the risk of VTE. In one study, smokers aged 18 to 39 who did not use COCs had double the risk of VTE compared with nonsmokers of the same age who did not use COCs. At even greater risk were smokers who did use COCs: their risk was 8.8 times higher than nonsmokers who did not use COCs.[118] The risks showed a dose response among young smokers, with higher doses of estrogen associated with greater risks of VTE.

Patients need to know the increase in VTE risk that they experience during COC use is a completely reversible risk. The risk of thrombosis usually disappears 30 days after discontinuation.

2. **Myocardial Infarction (MI).** In healthy, nonsmoking U.S. pill users, it is unlikely that the use of low-dose COCs (≤50 mcg EE) alone is associated with any significant risk of MI. One pooled analysis showed that the relative risk for MI with low-dose COC use was 1.0.[119] Although a meta-analysis of studies including high-dose COCs showed an overall risk of 2.48 for current users, there was no increased risk for those using 20 mcg formulations.[120] And the American College of Cardiology concluded that low-dose COC formulations pose no increased myocardial infarction risk for current users.[121] Similarly, in a more recent cohort study by Lidegaard et al., the risk of MI doubled in users of COCs containing 30 to 40 mcg of EE, but did not increase in users of COCs containing 20 mcg of EE.[122] In looking at various progestins contained in COCs, the EURAS study (with over 58,000 participants) found no difference in MI rates.[112] Duration of COC use likewise appears to cause no difference in MI risk.[123] Past COC users have no increased risk due to their prior COC use.

   The risks for MI increase with age, but are greatly magnified by the combination of age, smoking, and hypertension.[120,124] In one meta-analysis of COC users, smoking, hypertension, and dyslipidemia each were associated with a 9-fold increased risk for MI.[120] The attributable risk of death from MI in absolute terms with COC use itself is very low. Estimates are that among women age 20 to 24 who do not smoke and do not use COCs, 4 per 1 million die from MI: that risk rises to 10 per million among smokers who use COCs (Table 8-1).[104]

3. **Stroke.** Cerebrovascular disease is rare in young reproductive-age women but becomes more common in women in their 40s.

Table 8-1 Age-specific estimates of attributable MI deaths due to low-dose COC use per 1 million users in international studies: the effect of smoking and hypertension

	Risk of Myocardial Infarction/1,000,000 Users		
	Age Range (years)		
Risk Category	**20–24**	**30–34**	**40–44**
Healthy nonsmokers	4	6	20
With smoking	10	20	200
With hypertension	100	120	450

Source: Farley TM, et al. (1998).[125]

The risk of stroke attributable to current COC use is likely low with low-dose COCs. One meta-analysis concluded that use of low-dose COCs was associated with a significantly increased risk of ischemic stroke among non-smoking, non-hypertensive women (RR = 1.9; 95% CI 1.35–2.74).[126] A second meta-analysis concluded that the risk declines with decreasing doses of estrogen.[127] However, there is little evidence of the risk associated with use of COCs with less than 20 mcg EE.[128] There is no apparent increase in the risk of either type of stroke with increasing duration of COC use[129] or with past use of COCs.[130] Data are insufficient to make conclusions about how the type or dose of progestin might influence the risk of stroke.[131] COC use does not affect the risk of *subarachnoid* hemorrhage.[132]

Risk factors for stroke should be screened for, and if present, patients counseled to modify them if possible. Risk factors for *ischemic* stroke include smoking, hypertension, diabetes, overweight or obesity, lower socioeconomic status, and migraine headaches with aura. The risk factors for *hemorrhagic* stroke include age, hypertension, smoking, obesity, and heavy alcohol use. A recent systematic review found a significant increase in the risk of ischemic stroke among COC users who experienced migraine with aura but no significant increase overall among COC users who reported migraine without aura.[128] (See Chronic Medical Conditions: Migraine Headaches.) Most studies suggest there is no synergistic effect between COC use and hypertension or smoking on risk of ischemic stroke. However, increased risk of ischemic stroke was noted in one study among COC users who did not have blood pressure screening prior to use compared with those who did.[133] And one case-control study found that the risk of hemorrhagic stroke was further increased for COC users who were older than 35 years of age, hypertensive, or smokers.[134] Therefore, it is advisable to avoid estrogen-containing contraceptives if possible in individuals with significant risk factors for stroke.

4. **Hyperlipidemia.** Estrogen is known to decrease low-density lipoprotein (LDL), and to increase high-density lipoprotein (HDL), triglycerides, and total cholesterol. COC users are 2 to 4 times more likely to develop abnormal lipid levels compared with COC nonusers.[135] Hypertriglyceridemia is an independent risk factor for early cardiovascular disease. However, COC-induced lipid changes may not increase a patient's risk for atherosclerosis.[136] Although most modern COC formulations increase triglycerides by about 30%, these estrogen-induced triglycerides are different in size than endogenously produced triglycerides. And the alterations in lipids nevertheless result in a net decrease in the LDL:HDL ratio, which is a more accurate marker for risk than are absolute levels.[135] The androgen-derived progestins in COCs may be neutral or may reverse some of estrogen's stimulatory effects on high-density lipoprotein (HDL) and triglycerides and may increase low-density lipoprotein (LDL). The net effect depends upon the dose, potency, and estrogen/androgen balance of each formulation. If LDL levels rise or HDL levels drop significantly with COC use, change to a formulation with more estrogenic activity and less androgenic activity. Routine screening of lipid levels is not necessary before prescribing or continuing COCs unless a patient has pre-existing hyperlipidemia or a very strong family history of premature cardiovascular disease.[137]

5. **Cervical cancer.** Cervical dysplasia and cervical carcinoma are caused by the high-risk human papillomavirus (HPV), especially the high-risk subtypes HPV 16 and 18. A review of cross-sectional studies found no strong evidence for an association between ever using COCs and having HPV infection.[138] However, a large meta-analysis of 28 studies including 12,531 women with squamous cell and adenocarcinoma found only an RR 1.1 after 5 years of COC use, but the RR increased to 1.6 after 5 to 10 years, and to 2.2 after more than 10 years.[139] However, this COC-associated risk is lower than the risk that is associated with high parity; women with HPV infection who had 7 or more pregnancies had higher RR (8.29) for cervical cancer.[140] And increasing use of the HPV vaccine will likely decrease the clinical significance of this associated risk over time.[141] Despite this slight increase in risk, even long-term COC users do not need to have cervical cytology testing performed more frequently or with more sensitive tests than required by their other risk factors.

6. **Cervicitis.** A systematic review of the literature concluded that women who use COCs are at increased risk for acquiring Chlamydia cervicitis, although the authors noted that nearly all the studies failed to adjust for confounders, had relatively small sample sizes, and were given a "poor" quality rating. The pooled odds

ratio was 2.9 (95% CI, 1.86–4.55).[142] A previous meta-analysis had concluded that COC users may be more likely to have cervical ectopy and that COC users with cervical ectopy may be more likely to acquire chlamydial infection.[143] A prospective study found that cervical ectopy is a risk factor for cervicitis, but the presence of cervical ectopy did not change the association between COC use and cervicitis.[144] However, cervical ectopy may make the detection of chlamydial infection easier.[145] Studies of gonorrhea or herpes infection and COC use are conflicting. Studies have consistently shown no increased risk of HIV, trichomonas, or syphilis infection with COC use.[142,146]

7. **Breast cancer.** A population-based case-control study investigated the incidence of breast cancer among U.S. women aged 35 to 64 years and found no increased risk of breast cancer among ever-users of COCs compared to never-users (RR of 0.9; 95% CI 0.8–1.0) regardless of EE dose, duration of use,[147] or COC formulation.[148] In a recent prospective cohort of 1.8 million Danish women aged 15 to 49 years, current and recent users of any hormonal contraception (with the vast majority using low-dose COCs) had an RR of 1.20; 95% CI 1.14–1.26, for breast cancer compared to never-users.[149] This translates to an attributable risk of 13 diagnosed cases of breast cancer per 100,000 women using low-dose COCs per year. However, the cohort was limited to women no older than 49 even though the vast majority of breast cancer cases occur above this age. Furthermore, such a small RR in an observational study should be read with caution and not used to suggest causation.[150] Patients should ultimately be counseled on the data and be able to weigh the risks and benefits that meet their contraceptive goals. In regard to high-risk groups, women who carry mutations for BRCA1 or BRCA2 and use COCs do not experience any increase in their already high risk of developing breast cancer.[151] And women with a family history of breast cancer (unknown BRCA status) do not increase their risk of disease by using COCs.[152]

PROVIDING THE METHOD

MEDICAL ELIGIBILITY

The U.S. Medical Eligibility Criteria for Contraceptive Use (U.S. MEC) provides guidelines for practitioners to follow when assessing risks associated with the use of various contraceptive methods versus the risks of unintended pregnancy.[38] In summary, patients are candidates for COCs when their health risks from COC use are less than the health risks they

Table 8-2 **Medical conditions precluding COC use, as listed in the U.S. Medical Eligibility Criteria for Contraceptive Use**

Medical conditions precluding COC use	U.S. MEC Rating
Current venous thromboembolism	4
History of venous thromboembolism with high risk of recurrence	4
Cerebrovascular or coronary artery disease	4
Valvular heart disease with complications	4
Severe hypertension or with vascular disease	4
Diabetes mellitus with vascular disease or > 20 years' duration	4
Migraine headaches with aura	4
Major surgery with prolonged immobilization	4
Current breast cancer	4
Thrombogenic mutations	4
Systemic lupus erythematosus with + antiphospholipid antibodies	4
Solid organ transplant with complications	4
Peripartum cardiomyopathy with impaired cardiac function	4
Heavy smokers > 35 years of age	4
Hepatic adenoma or carcinoma	4
Severe cirrhosis or acute hepatitis	4
< 21 days postpartum	4
Multiple risk factors for atherosclerotic cardiovascular disease	3/4*

* Category 3 or 4 depending on number of major risk factors for cardiovascular disease.

Source: Centers for Disease Control and Prevention (2016).[38]

would face with pregnancy. Although the FDA-approved prescribing information also lists medical conditions that are not compatible with COC use, FDA package labeling for many drugs has been shown to be at least 20 years obsolete.[153] The U.S. MEC represents an up-to-date synthesis of the medical literature on the risks associated with COC use. Table 8-2 shows a list of medical conditions in which COC use is contraindicated. For a complete list of the U.S. MEC upon which to make your clinical decisions, go to www.cdc.gov, and see Chapter 18 on Contraception for Women with Medical Conditions for ways in which you can use the guidelines in your everyday practice. (See also the U.S. MEC summary chart insert in this book.)

Chronic Medical Conditions

In the past, patients who faced any significant health risks were prohibited from using COCs. This practice ignored the fact that pregnancy might pose even greater and more severe health threats. Many medical conditions present no contraindications to use of COCs; for these conditions,

COC use neither worsens disease progression nor increases risk of complications. These conditions are assigned "category 1" (use is not restricted) and "category 2" (benefits of use outweigh risks) in the U.S. MEC and include thyroid disorders, cystic fibrosis, and sickle cell anemia, among others. COCs can help treat abnormal uterine bleeding (AUB) associated with medical conditions like thyroid disorders or anticoagulation. In addition, patients with sickle cell or other pre-existing anemias benefit from decreased menstrual blood loss. However, sometimes the medications used to treat medical conditions, such as depression and epilepsy, may interact with and decrease the efficacy of COCs (see Medication Interactions). Use of an additional contraceptive method, or substitution of a locally acting method like an IUD, is therefore recommended.

The following are some of the more common medical conditions that present challenges for clinicians and their patients requesting COCs.

Hypertension

Patients with elevated blood pressure have an increased risk of MI and stroke, and COC use further increases this risk.[133] However, it is not as clear if well-controlled hypertension is equivalent to normotension. The estrogen component in COCs increases circulating levels of angiotensinogen. Some patients are sensitive to angiotensinogen metabolites (angiotensin) and experience increases in both systolic and diastolic blood pressures with COCs. Finally, estrogen, and to some extent progestin, enhance aldosterone activity, which may result in fluid retention and, in turn, an increase in blood pressure. The U.S. MEC recommends that COC use be contraindicated in patients with hypertension with uncontrolled blood pressure (Systolic Blood Pressure (SBP) ≥160, Diastolic Blood Pressure (DBP) ≥100) or advanced vascular disease such as retinopathy or nephropathy (category 4), and recommends caution for use of COCs with mildly elevated blood pressure (SBP 140-159, DBP 90-99) or well-controlled blood pressure, unless no other contraceptive method is available or acceptable (category 3). If you do prescribe COCs to a patient with treated hypertension, monitor her blood pressure carefully. If it rises due to COC use or due to nonadherence with her antihypertensives, she may become ineligible for COC use.[154] In these cases, effective progestin-only or nonhormonal methods are typically available. Patients with a history of gestational hypertension or pre-hypertension (120–139 systolic or 80–89 diastolic) have no restrictions to COC use.

Most studies find no increase in the incidence of hypertension with low-dose COCs, although a 3 to 5 mmHg rise in blood pressure during COC use is not uncommon.[155,156] One study found that elevated blood pressure occurred in only 41.5 cases per 10,000 COC users.[155] For patients who do experience increases in blood pressures consistent with new onset hypertension during COC use, stop her COC and switch her to a non-estrogenic contraceptive. Patients with hypertension attributable to COC use will normalize their blood pressures within 3 to 6 months of stopping estrogen-containing contraceptives.[121] Patients whose readings do not return to normal after stopping should undergo a standard work-up; most will be found to have essential hypertension.

Diabetes

Diabetes increases a patient's risk for microvascular (retinopathy, nephropathy, neuropathy) and macrovascular (coronary artery disease, peripheral artery disease) complications. However, the use of low-dose COCs by patients with diabetes mellitus does not appear to significantly alter glucose levels or increase risk of vascular complications.[157] COCs can also provide a diabetic patient the chance to achieve tight glucose control before conception and thereby decrease the risk for maternal and fetal complications including fetal malformation. Therefore, the U.S. MEC concluded that COCs may be used by patients with diabetes who do not have vascular disease because the benefits outweigh the risks (category 2). However, the U.S. MEC recommends against the initiation of COCs in patients with diabetes who have co-existing vascular disease or who have had diabetes for over 20 years, unless no other contraceptive method is available or acceptable (category 3). COC continuation is contraindicated in diabetic patients who develop micro- or macrovascular complications during COC use (category 4).[38] In each of these cases, the patient is still eligible for effective progestin-only or non-hormonal methods. Patients with a history of gestational diabetes have no restrictions to COC use. In these patients, more frequent screening may be needed because they are at higher risk of developing diabetes over time, but COC use does not appear to increase this risk.[158]

Thrombogenic Mutations

The increase in VTE risk seen with COC use is greatly magnified in the face of genetic thrombogenic mutation disorders, such as factor V Leiden mutation. The factor V Leiden mutation alone explains 30% of all cases of deep venous thromboses. In the United States, it is estimated that 5.3% of Caucasians, 2.2% of Hispanics, 1.2% of Blacks and Native Americans, and 0.5% of Asians carry this mutation. A WHO literature review reported that COC users with factor V Leiden mutations were 6.4 to 99.0 times more likely to form blood clots than were nonusers without the mutation. When a carrier uses COCs, her VTE risk rises 100 times higher than non-carriers who do not use COCs.[159] Genetic mutations in prothrombin also increase VTE risks. For patients with deficiencies in antithrombin, protein C, or protein S, the relative risks for VTE are 8 to 10, with an absolute risk of 120 to 150/100,000 a year. Despite the impact that these mutations may have on a patient's risk for thrombosis, routine laboratory screening of patients is not appropriate.[160]

Migraine Headaches

Before providing hormonal contraception to a patient with pre-existing headaches, characterize the type of headache she experiences. What a patient calls a "migraine" may actually be a severe non-migrainous headache. The International Headache Society[161] established guidelines for identifying headache type, including tension, cluster, and migraine headaches. *Tension* headaches are the most common; they are bilateral in location, throbbing in nature, and mild to moderate in intensity. They may be associated with mild or no nausea, and either photo- or phonophobia. *Cluster* headaches are unilateral, severe in intensity, and occur in "clusters" over several days. They may be associated with sympathetic symptoms like eye tearing, nasal congestion, or a feeling of restlessness. There is no contraindication to the use of combined hormonal contraceptives with tension or cluster headaches because there is no evidence to suggest that COC use causes any increased risk of complications.[64]

Migraine headaches are unilateral, throbbing in nature, moderate to severe in intensity, and last at least several hours in duration. They are exacerbated by physical activity and associated with nausea and vomiting or both photophobia and phonophobia. Migraines may be preceded by *aura*, which are reversible focal neurological symptoms that develop gradually, usually prior to onset of headache, and last no more than 60 minutes. Symptoms can include scotoma or flashing lights, loss of vision, numbness, tingling, or trouble speaking. A personal history of migraines is a risk factor for ischemic stroke, and the presence of aura further increases that risk. COC use increases stroke risk in users with migraines by 2- to 4-fold. The only study that evaluated COC use and stroke risk by migraine type (aura vs. no aura) found an elevated stroke risk only in users with migraine with aura.[128] Furthermore, the absolute risk of stroke in young women is very low (5 to 10 per 100,000 women-years).[64] And so while COCs may be prescribed to patients with migraines without aura (category 2), COCs are contraindicated in patients who experience migraines with aura (category 4).[162] These patients are still eligible for effective progestin-only or non-hormonal methods.

It is important to ask *when* in a menstrual cycle a patient experiences her headaches. Headaches due to estrogen withdrawal, whether related to menses or cyclic COC use, are called *menstrual migraines*. For menstrual migraines, extended-cycle COC use could provide relief. Although there is no evidence that a patient's stroke risk decreases if the migraines improve with extended COC use, the therapeutic relief in symptoms may provide enough benefit to outweigh the minimal risk of stroke.[64,162] If a patient develops new headaches while on COCs or has worsening of pre-existing headaches, provide prompt evaluation and possible discontinuation of estrogen-containing contraceptives. (See Managing Side Effects, Headaches.)

Tobacco Use

Although not a medical condition per se, smoking increases COC users' risk of MI at least 32-fold compared with users with neither risk factor. The risk attributable to smoking alone is greater than the risk attributable to COCs alone.[163] Indeed, women who smoke as few as 3 to 4 cigarettes a day have a 2.5-fold increased risk of coronary heart disease.[164] But 3 to 12 months after stopping smoking, past smokers have the same COC-related cardiovascular risks as nonsmokers. So the foremost clinical goal should be to help your patient stop smoking, though this can be challenging. Moderate and heavy smoking (i.e., at least 15 cigarettes a day) by patients over age 35 precludes the use of COCs (category 4). Light smoking by patients older than 35 merits caution (category 3). The older the smoker, the more cigarettes smoked, and the more comorbid cardiovascular risk factors present, the less likely the patient is to be a candidate for COCs. In otherwise healthy young patients, the absolute risk of cardiovascular disease is low, so use of COCs by young adults who smoke is still safer than pregnancy (category 2).

It is not clear which COC formulation is the best for smokers. On one hand, the ideal COC would have the lowest EE content (to reduce arterial thrombosis) and the lowest androgenic activity (to minimize any adverse impacts on lipids). On the other hand, the carcinogens in tobacco smoke induce the cytochrome P450 metabolism of EE (see Medication Interactions and the Impact on COC Effectiveness) so that smokers are 47% more likely to have spotting or bleeding than non-smokers using the same formulation. It is not clear whether this indicates a decrease in contraceptive effectiveness for smokers, but it likely contributes to increased COC discontinuation.[165] It may be prudent to start smokers and patients who use a nicotine replacement product on a 20-mcg EE formulation with an extended cycle. Vaginal contraceptive rings are another option for smokers who want good cycle control. Effective progestin-only and non-hormonal methods are still viable options.

HIV and AIDS

Worldwide, over 29 million adults are infected with HIV. New infections are concentrated among young adults, and more likely in women in this age group (15 to 24 years).[166] With the increased use of antiretroviral therapy (ART) that improves health and pregnancy outcomes, more HIV-infected patients are seeking reversible contraceptive methods. The most recent systematic review concluded that there is no association between COC use and disease progression or death among HIV-positive women.[167] Therefore, COCs may be safely used (category 1) by HIV-positive patients per the U.S. MEC, whether or not they are taking antiretrovirals or are diagnosed with AIDS.[38] Furthermore, COC use is not associated with an increased risk of HIV acquisition. A 2016 systematic review included 11 studies of COC use and HIV risk that found either no or marginally increased risk of HIV acquisition, even among discordant couples.[146] Correct and consistent use of condoms remains the first-line recommendation to prevent partner-to-partner transmission, so dual protection (i.e., condom and COC use) is recommended for HIV-discordant couples. In addition, several antiretrovirals can interact with COCs, resulting in a change in the serum level of either the antiretroviral or the COC. This is another possible reason for HIV-positive individuals to use condoms in addition to COCs. (See Medication Interactions)

Rheumatologic Disease

Four studies have shown that the incidence of disease flares does not increase in COC users with systemic lupus erythematosus (SLE), although patients with severe disease were not studied. Antiphospholipid antibodies in SLE patients are a known risk factor for thromboembolism, so COC use is contraindicated (category 4). However, patients with mild SLE may use COCs if they have no antiphospholipid antibodies, even if they are using immunosuppressive therapy (category 2).[168] Effective progestin-only and non-hormonal methods are still a reasonable and safe alternative for all patients with SLE. A review of six studies of COC use in patients with rheumatoid arthritis found no improvement or worsening of disease progression, whether or not they were using immunosuppressive therapy (category 2).[169]

Liver Disease

A systematic review found that COC use did not increase liver transaminase levels, hepatic inflammation, or fibrosis in patients with chronic hepatitis, though studies were all limited by short duration of follow-up. Only one small trial investigated COC use in patients with acute hepatitis and noted no increase in severity of disease. Patients with chronic hepatitis and mild cirrhosis may use COCs. In hepatitis carriers, COC use does not appear to precipitate liver failure or severe dysfunction. [170] U.S. MEC rates COC use as category 1 for both chronic viral hepatitis and carriers.[38] However, it is recommended that patients with acute hepatitis or with a severe flare or cirrhosis avoid COC use (category 4).[170]

Low-dose COCs do not appear to be associated with an increased risk of hepatocellular adenoma or other benign liver lesions, though this was noted in the past with high-dose COCs. Preexisting benign hepatic lesions do not appear to be affected by COC use: in patients who have focal nodular hyperplasia, a type of benign liver tumor, studies of COC use are limited but nonetheless show no effect on tumor size or number of lesions (category 2). Hepatocellular carcinoma risk is not increased with low-dose COC use,[171] even among high-risk patients (chronic hepatitis B or C, cirrhosis). Although use of COCs is not associated with a de novo increased risk of benign or malignant liver tumors, the hepatic metabolism of COCs is significant. Therefore, use of COCs in patients with hepatocellular adenoma or carcinoma is contraindicated (category 4).[172]

Gallbladder Disease

Low-dose COCs have not been associated with an increased risk of cholelithiasis or cholecystitis, as had been seen earlier with high-dose COCs. However, it may still be possible that low-dose COCs accelerate the course or development of symptomatic gallbladder disease in patients with preexisting gallstones or sludge. The EE in high-dose COCs was found to impair active transport of bile, resulting in cholestatic jaundice with pruritus. Patients who either have current gallbladder disease or a personal history but still have their gallbladder are at higher risk for recurrence and so should not be given COCs unless other methods are not available (category 3).[38] Patients who have a history of cholestasis treated with cholecystectomy are likely at lower risk, so the U.S. MEC rates their use as a category 2. COCs do not increase the risk of gallbladder cancer.[173]

Special Conditions

Adolescence

Adolescents are typically healthy, so the risks of unintended pregnancy generally far outweigh the health risks associated with COC use. Many states guarantee adolescents confidential access to reproductive health care, including contraception, so providing adolescent-friendly services in your office or clinic will increase access for this vulnerable population. If a parent is present, assure that you are directing your patient-centered counseling toward your adolescent patient, and that you also spend some time during the visit speaking to her confidentially. Targeted counseling is important. Adolescents may be more likely to abandon COCs because of minor side effects such as nausea or spotting, so actively listen to all her concerns about side effects.[174] Provide concrete counseling; studies show that adolescents anticipated having side effects at much higher rates than actually occur, and they expected to have no difficulty with consistent pill taking.[175] Anticipate that they may find it more challenging to use COCs correctly and consistently than do older patients. Practitioners and health educators may need to take more time instructing adolescents in what to do for missed pills, including use of condoms and emergency contraception for back-up. Studies have shown that women of all ages more successfully use the once-a-week or once-a-month methods instead of taking a pill once a day, but teens benefit most from less frequent dosing.[176] For this reason, be sure to also offer the full range of contraceptive methods.

Many adolescents can also benefit from taking COCs to treat anovulatory cycling, heavy menstrual bleeding, primary dysmenorrhea, or acne. If your patient is not sexually active or contemplating COC use for non-contraceptive benefits, reassure her that it is common among her peers to use hormonal contraception for noncontraceptive benefits. In particular, the cause for an adolescent's irregular or heavy menstrual bleeding is often anovulation from an immature hypothalamic-pituitary-ovarian axis. COCs can effectively and safely regulate menses in this circumstance. Low-dose COCs will not interfere with maturation of the hypothalamic-pituitary-ovarian axis nor stunt growth in height by prematurely closing her epiphyseal plates. Although adolescent COC users do not accumulate increases in bone mineral density as rapidly as non-users, this relative decrease is rapidly reversible after COC cessation.[177,178] Equally important, adolescent patients with AUB should be evaluated to rule out polycystic ovarian syndrome (PCOS), thyroid disorders, etc., when COC use is initiated. Clarify for her that when she stops taking her COCs, her menses may return to being abnormal, unless the primary cause of her menstrual disruption has resolved or been treated.

Perimenopause

Healthy patients without contraindications to estrogen can safely use COCs until they reach menopause. Specifically for perimenopausal patients, COCs can reduce irregular menstrual bleeding and the risk of endometrial hyperplasia associated with anovulatory cycling. However as patients get older, additional health issues may evolve that increase the risk of using an estrogen-containing contraceptive method.

COC users in their 40s or early 50s may not experience traditional symptoms of menopause while taking COCs. They will not experience menstrual irregularities or hot flashes, especially if COCs are used on an extended basis. In this context, it may be difficult to detect when menopause occurs. (See Chapter 19 on Contraception in the Later Reproductive Years.)

Postpartum

Pregnancy itself is a hypercoagulable state, and the postpartum period is the time that the risk of venous thromboembolism (VTE) is greatest.[113] As a result, it is recommended that postpartum patients delay use of estrogen-containing contraception that could further increase VTE risk until at least 21 days after delivery, when those pregnancy-induced changes in the coagulation system start to resolve. For patients with other risk factors for VTE (i.e., age over 35, obesity, cesarean delivery, postpartum hemorrhage, blood transfusion at delivery, preeclampsia, peripartum cardiomyopathy, smoking, immobility), it is advised to wait 42 days before initiating combined hormonal contraception.[38] (See Chapter 17 on Contraception After Pregnancy.)

COCs can be safely initiated immediately after first or second trimester abortion or early pregnancy loss (category 1).[38]

Breastfeeding

High-dose estrogen was once given to postpartum patients to inhibit breast milk formation. From this outdated practice, theoretical concerns persisted for years that COCs would adversely affect the quality or quantity of breast milk production at any time during breastfeeding. As reassuring evidence emerged, the American Academy of Pediatrics approved of estrogen-containing methods once some other source of nutrition (e.g., solid food) was added to the baby's diet. A thorough review of the world literature found that existing trials are insufficient to establish any effect of hormonal contraception on milk quality or its nutrients.[179] (See Chapter 17 on Contraception After Pregnancy.) The U.S. MEC concluded that the benefits of COC use outweigh the risks (i.e., category 2) in breastfeeding patients after 30 days postpartum when no other risk factors for VTE are present, when hypercoagulability is decreased, and when the milk flow is established.[38]

MYTHS

Surveys show that the vast majority of women rank COCs as more hazardous to health than pregnancy[180] when in truth COCs have decreased all-cause mortality in women.[5] Clinicians are partially responsible for this misperception as the informed consent process often focuses on risks and potential side effects rather than benefits.[181] Myths may also have originated from theoretical concerns but then continue to linger despite evidence to the contrary.

Table 8-3 lists several common myths that have been clearly refuted by existing evidence. The Population Reference Bureau also has a free

Table 8-3 Common COC myths 'debunked'

COC Myths	COC Facts
The pill causes infertility.	The pill is rapidly and completely reversible and has no impact on a patient's inherent fertility.[32] Return to fertility is very rapid following discontinuation of COCs. The 12-month conception rates ranged from 72% to 94%. The return to fertility is so rapid and consistent that no more than a 2-week delay in menses is expected following discontinuation of COCs.
The pill causes birth defects.	The pill will not harm the fetus even if the patient becomes pregnant accidentally while taking the pill. Patients who become pregnant while using COCs have no higher rates of spontaneous abortion, preterm deliveries, birth defects, or complications in the health of their offspring than do non-users.[182–186] The risks of significant congenital anomalies among infants of COC users is the same as that of the general population; patients who decided to continue a pregnancy following COC exposure need no special care or testing. Patients who experience spontaneous losses following COC use can be reassured that the COC did not contribute to the loss.
The pill causes cancer.	The pill protects against ovarian and endometrial cancer. Women who carry mutations for BRCA1 or BRCA2 and use COCs do not experience any increase in their already high risk of developing breast cancer.[151] Women with a family history of breast cancer (unknown BRCA status) do not increase their risk of disease by using COCs.[152]
After taking pills for several years, a patient should take a "break".	A healthy patient can take the pill for as long as she wants to and only needs a break if she would like a pregnancy.[5]
The pill causes depression.	The pill does not worsen the clinical course of a user's depression.[187]
The pill causes weight gain.	The pill does not appear to cause a change in weight.[188]
The pill causes acne.	The pill improves acne.[88]
The pill causes abortion.	The pill is contraceptive (prevents fertilization) but does not prevent implantation.
The pill kills your sex drive.	Studies have failed to find an association between libido and COC use.[189–191] Even though the pill changes androgen levels for reproductive-aged women, sexual desire and activity have been shown to be independent of serum testosterone levels.[192] The best evidence about the interactions between COCs and sexual desire comes from a study of using a COC with the anti-androgenic progestin drospirenone. Compared with their baselines, women using the drospirenone-containing COC had significant improvement in sexual enjoyment, sexual satisfaction, and frequency of orgasms, but no change in libido. Longer-term use was associated with significant increases in arousal and frequency of sexual activity.[193]

resource available called 'Contraceptive Evidence: Questions and Answers'(www.prb.org/Publications/Reports/2013/contraceptive-evidence.aspx). This document addresses additional COC myths (as well as other contraceptive methods). It is evidenced-based and arranged in a question/answer format that is useful not only for providers but patients too.

How to Prescribe COCs

Guiding patients in appropriate and safe decision-making is the key to safe COC use. Patients who desire a short-acting reversible method or seek the non-contraceptive benefits of combined hormonal contraception often choose COCs. The benefits of COCs generally far outweigh the risks of COCs. However, some patients have medical conditions or personal habits that increase their risk of complications or failure with use. Some patients will not choose COCs because they have underlying beliefs about the nature of hormones in contraceptives, a desire for "natural" contraception, or a lack of belief in their need to avoid pregnancy.[194] Patients seeking the most effective contraception may be better served by using IUDs, implants, or a permanent method. Those who have difficulty with daily pill administration should consider all of the long-acting methods as well as the intermediate acting hormonal methods: the injection, transdermal patch, or the vaginal ring.

Explore the patient's medical and reproductive health history and her family history to ensure that she has no conditions that would preclude her use of COCs. A comprehensive history will identify the vast majority of medical conditions in the U.S. MEC that are contraindications or cautions to COC use. In addition, the U.S. Selected Practice Recommendations for Contraceptive Use (U.S. SPR) provides guidelines for practitioners to follow when initiating contraceptive methods, switching from one method to another, and when screening tests are required before prescribing each method. Specifically, a blood pressure measurement is recommended before COC initiation.[137] An assessment of BMI before COC initiation might be helpful to inform counseling of patients who subsequently perceive that their COC use is causing weight gain. Otherwise, no other examinations or laboratory tests are required before initiating COCs in healthy patients.[195]

Although the need for a breast and pelvic examination may be indicated by the patient's history or symptoms, neither is needed before initiating COCs in an asymptomatic, healthy patient.[137,196] Wellness exams, including pap and STI testing, may or may not be done at the same time as COC initiation, per patient preference. No other screening tests are routinely needed unless the patient's medical history or blood pressure indicates a need for further assessment. The U.S. MEC provides guidance as to which medical conditions might require further assessment or follow up.[38] In particular, routine screening for thrombotic mutations is not recommended prior to prescribing COCs.[197]

Once your patient expresses a potential interest in using COCs, realize that despite the wide range of health *benefits,* attention in the public eye has been focused on possible health *risks* associated with COC use. Patients may have an inflated estimate of the health risks posed by COC use. Help them understand that their risks with unintended pregnancy are greater than their risks with using COCs. Discuss noncontraceptive benefits, as well as lifestyle issues to ensure they feel confident that they can take a pill each day. Anticipatory counseling about safety concerns or side effects may reduce later discontinuation. (See Chapter 2 on patient-centered counseling.)

When to Start COCs

COCs can be initiated on any day of the menstrual cycle, as long as it reasonably certain the patient is not pregnant. Guidelines for how to be reasonably certain a patient is not pregnant can be found in the U.S. SPR. (See Box 2-6 on How to be reasonably certain that a woman is not pregnant.) Initiating COCs on any day of the menstrual cycle is an easy instruction and allows a patient to be protected from unintended pregnancy as soon as possible. If she is not within the first 5 days of her menstrual cycle, advise her to use a back-up method of contraception for the first 7 days of COC use. If she needs emergency contraception (EC) that day and is using the levonorgestrel (LNG) pill, she can still start her COCs immediately. If she is using ulipristal acetate (UPA) for emergency contraception, then she should start her COCs 5 days after taking the UPA.[195] (See Chapter 10 on Emergency Contraception.)

This method of same-day contraceptive initiation was first studied as the "Quick Start" method. A systematic review found that pregnancy rates, unscheduled bleeding, and side effects were not increased when COCs were started on other days in the menstrual cycle.[198] It is also the easiest way to teach contraceptive initiation to patients, trainees, and staff. Quick Start is an off-label practice supported by good clinical research, so it's important to reassure your patient that she can start her COCs right away despite how the COC package may instruct her. As many as 25% of young women given prescriptions for COCs that used outdated Sunday or first-day start protocols failed to begin taking the COCs as instructed because they conceived in the interim, forgot the pill-taking instructions, failed to fill the prescription, or worried about taking the pills.[3,199] The Quick Start method improved continuation from the first pack of COCs to the second pack when compared with non-same day starts, although continuation rates were the same at 3 and 6 months.[200]

The next scheduled bleeding episode will likely not occur until the patient completes the active pills in the pack and starts the placebo pills.

If there is a possibility of an undetectable early pregnancy (i.e., less than 10–14 days), the patient can still start her COCs and take a urine pregnancy test at home (or return to your office or clinic to do so) in 2 weeks. Reassure patients that the hormones in the pills will not adversely affect an early pregnancy, and that rechecking a urine pregnancy test will detect a pregnancy early enough to allow them to pursue any pregnancy options they choose. Even if an early pregnancy is missed when COCs are initiated, fetuses inadvertently exposed in utero to COCs are not at any increased risk for birth defects than are unexposed fetuses.[201]

Switching From Other Methods

Patients who switch from other contraceptive methods can start COCs immediately, using the same guidelines just explained for same-day initiation.[195] For example, if a patient has her contraceptive implant removed, she should start her COCs that same day. If she is not within the first 5 days of her scheduled bleeding, advise her to use a back-up method of contraception for the first 7 days of COC use. The exception is after intrauterine device (IUD) removal. If she has had recent unprotected sex and is more than 5 days from the first day of her menstrual cycle, residual sperm in the genital tract may expose her to the risk of unintended pregnancy once the IUD is removed. In which case, she has three options:

- Start the COCs that day and return in 7 days for IUD removal
- Abstain or use a barrier method for the next 7days and then return for IUD removal and COC initiation
- Have the IUD removed that day and take emergency contraception. If she is using the LNG pill, she can start her COCs immediately. If she is using UPA, then she should start her COCs 5 days after taking the UPA.

Choosing a Formulation

Clinicians and patients in the United States have more than 70 COC formulations from which to choose. (See the color insert for photographs and formulations of COCs available in the United States). Select a COC based on the hormonal dose and on your patient's clinical picture, preferences, past experiences with COCs, availability, insurance coverage, and cost. Both WHO and the FDA recommend using the lowest dose COC to reduce potential side effects, especially in patients who have hormone sensitivity. Although studies have shown that several COCs containing 20 mcg EE (and generally 7 placebo pills) were associated with higher rates of unscheduled bleeding and discontinuation than COCs containing more than 20 mcg EE, the progestin components often differed among the COCs compared.[202] Whether the EE dose or the progestin type is responsible for the bleeding differences among COC formulations has yet to be answered.

Instructions for Taking COCs, Missed Pills

Instructions for COC use can effectively be provided by the practitioner, nurse, health educator, or written instructions, depending on the process that works best in your clinic or office setting.

- Remind your patient of the need to take COCs daily in order for them to remain effective. Although taking a COC at the same time every day is not required to maintain effectiveness, maintaining a daily routine will likely help her remember to take her COC consistently. Direct her to tools that may help her remember: a "pill app" for her smart phone, bedsider.org's texting service, or her alarm on her phone or watch.
- Instruct her to start her COC immediately, use a back-up method for the first 7 days if needed, and use a barrier method for dual protection thereafter if she is at risk for STIs.
- Determine if she wants to have monthly scheduled bleeding or if she would prefer less frequent scheduled bleeding episodes. If she chooses extended COC use, you can prescribe a formulation specifically packaged for this purpose. Alternatively, she can use other COC formulations for extended use by using the active pills, discarding the placebo pills, and starting a new packet right away. Patients who skip the placebo pills and start the next packet may not be able to get another packet of COCs until the usual refill time due to restrictive dispensing protocols required by third party-payers. Adjusting your prescription instructions or clinical documentation when extended use is indicated or desired may help in ensuring her coverage.
- Instruct your patient on the warning signs for complications with COC use. Even though they are rare, the sequelae of complications can be significant and even life-threatening. Using the pneumonic "ACHES" with the accompanying graphic might be easier for providers and patients to remember.

Managing Missed Pills

COC users commonly miss taking their pill daily.[1] After having taken at least 7 COCs at the correct time, patients are at little risk for ovulation until they subsequently miss 7 consecutive pills. Breakthrough ovulation and unintended pregnancy are more likely to occur if the patient missing

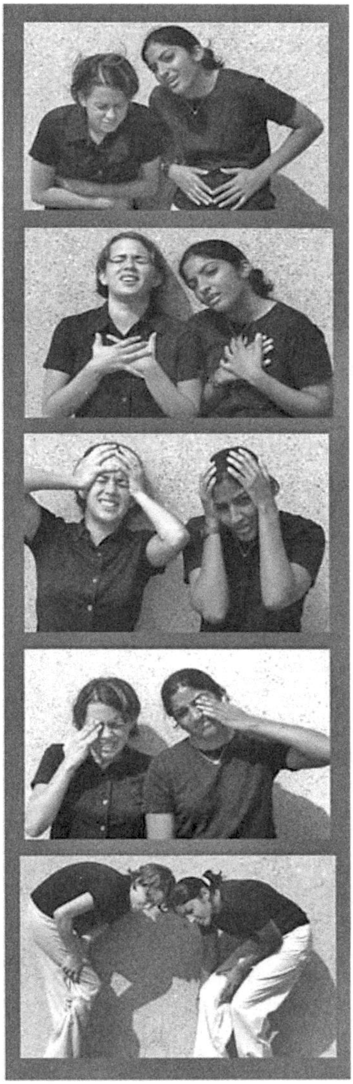

Abdominal Pain

- Blood clot in the pelvis or liver *[mesenteric or pelvic vein thrombosis]*
- Vomiting
- Cramping
- Weakness

Chest Pain

- Blood clot in the lung or heart vessels *[pulmonary embolism or myocardial infarction]*
- Heart attack, angina
- Chest or heart pain, left arm and shoulder pain
- Coughing and shortness of breath

Headaches

- Stroke
- Blurred vision, spots, zigzag lines, weakness, difficulty speaking
- Sudden intellectual impairment

Eye Problems

- Stroke or retinal vein thrombosis
- Complete or partial loss of vision

Severe Leg Pain

- Inflammation and blood clots of a leg in the leg *[thrombophlebitis]*
- Swelling, heat or redness, tenderness in leg

You should also return to the office if you develop severe mood swings or depression, become jaundiced (yellow-colored skin), miss 2 periods or have signs of pregnancy.

Source: Hatcher RA et al (2003), adapted with permission

Figure 8-1 Pill warning signs—ACHES

pills is using a 21/7 formulation.[20] COCs containing 20 mcg or less of EE are associated with more breakthrough ovulation with missed pills.[203] When initiating COCs, proactively instruct your patient in what to do after missing one or more of her pills:

For 1 late or missed active (hormonal) pill:

- Take 1 active pill as soon as possible.
- Continue taking your pills daily on time, which may mean taking 2 pills in one day.
- No back-up contraception is needed.
- EC is not typically needed unless pills were also missed earlier in the packet or at the end of the previous packet.

For 2 or more late or missed active (hormonal) pills:

- Take 1 active pill as soon as possible.
- Continue taking your pills daily on time, which may mean taking 2 pills in one day.
- Use condoms or abstain from vaginal sex until you have taken active pills for 7 days in a row.
- If pills were missed during the last week of active pills (days 15 through 21 of a packet), finish the active pills in the current packet and start a new packet the next day without using any placebo pills, OR use condoms or abstain from vaginal sex until you have taken active pills in the new packet for 7 days in a row.
- Use LNG emergency contraceptive pills if you missed COCs during the first week of a packet and you had any unprotected intercourse.

Patients who have vomiting or severe diarrhea within 24 hours of taking their COC should be treated as if they had missed pills.

Providing Adequate Supplies

To facilitate access to contraception, the CDC recommends providing up to 1 year's supply (pack or prescribed refills) of COCs when a patient initiates pill use.[195] For patients who obtain their COCs from a pharmacy, many commercial and Medicaid insurance plans will provide a 90-day supply (3 packs) at a time if the prescription is written as such. In light of updated cervical cancer screening guidelines, consider reasonable refill protocols for your office or clinic for patients who return less often than annually for a wellness visit. A systematic review of the literature found that COC continuation rates are greater when more pill packs are given at one time.[204] Finally, prescribe or provide condoms and emergency contraception for all COC users.

Follow-Up

Because side effects that may lead to COC discontinuation generally appear in the first few months of COC use,[174] encourage patients to return if problems develop or if they wish to change their method. Many patients discontinue COCs without consulting their clinicians. Although routine follow-up visits are not required, certain populations may benefit from follow-up visits, such as adolescents and adults with chronic medical conditions. At return visits for any reason (i.e., need for a COC refill or a wellness visit), responsiveness to patient concerns may increase patient continuation of COCs. Assess how well they are able to take their pills each day. Recognize how difficult it may be for patients to remember to take pills daily,[205] and remind them that such daily pill-taking is critical for COC effectiveness.

Managing Problems

How To Manage Side Effects And Bleeding Changes

Side effects are the most common reason for COC discontinuation. In one large study, 34% of women reported that side effects were the main reason for discontinuation of their COC.[174] Many of these side effects have been determined not to be caused by COCs (see Myths) while others remain difficult to determine causation or association—meaning, is it the COC? Or are these symptoms just common among individuals? In a population-based survey of approximately 2,500 Germans, 82% of respondents reported that at least one common symptom (fatigue, headache, muscle pain etc.) was causing mild impairment and 22% reported at least one symptom causing severe impairment.[206] Reported side-effects may occur more commonly in women than men when pre-conditioned to do so, such as by warning them that they might experience symptoms.[207]

However, perception is often everything. Active listening to and being supportive of patients in a nonjudgmental manner while still providing them the evidence about an issue may encourage continuation or the opportunity to switch to another method. Be clear that side effects are not adverse events and discuss what signs would be concerning. Advise patients that side effects are usually time-limited. Address the patient's main concerns about use of COCs directly. In the end, support them in their decision if they decide to switch to a different COC formulation or contraceptive method.

Amenorrhea Or Unscheduled Bleeding

Initial COC use is associated with unscheduled bleeding and the timing of initiation (i.e., Quick Start versus Sunday start) does not change the amount or duration of this bleeding.[208] Over time, bleeding should become more scheduled when using a COC that has a scheduled withdrawal week. Advise patients that overall the amount of bleeding they experience during a scheduled withdrawal is typically less than during natural menstruation. Likely the most common reason for unscheduled spotting or bleeding is missed or late pills.

As mentioned previously, extended-cycling formulations with skipped or delayed withdrawal can have a longer duration of unscheduled bleeding, but for most users that bleeding will improve over time.[22] If unscheduled bleeding becomes a nuisance with extended cycling, a 3 to 4 day break in COC use[24] or supplementing with a pill containing norethindrone acetate[25] may result in more days of amenorrhea.

Before changing COC type for complaints of unscheduled bleeding, rule out more likely or more serious causes, such as pregnancy, infection (vaginitis and cervicitis), or medications that interfere with COC metabolism (certain anticonvulsants, St. John's Wort, rifampin). Consider changing the patient's COC formulation if unscheduled spotting or bleeding persists after the first several months of use. Switch earlier if a patient is planning to discontinue due to the bleeding pattern. No research indicates that any specific COC formulation is best at eliminating unscheduled spotting or bleeding.

Experiencing amenorrhea during the time a scheduled withdrawal bleed should occur could be completely normal. The incidence likely varies for different individuals. COCs containing estradiol valerate combined with dienogest, as compared with an EE-levonorgestrel COC, appear to have shorter and less intense scheduled withdrawal bleeds as well as more likelihood of amenorrhea during the scheduled withdrawal week.[209] If there is cause for concern, the most obvious cause of amenorrhea—pregnancy—should be ruled out. Thyroid problems, prolactinoma, hypothalamic amenorrhea due to stress or excessive exercise, or anovulatory states (such as PCOS or obesity) are often masked by COCs. Other specific conditions, such as cervical stenosis, need to be evaluated if the patient has recently had cervical surgery (e.g., D&C, cone biopsy, LEEP, etc.). In general, reassurance can be given that they are not pregnant and, given the progestin-dominant effect on the endometrium, the lining of the uterus is not "building up." Additionally, the patient could consider intermittently using a home pregnancy test if that might be helpful to reduce anxiety around concerns about pregnancy. If the patient desires cyclic bleeding, consider switching to a different pill or a triphasic formulation.

Weight Changes

Randomized clinical trials have demonstrated that, on average, patients do *not* experience more weight gain with low-dose COCs than with placebo or no intervention.[188,210,211] In a prospective trial of women using triphasic COCs with daily weight measurements for 4 months, no changes in mean weight fluctuations were noted during the cycle.[212] A 9-year study showed that COC use by adolescents was *not* associated with either weight gain or increased body fat.[213] In clinical trials, women who use COCs do not typically gain more weight than they normally do in the same time interval without COCs. A Cochrane review confirmed that available evidence is insufficient to determine the effect of combination contraceptives on weight, but concluded that no large effect was evident.[188] However, it is important for clinicians to understand that what troubles a patient is her *perception* of weight changes and that often a patient's opinions about weight change in clinical trials may not correlate with measured changes on a scale.

The most common reason for weight gain in adults is simply age—as adults age, their metabolism changes and weight increases if no changes to diet or exercise are made. In addition, women have several events over their lifetime that can significantly act upon their metabolism and thus their weight, including puberty, each successive pregnancy, and menopause.[214–217] The hypothesized mechanisms for COC-related weight gain include changes to the renin-angiotensin-aldosterone system causing fluid retention and hypertrophy of adipose tissue. But as no clear clinical evidence has been found, it is unlikely that any of these mechanisms cause significant problems. Nonetheless, individual weight-changes to COC may exist and given that weight changes are an incredibly sensitive topic for many people, the most important thing is listen to a patient's concerns, briefly review what we know about COC and weight changes, and balance the pros / cons of changing methods.

Headaches

Headaches are common,[218] but if a patient develops new headaches while on COCs or has worsening of her pre-existing headaches, she deserves prompt evaluation and possible discontinuation of estrogen-containing contraceptives (see Chronic Medical Conditions, Headaches earlier in this chapter or Chapter 18 on Contraception for Women with Medical Conditions for more information on epidemiology and diagnosis and classification of headaches). Women report experiencing fewer headaches with extended regimens as compared with cyclic COCs.[22] For menstrual migraines, extended-cycle COC use could also provide relief. Although there is no evidence that a patient's stroke risk decreases if her migraines improve with extended COC use, the therapeutic relief in symptoms may provide enough benefit to outweigh the minimal risk of stroke.[64,162]

Headache complaints decrease with continued use of COCs. Patients experiencing headaches during the first cycle have only a 1 in 3 chance of having those headaches the second month of use. The risk drops to 1 in 10 by the third cycle. A systematic review of the literature found that there is no scientific evidence to support the common clinical practice of switching formulations to treat headache. However, the authors suggested that manipulation of the extent or duration of estrogen withdrawal might be beneficial, especially if her headaches worsen during bleeding.[219] Stepwise evaluation of the headache is necessary. For discussion on headache classification, see Chapter 18 Contraception for Women with Medical Conditions.

- **Confirm whether the headaches started or worsened in frequency or severity with the onset of COC use.** New or worsening symptoms prompt medical evaluation. Stop COCs during evaluation, especially if the headaches are severe or if the patient develops any aura with her headaches. Progestin-only pills may be used. If the headaches are not serious, consider lowering estrogen doses.
- **Rule out other causes.** Measure the patient's blood pressure. Obtain a personal history of medication use, caffeine intake, and other prescription, nonprescription, and recreational drug use. Inquire about recent trauma. Note if there are other associated problems with vision, sensation, or other functions. Evaluate for signs and symptoms of transient ischemic attacks, cerebrovascular accidents, temporal arteritis, sinusitis, viremia, sepsis, allergy, temporomandibular joint (TMJ) disorders, dental problems, drug use, alcohol or caffeine withdrawal, or central nervous system tumor.
- **Characterize the type of headache.** The consequences are different for different types of headaches. If a patient develops new-onset migraine or a worsening in the severity or frequency of her migraine headaches during her active pill days, she may no longer be a candidate for COCs. *If she develops associated neurological auras, stop the COCs immediately* and provide contraception without estrogen. On the other hand, if her symptoms develop or worsen only on the days she takes placebo pills (when her estrogen levels drop), it may be possible to offer her extended use, low-dose COCs to reduce her menstrual migraines.

Mood Swings and Depression

There is a common belief that COCs adversely impact mood but the published evidence is significantly flawed[220] and recent publications have been conflicting, either demonstrating a protective effect[221] or not.[222] It is important to note that the study reporting a risk of depression in COC users had a risk estimate well below 2, which is considered by epidemiologists not to be significant. In women with depression, COC use does not appear to worsen the disease.[187]

If patients do report an increase in depressive symptoms, moodiness, and other emotional states when on COCs, consider an empiric change to a lower dose pill or COC cessation. However, it is also important to identify when in a patient's cycle these symptoms develop. If the symptoms appear just before menses, then extended use of active pills may help to suppress or prevent cycle-related mood changes.[23] For those who suffer from premenstrual dysphoric disorder (PMDD), all COCs likely have the ability to suppress or reduce symptoms, and consideration should be given to extended dosing (eliminating the scheduled withdrawal week). The fourth-generation pill containing drospirenone/EE has an FDA indication for treatment of PMDD. A systematic review of drospirenone-containing pills for PMDD demonstrates that in the first 3 months of use, women experienced less severe symptoms, but data were insufficient to determine a longer impact.[70] In addition, the use of placebo had a significant beneficial impact on symptoms. (See Chapter 1 on the Menstrual Cycle and Chapter 23 on Mental Health and Contraception.)

If you have any concern about your patient suffering from an underlying depressive or anxiety disorder, perform or refer for an explicit evaluation and treatment. Stopping COC use is not adequate therapy and may not even be indicated. Suicidal patients need emergency treatment by specialists.

Changes in Libido

As mentioned previously in Myths, studies have failed to find a clear association between libido and COC use.[189–191] However, sexual desire and libido are not linear processes and can be influences by a variety of internal and external factors (see Chapter 22 on Sexuality and Contraception). A subset of individuals may be adversely affected by hormonal exposure, given that COCs can change the amount and consistency of vaginal lubrication. No clear guidance exists regarding what to do when patients experience these symptoms—it may be useful to switch to a lower dose pill. A study comparing a 30 mcg EE/LNG versus a 20 mcg EE/LNG pill demonstrated an increase in a sexual desire.[223] Given this evidence, its conceivable that other lower-dose hormonal methods might also provide improvement.

Skin Changes

Estrogen stimulates the production and activity of melanocytes, which can cause darkening of pigmented areas (linea nigra) or a dark patch on the face (melasma or chloasma). Patients with darker skin pigment are more susceptible. After discontinuation of estrogen, the melasma can fade over time but often incompletely. Progestin-only methods may be preferable for at-risk patients. In vitro studies have demonstrated that progesterone reduces the proliferation rate of melanocytes as compared with 17B-estradiol.[224] Recommend consistent use of sunscreen and hats in those at risk or if melasma has already occurred. If a patient is particularly bothered by these skin changes, refer to a dermatology specialist.

Estrogen can also stimulate the formation of telangiectasias, which are fine, dilated intracutaneous capillaries and small terminal arteries. Telangiectasias are not clinically significant, but may be cosmetically disturbing to a patient. Avoid the use of estrogen-containing hormonal methods in patients troubled by telangiectasia.

As mentioned earlier, COCs are universally used as treatment for acne.[88] If using COCs in the treatment of acne, the effect is not immediate and takes several months before benefits become apparent to the patient. Although certain COCs have received FDA approval for the treatment of acne, all COCs should have a similar effect given their ability to decrease free testosterone by increasing SHBG. If it appears the patient's COC may be contributing to acne, consider extended-use cycling or switch to a COC with a progestin component with low androgenicity formulation.[225]

Mastalgia

Breast tissue is dynamic and responsive to hormone exposure. For example, breast volume varies greatly during the menstrual cycle. An imaging study found that overall volume of the breast varies by 76 mL during the menstrual cycle![226] Mastalgia, or breast tenderness, is not an uncommon complaint, especially with initiation of COCs. A proper fitting bra is the first recommendation. A Cochrane review of COCs with different progestin types found that desogestrel-containing pills users complained less of breast tenderness than did those using a drospirenone-containing pill.[227] COC users with a lower EE component (20 mcg) also report less breast pain than do those using higher EE pills.[203] If the symptoms develop just before or during menses, extended-cycle COCs should also be helpful.

Gastrointestinal Complaints

Working at the level of the central nervous system, estrogen can induce nausea or vomiting. Progesterone slows gastric peristalsis and can increase constipation and sensations of bloating and distention. Most affected patients acclimate to the hormones, and nausea resolves within 1 to

3 months of use. If a patient complains of nausea, she can try taking her pills with food or at night. Patients with onset of severe gastrointestinal symptoms should be promptly evaluated for other causes, as this is likely unrelated to COC use.

If vomiting or diarrhea is related to taking the pill, try the following approaches:

- Switch to a progestin-only formulation.
- Decrease the dose of the estrogen-component.

USER INSTRUCTIONS FOR COMBINED ORAL CONTRACEPTIVES

Many high-quality resources now exist for providers in creating their own COC user instructions or in referring patients to use. One such site is Planned Parenthood's online resources: www.plannedparenthood.org/learn/birth-control/birth-control-pill. For additional resources, see the Appendix on Digital Resources for Health and Medical Information.

Author Disclosures—Cwiak: none. Edelman: consultant for World Health Organization, CDC, Gynuity Health Projects, Genzyme, Agile Therapeutics, HRA Pharma and FHI360; Nexplanon trainer for Merck; author for UptoDate (royalties received); research funding from Merck and National Institutes of Health (received NIH grant funding for several of the studies referenced in the chapter specific to obesity and contraceptive effectiveness).

REFERENCES

1. Potter L, Oakley D, de Leon-Wong E, Canamar R. Measuring compliance among oral contraceptive users. Fam Plann Perspect 1996;28:154–8.
2. Foster DG, Hulett D, Bradsberry M, Darney P, Policar M. Number of oral contraceptive pill packages dispensed and subsequent unintended pregnancies. Obstet Gynecol 2011;117:566–72.
3. Westhoff C, Kerns J, Morroni C, Cushman LF, Tiezzi L, Murphy PA. Quick start: novel oral contraceptive initiation method. Contraception 2002;66:141–5.
4. Tessler SL, Peipert JF. Perceptions of contraceptive effectiveness and health effects of oral contraception. Womens Health Issues 1997;7:400–6.
5. Hannaford PC, Iversen L, Macfarlane TV, Elliott AM, Angus V, Lee AJ. Mortality among contraceptive pill users: cohort evidence from Royal College of General Practitioners' Oral Contraception Study. BMJ 2010;340:c927.
6. Franks AL, Beral V, Cates W, Jr., Hogue CJ. Contraception and ectopic pregnancy risk. Am J Obstet Gynecol 1990;163:1120–3.
7. Marchbanks PA, Annegers JF, Coulam CB, Strathy JH, Kurland LT. Risk factors for ectopic pregnancy. A population-based study. JAMA 1988;259:1823–7.
8. Centers for Disease Control and Prevention. Ten great public health achievements—United States, 1900–1999. MMWR Morb Mortal Wkly Rep 1999;48:241–3.

9. Daniels K, Daugherty J, Jones J, Mosher W. Current contraceptive use and variation by selected characteristics among women aged 15–44: United States, 2011–2013. Natl Health Stat Report 2015:1–14.
10. Daniels K, Mosher WD. Contraceptive methods women have ever used: United States, 1982–2010. Natl Health Stat Report 2013:1–15.
11. Seidman L, Kroll R, Howard B, Ricciotti N, Hsieh J, Weiss H. Ovulatory effects of three oral contraceptive regimens: a randomized, open-label, descriptive trial. Contraception 2015;91:495–502.
12. Lewis RA, Taylor D, Natavio MF, Melamed A, Felix J, Mishell D, Jr. Effects of the levonorgestrel-releasing intrauterine system on cervical mucus quality and sperm penetrability. Contraception 2010;82:491–6.
13. Natavio MF, Taylor D, Lewis RA, et al. Temporal changes in cervical mucus after insertion of the levonorgestrel-releasing intrauterine system. Contraception 2013;87:426–31.
14. Stanczyk FZ, Archer DF, Bhavnani BR. Ethinyl estradiol and 17beta-estradiol in combined oral contraceptives: pharmacokinetics, pharmacodynamics and risk assessment. Contraception 2013;87:706–27.
15. Nelson A, Parke S, Mellinger U, Zampaglione E, Schmidt A. Efficacy and safety of a combined oral contraceptive containing estradiol valerate/dienogest: results from a clinical study conducted in North America. J Womens Health (Larchmt) 2014;23:204–10.
16. Stanczyk FZ. All progestins are not created equal. Steroids 2003;68:879–90.
17. Zimmerman Y, Eijkemans MJ, Coelingh Bennink HJ, Blankenstein MA, Fauser BC. The effect of combined oral contraception on testosterone levels in healthy women: a systematic review and meta-analysis. Hum Reprod Update 2014;20:76–105.
18. Han L, Jensen JT. Does the progestogen used in combined hormonal contraception affect venous thrombosis risk? Obstet Gynecol Clin North Am 2015;42:683–98.
19. Edelman A. Menstrual nirvana: amenorrhea through the use of continuous oral contraceptives. Curr Womens Health Rep 2002;2:434–8.
20. Dinger J, Minh TD, Buttmann N, Bardenheuer K. Effectiveness of oral contraceptive pills in a large U.S. cohort comparing progestogen and regimen. Obstet Gynecol 2011;117:33–40.
21. Sulak PJ, Scow RD, Preece C, Riggs MW, Kuehl TJ. Hormone withdrawal symptoms in oral contraceptive users. Obstet Gynecol 2000;95:261–6.
22. Edelman A, Micks E, Gallo MF, Jensen JT, Grimes DA. Continuous or extended cycle vs. cyclic use of combined hormonal contraceptives for contraception. Cochrane Database Syst Rev 2014:Cd004695.
23. Sulak PJ, Kuehl TJ, Ortiz M, Shull BL. Acceptance of altering the standard 21-day/7-day oral contraceptive regimen to delay menses and reduce hormone withdrawal symptoms. Am J Obstet Gynecol 2002;186:1142–9.
24. Sulak PJ, Kuehl TJ, Coffee A, Willis S. Prospective analysis of occurrence and management of breakthrough bleeding during an extended oral contraceptive regimen. Am J Obstet Gynecol 2006;195:935–41.
25. Edelman AB, Koontz SL, Nichols MD, Jensen JT. Continuous oral contraceptives: are bleeding patterns dependent on the hormones given? Obstet Gynecol 2006;107:657–65.
26. Winner B, Peipert JF, Zhao Q, et al. Effectiveness of long-acting reversible contraception. N Engl J Med 2012;366:1998–2007.
27. Foster DG, Parvataneni R, de Bocanegra HT, Lewis C, Bradsberry M, Darney P. Number of oral contraceptive pill packages dispensed, method continuation, and costs. Obstet Gynecol 2006;108:1107–14.
28. Potter L. Oral contraceptive compliance and its role in the effectiveness of the method. In: Cramer J, Spilker B, eds. Patient Compliance In Medical Practice And Clinical Trials. New York: Raven Press; 1991:195–207.
29. Nettleman MD, Chung H, Brewer J, Ayoola A, Reed PL. Reasons for unprotected intercourse: analysis of the PRAMS survey. Contraception 2007;75:361–6.
30. Jones RK. Change and consistency in US women's pregnancy attitudes and associations with contraceptive use. Contraception 2017;95:485–90.

31. Hou MY, Hurwitz S, Kavanagh E, Fortin J, Goldberg AB. Using daily text-message reminders to improve adherence with oral contraceptives: a randomized controlled trial. Obstet Gynecol 2010;116:633–40.
32. Barnhart KT, Schreiber CA. Return to fertility following discontinuation of oral contraceptives. Fertil Steril 2009;91:659–63.
33. Edelman AB, Carlson NE, Cherala G, et al. Impact of obesity on oral contraceptive pharmacokinetics and hypothalamic-pituitary-ovarian activity. Contraception 2009;80: 119–27.
34. Westhoff CL, Torgal AH, Mayeda ER, Pike MC, Stanczyk FZ. Pharmacokinetics of a combined oral contraceptive in obese and normal-weight women. Contraception 2010;81:474–80.
35. Lopez LM, Bernholc A, Chen M, et al. Hormonal contraceptives for contraception in overweight or obese women. Cochrane Database Syst Rev 2016:Cd008452.
36. Dinger JC, Cronin M, Mohner S, Schellschmidt I, Minh TD, Westhoff C. Oral contraceptive effectiveness according to body mass index, weight, age, and other factors. Am J Obstet Gynecol 2009;201:263 e1–9.
37. Yamazaki M, Dwyer K, Sobhan M, et al. Effect of obesity on the effectiveness of hormonal contraceptives: an individual participant data meta-analysis. Contraception 2015;92:445–52.
38. Centers for Disease C, Prevention. U S. Medical Eligibility Criteria for Contraceptive Use, 2010. MMWR Recomm Rep 2016;65.
39. American College of Obstetricians and Gynecologists. ACOG practice bulletin no. 105: bariatric surgery and pregnancy. Obstet Gynecol 2009;113:1405–13.
40. Sabers A, Buchholt JM, Uldall P, Hansen EL. Lamotrigine plasma levels reduced by oral contraceptives. Epilepsy Res 2001;47:151–4.
41. Dickinson BD, Altman RD, Nielsen NH, Sterling ML. Drug interactions between oral contraceptives and antibiotics. Obstet Gynecol 2001;98:853–60.
42. Murphy AA, Zacur HA, Charache P, Burkman RT. The effect of tetracycline on levels of oral contraceptives. Am J Obstet Gynecol 1991;164:28–33.
43. Neely JL, Abate M, Swinker M, D'Angio R. The effect of doxycycline on serum levels of ethinyl estradiol, norethindrone, and endogenous progesterone. Obstet Gynecol 1991;77:416–20.
44. Joshi JV, Joshi UM, Sankholi GM, et al. A study of interaction of low-dose combination oral contraceptive with Ampicillin and Metronidazole. Contraception 1980;22:643–52.
45. Maggiolo F, Puricelli G, Dottorini M, Caprioli S, Bianchi W, Suter F. The effect of ciprofloxacin on oral contraceptive steroid treatments. Drugs Exp Clin Res 1991;17:451–4.
46. Friedman CI, Huneke AL, Kim MH, Powell J. The effect of ampicillin on oral contraceptive effectiveness. Obstet Gynecol 1980;55:33–7.
47. Berry-Bibee EN, Kim MJ, Tepper NK, Riley HE, Curtis KM. Co-administration of St. John's wort and hormonal contraceptives: a systematic review. Contraception 2016;94:668–77.
48. Berry-Bibee EN, Kim MJ, Simmons KB, et al. Drug interactions between hormonal contraceptives and psychotropic drugs: a systematic review. Contraception 2016;94:650–67.
49. Mikkelsen EM, Riis AH, Wise LA, Hatch EE, Rothman KJ, Sorensen HT. Pre-gravid oral contraceptive use and time to pregnancy: a Danish prospective cohort study. Hum Reprod 2013;28:1398–405.
50. Davis A, Godwin A, Lippman J, Olson W, Kafrissen M. Triphasic norgestimate-ethinyl estradiol for treating dysfunctional uterine bleeding. Obstet Gynecol 2000;96:913–20.
51. Farquhar C, Brown J. Oral contraceptive pill for heavy menstrual bleeding. Cochrane Database Syst Rev 2009:CD000154.
52. ACOG Practice Bulletin No. 110: noncontraceptive uses of hormonal contraceptives. Obstet Gynecol 2010;115:206–18.
53. NICE Clinical Guidelines No. 44. Heavy menstrual bleeding: assessment and management. London: RCOG Press National Institute for health and Clinical Excellence, 2007. Available at www.nice.org.uk/guidance/cg44.
54. Davis AR, Westhoff C, O'Connell K, Gallagher N. Oral contraceptives for dysmenorrhea in adolescent girls: a randomized trial. Obstet Gynecol 2005;106:97–104.

55. Zahradnik HP, Hanjalic-Beck A, Groth K. Nonsteroidal anti-inflammatory drugs and hormonal contraceptives for pain relief from dysmenorrhea: a review. Contraception 2010;81:185–96.
56. Sangi-Haghpeykar H, Poindexter AN, 3rd. Epidemiology of endometriosis among parous women. Obstet Gynecol 1995;85:983–92.
57. Westhoff C, Britton JA, Gammon MD, Wright T, Kelsey JL. Oral contraceptive and benign ovarian tumors. Am J Epidemiol 2000;152:242–6.
58. Seracchioli R, Mabrouk M, Frasca C, et al. Long-term cyclic and continuous oral contraceptive therapy and endometrioma recurrence: a randomized controlled trial. Fertil Steril 2010;93:52–6.
59. Harada T, Momoeda M, Taketani Y, Hoshiai H, Terakawa N. Low-dose oral contraceptive pill for dysmenorrhea associated with endometriosis: a placebo-controlled, double-blind, randomized trial. Fertil Steril 2008;90:1583–8.
60. Parazzini F, Ferraroni M, Bocciolone L, Tozzi L, Rubessa S, La Vecchia C. Contraceptive methods and risk of pelvic endometriosis. Contraception 1994;49:47–55.
61. Nisolle-Pochet M, Casanas-Roux F, Donnez J. Histologic study of ovarian endometriosis after hormonal therapy. Fertil Steril 1988;49:423–6.
62. Edlow AG, Bartz D. Hormonal contraceptive options for women with headache: a review of the evidence. Rev Obstet Gynecol 2010;3:55–65.
63. Martin VT. Menstrual migraine: a review of prophylactic therapies. Curr Pain Headache Rep 2004;8:229–37.
64. Harris M, Kaneshiro B. An evidence-based approach to hormonal contraception and headaches. Contraception 2009;80:417–21.
65. Combination oral contraceptive use and the risk of endometrial cancer. The Cancer and Steroid Hormone Study of the Centers for Disease Control and the National Institute of Child Health and Human Development. JAMA 1987;257:796–800.
66. Schlesselman JJ. Risk of endometrial cancer in relation to use of combined oral contraceptives. A practitioner's guide to meta-analysis. Hum Reprod 1997;12:1851–63.
67. Sangthawan M, Taneepanichskul S. A comparative study of monophasic oral contraceptives containing either drospirenone 3 mg or levonorgestrel 150 microg on premenstrual symptoms. Contraception 2005;71:1–7.
68. Coffee AL, Kuehl TJ, Willis S, Sulak PJ. Oral contraceptives and premenstrual symptoms: comparison of a 21/7 and extended regimen. Am J Obstet Gynecol 2006;195:1311–9.
69. Halbreich U, Borenstein J, Pearlstein T, Kahn LS. The prevalence, impairment, impact, and burden of premenstrual dysphoric disorder (PMS/PMDD). Psychoneuroendocrinology 2003;28 Suppl 3:1–23.
70. Lopez LM, Kaptein AA, Helmerhorst FM. Oral contraceptives containing drospirenone for premenstrual syndrome. Cochrane Database Syst Rev 2012:Cd006586.
71. Freeman EW, Halbreich U, Grubb GS, et al. An overview of four studies of a continuous oral contraceptive (levonorgestrel 90 mcg/ethinyl estradiol 20 mcg) on premenstrual dysphoric disorder and premenstrual syndrome. Contraception 2012;85:437–45.
72. Lanes SF, Birmann B, Walker AM, Singer S. Oral contraceptive type and functional ovarian cysts. Am J Obstet Gynecol 1992;166:956–61.
73. Vessey M, Metcalfe A, Wells C, McPherson K, Westhoff C, Yeates D. Ovarian neoplasms, functional ovarian cysts, and oral contraceptives. Br Med J (Clin Res Ed) 1987;294: 1518–20.
74. Christensen JT, Boldsen JL, Westergaard JG. Functional ovarian cysts in premenopausal and gynecologically healthy women. Contraception 2002;66:153–7.
75. Holt VL, Cushing-Haugen KL, Daling JR. Oral contraceptives, tubal sterilization, and functional ovarian cyst risk. Obstet Gynecol 2003;102:252–8.
76. Young RL, Snabes MC, Frank ML, Reilly M. A randomized, double-blind, placebo-controlled comparison of the impact of low-dose and triphasic oral contraceptives on follicular development. Am J Obstet Gynecol 1992;167:678–82.
77. Chiaffarino F, Parazzini F, La Vecchia C, Ricci E, Crosignani PG. Oral contraceptive use and benign gynecologic conditions. A review. Contraception 1998;57:11–8.

78. Grimes DA, Godwin AJ, Rubin A, Smith JA, Lacarra M. Ovulation and follicular development associated with three low-dose oral contraceptives: a randomized controlled trial. Obstet Gynecol 1994;83:29–34.
79. MacKenna A, Fabres C, Alam V, Morales V. Clinical management of functional ovarian cysts: a prospective and randomized study. Hum Reprod 2000;15:2567–9.
80. Collaborative Group on Epidemiological Studies of Ovarian C, Beral V, Doll R, Hermon C, Peto R, Reeves G. Ovarian cancer and oral contraceptives: collaborative reanalysis of data from 45 epidemiological studies including 23,257 women with ovarian cancer and 87,303 controls. Lancet 2008;371:303–14.
81. Ness RB, Grisso JA, Klapper J, et al. Risk of ovarian cancer in relation to estrogen and progestin dose and use characteristics of oral contraceptives. SHARE Study Group. Steroid Hormones and Reproductions. Am J Epidemiol 2000;152:233–41.
82. Jensen JT, Speroff L. Health benefits of oral contraceptives. Obstet Gynecol Clin North Am 2000;27:705–21.
83. Brinton LA, Vessey MP, Flavel R, Yeates D. Risk factors for benign breast disease. Am J Epidemiol 1981;113:203–14.
84. Rohan TE, Miller AB. A cohort study of oral contraceptive use and risk of benign breast disease. Int J Cancer 1999;82:191–6.
85. Charreau I, Plu-Bureau G, Bachelot A, Contesso G, Guinebretiere JM, Le MG. Oral contraceptive use and risk of benign breast disease in a French case-control study of young women. Eur J Cancer Prev 1993;2:147–54.
86. Palatsi R, Hirvensalo E, Liukko P, et al. Serum total and unbound testosterone and sex hormone binding globulin (SHBG) in female acne patients treated with two different oral contraceptives. Acta Derm Venereol 1984;64:517–23.
87. Wishart JM. An open study of Triphasil and Diane 50 in the treatment of acne. Australas J Dermatol 1991;32:51–4.
88. Arowojolu AO, Gallo MF, Lopez LM, Grimes DA. Combined oral contraceptive pills for treatment of acne. Cochrane Database Syst Rev 2012:Cd004425.
89. Sullivan H, Furniss H, Spona J, Elstein M. Effect of 21-day and 24-day oral contraceptive regimens containing gestodene (60 microg) and ethinyl estradiol (15 microg) on ovarian activity. Fertil Steril 1999;72:115–20.
90. Redmond GP, Olson WH, Lippman JS, Kafrissen ME, Jones TM, Jorizzo JL. Norgestimate and ethinyl estradiol in the treatment of acne vulgaris: a randomized, placebo-controlled trial. Obstet Gynecol 1997;89:615–22.
91. Lucky AW, Henderson TA, Olson WH, Robisch DM, Lebwohl M, Swinyer LJ. Effectiveness of norgestimate and ethinyl estradiol in treating moderate acne vulgaris. J Am Acad Dermatol 1997;37:746–54.
92. Panzer C, Wise S, Fantini G, et al. Impact of oral contraceptives on sex hormone-binding globulin and androgen levels: a retrospective study in women with sexual dysfunction. J Sex Med 2006;3:104–13.
93. Dewis P, Petsos P, Newman M, Anderson DC. The treatment of hirsutism with a combination of desogestrel and ethinyl oestradiol. Clin Endocrinol (Oxf) 1985;22:29–36.
94. Lobo RA. The androgenicity of progestational agents. Int J Fertil 1988;33 Suppl:6–12.
95. De Leo V, Di Sabatino A, Musacchio MC, et al. Effect of oral contraceptives on markers of hyperandrogenism and SHBG in women with polycystic ovary syndrome. Contraception 2010;82:276–80.
96. Kriplani A, Periyasamy AJ, Agarwal N, Kulshrestha V, Kumar A, Ammini AC. Effect of oral contraceptive containing ethinyl estradiol combined with drospirenone vs. desogestrel on clinical and biochemical parameters in patients with polycystic ovary syndrome. Contraception 2010;82:139–46.
97. Shargil AA. Hormone replacement therapy in perimenopausal women with a triphasic contraceptive compound: a three-year prospective study. Int J Fertil 1985;30:15, 8–28.
98. Hergenroeder AC, Smith EO, Shypailo R, Jones LA, Klish WJ, Ellis K. Bone mineral changes in young women with hypothalamic amenorrhea treated with oral contraceptives, medroxyprogesterone, or placebo over 12 months. Am J Obstet Gynecol 1997;176:1017–25.

99. Grinspoon S, Thomas L, Miller K, Herzog D, Klibanski A. Effects of recombinant human IGF-I and oral contraceptive administration on bone density in anorexia nervosa. J Clin Endocrinol Metab 2002;87:2883–91.
100. Nappi C, Bifulco G, Tommaselli GA, Gargano V, Di Carlo C. Hormonal contraception and bone metabolism: a systematic review. Contraception 2012;86:606–21.
101. Lopez LM, Chen M, Mullins S, Curtis KM, Helmerhorst FM. Steroidal contraceptives and bone fractures in women: evidence from observational studies. Cochrane Database Syst Rev 2012:CD009849.
102. Sonfield A, Gold RB, Frost JJ, Darroch JE. U.S. insurance coverage of contraceptives and the impact of contraceptive coverage mandates, 2002. Perspect Sex Reprod Health 2004;36:72–9.
103. Shapiro S, Dinger J. Risk of venous thromboembolism among users of oral contraceptives: a review of two recently published studies. J Fam Plann Reprod Health Care 2010;36:33–8.
104. Cardiovascular disease and steroid hormone contraception. Report of a WHO Scientific Group. World Health Organ Tech Rep Ser 1998;877:i-vii, 1–89.
105. Effect of different progestagens in low oestrogen oral contraceptives on venous thromboembolic disease. World Health Organization Collaborative Study of Cardiovascular Disease and Steroid Hormone Contraception. Lancet 1995;346:1582–8.
106. Jick SS, Kaye JA, Russmann S, Jick H. Risk of nonfatal venous thromboembolism with oral contraceptives containing norgestimate or desogestrel compared with oral contraceptives containing levonorgestrel. Contraception 2006;73:566–70.
107. Romero A, Alonso C, Rincon M, et al. Risk of venous thromboembolic disease in women A qualitative systematic review. Eur J Obstet Gynecol Reprod Biol 2005;121:8–17.
108. Spitzer WO, Lewis MA, Heinemann LA, Thorogood M, MacRae KD. Third generation oral contraceptives and risk of venous thromboembolic disorders: an international case-control study. Transnational Research Group on Oral Contraceptives and the Health of Young Women. BMJ 1996;312:83–8.
109. van Hylckama Vlieg A, Helmerhorst FM, Vandenbroucke JP, Doggen CJ, Rosendaal FR. The venous thrombotic risk of oral contraceptives, effects of oestrogen dose and progestogen type: results of the MEGA case-control study. BMJ 2009;339:b2921.
110. Lidegaard O, Lokkegaard E, Svendsen AL, Agger C. Hormonal contraception and risk of venous thromboembolism: national follow-up study. BMJ 2009;339:b2890.
111. Seeger JD, Loughlin J, Eng PM, Clifford CR, Cutone J, Walker AM. Risk of thromboembolism in women taking ethinylestradiol/drospirenone and other oral contraceptives. Obstet Gynecol 2007;110:587–93.
112. Dinger JC, Heinemann LA, Kuhl-Habich D. The safety of a drospirenone-containing oral contraceptive: final results from the European Active Surveillance Study on oral contraceptives based on 142,475 women-years of observation. Contraception 2007;75:344–54.
113. Heinemann LA, Dinger JC. Range of published estimates of venous thromboembolism incidence in young women. Contraception 2007;75:328–36.
114. Manzoli L, De Vito C, Marzuillo C, Boccia A, Villari P. Oral contraceptives and venous thromboembolism: a systematic review and meta-analysis. Drug Saf 2012;35:191–205.
115. Heit JA, Kobbervig CE, James AH, Petterson TM, Bailey KR, Melton LJ, 3rd. Trends in the incidence of venous thromboembolism during pregnancy or postpartum: a 30-year population-based study. Ann Intern Med 2005;143:697–706.
116. Naess IA, Christiansen SC, Romundstad P, Cannegieter SC, Rosendaal FR, Hammerstrom J. Incidence and mortality of venous thrombosis: a population-based study. J Thromb Haemost 2007;5:692–9.
117. ACOG Committee on Practice Bulletins-Gynecology. ACOG practice bulletin. No. 73: Use of hormonal contraception in women with coexisting medical conditions. Obstet Gynecol 2006;107:1453–72.
118. Pomp ER, Rosendaal FR, Doggen CJ. Smoking increases the risk of venous thrombosis and acts synergistically with oral contraceptive use. Am J Hematol 2008;83:97–102.

COLOR PHOTOS

Combined and Progestin-Only Oral Contraceptives

www.managingcontraception.com

Pills which are pharmacologically exactly the same are grouped within black boxes.

Each year 5 to 10% of women using pills become pregnant. Each year there are 800,000 to 1 million pregnancies among women using pills and 40% of these women respond to their pregnancy by having an abortion performed. These are not good numbers. To reduce pill pregnancies:

1. Women can take pills continuously (no hormone-free days)
2. Women on pills can also use a condom if they have vaginal intercourse
3. Women on pills can switch to an IUD or an implant

* A 4th approach would be for women to take pills perfectly. Well, they have been trying to do this since 1960 when pills arrived on the scene. Sadly, for the past 57 years failure rates have continued to remain in the 5 to 10% range annually.

POSTERS showing all pills can be ordered on form at end of book or at the website: www.managingcontraception.com

PARAGARD
Copper T 380-A IUD
The most commonly used reversible contraceptive in the world

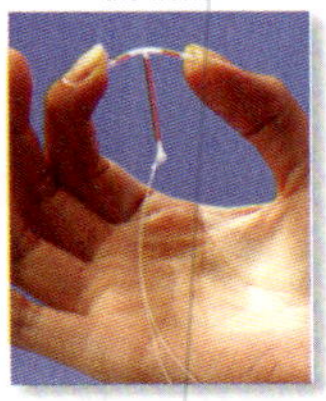

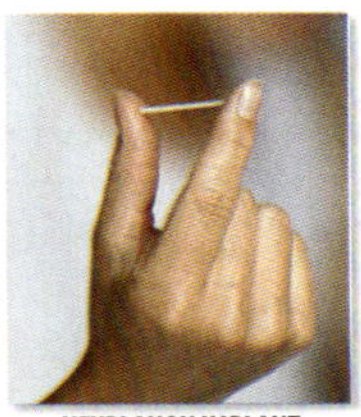

NEXPLANON IMPLANT
The Etonorgestrel Implant
Chosen by young teenagers more often than an IUD.

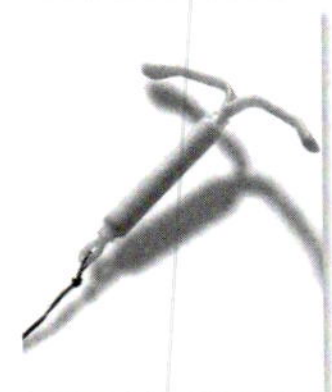

MIRENA/ LILETTA IUD
The Levonorgestrel IUD
The IUD choosen by 85% of IUD users in the United States.

Albert Einstein said that insanity is to do the same thing over and over again expecting different results. For pills to play the role they are designed to play, women must take one of the 3 steps above OR take their pills perfectly.

PROGESTIN - ONLY PILLS

0.35 mg norethindrone

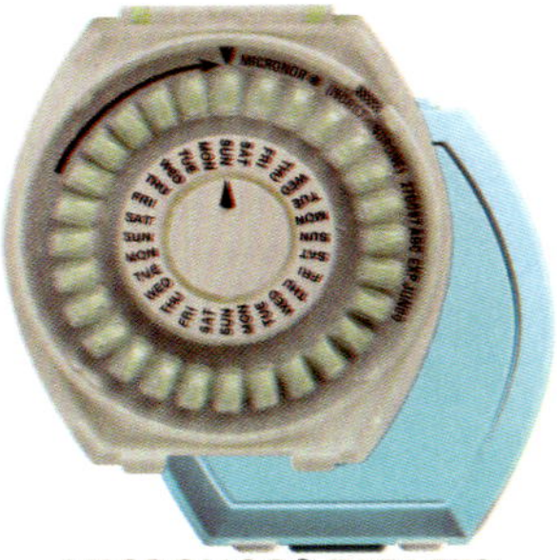

MICRONOR® TABLETS
28-DAY REGIMEN
Janssen

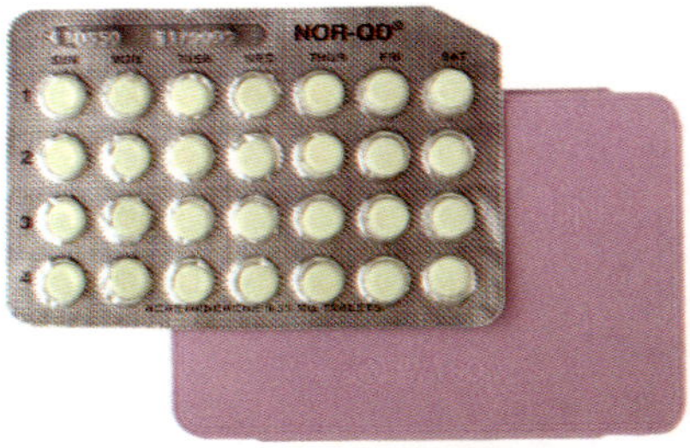

NOR-QD® TABLETS
Actavis

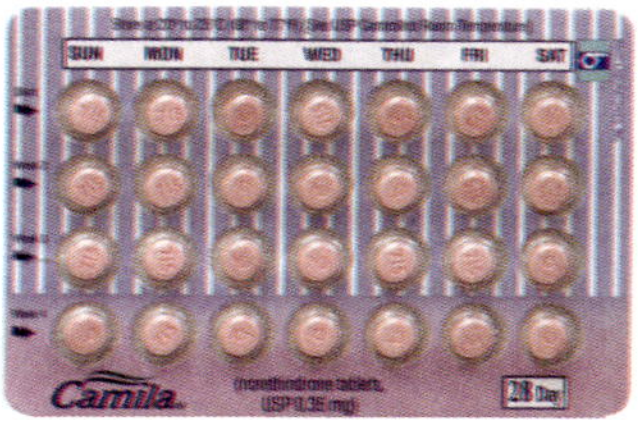

CAMILA®
Teva Pharmaceuticals USA

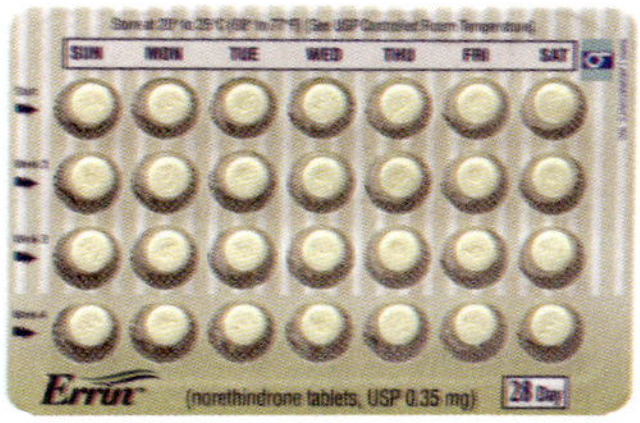

ERRIN®
Teva Pharmaceuticals USA

JOLIVETTE®
Actavis

NORA-BE®
Actavis

THE ONLY THREE 10 microgram PILLS

1 mg norethindrone acetate/10 mcg ethinyl estradiol/75 mg ferrous fumarate [7d]

MINASTRINE® FE 1/10 CHEWABLE
Actavis

(levonorgestrel/ethinyl estradiol/0.10mg/20 mcg and ethinyl estridol 0.01 mg

LoSEASONIQUE®
Duramed

CAMRESE®LO
Teva Women's Health

COMBINED PILLS - 20 microgram PILLS

NO SCHEDULED PERIODS - No inactive pills

90 mcg levonorgestrel/20 mcg ethinyl estradiol

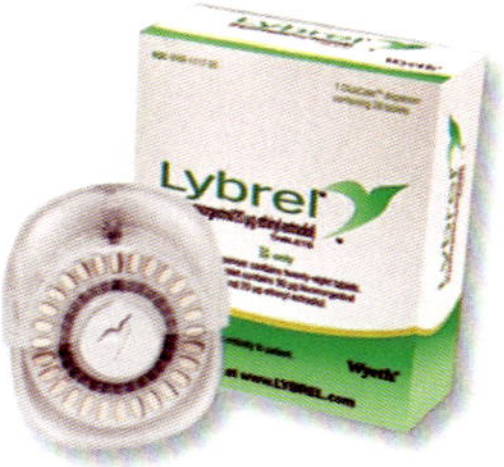

LYBREL™
Wyeth

3.0 mg drospirenone / 0.02 mg ethinyl estradiol

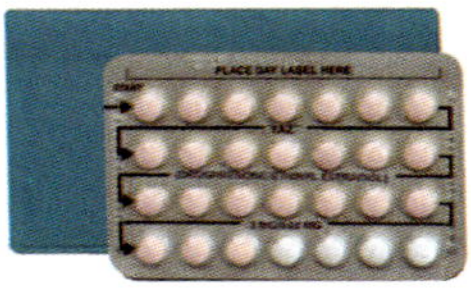

YAZ® 28 TABLETS
Bayer

→ **BEYAZ® 28 TABLETS**
Beyaz = Yaz + 451mcg folic acid
Bayer

GIANVI®
Teva Pharmaceuticals USA

YASMINELLE
BAYER

VESTURA® 3 X 28 TABLETS
ACTAVIS

0.1 mg levonorgestrel / 20 mcg ethinyl estradiol

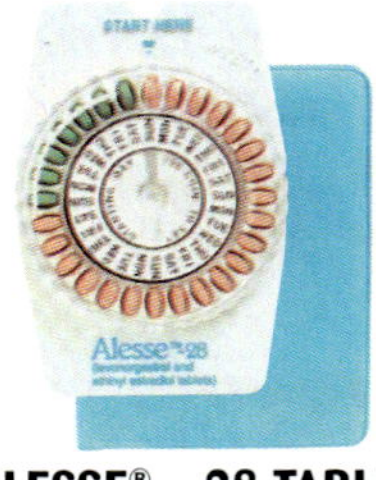

ALESSE® - 28 TABLETS
Wyeth

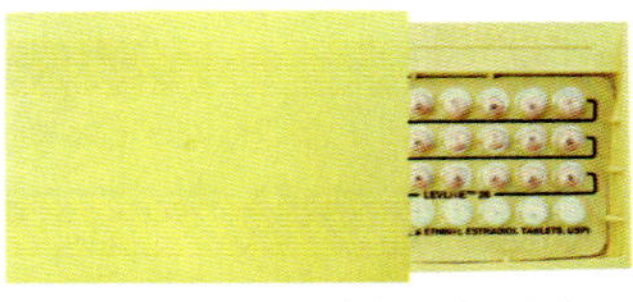

LEVLITE™ - 28 TABLETS
Bayer

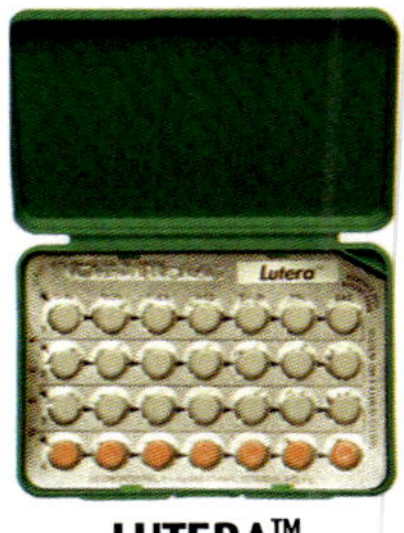

LUTERA™
Actavis

AMETHYST® - 28 TABLETS
ACTAVIS

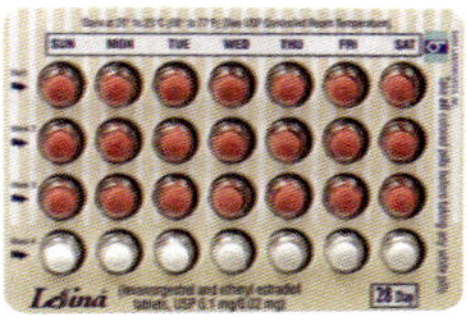

LESSINA®
Teva Pharmaceuticals USA

SRONYX®
Actavis

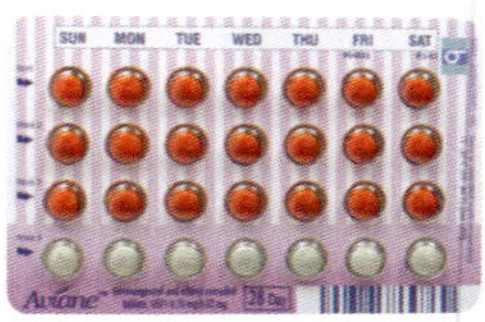

AVIANE®
Teva Pharmaceuticals USA

COMBINED PILLS - 20 microgram PILLS cont.

1 mg norethindrone acetate / 20 mcg ethinyl estradiol / 75 mg ferrous fumarate [7d]

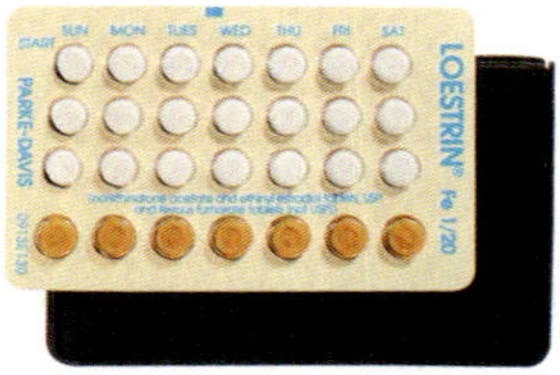

LOESTRIN® FE 1/20
Teva Pharmaceuticals USA

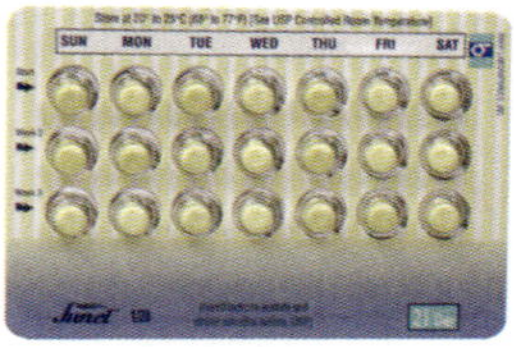

JUNEL ™
Teva Pharmaceuticals USA

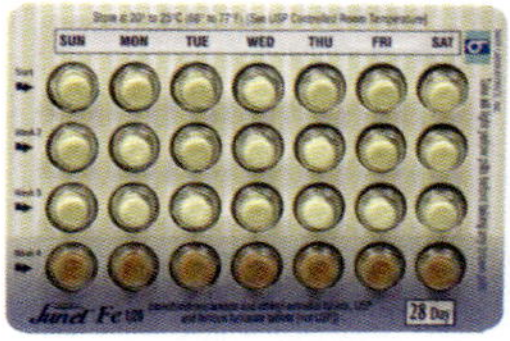

JUNEL ™ Fe
Teva Pharmaceuticals USA

MICROGESTIN® & MICROGESTIN FE®
Actavis

TILIA FE® - 28 TABLETS
Actavis

desogestrel / estradiol tablets 0.15 mg / 0.02 mg and ethinyl estradiol tablets 0.01 mg

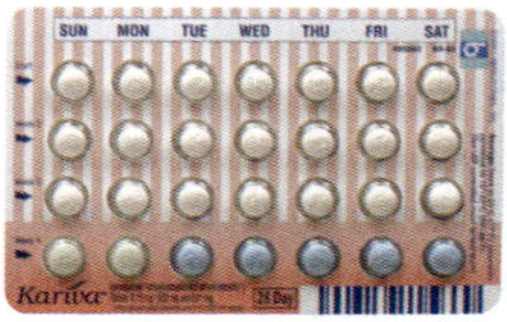

KARIVA®
Teva Pharmaceuticals USA

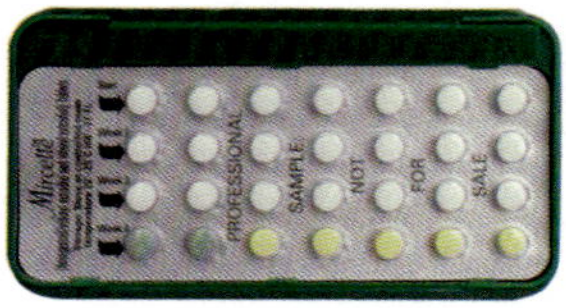

MIRCETTE® - 28 TABLETS
Duramed

MERCILON®
Merck

AZURETTE® - 28 TABLETS
ACTAVIS

COMBINED PILLS - ESTRODIAL VALERATE

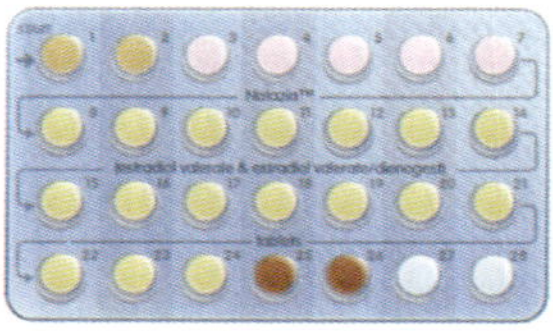

NATAZIA™

Natazia consists of 28 film-coated, unscored tablets in the following order:

- 2 dark yellow tablets each containing 3mg estradiol valerate
- 5 medium red tablets each containing 2mg estradiol valerate and 2mg dienogest
- 17 light yellow tablets each containing 2mg estradiol valerate and 3mg dienogest
- 2 dark red tablets each containing 1 mg estradiol valerate
- 2 white tablets (inert)

Bayer

COMBINED PILLS - 20 microgram ESTRADIOL PILL

norethindrone acetate and ethinyl estradiol and iron tabs

ZOELY
Teva Women's Health

COMBINED PILLS - 20 - 25 -30 microgram PILL

QUARTETTE

A 91 day ascending-dose, extended-regimen oral contraceptive for the prevention of pregnancy.
For each 91-day course, take in the following order:

1. Start the first light pink tablet (0.15 mg of levonorgestrel and 0.02 mg ethinyl estradiol) on the first Sunday after the onset of menstruation. take one light pink tablet once a day for a total of 42 consecutive days.
2. One pink tablet (0.15 mg of levonorgestrel and 0.025 mg ethinyl estradiol) once a day for 21 consecutive days.
3. One purple tablet (0.15 mg of levonorgestrel and 0.03 mg ethinyl estradiol) once a day for 21 days.
4. One yellow tablet (0.01 mg of ethinyl estradiol) once a day for 7 days. Bleeding should occur during yellow tablet use.

Teva Women's Health

COMBINED PILLS - 25 microgram PILL

CAZIANT™ 3X28 TABLETS
(0.1mg/0.025mg, 0.125mg/0.025mg, 0.15mg/0.025mg)

Each 28-day treatment cycle pack consists of three active dosing phases:

7 white tablets containing 0.100 mg desogestrel and 0.025 mg ethinyl estradiol;

7 light blue tablets containing 0.125 mg desogestrel and 0.025 mg ethinyl estradiol

7 blue tablets containing 0.150 mg desogestrel and 0.025 mg ethinyl estradiol.

ACTAVIS

COMBINED PILLS - 30 microgram PILLS

3.0 mg drospirenone / 30 mcg ethinyl estradiol

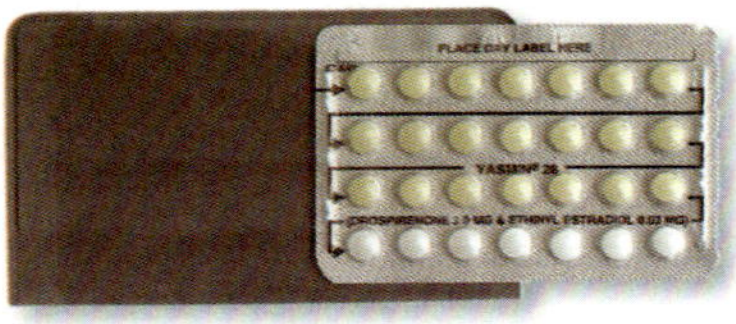

YASMIN® 28 TABLETS
BAYER

ZARAH™
Actavis

OCELLA™ 28 TABLETS
Teva Women's Health

SAFYRAL™
Safyral = Yasmin + 451mcg Folic Acid
BAYER

SCHEDULED PERIODS QUARTERLY

3.0 mg drospirenone / 30 mcg ethinyl estradiol

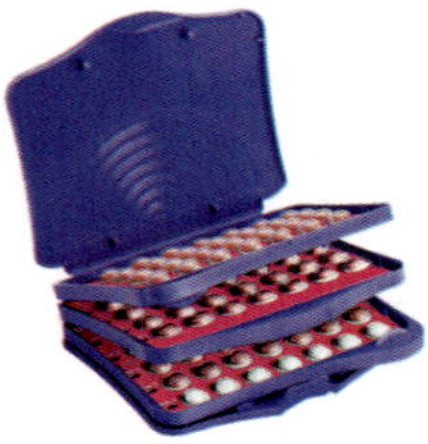

SEASONALE®
Duramed

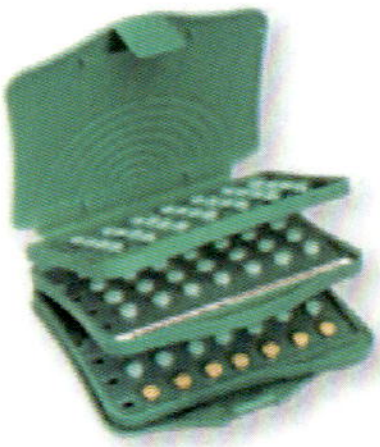

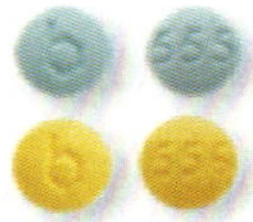

SEASONIQUE®
Teva Women's Health

JOLESSA™
Teva Women's Health

CAMRESE™
Teva Women's Health

0.15 mg levonorgestrel / 30 mcg ethinyl estradiol

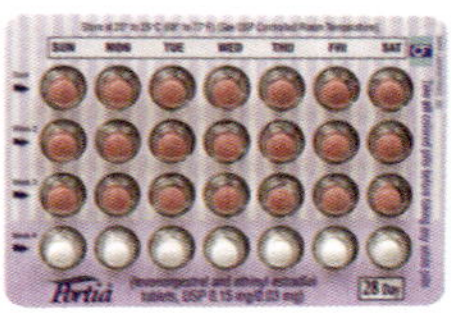

PORTIA®
Teva Pharmaceuticals USA

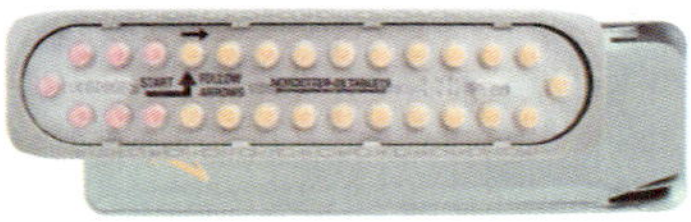

NORDETTE®-28 TABLETS
Wyeth

QUASENSETM
Actavis

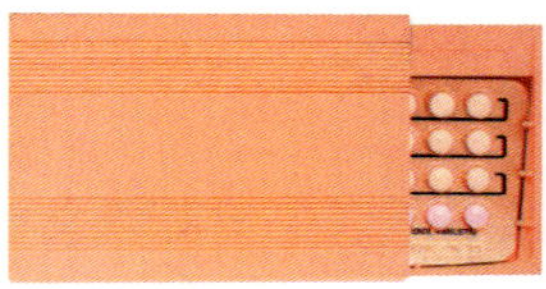

LEVLEN® 28 TABLETS
MK Drughouse

0.15 mg drospirenone / 30 mcg ethinyl estradiol

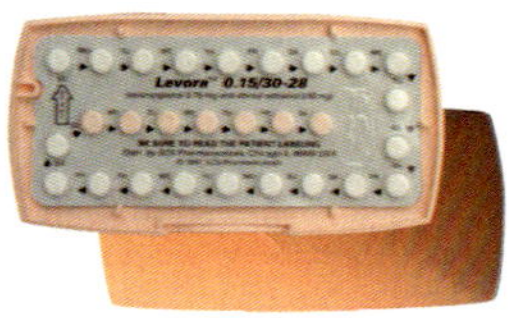

LEVORA TABLETS
Actavis

COMBINED PILLS - 30 microgram PILLS cont.

0.3 mg norgestrel / 30 mcg ethinyl estradiol

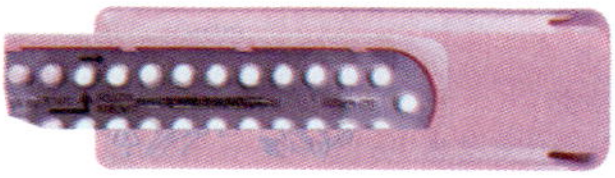

LO/OVRAL®-28 TABLETS
Wyeth

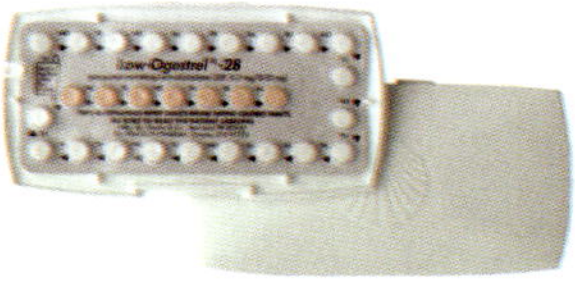

LOW-OGESTREL® - 28
Actavis

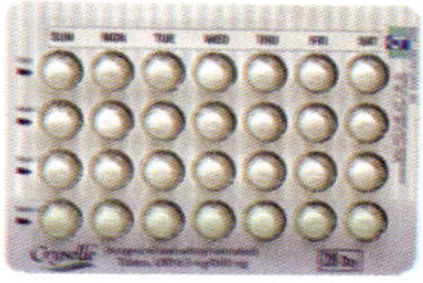

CRYSELLE®
Teva Pharmaceuticals USA

0.15 mg desogestrel/ 30 mcg ethinyl estradiol

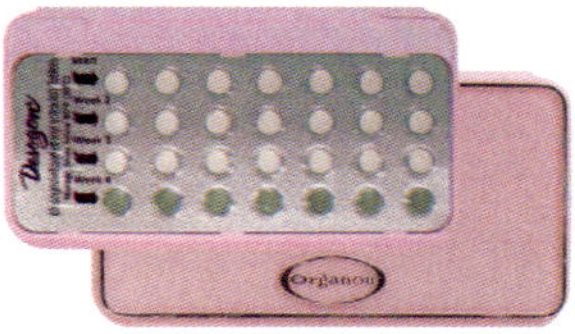

DESOGEN®
Merck

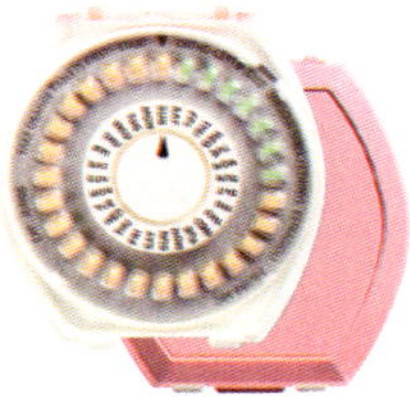

ORTHO-CEPT®
Jannsen

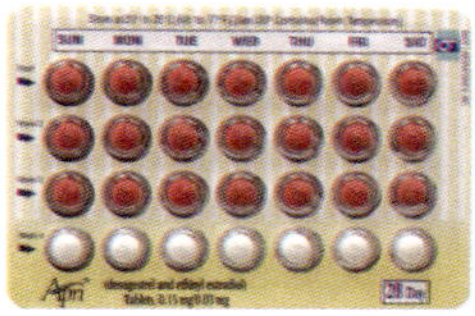

APRI®
Teva Pharmaceuticals USA

RECLIPSEN™
Actavis

SOLIA™
Prasco

1.5 mg norethindrone acetate / 30 mcg ethinyl estradiol

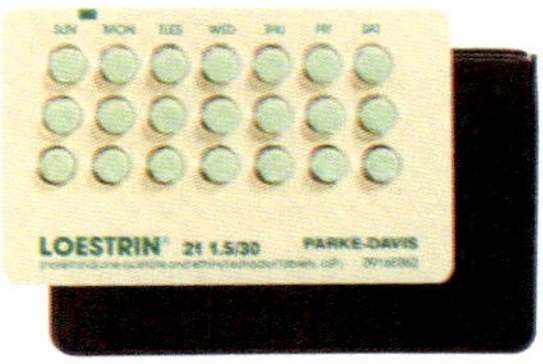

LOESTRIN® 21 1.5/30
Teva Pharmaceuticals USA

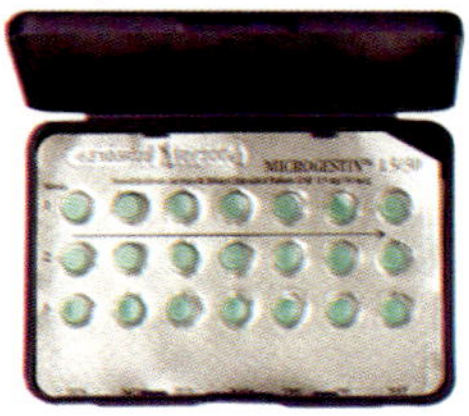

MICROGESTIN® 1.5/30 with or without Fe
Actavis

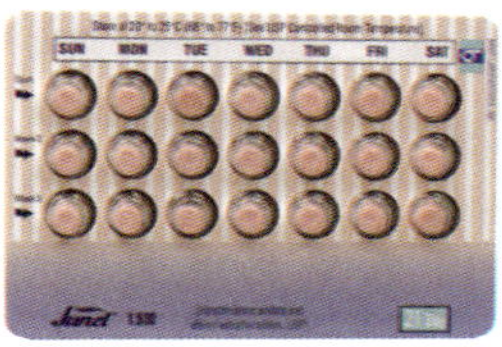

JUNEL ™
Teva Pharmaceuticals USA

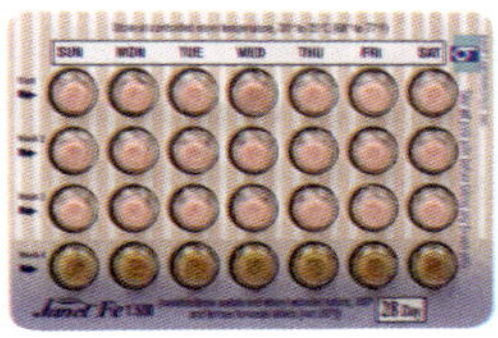

JUNEL ™ Fe
Teva Pharmaceuticals USA

COMBINED PILLS - 35 microgram PILLS

MONTHLY PERIODS

0.25 mg norgestimate / 35 mcg ethinyl estradiol

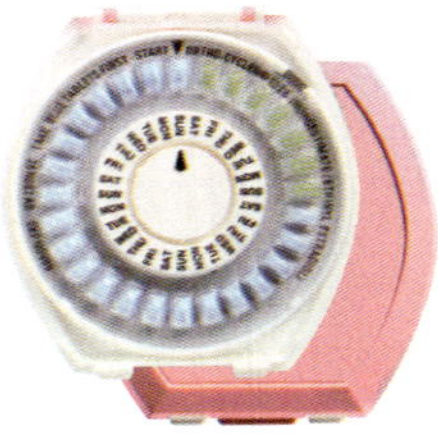

ORTHO-CYCLEN® 28 TABLETS
Jannsen

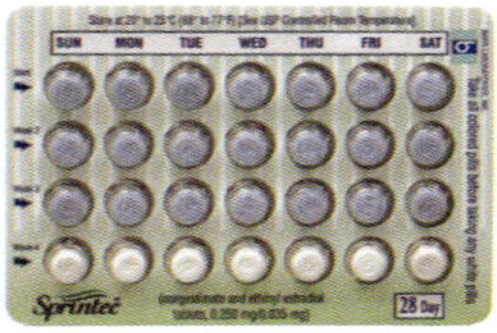

SPRINTEC®
Teva Pharmaceuticals USA

PREVIFEM™
Qualitest

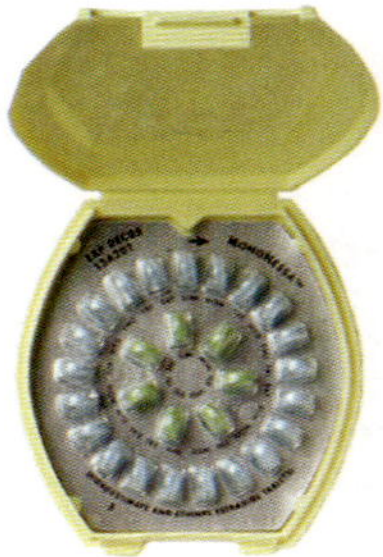

MONONESESSA®
Actavis

0.4 mg norethindrone / 35 mcg ethinyl estradiol

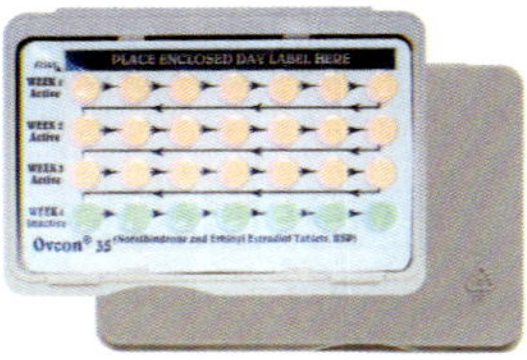

OVCON® 35 28-DAY
Actavis
Now there is a chewable
Ovcon-35 pill!

ZENCHENT®
Actavis

BALZIVA™ 1/35
Teva Pharmaceuticals USA

FEMCON FE™
Actavis

ZEOSA™
(chewable)
Actavis

COMBINED PILLS - 35 microgram PILLS cont.

MONTHLY PERIODS

1 mg norethindrone / 35 mcg ethinyl estradiol

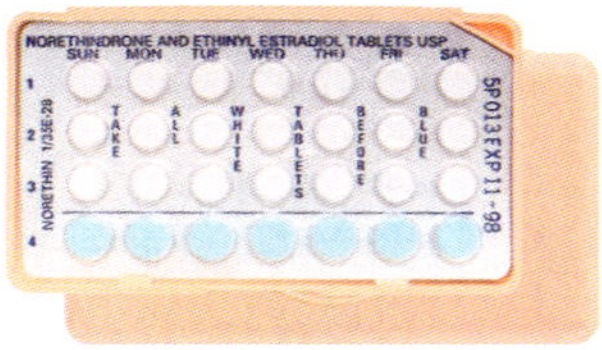

NORETHIN 1/35E–28
Shire

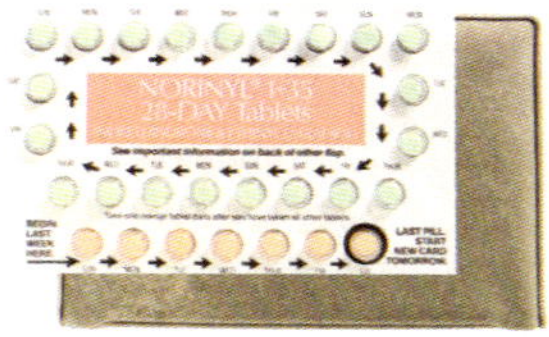

NORINYL® 1+35 28-DAY TABLETS
Actavis

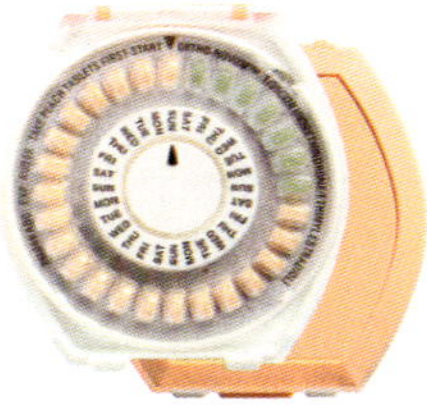

ORTHO-NOVUM® 1/35 28 TABLETS
Jannsen

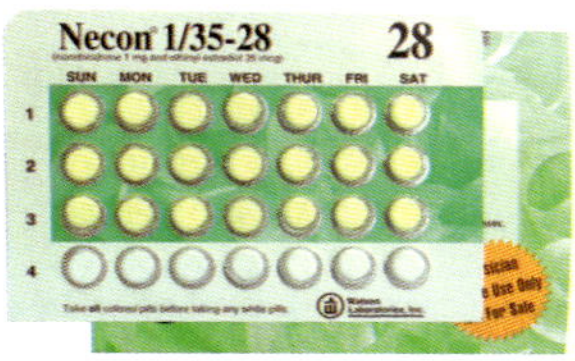

NECON® 1/35-28
Actavis

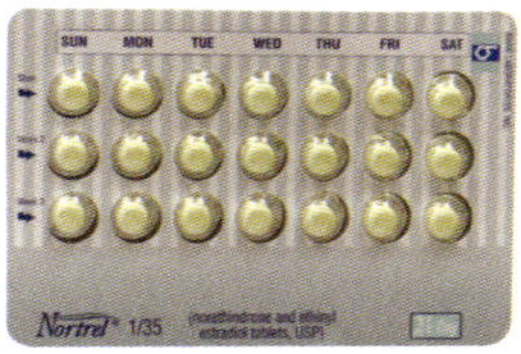

NORTREL®
Teva Pharmaceuticals USA

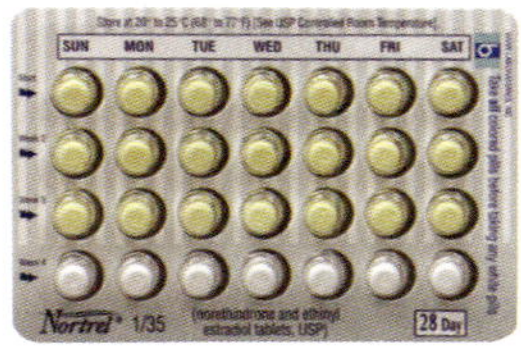

NORTREL®
Teva Pharmaceuticals USA

1 mg ethynodiol diacetate / 35 mcg ethinyl estradiol

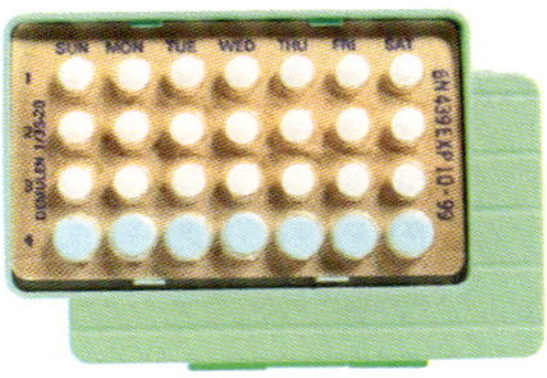

DEMULEN® 1/35-28
Pfizer

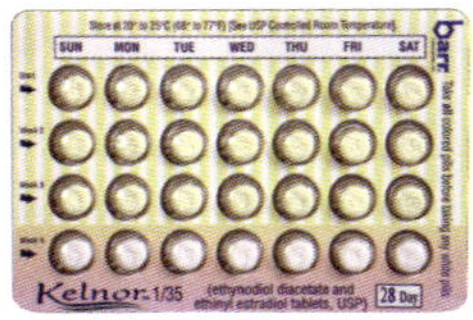

KELNOR™
Teva Pharmaceuticals USA

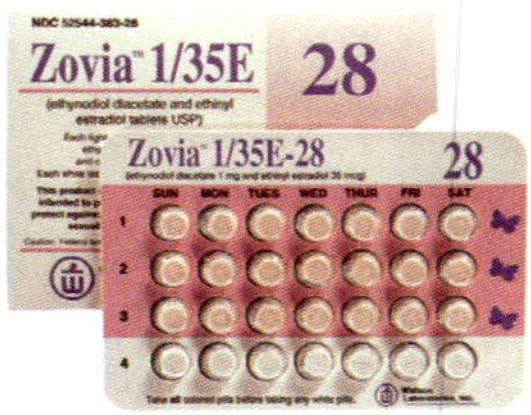

ZOVIA® 1/35E–28
Actavis

COMBINED PILLS - 35 microgram PILLS cont.

MONTHLY PERIODS

1 mg ethynodiol diacetate / 35 mcg ethinyl estradiol

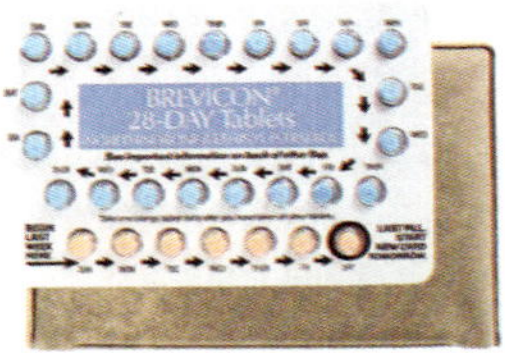

BREVICON® 28-DAY TABLETS
Actavis

NECON 0.5/35®
Actavis

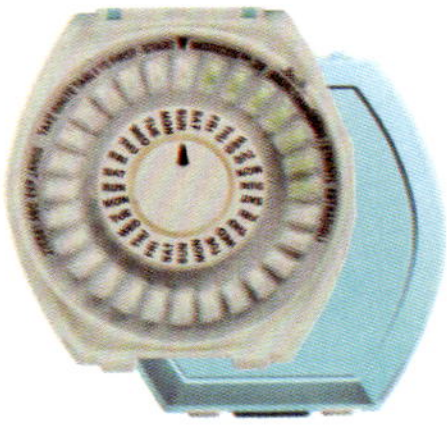

MODICON® TABLETS
Jannsen

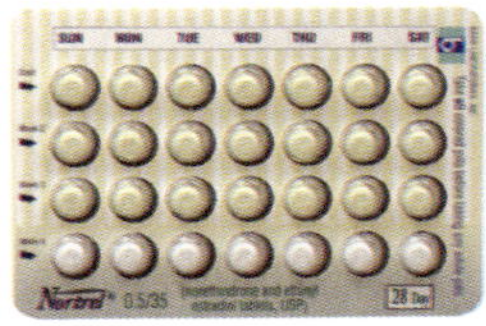

NORTREL®
Teva Pharmaceuticals USA

COMBINED PILLS - PHASIC PILLS

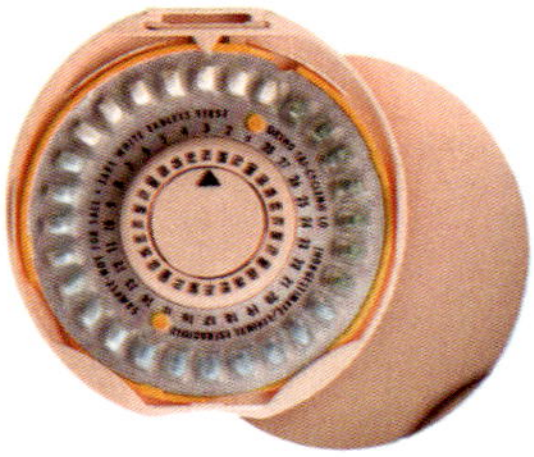

norgestimate / ethinyl estradiol
0.18 mg / 25 mcg (7d),
0.215 mg / 25 mcg (7d),
0.25 mg / 25 mcg (7d)

ORTHO TRI-CYCLEN® LO - 28 TABLETS
Jannsen

desogestrel / ethinyl estradiol–triphasic regimen
0.1 mg/25 mcg (7d),
0.125 mg/25 mcg (7d),
0.150 mg/25 mcg (7d)

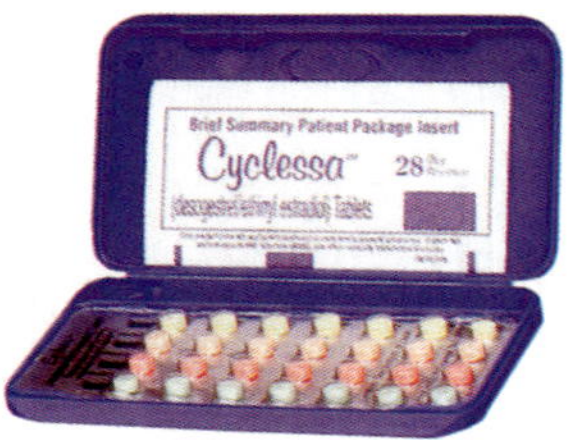

CYCLESSA®
Merck

CESIA™
Prasco

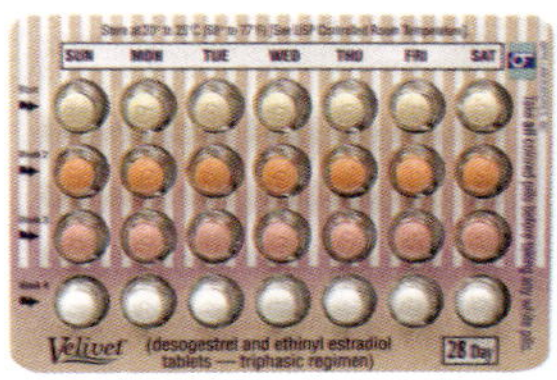

VELIVET™
Teva Pharmaceuticals USA

norethindrone / ethinyl estradiol
0.5 mg / 35 mcg (10d),
1 mg / 35 mcg (11d)

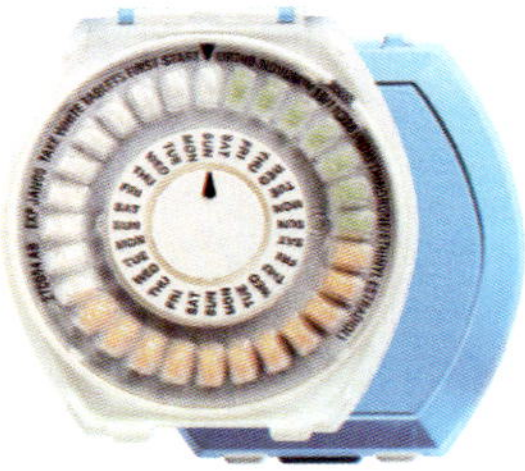

ORTHO-NOVUM® 10/11 - 28 TABLETS
Jannsen

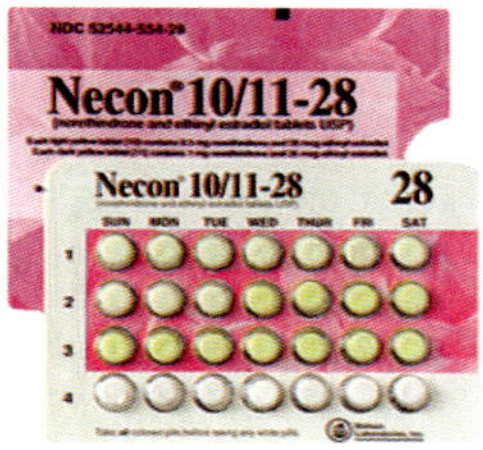

NECON® 10/11 - 28 TABLETS
Actavis

ARANELLE™
Teva Pharmaceuticals USA

TRI-NORINYL®
Actavis

LEENA®
Actavis

norethindrone acetate / ethinyl estradiol
1 mg / 20 mcg (5d),
1 mg/30 mcg (7d),
1 mg/35 mcg (9d),
75 mg ferrous fumarate (7d)

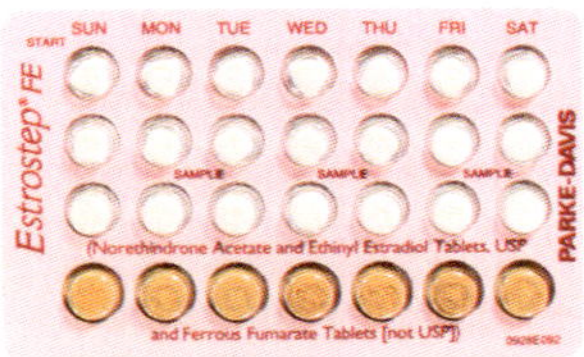

ESTROSTEP® FE - 28 TABLETS
Actavis

TRI-LEGEST® FE
Teva Pharmaceuticals USA

norethindrone /
ethinyl estradiol
0.5 mg / 35 mcg (7d),
1 mg / 35 mcg (14d)

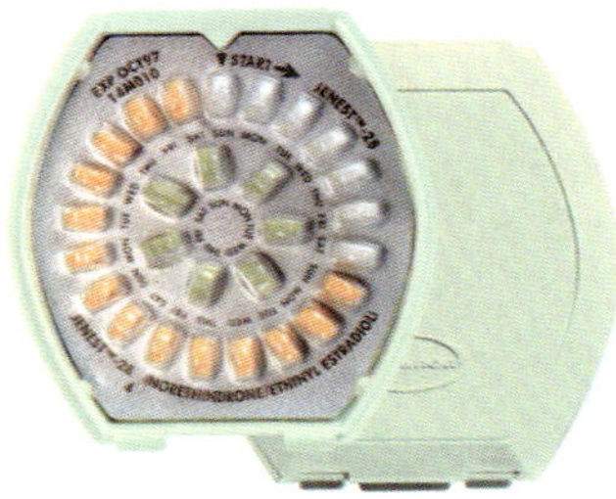

JENEST® 28 TABLETS
Organon

COMBINED PILLS - PHASIC PILLS cont.

levonorgestrel / ethinyl estradiol–triphasic regimen
0.050 mg / 30 mcg (6d),
0.075 mg / 40 mcg (5d),
0.125 mg / 30 mcg (10d)

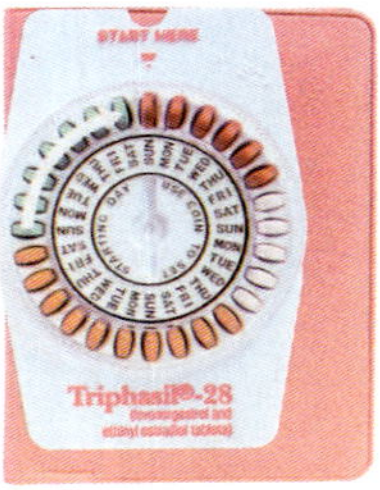

TRIPHASIL®- 28 TABLETS
Wyeth

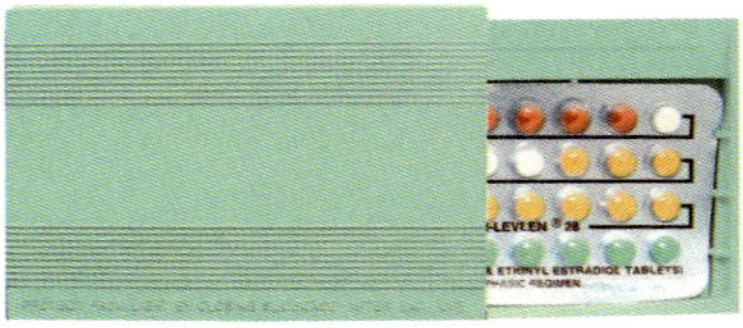

TRI-LEVLEN® 28 TABLETS
MK Drughouse

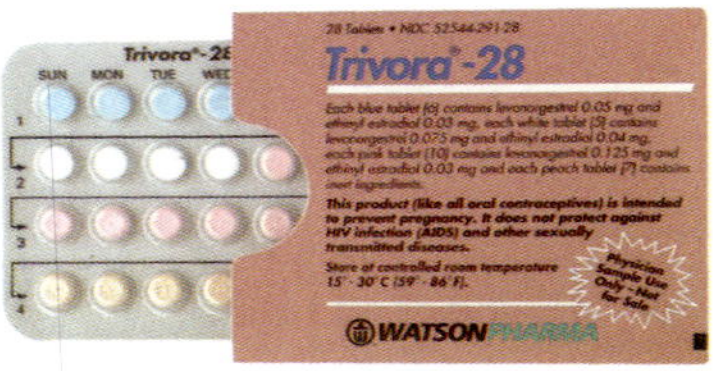

TRIVORA®
Actavis

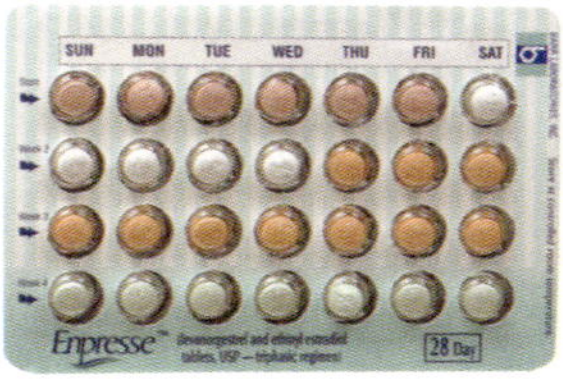

ENPRESSE®
Teva Pharmaceuticals USA

norgestimate / ethinyl estradiol
0.18 mg / 35 mcg (7d),
0.215 mg / 35 mcg (7d),
0.25 mg / 35 mcg (7d),
placebo (7d)

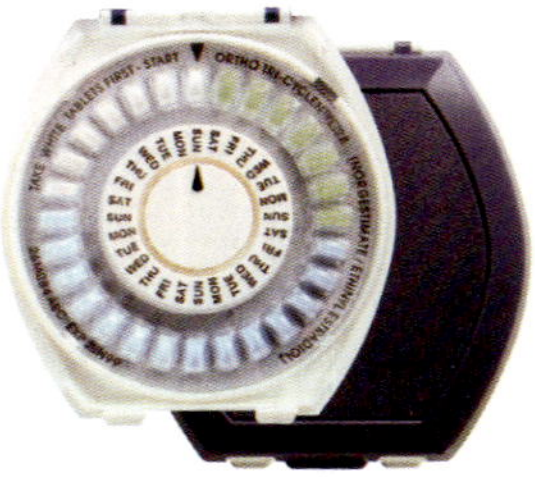

ORTHO TRI-CYCLEN® - 28 TABLETS
Jannsen

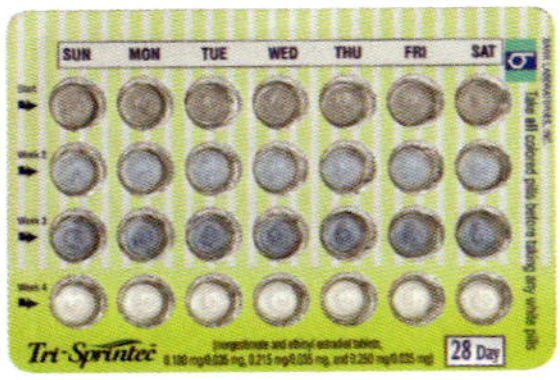

TRI-SPRINTEC®
Teva Pharmaceuticals USA

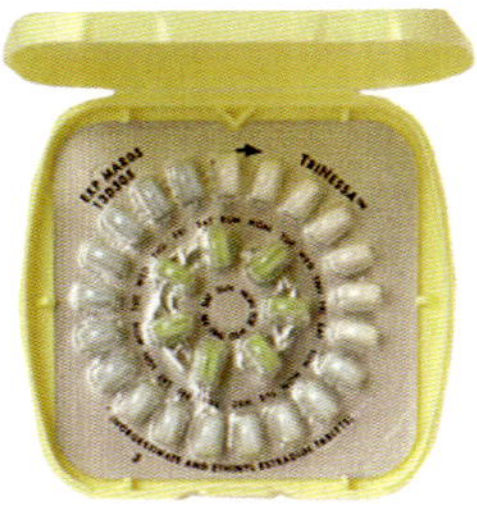

TRINESSA®
Actavis

TRI-PREVIFEM™ - 28 TABLETS
Qualitest

norethindrone / ethinyl estradiol
0.5 mg / 35 mcg (7d),
0.75 mg / 35 mcg (7d),
1 mg / 35 mcg (7d)

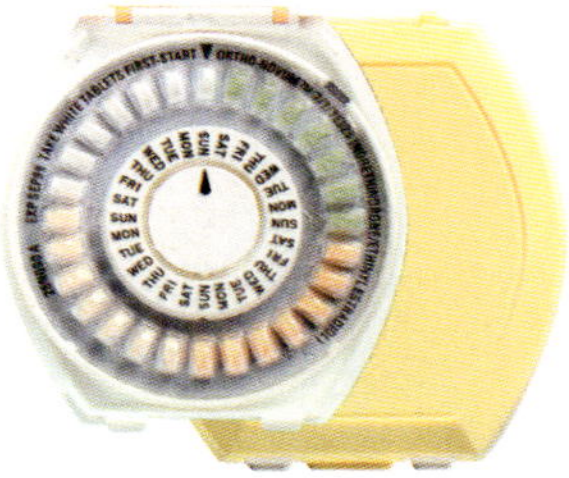

ORTHO-NOVUM® 7/7/7
28 TABLETS
Jannsen

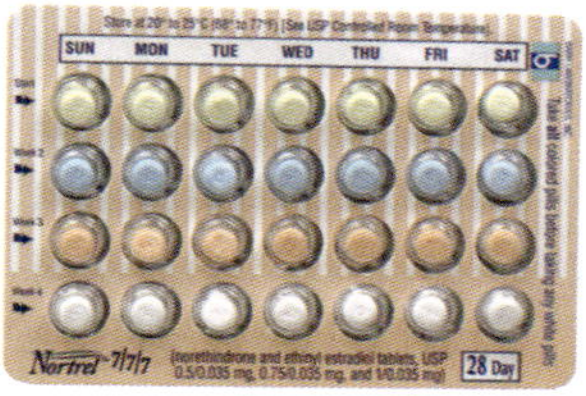

NORTREL® 7/7/7
Teva Pharmaceuticals USA

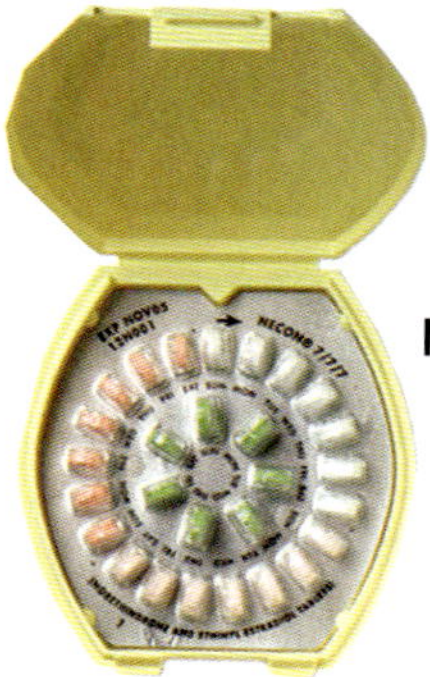

NECON® 7/7/7
Actavis

COMBINED PILLS - 50 microgram PILLS

MONTHLY PERIODS

Pills with 50 micrograms of mestranol are not as strong as pills with 50 micrograms of ethinyl estradiol

0.5 mg norgestrel / 50 mcg ethinyl estradiol

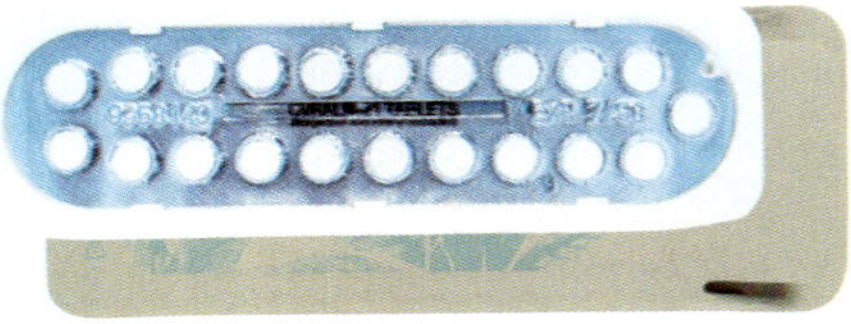

OVRAL® - 21 TABLETS
Wyeth

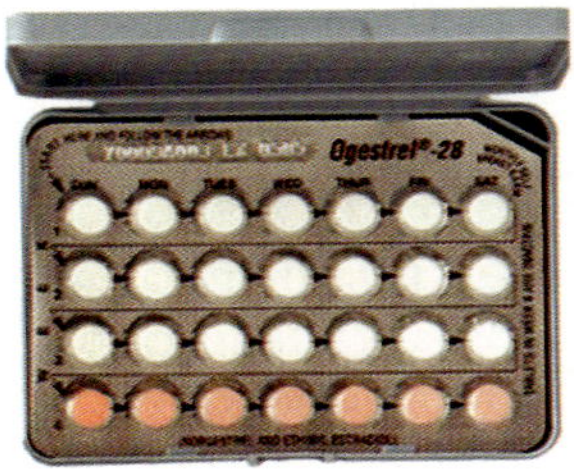

OGESTREL®
Actavis

1 mg norethindrone / 50 mcg mestranol

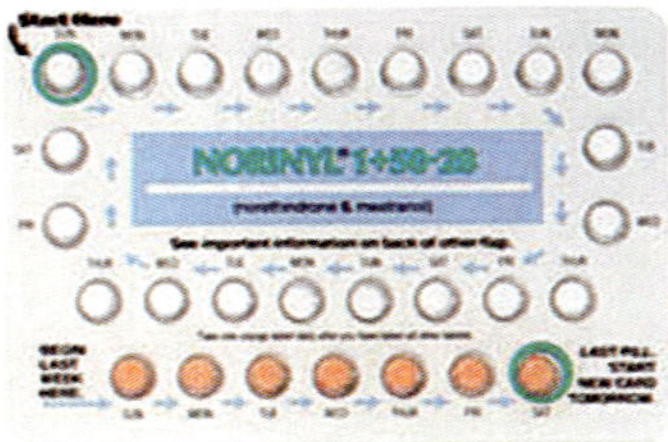

NORINYL® 1/50
Actavis

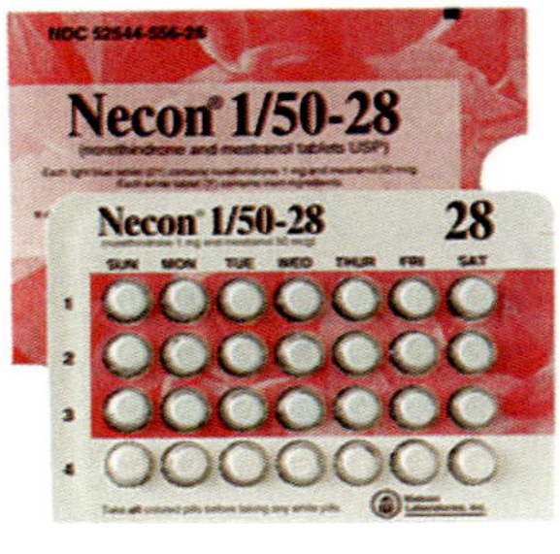

NECON® 1/50 - 28 TABLETS
Actavis

COMBINED PILLS - 50 microgram PILLS cont.

MONTHLY PERIODS

1 mg norethindrone / 50 mcg ethinyl estradiol

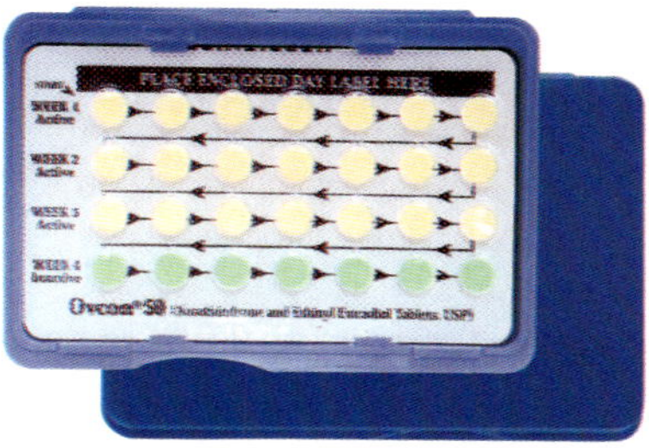

OVCON® 50 28-DAY
Warner-Chilcott

1 mg ethynodiol diacetate / 50 mcg ethinyl estradiol

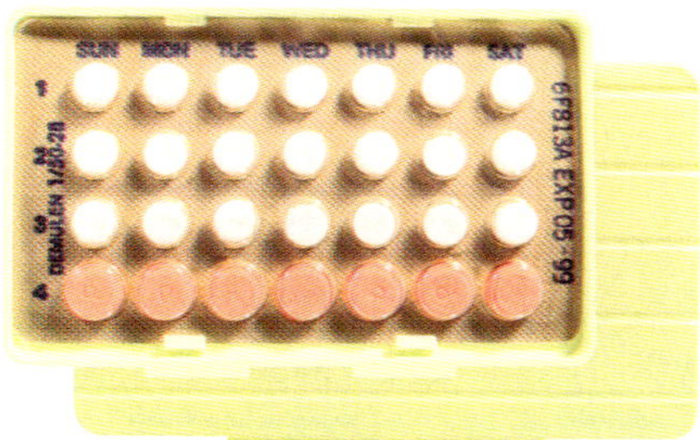

DEMULEN® 1/50-28
Pfizer

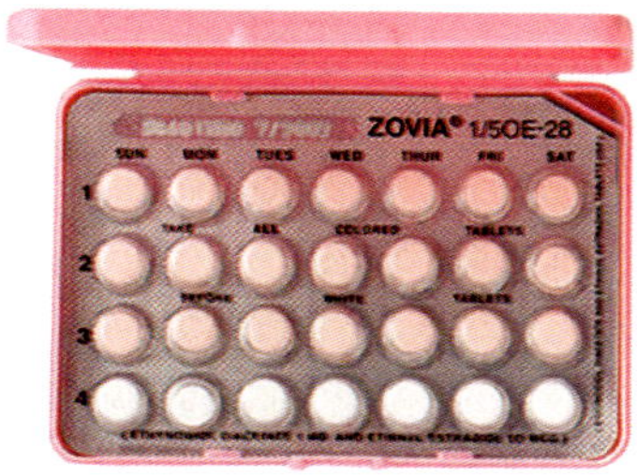

ZOVIA® 1/50
Actavis

NOTES

119. Petitti DB. Clinical practice. Combination estrogen-progestin oral contraceptives. N Engl J Med 2003;349:1443–50.
120. Khader YS, Rice J, John L, Abueita O. Oral contraceptives use and the risk of myocardial infarction: a meta-analysis. Contraception 2003;68:11–7.
121. Shufelt CL, Bairey Merz CN. Contraceptive hormone use and cardiovascular disease. J Am Coll Cardiol 2009;53:221–31.
122. Margolis KL, Adami HO, Luo J, Ye W, Weiderpass E. A prospective study of oral contraceptive use and risk of myocardial infarction among Swedish women. Fertil Steril 2007;88:310–6.
123. Acute myocardial infarction and combined oral contraceptives: results of an international multicentre case-control study. WHO Collaborative Study of Cardiovascular Disease and Steroid Hormone Contraception. Lancet 1997;349:1202–9.
124. Schwingl PJ, Ory HW, Visness CM. Estimates of the risk of cardiovascular death attributable to low-dose oral contraceptives in the United States. Am J Obstet Gynecol 1999;180:241–9.
125. Farley TM, Collins J, Schlesselman JJ. Hormonal contraception and risk of cardiovascular disease. An international perspective. Contraception 1998;57:211–30.
126. Gillum LA, Mamidipudi SK, Johnston SC. Ischemic stroke risk with oral contraceptives: A meta-analysis. JAMA 2000;284:72–8.
127. Xu Z, Li Y, Tang S, Huang X, Chen T. Current use of oral contraceptives and the risk of first-ever ischemic stroke: A meta-analysis of observational studies. Thromb Res 2015;136:52–60.
128. Tepper NK, Whiteman MK, Zapata LB, Marchbanks PA, Curtis KM. Safety of hormonal contraceptives among women with migraine: A systematic review. Contraception 2016;94:630–40.
129. Hannaford PC, Croft PR, Kay CR. Oral contraception and stroke. Evidence from the Royal College of General Practitioners' Oral Contraception Study. Stroke 1994;25:935–42.
130. Curtis KM, Chrisman CE, Peterson HB, Health WHO Programme for Mapping Best Practices in Reproductive Health. Contraception for women in selected circumstances. Obstet Gynecol 2002;99:1100–12.
131. Kemmeren JM, Tanis BC, van den Bosch MA, et al. Risk of Arterial Thrombosis in Relation to Oral Contraceptives (RATIO) study: oral contraceptives and the risk of ischemic stroke. Stroke 2002;33:1202–8.
132. Feigin VL, Rinkel GJ, Lawes CM, et al. Risk factors for subarachnoid hemorrhage: an updated systematic review of epidemiological studies. Stroke 2005;36:2773–80.
133. Curtis KM, Mohllajee AP, Martins SL, Peterson HB. Combined oral contraceptive use among women with hypertension: a systematic review. Contraception 2006;73:179–88.
134. Haemorrhagic stroke, overall stroke risk, and combined oral contraceptives: results of an international, multicentre, case-control study. WHO Collaborative Study of Cardiovascular Disease and Steroid Hormone Contraception. Lancet 1996;348:505–10.
135. Berenson AB, Rahman M, Wilkinson G. Effect of injectable and oral contraceptives on serum lipids. Obstet Gynecol 2009;114:786–94.
136. Walsh BW, Sacks FM. Effects of low dose oral contraceptives on very low density and low density lipoprotein metabolism. J Clin Invest 1993;91:2126–32.
137. Tepper NK, Steenland MW, Marchbanks PA, Curtis KM. Laboratory screening prior to initiating contraception: a systematic review. Contraception 2013;87:645–9.
138. Green J, Berrington de Gonzalez A, Smith JS, et al. Human papillomavirus infection and use of oral contraceptives. Br J Cancer 2003;88:1713–20.
139. Smith JS, Green J, Berrington de Gonzalez A, et al. Cervical cancer and use of hormonal contraceptives: a systematic review. Lancet 2003;361:1159–67.
140. Munoz N, Franceschi S, Bosetti C, et al. Role of parity and human papillomavirus in cervical cancer: the IARC multicentric case-control study. Lancet 2002;359:1093–101.
141. Ursin G, Peters RK, Henderson BE, d'Ablaing G, 3rd, Monroe KR, Pike MC. Oral contraceptive use and adenocarcinoma of cervix. Lancet 1994;344:1390–4.

142. Mohllajee AP, Curtis KM, Martins SL, Peterson HB. Hormonal contraceptive use and risk of sexually transmitted infections: a systematic review. Contraception 2006;73:154–65.

143. Cottingham J, Hunter D. Chlamydia trachomatis and oral contraceptive use: a quantitative review. Genitourin Med 1992;68:209–16.

144. Morrison CS, Bright P, Wong EL, et al. Hormonal contraceptive use, cervical ectopy, and the acquisition of cervical infections. Sex Transm Dis 2004;31:561–7.

145. Rahm VA, Odlind V, Gnarpe H. Chlamydia trachomatis among sexually active teenage girls: influence of sampling location and clinical signs on the detection rate. Genitourin Med 1990;66:66–9.

146. Polis CB, Curtis KM, Hannaford PC, et al. An updated systematic review of epidemiological evidence on hormonal contraceptive methods and HIV acquisition in women. AIDS 2016;30:2665–83.

147. Marchbanks PA, McDonald JA, Wilson HG, et al. Oral contraceptives and the risk of breast cancer. N Engl J Med 2002;346:2025–32.

148. Marchbanks PA, Curtis KM, Mandel MG, et al. Oral contraceptive formulation and risk of breast cancer. Contraception 2012;85:342–50.

149. Morch LS, Skovlund CW, Hannaford PC, Iversen L, Fielding S, Lidegaard O. Contemporary hormonal contraception and the risk of breast cancer . N Engl J Med 2017;377: 2228–39.

150. Grimes DA, Schulz KF. False alarms and pseudo-epidemics: the limitations of observational epidemiology. Obstet Gynecol 2012;120:920–7.

151. Figueiredo JC, Haile RW, Bernstein L, et al. Oral contraceptives and postmenopausal hormones and risk of contralateral breast cancer among BRCA1 and BRCA2 mutation carriers and noncarriers: the WECARE Study. Breast Cancer Res Treat 2010;120:175–83.

152. Gaffield ME, Culwell KR, Ravi A. Oral contraceptives and family history of breast cancer. Contraception 2009;80:372–80.

153. Mullen WH, Anderson IB, Kim SY, Blanc PD, Olson KR. Incorrect overdose management advice in the Physicians' Desk Reference. Ann Emerg Med 1997;29:255–61.

154. Lubianca JN, Faccin CS, Fuchs FD. Oral contraceptives: a risk factor for uncontrolled blood pressure among hypertensive women. Contraception 2003;67:19–24.

155. Chasan-Taber L, Willett WC, Manson JE, et al. Prospective study of oral contraceptives and hypertension among women in the United States. Circulation 1996;94:483–9.

156. Darney P. Safety and efficacy of a triphasic oral contraceptive containing desogestrel: results of three multicenter trials. Contraception 1993;48:323–37.

157. Visser J, Snel M, Van Vliet HA. Hormonal versus non-hormonal contraceptives in women with diabetes mellitus type 1 and 2. Cochrane Database Syst Rev 2013:CD003990.

158. Nelson AL, Le MH, Musherraf Z, Vanberckelaer A. Intermediate-term glucose tolerance in women with a history of gestational diabetes: natural history and potential associations with breastfeeding and contraception. Am J Obstet Gynecol 2008;198:699 e1–7; discussion e7–8.

159. Vandenbroucke JP, Koster T, Briet E, Reitsma PH, Bertina RM, Rosendaal FR. Increased risk of venous thrombosis in oral-contraceptive users who are carriers of factor V Leiden mutation. Lancet 1994;344:1453–7.

160. Vandenbroucke JP, van der Meer FJ, Helmerhorst FM, Rosendaal FR. Factor V Leiden: should we screen oral contraceptive users and pregnant women? BMJ 1996;313:1127–30.

161. Headache Classification Subcommittee of the International Headache S. The International Classification of Headache Disorders: 2nd edition. Cephalalgia 2004;24 Suppl 1: 9–160.

162. Curtis KM, Mohllajee AP, Peterson HB. Use of combined oral contraceptives among women with migraine and nonmigrainous headaches: a systematic review. Contraception 2006;73:189–94.

163. Chasan-Taber L, Stampfer M. Oral contraceptives and myocardial infarction—the search for the smoking gun. N Engl J Med 2001;345:1841–2.

164. Willett WC, Green A, Stampfer MJ, et al. Relative and absolute excess risks of coronary heart disease among women who smoke cigarettes. N Engl J Med 1987;317:1303–9.

165. Kroon LA. Drug interactions with smoking. Am J Health Syst Pharm 2007;64:1917–21.
166. Murray CJ, Ortblad KF, Guinovart C, et al. Global, regional, and national incidence and mortality for HIV, tuberculosis, and malaria during 1990–2013: a systematic analysis for the Global Burden of Disease Study 2013. Lancet 2014;384:1005–70.
167. Phillips SJ, Polis CB, Curtis KM. The safety of hormonal contraceptives for women living with HIV and their sexual partners. Contraception 2016;93:11–6.
168. Culwell KR, Curtis KM, del Carmen Cravioto M. Safety of contraceptive method use among women with systemic lupus erythematosus: a systematic review. Obstet Gynecol 2009;114:341–53.
169. Farr SL, Folger SG, Paulen ME, Curtis KM. Safety of contraceptive methods for women with rheumatoid arthritis: a systematic review. Contraception 2010;82:64–71.
170. Kapp N, Tilley IB, Curtis KM. The effects of hormonal contraceptive use among women with viral hepatitis or cirrhosis of the liver: a systematic review. Contraception 2009;80:381–6.
171. Combined oral contraceptives and liver cancer. The WHO Collaborative Study of Neoplasia and Steroid Contraceptives. Int J Cancer 1989;43:254–9.
172. Kapp N, Curtis KM. Hormonal contraceptive use among women with liver tumors: a systematic review. Contraception 2009;80:387–90.
173. Milne R, Vessey M. The association of oral contraception with kidney cancer, colon cancer, gallbladder cancer (including extrahepatic bile duct cancer) and pituitary tumours. Contraception 1991;43:667–93.
174. Westhoff CL, Heartwell S, Edwards S, et al. Oral contraceptive discontinuation: do side effects matter? Am J Obstet Gynecol 2007;196:412 e1–6; discussion e6–7.
175. Rosenthal SL, Cotton S, Ready JN, Potter LS, Succop PA. Adolescents' attitudes and experiences regarding levonorgestrel 100 mcg / ethinyl estradiol 20 mcg. J Pediatr Adolesc Gynecol 2002;15:301–5.
176. Archer DF, Cullins V, Creasy GW, Fisher AC. The impact of improved compliance with a weekly contraceptive transdermal system (Ortho Evra) on contraceptive efficacy. Contraception 2004;69:189–95.
177. Lopez LM, Grimes DA, Schulz KF, Curtis KM. Steroidal contraceptives: effect on bone fractures in women. Cochrane Database Syst Rev 2009:CD006033.
178. d'Arcangues C. WHO statement on hormonal contraception and bone health. Contraception 2006;73:443–4.
179. Lopez LM, Grey TW, Stuebe AM, Chen M, Truitt ST, Gallo MF. Combined hormonal versus nonhormonal versus progestin-only contraception in lactation. Cochrane Database Syst Rev 2015:CD003988.
180. Bongaarts J, Bruce J. The causes of unmet need for contraception and the social content of services. Stud Fam Plann 1995;26:57–75.
181. Grimes DA, Schulz KF. Nonspecific side effects of oral contraceptives: nocebo or noise? Contraception 2011;83:5–9.
182. Raman-Wilms L, Tseng AL, Wighardt S, Einarson TR, Koren G. Fetal genital effects of first-trimester sex hormone exposure: a meta-analysis. Obstet Gynecol 1995;85:141–9.
183. Lammer EJ, Cordero JF. Exogenous sex hormone exposure and the risk for major malformations. JAMA 1986;255:3128–32.
184. Bracken MB. Oral contraception and congenital malformations in offspring: a review and meta-analysis of the prospective studies. Obstet Gynecol 1990;76:552–7.
185. Cardy G. Outcome of pregnancies after failed hormonal postcoital contraception—an interim report. Brit J Fam Plan 1995;21:112–5.
186. Hemminki E, Gissler M, Merilainen J. Reproductive effects of in utero exposure to estrogen and progestin drugs. Fertil Steril 1999;71:1092–8.
187. Pagano HP, Zapata LB, Berry-Bibee EN, Nanda K, Curtis KM. Safety of hormonal contraception and intrauterine devices among women with depressive and bipolar disorders: a systematic review. Contraception 2016;94:641–9.
188. Gallo MF, Lopez LM, Grimes DA, Carayon F, Schulz KF, Helmerhorst FM. Combination contraceptives: effects on weight. Cochrane Database Syst Rev 2014:Cd003987.

189. Pastor Z, Holla K, Chmel R. The influence of combined oral contraceptives on female sexual desire: a systematic review. Eur J Contracept Reprod Health Care 2013;18:27–43.
190. Davis AR, Castano PM. Oral contraceptives and libido in women. Annu Rev Sex Res 2004;15:297–320.
191. Burrows LJ, Basha M, Goldstein AT. The effects of hormonal contraceptives on female sexuality: a review. J Sex Med 2012;9:2213–23.
192. Reed BG, Bou Nemer L, Carr BR. Has testosterone passed the test in premenopausal women with low libido? A systematic review. Int J Womens Health 2016;8:599–607.
193. Caruso S, Agnello C, Intelisano G, et al. Prospective study on sexual behavior of women using 30 microg ethinylestradiol and 3 mg drospirenone oral contraceptive. Contraception 2005;72:19–23.
194. Cheung E, Free C. Factors influencing young women's decision making regarding hormonal contraceptives: a qualitative study. Contraception 2005;71:426–31.
195. Curtis KM, Jatlaoui TC, Tepper NK, et al. U.S. Selected Practice Recommendations for Contraceptive Use, 2016. MMWR Recomm Rep 2016;65:1–66.
196. Stewart FH, Harper CC, Ellertson CE, Grimes DA, Sawaya GF, Trussell J. Clinical breast and pelvic examination requirements for hormonal contraception: Current practice vs evidence. JAMA 2001;285:2232–9.
197. Comp PC. Should coagulation tests be used to determine which oral contraceptive users have an increased risk of thrombophlebitis? Contraception 2006;73:4–5.
198. Brahmi D, Curtis KM. When can a woman start combined hormonal contraceptives (CHCs)? A systematic review. Contraception 2013;87:524–38.
199. Oakley D, Sereika S, Bogue EL. Oral contraceptive pill use after an initial visit to a family planning clinic. Fam Plann Perspect 1991;23:150–4.
200. Westhoff C, Heartwell S, Edwards S, et al. Initiation of oral contraceptives using a quick start compared with a conventional start: a randomized controlled trial. Obstet Gynecol 2007;109:1270–6.
201. Brent RL. Nongenital malformations following exposure to progestational drugs: the last chapter of an erroneous allegation. Birth Defects Res A Clin Mol Teratol 2005;73:906–18.
202. Gallo MF, Nanda K, Grimes DA, Lopez LM, Schulz KF. 20 microg versus >20 microg estrogen combined oral contraceptives for contraception. Cochrane Database Syst Rev 2013:CD003989.
203. Gallo MF, Nanda K, Grimes DA, Lopez LM, Schulz KF. 20 μg versus >20 μg estrogen combined oral contraceptives for contraception. Cochrane Database Syst Rev 2013:Cd003989.
204. Steenland MW, Rodriguez MI, Marchbanks PA, Curtis KM. How does the number of oral contraceptive pill packs dispensed or prescribed affect continuation and other measures of consistent and correct use? A systematic review. Contraception 2013;87:605–10.
205. Osterberg L, Blaschke T. Adherence to medication. N Engl J Med 2005;353:487–97.
206. Hiller W, Rief W, Brahler E. Somatization in the population: from mild bodily misperceptions to disabling symptoms. Soc Psychiatry Psychiatr Epidemiol 2006;41:704–12.
207. Klosterhalfen S, Kellermann S, Braun S, et al. Gender and the nocebo response following conditioning and expectancy. J Psychosom Res 2009;66:323–8.
208. Westhoff C, Morroni C, Kerns J, Murphy PA. Bleeding patterns after immediate vs. conventional oral contraceptive initiation: a randomized, controlled trial. Fertil Steril 2003;79:322–9.
209. Ahrendt HJ, Makalova D, Parke S, Mellinger U, Mansour D. Bleeding pattern and cycle control with an estradiol-based oral contraceptive: a seven-cycle, randomized comparative trial of estradiol valerate/dienogest and ethinyl estradiol/levonorgestrel. Contraception 2009;80:436–44.
210. Coney P, Washenik K, Langley RG, DiGiovanna JJ, Harrison DD. Weight change and adverse event incidence with a low-dose oral contraceptive: two randomized, placebo-controlled trials. Contraception 2001;63:297–302.

211. Goldzieher JW, Moses LE, Averkin E, Scheel C, Taber BZ. A placebo-controlled double-blind crossover investigation of the side effects attributed to oral contraceptives. Fertil Steril 1971;22:609–23.
212. Rosenberg M. Weight change with oral contraceptive use and during the menstrual cycle. Results of daily measurements. Contraception 1998;58:345–9.
213. Lloyd T, Lin HM, Matthews AE, Bentley CM, Legro RS. Oral contraceptive use by teenage women does not affect body composition. Obstet Gynecol 2002;100:235–9.
214. Flegal KM, Kruszon-Moran D, Carroll MD, Fryar CD, Ogden CL. Trends in obesity among adults in the United States, 2005 to 2014. JAMA 2016;315:2284–91.
215. Panotopoulos G, Raison J, Ruiz JC, Guy-Grand B, Basdevant A. Weight gain at the time of menopause. Hum Reprod 1997;12 Suppl 1:126–33.
216. Abraham S, Boyd C, Lal M, Luscombe G, Taylor A. Time since menarche, weight gain and body image awareness among adolescent girls: onset of eating disorders? J Psychosom Obstet Gynaecol 2009;30:89–94.
217. Phelan S. Pregnancy: a "teachable moment" for weight control and obesity prevention. Am J Obstet Gynecol 2010;202:135.e1–8.
218. Scher AI, Stewart WF, Liberman J, Lipton RB. Prevalence of frequent headache in a population sample. Headache 1998;38:497–506.
219. Loder EW, Buse DC, Golub JR. Headache as a side effect of combination estrogen-progestin oral contraceptives: a systematic review. Am J Obstet Gynecol 2005;193: 636–49.
220. Schaffir J, Worly BL, Gur TL. Combined hormonal contraception and its effects on mood: a critical review. Eur J Contracept Reprod Health Care 2016;21:347–55.
221. Keyes KM, Cheslack-Postava K, Westhoff C, et al. Association of hormonal contraceptive use with reduced levels of depressive symptoms: a national study of sexually active women in the United States. Am J Epidemiol 2013;178:1378–88.
222. Skovlund CW, Morch LS, Kessing LV, Lidegaard O. Association of hormonal contraception with depression. JAMA Psychiatry 2016;73:1154–62.
223. Strufaldi R, Pompei LM, Steiner ML, et al. Effects of two combined hormonal contraceptives with the same composition and different doses on female sexual function and plasma androgen levels. Contraception 2010;82:147–54.
224. Wiedemann C, Nagele U, Schramm G, Berking C. Inhibitory effects of progestogens on the estrogen stimulation of melanocytes in vitro. Contraception 2009;80:292–8.
225. Thorneycroft l H, Gollnick H, Schellschmidt I. Superiority of a combined contraceptive containing drospirenone to a triphasic preparation containing norgestimate in acne treatment. Cutis 2004;74:123–30.
226. Hussain Z, Roberts N, Whitehouse GH, Garcia-Finana M, Percy D. Estimation of breast volume and its variation during the menstrual cycle using MRI and stereology. Br J Radiol 1999;72:236–45.
227. Lawrie TA, Helmerhorst FM, Maitra NK, Kulier R, Bloemenkamp K, Gulmezoglu AM. Types of progestogens in combined oral contraception: effectiveness and side-effects. Cochrane Database Syst Rev 2011:Cd004861.

Progestin-Only Pills

9

Elizabeth G. Raymond, MD, MPH
Daniel Grossman, MD

- Progestin-only pills contain a progestin hormone and no estrogen. Currently marketed products require ingestion of one active tablet every day.
- Progestin-only pills are highly effective if taken as directed.
- Progestin-only pills are safe for almost all women, including many with contraindications to combined oral contraceptive pills.
- The most common complaint of progestin-only pill users is irregular bleeding.
- Distribution of progestin-only pills over the counter without a prescription could increase access to effective contraception without compromising safety.

Progestin-only pills (POPs), sometimes called *minipills,* contain a progestin hormone. As of May 2017, the progestin in all POP products sold in the United States is norethindrone, but POPs containing levonorgestrel, desogestrel, or other progestins are available in other countries. The amount of progestin in each POP tablet is lower than the amount in tablets of combined oral contraceptive pill (COC) products that contain the same compound together with an estrogen. (See the insert of color photos of combined and progestin-only oral contraceptives.) All currently marketed POP products consist of active pills that users take once every day without hormone-free breaks. A new POP product that uses a regimen of 24 daily pills containing drospirenone 4 mg followed by 4 days without hormone is under development and may be available within several years.[1]

MECHANISM OF ACTION

POPs may prevent pregnancy by the following mechanisms:

- Ovulation is inhibited in some proportion of cycles.
- Cervical mucus is thickened and decreased in amount, which may prevent sperm penetration.
- The activity of the cilia in the fallopian tube is reduced, which may prevent the sperm and the egg from meeting.
- The endometrium is altered, which may inhibit implantation of a fertilized egg.

The specific mechanism active in a particular cycle may vary among women and, in any single woman, between cycles.[2] POPs containing desogestrel 75 mcg inhibit ovulation more consistently than POPs containing levonorgestrel 30 mcg.[3]

EFFECTIVENESS

POPs can be a highly effective contraceptive method when taken as directed. They are included in the second tier of effectiveness, along with combined oral contraceptive pills, injectable contraceptives, and hormonal patches and rings (see Figure 3-1 in Chapter 3 on Efficacy, Safety, and Personal Considerations). In clinical studies, all of which were conducted at least 20 years ago, the proportion of women becoming pregnant in the first year of use ranged from 0.2-13.2% (see Table 26-11).[2] The quality of many of these studies was poor.

Scant data are available comparing efficacy of different POP products.[4] One randomized trial found no significant difference in efficacy between POPs containing norethindrone and POPs containing levonorgestrel.[5] Pregnancy rates in both POP groups in this trial were greater than 9% at one year, higher than in many other studies. Another randomized trial found fewer pregnancies among women using POPs containing desogestrel (0.41 pregnancies/100 woman-years) than among women using POPs containing levonorgestrel (1.17 pregnancies/100 woman-years), although the difference did not reach statistical significance.[6] A third randomized trial conducted nearly four decades ago found similar and relatively low pregnancy rates in users of three POPs containing different hormones (2 to 4 pregnancies/100 woman-years), and a higher rate in users of POPs containing a fourth hormone. However, none of these four regimens is currently available.[7] An observational study that included more than

3,000 woman-years of use of POPs found no appreciable difference in efficacy among users of different preparations.[8]

POPs are widely believed to be less effective than COCs, but this belief is not supported by rigorous evidence.[4] One randomized trial comparing 2 COC and 2 POP preparations found that the pregnancy rate was significantly lower in one group of COC users than the rates in the other three groups. Losses from the study for reasons other than pregnancy were very high in all the groups, which seriously compromised the comparisons.[5] Another small study comparing a POP to a COC (neither of which is currently marketed), found no pregnancies in either group, although the study contained only 43 women in each group who used the assigned method for only 6.7 and 9.2 cycles on average.[9]

In typical use, factors such as age, coital frequency, lactation, and compliance with pill-taking may influence pregnancy rates more than relatively minor differences in inherent method efficacy.[10] Guidelines on use of POPs emphasize that for maximum efficacy, the pills must be taken within several hours of the same time every day. This recommendation is based primarily on data about serum progestin levels, which peak shortly after pill ingestion and then decline to nearly undetectable levels 24 hours later.[2] However, no clinical data are available that correlate pregnancy rates with timeliness in taking POPs. One study suggests that POPs containing desogestrel 75 mcg may inhibit ovulation reliably even when pills are occasionally taken 12 hours late.[11] A study has found that an investigational POP containing drospirenone inhibited ovulation in nearly all women despite intentional 24-hour delays in pill intake and a planned four-day hormone hiatus.[12]

ADVANTAGES

POPs have numerous beneficial features, as described below.

1. **Safety.** Because POPs contain lower doses of progestin than COCs and do not contain estrogen, they are presumably at least as safe as COCs and are quite likely safer. However, rigorous data on safety of POPs as distinct from or in comparison to COCs are relatively scant. Without evidence to the contrary, expert bodies such as the World Health Organization (WHO) and the Centers for Disease Control and Prevention assume the risks of COCs also apply to POPs. However, in fact, this assumption may be overly conservative. In general, data suggest that POPs appear not to be associated with an overall clinically important increase in risk of hypertension,[13] cardiovascular disease and stroke,[14–17] breast cancer,[18,19] or blood clots.[20,21] POPs are not associated with birth

defects in babies of women who accidentally took them during pregnancy.[2,22]

2. **Few contraindications.** According to the both the WHO's Medical Eligibility Criteria for Contraceptive Use (WHO MEC)[23] and the corresponding United States document (U.S. MEC),[24] POPs can safely be used by almost all women. These criteria list many fewer contraindications to POPs than to COCs.
3. **Acceptable efficacy**, especially if the pills are taken as directed. See above.
4. **Improved menstrual symptoms for some women.** POPs cause menstrual cycle changes that are welcome to some women (see below under Disadvantages.) They may also reduce the severity of menstrual cramps.[25]
5. **Simple, fixed daily regimen.** Users of currently available POPs take the same type of pill every day (same color and hormone content).
6. **Immediate reversibility.** Limited data suggest that fertility is normal immediately after stopping use of POPs, regardless of the duration of POP use.[2]
7. **Non-contraceptive health benefits.** POPs may reduce the incidence of painful crises in women with sickle cell disease[26] and may relieve pelvic pain associated with endometriosis.[27,28] Some data suggest that POPs may reduce frequency and severity of migraines[28,29] and that they can be useful in treatment of endometriosis[27] and estrogen dermatitis related to the menstrual cycle.[30] A recent analysis suggested that POPs may protect against breast cancer mortality.[31]

DISADVANTAGES AND CAUTIONS

POPs also have disadvantages, as described below.

1. **Menstrual cycle disturbances.** POPs cause bleeding changes in many or most users. These changes are unpredictable and may include short cycles, irregular periods, intermenstrual bleeding and spotting, and less commonly, prolonged bleeding or amenorrhea. Analysis of bleeding patterns of women in six clinical trials studying various methods of contraception showed that POP users typically had less regular bleeding patterns and more total bleeding or spotting days over time than users of COCs.[32] Whether or not bleeding patterns tend to become more regular with increased

duration of POP use is unknown. Bleeding irregularities caused by POPs are not inherently dangerous, but they can complicate the detection of pregnancy if the pills fail or mask underlying pathologies and thus cause women to delay seeking care. They are also a common reason for discontinuing POPs, although some women consider the altered bleeding pattern, particularly if it constitutes less total bleeding than expected, to be a benefit of the method.

2. **Other side effects.** Complaints by POP users include headaches, nausea, weight gain or loss, breast tenderness, depression, fatigue, decreased libido, androgenic symptoms such as hirsutism and acne, and other side effects. However, the precise extent to which these common symptoms are actually caused by the pills cannot be determined from available data.[2]

3. **Possibly vulnerable efficacy.** To maximize contraceptive efficacy, POP users are advised to be especially careful (more careful than users of COCs) to take the pills at the same time each day and to use back-up methods such as condoms when taking drugs that may interact with the hormones in the pills or during periods of vomiting or diarrhea.

4. **Lower efficacy than some other methods in preventing ectopic pregnancy.** Rigorous data are not available about the effect of POPs on the absolute risk of ectopic pregnancy. One early report suggested that POP users may be at higher risk than users of no method or of other methods[33], but other data seem to refute that contention.[2] However, up to 10% of pregnancies that occur among POP users may be ectopic, a proportion higher than is seen in users of COCs or women who use no method at all. Thus, POPs appear not to prevent ectopic pregnancy as well as they prevent intrauterine pregnancy.[2,33]

5. **Possible increased risk of diabetes.** One study suggested that use of POPs during breastfeeding after a pregnancy complicated by gestational diabetes may increase the subsequent long-term risk of type II diabetes mellitus.[34] However, POPs are generally felt to be safe for use by diabetic women.[23,24]

6. **Ovarian cysts.** Unlike COCs, which substantially inhibit ovarian activity and reduce the risk of functional ovarian cysts, POPs may be associated with an increased incidence of functional ovarian cysts or persistent follicles.[35] Most ovarian cysts cause minor or no symptoms and resolve without treatment.

7. **Lack of protection against sexually transmitted infections (STIs).** Progestin-only contraceptives provide no known substantial protection against STIs, including HIV.

Special Issues

Breastfeeding: The physiologic effects of contraceptive steroids could, in theory, impair lactation. In addition, a small amount of the progestin in the pills passes into breast milk, which exposes a breastfeeding baby to the hormone. Although rigorous data on the effects of such exposure are limited, no strong or consistent evidence exists suggesting harm.[36–38] Both the WHO and U.S. MEC recommend that the benefits of initiating and using POPs at any point after delivery postpartum generally outweigh the risks. (See Chapter 17 on Contraception After Pregnancy.)

Drug interactions: Interactions between POPs and other drugs have not been well studied, but it is reasonable to suspect that they may be similar to interactions with COCs. Because POPs produce relatively low progestin levels even in the absence of other drugs, POPs may not be an especially good contraceptive option for women who are taking certain drugs on a chronic basis. These drugs include rifampicin, certain anticonvulsants, and some anti-retroviral drugs, which affect the metabolism of ingested steroid hormones.[24] However, even for women on these drugs, POPs may be more effective than some other contraceptive methods, particularly barrier methods or natural family planning. Combined use of a barrier method and POPs might be the best choice for women taking potentially interacting drugs if they cannot use other highly effective contraceptive methods. Advise POP users to use a back-up method while temporarily taking a potentially interacting drug, and possibly for some period of time after stopping it. Although some providers have proposed that POP users should increase the dose of POPs while taking a potentially interacting drug, no data are available on the efficacy or advisability of this idea.

Providing the Method

Almost all women can safely use POPs, including most women who are not eligible to take COCs. Neither the WHO MEC[23] nor the U.S. MEC[24] include any restriction on use of POPs based on age, smoking, hypertension, migraine without aura, uterine fibroids, diabetes, gall bladder disease, or sickle cell disease. No examination or laboratory test is needed to determine whether a woman is eligible to receive POPs.

The WHO MEC and the U.S. MEC list few category 3 or 4 contraindications to POPs (Table 9-1). Only one condition, current breast cancer, is classified as category 4, indicating that POPs pose an unacceptable health risk to women with this condition. (See the U.S. MEC summary chart insert in this book.)

In addition, both the WHO and U.S. MEC note that POPs should usually be stopped if the user develops ischemic heart disease or stroke (category 3).

Table 9-1 Contraindications to use of progestin-only pills

	WHO MEC	U.S. MEC
Current breast cancer	4	4
Current deep venous thrombosis or pulmonary embolus	3	
History of bariatric surgery (malabsorptive procedures)		3
Systemic lupus erythematosus with positive or unknown antiphospholipid antibodies	3	3
Severe (decompensated) cirrhosis, benign or malignant liver tumors	3	3
Past breast cancer and no evidence of current disease for 5 years	3	3
Certain anticonvulsants, (phenytoin, carbamazepine, barbiturates, primidone, topiramate, oxcarbazepine), rifampicin or rifabutin	3	3

The WHO MEC, but not the U.S. MEC, recommends that POPs should be stopped if the user develops migraine with aura while using POPs.

Immediate start of certain kinds of POPs following use of ulipristal acetate emergency contraceptive pills may counteract the ability of ulipristal to suppress ovulation, putting the user at risk of pregnancy from the act of intercourse that has already occurred.[39] Whether ulipristal counteracts the efficacy of POPs is not known, although one study showed that ulipristal did not interfere with the ability of combined oral contraceptive pills to induce ovarian quiescence.[40] Until more is known, POPs should not be initiated within 5 days after taking ulipristal, and women using POPs who need emergency contraceptives should be advised to use regimens that do not contain ulipristal. If a user of POPs takes ulipristal, she should use a back-up contraceptive if she has sex within the following 5 days, and she should be vigilant about the possibility of pregnancy. (See Chapter 10 on Emergency Contraception.)

POPs are not a good choice for women who cannot tolerate irregular bleeding or amenorrhea. Because they should be taken at close to the same hour each day, they may not be suitable for women whose schedules do not allow such consistency.

Counseling. Women considering POPs should be advised about their advantages and disadvantages, described above. (See Chapter 2 for more complete discussion of patient-centered contraception counseling.)

Timing of initiation. A woman may start taking POPs at any time (Quick Start) when it is reasonably certain that she is not pregnant, if she has not used ulipristal acetate emergency contraception within the last 5 days. (See Box 2-6 on how to be reasonably certain that a woman is not pregnant.)

The 2016 U.S. Selected Practice Recommendations for Contraceptive Use[41] indicate that no back-up method is needed if she starts POPs within the first 5 days after onset of menses, but otherwise, she should use a back-up method if she has vaginal sex within the first 2 days after starting POPs. A simpler approach, which we recommend here, is to use a back-up method for the first 2 days of use regardless of when in the cycle the method is initiated.

Distribution of commodities. Currently in the United States, POPs are available only by prescription. Provide or prescribe as many packs of POPs as the patient wants. Advise the patient to check with her insurance carrier about any limits on the number of packs that may be dispensed at one time under her policy.

The characteristics of POPs make them eminently suitable for distribution over the counter: they are safe, contraindications are rare[42] and readily recognizable by women themselves,[43] and the regimen is very simple. Consequently, efforts are now underway to apply to the U.S. Food and Drug Administration for approval to market POPs without a prescription. If that occurred, POPs would become the most effective contraceptive method available without a prescription. Research suggests that this change in status would increase access to and use of effective contraception in the United States.[44,45]

MANAGING PROBLEMS AND FOLLOW-UP

Abnormal bleeding in women using POPs can be managed by a number of approaches, including reassurance, prostaglandin inhibitors, estrogen supplementation, or a method switch. (See Chapter 1 on the Menstrual Cycle.)

If a woman becomes pregnant while using POPs, be vigilant for the possibility of ectopic pregnancy.

USER INSTRUCTIONS FOR PROGESTIN-ONLY PILLS*

To use POPs, follow these instructions:

1. Start taking the pills during the first 5 days of your normal menstrual period or on any day you are reasonably sure that you are not pregnant. If you are switching from estrogen-containing oral contraceptive pills (regular birth control pills), skip the inactive pills at the end of the pack, and instead start the POPs the day after the last active pill.

*These instructions are intended to guide providers in educating patients in how to use their method.

2. Use a back-up method such as condoms every time you have vaginal sex within 2 days after starting POPs.
3. Take 1 pill every day. Choose a time and take the pill at that time or within 3 hours after that time.
4. Start the next pack the day after the last pack is finished. Do not take any break or days off between packs. Always have your next pack ready *before* you finish each pack.
5. If you miss taking a pill during the 3-hour window, take it as soon as you remember, and continue taking 1 pill each day at the usual time, even if that means you will take 2 pills in one day. Use a back-up method such as condoms or abstain from vaginal sex during the next 48 hours. Take further pills at the usual time.
6. If you vomit or have severe diarrhea within 4 hours after taking a pill, your body might not properly absorb the medicine in the POPs. Keep taking the pills on schedule, but use a back-up method such as condoms every time you have sex, until 48 hours after the vomiting or diarrhea are over.
7. Get a pregnancy test if:
   - Your menstrual period is late, and you have not taken all your pills on time, and you had sex without a condom or other back up method.
   - You have not had any periods for 2 months.
   - You are concerned about pregnancy for any reason.

   Keep taking the pills daily until you know the pregnancy test result. If the result is positive, then stop taking the pills and consult your clinician about your options. If the result is negative, then the late or missed periods are probably due to the pills and are not dangerous. Consult your clinician about other possible causes and your options.
8. Certain medicines and some over-the-counter preparations can reduce the effectiveness of POPs. If you take any other drug while using POPs, ask your clinician whether it might interact with POPs. If so, you should use a back-up method (such as condoms) during the entire time you are taking the other drug and possibly for some time after you stop taking it. If you are planning to take the other drug for a long period of time, consult with your clinician about whether a contraceptive method other than POPs might be appropriate for you.
9. Changes in your menstrual periods (frequency and length and bleeding between periods) are common in women taking POPs. These changes are usually not dangerous. If you have unusual

bleeding, keep taking the POPs. If the bleeding lasts for more than 8 days or is particularly heavy, or if you want to switch to another contraceptive method that is less likely to cause bleeding irregularities, consult your clinician.

10. If you have other problems or questions while taking POPs, keep taking the pills according to schedule while you figure out what to do.
11. If you stop taking POPs and do not want to become pregnant, start using another contraceptive immediately, or abstain from vaginal sex. Your ability to become pregnant returns right away after you stop POPs.
12. If you have had sex that was not properly protected by POPs or another contraceptive method (that is, if you did not follow the instructions above), consider using emergency contraception. Choose a copper IUD or morning-after pills that contain levonorgestrel. Do not use emergency contraceptives containing ulipristal because that medication could interact with the hormone in POPs.

Emergency Contraceptives (EC): Emergency contraceptive pills or placement of a copper intrauterine contraceptive after unprotected intercourse substantially reduces the risk of pregnancy. POPs users should take EC regimens other than ulipristal, but if they do, they should use a back-up contraceptive if they have sex within the following 5 days, and be aware of the possibility of pregnancy.

Author Disclosures—Raymond: none. Grossman: none.

References

1. Archer DF, Ahrendt HJ, Drouin D. Drospirenone-only oral contraceptive: results from a multicenter noncomparative trial of efficacy, safety and tolerability. Contraception 2015;92:439–44.
2. McCann MF, Potter LS. Progestin-only oral contraception: a comprehensive review. Contraception 1994;50:S1–195.
3. Rice CF, Killick SR, Dieben T, Coelingh Bennink H. A comparison of the inhibition of ovulation achieved by desogestrel 75 micrograms and levonorgestrel 30 micrograms daily. Hum Reprod 1999;14:982–5.
4. Grimes DA, Lopez LM, O'Brien PA, Raymond EG. Progestin-only pills for contraception. Cochrane Database Syst Rev 2010:CD007541.
5. Sheth A, Jain U, Sharma S, et al. A randomized, double-blind study of two combined and two progestogen-only oral contraceptives. Contraception 1982;25:243–52.
6. Collaborative Study Group on the Desogestrel-containing Progestogen-only Pill. A double-blind study comparing the contraceptive efficacy, acceptability and safety of two progestogen-only pills containing desogestrel 75 micrograms/day or levonorgestrel 30 micrograms/day. Eur J Contracept Reprod Health Care 1998;3:169–78.

7. Vessey MP, Mears E, Andolšek L, Ogrinc-Oven M. Randomised double-blind trial of four oral progestagen-only contraceptives. Lancet 1972;299:915–22.
8. Vessey M, Lawless M, Yeates D, McPherson K. Progestogen-only oral contraception. Findings in a large prospective study with special reference to effectiveness. Brit J Fam Plan 1985;10:117–21.
9. Paulsen ML, Varaday A, Brown BW, Kalman SM. A randomized contraceptive trial comparing a daily progestogen with a combined oral contraceptive steroid. Contraception 1974;9:497–506.
10. Steiner M, Dominik R, Trussell J, Hertz-Picciott I. Measuring contraceptive effectiveness: a conceptual framework. Obstet Gynecol 1996;88:24S–30S.
11. Korver T, Klipping C, Heger-Mahn D, Duijkers I, van Osta G, Dieben T. Maintenance of ovulation inhibition with the 75-microg desogestrel-only contraceptive pill (Cerazette) after scheduled 12-h delays in tablet intake. Contraception 2005;71:8–13.
12. Duijkers IJ, Heger-Mahn D, Drouin D, Colli E, Skouby S. Maintenance of ovulation inhibition with a new progestogen-only pill containing drospirenone after scheduled 24-h delays in pill intake. Contraception 2016;93:303–9.
13. Hussain SF. Progestogen-only pills and high blood pressure: is there an association? A literature review. Contraception 2004;69:89–97.
14. Chakhtoura Z, Canonico M, Gompel A, Scarabin PY, Plu-Bureau G. Progestogen-only contraceptives and the risk of acute myocardial infarction: a meta-analysis. J Clin Endocrinol Metab 2011;96:1169–74.
15. Chakhtoura Z, Canonico M, Gompel A, Thalabard JC, Scarabin PY, Plu-Bureau G. Progestogen-only contraceptives and the risk of stroke: a meta-analysis. Stroke 2009;40:1059–62.
16. Heinemann LA, Assmann A, DoMinh T, Garbe E. Oral progestogen-only contraceptives and cardiovascular risk: results from the Transnational Study on Oral Contraceptives and the Health of Young Women. Eur J Contracept Reprod Health Care 1999;4:67–73.
17. Xu Z, Li Y, Tang S, Huang X, Chen T. Current use of oral contraceptives and the risk of first-ever ischemic stroke: A meta-analysis of observational studies. Thromb Res 2015;136:52–60.
18. Skegg DC, Paul C, Spears GF, Williams SM. Progestogen-only oral contraceptives and risk of breast cancer in New Zealand. Cancer Cause Control 1996;7:513–9.
19. Samson M, Porter N, Orekoya O, et al. Progestin and breast cancer risk: a systematic review. Breast Cancer Res Treat 2016;155:3–12.
20. Bergendal A, Odlind V, Persson I, Kieler H. Limited knowledge on progestogen-only contraception and risk of venous thromboembolism. Acta Obstet Gynecol Scand 2009;88:261–6.
21. Tepper NK, Whiteman MK, Marchbanks PA, James AH, Curtis KM. Progestin-only contraception and thromboembolism: A systematic review. Contraception 2016;94:678–700.
22. Simpson JL, Phillips OP. Spermicides, hormonal contraception and congenital malformations. Adv Contracept 1990;6:141–67.
23. World Health Organization. Medical Eligibility Criteria for Contraceptive Use, 5th Edition. Geneva, Switzerland; 2015.
24. Curtis KM, Tepper NK, Jatlaoui TC, et al. U.S. Medical Eligibility Criteria for Contraceptive Use, 2016. MMWR Recomm Rep 2016;65:1–103.
25. Ahrendt HJ, Karckt U, Pichl T, Mueller T, Ernst U. The effects of an oestrogen-free, desogestrel-containing oral contraceptive in women with cyclical symptoms: results from two studies on oestrogen-related symptoms and dysmenorrhoea. Eur J Contracept Reprod Health Care 2007;12:354–61.
26. de Abood M, de Castillo Z, Guerrero F, Espino M, Austin KL. Effect of Depo-Provera or Microgynon on the painful crises of sickle cell anemia patients. Contraception 1997;56:313–6.
27. Casper RF. Progestin-only pills may be a better first-line treatment for endometriosis than combined estrogen-progestin contraceptive pills. Fertil Steril 2017;107:533–6.

28. Morotti M, Remorgida V, Venturini PL, Ferrero S. Progestogen-only contraceptive pill compared with combined oral contraceptive in the treatment of pain symptoms caused by endometriosis in patients with migraine without aura. Eur J Obstet Gynecol Reprod Biol 2014;179:63–8.
29. Merki-Feld GS, Imthurn B, Dubey R, Sandor PS, Gantenbein AR. Improvement of migraine with change from combined hormonal contraceptives to progestin-only contraception with desogestrel: How strong is the effect of taking women off combined contraceptives? J Obstet Gynaecol 2017;37:338–41.
30. Randall K, Steele R. Estrogen dermatitis: treatment with progestin-only pill. Arch Dermatol 2005;141:792–3.
31. Samson ME, Adams SA, Mulatya CM, et al. Types of oral contraceptives and breast cancer survival among women enrolled in Medicaid: A competing-risk model. Maturitas 2017;95:42–9.
32. Belsey EM. Vaginal bleeding patterns among women using one natural and eight hormonal methods of contraception. Contraception 1988;38:181–206.
33. Bergsjo P, Langengen H, Aas J. Tubal pregnancies in women using progestagen-only contraception. Acta Obstet Gynecol Scand 1974;53:377–8.
34. Kjos SL, Peters RK, Xiang A, Thomas D, Schaefer U, Buchanan TA. Contraception and the risk of type 2 diabetes mellitus in Latina women with prior gestational diabetes mellitus. JAMA 1998;280:533–8.
35. Tayob Y, Adams J, Jacobs HS, Guillebaud J. Ultrasound demonstration of increased frequency of functional ovarian cysts in women using progestogen-only oral contraception. Br J Obstet Gynaecol 1985;92:1003–9.
36. Lopez LM, Grey TW, Stuebe AM, Chen M, Truitt ST, Gallo MF. Combined hormonal versus nonhormonal versus progestin-only contraception in lactation Cochrane Database Syst Rev 2015:CD003988.
37. Kapp N, Curtis K, Nanda K. Progestogen-only contraceptive use among breastfeeding women: a systematic review. Contraception 2010;82:17–37.
38. Bhardwaj NR, Espey E. Lactation and contraception. Curr Opin Obstet Gynecol 2015;27:496–503.
39. Brache V, Cochon L, Duijkers IJ, et al. A prospective, randomized, pharmacodynamic study of quick-starting a desogestrel progestin-only pill following ulipristal acetate for emergency contraception. Hum Reprod 2015;30:2785–93.
40. Cameron ST, Berger C, Michie L, Klipping C, Gemzell-Danielsson K. The effects on ovarian activity of ulipristal acetate when 'quickstarting' a combined oral contraceptive pill: a prospective, randomized, double-blind parallel-arm, placebo-controlled study. Hum Reprod 2015;30:1566–72.
41. Curtis KM, Jatlaoui TC, Tepper NK, et al. U.S. Selected Practice Recommendations for Contraceptive Use, 2016. MMWR Recomm Rep 2016;65:1–66.
42. White K, Potter JE, Hopkins K, Fernandez L, Amastae J, Grossman D. Contraindications to progestin-only oral contraceptive pills among reproductive-aged women. Contraception 2012;86:199–203.
43. Grossman D, Fernandez L, Hopkins K, Amastae J, Garcia SG, Potter JE. Accuracy of self-screening for contraindications to combined oral contraceptive use. Obstet Gynecol 2008;112:572–8.
44. Grossman D. The potential impact of over-the-counter access to oral contraceptives to reduce unintended pregnancy. Am Fam Physician 2015;92:968–9.
45. Foster DG, Biggs MA, Phillips KA, Grindlay K, Grossman D. Potential public sector cost-savings from over-the-counter access to oral contraceptives. Contraception 2015;91:373–9.

10 Emergency Contraception

James Trussell, PhD
Kelly Cleland, MPA, MPH
Eleanor Bimla Schwarz, MD, MS

- Emergency contraception (EC) substantially reduces the chance of pregnancy after an episode of unprotected intercourse.
- Placement of a copper IUD within 5 (or 7 or even 10) days after unprotected intercourse reduces the risk of pregnancy by more than 99%.
- Emergency contraceptive pills (ECPs) taken within 5 days of unprotected intercourse are effective but less effective than a copper IUD. From most to least effective, these pills contain:
  - 30 mg ulipristal acetate (UPA) (*ella*)
  - 1.5 mg levonorgestrel (LNG) (*Plan B One-Step and several generic versions*)
  - A combination of ethinyl estradiol and either levonorgestrel or norgestrel (the previous dedicated combined product, *Preven,* is no longer marketed).
- EC is safe for everyone; if someone is already pregnant, EC pills are ineffective but will not harm the pregnancy.

Emergency contraceptives are methods that can be used after intercourse to prevent pregnancy.[1] Two types of dedicated emergency contraceptive pills (ECPs) are currently available for use in the United States:

- *ella,* a single 30 mg ulipristal acetate (UPA) pill, was approved by the FDA in 2010.
- *Plan B One-Step,* a single 1.5 mg levonorgestrel (LNG) pill, replaced the previously available *Plan B* (two 0.75 mg tablets of LNG) product in 2009. Several generic versions are available, including *My Way, Take Action, Fallback Solo, Opcicon One-Step* and *Aftera.*

Plan B One-Step and its generic forms are available without prescription from pharmacies to anyone of any age. Until August 2013 (for Plan B One-Step, and February 2014 for one-dose generic LNG ECPs) a prescription was required for women under age 17, but this restriction has been removed. The two-dose version of LNG ECPs (Plan B and its generic forms) is no longer sold in the United States.

There are no contraindications to use of any ECP by anyone of any age except pregnancy, because the EC will not work. A prescription is still required for U.S. patients of any age to use ella (although in January 2015, the European Medicines Agency decided that UPA ECPs should be available from a pharmacist without a prescription). Placement of a copper IUD has also proved highly effective as emergency contraception (EC).[2,3]

Less-effective options for EC include use of combined oral contraceptive pills containing ethinyl estradiol and either norgestrel or LNG, sometimes called the Yuzpe regimen. (See Table 10-1 for a list of pills that can be used for EC.) Preven, a dedicated product containing two doses of 0.1 mg ethinyl estradiol and 0.5 mg LNG, was approved for use in 1998 but withdrawn from the market in 2004, as more effective ECPs with fewer side effects were available. Emergency use of combined pills containing norethindrone was found in one study to have an efficacy slightly lower than that for combined pills containing LNG.[4] No published studies are available for emergency contraceptive use of combined pills containing gestodene, etonorgestrel, or other progestins; such pills should therefore not be used for EC.

In the United States, access to mifepristone remains constrained by individuals who seek to limit access to abortion services. However, in Armenia, China, Russia, Moldova, Ukraine, and Vietnam, mifepristone in doses of 10 to 25 mg is available as an ECP. Mifepristone prevents ovulation by blocking the effects of progesterone by binding to its receptors. Depending on whether the drug is administered before or after ovulation, it can also disrupt luteal-phase events and endometrial development.[5] Mifepristone is more effective and causes less nausea and vomiting and fewer side effects than do the Yuzpe regimen[3,6–8] and LNG EC[3]; it has not been directly compared to UPA.

Meloxicam (a COX-2 inhibitor) given for 5 consecutive days in the late follicular phase at a dose of 30 mg may also be an effective option for EC. This regimen does not alter the endocrine profile of the cycle and causes no menstrual disturbance.[9,10] (In contrast, celecoxib, another COX-2 inhibitor, appears to have no potential for EC.[11]) However, the effectiveness of meloxicam has yet to be compared to other EC options in a randomized controlled fashion, and it is not sold as an emergency contraceptive.

Table 10-1 Pills that can be used for EC in the United States[a]

Brand	Company	First Dose	Second Dose (12 hours later)	Ulipristal Acetate (UPA) per Dose (mg)	Ethinyl Estradiol per Dose (mcg)	Levonorgestrel (LNG) per Dose (mg)
			UPA (Dedicated ECPs)			
ella	Afaxys	1 white pill	None	30	—	—
			LNG (Dedicated ECPs)			
Aftera[b]	Teva	1 white pill	None	—	—	1.5
AfterPill[c]	Syzygy	1 white pill	None	—	—	1.5
Athentia Next	Aurobindo	1 white pill	None	—	—	1.5
EContra Ez[d]	Afaxys	1 white pill	None	—	—	1.5
Fallback Solo	Lupin	1 white pill	None	—	—	1.5
My Way	Gavis	1 white pill	None	—	—	1.5
Next Choice One Dose	Actavis	1 peach pill	None	—	—	1.5
Opcicon One-Step	Sun Pharma	1 white pill	None	—	—	1.5
Option 2	Perrigo	1 white pill	None	—	—	1.5
Plan B One-Step	Teva	1 white pill	None	—	—	1.5
Take Action	Teva	1 white pill	None	—	—	1.5
		Combined progestin and estrogen pills (Regular oral contraceptive pills)				
Afirmelle	Aurobindo	5 white pills	5 white pills	—	100	0.50
Altavera	Sandoz	4 peach pills	4 peach pills	—	120	0.60
Amethia	Actavis	4 white pills	4 white pills	—	120	0.60
Amethia Lo	Actavis	5 white pills	5 white pills	—	100	0.50

(continued)

Table 10-1 Pills that can be used for EC in the United States[a]—*(continued)*

Brand	Company	First Dose	Second Dose (12 hours later)	Ulipristal Acetate (UPA) per Dose (mg)	Ethinyl Estradiol per Dose (mcg)	Levonorgestrel (LNG) per Dose (mg)
Amethyst	Actavis	6 white pills	6 white pills	—	120	0.54
Aubra	Afaxys	5 white pills	5 white pills	—	100	0.50
Ayuna	Aurobindo	4 orange pills	4 orange pills	—	100	0.50
Aviane	Teva	5 orange pills	5 orange pills	—	100	0.50
Camrese	Teva	4 light blue-green pills	4 light blue-green pills	—	120	0.60
CamreseLo	Teva	5 orange pills	5 orange pills	—	100	0.50
Chateal	Afaxys	4 white pills	4 white pills	—	120	0.60
Cryselle[e]	Teva	4 white pills	4 white pills	—	120	0.60
Elinest[e]	Novast	4 orange pills	4 orange pills	—	120	0.60
Enpresse	Teva	4 orange pills	4 orange pills	—	120	0.50
Falmina	Novast	5 orange pills	5 orange pills	—	100	0.50
Introvale	Sandoz	4 peach pills	4 peach pills	—	120	0.60
Jolessa	Teva	4 pink pills	4 pink pills	—	120	0.60
Kurvelo	Lupin	4 peach pills	4 peach pills	—	120	0.60
Lessina	Teva	5 pink pills	5 pink pills	—	100	0.50
Levonest	Novast	4 light brown pills	4 light brown pills	—	120	0.50
Levora	Actavis	4 white pills	4 white pills	—	120	0.60
LoSeasonique	Teva	5 orange pills	5 orange pills	—	100	0.50
Low-Ogestrel[e]	Actavis	4 white pills	4 white pills	—	120	0.60
Lutera	Actavis	5 white pills	5 white pills	—	100	0.50
Marlissa	Glenmark	4 peach pills	4 peach pills	—	120	0.60

(continued)

Table 10-1 Pills that can be used for EC in the United States[a]—*(continued)*

Brand	Company	First Dose	Second Dose (12 hours later)	Ulipristal Acetate (UPA) per Dose (mg)	Ethinyl Estradiol per Dose (mcg)	Levonorgestrel (LNG) per Dose (mg)
Myzilra	Novast	4 yellow pills	4 yellow pills	—	120	0.50
Nordette	Teva	4 light-orange pills	4 light-orange pills	—	120	0.60
Orsythia	Vintage	5 pink pills	5 pink pills	—	100	0.50
Portia	Teva	4 pink pills	4 pink pills	—	120	0.60
Quasense	Actavis	4 white pills	4 white pills	—	120	0.60
Seasonale	Teva	4 pink pills	4 pink pills	—	120	0.60
Seasonique	Teva	4 light-blue-green pills	4 light-blue-green pills	—	120	0.60
Setlakin	Novast	4 pink pills	4 pink pills	—	120	0.60
Sronyx	Actavis	5 white pills	5 while pills	—	100	0.50
Triphasil	Wyeth	4 yellow pills	4 yellow pills	—	120	0.50
Trivora	Actavis	4 pink pills	4 pink pills	—	120	0.50
Vienva	Sandoz	5 white pills	5 white pills	—	100	0.50

Notes:

[a]ella and the LNG EC products listed in the top section are dedicated products specifically marketed for emergency contraception. The regular oral contraceptives listed above have been declared safe and effective for use as ECPs by the United States Food and Drug Administration. In the United States, LNG EC, like Plan B One-Step and Take Action, is available on the shelf with no restrictions. ella is available by prescription only.

[b]Aftera is sold exclusively at CVS stores

[c]Afterpill is sold online at www.afterpill.com

[d]EContra EZ is sold at family planning clinics and online at www.kwikmed.com

[e]The progestin in Cryselle, Elinest, and Low-Ogestrel is norgestrel, which contains two isomers, only one of which (LNG) is bioactive; the amount of norgestrel in each tablet is twice the amount of LNG.

Older methods of EC, which are no longer recommended, include the following:

- High-dose estrogen. Ethinyl estradiol, 5 mg to 10 mg given daily for 5 days, provides efficacy similar to the Yuzpe method[12,13] but with a high incidence of nausea and vomiting.
- Danazol. Studies of danazol, an androgenic and progestogenic steroid, were initially promising,[14] but this approach was abandoned when a subsequent study found an unacceptably low efficacy.[7]
- Diethylstilbestrol (DES), 25 mg to 50 mg.

Barriers to Use

The major barriers to use of EC are awareness and access. None of the companies that have marketed ECPs have made significant investments in direct-to-consumer advertising. Without commercial marketing, many couples still may not know that EC is available, effective, and safe. Nevertheless, among U.S. women aged 15 to 44 who have ever had intercourse, the fraction that had ever used ECPs increased from 2% in 2002 to 18% in 2011-2013.[15] In addition, many healthcare providers have limited knowledge of EC.[16]

Even in cases of rape, many hospital emergency departments do not provide emergency contraceptive services,[17–20] despite the fact that legal precedent indicates that failure to provide EC constitutes inadequate care and provides grounds to sue the hospital.[21] It is estimated that thousands of pregnancies resulting from rape each year could be prevented by use of EC.[22] However, until 2012, the Department of Justice made no mention of EC in its 130-page *National Protocol for Sexual Assault Medical Forensic Examinations*;[23] this omission was fully rectified in April 2013.[24]

Promoting Awareness and Use

Multiple initiatives have encouraged greater awareness and use of EC (see Additional Information and Materials). One concern often voiced about making ECPs more widely available has been that individuals who know they can use ECPs may become less diligent with other contraception. However, to date, 18 studies have demonstrated that making ECPs more widely available did not increase sexual risk-taking.[25–42]

In the four studies that examined the impact of easier access to ECPs on rates of sexually transmitted infections (STIs), access to ECPs did not affect incidence of STIs.[29,37,40,42] Another study demonstrated that educating teens about ECPs did not increase their level of sexual activity or use of EC but did increase their knowledge about proper administration of ECPs.[43] Reanalysis of one randomized trial suggested that providing free, unlimited access to ECPs may have increased the frequency of coital acts with the potential to lead to pregnancy, compared with women who purchased ECPs.[44] Women in the free access group were significantly more likely than those who purchased ECPs to report that they had ever used emergency contraception because they did not want to use either condoms or another contraceptive method.[45] More recently, ecological studies comparing outcomes before and after ECPs became available without a prescription in the United States have provided conflicting information about whether increased access to ECPs is associated with changes in behavior: one study that was not able to control for secular trends found that women were 5% more likely to report multiple sexual partners after ECPs became available without a prescription,[46] but another more robust study by the same author, that was able to control for state-level policy changes, found exactly the opposite effect.[47] A third study suggested that condom use among public school students declined by 5% to 7% over the same time period that ECPs became available without a prescription;[48] although this study was not able to demonstrate a causal relationship between access to EC and condom use, it highlights the continued importance of facilitating teen access to condoms and education about STI transmission.

Over-the-Counter (OTC) Availability

There are no medical reasons for ECPs to require a prescription.[49,50] However, changing Plan B from prescription to OTC status in the United States was a long and politically charged process. Following recommendations by respected reproductive health leaders[51,52] and endorsements by many professional organizations including the American College of Obstetricians and Gynecologists and the American Medical Association,[53] in December 2003 an FDA advisory committee voted 23 to 4 to approve a switch for Plan B from prescription to OTC. Unfortunately, despite this recommendation, the FDA rejected an OTC switch in May 2004 in unprecedented disregard for such an overwhelmingly positive advisory committee recommendation. LNG ECPs finally became available OTC in the United States with age restrictions beginning in August 2006. In August 2013, the age restriction was finally removed for Plan B One-Step. In most pharmacies, ECPs are now located on the shelf in the family planning aisle. Given concerns about potential shoplifting, some pharmacies choose to keep ECPs and other relatively expensive medications in a locked cabinet.

Two unintended, negative outcomes of OTC access to EC in the United States include an increase in price, from about $25 per treatment to about $45, coupled with a loss of insurance coverage for ECPs for most Americans whose drug insurance covers only prescription drugs. In addition, OTC access may reduce opportunities for physicians to counsel patients about use of more effective, longer-term contraceptive methods when they present for EC,[54] such as the copper IUD.

Cost Effectiveness

Studies based on economic models have shown that EC has the potential to be cost-effective by preventing unintended pregnancies, which are very costly. In the United States, placement of a copper T IUD is cost-saving as long as the IUC is used as an ongoing method of contraception for at least 4 months after emergency placement[55] and can provide continuous contraceptive protection for at least 12 years thereafter.[56] ECPs have also been shown to be cost effective, regardless of whether they are provided when needed or provided in advance of need.[57–64] However, all of the above studies have assumed that ECPs would actually be used after unprotected intercourse. Unfortunately, studies have not yet demonstrated that increasing access to ECPs reduces pregnancy or abortion rates at the population level. Although an ecological study from Chile reported an association between access to EC pills and lower rates of pregnancy, the study was unable to control for use of other contraceptives, which may have also varied between communities.[65] Therefore, while ECP are cost-effective when used by women seeking EC, at the population level, advance provision of ECPs is not cost effective, because women provided ECPs in advance of need use the ECPs so rarely.

MECHANISM OF ACTION

Copper-Releasing IUDs

When used as a regular or emergency method of contraception, copper IUDs act primarily to prevent fertilization. Emergency placement of a copper IUD is significantly more effective than use of ECPs, reducing the risk of pregnancy following unprotected intercourse by 99% (10 failures with 7,034 placements).[66] This very high level of effectiveness implies that emergency placement of a copper IUD must prevent some pregnancies after fertilization. The important point is that effectiveness and mechanism of action are not independent;[96] a regimen without a post-fertilization effect could not be 100% effective in typical populations, which inevitably include some users who take ECPs after ovulation, and potentially fertilization, have already occurred. (See Chapter 5 on IUDs.)

ECPs

The best available evidence indicates that LNG and UPA ECPs prevent pregnancy without any post-fertilization effects. ECPs—as with the birth control pill, patch, ring, shot, and implant,[67] and even breastfeeding[68]—prevent pregnancy primarily by delaying or inhibiting ovulation, thereby preventing fertilization. As there is no scientific method to test for fertilization, it is not possible to definitively rule out the possibility that any contraceptive methods, including breastfeeding, inhibit implantation of a fertilized egg in the endometrium.

ECPs do not cause abortion[69] or harm an established pregnancy, which begins with implantation, according to medical authorities such as the U.S. FDA, the National Institutes of Health[70] and the American College of Obstetricians and Gynecologists (ACOG).[71]

Ulipristal acetate (UPA). A number of studies have demonstrated that UPA can delay ovulation.[72–74] Timing of treatment can make a difference. In one study, 34 women were treated when the size of the leading follicle was 18 to 22 mm.[75] Each woman contributed one cycle treated with placebo and another with UPA. Follicular rupture failed to occur within 5 days following UPA treatment in 20 (59%) subjects while normal ovulation was observed in all women within 5 days after placebo intake. Follicular rupture failed to occur within 5 days after treatment with UPA in all women treated before onset of the luteinizing hormone (LH) surge, in 79% of women treated after the onset of the LH surge but before the LH peak, and in 8% of women treated after the LH peak. Another study was designed to assess whether UPA EC has similar efficacy when used before and after ovulation. The researchers measured pregnancy rates in women who took UPA within 120 hours of unprotected sex. The women were classified as pre-ovulatory or post-ovulatory based on several parameters, including serum LH, estradiol and progesterone levels, presence and size of a lead ovarian follicle >10 mm in mean diameter, and self-reported cycle length. Among women in the pre-ovulatory group, 77.6% of expected pregnancies were prevented, while in women who took UPA EC on the day of ovulation or after 36.4% of pregnancies were prevented. The pregnancy rate in the pre-ovulatory group was significantly lower than would be expected without the use of EC, while the rate in the post-ovulatory group was not different than would have been expected without any use of EC.[76] This result builds on earlier work suggesting that the primary mechanism of action of UPA EC is interference with ovulation. Other studies have focused on potential effects of UPA on the endometrium: one found that UPA altered the endometrium, but whether this change would inhibit implantation is unknown.[77] An in vitro study found that UPA, at the dosage used for EC, does not affect human embryo implantation process.[78] UPA does not impair sperm function.[79]

Levonorgestrel ECPs. LNG used as EC does not appear to interfere with implantation. Rather, early treatment with ECPs containing only the progestin LNG has been shown to impair the ovulatory process and luteal function.[80–84] No effect on the endometrium was found in two studies,[81,82] but in another study LNG taken before the LH surge altered the luteal phase secretory pattern of glycodelin in serum and the endometrium.[85] Glycodelin is a protein that the endometrium produces that reduces sperm capacitation and inhibits sperm egg binding.[86] However, two later studies explicitly designed to assess endometrial glycodelin expression found no alteration in the secretory pattern.[87,88] The second of these studies also found no effect on other endometrial receptivity biomarkers or progesterone receptors. In another study, LNG taken before the LH surge increased serum and intrauterine concentrations of glycodelin at the time of ovulation, implying the possibility of an additional mechanism of action of LNG in inhibiting sperm-egg binding.[89] LNG does not impair the attachment of human embryos to in vitro endometrial models and has no effect on the expression of endometrial receptivity markers.[90,91] In a study conducted more than 30 years ago, LNG was found to interfere with sperm migration and function, at all levels of the genital tract;[92] however, another study designed to assess this issue found that 1.5 mg LNG had no effect on the quality of cervical mucus, or on the penetration of spermatozoa in the uterine cavity,[87] and a recent study found an effect on sperm function only with much higher levels of LNG than are used for emergency contraception.[93]

The reduced efficacy of LNG ECP, after a delay in use, even when use is adjusted for cycle day of unprotected intercourse,[94] suggests that interference with implantation is likely not an effect of ECPs. If ECPs did prevent implantations, then delays in use should not reduce their efficacy as long as they are used before implantation.[95] Results of a simulation model demonstrated that, without a post-fertilization effect, the LNG regimen could not be effective when started after 96 hours, because with increasing delay, a greater proportion of women would be too near to ovulation.[96] Studies in the rat and the Cebus monkey demonstrate that LNG administered in doses that inhibit ovulation has no post-fertilization effect that impairs fertility.[97–99] However, the extent to which these results can be extrapolated to humans is unknown.

Croxatto and colleagues have argued that most, if not all, of the contraceptive effect of LNG ECPs can be explained by inhibited or dysfunctional ovulation, based on the existing animal and human studies, including two human studies comparing observed and expected pregnancies when LNG ECPs were administered before and after ovulation. In the first study, 0 pregnancies were observed when LNG ECPs were taken on or before the day of ovulation (in contrast to the 4 pregnancies that would have been expected without use of ECPs), whereas 3 pregnancies occurred when ECPs were taken after the day of ovulation (versus 3.5 expected pregnancies).[100] In a follow-up study, 0 pregnancies were observed when LNG ECPs were taken before the day of ovulation (in contrast to the 16 pregnancies that would have been expected without use of ECPs, whereas when ECPs were taken on or after the day of ovulation, 8 pregnancies occurred (versus 8.7 expected pregnancies).[101] While some find the existing human and animal studies adequate to conclude that ECPs have no post-fertilization effect,[101–103] others may feel that this question has not been answered until it is scientifically possible to determine whether fertilization has occurred prior to implantation.

Combined ECPs. Several clinical studies have shown that combined ECPs containing ethinyl estradiol and LNG can inhibit or delay ovulation.[104–107] This mechanism of action may explain the effectiveness of combined ECPs when used during the first half of the menstrual cycle, before ovulation has occurred. Some studies have shown histologic or biochemical alterations in the endometrium after treatment with the regimen, leading to the conclusion that combined ECPs may act by impairing endometrial receptivity to subsequent implantation of a fertilized egg.[105–110] However, other more recent studies have found no such effects on the endometrium.[104,111,112] Additional possible mechanisms include interference with corpus luteum function; thickening of the cervical mucus resulting in trapping of sperm; alterations in the tubal transport of sperm, egg, or embryo; and direct inhibition of fertilization.[97,113–115] No clinical data exist regarding direct inhibition of fertilization.

EFFECTIVENESS

Intrauterine Devices

More than 7,000 postcoital placements of copper-bearing IUDs have been reported in the literature since the practice was introduced in 1976. With only 10 known failures, this approach has a pregnancy rate of 0.1%.[66] In a review of this literature, IUDs were placed up to 7 days after unprotected intercourse (UPI) in three studies, up to 10 days after UPI in one study, and up to 10+ days after UPI in one study; there were 0 pregnancies. There was one pregnancy (0.1%) in one study in which IUDs were placed up to 5+ days after UPI. A reanalysis of Chinese data found 0 pregnancies in 52 women when the IUD was placed >5 days after UPI.[116] Recently, a study compared copper IUDs and oral LNG ECPs with concomitant placement of an LNG IUD;[117] more women in this study chose oral LNG EC plus LNG IUD (121 women) over the copper IUD (67 women) at the time of their visit. There were 0 pregnancies in the copper IUD group, and 1 pregnancy in the LNG group, which was determined to be an existing luteal phase pregnancy rather than a failure. For patients who need EC and wish to use a LNG IUD as their ongoing method of contraception, there is no need to delay IUD placement until patients report they have had no unprotected intercourse since their last menses. Studies are now underway to assess the efficacy of the LNG IUD as EC (without concomitant use of ECP).

ECPs

Using ECPs lowers the user's risk of pregnancy; however, the method's effectiveness may be lower than previously reported. The effectiveness of a preventive therapy is best measured by comparing the probability that the condition will occur if the therapy is used to the probability that it will occur without treatment. For many preventive therapies, effectiveness is determined by randomized clinical trials comparing treatment to a placebo. In the case of EC, however, efficacy was demonstrated initially by noncomparative observational studies, and, thereafter, use of a placebo was felt to be unethical. Therefore, the chance that pregnancy would occur in the absence of EC is estimated indirectly using published data on the probability of pregnancy on each day of the menstrual cycle.[118,119] This estimate is compared to the actual number of pregnancies observed after treatment in observational treatment trials. Effectiveness is calculated as 1-[O/E], where O and E are the observed and expected number of pregnancies, respectively.

Calculation of effectiveness involves many assumptions that are difficult to validate including accurate estimates of timing of intercourse and cycle day (which affects estimates of the timing of ovulation). One study compared self-report of cycle day with urinary pregnanediol concentrations to demonstrate that over 30% of women presenting for ECPs had inaccurately dated their own menstrual cycles, believing themselves to be in the fertile phase of their cycle when they were not.[120] Another study found that 99 women were between five days before and one day after the day of ovulation, which was estimated as usual cycle length minus 13 days. However, hormonal data indicated that only 51 of these 99 (56%) were in fact in this fertile window.[121] In another study, cervical smears showed that more than one-third of women requesting ECPs had no sperm present in the vagina, and those with sperm present had fewer sperm than women attempting to become pregnant.[122] Thus, the risk of pregnancy for users of ECPs appears to be lower than initially assumed in estimates of ECP efficacy, which are consequently likely to be overestimates. Yet, precise estimates of efficacy may not be highly relevant to many individuals who have had unprotected intercourse, since ECPs are often the only available treatment. A more important consideration for most ECP clients may be the fact that studies clearly show that both LNG and UPA ECPs are more effective than doing nothing.[123]

Ulipristal acetate. The antiprogestin UPA (30 mg in a single dose) is the most effective EC pill available in the United States, with reported estimates of effectiveness ranging from 62% to 85% risk reduction.[76,124–126] Two randomized trials compared the efficacy of LNG and UPA, one up to 72 hours after unprotected intercourse[125] and the second up to 120 hours after intercourse.[124] When these two studies were combined in a meta-analysis, the odds of pregnancy were 42% lower for UPA taken within 72 hours and 65% lower when taken within the first 24 hours.[124] In the second randomized study, UPA prevented significantly more pregnancies than did LNG in the 72 to 120 hour subgroup. The reason seems to be that UPA is more effective than LNG in postponing imminent ovulation. LNG is no more effective than a placebo in preventing ovulation when the leading follicle reaches 15-17 mm.[84] In contrast, by the time the follicle reaches 18 to 20 mm (which indicates that ovulation should occur within the next 48 hours) and the probability of conception without medication is >30%, UPA delayed ovulation for at least 5 days in 59% of cycles (versus 0% for the placebo).[72]

Mifepristone. Three randomized trials compared the efficacy of 1.5 mg LNG and 10 mg mifepristone for use as EC. Two trials found no significant difference in efficacy of the two-dose (0.75 mg each) LNG regimen and mifepristone; pregnancy rates for the two regimens were respectively 1.8% and 1.5% in the first trial[127] and 2.0% and 1.3% in the second.[128] The first trial also included a one-dose (1.5mg) LNG regimen, which yielded a pregnancy rate of 1.5%. An earlier trial showed a significant difference between pregnancy rates for the two-dose LNG regimen (3.1%) and the 10 mg mifepristone regimen (1.4%).[129] It is possible that the divergent results from this trial are due to differences in the study population as well as differences in the composition of the study drugs themselves, which were manufactured in China. A meta-analysis of 20 Chinese randomized trials found that a mid-dose (25 mg or 50 mg) of mifepristone had a lower failure rate than LNG; for the 13 trials that reported side effects, mifepristone was more tolerable but the delay in menses was greater for mifepristone.[3] A meta-analysis of 11 randomized trials (9 Chinese, 1 United Kingdom[128] and one multinational[127]) found that low dose (<25mg) mifepristone was more effective than LNG, but when only the 4 high-quality studies were included, mifepristone was not superior.[3] Another Chinese trial found that the antiprogestin gestrinone was as effective as 10 mg mifepristone.[130] As yet, mifepristone has not been directly compared to UPA for EC.

Progestin-only (LNG) and combined regimens. Twelve studies of the LNG regimen, which together included more than 13,500 women, reported estimates of effectiveness between 52% and 100%; that is, this regimen reduced the chance of pregnancy by that amount.[127–136] A meta-analysis of eight studies of the combined regimen, which in total included more than 3,800 women, concluded that the regimen prevents about 74% of expected pregnancies; the proportion ranged from 56% to 89% in the different studies.[137] A more recent analysis using possibly improved methodology found effectiveness rates of 53% and 47% in two of the largest trials of the combined regimen.[138] Combined data from two randomized trials that directly compared the LNG and combined regimens showed a relative risk of pregnancy of 0.51 (95% confidence limits 0.31, 0.83), indicating that the chance of pregnancy among women who received the LNG regimen was about half the chance among those who received the combined regimen.[123,133,134] This estimate makes *no* assumption about the number of pregnancies that would have been observed in the absence of treatment. The results imply that (1) if the Yuzpe regimen is completely inefficacious, then the LNG regimen has an efficacy of 49% and (2) for every additional 2 percentage points of efficacy of the Yuzpe regimen, 1 percentage point of efficacy is added to the LNG regimen.

Studies have shown that a single dose of 1.5 mg LNG is as effective as (and causes no more side effects than) taking two 0.75 mg doses 12 hours apart.[127,131] Another study found that two 0.75 mg doses taken 24 hours apart were just as effective as two 0.75 mg doses taken 12 hours apart.[132] A pilot study of 41 women found that adding a COX-2 inhibitor (meloxicam 15 mg) to 1.5 mg LNG significantly increased the proportion of cycles with no follicular rupture or with ovulatory dysfunction (88% vs. 66%, $p = 0.012$), and that COX-2 inhibitors can disturb the ovulatory process after the onset of the LH surge.[139]

Treatment delay. Several studies have indicated that both the combined and LNG regimens are more effective the sooner after sex the pills are taken.[8,94,127,131,134,135,140] Other studies have not found that delays in use have this effect,[4,125,128,129,132,133,141–143] although sample sizes were often small. The initial studies showed that these regimens are effective when used up to 72 hours after intercourse.[134,144] Consequently, U.S. product package instructions for LNG ECPs advise use only within that time frame. Recent studies indicate that the regimens continue to be moderately effective if started between 72 and 120 hours.[127,132,135,142,143] However, a pooled analysis of four WHO trials of the LNG regimen shows no decline in efficacy until day 5, when it may offer no protection at all.[145] Analysis of the pooled data from the two Phase III trials of UPA showed no statistically significant effect of treatment delay (0 to 24 hours, 25 to 48 hours, 49 to 72 hours, 73 to 96 hours, 97 to 120 hours) on pregnancy rates ($p = 0.91$).[146] No data are available establishing efficacy if ECPs are taken more than 120 hours after intercourse.

Body Mass Index (BMI). Analysis of data from the two randomized trials of the UPA and LNG regimens found that heavier women taking ECP had a significantly higher risk of pregnancy than did thinner women. In fact, women were as likely to experience a pregnancy as those who had taken no ECP, if they had a BMI of ≥26 and took LNG EC, or a BMI≥35 and took UPA.[147] The label for NorLevo (1.5 mg LNG) in Europe was changed in November 2013 to reflect additional analyses of these data; the label stated: "In clinical trials, contraceptive efficacy was reduced in women weighing 75 kg or more and LNG was not effective in women who weighed more than 80 kg."[148] However, the European Medicines Agency, after reviewing additional data from three WHO trials[127,134,135] that did not find reduced efficacy with increasing weight or BMI, removed that statement from the Norlevo label in July 2014.[149] In May 2016, the U.S. FDA similarly announced that the evidence was too limited to merit a label change, and encouraged EC manufacturers to further study the relationship between obesity and the effectiveness of ECP.[150] WHO recently published a report with data from four studies (the three above plus one more) that did find a higher failure rate for obese women, but only after controlling for other factors in a regression model. It is notable that there was no effect of weight in contrast to BMI; the rate was not higher among women weighing >80 kg.[151]

This issue remains an active area of pharmacokinetic research: one recent study found that the serum concentration of LNG 1.5 mg was about 50% lower in obese women compared with normal-BMI women.[152] The same study found that doubling the dose of LNG EC (from 1.5 mg to 3.0 mg) appeared to produce serum concentration levels similar to those in normal-BMI women who had taken the regular dose (1.5 mg). This is a small pharmacokinetic study that did not measure endpoints more directly related to effectiveness (ovulation or pregnancy), but it suggests that obesity does affect the bioavailability of LNG EC. Another pharmacokinetic study (involving 32 women) similarly found that 24 hours after the women ingested LNG, serum concentration levels were 50% lower among obese women.[153] Following use of UPA, however, blood levels were similar among obese and normal-BMI women. The effect of weight on the efficacy of combined ECPs has not been studied. When acceptable, the copper IUD is always the most effective option for EC, especially for patients who are obese. Recent U.K. EC guidelines state that when a copper IUD is not indicated or acceptable, and UPA is not available or acceptable "Consider double-dose (3 mg) LNG if BMI >26 kg/m2 or weight >70 kg."[154]

Repeated Use Repeated use of ECPs is far less effective than most other contraceptive methods. For a typical individual who repeatedly used LNG ECPs, the chance of pregnancy after 1 year would be 20%.[155] In a recent study of women with infrequent intercourse (up to six times a month) using LNG ECPs, the pregnancy rate was 11 per 100 women-years.[156]

Population Impact of ECPs Only one[39] of 15 published studies has demonstrated that increasing access to ECPs reduces pregnancy or abortion rates,[157,158] although one demonstration project[159] and four clinical trials[39–42] were specifically designed to address this issue. One explanation for this result is that even when provided with ECPs in advance of need, most individuals use ECPs too rarely after unprotected sex to result in a substantial population impact. In the San Francisco trial, 45% of the women in the advance provision group who had unprotected intercourse during the study period did not use ECPs.[40] In the Nevada/North Carolina trial, 33% of women in the advance provision group had unprotected intercourse at least once without using ECPs[42]. In this trial, increased access to EC increased use of ECPs most among women who were at lower baseline risk of pregnancy.[160] This may explain in part why increased access to EC has increased use of EC without measurable effect on pregnancy rates in clinical trials. The single exception occurred among women using the lactational amenorrhea method in Egypt.[39] Those in the advance provision group had a lower pregnancy rate (0.8% versus 5.0%, $p = 0.0002$) in the first six months postpartum, but the reason is that these women were far more likely to start using an ongoing contraceptive; the authors argue that using ECPs allowed the women time to get to a clinic for ongoing contraception.

Reproductive Coercion and Emergency Contraception

For some individuals, such as those facing reproductive coercion, repeated use of ECPs may be the best pregnancy prevention strategy they are aware of, or the one they feel best suits their needs.[161] Thus, patients identified as repeatedly using ECPs should not be condemned, but rather compassionately screened for contraceptive challenges. For those facing reproductive coercion, a copper IUD with the strings trimmed so they don't exit the cervix is often an ideal option, as it offers long-term, highly effective contraception, without menstrual changes or the need to store contraceptive supplies at home.

ADVANTAGES AND INDICATIONS

Emergency contraceptives can prevent pregnancy after unprotected sexual intercourse or after a contraceptive "accident." This makes EC an essential part of treatment following sexual assault.[162] EC may also be appropriate in the following circumstances:[69,163]

- No contraceptive was used at the time of intercourse.
- A male condom slipped, broke, or leaked.
- A female condom, diaphragm, or cervical cap was placed incorrectly, dislodged during intercourse, removed too early, or found to be torn.
- A patient missed too many combined oral contraceptive pills (e.g. 3+ consecutive pills containing 0.03 to 0.035 mg ethinyl estradiol or 2+ consecutive pills containing 0.02 mg or less ethinyl estradiol). Note: Missed pills during the first week of a pill pack pose the greatest risk of pregnancy.

- A breastfeeding patient is incompletely protected by lactational amenorrhea (because menses have returned, or baby has received feedings other than breast milk).
- Contraceptive use was delayed:
  - 3 or more hours late for a progestin-only pill.
  - More than 14 days late for a Depo-Provera injection.
  - 2 or more days late starting a new vaginal ring cycle.
  - 2 or more days late starting a new patch cycle.
- A female condom was placed or removed incorrectly leading to spillage of semen, or the penis was inserted mistakenly between the female condom and the vaginal wall resulting in intravaginal ejaculation.
- An attempt at coitus interruptus resulted in ejaculation in the vagina or on external genitalia.
- A couple, attempting to practice periodic abstinence, inadvertently had intercourse on a fertile day of the cycle.
- A patient cannot feel the IUD string, or the IUD was removed less than 7 days after the last act of intercourse.
- A patient was exposed to a possible teratogen such as Zika virus or isotretinoin when not protected by effective contraception.

The copper IUD may be an especially useful option for patients who present 4 or 5 days after unprotected intercourse, because it provides extremely high emergency contraceptive efficacy for at least 5 days after intercourse, and it is an excellent choice for those who wish to continue using an IUD as a long-term method of contraception.

Side Effects

Copper-Releasing IUD

Side effects after emergency placement of an IUD are similar to those seen after routine placement and may include abdominal discomfort and vaginal bleeding or spotting. (See Chapter 5 on IUDs.)

ECPs

Nausea and vomiting. These side effects affect about 13% to 29% of patients treated with either LNG or UPA ECPs;[124,125] the incidence of nausea was significantly higher with UPA than LNG in one randomized trial[125] but not in the other.[124] In contrast, following treatment with combined estrogen-progestin ECPs, nausea occurs in about 50% of women, and vomiting in about 20%. Other reported complaints include fatigue, breast tenderness, headache, lower abdominal pain, dizziness, and diarrhea. Side effects are similar for the LNG and UPA regimens.[124,125] Side effects subside within a day or two after treatment is completed. Routine use of the anti-nausea medication meclizine 1 hour before the first ECP dose may help reduce nausea and vomiting,[164] but is generally unnecessary with use of either LNG or UPA ECPs.

There is no research to indicate whether it is necessary to repeat the ECP dose if vomiting occurs within 2 hours after taking ECPs. Some practitioners take the view that a replacement dose should be given orally, or vaginally to prevent the tablets from being vomited a second time. Other providers, believing that nausea and vomiting are evidence of hormonal effects on the central nervous system and thus of absorption of the drugs, conclude that a replacement dose is not necessary unless an ECP tablet is visible in the vomitus.

Effects on future fertility and inadvertently exposed pregnancies. There is no evidence that ECPs have any long-term or adverse effects on fertility. One study of 332 pregnant women who had used LNG ECPs in the conception cycle found no increased risk of birth defects.[165] Combined data from post-marketing surveillance and clinical trials of UPA found no teratogenic effects among 232 pregnancies with a known outcome in which the woman and conceptus were exposed to UPA.[166] Moreover, two observations provide reassurance for any concern about birth defects.[113] First, in the event of treatment failure, ECPs are taken long before organogenesis starts so, they should not have a teratogenic effect. Second, studies that have examined births to individuals who inadvertently continued to take combined oral contraceptives (including high-dose formulations) without knowing they were pregnant have found no increased risk of birth defects.[167–169] For this reason, the FDA removed warnings about adverse effects of combined oral contraceptives on the fetus from contraceptive package inserts years ago.[170]

Available evidence suggests that ECPs do not increase the chance that a pregnancy following ECP use will be ectopic; moreover, like all contraceptive methods, ECPs reduce the absolute risk of ectopic pregnancy by preventing ovulation, and thus pregnancy.[171,172] However, ectopic pregnancy can occur following ECP treatment, and it is important to keep this possibility in mind whenever a treatment failure occurs.

Menstrual changes. Three studies have been specifically designed to assess the effects of LNG ECPs on bleeding patterns. Outcomes examined included length of the treatment and post-treatment cycles (where the first day of bleeding is cycle day 1), duration of bleeding during the menstrual period, and unscheduled bleeding. All three found that the length of the menstrual cycle can be shortened when treatment occurs early in the cycle.

The first study found that when taken in the first 3 weeks of the cycle, 1.5 mg LNG in a single dose significantly shortened that cycle as compared both to the usual cycle length and to the cycle length in a comparison group of similar women who had not taken ECPs. The magnitude of this effect was greater the earlier the pills were taken. However, when this regimen was taken later in women's cycles it had no effect on cycle length, but it did cause prolongation of bleeding during the next menstrual period. The ECPs had no effect on the length of the post-treatment cycle, but bleeding during the second period was prolonged. Unscheduled bleeding was uncommon after ECP use, although more common than among women who had not taken ECPs.[173]

The second study compared the baseline cycle with the treatment and post-treatment cycles when 1.5 mg LNG was administered in a single dose. Cycle length was significantly shortened by 1 day when ECPs were taken in the preovulatory phase of the cycle and was significantly lengthened by 2 days when ECPs were taken in the postovulatory phase. No difference in cycle length was observed for women who took ECPs during the periovulatory phase of the cycle (from 2 days before to 2 days after the expected day of ovulation). In both the treatment and post-treatment cycles, the duration of bleeding during the menstrual period increased significantly when ECPs were taken in the periovulatory or postovulatory phase. The length of the post-treatment cycle remained significantly longer when ECPs were taken in the postovulatory phase. During the treatment cycle, 15% of women experienced unscheduled bleeding; this was significantly more common when ECPs were taken in the preovulatory phase.[174]

The third study examined the effects of two 0.75 mg LNG pills taken 12 hours apart.[175] When taken in the follicular phase, ECPs significantly shortened the cycle when compared with usual cycle length; no effect on cycle length was found when ECPs were taken in the periovulatory or luteal phase. The post-treatment cycle length was the same as the usual cycle length.

Cautions

There are no contraindications to the use of any ECPs, with the exception of pregnancy.[176] In the United States, the labeling for LNG and UPA ECPs includes only one contraindication: known or suspected pregnancy. The reason ECPs should not be used in pregnancy is not because they are harmful, but because they are ineffective. The advantages of ECP use generally outweigh the risks even in the presence of one or more contraindications to the ongoing use of estrogen-containing contraceptives, such as vascular disease or migraine with aura. In such cases, use of UPA or LNG only ECPs, however, is preferable to use of combined estrogen-progestin ECPs.

Few adverse events have been reported for individuals using EC. The Committee on Safety of Medicines in the United Kingdom reviewed all problems reported during the first 13 years of use of the combination estrogen-progestin ECP product (called PC4) available in the United Kingdom. Among 4 million uses, the review found 61 pregnancies, 3 cases of venous thrombosis (including 1 death), and 3 cases of cerebrovascular disorder. The Committee concluded that none of the 6 vascular cases could be definitely linked to ECP use because of the significant delay between ECP use and the onset of symptoms.[113]

Breastfeeding. During the first 6 months postpartum, individuals who are exclusively breastfeeding and amenorrheic have little risk of pregnancy. There are no restrictions on use of any ECPs based on breastfeeding status.[176] One study has examined LNG pharmacokinetics in plasma and milk of lactating women who take 1.5 mg for EC. The authors conclude that to limit infant exposure to the period of maximum LNG excretion in milk, mothers may consider avoiding nursing for 8 hours after they take ECP;[177] however, the U.S. Medical Eligibility Criteria for Contraceptive Use (U.S. MEC) recommends no change in breastfeeding patterns. One study compared outcomes among women who took LNG ECPs (after a breastfeed) and among women who used progestin-only oral contraceptives; no adverse effects were noted on maternal or infant health or continued lactation among the women who took ECPs.[178] The label for ella states "It is not known if UPA is excreted in human milk. However, UPA is detected in milk of lactating rats. Because many drugs are excreted in human milk, risk to the breast-fed child cannot be excluded. Use of ella by breastfeeding women is not recommended."[179] However, the U.S. Medical Eligibility Criteria for Contraceptive Use states that there is no restriction on use of ella by breastfeeding women but recommends that breastfeeding women refrain from breastfeeding and discard pumped milk for 24 hours.[176]

Drug interactions. Although medications that induce hepatic enzymes (such as phenytoin, rifampin, or efavirenz) could theoretically reduce the effectiveness of ECPs, whether such medications reduce the effectiveness of ECPs has not been directly studied. Nonetheless, caution is warranted, and patients taking such medications should be offered prompt access to placement of a copper IUD. Recent U.K. EC Guidelines suggest "consider double-dose (3 mg) LNG if taking an enzyme inducer," but studies have not been conducted to inform this recommendation. Similarly, there is no clear guidance available regarding adjustment of dosing UPA for women taking hepatic enzyme inducing agents.[154] No significant interactions have been found with concurrent use of ECP and most antibiotics (see Chapter 8 on Combined Oral Contraceptives).

UPA is an antiprogestin. Therefore there are implications for immediately starting progestin-containing contraceptives after taking UPA (or using UPA after recently taking a progestin). One randomized double-blind placebo controlled study found no difference in the time (14 days) to achieve ovarian quiescence after taking UPA and starting a daily pill between the placebo group and the group who took a combined oral contraceptive starting the day after taking UPA.[180] A second randomized cross-over study examined women who quick-started a desogestrel progestin-only oral contraceptive (75 mcg desogestrel, not available in the US) after taking UPA or a placebo,[181] and found that initiating desogestrel the day after UPA significantly reduced UPA's ability to delay ovulation, from 97% to 55%. However, no significant differences were found in time to ovarian quiescence or cervical mucus penetrability with continued use of desogestrel. The FDA updated the ella package label to include warnings regarding the coadministration of ella and hormonal contraception. The label now states that if a patient wishes to use hormonal contraception after using ella, the ongoing method should be initiated no sooner than 5 days after taking ella, and that a reliable barrier method should be used until the next menstrual period. The label also now states that because ella and the progestin component of hormonal contraceptives both bind to the progesterone receptor, using them together may impair the ability of ella to delay ovulation. Although further research is needed on the effects of taking hormonal contraception within 5 days of ella, some researchers and providers endorse a more flexible protocol for providing ongoing contraception after EC as shown in Figure 10-2.

Eligibility criteria and contraindications for emergency placement of an IUD are the same as for all IUD placements. (See Chapter 5 on IUDs.) If concern exists about sexually transmitted infection (STI) (e.g. after unprotected intercourse with a new sexual partner or sexual assault), testing for STIs should occur at the time of IUD placement; if clinical suspicion of STI is high, empiric antibiotics may be given. Patients who are found to harbor an STI after an IUD has been placed can be effectively treated with antibiotics with the IUD in place.

Providing Emergency Contraception

Although pregnancy can result from intercourse only during the fertile phase of the menstrual cycle, anyone requesting EC within 120 hours of unprotected intercourse should be offered treatment.[124,127,132,142,143]

It is important to remember that determining pregnancy risk is rarely straightforward. Although the probability of conception is low except for the 5 days just before ovulation and on the day of ovulation (see Figure 10-1, graph 1),[182] neither the patient nor the clinician is likely to actually know

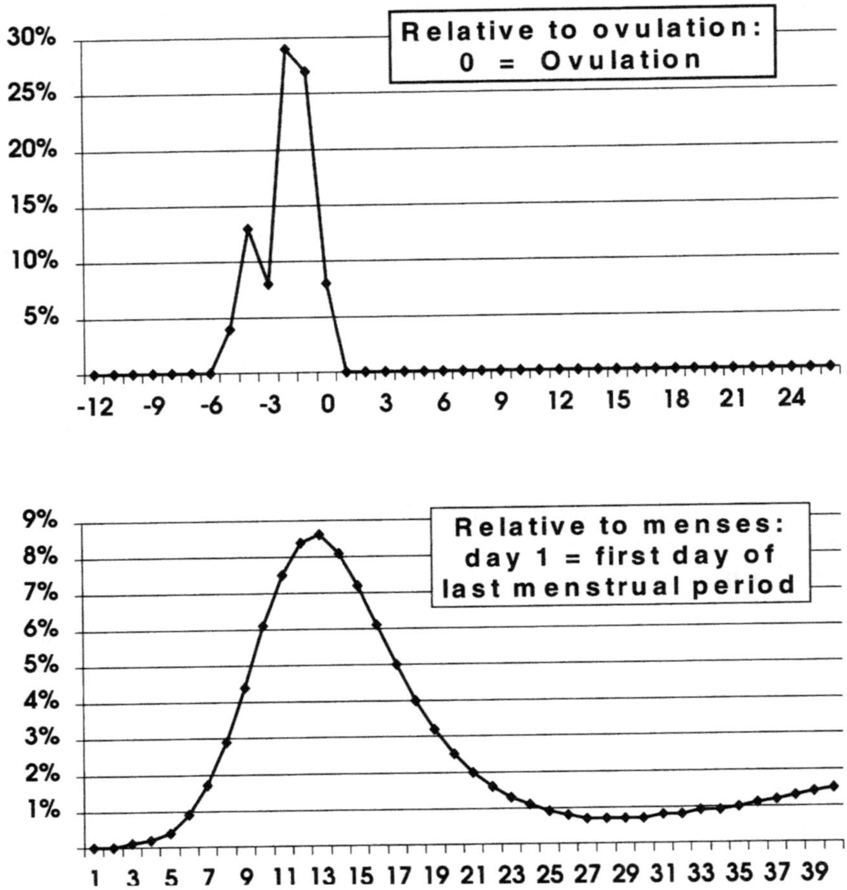

Source: Adapted from Wilcox et al. (2001)[182]

Figure 10-1 Pregnancy probability by cycle day

which day ovulation occurs. What may be known is prior menstrual period dates. Plotting the probability of pregnancy versus menstrual period dates (see Figure 10-1, graph 2) shows that late (or early) ovulation is common enough that pregnancy risk is above 1% beginning as early as cycle day 7 and continuing until at least day 39.[182]

Counseling

In counseling patients who seek emergency contraceptive treatment, remember that those in need of EC are often facing a difficult and stressful situation. Be respectful of such patients and responsive to their needs.

Patients may feel embarrassed about failing to use regular contraception effectively. Rape survivors may feel traumatized. Patients may be very concerned about possible infection, especially in cases of rape. Counsel patients and provide STI diagnostic services (or referrals) and information about preventive measures. If appropriate, explain reporting requirements regarding statutory rape. Be as supportive as possible of the patient's choices and refrain from making judgmental comments or indicating disapproval through body language or facial expressions. Supportive attitudes will help improve adherence to contraceptive plans and set the stage for effective follow-up counseling about regular contraceptive use and STI prevention. (See Chapter 2 on patient-centered counseling.) Everyone must understand that EC offers no protection against STIs, including infection with the human immunodeficiency virus (HIV). Therefore, post-exposure HIV prophylaxis, and emergency treatment of other infections, may also be needed. (See Chapter 20 on Reproductive Tract Infections, Including HIV/AIDS.)

Patients who would not have an abortion if EC treatment fails can be reassured that pregnancies occurring despite EC treatment do not have an increased risk of birth defects or other adverse outcomes.

Frequent use. Emphasize that ECPs are less effective than other contraceptives. However, repeated use of combined or LNG ECPs is not known to pose health risks to users other than pregnancy. The label for ella states that "Repeated use of ella within the same menstrual cycle is not recommended, as safety and efficacy of repeat use within the same cycle has not been evaluated."[179] However, a pharmacodynamic study of repeated use of UPA EC (every 7 days for 8 weeks) showed no safety concerns, indicating that UPA can be safely used more than once per cycle. However, the same study found that the majority of women in a smaller subgroup ovulated at least once during this period, suggesting that this may not be an effective longer-term method.[183]

Use after 72 hours. Although most studies of ECP treatment have specified that treatment be administered within 72 hours, more recent studies have demonstrated the efficacy of ECPs up to 120 hours after unprotected intercourse.[127,132,142,143] However, a re-analysis of WHO studies concluded that LNG might not be effective at all after 96 hours.[145] Nonetheless, ella is labeled for use up to 120 hours after intercourse.[124,126,179] The copper IUD remains the most effective form of EC, even when placed more than a week after unprotected intercourse.

Use after multiple acts of unprotected intercourse. If more than 120 hours have elapsed since the time of the first unprotected act of intercourse, ECPs may be less effective in preventing pregnancy that resulted from that first exposure. Providing ECPs, however, would not be expected to disrupt or harm subsequent pregnancy development and would reduce the risk that pregnancy would result from later acts of intercourse that occurred within the preceding 120 hours.

Ongoing contraception. Patients requesting EC should be offered information and services for regular contraception. However, not everyone will want extensive contraceptive counseling or feel able to use other contraceptives. Thus, while counseling about regular contraceptives is recommended, adoption of a regular method of contraception should not be a prerequisite for providing EC. If the reason for requesting EC is that the regular contraceptive method failed, discuss reasons for failure and how this might be prevented in the future. Note that, given the interactions between UPA and progestin-containing contraceptives, some suggest waiting 5 days after UPA to start a progestin-containing contraceptive, while others endorse the protocol shown in Figure 10-2.

Preferred ongoing contraceptive	Prefers this EC*	Start ongoing method	Back up method needed after starting routine method**
Condoms, barrier, or behavioral method	UPA or LNG	Same day	None
Combined pills, patch, or ring	UPA	At least one day after UPA and 5+ days after last UPI	7 days
	LNG ****	Same day	7 days
Progestin only pill	UPA	At least one day after UPA and 5+ days after last UPI	2 days
	LNG ****	Same day	2 days
DMPA shot	UPA	At least one day after UPA and 5+ days after last UPI	7 days
	LNG ****	Same day	7 days
LNG IUD*** *	UPA	At least one day after UPA and 5+ days after last UPI	7 days
	LNG ****	Same day	7 days
Copper IUD*** *	Copper IUD ****	Same day	None
Implant	UPA	At least one day after UPA and 5+ days after last UPI	7 days
	LNG ****	Same day	7 days

UPI = unprotected intercourse

*Preferences for EC pills are often shaped by cost, availability, and the potential effects of their weight/BMI on the effectiveness of LNG and UPA EC pills

**Need to abstain or use a condom between taking ECP and starting routine method

***Consider double-dose (3 mg) LNG if BMI >26 kg/m2 or weight >70 kg or if taking an enzyme inducing medication

****If reasonably certain the patient is not pregnant (see Chapter 5 on IUDs.)

Source: Derived from American Society for Emergency Contraception (2016)[185]

Figure 10-2. Guidance for EC users, by preference for ongoing contraception

Before Providing Emergency Contraceptive Treatment

Make certain the patient does not want to become pregnant and understands there is still a chance of pregnancy after treatment. Describe common side effects; advance counseling about possible side effects helps patients know what to expect and may lead to greater tolerance. If the patient has no option but to use a combined estrogen-progestin ECP option, consider offering 50 mg meclizine 1 hour before starting ECP treatment.[155]

A pregnancy test may be helpful if there is some doubt about whether the patient may have become pregnant after previous episodes of unprotected sex earlier in the month. If this is not the case, pregnancy testing is unnecessary. If the patient is pregnant, ECP treatment will not be effective. Those with negative pregnancy tests can use ECPs to reduce their risk of becoming pregnant. Patients who do not have a period within 3 weeks of taking ECPs should be instructed to take a pregnancy test to see if they have become pregnant.[184]

Make sure patients understand that ECPs will not protect them from pregnancy if they engage in unprotected intercourse in the days or weeks following treatment. Because ECPs, especially UPA, can delay ovulation, a patient could be at risk of pregnancy if unprotected intercourse occurs within the first few days of ECP treatment. Individuals using LNG ECPs can start an ongoing hormonal method immediately, but those who use UPA should wait to start an ongoing method for 5 days after the last episode of unprotected sex before starting or resuming a hormonal method. Anyone who needs EC because of missed or late pills, patch or ring should be advised to consider a copper IUD or use LNG EC, and then resume their method. Patients who would like to start ongoing contraception should be counseled to determine the most appropriate EC method, taking into consideration which ongoing method they would like to use, and whether they are at greater risk of pregnancy from the previous act of intercourse or future acts of intercourse. The American Society for Emergency Contraception offers a flexible algorithm for providing EC for patients who want to begin or resume an ongoing contraceptive method, taking into account these complex factors (see Figure 10-2).[185] EC users should abstain from intercourse or use a barrier method of contraception for seven days after taking LNG or UPA.

EC Treatment Regimens

ECPs. For maximum effectiveness, ECP treatment should be started as soon as possible after unprotected intercourse, and within 120 hours. Treatment with UPA (one 30 mg tablet) is the most effective ECP option. LNG ECP treatment (1.5mg LNG tablet) is more effective and causes significantly less nausea and vomiting than treatment with combined estrogen-progestin ECP options (e.g., 0.1 to 0.12 mg ethinyl estradiol and 0.5 to 0.6 mg LNG in each dose).

Combined estrogen-progestin treatment involves two doses taken 12 hours apart. If necessary, adjust the timing for the second dose by a few hours to avoid a middle-of-the-night dose. Drugs and doses are shown in Table 10-1.

Intrauterine devices. Implantation occurs 6 to 12 days following ovulation.[186] Therefore, a copper IUD can be provided as a method of EC up to 5 days after ovulation. Thus, in the case of unprotected intercourse 3 days before the day ovulation is estimated to have occurred, the IUD could, in principle, be placed up to 8 days after intercourse. Most family planning providers, however, limit placement to the first 5 days after intercourse because it is difficult to reliably estimate the day of ovulation. If emergency IUD placement is planned, but cannot be carried out immediately, provide ECP treatment right away. If possible, UPA should be offered, because it is the most effective ECP, especially if the interval since unprotected intercourse is longer than 72 hours. However, even if UPA is not available, LNG ECPs should still be used, as they may help reduce the risk of pregnancy.

After Providing EC Treatment

Review all available contraceptive options, highlighting the potential benefits of using a highly effective reversible method such as an IUD or implant. If the patient wishes to continue to use a previously selected method of routine contraception, no follow-up is needed unless a normal menstrual period does not occur within 3 weeks, the patient suspects pregnancy, or if there are other reasons for concern. If there is any concern of pregnancy, perform a pregnancy test.

If EC has failed and the patient is pregnant, provide appropriate services or referrals. Recent use of UPA does not preclude subsequent use of mifepristone as needed to end an undesired pregnancy. For patients who decide to continue the pregnancy, reassure them that there is no evidence of any teratogenic effect following the use of ECPs. Pregnancy following emergency placement of a copper IUD should be managed with prompt counseling about and a discussion of the pros and cons of immediately removing the IUD. (See Chapter 5 on IUDs.)

Advance Prescription of ella

Provide a prescription in advance of need to interested patients for use when needed in the coming year. Alternatively, those who need EC can order ella online (with overnight delivery in the United States) from Prjkt Ruby (www.prjktruby.com/emergency-contraception).

Additional Information and Materials

Additional information and materials are available from the following sources:

- The Office of Population Research at Princeton University and the Association of Reproductive Health Professionals maintain the Emergency Contraception Website (www.not-2-late.com or ec.princeton.edu). Detailed information about EC is available on this website, which now receives more than 750,000 visitors each month. The website is completely confidential, available 24 hours a day, and offers names and telephone numbers of providers of EC located near the user's zip code. The website is available in English, Spanish, and Arabic.
- The American Society for Emergency Contraception (www.americansocietyforec.org) offers clinical guidance about EC and information about EC access in the United States.
- ACOG Practice Bulletin No. 152: Emergency Contraception. *Obstet Gynecol* 2015;126:e1-e11.

INSTRUCTIONS FOR USING EC*

ECP users should receive medication labeling that identifies the specific product prescribed and the number of tablets needed for each dose (see Table 10-1). Give the following instructions to ensure correct use.

1. **Take your ECP as directed:**
   a. **ella.** Swallow the tablet as soon as possible within 120 hours after unprotected sex. Taking more pills will not make you less likely to become pregnant; taking in combination with LNG ECP will paradoxically increase your risk of pregnancy.
   b. **LNG ECPs.** Swallow the one *Plan B One-Step* pill (or generic equivalent such as *My Way, Take Action or Aftera)* as soon as possible within 120 hours after unprotected sex. Taking more pills will not make you less likely to become pregnant.
   c. **Combined estrogen-progestin ECPs.** Swallow the first dose as soon as possible within 120 hours after unprotected sex. Do not take any extra pills. Taking more pills will not make you less likely to become pregnant but may make you more nauseated and cause vomiting. Swallow the second dose 12 hours after taking the first dose. If necessary, you can delay the second dose by a few hours to avoid having to take your second dose in the middle of the night.

*These instructions are intended to guide providers in educating patients in how to use emergency contraceptive methods.

Consider taking anti-nausea medication (two 25 mg tablets of meclizine) 1 hour before the first dose. About one half of those who use combined ECPs have temporary nausea. It is usually mild and should stop in a day or so. If you vomit within 2 hours after taking a dose, call your clinician. You may need to repeat a dose of ECP.

2. **If your period does not start within 3 weeks, take a pregnancy test and/or see your clinician.** Your next period may start a few days earlier or later than usual. If you think you may be pregnant, see your clinician as soon as possible, whether or not you plan to continue the pregnancy.
3. **Do not have intercourse without a condom until you are protected by another method of birth control (most hormonal contraception must be taken for a week before it protects you).** ECPs will not protect you from more than one episode of unprotected intercourse. See Figure 10-2 for guidance on when hormonal contraception can be started and how long back-up contraception (barrier method) or abstinence is required.
4. **Discuss with your clinician which birth control method may work best for you over the long term and when you can start it.**

Instructions for patients who have emergency placement of an IUD are the same as for anyone who has an IUD placed (see Chapter 5 on IUDs).

Author Disclosures—Trussell: none. Cleland: none. Schwarz: none.

References

1. Consensus statement on emergency contraception. Contraception 1995;52:211–3.
2. Trussell J, Ellertson C. Efficacy of emergency contraception. Fertility Control Reviews 1995;4:8–11.
3. Shen J, Che Y, Showell E, Chen K, Cheng L. Interventions for emergency contraception. Cochrane Database Syst Rev 2017, Issue 7.
4. Ellertson C, Webb A, Blanchard K, Bigrigg A, Haskell S, Shochet T, Trussell J. Modifying the Yuzpe regimen of emergency contraception: a multi-center randomized, controlled trial. Obstet Gynecol 2003;101:1160–7.
5. Van Look PF, von Hertzen H. Clinical uses of antiprogestogens. Hum Reprod Update 1995;1:19–34.
6. Glasier A, Thong KJ, Dewar M, Mackie M, Baird DT. Mifepristone (RU 486) compared with high-dose estrogen and progestogen for emergency postcoital contraception. N Engl J Med 1992;327:1041–4.
7. Webb AM, Russell J, Elstein M. Comparison of Yuzpe regimen, danazol, and mifepristone (RU486) in oral postcoital contraception. BMJ (Clinical Research Ed.) 1992;305:927–31.
8. Ashok PW, Stalder C, Wagaarachchi PT, Flett GM, Melvin L, Templeton A. A randomised study comparing a low dose of mifepristone and the Yuzpe regimen for emergency contraception. BJOG 2002;109:553–60.

9. Hester KE, Harper MJK, Duffy DM. Oral administration of the cyclooxygenase-2 (COX-2) inhibitor meloxicam blocks ovulation in non-human primates when administered to simulate emergency contraception. Hum Reprod 2010;25:360–7.
10. Jesam C, Salvatierra AM, Schwartz JL, Croxatto HB. Suppression of follicular rupture with meloxicam, a cyclooxygenase-2 inhibitor: potential for emergency contraception. Hum Reprod 2010;25:368–73.
11. Edelman AB, Jensen JT, Doom C, Hennebold JD. Impact of the prostaglandin synthase-2 inhibitor celecoxib on ovulation and luteal events in women. Contraception 2013;87:352–7.
12. Morris JM, Van Wagenen G. Postcoital oral contraception. In: Hankinson R, Kleinman R, Esckstein P, Romero H, (eds). Proceedings of the Eighth International Conference of the International Planned Parenthood Federation: 1967 Apr 9–15; Santiago, Chile. London: International Planned Parenthood Federation; 1967.
13. Van Look F. Postcoital contraception: a cover-up story. In: Diczfalusy E, Bygdeman M, (eds). Fertility regulation today and tomorrow. Serono symposia publications; vol 36. New York: Raven Press, 1987.
14. Zuliani G, Colombo UF, Molla R. Hormonal postcoital contraception with an ethinylestradiol-norgestrel combination and two danazol regimens. Europ J Obstet Gynecol Reprod Biology 1990;37:253–60.
15. National Center for Health Statistics. Special tabulation. Available at: Available at: www.cdc.gov/nchs/nsfg/key_statistics/e.htm
16. Batur P, Cleland K, McNamara M, Wu J, Pickle S, EC Survey Group. Emergency contraception: A multispecialty survey of clinician knowledge and practices. Contraception 2016;93:145–52.
17. Patel A, Tilmon S, Bhogireddy V, Chor J, Patel D, Keith L. Emergency contraception after sexual assault: changes in provision from 2004 to 2009. J Reprod Med 2012;57:98–104.
18. Patel A, Panchal H, Piotrowski ZH, Patel D. Comprehensive medical care for victims of sexual assault: a survey of Illinois hospital emergency departments. Contraception 2008;77:426–30.
19. Kavanaugh ML, Saladino RA, Gold MA. Emergency contraception services for adolescents: a national survey of children's hospital emergency department directors. J Pediatr Adolesc Gynecol 2009;22:111–9.
20. Goyal M, Zhao H, Mollen C. Exploring emergency contraception knowledge, prescription practices, and barriers to prescription for adolescents in the emergency department. Pediatrics 2009;123:765–70.
21. Goldenring JM, Allred G. Post-rape care in hospital emergency rooms. Am J Public Health 2001;91:1169–70.
22. Stewart FH, Trussell J. Prevention of pregnancy resulting from rape: a neglected preventive health measure. Am J Prevent Med 2000;19:228–9.
23. National Protocol for Sexual Assault Medical Forensic Examinations: Adults/Adolescents. Washington (DC): US Dept of Justice, Office on Violence Against Women; 2004 Sep.
24. National Protocol for Sexual Assault Medical Forensic Examinations: Adults/Adolescents, Second Edition. Washington (DC): US Dept of Justice, Office on Violence Against Women; 2013 Apr.
25. Glasier A, Baird D. The effects of self-administering emergency contraception. N Engl J Med 1998;339:1–4.
26. Raine T, Harper C, Leon K, Darney P. Emergency contraception: advance provision in a young, high-risk clinic population. Obstet Gynecol 2000;96:1–7.
27. Hazari K. Use of emergency contraception by women as a back-up method. Health Popul 2000;23:115–122.
28. Jackson RA, Schwarz EB, Freedman L, Darney P. Advance supply of emergency contraception: effect on use and usual contraception—a randomized trial. Obstet Gynecol 2003;102:8–16.
29. Gold MA, Wolford JE, Smith KA, Parker AM. The effects of advance provision of emergency contraception on adolescent women's sexual and contraceptive behaviors. J Pediatr Adolesc Gynecol 2004;17:87–96.

30. Lo SS, Fan SYS, Ho PC, Glasier AF. Effect of advanced provision of emergency contraception on women's contraceptive behavior: a randomized controlled trial. Hum Reprod 2004;19:2404–10.
31. Belzer M, Sanchez K, Olson J, Jacobs AM, Tucker D. Advance supply of emergency contraception: a randomized trial in adolescent mothers. J Pediatr Adolesc Gynecol 2005;18:347–54.
32. Trussell J, Raymond E, Stewart FH. Letter to the editor. J Pediatr Adolesc Gynecol 2006;19:251. Comment on: Advance supply of emergency contraception. J Pediatr Adolesc Gynecol 2005 Oct;18(5):347–54.
33. Walsh TL, Frezieres RG. Patterns of emergency contraception use by age and ethnicity from a randomized trial comparing advance provision and information only. Contraception 2006;74:110–7.
34. Marston C, Meltzer H, Majeed A. Impact on contraceptive practice of making emergency hormonal contraception available over the counter in Great Britain: repeated cross sectional surveys. BMJ 2005;331(7511):271–3.
35. Moreau C, Bajos N, Trussell J. The impact of pharmacy access to emergency contraceptive pills in France. Contraception 2006;73:602–8.
36. Schwarz EB, Gerbert B, Gonzales R. Computer-assisted provision of emergency contraception: a randomized controlled trial. J Gen Intern Med 2008;23:794–9.
37. Ekstrand M, Larsson M, Darj E, Tydén T. Advance provision of emergency contraceptive pills reduces treatment delay: a randomised controlled trial among Swedish teenage girls. Acta Obstet Gynecol Scand 2008;87:354–9.
38. Ekstrand M, Tydén T, Darj E, Larsson M. Twelve-month follow-up of advance provision of emergency contraception among teenage girls in Sweden-a randomized controlled trial. Ups J Med Sci 2013;118:271–5.
39. Shaaban OM, Hassen SG, Nour SA, Kames MA, Yones EM. Emergency contraceptive pills as a backup for lactational amenorrhea method (LAM) of contraception: a randomized controlled trial. Contraception 2013;87:363–369.
40. Raine TR, Harper CC, Rocca CH, Fischer R, Padian N, Klausner JD, Darney PD. Direct access to emergency contraception through pharmacies and effect on unintended pregnancy and STIs: a randomized controlled trial. JAMA 2005;293:54–62.
41. Hu X, Cheng L, Hua X, Glasier A. Advanced provision of emergency contraception to postnatal women in China makes no difference in abortion rates: a randomized controlled trial. Contraception 2005;72:111–6.
42. Raymond EG, Stewart F, Weaver M, Monteith C, Van Der Pol B. Randomized trial to evaluate the impact of increased access to emergency contraceptive pills. Obstet Gynecol 2006;108:1098–106.
43. Graham A, Moore L, Sharp D, Diamond I. Improving teenagers' knowledge of emergency contraception: cluster randomized controlled trial of a teacher led intervention. BMJ 2002;234:1179–84.
44. Raymond EG, Weaver MA. Effect of an emergency contraceptive pill intervention on pregnancy risk behavior. Contraception 2008;77:333–6.
45. Weaver MA, Raymond EG, Baecher L. Attitude and behavior effects in a randomized trial of increased access to emergency contraception. Obstet Gynecol 2009;113:107–16.
46. Atkins D. Association between increased availability of emergency contraceptive pills and the sexual and contraceptive behaviors of women. Journal of Public Health Policy 2014;35:292–310.
47. Atkins DN, Bradford WD. Association between increased emergency contraception availability and risky sexual practices. Health Serv Res 2015;50:809–29.
48. Atkins D, Bradford WD. The effect of changes in state and federal policy for non-prescription access to emergency contraception on youth contraceptive use: a difference-in-difference analysis across New England states. Contemporary Economic Policy 2015;33:405–417.
49. Ellertson C, Trussell J, Stewart F, Winikoff B. Should emergency contraceptive pills be available without prescription? J Am Med Wom Assoc 1998;53 Suppl 2:S226–9, 232.

50. Grimes DA, Raymond EG, Scott Jones B. Emergency contraception over-the-counter: the medical and legal imperatives. Obstet Gynecol 2001;98:151–5.
51. Grimes DA. Emergency contraception and fire extinguishers: a prevention paradox. Am J Obstet Gynecol 2002;187:1536–8.
52. Grimes DA, Raymond EG, Scott Jones B. Emergency contraception over-the-counter: the medical and legal imperatives. Obstet Gynecol 2001;98:151–5.
53. Association of Reproductive Health Professionals. ARHP sign-on letter: switch status of emergency contraceptive from Rx to OTC; Available from: www.arhp.org/uploadDocs/ec_signon.pdf. Accessed 9 February 2017.
54. Trussell J, Guthrie KA. Talking straight about emergency contraception. J Fam Plan Reprod Health Care 2007;33:139–42.
55. Trussell J, Leveque JA, Koenig JD, et al. The economic value of contraception: a comparison of 15 methods. Am J Public Health 1995;85:494–503.
56. Sivin I. Utility and drawbacks of continuous use of a copper T IUD for 20 years. Contraception 2007;75:Suppl S70–5.
57. Trussell J, Koenig J, Ellertson C, Stewart F. Preventing unintended pregnancy: the cost-effectiveness of three methods of emergency contraception. Am J Public Health 1997;87:932–7.
58. Trussell J, Koenig J, Stewart F, Darroch JE. Medical care cost savings from adolescent contraceptive use. Fam Plann Perspect 1997;29:248–55, 295.
59. Trussell J, Wiebe E, Shochet T, Guilbert É. Cost savings from emergency contraceptive pills in Canada. Obstet Gynecol 2001;97:789–93.
60. Trussell J, Shochet T. Cost-effectiveness of emergency contraceptive pills in the public sector in the USA. Expert Rev Pharmacoeconomics Outcomes Res 2003;3:433–40.
61. Trussell J, Calabretto H. Cost savings from use of emergency contraceptive pills in Australia. Aust N Z J Obstet Gynaecol 2005;45:308–11.
62. Foster DG, Rostovtseva DP, Brindis CD, Biggs MA, Hulett D, Darney PD. Cost savings from the provision of specific methods of contraception in a publicly funded program. Am J Public Health 2009;99:446–51.
63. Foster DG, Raine TR, Brindis C, Rostovtseva DP, Darney PD. Should providers give women advance provision of emergency contraceptive pills? A cost-effectiveness analysis. Womens Health Issues 2010;20:242–7.
64. Bayer LL, Edelman AB, Caughey AB, Rodriguez MI. The price of emergency contraception in the United States: what is the cost-effectiveness of ulipristal acetate versus single-dose levonorgestrel? Contraception 2013;87:385–90.
65. Bentancor A, Clarke D. Assessing Plan B: the effect of the morning after pill on children and women. Econ J 2017;127:2525–2.
66. Cleland K, Hoaping Z, Goldstruck N, Cheng L, Trussell J. The efficacy of IUDs for emergency contraception: a systematic review of 35 years of experience. Hum Reprod 2012;27:1994–2000.
67. Statement on Contraceptive Methods. Washington (DC): American College of Obstetricians and Gynecologists; July 1998.
68. Díaz S, Cárdenas H, Brandeis A, Miranda P, Salvatierra AM, Croxatto HB. Relative contributions of anovulation and luteal phase defect to the reduced pregnancy rate of breastfeeding women. Fertil Steril 1992;58:498–503.
69. Levonorgestrel for emergency contraception [Fact sheet]. Geneva (Switzerland): World Health Organization; 2005 March.
70. Protection of Human Subjects, 45 C.F.R. Sect. 46.202 (2009).
71. Hughes EC (ed). Committee on Terminology, The American College of Obstetricians and Gynecologists, Obstetric-Gynecologic Terminology. Philadelphia (PA): F.A. Davis Company; 1972.
72. Brache V, Cochon L, Deniaud M, Croxatto HB. Ulipristal acetate prevents ovulation more effectively than levonorgestrel: analysis of pooled data from three randomized trials of emergency contraception regimens. Contraception 2013;88:611–8.

73. Stratton P, Hartog B, Hajizadeh N, et al. A single mid-follicular dose of CDB-2914, a new antiprogestin, inhibits folliculogenesis and endometrial differentiation in normally cycling women. Hum Reprod 2000;15:1092–9.
74. Nallasamy S, Kim J, Sitruk-Ware R, Bagchi M, Bagchi I. Ulipristal blocks ovulation by inhibiting progesterone receptor-dependent pathways intrinsic to the ovary. Reprod Sci 2013;20:371–81.
75. Brache V, Cochon L, Jesam C, et al. Immediate preovulatory administration of 30 mg ulipristal acetate significantly delays follicular rupture. Hum Reprod 2010;25:2256–63
76. Li HW, Lo SS, Ng EH, Ho PC. Efficacy of ulipristal acetate for emergency contraception and its effect on the subsequent bleeding pattern when administered before or after ovulation. Hum Reprod 2016;31:1200–7.
77. Stratton P, Levens ED, Hartog B, Piquion J, Wei Q, Merino M, Nieman LK. Endometrial effects of a single early luteal dose of the selective progesterone receptor modulator CDB-2914. Fertil Steril 2010;93:2035–41.
78. Berger C, Boggavarapu NR, Menezes J, Lalitkumar PG, Gemzell-Danielsson K. Effects of ulipristal acetate on human embryo attachment and endometrial cell gene expression in an in vitro co-culture system. Hum Reprod 2015;30:800–11.
79. Zumoffen C, Gómez-Elías MD, Caille AM, Bahamondes L, Cuasnicú PS, Cohen DJ, Munuce MJ. Study of the effect of ulipristal acetate on human sperm ability to interact with tubal tissue and cumulus-oocyte-complexes. Contraception 2017;95:586–91.
80. Hapangama D, Glasier AF, Baird DT. The effects of peri-ovulatory administration of levonorgestrel on the menstrual cycle. Contraception 2001;63:123–9.
81. Durand M, del Carmen Cravioto M, Raymond EG, et al. On the mechanisms of action of short-term levonorgestrel administration in emergency contraception. Contraception 2001;64:227–34.
82. Marions L, Hultenby K, Lindell I, Sun X, Ståbi B, Gemzell Danielsson K. Emergency contraception with mifepristone and levonorgestrel: mechanism of action. Obstet Gynecol 2002;100:65–71.
83. Marions L, Cekan SZ, Bygdeman M, Gemzell-Danielsson K. Effect of emergency contraception with levonorgestrel or mifepristone on ovarian function. Contraception 2004;69:373–7.
84. Croxatto HB, Brache V, Pavez M, et al. Pituitary-ovarian function following the standard levonorgestrel emergency contraceptive dose or a single 0.75-mg dose given on the days preceding ovulation. Contraception 2004;70:442–50.
85. Durand M, Séppala M, del Carmen Cravioto M, et al. Late follicular phase administration of levonorgestrel as an emergency contraceptive changes the secretory pattern of glycodelin in serum and endometrium during the luteal phase of the menstrual cycle. Contraception 2005;71:451–7.
86. Seppälä M, Taylor RN, Koistinen H, Koistinen R, Milgrom E. Glycodelin: a major lipocalin protein of the reproductive axis with diverse actions in cell recognition and differentiation. Endocr Rev 2002;23:401–30.
87. do Nascimento JA, Seppala M, Perdigao A, et al. In vivo assessment of the human sperm acrosome reaction and the expression of glycodelin-A in human endometrium after levonorgestrel-emergency contraceptive pill administration. Hum Reprod 2007;22: 2190–5.
88. Palomino WA, Kohen P, Devoto L. A single midcycle dose of levonorgestrel similar to emergency contraceptive does not alter the expression of the L-selectin ligand or molecular markers of endometrial receptivity. Fertil Steril 2010;94:1589–94.
89. Durand M, Koistinen R, Chirinos M, Rodríguez JL, Zambrano E, Seppälä M, Larrea F. Hormonal evaluation and midcycle detection of intrauterine glycodelin in women treated with levonorgestrel as in emergency contraception. Contraception 2010;82:526–33.
90. Lalitkumar PG, Lalitkumar S, Meng CX, et al. Mifepristone, but not levonorgestrel, inhibits human blastocyst attachment to an in vitro endometrial three-dimensional cell culture model. Human Reprod 2007;22:3031–7.

91. Meng CX, Andersson KL, Bentin-Ley U, Gemzell-Danielsson K, Lalitkumar PG. Effect of levonorgestrel and mifepristone on endometrial receptivity markers in a three-dimensional human endometrial cell culture model. Fertil Steril 2009;91: 256–64.
92. Kesserü E, Garmendia F, Westphal N, Parada J. The hormonal and peripheral effects of d-norgestrel in postcoital contraception. Contraception 1974;10:411–24.
93. Yeung WS, Chiu PC, Wang CH, Yao YQ, Ho PC. The effects of levonorgestrel on various sperm functions. Contraception 2002;66:453–7.
94. Piaggio G, von Hertzen H, Grimes DA, Van Look PFA. Timing of emergency contraception with levonorgestrel or the Yuzpe regimen. Lancet 1999;353:721.
95. Davidoff F, Trussell J. Plan B and the politics of doubt. JAMA 2006;296:1775–8.
96. Mikolajczyk RT, Stanford JB. Levonorgestrel emergency contraception: a joint analysis of effectiveness and mechanism of action. Fertil Steril 2007;88:565–71.
97. Croxatto HB, Devoto L, Durand M, et al. Mechanism of action of hormonal preparations used for emergency contraception: a review of the literature. Contraception 2001;63:111–21.
98. Müller AL, Llados CM, Croxatto HB. Postcoital treatment with levonorgestrel does not disrupt postfertilization events in the rat. Contraception 2003;67:415–19.
99. Ortiz ME, Ortiz RE, Fuentes MA, Parraguez VH, Croxatto HB. Postcoital administration of levonorgestrel does not interfere with post-fertilization events in the new-world monkey Cebus apella. Hum Reprod 2004;19:1352–6.
100. Novikova N, Weisberg E, Stanczyk FZ, Croxatto HB, Fraser, IS. Effectiveness of levonorgestrel emergency contraception given before or after ovulation—a pilot study. Contraception 2006;74:349–50.
101. Noé G, Croxatto HB, Salvatierra AM, et al. Contraceptive efficacy of emergency contraception with levonorgestrel given before or after ovulation. Contraception 2011;84: 486–92.
102. Emergency contraception's mode of action clarified. Popul Briefs 2005;11:2. Available from: www.popcouncil.org/uploads/pdfs/pbmay05.pdf. Accessed 9 February 2017.
103. Gemzell-Danielsson K, Berger C, Lalitkumar PGL. Emergency contraception - mechanisms of action. Contraception 2013;87:300–308.
104. Swahn ML, Westlund P, Johannisson E, Bygdeman M. Effect of post-coital contraceptive methods on the endometrium and the menstrual cycle. Acta Obstet Gynecol Scand 1996;75:738–44.
105. Ling WY, Robichaud A, Zayid I, Wrixon W, MacLeod SC. Mode of action of dl-norgestrel and ethinylestradiol combination in postcoital contraception. Fertil Steril 1979;32: 297–302.
106. Rowlands S, Kubba AA, Guillebaud J, Bounds W. A possible mechanism of action of danazol and an ethinylestradiol/norgestrel combination used as postcoital contraceptive agents. Contraception 1986;33:539–45.
107. Croxatto HB, Fuentalba B, Brache V, Salvatierra AM, Alvarez F, Massai R, Cochon L, Faundes A. Effects of the Yuzpe regimen, given during the follicular phase, on ovarian function. Contraception 2002;65:121–8.
108. Kubba AA, White JO, Guillebaud J, Elder MG. The biochemistry of human endometrium after two regimens of postcoital contraception: a dl-norgestrel/ethinylestradiol combination or danazol. Fertil Steril 1986;45:512–6.
109. Ling WY, Wrixon W, Zayid I, Acorn T, Popat R, Wilson E. Mode of action of dl-norgestrel and ethinylestradiol combination in postcoital contraception. II. Effect of postovulatory administration on ovarian function and endometrium. Fertil Steril 1983;39:292–7.
110. Yuzpe AA, Thurlow HJ, Ramzy I, Leyshon JI. Post coital contraception—a pilot study. J Reprod Med 1974;13:53–8.
111. Taskin O, Brown RW, Young DC, Poindexter AN, Wiehle RD. High doses of oral contraceptives do not alter endometrial α1 and ανβ3 integrins in the late implantation window. Fertil Steril 1994;61:850–5.

112. Raymond EG, Lovely LP, Chen-Mok M, Seppälä M, Kurman RJ, Lessey BA. Effect of the Yuzpe regimen of emergency contraception on markers of endometrial receptivity. Hum Reprod 2000;15:2351–5.
113. Glasier A. Emergency postcoital contraception. N Engl J Med 1997;337:1058–64.
114. Ling WY, Wrixon W, Acorn T, Wilson E, Collins J. Mode of action of dl-norgestrel and ethinylestradiol combination in postcoital contraception. III. Effect of preovulatory administration following the luteinizing hormone surge on ovarian steroidogenesis. Fertil Steril 1983;40:631–6.
115. Croxatto HB, Ortiz ME, Müller AL. Mechanisms of action of emergency contraception. Steroids 2003;68:1095–8.
116. Turok DK, Godfrey EM, Wojdyla D, Dermish A, Torres L, Wu SC. Copper T380 intrauterine device for emergency contraception: highly effective at any time in the menstrual cycle. Hum Reprod 2013;28:2672–6.
117. Turok DT, Sanders JN, Thompson IS, Royer PA, Eggebroten J, Gawron L. Preference for and efficacy of oral levonorgestrel for emergency contraception with concomitant placement of a levonorgestrel IUD: a prospective cohort study. Contraception 2016;93:526–32.
118. Dixon GW, Schlesselman JJ, Ory HW, Blye RP. Ethinyl estradiol and conjugated estrogens as postcoital contraceptives. JAMA 1980;244:1336–9.
119. Wilcox AJ, Weinberg CR, Baird DD. Timing of sexual intercourse in relation to ovulation. Effects on the probability of conception, survival of the pregnancy, and sex of the baby. N Engl J Med 1995;333:1517–21.
120. Stirling A, Glasier A. Estimating the efficacy of emergency contraception–how good are the data? Contraception 2002;66:19–22.
121. Espinos JJ, Rodriguez-Espinosa J, Senosiain et al. The role of matching menstrual data with hormonal measurements in evaluating effectiveness of postcoital contraception. Contraception 1999;60:243–7.
122. Espinos-Gomez JJ, Senosiain R, Mata A, Vanrell C, Bassas L, Calaf J. What is the seminal exposition among women requiring emergency contraception? A prospective, observational comparative study. Eur J Obstet Gynecol Reprod Bio 2007;131:57–60.
123. Raymond E, Taylor D, Trussell J, Steiner MJ. Minimum effectiveness of the levonorgestrel regimen of emergency contraception. Contraception 2004;69:79–81.
124. Glasier AF, Cameron ST, Fine PM, et al. Ulipristal acetate versus levonorgestrel for emergency contraception: a randomised non-inferiority trial and meta-analysis. Lancet 2010;375:555–62.
125. Creinin MD, Schlaff W, Archer DF, et al. Progesterone receptor modulator for emergency contraception: a randomized controlled trial. Obstet Gynecol 2006;108:1089–97.
126. Fine P, Mathé H, Ginde S, Cullins V, Morfesis J, Gainer E. Ulipristal acetate taken 48–120 hours after intercourse for emergency contraception. Obstet Gynecol 2010;115:257–63.
127. von Hertzen H, Piaggio G, Ding J, et al. Low dose mifepristone and two regimens of levonorgestrel for emergency contraception: a WHO multicentre randomised trial. Lancet 2002;360:1803–10.
128. Hamoda H, Ashok PW, Stalder C, Flett GM, Kennedy E, Templeton A. A randomized trial of mifepristone (10 mg) and levonorgestrel for emergency contraception. Obstet Gynecol 2004;104:1307–13.
129. Wu S, Wang C, Wang Y, et al. A randomized, double-blind, multicenter study on comparing levonorgestrel and mifepristone for emergency contraception. J Reprod Med (Sheng Zhi Yi Xue Za Zhi) 1999;**8**(suppl 1):43–46. (In English).
130. Wu S, Dong J, Cong J, Wang C, VonHertzen H, Godfrey EM. Gestrinone compared with mifepristone for emergency contraception: a randomized controlled trial. Obstet Gynecol 2010;115:740–4.
131. Arowojolu AO, Okewole IA, Adekunle AO. Comparative evaluation of the effectiveness and safety of two regimens of levonorgestrel for emergency contraception in Nigerians. Contraception 2002;66:269–73.
132. Ngai SW, Fan S, Li S, et al. A randomized trial to compare 24h versus 12h double dose regimen of levonorgestrel for emergency contraception. Hum Reprod 2004;20:307–11.

133. Ho PC, Kwan MS. A prospective randomized comparison of levonorgestrel with the Yuzpe regimen in post-coital contraception. Hum Reprod 1993;8:389–92.
134. Task Force on Postovulatory Methods of Fertility Regulation. Randomised controlled trial of levonorgestrel versus the Yuzpe regimen of combined oral contraceptives for emergency contraception. Lancet 1998;352:428–33.
135. Dada OA, Godfrey EM, Gilda Piaggio G, von Hertzen H. A randomized, double-blind, noninferiority study to compare two regimens of levonorgestrel for emergency contraception in Nigeria. Contraception 2010;82:373–8.
136. Farajkhoda T, Khoshbin A, Enjezab B, Bokaei M, Karimi Zarchi M. Assessment of two emergency contraceptive regimens in Iran: levonorgestrel versus the Yuzpe.Niger J Clin Pract 2009;12:450–2.
137. Trussell J, Rodríguez G, Ellertson C. Updated estimates of the effectiveness of the Yuzpe regimen of emergency contraception. Contraception 1999;59:147–51.
138. Trussell J, Ellertson C, von Hertzen H, et al. Estimating the effectiveness of emergency contraceptive pills. Contraception. 2003;67:259–65.
139. Massai MR, Forcelledo ML, Brache V, Tejada AS, Salvatierra AM, Reyes MV, Alvarez F, Faúndes A, Croxatto HB. Does meloxicam increase the incidence of an ovulation induced by single administration of levonorgestrel in emergency contraception? A pilot study. Hum Reprod 2007;22:434–9.
140. Kane LA, Sparrow MJ. Postcoital contraception: a family planning study. N Z Med J 1989;102:151–3.
141. Trussell J, Ellertson C, Rodríguez G. The Yuzpe regimen of emergency contraception: how long after the morning after? Obstet Gynecol 1996;88:150–4.
142. Rodrigues I, Grou F, Joly J. Effectiveness of emergency contraception pills between 72 and 120 hours after unprotected sexual intercourse. Am J Obstet Gynecol 2001;184:531–7.
143. Ellertson C, Evans M, Ferden S, Leadbetter C, Spears A, Johnstone K, Trussell J. Extending the time limit for starting the Yuzpe regimen of emergency contraception to 120 hours. Obstet Gynecol 2003;101:1168–71.
144. Yuzpe AA, Lancee WJ. Ethinylestradiol and dl-norgestrel as a postcoital contraceptive. Fertil Steril 1977;28:932–6.
145. Piaggio G, Kapp N, von Hertzen H. Effect on pregnancy rates of the delay in the administration of levonorgestrel for emergency contraception: a combined analysis of four WHO trials. Contraception 2011;84:35–39.
146. Moreau C, Trussell J. Results from pooled phase III studies of ulipristal acetate for emergency contraception. Contraception 2012;86:673–680.
147. Glasier A, Cameron ST, Blithe D, et al. Can we identify women at risk of pregnancy despite using emergency contraception? Data from randomized trials of ulipristal acetate and levonorgestrel. Contraception 2011;84:363–7.
148. www.ema.europa.eu/docs/en_GB/document_library/Referrals_document/Emergency_contraceptives_31/WC500176384.pdf. Accessed 9 February 2017.
149. www.ema.europa.eu/ema/index.jsp?curl=pages/news_and_events/news/2014/07/news_detail_002145.jsp&mid=WC0b01ac058004d5c1 Accessed 9 February 2017.
150. United States Food and Drug Administration. FDA communication on levonorgestrel emergency contraceptive effectiveness and weight. Available at: www.fda.gov/Drugs/DrugSafety/PostmarketDrugSafetyInformationforPatientsandProviders/ucm109775.htm. Accessed 9 February 2017.
151. Festin MP, Peregoudov A, Seuc A, Kiarie J, Temmerman M. Effect of BMI and body weight on pregnancy rates with LNG as emergency contraception: analysis of four WHO HRP studies. Contraception 2017;95:50–54.
152. Edelman A, Cherala G, Blue S, Erikson D, Jensen J. Impact of obesity on the pharmacokinetics of levonorgestrel-based emergency contraception: single and double dosing. Contraception. 2016 ;94:52–57.
153. Praditpan P, Hamouie A, Basaraba CN, et al. Pharmacokinetics of levonorgestrel and ulipristal acetate emergency contraception in women with normal and obese body mass index. Contraception 2017;95:464–9.

154. Faculty of Sexual & Reproductive Healthcare. FSRH Guideline: Emergency Contraception. London: March 2017. Available at www.fsrh.org/standards-and-guidance/documents/ceu-clinical-guidance-emergency-contraception-march-2017/fsrh-guideline-emergency-contraception-17mar2017.pdf. Accessed 2 April 2017.

155. Trussell J, Ellertson C, Stewart F, Raymond EG, Shochet T. The role of emergency contraception. Am J Obstet Gynecol 2004;190:S30–8.

156. Festin MP, Bahamondes L, Nguyen TM, et al. A prospective, open-label, single arm, multicentre study to evaluate efficacy, safety and acceptability of pericoital oral contraception using levonorgestrel 1.5 mg. Hum Reprod 2016;31:530–40.

157. Raymond EG, Trussell J, Polis C. Population effect of increased access to emergency contraceptive pills: a systematic review. Obstet Gynecol 2007;109:181–8.

158. Polis CB, Grimes DA, Schaffer K, Blanchard K, Glasier A, Harper C. Advance provision of emergency contraception for pregnancy prevention. Cochrane Database of Systematic Reviews 2010, Issue 3. Art. No.: CD005497. DOI: 10.1002/14651858.CD005497.pub2.

159. Glasier A, Fairhurst K, Wyke S, Ziebland S, Seaman P, Walker J, Lakha F. Advanced provision of emergency contraception does not reduce abortion rates. Contraception 2004;69:361–6.

160. Baecher L, Weaver MA, Raymond EG. Increased access to emergency contraception: why it may fail. Hum Reprod 2009;24:815–9.

161. Raymond EG, Shochet T, Drake JK, Westley E. What some women want? On-demand oral contraception. Contraception 2014;90:105–10.

162. Feldhaus KM. A 21st-century challenge: improving the care of the sexual assault victim. Ann Emerg Med 2002;39:653–5.

163. Selected practice recommendations for contraceptive use. 2nd ed. Geneva (Switzerland): World Health Organization; 2005.

164. Raymond EG, Creinin MD, Barnhart KT, Lovvorn AE, Rountree RW, Trussell J. Meclizine for prevention of nausea associated with use of emergency contraceptive pills: a randomized trial. Obstet Gynecol 2000;95:271–7.

165. Zhang L, Chen J, Wang Y, Ren F, Yu W, Cheng L. Pregnancy outcome after levonorgestrel-only emergency contraception failure: a prospective cohort study. Hum Reprod 2009;24:1605–11.

166. Levy DP, Jager M, Kapp N, Abitbol JL. Ulipristal acetate for emergency contraception: postmarketing experience after use by more than 1 million women. Contraception 2014; 89:431–3.

167. Raman-Wilms L, Tseng AL, Wighardt S, Einarson TR, Koren G. Fetal genital effects of first-trimester sex hormone exposure: a meta-analysis. Obstet Gynecol 1995;85:141–9.

168. Bracken MB. Oral contraception and congenital malformations in offspring: a review and meta-analysis of the prospective studies. Obstet Gynecol 1990;76:552–7.

169. Simpson JL, Phillips OP. Spermicides, hormonal contraception and congenital malformations. Adv Contraception 1990;6:141–67.

170. Food and Drug Administration. Prescription drug products; certain combined oral contraceptives for use as postcoital emergency contraception. Federal Regist 1997;62:8610–2.

171. Trussell J, Hedley A, Raymond E. Ectopic pregnancy following use of progestin-only ECPs [letter]. J Fam Plann Reprod Health Care 2003;29:249.

172. Cleland K, Raymond E, Trussell J, Cheng L, Zhu H. Ectopic pregnancy and emergency contraception: a systematic review. Obstet Gynecol 2010;115:1263–6.

173. Raymond EG, Goldberg A, Trussell J, Hays M, Roach E, Taylor D. Bleeding patterns after use of levonorgestrel emergency contraceptive pills. Contraception 2006;73:376–81. Erratum in: Contraception 2006;74:349–50. Erratum in: Contraception 2007;75:476–7.

174. Gainer E, Kenfack B, Mboudou E, Doh AS, Bouyer J. Menstrual bleeding patterns following levonorgestrel emergency contraception. Contraception 2006;74:118–24.

175. Tirelli A, Cagnacci A, Volpe A. Levonorgestrel administration in emergency contraception: bleeding pattern and pituitary-ovarian function. Contraception 2008;77;328–32.

176. Centers for Disease Control and Prevention. U.S. Medical Eligibility Criteria for Contraceptive Use, 2016. MMWR 2016;65:1–108.

177. Gainer E, Massai R, Lillo S, et al. Levonorgestrel pharmacokinetics in plasma and milk of lactating women who take 1.5 mg for emergency contraception. Hum Reprod 2007;22:1578–84.

178. Polakow-Farkash S, Gilad O, Merlob P, Stahl B, Yogev Y, Klinger G. Levonorgestrel used for emergency contraception during lactation-A prospective observational cohort study on maternal and infant safety. J Matern Fetal Neonatal Med 2013;26:219–21.

179. Available from www.accessdata.fda.gov/drugsatfda_docs/label/2015/022474s007lbl.pdf Accessed 2 February 2017.

180. Cameron ST, Berger C, Michie L, Klipping C, Gemzell-Danielsson K. The effects on ovarian activity of ulipristal acetate when 'quickstarting' a combined oral contraceptive pill: a prospective, randomized, double-blind parallel-arm, placebo-controlled study. Hum Reprod 2015;30:1566–72.

181. Brache V, Cochon L, Duijkers IJM, et al. A prospective, randomised pharmacodynamic study of quick-starting desogestrel progestin-only pill following ulipristal acetate for emergency contraception. Hum Reprod 2015;30:2785–93.

182. Wilcox AJ, Dunson DB, Weinberg CR, Trussell J, Baird DD. Likelihood of conception with a single act of intercourse: providing benchmark rates for assessment of post-coital contraceptives. Contraception 2001;63:211–5.

183. Jesam C, Cochon L, Salvatierra AM, et al. A prospective, open-label, multicenter study to assess the pharmacodynamics and safety of repeated use of 30 mg ulipristal acetate. Contraception 2016 ;93:310–16.

184. Grimes DA, Raymond EG. Bundling a pregnancy test with the Yuzpe regimen of emergency contraception. Obstet Gynecol 1999;94:471–3.

185. American Society for Emergency Contraception. Providing Ongoing Hormonal Contraception after Use of Emergency Contraceptive Pills. November 2016. Available at: americansocietyforec.org/uploads/3/4/5/6/34568220/asec_fact_sheet-_hormonal_contraception_after_ec.pdf

186. Wilcox AJ, Baird DD, Weinberg CR. Time of implantation of the conceptus and loss of pregnancy. N Engl J Med 1999;340:1796–9.

Vaginal Barriers and Spermicides

11

Anita Nelson, MD
Bryna Harwood, MD, MS

- These are nonhormonal, "on demand" methods.
- Only spermicides are available over-the-counter or online without clinician consultation.
- Many can be combined with each other or other methods to increase contraceptive efficacy or to provide noncontraceptive benefits.
- Typical use failure rates for these methods are generally higher than for other methods, but they still significantly reduce the user's risk for unintended pregnancy compared to unprotected intercourse.
- All are rapidly reversible.
- Offer prescription for emergency contraception in advance of need for users of all these methods.

As a class, vaginal barrier methods and spermicides have features that appeal to many potential users in the United States. All of these methods are controlled by the person at risk for becoming pregnant. Use is episodic, that is, these methods need to be used only at the time of coitus.[1] There is no need for ongoing exposure to contraception. They are all nonhormonal methods, which can be used by patients with a wide range of medical conditions or other health risks. Some are available over-the-counter or online, eliminating the need to get a prescription. Many are modestly priced and do not need to be purchased until the need arises, although being prepared by having the chosen method available in advance is optimal. All vaginal barriers and spermicides are rapidly reversible. Additionally, most reduce transmission of at least some sexually transmitted infections (STIs). For those methods that use spermicide, exposure even in early pregnancy is not associated with increased risk of birth defects in the fetus.[2]

Vaginal barriers and spermicidal agents are among some of the oldest recorded methods of birth control. Egyptian papyri described vaginal plugs of honey, gum, acacia and crocodile dung, as well as sponges. Different societies used local products such as bamboo paper, seaweed, and willow leaves. In early second century Rome, soft wool balls combined with acidic fruit and nuts were described.

In the last few years, there has been renewed interest in contraceptive methods in this category. Older barrier methods that had been taken off the market have been reintroduced, such as the Today contraceptive sponge. Others have been retooled and reintroduced: the original female condom (Reality) has returned as FC2, and the Caya diaphragm has effectively replaced the older, more specifically sized diaphragms. The FemCap was redesigned slightly and is the only cervical cap available in the United States. Over a decade of research has yet to find an effective replacement for nonoxynol-9 (N-9) spermicides, especially one that will also have microbicidal activity to stem the spread of HIV.[3,4] See Table 11-1 for summary of characteristics of vaginal barrier methods available in the United States.

Vaginal barriers and spermicides may be used alone or in combination with each other to enhance efficacy. Spermicide is always used with the cervical cap and diaphragm, but it can also be used with the male and female condoms. Vaginal barriers and spermicides can be combined with most other methods, from IUDs to coitus interruptus, to enhance pregnancy protection or to provide better STI protection. Some exceptions exist. The male and female condoms should never be used together; diaphragms and female caps should not be used with IUDs. Because of the large gap between failure rates with consistent and correct use and the rates with typical use, anticipate accidents. Offer all patients who select these methods a prescription (with refills) for emergency contraception. (See Chapter 10 on Emergency Contraception.)

MECHANISM OF ACTION

All vaginal barriers and spermicides prevent fertilization by blocking sperm transport into the upper genital tract. The female condom provides a physical barrier that lines the vagina and partially shields the perineum and does not require use of a spermicidal agent. All other vaginal barriers combine both a physical barrier, to prevent sperm entry into the cervical canal, and a spermicide agent, to kill sperm. The diaphragm and the cervical cap hold the spermicide in place in front of the cervix.

Spermicidal preparations consist of two components: 1) a carrier/base (gel, foam, sponge, cream, film, suppository, or tablet) and 2) a chemical

Table 11-1 Summary of characteristics of vaginal barrier methods

Device	Description	Mechanism	1st Year Failure Rates With: Correct and Consistent Use	1st Year Failure Rates With: Typical Use	Availability	Special Features
FC2 (female condom) Scented Unscented	Nitrile sheath with an unattached flexible ring at top to aid in placing and stabilizing ring in vaginal vault and a second ring attached at bottom lying outside the introitus	Barrier	5%	21%	Requires prescription from clinician or online provider	• Single use protection • Can be placed early • One size • No need for spermicide
Caya (contraceptive diaphragm)	Silicone rubber molded device with circular nylon spring to stabilize against vaginal walls; spermicide-filled cup fits over cervix	Barrier & spermicide	6–12.5%	12–18%	Requires prescription Clinician needs to check size and placement	• Reusable • Can be used for up to 2 years. • Single size can accommodate 65–80 mm vaginal measurement. • Used with spermicidal gel. • May be used for multiple acts of intercourse by adding more spermicide vaginally

(continued)

Table 11-1 Summary of characteristics of vaginal barrier methods—*(cont'd)*

Device	Description	Mechanism	1st Year Failure Rates With: Correct and Consistent Use	1st Year Failure Rates With: Typical Use	Availability	Special Features
FemCap (cervical cap)	• Silicone rubber 'sailor hat' • Spermicide placed inside and outside dome, which covers cervix • Brim to stabilize the cap against vaginal walls	Barrier & spermicide	13.5% at 6 months		Available online with prescription	• Reusable for up to 1 year. • Sized by obstetric history with clinician confirmation. • Used with spermicidal gel • May be used for up to 48 hours for multiple acts without adding more spermicide
Today (contraceptive sponge)	• Pillow-shaped polyurethane sponge containing 1g of N-9 • Concave indentation to cover the cervix	Spermicide with some barrier activity	Nulliparous users 9% Parous users 20%	Nulliparous users 12% Parous users 29%	Over-the-counter and online	• Single use • Disposable • Single size • Requires liquid to activate spermicide just before placement • Tidy—absorbs the ejaculate
Spermicides*	• Foams, films, gels, creams, suppositories releasing nonoxonyl-9	Spermicide	18%	28%	Over-the-counter	Different formulations may need different lead times to activate within the vagina, but all are active as single agents for only 1-hour of use

*For more details on different types of spermicides, see Table 11-2.

available in different doses and concentrations to kill the sperm. The sponge additionally absorbs and traps sperm in its spongy matrix. For spermicidal products, the formulation helps disperse the spermicide in the vagina. In the case of viscous gel and foam, the formulation itself may provide both lubrication and an additional barrier effect. When combined with other barriers (cervical cap, diaphragm, or condoms), spermicide boosts the effectiveness of those methods.[5] The active chemical agent in spermicidal products available in the United States is N-9. It is a surfactant that destroys the membrane of the sperm body and flagella. The detergent action of N-9 also can disrupt epithelial cells of the vagina and the rectum, potentially increasing risk of HIV transmission. Newer spermicides that avoid surfactant activity are being studied as replacements for N-9.

Advantages

For Barrier Contraceptives As a Group

1. **User-controlled.** In general, these methods are controlled by the person at risk of becoming pregnant, including initiation and discontinuation. No partner action is needed, especially for those methods that can be applied far in advance of coitus. However, negotiation with the partner may be required for the visible methods, as well as for those that need to be placed at the time of coitus.

2. **Available if male condom not an option.** Vaginal barriers may be used by couples desiring barrier methods when the male condom cannot or will not be used.

3. **Nonhormonal.** Neither vaginal barriers nor spermicides affect endogenous hormone production or menstrual cycling. May be used by people who desire to avoid the use of synthetic hormones or who have medical contraindications to their use.

4. **On-demand contraception.** These methods are used only at the time of coitus. For couples with infrequent intercourse, this may significantly reduce costs and the burden of maintaining ongoing contraceptive methods.

5. **Immediately reversible.** All of these methods are immediately reversible simply by discontinuing their use.

6. **Portable.** Generally, these methods are portable. They can fit into a bag to be carried with the user.

7. **May be combined.** Many of these methods can be combined with most of the Tier 1 and Tier 2 methods or with other barrier methods

to enhance efficacy or to provide other non-contraceptive benefits. They may also be used during at-risk days identified by fertility awareness methods.

DISADVANTAGES

FOR BARRIER CONTRACEPTIVES AS A GROUP

1. **Must be used with every act of intercourse without exception to achieve efficacy.** Intermittent or inconsistent use greatly increases failure rates.

2. **Requires comfort and proficiency with vaginal or rectal placement.** The user must be comfortable placing the method in the vagina or rectum (for STI protection) or to have a willing partner place it. Comfort with touching one's own genitals or placing materials into the vagina or rectum vary with the user's age and culture.[6]

3. **Coitally dependent use.** The user needs time to place the method prior to genital-to-genital contact. This may diminish spontaneity, especially with unexpected sexual encounters.

4. **Higher failure rates.** As a group, these methods can significantly reduce the chance of pregnancy, but in typical use they have the highest failure rates of any method with the possible exception of behavioral methods, such as coitus interruptus or fertility awareness methods.

5. **Subject to partner sabotage.** Because these methods may be evident to a partner, negotiation with the partner may be required for their use. Their effectiveness is reduced in the presence of reproductive coercion.

6. **Increased risks with high-risk behavior.** People who have multiple acts of intercourse per day, particularly with different partners, are at increased risk of HIV transmission with frequent and repeated use of nonoxyonol-9, which can disrupt the vulvovaginal epithelium. All the barriers that use spermicide require that the device be kept in place in the vagina for at least 6 hours following coitus. Adherence to this rule would limit the number of acts of intercourse. Noncompliance would decrease the efficacy of the method.

7. **Local irritation or allergy.** Spermicide may cause local irritation.

8. **May increase risk of toxic shock syndrome (TSS).** To date, only diaphragms and contraceptive sponges have been reported to have caused TSS, but that potential risk is theoretically possible for any vaginal method.

FEMALE CONDOM (FC2)

The female condom currently available in the United States is called FC2. It is a single use, soft, loose-fitting, tapered nitrile sheath that measures 180 mm in length. The sheath is shaped to fit the anatomy of the vagina. The outer ring is oval with a diameter of 72 mm. The mid-body diameter of the sheath is 66 cm, while the inner ring that ultimately rests at the vault has a 58-mm diameter. This inner ring is made of polyurethane and floats freely within the device. This ring helps to introduce the sheath through the introitus and to guide the condom to the top of the vagina. Once the condom is in position, the inner ring is rotated around to help stabilize the device during intercourse. The inner ring should be placed above the pubic bone; it may cover the cervix or it may be positioned above the cervix in the vault. The outer polyurethane ring is attached to the edge of the condom and folds over on itself slightly to partially or completely cover the user's external genitalia. The nitrile sheath is coated internally and externally with a silicone-based lubricant to ease placement and to reduce friction during coitus. This lubricant does not have any spermicidal activity. Nitrile is a synthetic (not natural) rubber latex, and can be used by those with allergies to natural latex. Nitrile is an impermeable material that effectively transmits body heat but blocks passage of microbes. Petroleum and silicone based products can be used as lubricants without threatening the integrity of the condom. FC2 can be stored anywhere at a wide range of temperatures. The FC2 is available over-the-counter and online.

In 2007, about 25 million female condoms were distributed globally; by 2012, that number increased to over 60 million units.[7] However impressive that growth appears, it pales in comparison to the male condom. Female condoms comprise only 0.19% of global condom products.[7] However, a global coalition of public, private, and nongovernment organizations called the Reproductive Health Supplies Coalition has identified the female condom as one of several underutilized reproductive health technologies; it has the potential to expand choice in reproductive health and family planning programs, add value to the method, and respond to the needs of a range of clients.[7] Other female condoms are used in other countries and have clinical pregnancy rates and nonclinical failure measures similar to FC2. If demand continues to increase for female condoms in the United States, newer options in this category may become available.

EFFECTIVENESS

The FDA quotes FC2 first-year failure rates as being the same as its predecessor, the Reality female condom. Those rates are 5% with perfect use and 21% in typical use. Clinical experience shows that there is an early learning curve. Rates of functional failures, such as breakage, slippage, invagination, and misdirection, were highest in the first 5 uses of female condoms (7.7% with the first condom decreasing to 1.2% with the fifth one). The lower steady-state functional failure rates were not generally achieved until the person had used it 20 times.[8] For this reason, some experts advise that the couple not rely on the female condom for their first several uses of the method. It is recommended that users be prescribed emergency contraception in advance of need to have it available when some difficulty is encountered with FC2 use. (See Chapter 10 on Emergency Contraception.)

ADVANTAGES

In addition to the general advantages for vaginal barrier methods listed above, the female condom has specific features that many users can appreciate.

1. **STI protection.** The nitrile material is a synthetic rubber latex that blocks passage of even the smallest pathogens, either into or out of the condom, thus providing protection to both the user and the partner. The FDA-approved labeling states that FC2 is indicated for the prevention of HIV/AIDS and other STIs with vaginal use. The female condom can be used off-label for protection during anal sex, but it is recommended that the inner ring be removed after placement and before beginning anal intercourse. In some studies, focus groups have found that users perceive the female condom as an improvement over the male condom for STD protection, because it is in the user's control.[9]
2. **Can be used by couples who cannot use male condoms**—either due to issues of erectile dysfunction or because the penis cannot be fitted with any of the currently available male condoms.[10] Studies show that placement of the male condom is associated with softening or complete loss of erection in nearly one third of condom users.[11] This is not an issue with the female condom. In fact, some couples find that if the male partner places the female condom, it can be sexually exciting for both people.
3. **Can be used during menses.** The female condom does not interfere with menstrual flow, but it does not control it.
4. **May be used in the postpartum period.** Sizing is not needed.
5. **Potential insurance coverage.** Medicaid insurance programs in 36 states now cover the cost of FC2, most at "high rates."[12] Some commercial insurance companies may also cover the cost.

6. **Additional attractive features.** Nitrile warms to body temperature and avoids the cold shock that can be associated with latex condoms. The female condom can be placed up to 8 hours before coitus, avoiding disruption during the arousal/excitement phase. If the silicone lubricant on the female condom does not provide satisfactory lubrication, the user can add more lubricants that are silicone, petroleum-based, or water-soluble. There is a potential for the female condom to increase sexual pleasure at several points. The pressure of the inner ring along the vaginal wall, the stimulation of the outer ring against the clitoris, and the pressure of the inner ring against the head of the penis have all been reported as sources of heightened sexual pleasure with use.

Disadvantages

1. **Proper placement required for efficacy.** The placement procedure requires some practice. Many women in focus groups described the placement procedure as "too complicated" with the two rings.[13] Even those experienced with diaphragm use have commented that the female ring is slippery. The relatively high rates of early functional failures can be discouraging, but those errors diminish rapidly and after 20 uses, technical problems are very rare. The penis must be guided (usually manually) into the condom to insure the penis is not misdirected and enters into the space between the vaginal wall and the outer surface of the condom. For some couples, guiding the penis can be enjoyable, but for others it might be embarrassing, unnatural, or disruptive.
2. **Vaginal placement.** The female condom requires users to be willing and able to place the condom vaginally. Most patients are unfamiliar with the anatomy of the vagina. They do not know that the vagina is potentially a capacious space that is between 6.5 cm to 12.5 cm in length and is capable of expanding naturally to accommodate anything (including a fetus) that passes through that canal.[14] This unfamiliarity raises two concerns that affect acceptance of the female condom:

   a. Some potential users surveyed were very concerned about the size and shape of the female condom. In one study, a participant was quoted as saying, "By (just) looking at it, (FC2) it was scary and even the shape looks horrible." Another said, "The ring looked scary, in fact, the entire structure of FC2 is very scary." Another added that "it is not only scary, but also ugly."[13]

b. Many of the potential users seemed to think that they needed to advance the condom to the level of the cervix to cover it, like a diaphragm. They did not appreciate that coverage of the cervix is automatic. The inner ring just needs to rest in an area that will not apply pressure to internal structures.

3. **Visible.** The female condom is quite obvious to the partner. Negotiation for its use may not be successful.[9]

4. **Potential discomfort with use.** Incorrect introduction or misplacement of the female condom introduces the possibly of discomfort or pain with its use.[13]

5. **Local irritation.** Some users have reported a burning sensation, rash, or pruritus during use of the FC2 or for hours following its removal.

6. **Relatively expensive.** The cost of this single-use condom may present challenges for users who have to pay out-of-pocket for the condoms and who may have frequent acts of intercourse.

7. **Only available by prescription.** The manufacturer has announced that it will move FC2 out of over-the-counter availability and make it available only in 12-packs and only by prescription. However, in many states, users can use the Hey Doctor App to get a prescription for FC2 for a nominal fee to avoid a doctor's appointment. However, there is still the concern that this move will limit access to the condom for noncontraceptive uses, such as STI protection with anal intercourse.

Instructions for Use*

Users should be reminded to place the FC2 with every act of intercourse. The FC2 can be placed up to 8 hours before intercourse, so there is no interruption as passion increases. These are single-use devices. Although one study found that, in monogamous relationships, carefully washing and disinfecting the device enabled reuse of a single female condom for up to 10 times, this practice is not recommended at this time.[15,16] Before removal, the outer ring of the sheath should be twisted closed to contain the ejaculate. The used condom should be disposed of in the solid waste garbage. Caution users not to combine female condoms with male condoms.

Figure 11-1 displays step-by-step instructions for use of FC2 that are included in the packaging. Additional information is available at www.totalaccessgroup.com/FC2-Condom-how-to-use—Step-by-Step_ep_125-1.html.

*These instructions are intended to guide providers in educating patients in how to use their method.

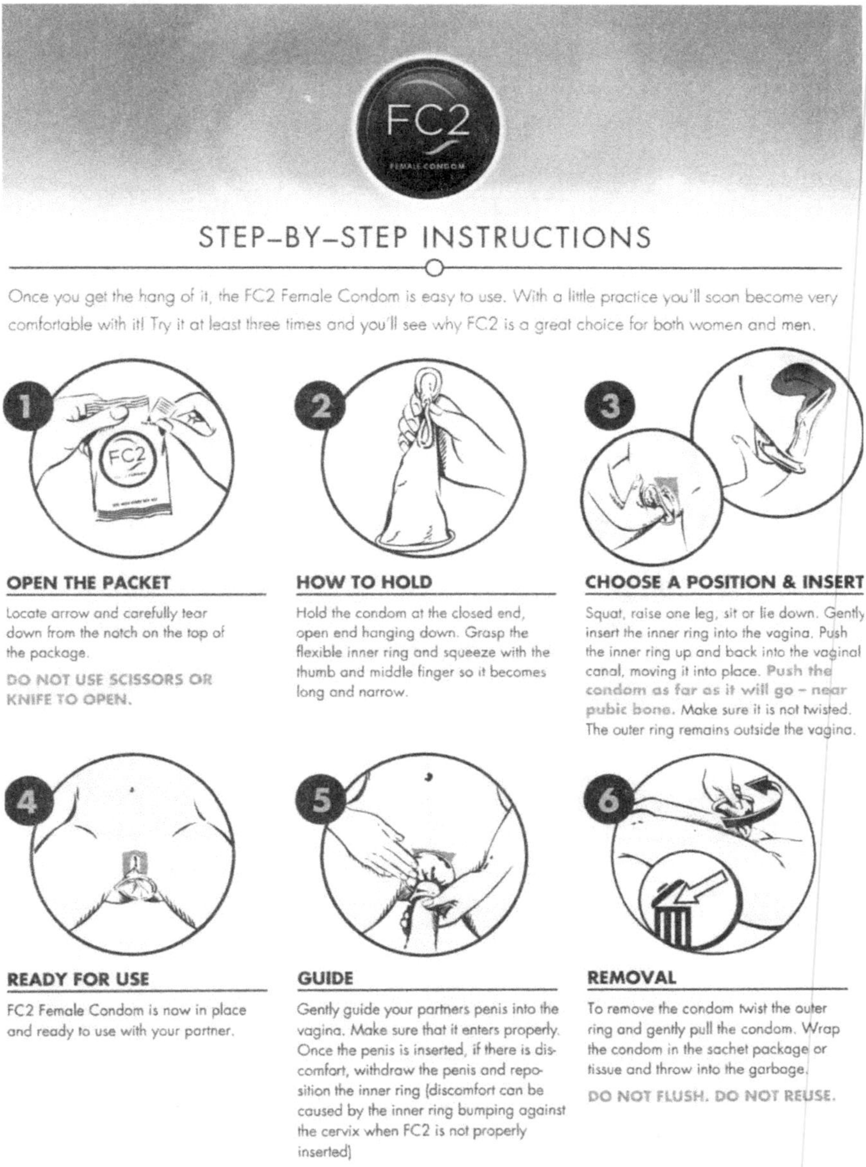

Source: FC2, 2017, with permission

Figure 11-1 FC2 Step-by-Step Detailed Instructions

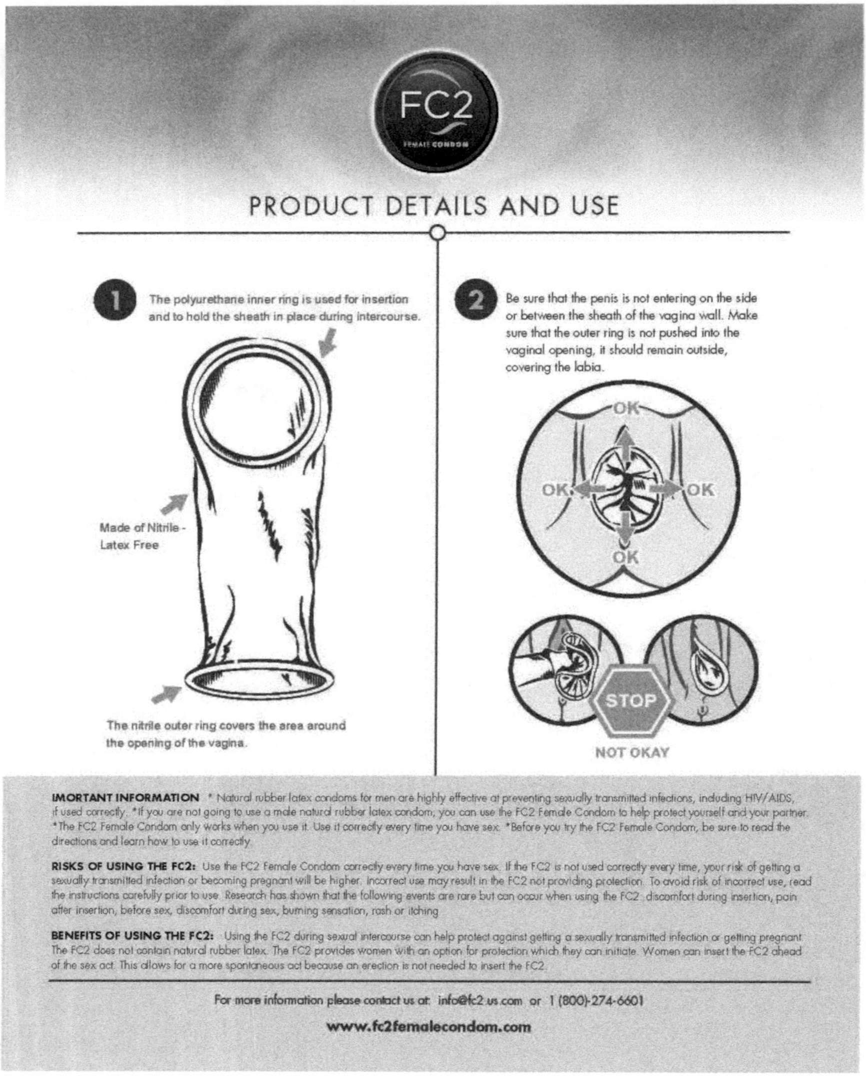

Figure 11-1 *(continued)*

The most important points are:

1. Direct the condom as high in the vagina as comfortably possible and rotate the inner ring to keep it out of the partner's way.
2. Ensure that the penis enters into the condom and stays within the condom during intercourse.

3. After the penis has exited the condom, grasp the outer ring of FC2 and twist it around to seal the fluids inside the condom before removing it.
4. Use a new condom with each act of intercourse.

CAYA DIAPHRAGM

The Caya diaphragm has essentially replaced earlier dome-shaped fitted diaphragms in the United States. Caya (previously known as the SILCs diaphragm) is a reusable lightweight, silicone rubber device molded with a circular nylon spring. It measures 75 mm in length and 67 mm in maximum width. Its spring enables Caya to be used for a variety of vaginal and cervical sizes and in users who have different degrees of vaginal support. Caya can be used by patients who would have been fitted with older diaphragms ranging in size from 65–80 mm. About 80% of potential users meet that criterion. The Caya has two cuplike structures. The large, oval dome-shaped cervical cup fits over cervix and holds spermicide in place over the cervical os. The smaller, everted removal dome tucks behind the symphysis and facilitates later digital removal of the device. The rim is flexible and eases placement through the introitus. Grip dimples on the sides of the rim help the user identify the best position to grasp the unit during placement. Caya has a notch in the anterior edge of the rim to reduce pressure against the urethra. (See Figure 11-2.) Caya fits people with a range of weights and BMIs. The user must be willing and able to place and remove the device or be able to arrange for the partner to perform those tasks.

The Caya diaphragm is used with spermicide.[17] About 1 teaspoon of spermicide should be put into the larger cup and spread around the rim just before placement. If additional acts of coitus are anticipated, Caya should be left in place and additional spermicide should be added into the vagina. Caya should be kept in place for at least 6 hours after the last act of coitus, but it should not be left in the vagina for more than a total of 24 hours. One Caya can be reused for up to 2 years before it needs to be replaced.

While the Caya is available in only one size and does not need to be sized as specifically as earlier diaphragms were, it is still available only by prescription. Professional examination is needed to ensure proper fitting and to confirm the patient's ability to use, place, and remove it correctly. The clinician needs to have clean models in the office available to verify the fit. "Test fit" units are available online for clinicians to use for this function.

CAYA® Contoured Diaphragm

Intravaginal Barrier Device Product Description

Product Benefits:

- Easy insertion and removal
- Easy fit (one size fits most)
- Comfortable for both partners
- Eliminates latex-related odors
- Hormone-Free Contraceptive

Product Specifications:

Elastic body:	50 shore-A durometer medical-grade silicone
Core:	Contoured, one-piece polymer spring
Overall length:	75 mm
Overall width:	67 mm
Membrane:	0.010" nominal thickness

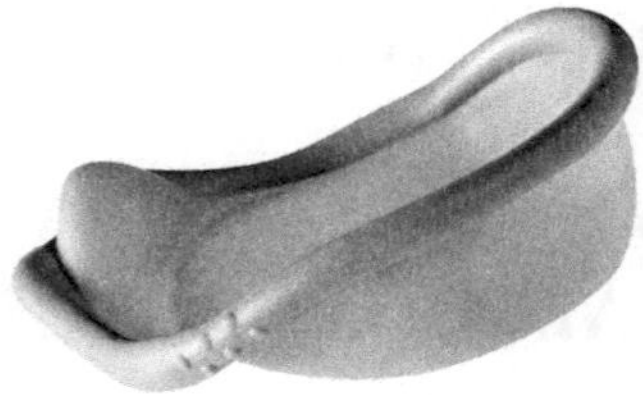

Product Features:

Dynamic contours
- Folds in optimal insertion shape
- Embeds gently in supportive tissue

Gentle folding dynamics
- Soft, easy folding during insertion and removal
- Slides gently out of the vagina

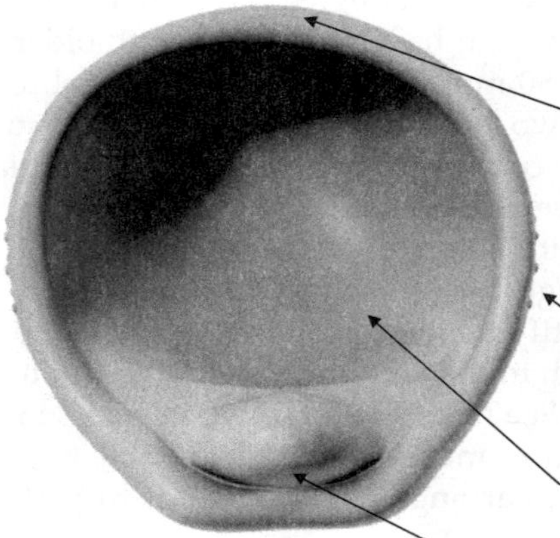

HPSRX ENTERPRISES

Distributed by
HPSRx Enterprises Inc.
Phone (800) 850-1657
Fax (800) 361-6984
www.hpsrx.com

caya® contoured diaphragm
www.caya.us.com

Source: Caya US, 2017, with permission

Figure 11-2 CAYA Diaphragm

Studies show that 75% of interested patients easily placed Caya correctly following instructions. With additional instruction, 94% are able to place, position and remove this diaphragm.[18] After the patient has placed Caya, perform a bimanual exam to confirm correct fit and correct placement. Check to see that—

- The larger dome completely covers the cervix.
- The back rim of Caya is past the cervix and pressed comfortably against the posterior fornix.
- There is no buckling of the rim. Such buckling would suggest that the Caya is too large.
- There is no spinning of Caya when you attempt to rotate it in place. Such spinning would demonstrate that Caya is too small for this user.
- The front rim tucks behind the symphysis pubis.

Also verify that the patient is able to place and remove Caya while in the office.

> It is still possible to order a silicone Milex wide-seal diaphragm in either an arching or omniflex style from the manufacturer. These silicone diaphragms are available in eight sizes ranging from 60–95 mm in 5 mm increments. The use of these more traditional dome-shaped diaphragms has diminished in part because very few practitioners have fitting rings to enable formal sizing (fitting) of diaphragms. However, it is feasible to size someone reasonably well on bimanual exam by measuring the distance between the tip of your middle finger of your examining hand when it is placed against the posterior vaginal fornix and the mark on the upper edge of your index finger where it touches the inferior edge of the pubic arch. This is much like measuring the conjugate angle in obstetrics. The number of millimeters in length to the nearest 5 mm gives you the size of diaphragm needed. After the patient purchases the diaphragm, you would test it in place using all the same maneuvers you used to check Caya to confirm correct sizing prior to having the patient use it for birth control.

Effectiveness

In the Caya clinical trial with 450 diaphragm users in which 150 used Caya with N-9 spermicide, the total 6-month Kaplan-Meier cumulative pregnancy rate for Caya was 12.5% (95% CI, 5.4–19.5%). This rate was annualized to 14% with correct and consistent use and 17.8% total failure rate with use seen in that trial (not equivalent to "typical use" failure rates quoted for other methods). This compared to the 6-month pregnancy rate of 10.7% with the older standard fitted round domed diaphragms.[18] Reanalysis of these data for this book yielded estimates that varied slightly from published estimates—failure rates with perfect use of 16.3% and total failure rate of 17.4%. It is generally recommended that users be prescribed emergency contraception in advance of need to have it available when difficulties are encountered with Caya use. (See Chapter 10 on Emergency Contraception.)

Advantages

In addition to the general advantages offered by barrier methods, Caya offers the following advantages:

1. **Reusable.** The diaphragm is reusable for up to 2 years. The only element that needs to be periodically resupplied is the spermicide, which is available over-the-counter.
2. **Some STD risk reduction.** Diaphragms traditionally have been associated with lower risks for transmitting cervical infection, such as gonorrhea and chlamydia.[19] However, no confirmation of that protection with the newer diaphragms has been published.
3. **Can be used with many other methods.** The Caya diaphragm can be combined with methods except the IUD and female cap to enhance pregnancy protection.
4. **Diaphragm is not often detected** by the partner during coitus and usually does not bother the partner.
5. **Multiple acts of intercourse possible.** More spermicide must be added in the vagina in front of device before each act.
6. **Easy to clean.** The material does not absorb orders.
7. **Additional attractive features.** The spermicide may provide vaginal lubrication. The diaphragm can be placed in advance of coitus, so sex is not interrupted.

Disadvantages

1. **Proper placement required for efficacy.** Users need practice to learn correct placement and removal. Placement of the Caya diaphragm is generally quickly mastered, but over 5% of potential users are not able to learn how to place the device, even with extra instruction and extensive encouragement. The product instructions suggest that the user practice placement a few times before relying on it for pregnancy protection.
2. **Initiation requires clinician visit.** Caya must be professionally fitted and is available only by prescription.
3. **May interrupt sex.** If the Caya is not placed in advance, the need to do so before intercourse may disrupt sexual pleasure.

4. **Postcoital delays.** Caya must be left in place for 6 hours following last act of coitus.
5. **24-hour limit.** Caya must be removed within 24 hours of placement.
6. **Not for immediate postpartum use.** Caya should not be used in the immediate (6 week) postpartum period. Wait until the cervix and vagina normalize and correct sizing can be reconfirmed.
7. **Potential risk of toxic shock syndrome (TSS).** Use during menses is not advised.

INSTRUCTION FOR USE†

Instructions for use of Caya diaphragm are clearly outlined in English and Spanish in the manufacturer's 10-step illustrated guidelines. We have reprinted the English language instructions in Figure 11-3. The website www.caya.eu/use/ has a video that also helps instruct patients in detail, in English and Spanish, on how to use this device.

After removal, the diaphragm should be rinsed clear, dried and stored in a clean, dry container.

FEMCAP CERVICAL CAP

FemCap is a reusable, surgical-grade silicone device shaped like a sailor's hat or a sombrero with a bowl that fits over the cervix, a rim that fits high into the vaginal vault and a variable size brim that stabilizes the unit against the vaginal walls. The wider brim fits against the posterior vaginal wall and the narrower brim fits anteriorly. Spermicide is placed into the bowl, in the space between the brim, on the outside of the bowl and along the outer surface of the brim. There is a thin loop of silicone over the bowl that facilitates removal of the cap. The FemCap can be used for multiple acts of intercourse for up to 48 hours. Some authorities recommend adding extra spermicide into the vagina prior to repeat episodes of intercourse, but the manufacturer states that is not necessary. However, the user must wait six hours after the last act of coitus to remove the cap. The cap is available in three sizes that can generally be determined by the user's obstetrical history. (See Table 11-2)

†These instructions are intended to guide providers in educating patients in how to use their method.

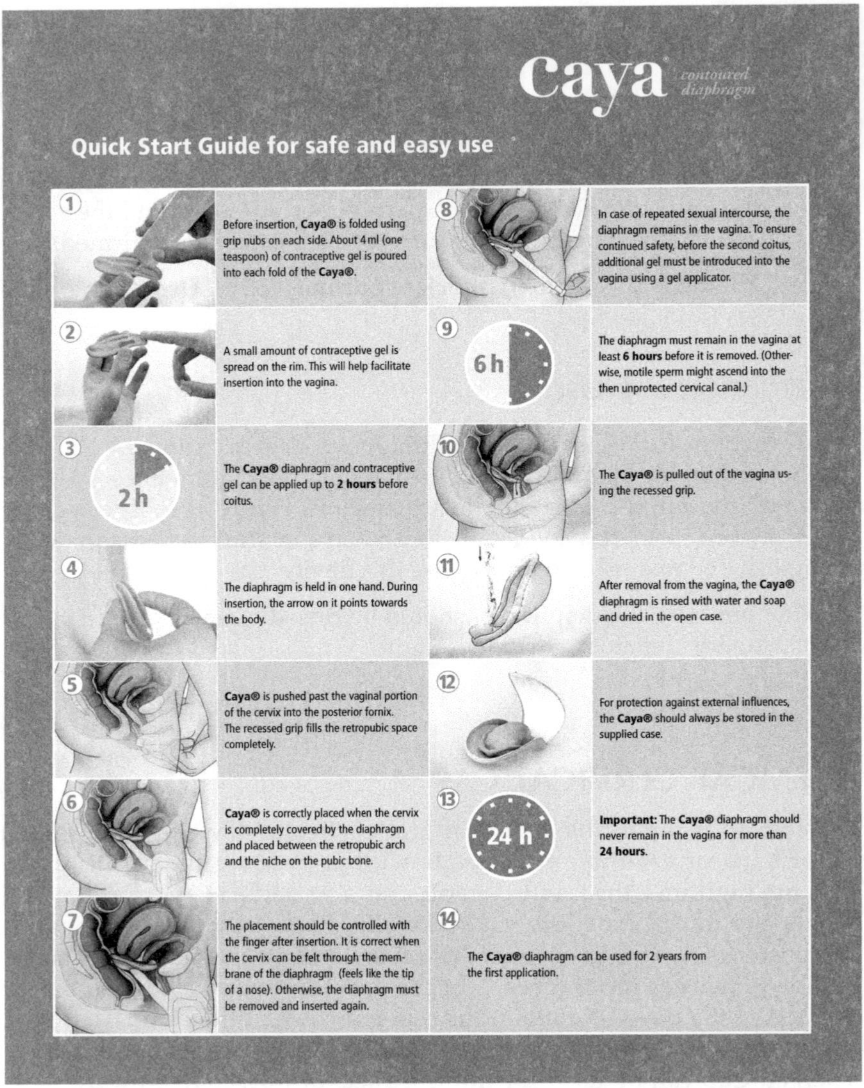

caya
contoured diaphragm
Quick Start Guide for safe and easy use
1
Before insertion, Caya® is folded using grip nubs on each side. About 4 ml (one teaspoon) of contraceptive gel is poured into each fold of the Caya®.
2
A small amount of contraceptive gel is spread on the rim. This will help facilitate insertion into the vagina.
3
2 h
The Caya® diaphragm and contraceptive gel can be applied up to 2 hours before coitus.
4
The diaphragm is held in one hand. During insertion, the arrow on it points towards the body.
5
Caya® is pushed past the vaginal portion of the cervix into the posterior fornix. The recessed grip fills the retropubic space completely.
6
Caya® is correctly placed when the cervix is completely covered by the diaphragm and placed between the retropubic arch and the niche on the pubic bone.
7
The placement should be controlled with the finger after insertion. It is correct when the cervix can be felt through the membrane of the diaphragm (feels like the tip of a nose). Otherwise, the diaphragm must be removed and inserted again.
8
In case of repeated sexual intercourse, the diaphragm remains in the vagina. To ensure continued safety, before the second coitus, additional gel must be introduced into the vagina using a gel applicator.
9
6 h
The diaphragm must remain in the vagina at least 6 hours before it is removed. (Otherwise, motile sperm might ascend into the then unprotected cervical canal.)
10
The Caya® is pulled out of the vagina using the recessed grip.
11
After removal from the vagina, the Caya® diaphragm is rinsed with water and soap and dried in the open case.
12
For protection against external influences, the Caya® should always be stored in the supplied case.
13
24 h
Important: The Caya® diaphragm should never remain in the vagina for more than 24 hours.
14
The Caya® diaphragm can be used for 2 years from the first application.

Source: Caya US, 2017, with permission

Figure 11-3 Detailed instructions on placement and removal of Caya diaphragm.

Effectiveness

In a small randomized 6-month trial, the pregnancy rate with FemCap was nearly twice that of the All-flex diaphragm (13.5% vs 7.9%).[20] (Because of small number of users in the United States, the FemCap was not included among the methods assessed in Chapter 26 on Contraceptive Efficacy.)

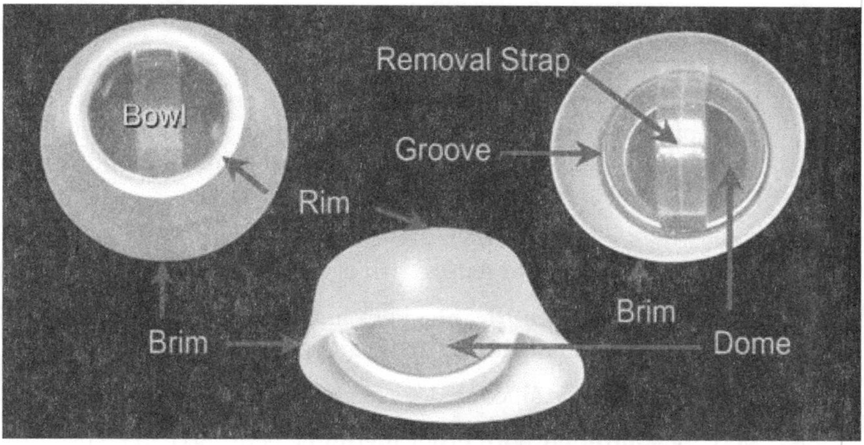

Source: Shihata A, FemCap, Inc., 2017, with permission

Figure 11-4 FemCap

The Planned Parenthood website quotes a 14% failure rate for nulliparous users and a 29% failure rate for those who have given birth, but it is not clear that those data are for this cervical cap or earlier versions such as the Prentif Cervical Cap. It is generally recommended that the user also be prescribed emergency contraception in advance of need to have it available when any difficulties are encountered with FemCap use. (See Chapter 10 on Emergency Contraception.)

Advantages

1. **Easy to fit (clinician benefit).** Size is determined by obstetric history.
2. **Well tolerated.** The FemCap has fewer side effects than seen with older cervical caps or diaphragms: fewer urinary tract infections and no increase in cervical dysplasia.

Table 11-2 Sizing of FemCap

Size	Obstetrical History
22 mm	Nulligravida
26 mm	Has been pregnant, but has not delivered full term baby vaginally
30 mm	Has delivered a term baby vaginally

3. **Advance placement possible.** The user may place the device in advance of coitus, so sex is not interrupted.
4. **Multiple acts possible with one use.** Users can participate in multiple acts of intercourse for up to 48 hours with no additional spermicide needed, but some users report unpleasant odor with such prolonged use.
5. **Reusable.** One FemCap can be used for 1 year. Annual replacement is encouraged to reduce risk of recurrent vaginal infection.
6. **Compatible with lubricants.** Petroleum-based lubricants as well as water-based and silicone ones can be used.
7. **Easy to clean.** The silicone does not absorb odors.
8. **May be combined with other methods.** FemCap can be used together with other methods except IUD, diaphragm or sponge.

Disadvantages

1. **Clinician exam required.** FemCap requires a pelvic exam and a prescription.
2. **Will not fit all interested potential users.** Only 80% of potential users can be fit. Will not work if cervix is adherent to or is flat against the vaginal wall.
3. **Vaginal placement.** Users need to be willing and able to place device vaginally. New users need to practice correct placement.
4. **May interrupt sex.** If it has not been placed in the vagina in advance, placement may interrupt sex.
5. **Postcoital delays.** Users must leave the cap in place for 6 hours after last coitus.
6. **Resizing needed.** The cap needs to be resized after the user has a baby, miscarriage or abortion.
7. **Potential discomfort or problems with use.** Users and their partners may feel discomfort or pain, especially if the cap is misplaced.[21]
8. **Potential for cervical trauma.** Some users have reported blood on the cap, indicating some degree of cervical trauma—usually with removal. However, there have been no reports of increased infection or dysplasia with FemCap use.
9. **May be difficult to remove.** The addition of removal strap did not increase ease of removal. Some patients need directed counselling to apply pressure directly against the dome to break suction before trying to remove the cap.

10. **Limitations on use.** FemCap should not be used during menses, in the immediate (6 week) postpartum period until cervix normalizes, or with cervicitis, PID or history of TSS.

Instructions for Use‡

1. Place the FemCap at least 15 minutes in advance of coitus.
2. Wash your hands and genitalia.
3. Place ½ teaspoon of spermicide into the inside of the bowl and ¼ teaspoon in the groove between the brim and outside of the bowl. Spread spermicide over brim.
4. Find a comfortable position (standing with one leg elevated, lying on back, or squatting). Feel for your cervix.
5. Squeeze the sides of the cap together to make it thin for introduction into your vagina.
6. Slide the FemCap through the opening to your vagina with the longer brim placed against the lower side of your vagina (the side closer to your anus).
7. Advance the cap inside your vagina in a downward angle toward your anus and upward deeper into your vagina, until it reaches your cervix.
8. Rotate the cap to cover your cervix. Tug on strap for ten seconds to make sure it will stay in place during intercourse.
9. Leave the cap in place for 6 hours after last intercourse. Do not use the cap for longer than 48 hours for any one use.

Removal

1. Wait 6 hours after last act of sex to remove FemCap.
2. Assume a position that allows you to feel your cervix.
3. Introduce 1 or 2 fingers into your vagina.
4. Slip your finger under the strap and press against dome of the cap to break the suction (make a dimple in the dome of the cap covering your cervix).
5. Hook the strap with your finger, rotate it slightly and gently pull the cap down toward the opening of your vagina.
6. Check for blood. Rinse the cap with soap and water. Dry. Store in clean dry container.

‡These instructions are intended to guide providers in educating patients in how to use their method.

SPERMICIDES

Spermicides are available over-the-counter without a prescription in a variety of formulations. Spermicides are available as gels and creams (usually for use with other barrier methods), foams (used as single agents or as the agent used before additional acts of intercourse with diaphragms), sponges (need to add liquid to activate spermicide), foaming suppositories, and films (which need 15 minutes to melt within vagina). (See Table 11-3.)

All spermicides currently available in the United States use N-9 as their active ingredient, which limits the patients who may be candidates for spermicides. Those who are at risk for HIV transmission and those who experience skin irritation are not appropriate candidates. Most formulations provide protection if sperm is released within 60 minutes of use. Later acts of intercourse generally require that additional spermicide be added to the vagina before intromission.

Spermicidal gels, creams, and foam are commonly marketed for use with a diaphragm, but they can also be used alone for contraception. One application delivers 52.5 mg to 150 mg of N-9, depending on the product: the spermicide concentration ranges from 8% to 12.5% in foams, and from 2% to 4% in gels and creams. Foams are useful for immediate application in case another method malfunctions (condom slipped off, etc.).

Spermicidal suppositories can be used alone for contraception or with a male or female condom. Suppositories have a spermicide concentration of 3% to 5% and provide 100 mg to 125 mg of N-9. Adequate time between placement and intercourse (10 to 15 minutes depending on the product)

Table 11-3 Spermicides used as a single agent

Base or Carrier	Onset of Action	Duration of Action	Spermicide
Foam	Immediate	≤60 min.	N-9
• Aerosol container			
Creams and gels	Immediate	≤60 min.	N-9
• Single-use packets			
• Reusable applicator			N-9
Suppositories	10–15 min.	<60 min.	N-9
Film	15 min.	<60 min.	N-9

is essential for the spermicide to dissolve and disburse. Incomplete dissolution of the suppository may reduce its contraceptive efficacy and may cause an uncomfortable gritty sensation or friction for one or both partners.

Spermicidal film containing N-9 can be used alone for contraception or with condoms, or, more rarely, with diaphragms or cervical caps. Each paper-thin sheet of film has a spermicide concentration of 28% and contains 72 mg to 100 mg of N-9. The sheet must be introduced into the vagina on or near the cervix at least 15 minutes before intercourse to allow time for the sheet to melt and disperse. Placing film on the tip of the penis for insertion is not recommended; the film will not have adequate time to dissolve, and it may not be properly placed so as to cover the cervical os.

The ***contraceptive sponge*** is a single use vaginal spermicide. This small, pillow-shaped polyurethane sponge contains 1 gram of N-9 spermicide. The concave dimple on one side is designed to fit over the cervix and decrease the chance of dislodgement during intercourse (see Figure 11-5). The other side of the sponge is covered with a woven polyester loop to facilitate removal. The sponge, made in one size, is available over-the-counter. It is moistened with tap water or other available liquid prior to use to activate the spermicide. It is then placed deep into the vagina to cover the cervix. It is immediately effective. There is no need to delay coital activity once it is in place.

The sponge protects for up to 24 hours, no matter how many times intercourse occurs. After the last act of intercourse, the sponge must be left in place for at least six hours before it is removed and discarded. Wearing the sponge for longer than 24 hours is not recommended because of the rare risk of toxic shock syndrome.

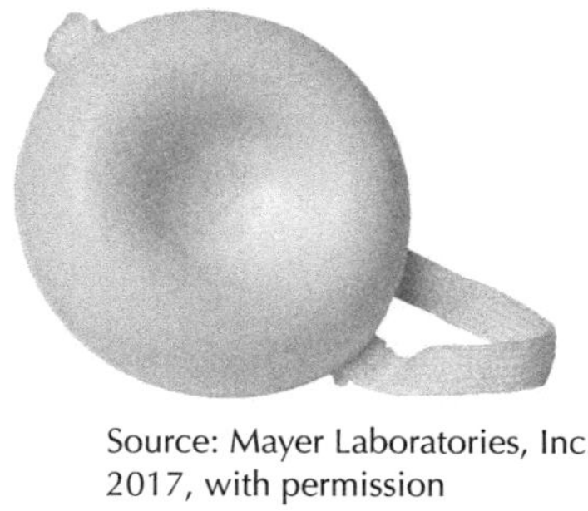

Source: Mayer Laboratories, Inc., 2017, with permission

Figure 11-5 Today contraceptive sponge

Effectiveness

Spermicides are considered to be among the least effective of all modern methods of family planning.[22] With correct and consistent use, spermicides as a single agent have a 16% first-year failure rate. With typical use, that rate rises to 21%, again demonstrating that methods requiring initiation at or around the time of coitus will have larger gaps between potential protection offered and actual protection achieved. Formulations with higher concentrations of N-9 are more effective.[23] There do not appear to be any differences in efficacy by delivery system for the same dose of spermicide.[25] It is recommended that emergency contraceptives be prescribed for users to have on hand if they have any problem with correctly using spermicide with any act of coitus. (See Chapter 10 on Emergency Contraception.)

Some researchers have attributed the relatively higher rates of pregnancy with spermicides to the user instructions that are provided in these over-the-counter methods. In one analysis, the "how to use" sections were found to be hard to understand, with reading levels that ranged from 8th to 12th grade and with line drawing illustrations that were fairly small. Overall, none of the products had instructions that scored high on all the features that make instructions user-friendly.[24] Researchers have developed models that can predict patients who will have <5% pregnancy risk with spermicides. For example, users aged over 35 who engage infrequently in intercourse and have low parity are more likely to use spermicides more successfully.[25] In general, it has been difficult to develop meaningful estimates of efficacy for these methods because of the widely varying failure rates in different studies.[24]

Sponge effectiveness. The efficacy of the contraceptive sponge has been analyzed separately from the other types of spermicides. The failure rates for the sponge are similar to those seen with other spermicides—12% with correct and consistent use and 17% with typical use. However, some studies seem to indicate higher failure rates with parous users (20% perfect use and 27% typical use) compared to nulliparous users (9% perfect use and 14% typical use). A Cochrane systematic review found two studies to compare the efficacy of the contraceptive sponge to the traditional fitted, domed diaphragms. A U.S. study found 12-month pregnancy rates for the sponge vs diaphragm were 17.4% vs 12.8%. In a U.K. study, those rates were 24.5% vs 10.9%.[26]

Mechanisms of Action

N-9 acts as a detergent to disrupt the membranes of the sperm's flagella and body to immobilize or destroy it. However, N-9 can have the same disruptive effect on the epithelial cells of the vagina, cervix, and rectum, which can increase the transmission of HIV. Therefore, patients at high risk for HIV should not use spermicides alone or in combination with other methods.[27] That recommendation would apply to those who have multiple acts of intercourse with multiple partners in a short time period as well as couples who are HIV-serodiscordant. Even in patients with low risk for STDs, the detergent action of N-9 can cause vaginal or penile irritation that can preclude its use.

Advantages

1. **Readily available.** Spermicidal products are available over-the-counter without prescription and can be purchased online or in stores.
2. **Lubricating.** Spermicide provides additional lubrication with intercourse.
3. **Rapid onset of activity.** Spermicidal foams, gels and contraceptive sponge are all immediately active upon placement.
4. **Postpartum use allowed.** Spermicidal products can be used postpartum, but only after lochia has stopped.
5. **Can enable multiple acts of intercourse.** Users can apply additional doses (foam, gel, film, suppository) for multiple acts of intercourse with the same partner (not recommended for use with multiple partners).
6. ***For sponge only.*** The sponge material absorbs ejaculate and is tidier postcoitally.

Disadvantages

1. **Higher failure rates.** High failure rates make this method less attractive for those who need more reliable pregnancy protection, but spermicides are clearly more effective than using no method.
2. **Out-of-pocket cost.** Only a limited number of Medicaid-waiver programs will pay for spermicides, and those programs generally limit the formulations offered and the numbers of uses covered.
3. **Limited candidates.** Spermicidal products cannot be used by those at high risk for HIV or those who have multiple acts of intercourse with multiple partners over a short period of time. Also, those with allergies to the ingredients cannot use the products.
4. **May require negotiation with partner.** The limited 1-hour duration of action often prevents opportunities for advance placement. Placement may interrupt sex.

5. **Delayed onset of activity.** Spermicidal suppository and film require 15 minutes to melt and activate, which may further interrupt coitus.
6. **May be messy.** Some forms (foams, gel) may be messy during and after coitus. Douching and perhaps bathing is to be discouraged for at least 6 hours following coitus. (Douching is discouraged in virtually all situations because it disrupts the vaginal defense system. Here it could also diminish the effectiveness of the spermicide.)
7. **Can cause local reaction.** Spermicide ingredients can cause irritation, allergic-type reactions, or dermatitis affecting the vagina, vulva, penis, anus, oral cavity.
8. **Taste may be unpleasant**.
9. **Failure rates in parous women may be higher.** Parous sponge users may have even higher failure rates with the sponge than with other forms of spermicides, but effectiveness has not been analyzed by parity for those other methods.
10. ***For sponge only:***
    - Must be left in place 6 hours after coitus.
    - May increase risk of TSS.
    - Should not be used first 6 weeks postpartum until the cervix normalizes in size.

For Use

The product packaging provides some insight into usage. Foams are placed by an applicator into the vagina and are immediately active. If possible, try to put the spermicide as close to your cervix as possible. Suppositories and films also need to be placed as close to your cervix as possible, but must be put in your vagina 10 to15 minutes prior to intercourse. Avoid douching for at least 6 hours after intercourse. Follow the specific instructions on the package.

Author Disclosures—Nelson: none. Harwood: none.

References

1. Aitken RJ, Hughes LM, Griffith R, Baker MA. Bridging the gap between male and female fertility control; contraception-on-demand. Contraception 2008;78:S28–35.
2. Gallaway MS, Waller DK, Canfield MA, Scheuerle A.; National birth defects prevention study. The association between use of spermicides or male condoms and major structural birth defects. Contraception 2009;80:422–9.

3. Guffey MB, Richardson B, Husnik M, et al. HPTN 035 phase II/IIb randomised safety and effectiveness study of the vaginal microbicides BufferGel and 0.5% PRO 2000 for the prevention of sexually transmitted infections in women. Sex Transm Infect 2014;90:363–9.
4. Obiero J, Mwethera PG, Wiysonge CS. Topical microbicides for prevention of sexually transmitted infections. Cochrane DB Syst Rev 2012;6:CD007961.pub2.
5. Bounds W, Guillebaud J, Dominik R, Dalberth BT. The diaphragm with and without spermicide. A randomized, comparative efficacy trial. J Reprod Med 1995;40:764–74.
6. van der Straten A, Sahin-Hodoglugil N, Clouse K, Mtetwa S, Chirenje MZ. Feasibility and potential acceptability of three cervical barriers among vulnerable young women in Zimbabwe. J Fam Plann Reprod Health Care 2010;36:13–9.
7. Beksinska M, Greener R, Kleinschmidt I, Pillay L, Maphumulo V, Smit J. A randomized noninferiority crossover controlled trial of the functional performance and safety of new female condoms: an evaluation of the Velvet, Cupid2, and FC2. Contraception 2015;92:261–7.
8. Beksinska M, Smit J, Greener R, Piaggio G, Joanis C. The female condom learning curve: patterns of female condom failure over 20 uses. Contraception 2015;91:85–90.
9. Hart GJ, Pool R, Green G, Harrison S, Nyanzi S, Whitworth JA. Women's attitudes to condoms and female-controlled means of protection against HIV and STDs in south western Uganda. AIDS Care 1999;11:687–98.
10. Cecil M, Nelson AL, Trussell J, Hatcher R. If the condom doesn't fit, you must resize it. Contraception 2010;82:489–90.
11. Crosby RA, Sanders SA, Yarber WL, Graham CA, Dodge B. Condom use errors and problems among college men. Sex Transm Dis 2002;29:552–7.
12. Witte SS, MacPhee C, Ginsburg N, Deshmukh N. Medicaid reimbursement for the female condom. Am J Public Health 2017;107:1633–1635.
13. Mogale R, Mulaudzi FM, Peu MD, Mataboge MS, Ngunyulu R, Phiri SS. The constraints and concerns regarding the size and/or shape of the second generation female condom: The narratives from the healthcare providers. Afr J Prim Health Care Fam Med 2016;8:e1–7.
14. Soo MJ, Bharwani N, Rockall AG. Vagina and vulva: Imaging techniques, normal anatomy and anatomical variants. Abdom Imaging 2014:2201–10.
15. Philpott A. Re-use of the female condom: now for the practical realities. Reprod Health Matters 2003;11:185–6.
16. Potter B, Gerofi J, Pope M, Farley T. Structural integrity of the polyurethane female condom after multiple cycles of disinfection, washing, drying and relubrication. Contraception 2003;67:65–72.
17. Mauck CK, Brache V, Kimble T, et al. A phase I randomized postcoital testing and safety study of the Caya diaphragm used with 3% Nonoxynol-9 gel, ContraGel or no gel. Contraception 2017;96:124–130.
18. Schwartz JL, Weiner DH, Lai JJ, et al. Contraceptive efficacy, safety, fit, and acceptability of a single-size diaphragm developed with end-user input. Obstet Gynecol 2015;125:895–903.
19. d'Oro LC, Parazzini F, Naldi L, La Vecchia C. Barrier methods of contraception, spermicides, and sexually transmitted diseases: a review. Genitourin Med 1994;70:410–7.
20. Mauck C, Callahan M, Weiner DH, Dominik R. A comparative study of the safety and efficacy of FemCap, a new vaginal barrier contraceptive, and the Ortho All-Flex diaphragm. The FemCap Investigators' Group. Contraception 1999;60:71–80.
21. Mauck CK, Weiner DH, Creinin MD, et al. FemCap with removal strap: ease of removal, safety and acceptability. Contraception 2006;73:59–64.
22. Raymond EG, Trussell J, Weaver MA, Reeves MF. Estimating contraceptive efficacy: the case of spermicides. Contraception 2013;87:134–7.
23. Grimes DA, Lopez LM, Raymond EG, Halpern V, Nanda K, Schulz KF. Spermicide used alone for contraception. Cochrane DB Syst Rev. 2013;12:CD005218.pub4.

24. Zite NB, Wallace LS. Do instructions for over-the-counter pre-coital female contraceptives promote "perfect use"? Contraception 2009;79:211–5.
25. Schreiber CA, Ratcliffe SJ, Sammel MD, Whittaker PG. A self-assessment efficacy tool for spermicide contraceptive users. Am J Obstet Gynecol 2016;214:264.e1–264.e7.
26. Kuyoh MA, Toroitich-Ruto C, Grimes DA, Schulz KF, Gallo MG. Sponge versus diaphragm for contraception. Cochrane Database Syst Rev 2002;3:CD003172.
27. Summary chart of US Medical Eligibility Criteria (US MEC) Contraceptive Use. Available at: www.cdc.gov/reproductivehealth/contraception/mmwr/mec/summary.html. Last accessed 8/30/2017.

Fertility Awareness-Based Methods

12

Victoria H. Jennings, PhD
Chelsea B. Polis, PhD

- Fertility awareness based methods (FABMs) help couples understand how to avoid pregnancy or how to become pregnant by teaching them to predict high fertility and low fertility days.
- Regardless of whether they use family planning, or which method they use, most people can find value in learning fertility awareness.
- There are several different kinds of FABMs, and they use one or more different indicators of fertility.
- FABMs can address preferences of some people to use a method that has no side effects, can be used together with their partners, and can be used to achieve or avoid pregnancy.

Fertility Awareness-Based methods (FABMs) of family planning depend on identifying the "fertile window," or the days in each menstrual cycle when intercourse is most likely to result in a pregnancy. Some FABMs simply involve keeping track of cycle days to understand which days of the menstrual cycle are most likely to be fertile. Other FABMs involve observing, recording, and interpreting the body's fertility signs.[1]

FABMs rely on five biological facts:[2]

- The periodicity of fertility and infertility that occurs during each menstrual cycle
- A single ovulatory event each cycle
- The limited lifespan of the ovum (which can be fertilized only in the short time span of 12–24 hours after release)[3]

- The limited lifetime of sperm in cervical mucus and the upper genital tract (3 to 5 days)[4]
- The ability of a person using FABM to monitor cycle length or cycle-related symptoms and signs

To avoid pregnancy, couples either use a barrier method or do not have vaginal intercourse during the fertile time. Although terminology varies, couples who use a barrier method on fertile days are often described as using a "fertility awareness-based method (FABM)" while those who abstain are often described as using "natural family planning."[5] This chapter uses the term FABM to indicate that the client can choose to abstain or use an alternative method on fertile days. Studies suggest that many people seeking family planning services would be interested in an FABM if it were explained to them appropriately[6] regardless of their intention to abstain or use a barrier method. Data from the U.S. National Survey of Family Growth between 2006 and 2010 suggest that about 22% of American couples have used periodic abstinence or natural family planning at least once, and 2-3% of contraceptive users are doing so currently; ever use increased with educational attainment.[7]

MECHANISM OF ACTION

FABMs use one or more indicators to identify the beginning and end of the fertile time during the menstrual cycle. FABMs discussed throughout this chapter include methods based on tracking of days of the menstrual cycle (e.g., the Standard Days Method, the Calendar Rhythm Method), methods based on observation of cervical secretions (e.g., the TwoDay Method, the Billings Ovulation Method, the Creighton Model), methods based on tracking of multiple indicators of fertility (e.g., symptothermal methods), and symptohormonal methods (e.g., the Marquette Model). Methods that rely upon mini-computers (which use predictive algorithms to identify the fertile time) as well as smartphone applications (apps) are discussed. Some FABMs can be effective for preventing pregnancy when they are used correctly. However, with incorrect use, unprotected intercourse takes place precisely on the days that are potentially fertile.

In most cycles, ovulation occurs at or very near the middle of the cycle.[8] There are only about 6 days during the cycle when unprotected intercourse can actually result in pregnancy (the 5 days preceding ovulation and the day of ovulation), related to the lifespan of the gametes.[9,10] Even though ovulation does not occur on the same day each cycle, in cycles that range between 26 and 32 days long (approximately 78% of cycles) the fertile window is highly likely to fall within cycle days 8 to 19.[11] In shorter or longer cycles, the fertile window shifts accordingly.

Two FABMs, the Standard Days Method and the Calendar Rhythm Method, involve counting the days in the menstrual cycle to identify the fertile days. The Standard Days Method requires only that menstrual cycles are between 26 and 32 days long and the first day of the menstrual cycle is tracked, noting potential fertility on days 8 through 19. It is important to have a record of the length of the previous 6 to 12 menstrual cycles prior to starting the Calendar Rhythm Method in order to identify the longest and shortest of these cycles. Once these are collected, calculations are performed to identify the probable days of fertility during the current cycle. (See Instructions for Use below.) While survey results show that, in many countries, a substantial number of couples state that they are using the "rhythm" or "calendar rhythm" method, as many as half of these couples have little understanding of its proper use and simply abstain from intercourse on a few days of the menstrual cycle when they believe, often erroneously, that pregnancy is most likely to occur.[12] It appears in these situations that "calendar rhythm" has become a generic term for "occasional abstinence."

Other FABMs, such as the TwoDay Method, the Billings Ovulation Method (and variants such as the Creighton Model),[13] involve actual observation of the presence or absence of cervical secretions or changes in their characteristics to identify the beginning and end of the fertile phase of the cycle. The Creighton Model is not discussed in depth, given the lack of comparable contraceptive effectiveness data due to the way analyses of this method have been conducted to date. Symptothermal methods involve observation of at least two fertility indicators: cervical secretions and basal body temperature. Some symptothermal method protocols also involve observation of changes in cervical position, a calendar calculation, or both. Changes in all these signs are caused by fluctuations in circulating hormone levels during the cycle.

The Marquette Model, a symptohormonal method, utilizes a self-test device, the Clearblue Fertility Monitor, which measures urinary hormones to detect the fertile phase of the menstrual cycle, and also relies upon information from cervical secretion, temperature observations, or both. Clearblue is approved in the U.S. for planning pregnancy; a similar product, Persona, has been studied in clinical trials and is available in Europe for planning or avoiding pregnancy.[14,15]

Over 1,000 smartphone applications are currently available to help people track their menstrual cycles.[16] Most are not appropriate for pregnancy prevention,[17] although the millions of people who have downloaded them do not necessarily understand this.[18] Thus, providers should be prepared to guide their patients in identifying and selecting which apps provide accurate information and are appropriate for their particular needs. Some apps facilitate use of an existing FABM (such as a symptothermal method, the Billings Ovulation Method, or the Standard

Days method) by providing a digital platform that serves as an alternative to traditional paper and pencil charts or other tools used to track fertility signs. In order to determine which days are fertile or non-fertile, the person using the app is primarily responsible for interpreting the information they enter into these apps, but those who choose an existing FABM app often find it a convenient tool.

Another category of smartphone apps requires input of information about fertility signs but uses a predictive algorithm embedded within the app itself to determine the fertile time—meaning that the user is not primarily responsible for determining which days are fertile or non-fertile.

Finally, we discuss mini-computers, which are usually linked to basal body temperature thermometers, may require the user to enter data about menses, and employ predictive algorithms to identify the fertile time.

EFFECTIVENESS

Successful use of FABMs for avoiding pregnancy depends on (1) the accuracy of the method in identifying the actual fertile window, (2) the ability of the person using the method to correctly interpret the information to identify the fertile window, and (3) the ability of the couple to follow the instructions of the method—that is, to use a barrier method or to avoid vaginal intercourse on the days the method identifies as fertile. Motivation of both members of the couple to avoid pregnancy also is a factor in successful use.[19]

The probability of pregnancy with typical use is approximately 15% across all women in the United States who self-report use of either "rhythm or safe period by calendar" or a "safe period by temperature or cervical mucus test, natural family planning" as their contraceptive method,[20] based upon an unpublished estimate from an analysis of the 2006–2010 NSFG (which is adjusted for underreporting of abortion).[21] The estimate was not published because the number of segments of use (257) did not meet the pre-specified minimum of observations (50) at each month for the first 12 months, so the estimate should be interpreted with caution. This estimate of 15% is substantially lower than that derived from the previous (2002) NSFG[22] (24%); it is unclear if this change relates to instability in the estimates given the small number of women reporting use of these methods, to improved use of these methods between the two survey periods, or to other factors.

However, use of this estimate—which "lumps" together a range of FABMs, has been controversial, and warrants additional explanation. National surveys in the United States can theoretically be used to estimate typical-use effectiveness of FABMs, but this is challenging in practice, given low use of all FABMs. Small numbers of users can lead to instability in estimates. For this reason, estimation of typical effectiveness for *individual* FABMs has not been possible in U.S. surveys to date. To overcome this statistical limitation, analyses of NSFG data have "lumped" various FABMs together to enable generation of an overall typical-use estimate across all women who self-report using an FABM. However, greater than 80% of FABM use in recent NSFG surveys consists of women self-reporting use of calendar rhythm. Furthermore, given colloquial use of terms such as "rhythm" (as described above), individuals self-reporting use of these methods may include women not following formal rules for calendar rhythm but instead attempting to time intercourse based on their own (correct or incorrect) understanding of the fertile period. Thus, such "lumped" estimates may not be applicable to individual FABMs but are provided to shed light on the typical experience of women in the United States who report using these methods.

Population-based survey data from the NSFG or other surveys have been used by experts to estimate typical-use failure rates for most other contraceptive methods. (See Figure 3-1 and Table 3-2 in Chapter 3.) These surveys allow experts to monitor the actual experience across a range of contraceptive users with differing demographic characteristics. Typical- (and perfect-) use rates derived from clinical trials can also be considered, but they should be interpreted differently. Participants in clinical trials are more highly selected (and thus, less generalizable) than those in population-based surveys. In addition, their behaviors may be influenced by frequent contact with investigators and study staff, which may be particularly important for methods that are highly user-dependent, such as FABMs. Furthermore, numerous FABM clinical trials have used inappropriate methodological approaches,[23] and estimates vary substantially by FABM studied, study quality, and country context.[24] A systematic review is underway to comprehensively summarize the best available evidence on FABM effectiveness derived from clinical trials.[25] Examples of estimated perfect- and typical-use pregnancy probabilities for individual FABMs are summarized below, although in the absence of a comprehensive systematic review, these estimates have not yet been systematically evaluated for quality or comprehensiveness. Furthermore, these are largely derived from clinical trials, and should thus be interpreted as "best case scenarios." FABMs that have not yet been tested in standard contraceptive effectiveness studies are described separately.[23]

Methods Based on Tracking Days of the Menstrual Cycle

Standard Days Method. The first-year probabilities of pregnancy for typical use is estimated at 12% and for perfect use at 5%, based on a prospective, multicountry study.[26] Similar typical-use probabilities were found when SDM was offered in regular service delivery (10% in Peru, 13% in Turkey,[27] and 14% in a meta-analysis of data from 14 countries).[28,29]

Calendar Rhythm. Estimated pregnancy probabilities for Calendar Rhythm vary widely, partially because the estimates come from flawed studies. Estimated first-year pregnancy probabilities for typical use were between 15% and 19% in a meta-analysis.[30] This estimate corresponds with those from national survey data domestically and internationally. In addition to estimates described above from NSFG data (composed largely of women reporting use of calendar rhythm), a study pooling Demographic and Health Survey data from 43 countries estimated a first-year typical-use pregnancy probability of 14% for periodic abstinence (also largely composed of women reporting use of calendar rhythm).[31]

Methods Based on Observation of Cervical Secretions

TwoDay Method. As estimated by a prospective multi-country study, this method has a first-year typical-use pregnancy probability of 14%, while the first-year perfect-use probability is between 4% and 6%.[32]

Billings Ovulation Method. Currently available studies suggest that the first-year probability of pregnancy for the Billings Ovulation Method is about 3% among perfect users and up to 23% among all users in studies.[33–35]

Methods Based on Tracking Multiple Indicators of Fertility

Symptothermal methods. A large German study estimated a first-year typical-use probability of pregnancy of about 2%, while perfect-use pregnancy probabilities were estimated at 0.4% (for women who abstained during the fertile period) or 0.6% (for women who had protected intercourse during the fertile period).[36] However, multiple other studies of symptothermal methods generated substantially higher estimates, up to 33% for typical use, although study quality and setting varied, as did rules utilized for identifying the fertile time.[37–41]

Marquette Method. A retrospective study of this symptohormonal method, which measures hormonal changes during the cycle as well as changes in cervical secretions, was conducted in several centers in the United States and found a first-year typical-use probability of pregnancy of 11%.[42] A subsequent randomized study found that women who used the Clearblue Fertility Monitor without monitoring cervical secretions had a typical-use probability of pregnancy of 7%.[43]

Fabms and Digital Technologies

Smartphone Apps that Facilitate Use of An Existing Method

In theory, apps that replace pencil and paper charts (or other tools) are intended to maintain fidelity with the methods themselves. That is, if an app accurately represents the FABM on which it is based, effectiveness for pregnancy avoidance could be the same as that for the underlying method, although this has not been empirically tested for any of the above-listed methods.

Smartphone Apps Based Upon Predictive, Embedded Algorithms

One of these apps, Natural Cycles, involves temperature monitoring, with the user entering her basal body temperature into the app daily. Users also enter information about menses and, as an option, urinary hormones. The app stores and analyzes this information over time and provides the user with an assessment of her fertility status. A study found a perfect-use annual probability of pregnancy of approximately 1% and an upper limit (i.e., when participants with unknown pregnancy status were considered pregnant) typical-use probability of 9.8%.[44,45] The app has been certified in the European Union to be legally sold and used for contraception.

Another app, Dynamic Optimal Timing (Dot) is based on an algorithm developed from a statistical analysis linking cycle length, timing of ovulation, and variable fecundability of the sperm and ovum to identify fertility status.[46] Theoretical efficacy based on this analysis, though not on actual use, is estimated at 1% to 3%. A prospective efficacy study to assess perfect and typical use has been registered and is underway.[47,48]

Mini-Computers with Predictive Algorithms

Neither of two mini-computers (LadyComp or Daysy) have been assessed through standard prospective effectiveness studies (though some manufacturers do make unsubstantiated claims about effectiveness).[49]

Advantages and Indications

Studies in several countries have shown that characteristics of FABMs perceived by some to be advantages may be perceived by others as disadvantages. For example, the importance of the partner's participation in method use is positive for some couples,[29] but it is difficult to achieve for others. Some people choose FABMs precisely because of the opportunity for daily awareness of fertility signs or cycle day, while others find this burdensome. For some, the lack of side effects of FABMs offsets their higher failure rates (as compared to other methods of family planning).[29] Indeed, studies have shown that most people who choose FABMs either began practicing family planning for the first time or stopped using another method several months before initiating FABM use—mostly because of their concerns about side effects with other methods.[29]

Fertility awareness is important for all people, regardless of which family planning method they use or whether they choose to use family planning at all. Fertility awareness information can be used for a number of purposes:

- ***To avoid pregnancy.*** For maximum effectiveness, couples should abstain from vaginal intercourse or use a barrier method during the entire fertile time.
- ***To become pregnant.*** Couples have intercourse on the days that are potentially fertile. Depending on the method used, these may include days 8 to 19 of the cycle, or the days cervical secretions are observed. Pregnancy is most likely to occur if they have intercourse within 1 to 2 days prior to ovulation.[3] A 2015 Cochrane review concluded that there are insufficient data available to draw conclusions on the effectiveness of timed intercourse for the outcomes of live birth, adverse events, and clinical pregnancy. Timed intercourse may improve (clinical or self-reported) pregnancy rates compared to intercourse without ovulation prediction, but the quality of evidence is low to very low and should be regarded with caution.[50] FABMs can also be used by couples in HIV serodiscordant relationships who desire a pregnancy, in order to maximize the chances of pregnancy using timed intercourse, while minimizing unnecessary exposure of the HIV-uninfected partner to the virus.[51]
- ***To detect pregnancy.*** A postovulatory temperature rise (see the section on Basal Body Temperature Charting) sustained for 18 or more days is an excellent early indicator that pregnancy is underway.[52]
- ***To detect impaired fertility.*** Charting fertility signs costs relatively little and can aid in diagnosing and treating fertility problems due to infrequent or absent ovulation. People who menstruate but do not ovulate tend to have a meandering basal body temperature pattern throughout the cycle, rather than the typical pattern (lower in the first part of the cycle and higher in the second). Similarly, cervical secretions may be absent or not conform to the typical pattern.
- ***To detect a need for medical attention.*** Changes in cervical and vaginal secretions, abdominal pain, and other signs or symptoms may indicate the need for medical attention. (See Chapter 20 on Reproductive Tract Infections.)

DISADVANTAGES AND CAUTIONS

FABMs are unforgiving of incorrect or inconsistent use, leading to higher typical-use pregnancy rates than for hormonal methods, intrauterine contraceptives, or sterilization. While FABMs produce no physical side effects, they offer no protection against sexually transmitted infections (STIs), including infection with the human immunodeficiency virus (HIV). Also, lack of the partner's cooperation will be an obstacle for some who wish to practice abstinence or use an alternative method during the fertile time. Certain conditions that increase the likelihood of irregular cycles may make FABMs more difficult to use, and patients with these conditions require more extensive counseling and follow-up:

- Recent childbirth
- Current breastfeeding
- Recent menarche
- Anovulatory cycling as with PCOS or obesity-related infrequent cycles
- Recent discontinuation of hormonal contraceptive methods
- Approaching menopause

FABMs are also not recommended for persons who are unable to abstain or use other contraceptive methods during the fertile days, for personal, partner, or cultural reasons. See Table 12-1.

Table 12-1 Reasons for which particular FABMs are contraindicated

Reasons	Billings Ovulation Method	Symptothermal Methods	TwoDay Method	Standard Days Method
Irregular cycles, including postpartum until cycle regularity returns				⊘
Inability to interpret fertility signs correctly	⊘	⊘	⊘	
Reproductive tract infections or vaginitis that affect fertility signs	⊘	⊘	⊘	
Intermenstrual bleeding not distinguishable from menstruation or that masks secretions	⊘	⊘	⊘	⊘
Reluctance to observe secretions	⊘	⊘	⊘	
Clinical detection of female genital cutting[53]	⊘	⊘	⊘	

Special Issues

Acceptability

Studies have shown that in their discussions with patients, family planning providers are less likely to routinely include information about FABMs than about other contraceptive methods. A survey of approximately 500 physicians in the United States found that 46% of responding physicians mentioned FABMs to at least some patients when discussing family planning. When asked by a patient for information about an FABM, most physicians described either calendar rhythm or basal body temperature methods.[54] A recent study in Canada shows that most physicians underestimate efficacy of FABMs and only a small proportion provide information about them.[55]

Recent development of FABMs that are easy to use may increase interest and availability. In addition, it is relatively easy to incorporate a discussion of the simpler methods into the context of regular clinical or community-based services, thus making the methods more widely available.[29,56] (See Chapter 2 for more complete discussion of patient-centered contraception counseling.)

Some couples, providers, and program managers worry that using an FABM will hamper a couple's sexual life, making the method less acceptable and leading to discontinuation of use. Analysis of intercourse patterns of users of the Standard Days Method and of the TwoDay Method show that people who use these methods have intercourse almost as frequently as do those who use other methods (5.6 and 5.5 coital acts per month, respectively). The pattern differs, however, as the couples who use these two FABMs tend to have sex more frequently during the infertile days before and after the fertile window and avoid sex during their fertile days.[54]

Safety

Because unintended pregnancies among couples who use FABMs usually result from having intercourse at the beginning or end of the fertile time, concerns have been raised about the risk of birth defects or poor pregnancy outcomes due to aged ovum or sperm. Research has shown that no such increased risks exist.[57,58] An exception is that, in one prospective study, women with a history of spontaneous abortion had a greater chance of having another spontaneous abortion when conception occurred very early or late in the fertile time (23% of women with a previous spontaneous abortion compared with 10% to 15% of women who had not experienced a previous spontaneous abortion).[57] Providers should reassure any concerned patients that FABMs do not pose a threat to the health of mothers and their children.

Sex Selection

A study of about 1,000 births showed no association between the timing of conception and the sex ratio at birth.[59] These results do not substantiate claims that couples can select the sex of their child by timing intercourse.

Traditional/Modern

The classification of contraceptive methods into "traditional" and "modern" categories is common in surveys in low-resource settings where the use of traditional practices is higher than in most other countries. Noting that certain methods, primarily FABMs, were categorized in some surveys as "traditional" and in others as "modern," the WHO and USAID convened a consultation in 2014 to attempt to harmonize definitions,[60,61] As an outcome of this consultation, both the WHO and USAID published articles defining modern and traditional methods and categorizing certain specific FABMs as modern.[60,61] This has sparked further discussion in the literature. One response article stated that any method that required couples to avoid sex or use another method when they do so was not modern.[62] Another stated that FABMs were "inferior" and not "rights-based" but rather were being promoted because of a particular policy agenda.[63] While the discussion continues, both WHO and USAID include specific FABMs in their guidance documents as modern methods.[64–68]

PROVIDING FERTILITY AWARENESS-BASED METHODS

A critical component of providing FABMs is helping patients and couples decide how they want to handle their fertile days (i.e., by abstaining or using another method) to avoid pregnancy. Those who choose to use a barrier method (a fertility awareness-combined method) on those days should be instructed on correct use of the method and counseled accordingly.

Studies have shown that it takes less than 20 minutes to learn that fertility should be considered likely on days 8 to 19 of the cycle and to keep track of cycle days (to use the Standard Days Method) or to learn how to notice the presence or absence of secretions (to use the TwoDay Method).[32] Counseling may be needed to foster correct method use. Couples using other FABMs need an instructor's teaching to observe, record, and interpret the fertility signs and patterns. Based on general medical practice within the National Health Service in Great Britain, it takes approximately 4 to 6 hours to teach fertility awareness skills, including charting fertility signs (cervical secretions and basal body temperature) and identifying the fertile time.[69] Most instruction in FABMs involves multiple sessions over several cycles, especially for those that involve observing, recording, and interpreting fertile signs.

> **Emergency Contraceptives (EC):** Emergency contraceptive pills or placement of a copper intrauterine contraceptive after unprotected intercourse substantially reduces the risk of pregnancy. (See Chapter 10 for more information.) Persons who use EC while using an FABM should be advised that EC could result in changes in cycle length and timing of ovulation in the forthcoming cycle.[70]

USER INSTRUCTIONS FOR FERTILITY AWARENESS-BASED METHODS

Instructions are presented here for a sample of FABMs: Standard Days Method, Calendar Rhythm, TwoDay Method, Billings Ovulation Method, and symptothermal methods. Instructions on use of the Marquette Method, the Creighton Model, app-based methods, and mini-computer-based methods are available online. Please note: some of these methods, such as the Billings Ovulation method and symptothermal methods, should be taught by a well-trained provider. The instructions below are not intended to replace formal instruction in proper use of these methods, and are provided for illustrative purposes only.

CYCLE DAY TRACKING METHODS

Standard Days Method

The Standard Days Method is most appropriate for people with menstrual cycles between 26 and 32 days long. Approximately 78% of people who are menstruating can expect to meet this requirement at any time.[26] Your cycle length should be reassessed as you age. To use the Standard Days Method, you will need to track the days of your menstrual cycle, starting with the day your menstrual bleeding begins. If you have more than 1 cycle in 1 year that is shorter than 26 days or longer than 32 days, you should contact your provider to discuss the possibility of using another method.

1. Count the first day of your menstrual bleeding as day 1.
2. Continue counting every day.
3. On days 1 to 7, you can have unprotected intercourse. (You may be bleeding on these days.)

4. **To prevent pregnancy.** Unprotected intercourse is permitted on days 1 to 7 and from day 20 until the end of your cycle. On days 8 to 19, use a barrier method or avoid vaginal intercourse.
5. **To become pregnant.** Unprotected intercourse is suggested frequently, as often as every day, between days 8 and 19 of your cycle.
6. From day 20 through the end of your cycle, you can have unprotected intercourse.

Many people who use the Standard Days Method use CycleBeads to help them keep track of their cycle days. This color-coded string of beads with a ring the user moves daily allows you to identify whether it is a fertile or infertile day and whether your cycle length is appropriate for using this method. More recently, people are using the CycleBeads app on their smartphones. To do so, enter your period start date, and the app tells you your daily fertility status and cycle length appropriateness. See Figure 12-1 for an illustration of the CycleBeads app and instructions for use.

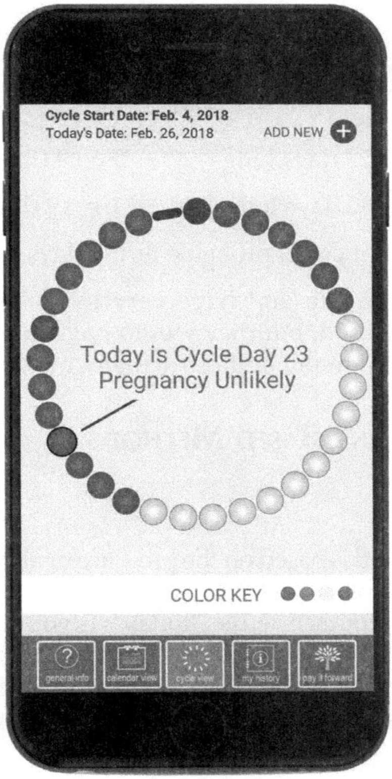

Source: Aksel S, et al. (2012)[53]

Figure 12-1 CycleBeads app for Standard Days Method

Calendar Rhythm Method

The Calendar Rhythm Method is rarely taught today, and thus is not described here in detail. To use this method, you will need to follow these steps:

1. Keep a record of the lengths of your past 6 menstrual cycles.
2. Find the longest and shortest of your past menstrual cycles.
3. To find the first fertile day in your current cycle, subtract 18 from the number of days in your shortest cycle.
4. To find the last fertile day in your current cycle, subtract 11 from the number of days in your longest cycle.
5. **To prevent pregnancy.** From the first through the last days identified as fertile, you should use a barrier method or avoid vaginal intercourse.
6. **To become pregnant.** Intercourse is suggested, frequently, as often as every day, on the days identified as fertile.
7. Update the calculation every cycle to determine your fertile days.

Example: If the lengths of the past six cycles were 29, 27, 30, 28, 29 and 27 days,

Shortest cycle was 27 days long→27 − 18 = 9 (first fertile day)

Longest cycle was 30 days long→30 − 11 = 19 (last fertile day)

Thus, for the current cycle, probable fertile days are 9 through 19.

People who menstruate and have very irregular cycles can use the Calendar Rhythm method, but they would have many days identified as potentially fertile, with many of those actually not fertile.

Cervical Secretions-Based Methods

TwoDay Method

The TwoDay Method is based on the presence or absence of cervical secretions. Cervical secretions of any type "today" or "yesterday" are a sign that you should consider yourself fertile "today." If you did not notice any secretions "today" or "yesterday," consider yourself not fertile "today."[71] This algorithm is illustrated in Figure 12-2. There are a variety of approaches to keep track of cervical secretions, e.g., a calendar, a chart, a smartphone app.

To use the TwoDay Method:

1. Check for secretions every time before you urinate. You can:
   — Look at the secretions in your underwear or in toilet paper,

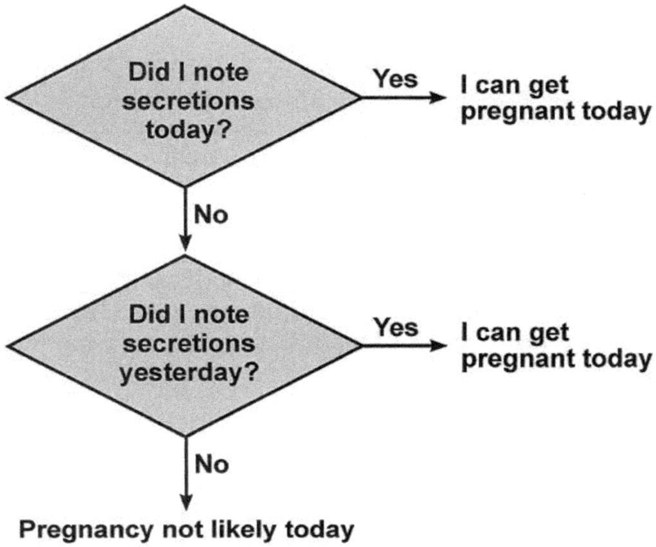

Did I note secretions today?
Yes
I can get pregnant today
No
Did I note secretions yesterday?
Yes
I can get pregnant today
No
Pregnancy not likely today

Figure 12-2 TwoDay Method algorithm

— Touch the secretions in your vulva, or

— Feel the sensation of wetness at your vulva.

2. Determine whether you are fertile or not TODAY based on the presence or absence of secretions. You can ask yourself these two questions:

— Did I notice ANY secretions of any type TODAY?

— Did I notice ANY secretions of any type YESTERDAY?

If you noticed ANY secretions TODAY or YESTERDAY, you can become pregnant if you have sex today. If you did not notice secretions of any type today or yesterday, you are not likely to get pregnant if you have sex today.

3. **To prevent pregnancy.** Avoid unprotected vaginal intercourse if you noticed any secretions of any type either today or yesterday.
4. **To become pregnant.** Unprotected intercourse is suggested every other day on days with secretions.
5. If you have continuous secretions for more than two weeks, or if your secretions are malodorous or irritating, you may have an infection that requires medical attention and should contact your healthcare provider. (See Chapter 20 on Reproductive Tract Infections.)

Billings Ovulation Method

Changes in the characteristics of cervical mucus signal the beginning, and later the end of the fertile time, even among those who have irregular cycles. When they first appear, the secretions may be scant but sticky and thick, with a cloudy or whitish color. Highly fertile secretions are abundant, clear, stretchy, wet, and slippery. Ovulation most likely occurs within 1 day before, during, or 1 day after the last day of abundant, clear, stretchy, slippery cervical secretions (peak day). If your secretions do not follow this pattern, you may have an infection that requires medical attention and should contact your healthcare provider. (See Chapter 20 on Reproductive Tract Infections.) Avoid douching, which can wash out the secretions and make it very difficult to notice changes.

Assistance of a trained instructor is necessary for correct use of the Billings Ovulation Method. A number of charts have been developed to help track observations of cervical secretions. Smartphone apps (e.g., MyFertilityMD) may also serve this purpose. People who use these apps enter their daily observations into the app, which stores this information so they can identify their fertility status according to method instructions.

To use the Billings Ovulation Method:

Observe your cervical secretions by 'the look, the touch, and the feel':

- *Look* at the secretions on your underwear, fingers, or toilet paper to determine color and consistency.
- *Touch* the secretions to determine their stretch and slipperiness.
- *Feel* how wet the sensation is at your vulva.
- Observe your cervical secretions every day, beginning the day after your menstrual bleeding has stopped, and record them daily on a special chart (Figure 12-3). To help you avoid confusing cervical secretions with semen and normal sexual lubrication, some counselors advise complete sexual abstinence throughout the first cycle. Alternatively, you can use a condom every time you have sex during that cycle. Remember, your own lubrication can increase the secretions you find when you check after sex.

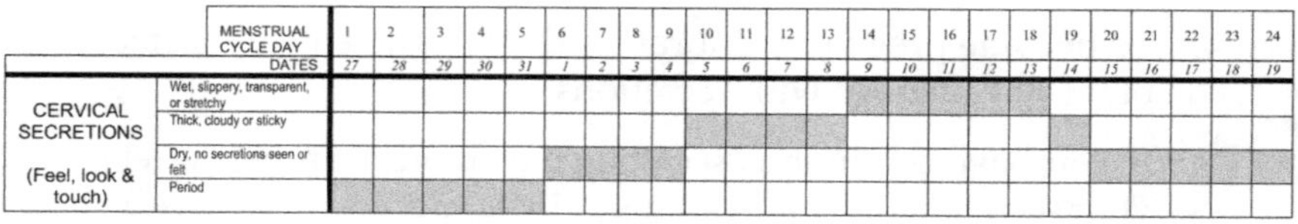

Figure 12-3 Cervical secretion variations during a model menstrual cycle

- Check secretions each time before and after you urinate by wiping (front to back) with tissue paper. Note and record the color and appearance (yellow, white, clear, or cloudy) and feel (dry, wet, or slippery), and consistency (thick, sticky, or stretchy) of the secretions by pulling it between your thumb and index finger. Also, note and chart the sensations of dryness, moistness, or wetness at your vulva. Always record the 'most fertile' observations you see during the day. (Reminder: *Most fertile* means abundant, clear, stretchy, and slippery.)
- **To prevent pregnancy.** Check for secretions as soon as your menses ends. (Some counselors recommend avoiding vaginal intercourse or using a barrier method during menses because it is difficult to detect secretions when they are mixed with menstrual blood.) You can have sexual intercourse on preovulatory days if no secretions are present. The fertile time begins when cervical secretions are first observed and ends on the 4th day after the *peak day* (see above).
- **To become pregnant.** Intercourse is suggested every day when cervical secretions are present. The probability of pregnancy is greatest when the secretions are abundant, clear, stretchy, and slippery. Most people need help in the first few cycles to interpret their cervical secretion patterns and charts to determine the fertile time.

Multiple Indicators

Symptothermal Methods

Some people who are using an FABM prefer to observe more than one indicator of fertility. Most couples who use a combined, or symptothermal, approach use both cervical secretions and basal body temperature (BBT) to identify the fertile time; some people additionally track cervical position, and some include monitoring cycle length. There are several variants of the symptothermal method (e.g., Sensiplan, or others taught by provider groups).[72,73] This section provides general instructions for an overview of characteristics common to many symptothermal method variants, and should be augmented by assistance of a trained instructor. Traditionally, people using a symptothermal method recorded their observations with a paper and pencil chart. More recently, apps such as Kindara, Sympto, and Lady Cycle, serve this purpose; clients record their observations, including their temperature, directly into the app, which stores this information so fertility status can be assessed according to the instructions of the method.

The BBT is the temperature of the body at rest. It is lower in the first part of the cycle, rises to a higher level beginning around the time of ovulation, and remains at the higher level for the rest of the cycle. By taking your temperature when you first wake in the morning and recording your temperature on a chart each day of your menstrual cycle, you can retrospectively identify whether you have ovulated and, thus, calculate the end of your fertile time. However, temperature alone is not sufficient to identify the beginning of the fertile time of the cycle.

In general, to use a symptothermal method, follow the steps for the Billings Ovulation Method. In addition, take and record your BBT as follows to determine the postovulatory infertile time:

1. Take your BBT every morning at the same time each day before getting out of bed or before having any activity in bed (after at least 3 hours of sleep). A special calibrated thermometer makes temperature reading easier. Take the BBT orally, rectally, or vaginally, but take it at the same site each day so changes in temperature can be detected accurately.

2. Record your BBT readings daily on a chart (Figure 12-4). Connect the dots for each day to make a line between successive days (day 2 to day 3, and so on).

3. Your temperature will probably rise at least 0.4 degrees F° around the time of ovulation and remain elevated until the next menses begins. Your actual temperature and maximum temperature are not important, just the rise over the baseline (preovulatory) temperatures.

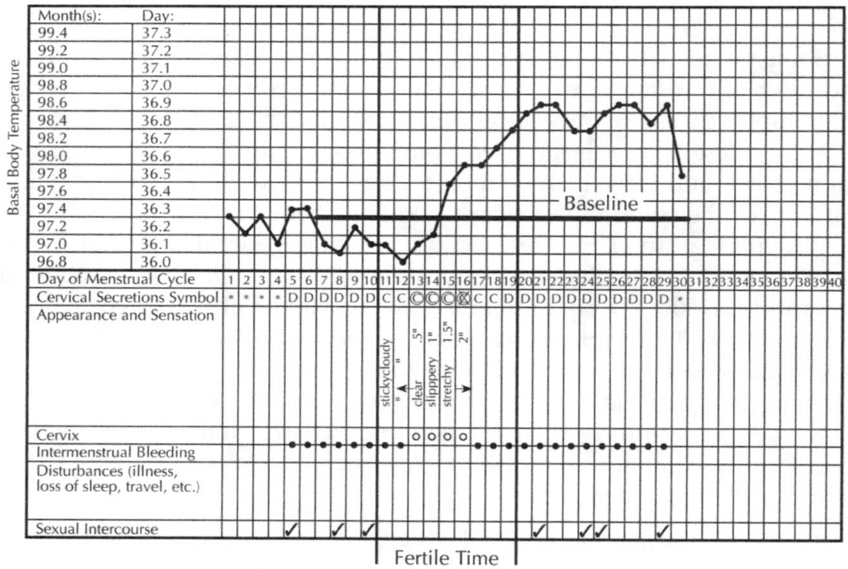

Figure 12-4 Symptothermal variations during a model menstrual cycle

4. If you have 3 continuous days of higher temperatures (above the baseline) following 6 days of lower temperatures, you have probably ovulated and your postovulatory infertile time has begun. To see the baseline and rise clearly on the chart, highlight the chart at the 0.1 degree line just above the lower (preovulatory) temperatures. When you record 3 continuous temperatures above this line, and the last temperature is 0.4 degrees higher than this line, your postovulatory infertile time has begun.

5. If you cannot detect a sustained rise in BBT, you may not have ovulated in that cycle. A true postovulatory BBT rise usually persists 10 days or longer.

6. Some people notice a temperature drop about 12 to 24 hours before it begins to rise after ovulation, whereas others have no drop in temperature at all. A drop in your BBT probably means ovulation will occur the next day.

7. **To prevent pregnancy.** Rely on your cervical secretions to identify the beginning of your fertile time. Your BBT can help you identify the end of your fertile time. You should use another method or not have vaginal intercourse during the fertile time if you do not want to become pregnant.

8. **To become pregnant.** It is often difficult to predict fertile days using BBT. By the time the rise is detected, you are probably in the infertile phase of your menstrual cycle and have missed the opportunity to become pregnant. To become pregnant, you should rely on your cervical secretions.

Author Disclosures—Jennings: grantee of the United States Agency for International Development and several foundations to conduct research on Fertility Awareness-Based Methods; related to but receiving no income from the owner of Cycle Technologies (company sells CycleBeads and is patenting Dynamic Optimal Timing).; Polis: none.

REFERENCES

1. World Health Organization. Family Planning: A global handbook for family providers. Geneva: World Health Organization 2011.Available at www.info.k4health.org/globalhandbook/#msword. Last accessed March 7 2017.
2. Freundl G, Godehardt E, Kern PA, Frank-Hermann P, Koubenec HJ, Gnoth C. Estimated maximum failure rates of cycle monitors using daily conception probabilities in the menstrual cycle. Human Reproduction 2003;18:2628–2633.
3. Wilcox AJ, Weinberg CR, Baird DD. timing of sexual intercourse in relation to ovulation — effects on the probability of conception, survival of the pregnancy, and sex of the baby. N Engl J Med 1995; 333:1517–1521.
4. Zinaman M, Drobnis EZ, Morales P, et al. The physiology of sperm recovered from the human cervix: acrosomal status and response to inducers of the acrosome reaction. Biol Reprod 1989; 41:790–797.

5. World Health Organization. Natural family planning: a guide to provision of services. Geneva: WHO, 1988.
6. Leonard CJ, Chavira W, Coonrod DV, Hart KW, Bay RC. Survey of attitudes regarding natural family planning in an urban Hispanic population. Contraception 2006; 74:313–331.
7. Daniels K, Mosher, WD, Jones J. Contraceptive methods women have ever used: United States, 1982–2010. National Health Statistics Reports 2013; 62:1–15.
8. Lamprecht VM, Grummer-Strawn L. Development of new formulas to identify the fertile time of the menstrual cycle. Contraception 1996;54:339–343.
9. Wilcox AJ, Weinberg CR, Baird DD. Timing of sexual intercourse in relation to ovulation. N Engl J Med 1995;333:1517–1521.
10. Wilcox AJ. Dunson D, Baird DB. The timing of the "fertile window" in the menstrual cycle: day specific estimates from a prospective study. BMJ 2000;321:1259–1262.
11. Arévalo M, Sinai I, Jennings V. A fixed formula to define the fertile window of the menstrual cycle as the basis of a simple method of natural family planning. Contraception 2000;60:357–360.
12. Che Y, Cleland JG, Ali MM. Periodic abstinence in developing countries: an assessment of failure rates and consequences. Contraception 2004;69:15–21.
13. Fehring RJ, Lawrence D, and Philpot C: Use effectiveness of the Creighton Model Ovulation Method of natural family planning. J Obstet Gynecol, and Neonat Nurs 1994;23:303–309.
14. Bonnar J, Flynn A, Freundl G, Kirkman R, Royston R, Snowden R. Personal hormone monitoring for contraception. Br J Fam Plan 2000; 26:178–9
15. Guida M, Bramante S, Acunzo G, Pellicano M, Cirillo D, Nappi C. Diagnosis of fertility with a personal hormonal evaluation test. Minerva Ginecol 2003; 55:167–73
16. Moglia ML, Nguyen HV, Chyjek K, Chen KT, Castano PM. Evaluation of smartphone menstrual cycle tracking applications using an adapted APPLICATIONS scoring systems. Obstet Gynecol 2016 Jun;127:1153–1160.
17. Duane M, Contreras A, Jensen ET, White A. The performance of fertility awareness-based method apps marketed to avoid pregnancy. J Am Board Fam Med 2016;29:508–511.
18. Simmons RG, Jennings VH, Haile L. Fertility apps: what do women want & need? Presentation at: United States Agency for International Development on App Classification; January 26 2017; Washington, DC.
19. Fehring R, Schneider M, Barron ML, Pruszynski J. The influence of motivation on the efficacy of natural family planning. Am J Matern Child Nurs 2013;38: 352–358.
20. Personal communication from Aparna Sundaram, March 13 2017.
21. Sundaram A, Vaughan B, Kost K, Bankole A, Finer L, Singh S, Trussell J. Contraceptive failure in the United States: Estimates from the 2006–2010 National Survey of Family Growth. Perspect Sex Reprod Health 2017 Mar;49:7–16.
22. Kost K, Singh S, Vaughan B, Trussell J, Bankole A. Estimates of contraceptive failure from the 2002 National Survey of Family Growth. Contraception 2008 Jan;77:10–21.
23. Trussell J, Kost K. Contraceptive failure in the United States: A critical review of the literature. Stud Fam Plann 1987;18:237–283.
24. Freundl G, Sivin I, Batár I. State of the art of non-hormonal methods of contraception: IV. Natural family planning. Eur J Contracept Reprod Health Care 2010;15:113–23.
25. Urrutia R, Polis C, Jensen E, Greene M, Stanford J. Efficacy of fertility awareness-based methods of family planning and modifying behavioral factors. PROSPERO 2015:CRD42015017760
26. Arevalo M, Jennings V, Sinai I. Efficacy of a new method of family planning: the Standard Days Method. Contraception 2002; 65:333–8.
27. Kursun Z, Cali S, Sakarya S. The Standard Days Method: Efficacy, satisfaction and demand at regular family planning service delivery settings in Turkey. Eur J Contracept Reprod Health Care 2014;19:203–210.
28. Arévalo M, Yeager B, Sinai I, Panfichi R, Jennings V. Adding the Standard Days Method® to the contraceptive method mix in a high-prevalence setting in Peru. Rev Panam Salud Publica 2010:28:80–85.

29. Gribble JN, Lundgren RI, Velasquez C, Anastasi EE. Being strategic about contraceptive introduction: the experience of the Standard Days Method®. Contraception 2008;77: 147–154.
30. Kambic RT, Lamprecht V. Calendar rhythm efficacy: a review. Adv Contracept 1996;12:123–128.
31. Polis CB, Bradley SEK, Bankole A, Onda T, Croft T, Singh S. Contraceptive failure rates in the developing world: an analysis of demographic and health survey data in 43 Countries, New York: Guttmacher Institute 2016, www.guttmacher.org/report/contraceptive-failure-rates-in-developing-world
32. Arevalo M, Jennings V, Nikula M, Sinai I. Efficacy of the new TwoDay Method of family planning. Fertility and Sterility 2004;82:885–892.
33. Trussell J, Grummer-Strawn L. Contraceptive failure of the ovulation method of periodic abstinence. Fam Plann Perspect 1990;22:65–75.
34. World Health Organization. A prospective multicentre trial of the ovulation method of natural family planning. II. The effectiveness phase. Fertil Steril 1981; 36:591–598.
35. Bhargava H, Bhatia JC, Ramachandran L, Rohatgi P, Sinha A. Field trial of Billings ovulation method of natural family planning. Contraception 1996;53:69–74.
36. Frank-Herrmann P, Heil J, Gnoth C, Toledo E, et al. The effectiveness of a fertility awareness based method to avoid pregnancy in relation to a couple's sexual behaviour during the fertile time: a prospective longitudinal study. Hum Reprod 2007;22:1310–9.
37. Medina JE, Cifuentes A, Abernathy JR, Spieler JM, Wade ME. Comparative evaluation of two methods of natural family planning in Columbia. Am J Obstet Gynecol 1980;138:1142–1147.
38. Wade ME, McCarthy P, Braunstein GD, et al. A randomized prospective study of the use-effectiveness of two methods of natural family planning. American Journal of Obstetrics and Gynecology 1981;141: 368–376.
39. Rice FJ, Lanctot CA, Garcia-Devesa C. Effectiveness of the symptothermal method of natural family planning: an international study. Int J Fertil 1981;26:222–230.
40. Ecochard R, Pinguet F, Ecochard I, De Gouvello R, Guy M, Huy F. Analysis of natural family planning failures. In 7007 cycles of use. Contracept Fertil Sex 1998;26:291–296.
41. The European Natural Family Planning Study Groups. European multicenter study of natural family planning (1989–1995): efficacy and drop-out. Adv Contracept 1999;15: 69–83.
42. Fehring R, Schneider M, Marron ML. Retrospective efficacy of the Marquette Model of natural family planning. Am J Matern Child Nurs 2008;33:348–354.
43. Fehring R, Schneider M, Raviele K, Rodrigues D, Prusynski J. Randomized comparison of two internet-supported fertility awareness based methods of family planning, Contraception, 2013;88:24–30.
44. Berglund SE, Gemzell DK, Sellberg JA, Scherwitzl R. Fertility awareness-based mobile application for contraception. Eur J Contracept Reprod Health Care 2016 Jun;21:234–241
45. Berglund Scherwitzl E, Lundberg O, Kopp Kallner H, Trussell J, Scherwitzl R. Perfect-use and typical-use Pearl Index of a contraceptive mobile app. Contraception 2017;96:420–425.
46. Li D, Heyer L, Jennings VH, Smith CA, Dunson DB. Personalised estimation of a woman's most fertile days. Eur J Contracept Reprod Health Care 2016;21:323–328
47. Clinicaltrials.gov (NCT02833922)
48. Simmons R, Shattuck D, Jennings V. Assessing the efficacy of an app-based method of family planning: the Dot Study protocol. JMITResearch Protocol, January 2017; 6(10)e5.
49. Demianczyk A, Michaluk K. Evaluation of the effectiveness of selected natural fertility symptoms used for contraception: estimation of the Pearl Index of Lady-Comp, Pearly and Daysy cycle computers based on 10 years of observation in the Polish market. Ginekologia Polska 2016;87(12):793–797.
50. Manders M, McLindon L, Schulze B, Beckmann MM, Kremer JAM, Farquhar C. Timed intercourse for couples trying to conceive. Cochrane Database of Systematic Reviews 2015;3.

51. Liao C, Wahab M, Anderson J, Coleman JS. Reclaiming fertility awareness methods to inform timed intercourse for HIV serodiscordant couples attempting to conceive. J Int AIDS Soc 2015;18:19447.
52. Kotz, H. Basal body temperature record: a multipurpose diagnostic tool. J Obstet Gynecol Neonatal Nurs 1973:2:43–48.
53. Aksel S, Sinai I, Yee KA. Female genital cutting and other intra-vaginal practices: implications for TwoDay Method use. J Biosoc Sci 2012;44:631–5
54. Stanford JB, Thurman PB, Lemaire JC. Physicians' knowledge and practices regarding natural family planning. Obstet Gynecol 1999;94:672–678.
55. Choi J, Chan S, Wiebe E. Natural Family Planning: Physicians' knowledge, attitudes, and practice. J Obstet Gynecol Canada 2010; 32:673–678.
56. Sinai I, Arevalo M. It's all in the timing: coital frequency and fertility awareness-based methods of family planning. J Biosoc Sci 2006;38:763–77.
57. Gray RH, Simpson JL, Kambic RT, Queenan JT, Mena P, Perez A, Barbato M. Timing of conception and the risk of spontaneous abortion among pregnancies occurring during use of natural family planning. Am J Obstet Gynecol 1995;172:1567–1572.
58. Simpson JL, Gray R, Perez A, et al. Fertilization involving aging gametes, major birth defects and Down's syndrome. Lancet 2002; 359:1670–1671.
59. Gray RH, Simpson JL, Bitto AC, Queenan JT, Chuanjun L. Sex ratio associated in timing of insemination and length of the follicular phase in planned and unplanned pregnancies during use of NFP. Hum Reprod 1998;13:1397–1400.
60. Malarcher S, Spieler J, Short Fabic M, Jordan S, Starbird EH, Kenon C. Fertility awareness methods: distinctive modern contraceptives. Global Health Science and Practice 2016;13–15.
61. Festin MPR, Kiariea J, Solo J, et al. Moving towards the goals of FP2020—classifying contraceptives. Contraception 2016;94:289–294.
62. Hubacher D, Trussell J. A definition of modern contraceptive methods. Contraception 2015;92:420–421.
63. Austad K, Chary A, Colom A, et al. Fertility awareness methods are not modern contraceptives: defining contraception to reflect our priorities. Global Health Science and Practice 2016;4:342–345.
64. Malarcher S, Short Fabic M, Spieler J, Starbird EH, Kenon C, Jordan S. Response to Austad: offering a range of methods, including fertility awareness methods, facilitates method choice. Global Health Science and Practice 2016;4:346–9.
65. Wright K, Townsend JW. The pitfalls of using selective data to represent the effectiveness, relevance and utility of the Standard Days Method (SDM) of contraception. [Letter to the Editor] Contraception 2016;94:374–383.
66. Sinai I. Standard Days Method effectiveness: opinion disguised as scientific review. [Letter to the Editor] Contraception 2016;94:374–383.
67. Marston CA, Church K. Does the evidence support global promotion of the calendar-based Standard Days Method® of contraception? Contraception 2016;93:492–497.
68. Marston CA, Church K. Response to Letters to the Editor from Irit Sinai "Standard Days Method Effectiveness: opinion disguised as scientific review" and Kelsey Wright, Karen Hardee, and John Townsend "The pitfalls of using selective data to represent the effectiveness, relevance and utility of the Standard Days Method of contraception." Contraception 2016;94:374–383.
69. Knight J. The complete guide to fertility awareness. Rutledge, London 2017; p364.
70. Gainer E, Kenfack B, Mboudou E, Doh AS, Bouyer J. Menstrual bleeding patterns following levonorgestrel emergency contraception. Contraception 2006;74:118–24.
71. Sinai I, Arevalo M, Jennings V. The TwoDay algorithm: a new algorithm to identify the fertile time of the menstrual cycle. Contraception 1999;60:65–70.
72. Couple to Couple League www.ccli.org/
73. Weschler T. Taking charge of your fertility: The definitive guide to natural birth control, pregnancy achievement, and reproductive health. William Morrow Paperbacks 1995.

13

Abstinence, Noncoital Sex, and Sexual Health: What Every Clinician Needs to Know

John S. Santelli, MD, MPH
Melissa Kottke, MD, MPH, MBA
Stephanie Grilo, MA

- Abstinence can be a wise and healthy choice at any life stage, particularly when a person does not feel ready for sexual involvement or a relationship. Sexual activity should always be mutually agreed upon; sexual coercion is unhealthy at any age.
- In real-life practice, abstinence from penile-vaginal sexual intercourse appears to be relatively ineffective against pregnancy (and sexually transmitted infections), as abstinence intentions can fail. A back-up method should always be planned.
- Engaging in noncoital sexual behaviors may effectively prevent an unwanted pregnancy but may not prevent sexually transmitted infections (STIs).
- The health care provider's role should be supportive: assessing relationship history and sexual practices, screening for sexual coercion, providing counseling about pregnancy and STI risk, and providing support for patient choices and the development of healthy and satisfying sexuality.

This chapter addresses several subjects: sexual rights and sexual expression, the demography and definitions of abstinence and noncoital sex, the effectiveness of abstinence in preventing pregnancy and STIs, sexual assault, clinical assessment and counseling, clinicians and comprehensive sexuality education, user instructions for abstinence, and web-based resources for adolescent and adult patients.

Individuals at every lifestage may pass through periods of abstinence from sexual intercourse. Likewise, women in particular may experience sexual coercion at every age, which has implications for the ability to rely on abstinence to prevent pregnancy and STIs. Thus, be alert to these realities and ready to provide education, counseling, support and referrals, as needed.

Sexual Rights and Sexual Expression

Although abstinence has become associated with saying "no," viewed from another perspective, abstinence can mean saying "yes" to a number of other sexual activities and personal priorities. For some people, only penile penetration of the vagina equals intercourse. Not only does this definition fall short in its heteronormity [*the restrictive societal norm of heterosexuality*], but also most people have a more expansive view of sexual expression, and other activities give them pleasure and meaning. Holding hands, kissing, massage, solo masturbation, mutual masturbation, dancing, oral-genital sex, fantasy, and erotic books and movies all fit along the sexual continuum, as do many other activities. Taste, smell, vision, and hearing may matter as much as touch for erotic pleasure. All human beings need touching—for nurture, for solace, for communication, for simple affection. Most human beings enjoy erotic touching, a specialized language of sexual gratification, and more intimate forms of affection.

A large group of experts convened by the World Health Organization and the World Association for Sexology to address the state of sexual health globally suggested that "Sexual health is a state of physical, emotional, mental and social well-being in relation to sexuality; it is not merely the absence of disease, dysfunction or infirmity. Sexual health requires a positive and respectful approach to sexuality and sexual relationships, as well as the possibility of having pleasurable and safe sexual experiences, free of coercion, discrimination and violence. For sexual health to be attained and maintained, the sexual rights of all persons must be respected, protected and fulfilled."[1]

Sexual rights must also include the right to abstain from specific sexual practices and to feel satisfaction in that choice. In our culture of highly sexualized media messages and a changing environment that has become not only more accepting but also more vocal about who is doing what with whom, some clients may benefit from counseling that explores abstinence as a healthy personal choice. All individuals should be encouraged to explore the range of sexual expression they find acceptable and pleasurable. (See Chapter 22 on Sexuality & Contraception.)

DEFINITIONS AND DEMOGRAPHICS: ABSTINENCE AND NONCOITAL SEX

In the United States of the 21st century, there is a lack of consensus about what abstinence does, and does not, entail. Some people define abstinence as refraining from all sexual behavior, including masturbation. Some people define abstinence as refraining from sexual behavior involving genital contact. Others define it as refraining from penetrative sexual practices. Still others would offer different definitions. Federal sexuality education policy from 1998 to 2008 focused on abstinence-only-until-marriage (AOUM) which focuses on abstaining from all sexual contact; the U.S. government and many states still provide considerable funding for AOUM programs.[2] Understanding how clients view abstinence has important clinical implications. Of note, clients will use a variety of terms for abstinence and sexual activity, so these terms need careful exploration when a client uses them.

Persons who are abstaining from penile-vaginal intercourse may engage in a variety of other sexual behaviors. In a study of high-school students who consider themselves virgins, 30% had engaged in heterosexual masturbation of or by a partner, 9% had engaged in fellatio (oral-penile contact) with ejaculation, and 10% had engaged in cunnilingus (oral-female genital contact).[3] More than half (59%) of college undergraduates in another study responded that oral-genital contact did not constitute having "had sex" with a partner, and 19% said the same about penile-anal intercourse.[4]

While allowing that individuals have personal definitions regarding what is meant by abstinence, it is important to also understand specifically the client's risk for pregnancy and STIs. For purposes of contraception, abstinence may be defined as refraining from penile-vaginal intercourse. For purposes of protection from sexually transmitted infections (STIs), abstinence should be defined as refraining from those acts that result in transmission of an STI and development of disease or continued transmission. These other sexual acts (particularly oral and anal sex) vary greatly in their STI risk (see below).

Abstinence can be primary or secondary. *Primary abstinence* occurs when a person has never had sexual intercourse with another person. First penile-vaginal intercourse generally occurs between ages 12 and 25,[5] so that primary abstinence is common among younger teens and not uncommon among young adults. Primary abstinence among women declines from 45% at age 15 to 19 years to 0.6% at age 40 to 44 (Table 13-1). Similarly, primary abstinence among males declines from 43% among 15 to 19 year olds to 1.6% among 40 to 44 year olds (Table 13-1).[6]

Table 13-1 Percentage of U.S. women age 15–44 who report primary abstinence, secondary abstinence and ever having oral, anal or vaginal sex with an opposite sex-partner, 2011–15 NSFG

Age	15–19	20–24	25–29	30–34	35–39	40–44	15–44
Primary Abstinence (Never had sexual contact, not oral, vaginal or anal sex)	45.3	9.8	3.3	1.8	1.1	0.6	9.8
Secondary Abstinence (Has had sexual contact, but not in the 12 months prior to the interview)	7.3	6.3	6.1	6.0	10.0	12.3	8.0
Ever had vaginal sex	47.6	87.3	96.2	98.0	98.8	99.3	88.4
Ever had oral sex	45.3	80.8	88.0	87.2	87.2	86.1	79.6
Ever had anal sex	10.9	31.6	40.5	35.8	38.6	40.8	33.3

Source: NSFG 2011–2015[6]

Another way to look to look at the demographic data examines exact ages.[5] Thus, at age 12, 97% of girls and boys report primary abstinence from penile-vaginal intercourse. This decreases to 84% at age 15, 23% at age 20, and 5% at age 25. These analyses find that abstinence until marriage is extremely rare (and gets rarer as people age, with more than 90% of people in one survey reporting premarital sex prior to age 30 and 97% reporting premarital sex by age 44).[5]

From the mid 1960s through about 1990, sexual activity among teens increased—with the median age for first sex declining from age 19 to age 17; age at first sex then rose to 17.6 years by 2003.[5] (The median age for first penile-vaginal intercourse in much of the developed world is between 17.5 and 18.5 years for young women and between 16.5 and 18.5 years for young men.)[7] Paralleling these changes in the median age at first sex since 1990, the percentage of adolescent women (15 to 19 years of age) in the United States who are sexually experienced declined from 51% in 1988 to 42% in 2006–2010; among adolescent men of the same age, the percentage declined from 60% to 44%.[8] The most recent data from 2011–2015 finds that this downward trend has plateaued.[8] Among young women age 18 to 24 years who first had sex as a teenager, 10% reported that their first sex was not voluntary. Young women also reported on the degree to which their first sex was wanted or not: 13% reported that they did not want it to happen at the time, and 52% reported having mixed feelings.[9]

Initiation of oral sex is closely linked in time with initiation of penile-vaginal intercourse;[10] presumably oral sex commonly occurs with the same sexual partner with whom one initiates penile-vaginal intercourse. Almost 90% of 25 to 44 year old men and 87% of women have had oral sex with an opposite sex partner (See Table 13-1 and

Table 13-2); at age 15 to 19 years 51% of men and 45% of women have had oral sex.[6]

Heterosexual anal sex is less common than oral sex and penile-vaginal intercourse and generally initiated later. Among 25 to 44 year olds, anal sex with an opposite sex partner is reported by 39% of women and 46% of men; among 15 to 19 year olds, these percentages are 11% and 11% (see Tables).[6]

Most lesbian, gay, bisexual, transgendered and questioning (LGBTQ) youth also initiate sexual activity in their teens and early 20s. Because the development of sexual identity may be gradual and nonheterosexual identity is often highly stigmatized, LGBTQ youth may engage in heterosexual activities including penile-vaginal intercourse.[11] Many LGBTQ young women are at risk of unintended pregnancy because of engagement in heterosexual activity.

Secondary abstinence occurs when individuals who have had sexual intercourse do not engage in behaviors they consider as "having sex." Among sexually experienced women age 15 to 44 years, 6.0% to 12.3%, depending on age group, report that they had not had sexual contact with a man in the 12 months prior to the interview (Table 13-1).[6] Among men, those percentages are 5.5% to 8.2%.[6] (See Table 13–2.) Many of these secondary abstainers are not currently in a relationship for a variety of reasons. While some may choose long-term abstinence, many desire a new sexual relationship or may resume sexual activity outside the context of a relationship. With re-initiating sexual activity, they are potentially at risk for unintended pregnancy and STIs. Thus, clinical counseling among secondary abstainers should address formation of new relationships, renewed sexual activity, contraception, and protection from STIs.

Table 13-2 Percentage of U.S. men age 15–44 who report primary abstinence, secondary abstinence and ever having oral, anal or vaginal sex with an opposite sex-partner, 2011–15 NSFG

Age	15–19	20–24	25–29	30–34	35–39	40–44	15–44
Primary Abstinence (Never had sexual contact, not oral, vaginal or anal sex)	42.5	12.1	4.4	2.2	1.1	1.6	10.7
Secondary Abstinence (Has had sexual contact, but not in the 12 months prior to the interview)	6.3	8.2	6.7	6.4	5.5	7.5	6.8
Ever had vaginal sex	45.0	85.6	94.8	97.3	98.8	97.8	86.6
Ever had oral sex	51.3	80.8	88.4	90.3	89.4	90.2	81.7
Ever had anal sex	10.5	33.6	45.1	47.3	45.0	45.0	37.7

Source: NSFG 2011–2015[6]

EFFECTIVENESS

As an action, abstinence prevents pregnancy or STI at the moment of abstaining. As an ongoing contraceptive method, abstinence should *in theory* be highly effective; *in reality*, however, abstinence intentions often fail.[12] Many primary abstainers do not anticipate first penile-vaginal intercourse; many report, "It just happened." Programs to promote abstinence until marriage among youth are generally not effective (see below). Abstinence intentions among youth (*primary abstainers*) as exemplified by virginity pledges generally provide, at best, short-term benefits in delaying initiation of penile-vaginal intercourse and may increase initiation of noncoital activity.[13] Likewise, *secondary abstainers* may see intentions to abstain derailed by situational factors such as a non-supportive partner or the development of a new romantic relationship. Clinician counseling should address these issues, and a back-up method to prevent pregnancy should always be planned.

SEXUAL ASSAULT

Not all sexual activity is voluntary. Screening and counseling regarding sexual coercion and assault are important aspects of reproductive health care. Sexual coercion and sexual assault happen at every age, and they have implications on individual's ability to rely on abstinence to prevent pregnancy and other STIs. Further, the trauma of sexual assault may be related to a woman's decision-making regarding abstinence. About 1 in 3 women and 1 in 6 men have experienced violent sexual contact in their lifetimes.[14] Among female victims of rape in the United States, 80% experienced their first rape before the age of 25 and 42% before the age of 18 years; among men, 28% experienced their first rape before age 10.[14] Risk factors for sexual assault include younger age, gender (with women and gender nonconforming persons experiencing rape and sexual assault at the highest rates), sexual orientation, and factors related to partners such as power dynamics and prior experience of violence within the relationship).[15,16] Adolescents who have initiated sex very early (before age 13) are at increased risk for their first sexual experience to have been sexual assault and are also at an increased risk for sexual assault later in life. Women who have already experienced sexual assault may have different counseling and clinical needs in reference to their sexual health, contraception and other protective and preventive care. Women and men who have experienced sexual violence should be offered counseling and referrals, as indicated.

CLINICAL ASSESSMENT AND COUNSELING REGARDING ABSTINENCE OR OTHER FORMS OF SEXUAL EXPRESSION

Consider discussing abstinence even with patients who currently engage in intercourse and other sexual behaviors. Many women and men abstain from all or some sexual activities at some time in their lives, both as primary and later as secondary abstainers. At some point, they may choose abstinence, removing themselves at least for a while from the health risks of intercourse.

Primary abstainers tend to be young and may choose to avoid certain sexual activities because of their youth, personal beliefs that suggest it is better to delay sexually intimate relationships until a given set of conditions is achieved, a desire to abide by the wishes of their adult guardians, a lack of interest, or any number of reasons.

For sexually experienced persons, abstinence may also make sense for variety of reasons. For example, the idea of *abstinence "for a while"* may be useful until a couple in a new relationship feels they are both ready, until effective contraception is achieved, while waiting for tests for STIs and agreement about protection, or during early the postpartum period. Short-term abstinence is also common among sexually experienced adolescents, who may engage in sex intermittently.

For many individuals, *abstinence "right now, tonight, or today"* is the ever-available back-up method of contraception and protection. For couples who are seeking pregnancy prevention, abstinence is immediately available as is engagement in a variety on noncoital behaviors that they find sexually satisfying (e.g. kissing, mutual masturbation, *outercourse* (nonpenetrative sexual stimulation), or oral sex).

For those who choose to abstain as a contraceptive method, your role as care provider is to understand the individual's long- and short-term goals, to support healthy choices and counsel about risks associated with different choices, to teach negotiation and planning skills to achieve goals for establishing or maintaining abstinence, and to provide counseling and referrals as needed. Reaffirm that participating in penile-vaginal intercourse is not a requirement for being a sexually fulfilled human. (See Chapter 22 for more on Sexuality & Contraception.)

Contraception. When the only goal of abstinence is to avoid unwanted pregnancy, then all forms of sexual expression are available to a couple except for penile-vaginal intercourse.

Because opportunities may arise for having sex and because intentions may change, educate all abstemious persons about the other methods of contraception and safer sex available to them, including the following:

- Effective over-the-counter products, including emergency contraception
- Prescription methods
- Safer-sex practices
- Options for managing an unintended pregnancy

STI protection. Engaging effectively in sexual behaviors, other than penile-vaginal intercourse, prevents pregnancy but may have implications for STI prevention. In considering STI risk, it is important to understand that most people engage in a variety of coital and noncoital behaviors with the same partner. These practices include mutual masturbation, oral-genital sex, and anal intercourse. Among these noncoital behaviors, anal intercourse carries considerably greater risk for transmission of HIV. For HIV, oral sex is generally safer than vaginal sex, which in turn is safer than anal sex. However, herpes and HPV infection are commonly transmitted via oral-genital contact, and HPV may cause oral cancer. Herpes is also readily transmitted via kissing. HPV may be transmitted via digital-genital contact. (See Chapter 20 on Reproductive Tract Infections.)

In clinical assessment and counseling, consider infection risk from partner factors (e.g. multiple partners) and the community prevalence of specific STIs.[17] The most important risk factor for becoming infected with an STI is having sexual contact with an infected partner. A person's history of multiple sexual partners and the history of one's partner(s) having multiple partners are predictors of being infected. Because most people engage in noncoital sex with the same partner with whom they engage in penile-vaginal intercourse, evaluate whether noncoital behaviors add additional risk beyond that posed by penile-vaginal intercourse. Clinical counseling should focus on reducing STI risks such as multiple partners, which may be more effective than discouraging noncoital sex.[10,17] Also suggest the use of condoms, latex dams, or other barriers to inhibit STI transmission during oral and anal sex. The care provider's role is to offer factual, explicit guidance on safer-sex options.

Lack of partner. Patients may be abstinent if they lack a partner or their partner becomes celibate. Give these individuals permission to engage in masturbation or other ways fulfill their sexual needs. They may also benefit from counseling (couples or individual) if abstinence is a dissatisfying situation. (For more information, see Chapter 22 on Sexuality & Contraception.)

Medical reasons. There are some medical situations that warrant encouraging abstinence from penile-vaginal sex:

- Known or suspected STI, which also calls for avoiding other sexual practices that transmit body fluids such as semen, cervical-vaginal secretions, and blood
- Post-operative pain or tenderness, such as from episiotomy, hemorrhoidectomy, vasectomy, and other procedures
- Dyspareunia or other pelvic pain (While providers may not encourage abstinence in these circumstances, it is important to explore if pain with sex is a reason for the choice of abstinence. It is the provider's role to identify the source of pain and to try to resolve the symptoms. For example, pain may be secondary to pelvic, vaginal, or urinary tract infection, which require urgent diagnosis and treatment.)
- Certain pregnancy conditions such as placenta previa and preterm labor
- Immediately postpartum
- Post-myocardial infarction
- Other physical conditions when one is not healthy enough for sex

Sex therapy. Therapy for a variety of sexual problems may include exploration of avenues of sexual gratification other than intercourse. Temporarily forbidding intercourse takes performance pressure off couples struggling with erection difficulty, orgasm difficulty, or rapid ejaculation.

CLINICIAN ROLES IN COMPREHENSIVE SEXUALITY EDUCATION PROGRAMS

Sexuality education is important for promoting sexual health and an informed use of abstinence. Thus, as a clinician, you have an important role to play in supporting young people's access to medically accurate, developmentally appropriate, and evidence-based sexuality education. Professional associations have been crucial supporters of sex education through the public schools.[12,18] Clinicians have been strong and steady supporters of comprehensive sexuality education as they often see the consequences of sexual ignorance and misinformation. Informed young people are better able to understand medical advice and to practice effective pregnancy and STI prevention.

Comprehensive sexuality education has been shown to have multiple positive behavioral outcomes, including helping youth delay initiation of intercourse, reduce STI risk, and improve contraceptive use.[19] *In contrast, abstinence-only-until-marriage programs have generally been a colossal failure, providing virtually no behavioral benefit.*[12] Two recent meta-analyses of abstinence interventions and comprehensive intervention by the CDC-sponsored Task Force on Community Preventive Services found "insufficient evidence" for the effectiveness of abstinence interventions in terms of behavioral impact on sexual initiation and other sexual behaviors.[20] In contrast, the Task Force found evidence of effectiveness and recommended comprehensive risk-reduction interventions for adolescents to promote behaviors that prevent or reduce the risk of pregnancy, HIV, and other STIs. Moreover, abstinence-only-until-marriage programs often promote misinformation about sexual health and contraception.[21] States such as California which have refused federal abstinence money and which have emphasized contraceptive access have been more effective in reducing teen pregnancy than states such as Texas that focused on abstinence promotion.[22] By restricting access to health promotion and life-saving information, abstinence-until-marriage programs violate the principles of medical ethics and human rights. Clinicians should support science-based policies and oppose nonsensical policies promoting ideas that are medically inaccurate and ineffective.

Comprehensive sexuality education should contain clear messages about the health benefits and health risks of both abstinence and sexual activity. Young people who are not ready for sexual intercourse need the social skills to refuse unwanted sexual advances—information they can use to protect themselves throughout their adult lives, including during periods of abstinence and sexual activity.

The internet has become an important source for information on sexual health. Help guide patients to websites that provide accurate and useful information by providing information in the office about these and providing social endorsement for their use. See the Appendix for a listing of helpful websites and apps.

USER INSTRUCTIONS FOR ABSTINENCE—FOR CONTRACEPTION OR STI PROTECTION*

1. **Planned abstinence.** Decide what you want to do about sex at a time when you feel clear-headed. If you have a partner, discuss your preferences and values. Be clear about your needs.

2. **Spontaneous abstinence.** The wrong partner? The wrong situation? Abstain now—today, tonight—for whatever reason.

*These instructions are intended to guide providers in educating patients in how to use their method.

3. **Decide in advance** what sexual activities you will say "yes" to and discuss these with your partner.
4. **Discuss with your partner,** very clearly and in advance what activities you will not do.
5. **Avoid high-pressure sexual situations.** Avoid drinking to excess and using drugs that may cloud judgment and decision-making
6. **You can choose abstinence** even if you have had sex in the past. You can choose abstinence even if you have had sex in the past with a partner who may expect that your past actions dictate your current actions.
7. **If you say "no,"** say it so it is clear that you mean it. This advice is meant to help you communicate more effectively; it is not meant to suggest you are to blame if a partner claims not to have understood what you were saying. Under no circumstances is it acceptable for a partner to pressure or force you to have sex.
8. **Learn more** about your body, sexual health, contraception, and how to keep yourself healthy.

   Good online resources include:

   - WebMD—www.webmd.com/sex-relationships/default.htm
   - American Sexual Health Association—www.ashasexualhealth.org/sexual-health
   - CDC—www.cdc.gov/sexualhealth
   - Planned Parenthood—www.plannedparenthood.org/learn

Good resources specifically for young people can be found at:

• Ask Alice	www.goaskalice.columbia.edu
• Sex, Etc.	www.sexetc.org
• Scarleteen	www.scarleteen.com
• Bedsider	www.bedsider.org
• Answer	answer.rutgers.edu (for teens and parents)
• Iwannaknow	www.iwannaknow.org/teens/sexualhealth.html

9. Learn about contraception and safer sex, so you will be ready if you change your mind. Always keep condoms on hand.

10. Refrain from intercourse if you do not have a contraceptive method available. Learn about emergency contraception in case you have intercourse when you do not expect it or you experience a contraceptive failure. If you need information about emergency contraception, visit www.not-2-late.com.

Emergency Contraceptives: Emergency contraceptive pills or placement of a copper intrauterine contraceptive after unprotected intercourse substantially reduces the risk of pregnancy.

Author Disclosures—Santelli: none. Kottke: none. Grilo: none.

Acknowledgements: A special thanks to Laura D. Lindberg and Isaac Maddow-Zimet for the running the special analyses of the 2011–2015 National Survey of Family Growth in Tables 13-1 and 13-2.

References

1. World Health Organization. Defining sexual health: report of a technical consultation on sexual health, 28–31 January 2002, Geneva: WHO, 2006.
2. Santelli JS, Grilo SA, Lindberg LD, al. Abstinence-only-until-marriage policies and programs: An updated position paper of the Society for Adolescent Health and Medicine. J Adolescent Health 2017; 61; 400–403.
3. Schuster MA, Bell RM, Kanouse DE. The sexual practices of adolescent virgins: genital sexual activities of high school students who have never had vaginal intercourse. Am J Public Health 1996; 86:1570–1576.
4. Sanders SA, Reinisch JM. Would you say you "had sex" if . . .? JAMA 1999; 281:275–277.
5. Finer LB. Trends in premarital sex in the United States, 1954–2003. Public Health Rep 2007; 122:73–8.
6. Lindberg, LD, Maddow-Zimet, I. Special analyses of the 2011–2015 National Survey of Family Growth. June 2017.
7. Wellings K, Collumbien M, Slaymaker E, et al. Sexual behaviour in context: a global perspective. The Lancet 2006;368(9548), 1706–1728.
8. Martinez GM, Abma JC. Sexual activity, contraceptive use, and childbearing of teenagers aged 15–19 in the United States. NCHS data brief, no 209. Hyattsville, MD: National Center for Health Statistics. 2015.
9. Abma JC, Martinez, GM, Mosher, WD, Dawson, BS. Teenagers in the United States: Sexual activity, contraceptive use, and childbearing, 2002. National Center for Health Statistics. Vital Health Stat 2004; 23(24).
10. Lindberg LD, Jones R, Santelli JS. Noncoital sexual activities among adolescents. J Adolescent Health 2008; 43: 231–238.
11. Coker TR, Austin B, Schuster MA. The health and health care of lesbian, gay, and bisexual adolescents. Ann Rev Public Health 2010; 31:457–77.
12. Santelli JS, Kantor, LM, Grilo, SA et al. Abstinence-only-until-marriage: an updated review of U.S. policies and programs and their impact. J Adolescent Health 2017; 61, 273–280.
13. Bearman PS and Bruckner H. Promising the future: virginity pledges and first intercourse. Am J Sociol 2001; 106:859–912.
14. Black MC, Basile KC, Breiding M, et al. The national intimate partner and sexual violence survey (NISVS): 2010 summary report. Atlanta, GA: National Center for Injury Prevention and Control, Centers for Disease Control and Prevention 2011:25.

15. Tharp AT, Simon TR, Saul J. Preventing violence against children and youth. J Safety Res 2012;43:291–298.
16. Carey KB, Durney, SE, Shepardson, RL, Carey MP. Incapacitated and forcible rape of college women: Prevalence across the first year. J Adolescent Health 2015; 56:678–680.
17. ACOG Committee Opinion No. 582: Addressing health risks of noncoital sexual activity. Obstet Gynecol 2013;122:1378–83.
18. Ott MA and Santelli JS. Abstinence and abstinence-only education. Curr Opin Obstet Gynecol 2007;19:446–452.
19. Kirby, D. Emerging Answers 2007: research findings on programs to reduce teen pregnancy and sexually transmitted diseases. Washington, DC: The National Campaign to Prevent Teen and Unplanned Pregnancy. At www.thenationalcampaign.org/sites/default/files/resource-primary-download/EA2007_full_0.pdf. Accessed 08/01/2017.
20. Chin HB, Sipe, TA, Elder R, et al. The effectiveness of group-based comprehensive risk-reduction and abstinence education interventions to prevent or reduce the risk of adolescent pregnancy, human immunodeficiency virus, and sexually transmitted infections: two systematic reviews for the Guide to Community Preventive Services. Am J Prev Med 2012;42:272–294
21. Santelli JS. Medical accuracy in sexuality education: Ideology and the scientific process. Am J Public Health 2008; 98:1786–1792.
22. Santelli JS, Kirby D. State policy effects on teen fertility and evidence-based policies. J Adol Health 2010; 46:515–516.

Male Condoms

14

Lee Warner, PhD, MPH
Markus J. Steiner, PhD, MSPH

- When used consistently and correctly, male latex condoms can reduce the risk of pregnancy and many sexually transmitted infections (STIs), including human immunodeficiency virus (HIV).
- Condoms are inexpensive, available without a prescription, and easy to use.
- By preventing STIs and their long-term sequelae, condoms help protect future fertility.
- Clients at risk for STIs, particularly those in a new sexual relationship, should be encouraged to use condoms even if they already rely on more effective methods of contraception, because many infections are asymptomatic.
- Condom use remains low in most populations at risk for pregnancy and STI, and new approaches to increasing use are urgently needed.

Male latex condoms remain among the most widely available and commonly used contraceptive methods in the United States. When used consistently and correctly, male condoms reduce the risk of both pregnancy and most sexually transmitted infections (STIs), including human immunodeficiency virus (HIV), based on results from laboratory and clinical studies. This multi-purpose role for condoms was recognized in a recent position statement developed by UNFPA, WHO, and UNAIDS.[1]

In the United States, condom use increased markedly during the late 1990s and early 2000s, largely in response to the HIV and STI epidemics, but has since leveled off, according to national surveys of adolescents and adults.[2,3,4,5] For example, according to the National Youth Risk Behavior Survey (YRBS),[5] the prevalence of condom use at last intercourse increased by one third among sexually active high school students between 1991 and 2003, from 46% to a peak of 63%; however, condom use has since gradually declined, most recently to 57% in 2015.

Similarly, condom use among reproductive-aged women appears to have stabilized over the last decade, according to the National Survey of Family Growth (NSFG). The most recent data from the 2013–2015 NSFG revealed that 20% of reproductive-age women in the United States currently used condoms for protection from both pregnancy and STIs,[6] a figure identical to that reported from the 2006–2008 survey.[7] Among women using any contraceptive, 13% reported currently using condoms for prevention of pregnancy alone, making it the third most popular method. Condom use thus continues to be an important part of public health efforts to prevent unintended pregnancy as well as new cases of infection with HIV and other STIs.

MECHANISM OF ACTION

The male condom acts as a physical barrier by covering the penile glans and shaft. The condom prevents pregnancy by blocking the passage of semen; it prevents infections by covering the major portals of entry and exit for many STI pathogens. Because of their coitally-dependent nature, condoms must be used consistently and correctly with each act of intercourse to be effective. Among contraceptive methods that are physical barriers, condoms provide the most protection of the genital tract and effective protection against many STIs (see section on Special Issues).

A sheath worn over the penis can be traced as far back as 1350 B.C., when Egyptian men wore decorative covers for their penises. In 1564 A.D., Fallopius first described linen sheaths used to protect against syphilis.[8] Protective sheaths were made from dried animal intestines in the 18th century, when according to some sources, they were first given the name "condom," presumably after inventor Colonel Cundum. The advent of vulcanized rubber in 1843 led to the mass production of condoms made from natural rubber latex.[9] During the past three decades, manufacturers increasingly began to use synthetic materials (e.g., polyurethane and polyisoprene) to develop new condom options for both men and women. (For more information on female condoms, see Chapter 11, Vaginal Barriers and Spermicides.)

CONDOM OPTIONS

Male condoms are available in a variety of shapes, sizes, colors, and thicknesses, as well as with or without lubricants or spermicides, and with or without reservoir-tip or nipple-ends. Condoms can be straight-sided or tapered toward the closed end, textured (e.g., ribbed) or smooth, solid-colored or nearly transparent, and odorless or scented or flavored.

Most condoms commercially available in the United States are about 7 inches (180 mm) long, 2 inches (52 mm) wide, and approximately 0.003 inches (0.08 mm) thick.

Male condoms are made from three types of material—latex, natural membrane, and synthetic (Table 14-1). More than 80% of male condoms commercially available in the United States are manufactured from natural rubber latex ("rubber" condoms).[10] A small proportion (<5%) is made from the intestinal caecum of lambs ("natural skin," "natural membrane," or "lambskin" condoms). Unlike latex condoms, natural membrane condoms contain small pores that may permit the passage of viruses (but not sperm), including hepatitis B virus, herpes simplex virus, and HIV.[11,12] Because of this porosity, natural membrane condoms may not provide the same level of protection against STIs as latex condoms and are thus not recommended for this purpose. No clinical data are available on the effectiveness of natural membrane condoms for STI prevention, however. The remaining 15% or so of male condoms are manufactured from synthetic materials, such as polyurethane and, more recently, polyisoprene. Compared with latex condoms, synthetic condoms are generally more resistant to deterioration, have a longer shelf-life, are compatible with use of both oil-based and water-based lubricants, and offer an option for couples who may be allergic or sensitive to latex. For pregnancy prevention, synthetic male condoms have rates of clinical failure that are comparable to their latex counterparts.[13] The effectiveness of synthetic male condoms to prevent STIs, including HIV, has not been extensively studied; however, based on their physical properties and laboratory testing, synthetic condoms are believed to provide contraception and STI protection similar to latex male condoms.[14]

Table 14-1 Characteristics of latex, natural membrane, and synthetic male condoms

	Material		
Characteristic	**Latex**	**Natural Membrane**	**Synthetic**
Material	Natural rubber	Lamb caecum	Polyurethane or polyisoprene*
Lubricant use	Water-based or silicone-based**	Any	Any
Cost	Low	Moderate	Moderate/high
Recommended for prevention of pregnancy	Yes	Yes	Yes***
Recommended for prevention of STIs and HIV	Yes	No	Yes***

*Most synthetic condoms currently available are made from polyurethane or polyisoprene

**Users should consult package labeling to ensure compatibility of silicone-based lubricants with latex condoms

***For latex sensitive or allergic persons

Spermicidal Condoms

Despite still being commercially available in the United States, use of condoms lubricated with the spermicide nonoxynol-9 (N-9) is not recommended because of their higher cost, shorter shelf life, and lack of additive benefit as compared with other lubricated condoms.[15] Concerns have also been raised about genital ulceration and irritation resulting from high-frequency use of vaginal spermicidal N-9 products and the potential for facilitating transmission of STIs including HIV.[16] (See Chapter 11 on Vaginal Barriers and Spermicides.) Because the amount of N-9 contained in spermicidal condoms is much lower than that found in separately applied vaginal products,[17] spermicidal condoms are probably less likely to cause adverse effects; however, their use was associated with increased risk of urinary tract infections among young women in one study.[18]

EFFECTIVENESS AGAINST PREGNANCY

Method failure of the male condom resulting in unintended pregnancy is uncommon. Of 100 couples using condoms, 2% are estimated to become pregnant during consistent and correct use during the first 12 months of use. (A summary of studies of contraceptive failure for the male condom, as well as a detailed discussion of the estimates used to derive these rates, can be found in Chapter 26 on Contraceptive Efficacy.)

Couples vary widely in their ability to use male condoms consistently and correctly. Among couples using condoms for contraception, about 13 of every 100 will become pregnant during the first year of typical use. The marked difference between the probabilities of pregnancy during typical use versus perfect use of condoms generally reflects errors in use, most notably the failure of couples to use condoms consistently and correctly during every act of sexual intercourse. Several user behaviors, described later, likely contribute to the risk of unintended pregnancy and the transmission of infection despite condom use. Detailed instructions for condom use are provided at the end of this chapter.

CONDOM TESTING

Condoms are regulated as medical devices by the U.S. Food and Drug Administration (FDA), and manufacturing standards have become more stringent in recent years. Every condom is tested electronically for holes and weak spots before it is packaged and released for sale. Samples of condoms also undergo a series of additional laboratory tests for leakage, strength, dimensional requirements, and package integrity.[19] If the sample condoms fail any of these tests, the entire lot is rejected and destroyed. Imported condoms are required to comply with the same performance requirements as domestic condoms. The most recent Consumer Reports (CR) Survey in 2009 showed that nearly all latex condoms tested met industry standards,[20] noting that test performance does not vary with price, thickness, or country of manufacture.

ADVANTAGES AND INDICATIONS

Male condoms offer several contraceptive and non-contraceptive benefits to users.

1. **Protection against STIs.** When used consistently and correctly, condoms reduce the risk of many STIs, including HIV (see Special Issues). By preventing STIs and their long-term sequelae, condoms also protect fertility.
2. **Accessibility.** Condoms are widely available and typically over the counter. Usage does not require medical examination, prescription, or fitting.
3. **Low cost.** Condoms are among the most inexpensive and cost-effective contraceptives, especially considering the added protection offered against STIs. Condoms are available at low cost in both the private and public sectors and often for free from publicly funded programs and many colleges and universities.
4. **Delayed ejaculation.** For some men, condom use may help prolong intercourse and also prevent premature ejaculation.
5. **Portability.** Condoms can be easily and discretely carried by men or women, for example, in wallets or purses.
6. **Minimal side effects.** Because condoms are non-hormonal, they rarely cause medical problems among users. The most frequent side effect is most likely latex sensitivity or allergy; men or women with this condition can be directed to use synthetic condoms (see the section on Managing Problems and Follow-up in this chapter as well as chapter 11).

DISADVANTAGES AND CAUTIONS

Male condoms also have disadvantages that may result in inconsistent or nonuse of the method.

1. **Reduced sensation.** Many men and their partners complain that condoms reduce sensitivity. Men should be encouraged to experiment with different types of condoms (and lubricants) to find ones that are most suitable for them.

2. **Lack of spontaneity.** Some men and their partners dislike interrupting foreplay to put on the condom and may find the coitally-dependent nature of condom use to be inconvenient.

3. **Problems with erection.** Some men cannot consistently maintain an erection during condom use, so condom use becomes unacceptable. In these cases, if culturally acceptable, involving the partner in putting the condom on as part of foreplay may be helpful. Female condom use also may be an appropriate alternative for some couples (see Chapter 11 on Vaginal Barriers and Spermicides). While occasional erectile difficulties are normal (yet nonetheless embarrassing) for males, frequent difficulties may be an early warning sign of an underlying medical problem and should be evaluated by a clinician.

4. **Embarrassment and mistrust.** Some men and their partners may be embarrassed to obtain condoms or to suggest or initiate condom use because they perceive condom use implies a lack of trust or intimacy. Counsel clients (and partners, when possible) about their embarrassment and teach clients about condoms and how to negotiate their use. (See section on Providing Condoms—Counseling). Encouraging clients to involve their partner in putting on the condom may help facilitate use.

5. **Lack of cooperation.** In some instances, men will not accept responsibility for contraception or prevention of infection, thus making male condom use impossible.

6. **Latex allergy or sensitivity**. A small proportion of men and their partners, especially health care workers repeatedly exposed to latex, may be allergic or sensitive to latex and thus unable to use latex condoms. Synthetic condoms are excellent alternatives.

Special Issues

Protection Against STIs, Including HIV

The primary noncontraceptive benefit of condom use is the protection conferred against STIs. When placed on the penis before any genital contact and used throughout intercourse, condoms prevent direct contact with semen; genital lesions and subclinical viral shedding on the glans and shaft of the penis; and penile, vaginal, or anal discharges or infectious fluids. Condoms thus greatly reduce the risk of STIs that are transmitted primarily to or from the penile urethra (such as gonorrhea, chlamydia, trichomoniasis, hepatitis B infection, and HIV). Condoms also provide protection against STIs that are transmitted primarily through skin-to-skin contact or contact with mucosal surfaces (such as genital herpes, human papillomavirus [HPV] and HPV-associated diseases, syphilis, and chancroid) to the extent that these areas are covered by the condom. Protection may be less when these STIs involve areas not covered by the condom.[14,17,21,22] In vitro laboratory studies indicate that latex condoms provide an effective physical barrier against passage of even the smallest sexually transmitted pathogen (hepatitis B).[23-29]

The level of protection for condoms is likely to vary for different STIs because STIs differ in their routes of transmission, as well as in their infectivity and prevalence.[30-32] Well-designed clinical studies of discordant couples (where one partner is infected and the other is not) have shown consistent use of latex condoms to be highly effective against heterosexual transmission of HIV infection, the most serious STI; thus, for this reason alone, male condoms should be promoted to sexually active clients at risk for STIs.[33] Two meta-analyses of these studies place the estimated effectiveness of consistent (though not necessarily correct) condom use between approximately 80% and 95%.[34,35] Very limited evidence exists concerning the protection provided against HIV during anal intercourse. One well-designed study of gay HIV-discordant couples, however, estimated the protective effect of consistent condom use to be in the same range.[36]

Clinical studies of effectiveness against most other STIs suggest inconsistent protective effects for condoms.[21,23,32,37-40] Much of this inconsistency in estimates of the effectiveness of condom use can be attributed to limitations in study design, as the overall quality of clinical studies for these STIs is considerably weaker than for the HIV studies. Specifically, limitations in measurement of self-reported condom use and exposure to infected partners complicate interpretation of condom effectiveness estimates.[21,23,32,40-50] Well-conducted studies and analyses[43,46,47,51-55] have empirically documented that effectiveness against many STIs is underestimated because of limitations in study design. Despite these limitations, studies and systematic reviews have nevertheless found condom use to be associated with reduced risk of many STIs in addition to HIV, including gonorrhea, chlamydia, trichomoniasis, syphilis, genital herpes, HPV infection, and HPV-associated conditions.[32,37-40,50,56-73] We refer readers elsewhere for more extensive discussion of condom effectiveness for STI prevention.[21,32,40,42,72]

Condom Use During Anal and Oral Intercourse

Latex and synthetic condoms also can be used during anogenital and orogenital intercourse to reduce the risk of STIs, including HIV[14] though, to date, FDA has not officially cleared any condoms for such use.

Household plastic wrap (including the microwaveable variety) is another option for cunnilingus and anilingus, although it has not been manufactured or cleared by the FDA for medical applications, and no effectiveness data are available. Latex or polyurethane dental dams (or oral dams), as well as condoms adapted to form a barrier sheet, have also been proposed as barriers for cunnilingus and anilingus;[74] however, their limited size may allow potentially infectious fluids to roll onto adjacent tissues.

Condom Promotion

Though general consensus holds that male condoms must play a central role in any STI/HIV prevention program,[75] the appropriate mix of condom promotion versus other prevention strategies (e.g., abstinence and mutual monogamy) remains a concern within specific settings and populations (e.g., adolescents) in many countries, including the United States.[76] Concerns also have been raised about the potential negative consequences of condom promotion[77,78] because increased availability of condoms may not necessarily translate into sufficient use for effective STI prevention. For example, even among studies of heterosexual couples discordant for HIV or genital herpes simplex virus (HSV) for whom there is known risk for infection, fewer than half of couples report regular use of condoms.[34,35] Of increasing interest is whether interventions promoting condom use may result, paradoxically, in the onset or increased frequency of high-risk sexual activity, as hypothesized in some studies.[79,80] Few randomized controlled trials have evaluated whether such an effect exists or whether it outweighs the protective effects of condom use for persons at risk. One trial of female STI clinics patients being treated for reproductive tract infections, however, found no difference between counseling messages that promoted abstinence only and those that promoted abstinence backed up by condom use on rates of unprotected intercourse.[81] Moreover, a review of 174 condom-related prevention approaches concluded that interventions designed to reduce the risk of HIV infection do not increase unsafe sexual behavior.[82]

Providing Condoms—Counseling

All clients should understand when to use condoms, how to use them most effectively, how to discuss condom use with their partner(s), and how to integrate condom use into intercourse.

Unintended pregnancy prevention. Advise men and their partners that condoms should be used with every act of intercourse regardless of cycle day because ovulation can occur on any cycle day.[83]

STI protection. Emphasize the need for consistent and correct condom use during sexual activities that can transmit STIs and HIV. Recommend that clients use a new condom for each act of anal, vaginal, or oral intercourse that involve penile contact when any risk of infection exists.[74] (See the section on Effectiveness against STIs and HIV.)

Dual method use. Encourage clients to use a condom plus another contraceptive, which could dramatically reduce the risk of both pregnancy and STIs.[84] Use caution when recommending dual method use to clients, however, because simultaneous use of multiple methods may be overly cumbersome for some couples; instead they may opt to use no method of contraception at all. Follow the client's lead and perhaps suggest a brief trial period of dual method use. If this proves difficult for the client, consider recommending consistent and correct use of condoms alone to provide adequate protection against both pregnancy and infection. Emergency contraception can be used as a backup method against pregnancy in case a condom breaks, falls off, or is not used.

Tailored counseling. Adapt counseling messages on condom use to each client's needs and preferences for contraceptive method characteristics. Clients may have formed their own attitudes about condom use and may have had varying experiences with condoms. Tailor the counseling session to each client's risk factors, abilities, needs, and readiness to change.[85]

Communication of pregnancy rates. Ensure clients choosing contraceptive methods (including condoms) understand the risks and benefits of the range of methods available. Although the ability to prevent pregnancy is often mentioned as the single most important criterion considered when choosing a method,[86-88,] clients may have difficulty understanding typical use and perfect use pregnancy rates across various methods.[88] Because clients may find it difficult to understand contraceptive failure rates, show them a scale of the relative effectiveness of contraceptives, as shown in Figure 3–1 (see Chapter 3 on Efficacy, Safety, and Personal Considerations). Consider using a similar approach when counseling clients about the ability of condoms to prevent STIs, including HIV (see the section on Protection Against STIs and HIV).

Personal benefits. Make sure clients understand how condom use benefits them personally. Explain that condoms protect future fertility by preventing long-term sequelae of STIs. (See Chapter 20 on Reproductive Tract Infections.) Strongly encourage pregnant women at high risk for STIs to use condoms consistently and correctly to protect their fetus, their partner(s), and themselves.

Partner negotiation. Teach clients how to negotiate condom use with partners. Many clients may have contemplated using condoms but may be uncomfortable suggesting condom use to their partners. Teach clients how to negotiate condom use with their partner(s), and help them develop replies they can use when a partner objects to condoms. Assess the likelihood of a partner's negative reaction to the suggestion of condom use; some clients fear that they will be abused or abandoned if they insist on using condoms. Counsel or refer as appropriate if you detect intimate partner violence.

Effective use. Make sure clients understand how to use condoms effectively. Emphasize that condoms are most effective when used correctly during every act of intercourse. Assessing condom use among clients is a two-tiered process. First ask clients how often they are using condoms (e.g., always, mostly, sometimes, never) and explore their barriers to use. Then, to recognize potential misuse, ask clients to explain (and perhaps demonstrate on an appropriate model of a penis) how they use condoms. (See sections on Increasing Effective Use and Instructions for Condom Use.) Encourage clients to use condoms consistently and correctly with every act of anal, vaginal, and oral intercourse.

Suitability. Offer to help clients select the condom most suitable to their needs, which may include a non-latex condom or a female condom. Some clinics now provide a variety of condoms to clients, although one study[90] found that providing a choice of condoms increased acceptability but had no impact on levels of use or STIs.

Practice. Encourage clients to practice using condoms. Many problems that occur during condom use can be attributed to inexperience[89] and can be overcome with practice. Users who have had negative experiences with condoms may be at risk of discontinuing condom use altogether[91]; encourage them to continue practicing with condoms. When providing instruction on how to use condoms, have the client unroll a condom onto a model of a penis or similarly shaped object (e.g., banana), both with eyes open and then again in the dark.

Provision of condoms. Provide each client a large number of condoms at low or no cost. Providing clients with a few condoms is only a short-term solution for clients who find the health care system inaccessible or who find it embarrassing to return repeatedly for condoms. Selling condoms, even at a low cost, dramatically reduces the number of condoms clients will obtain from a clinic compared with the number of free condoms they will take.

Strategies for Increasing Effective Condom Use

Condom effectiveness depends heavily on the skill level and experience of the user.[21] Studies have documented relatively high levels of problems with condom use that may reduce their effectiveness, many of which can be minimized with appropriate counseling and practice. Interventions promoting condom use should address user-related behaviors that result in exposure to STIs and pregnancy, including the following:

1. **Failure to use condoms with every act of intercourse.** Non-use of condoms, rather than poor condom quality or other condom-related problems, is the most common problem.[92,93] The highest single priority for any prevention program should be to address factors that lead to nonuse of condoms, including lack of device acceptability, poor skills for negotiating use with partners, and latex allergy or sensitivity. New strategies that emphasize condom use for contraception in addition to disease prevention may help decrease nonuse.[1] Persons at risk should be provided with an adequate supply of condoms at low or no cost.

2. **Failure to use condoms throughout intercourse.** Recent studies have documented that some men put condoms on after starting intercourse or remove condoms prior to ejaculation.[45,54,55,94-96] These behaviors represent product misuse and could expose partners to risk of pregnancy or STIs despite condom use. Clients should be counseled to use condoms every time throughout intercourse, from beginning to end.

3. **Condom breakage and slippage.** Although users often fear that the condom will break or fall off during use, these events are rare with proper use and tend to be concentrated among a small proportion of users.[89] Most studies show that during vaginal sex, condoms break approximately 2 percent of the time during intercourse or withdrawal and a similar proportion slip off completely.[55,97-101] However, higher rates of breakage and slippage have been reported in a few studies.[102,103] Reviews of studies evaluating breakage and slippage during anal intercourse indicate that the rates may be slightly higher than during vaginal intercourse.[104-106] Advise users to have several condoms available in case a condom is torn or put on incorrectly, or repeated intercourse is desired.

4. **Improper lubricant use with latex condoms.** Unlike water-based (e.g., K-Y Jelly) and most silicone-based lubricants, oil-based lubricants (e.g., petroleum jelly, baby oil, and hand lotions) reduce latex condom integrity[107] and may facilitate breakage (See Table 14–2). People may mistakenly believe oil-based products that readily wash off with water to be water-based lubricants. Because vaginal medications (e.g., for yeast infections) often contain oil-based ingredients that can damage latex condoms, advise clients to remain abstinent or use synthetic condoms until the medication is fully completed and the infection is cured. Note that oil-based products in general can be safely used as lubricants with currently available polyurethane and polyisoprene condoms.

Table 14-2 Examples of lubricant products that should and should not be used with latex condoms

Safe	Not safe
Egg whites	Baby oil
Glycerine	Cold creams
Saliva	Edible oils (olive, peanut, corn, sunflower)
Silicone	Hand and body lotions
S-s	Massage oil
Water	Petroleum jelly
Water-based lubricants (e.g., K-Y Jelly, Astroglide)	Rubbing alcohol Suntan oil and lotions
Silicone-based lubricants	Vegetable or mineral oil
	Vaginal infection medications in cream or suppository form

MANAGING PROBLEMS AND FOLLOW-UP

Persons sensitive or allergic to natural rubber latex may experience irritation, allergic contact dermatitis, or systemic anaphylactic symptoms when exposed to latex-containing products.[108,109] While 1% to 6% of the U.S. population are estimated to be allergic to latex, the prevalence of latex sensitivity is thought to be much higher (8% to 12%) among health care and laboratory workers who have repeated exposure to latex-containing medical devices (e.g., surgical and examination gloves, catheters, intubation tubes, anesthesia masks, and dental dams).[110,111] Proteins in the latex appear to be the primary source of allergic reactions. All clients should be questioned for potential latex allergy.

Ask whether the client experiences itching, rash, or wheezing after wearing latex gloves or inflating a balloon. If you suspect a client has generalized latex sensitivity, consider recommending synthetic condoms and refer the client for allergy skin testing.[112] While latex condom use is contraindicated for clients with general latex sensitivity, both synthetic and natural membrane condoms can be recommended for prevention of pregnancy, while only synthetic condoms should be recommended for prevention of STIs, including HIV.

Allergic reactions that occur only after exposure to latex condoms and not after exposure to other latex-containing products may be attributable to brand-specific condom attributes such as spermicides, lubricants, perfumes, local anesthetics, or other chemical agents added during the manufacturing process.[113] Advise clients to try different brands of latex and synthetic condoms. In any case, clients should immediately contact their health care provider for follow-up if they or their partner(s) experience a severe allergic reaction while using latex condoms or spermicides. Additional comprehensive information on latex allergy can also be obtained from the American Latex Allergy Association (see www. latexallergyresources.org). When counseling men and their partners about condom use, providers should bear in mind the possibility that client reports of latex sensitivity or allergy may in fact represent a simple dislike for condoms.

USER INSTRUCTIONS FOR CONDOMS

Instructions for condom use are often overcomplicated and may have no scientific basis.[114] During a World Health Organization Experts Meeting (Geneva, June 22–24, 2005) to develop a Global Handbook for Family Planning Providers, consensus was reached on five key condom instructions.

Five Key Instructions for Condom Use

1. Use a new condom for each act of intercourse if any risk of pregnancy or STIs exists.
2. Before any genital contact, place the condom on the tip of the erect penis with the rolled side out.
3. Unroll the condom all the way to the base of the erect penis.
4. Immediately after ejaculation, hold the rim of the condom and withdraw the penis while it is still erect.
5. Throw away the used condom safely.

Updated, more detailed instructions for using condoms are included below and can be found elsewhere (www.cdc.gov/condomeffectiveness/male-condom-use.html):

Before Intercourse

1. Have on hand an adequate supply of latex or synthetic condoms and lubricant if you think you may need to use a condom, even if you plan to use another contraceptive. Have extra condoms available in case the first is damaged, torn before use, or put on incorrectly. You will need a new condom if you have repeated intercourse.
2. Discuss condom use with your partner before you have intercourse.

At Time of Intercourse

1. Open the condom package carefully to avoid damaging it with fingernails, teeth, or other sharp objects.
2. Before any genital contact, put the condom on the erect penis.
3. Unroll the condom a short distance to make sure the condom is being unrolled in the correct direction. Then hold the tip of the condom and unroll it down to the base of the erect penis. If the condom does not unroll easily, it probably has been put on inside-out. Discard the condom and begin with a new one, because flipping it over and using it could expose your partner to infectious organisms contained in the pre-ejaculate.
4. Adequate lubrication is important. For latex condoms, use only water-based lubricants, like water, lubricating jellies (e.g., K-Y Jelly), and spermicidal lubricants, jellies, foam, or suppositories, or silicone-based lubricants. Avoid oil-based lubricants (like cold cream, mineral oil, cooking oil, petroleum jelly, body lotions, massage oil, or baby oil) that can damage latex condoms (see Table 14–2).
5. Keep the condom on the penis until after intercourse. If the condom breaks or falls off during intercourse but before ejaculation, stop and put on a new condom. Use a new condom when you have prolonged intercourse, and when you have different types of intercourse within a single session (e.g., after anal sex, change the condom before having vaginal sex to decrease the risk of urinary tract infection).

After Intercourse

1. Soon after ejaculation, withdraw the penis while it is still erect. Hold the condom firmly against the base of the penis to prevent slippage and leakage of semen.
2. Check the condom for visible damage such as holes, then wrap it in tissue and discard. Do not flush condoms down the toilet.
3. If the condom breaks, falls off, leaks, is damaged, or is not used, the following may help:
   - Discuss the possibility of pregnancy or infection with your partner and contact your health care provider as soon as you can. Do not douche. Emergency contraception, now available without a prescription, may be used to prevent pregnancy if it is started within 5 days (120 hours) of having unprotected intercourse. (See Chapter 10 on Emergency Contraception.)

— Gently wash the penis, vulva, anus, and adjacent areas with soap and water immediately after intercourse to help reduce the risk of acquiring an STI. Then insert an applicator full of spermicide into the vagina as soon as possible.

Repeated Intercourse

1. Use a new condom from "beginning to end" with each act of anal, vaginal, or oral intercourse. Do not reuse condoms.

Taking Care of Supplies

1. Store condoms in a cool and dry place out of direct sunlight (excessive heat will weaken latex). Latex condoms can probably be stored in a wallet for a short period of time (e.g., up to 1 month) when kept away from heat and sunlight.[115]
2. Check the expiration or manufacture date on the box or individual package of condoms. Expiration dates are marked as "Exp"; otherwise, the date is the manufacture date (MFG). Latex condoms should not be used beyond their expiration date or more than 5 years after the manufacturing date. Condoms in damaged packages or that show obvious signs of deterioration (e.g., brittleness, stickiness, or discoloration) should not be used regardless of their expiration date.

References

1. UNFPA, WHO and UNAIDS: Position statement on condoms and the prevention of HIV, other sexually transmitted infections and unintended pregnancy. 2015. Available from www.unaids.org/en/resources/presscentre/feature stories/2015/july/20150702_condoms_prevention. Accessed September 10, 2017
2. Anderson J, Warner L, Macaluso M. Condom use among U.S. adults at last sexual intercourse, 1996–2008: an analysis of General Social Survey (GSS) data. Sex Transm Dis 2011;38:919–21.
3. Abma JC, Martinez GM. Sexual activity and contraceptive use among teenagers in the United States, 2011–2015. National health statistics reports; no 104. Hyattsville, MD: National Center for Health Statistics. 2017.
4. Daniels K, Abma JC. Unmarried men's contraceptive use at recent sexual intercourse: United States, 2011–2015. NCHS data brief, no 284. Hyattsville, MD: National Center for Health Statistics. 2017.
5. Kann L, McManus T, Harris WA, et al. Youth Risk Behavior Surveillance – United States, 2015. MMWR, 2016;65:1–174.
6. Daniels K, Abma J, Personal communication to James Trussell, April 3, 2017.
7. Trussell J, Guthrie KA. Choosing a Contraceptive: Efficacy, Safety, and Personal Considerations. In: Hatcher RA, Guest F, Stewart F, Stewart G, Kowal D, Trussell J, Cates W, Policar M. *Contraceptive Technology (20th edition)*. New York, NY: Ardent Media, Inc., 2011.

8. Valdiserri RO. Cum hastis sic clypeatis: the turbulent history of the condom. Bull NY Acad Med. 1988;64:237–245.
9. Murphy JS. The condom industry in the United States, 1990. Jefferson NC: McFarland & Company, Inc., Publishers, 1990.
10. Global Industry Analysts, Inc. Condoms: A global business strategic report. San Jose, CA, March 2008, Publication # MCP-3209.
11. Carey RF, Lytle CD, Cyr WH. Implications of laboratory tests of condom integrity. Sex Transm Dis. 1999;26:216–220.
12. Lytle CD, Routson LB, Seaborn GB, et al. An in vitro evaluation of condoms as barriers to a small virus. Sex Transm Dis. 1997;24:161–164.
13. Gallo M, Grimes D, Lopez L, Schulz K. Non-latex versus latex male condoms for contraception. Cochrane Database Syst Rev. 2006;1:CD003550.
14. Workowski K, Bolan G. Sexually Transmitted Diseases Treatment Guidelines 2015 MMWR Recomm Rep 2015;64(No. RR-3):pp. 1–140.
15. Centers for Disease Control and Prevention. Nonoxynol-9 spermicide contraception use—United States 1999. MMWR. 2002;51:389–92.
16. Centers for Disease Control and Prevention. CDC statement on study results of products containing nonoxynol-9. MMWR. 2000;49:717–718.
17. Centers for Disease Control and Prevention. Sexually transmitted diseases treatment guidelines 2002. MMWR. 2002;51(No. RR-6).
18. Fihn SD, Boyko EJ, Normand EH, et al. Association between use of spermicide coated condoms and Escherichia coli urinary tract infection in young women. Am J Epidemiol. 1996;144:512–20.
19. American Society for Testing Materials. Annual book of ASTM standards: Easton MD: ASTM: section 9, rubber. Volume 09.02 Rubber products; standard specifications for rubber contraceptives (male condoms-D3492). West Conshohocken, PA: American Society for Testing Materials, 1996.
20. Consumers Union: Seven of 20 condoms tested earn perfect score: Extra protection. Consumer Reports. 2009; December.
21. Steiner MJ, Warner L, Stone KM, Cates W Jr. Condoms and other barrier methods for prevention of STD/HIV infection, and pregnancy. In: Holmes KK, Sparling PF, Mardh P-A (editors). Sexually Transmitted Diseases, 4th ed. New York, NY: MacGraw-Hill, 2008.
22. Stone KM, Thomas E, Timyan J. Barrier methods for the prevention of sexually transmitted diseases. In: Holmes KK, Sparling FP, Mardh P-A (editors). Sexually Transmitted Diseases, 3rd edition. New York: McGraw-Hill, 1998.
23. National Institute of Allergy and Infectious Diseases. Workshop summary: scientific evidence on condom effectiveness for sexually transmitted diseases prevention. July 20, 2001. www.niaid.nih.gov/dmid/stds/condomreport.pdf [Accessed October 27, 2010.]
24. Carey RF, Herman WA, Retta SM, et al. Effectiveness of latex condoms as a barrier to human immunodeficiency virus-sized particles under conditions of simulated use. Sex Transm Dis. 1992;19:230–4.
25. Conant MA, Spicer DW, Smith CD. Herpes simplex virus transmission: condom studies. Sex Transm Dis. 1984;11:94–5.
26. Katznelson S, Drew WL, Mintz L. Efficacy of the condom as a barrier to the transmission of cytomegalovirus. J Infect Dis. 1984;150:155–7.
27. Rietmeijer CA, Krebs JW, Feorina PM, et al. Condoms as physical and chemical barriers against human immunodeficiency virus. JAMA. 1988;259:1851–1853.
28. Van de Perre P, Jacobs D, Sprecher-Goldberger S. The latex condom, an efficient barrier against sexual transmission of AIDS-related viruses. AIDS. 1987;1:49–52
29. Judson FN, Ehret JM, Bodin GF, Levin MJ, Rietmeijer CA. In vitro evaluations of condoms with and without nonoxynol 9 as physical and chemical barriers against Chlamydia trachomatis, herpes simplex virus type 2, and human immunodeficiency virus. Sex Transm Dis. 1989;16:51–6.

30. Cates W Jr. The condom forgiveness factor: the positive spin. Sex Transm Dis. 2002;29:350–2.
31. Mann JR, Stine CC, Vessey J. The role of disease-specific infectivity and number of disease exposures on long-term effectiveness of the latex condom. Sex Transm Dis. 2002;29:344–9.
32. Warner L, Stone KM, Macaluso M, Buehler J, Austin HD. A systematic review of design factors assessed in epidemiologic studies of condom effectiveness for preventing gonorrhea and chlamydia. Sex Transm Dis. 2006;33:36–51.
33. Cates W Jr. The NIH condom report: the glass is 90% full. Fam Plann Perspect. 2001;33:231–3.
34. Weller S, Davis K. Condom effectiveness in reducing heterosexual HIV transmission. Cochrane Database Syst Rev 2002;(3):CD003255.
35. Pinkerton SD, Abramson PR. Effectiveness of condoms in preventing HIV transmission. Soc Sci Med. 1997;44:1303–1312
36. Smith DK, Herbst JH, Zhang X, Rose CE. Condom effectiveness for HIV prevention by consistency of use among men who have sex with men in the United States. J Acquir Immune Defic Syndr 2015;68:337–344.
37. d'oro LC, Parazzini F, Naldi L, et al. Barrier methods of contraception, spermicides, and sexually transmitted diseases: A review. Genitourin Med. 1994;70:410.
38. Manhart LE, Koutsky LA. Do condoms prevent genital HPV infection, external genital warts, or cervical neoplasia? A meta-analysis. Sex Transm Dis. 2002;29:725–35.
39. Centers for Disease Control and Prevention. Report to Congress: prevention of genital human papillomavirus infection, January 2004.
40. Holmes KK, Levine R, Weaver M. Effectiveness of condom in preventing sexually transmitted infections. Bull WHO. 2004;84:454–461.
41. Aral SO, Peterman TA. Measuring outcomes of behavioural interventions for STD/HIV prevention. Int J STD AIDS. 1996;7 Suppl 2:30–8.
42. Crosby R, DiClemente RJ, Holtgrave DR, Wingood GM. Design, measurement, and analytical considerations for testing hypotheses relative to condom effectiveness against non-viral STIs. Sex Transm Inf. 2002;78:228–31.
43. Devine OJ, Aral SO. The impact of inaccurate reporting of condom use and imperfect diagnosis of sexually transmitted disease infection in studies of condom effectiveness: a simulation-based assessment. Sex Transm Dis. 2004;31:588–95.
44. Steiner MJ, Feldblum PJ, Padian N. Invited commentary: condom effectiveness—will Prostate specific antigen shed new light on this perplexing problem: Am J Epidemiol. 2003;157:298–300.
45. Warner L, Clay-Warner J, Boles J, Williamson J. Assessing condom use practices. Implications for evaluating method and user effectiveness. Sex Transm Dis. 1998;25:273–7.
46. Warner L, Macaluso M, Austin HD, et al. Application of the case-crossover design to reduce unmeasured confounding in studies of condom effectiveness. Am J Epidemiol. 2005;161:765–73.
47. Warner L, Newman DR, Austin HD, et al. Condom effectiveness for reducing transmission of gonorrhea and chlamydia: the importance of assessing partner infection. Am J Epidemiol 2004;159:242–51.
48. Warner L, Macaluso M, Newman DR, et al. Re: Condom effectiveness for prevention of chlamydia trachomatis infection. Sex Transm Inf. 2006;82:265.
49. Zenilman JM, Weisman CS, Rompalo AM, et al. Condom use to prevent incident STDs: the validity of self-reported condom use. Sex Transm Dis. 1995;22:15–21.
50. Koss CA, Dunne EF. Warner L. A systematic review of epidemiologic studies assessing condom use and risk of syphilis. Sex Transm Dis. 2009;36:401–5.
51. Niccolai L, Rowhani-Rahbar A, Jenkins H, et al. Condom effectiveness for prevention of chlamydia trachomatis infection. Sex Transm Inf. 2005;81:323–5.
52. Shlay JC, McClung MW, Patnaik JL, Douglas JM Jr. Comparison of sexually transmitted disease prevalence by reported condom use: errors among consistent condom users seen at an urban sexually transmitted disease clinic. Sex Transm Dis. 2004;31:526–32.

53. Shlay JC, McClung MW, Patnaik JL, Douglas JM Jr. Comparison of sexually transmitted disease prevalence by reported level of condom use among patients attending an urban sexually transmitted disease clinic. Sex Transm Dis. 2004;31:154–160.

54. Paz-Bailey G, Koumans EH, Sternberg M, et al. The effect of correct and consistent condom use on chlamydial and gonococcal infection among urban adolescents. Arch Pediatr Adolesc Med. 2005;159:536–42

55. Warner L, Newman DR, Kamb ML, et al., Project RESPECT Study Group. Problems with condom use among patients attending sexually transmitted disease clinics: prevalence, predictors, and relation to incident gonorrhea and chlamydia. Am J Epidemiol. 2008; 167:341–49.

56. Winer RL, Hughes JP, Feng Q, et al. Condom use and the papillomavirus infection in young women. N Engl J Med. 2006;354:2645–2654.

57. Casper C, Wald A. Condom use and the prevention of genital herpes acquisition. Herpes. 2002;9:10–4.

58. Wald A, Langenberg AG, Krantz, et al. The relationship between condom use and herpes simplex virus acquisition. Ann Intern Med. 2005;143:707–713.

59. Wald A, Langenberg AG, Link K, et al. Effect of condoms on reducing the transmission of herpes simplex virus type 2 from men to women. JAMA. 2001;285:3100–6.

60. Barlow D. The condom and gonorrhoea. Lancet. 1977;222:811–812.

61. Ramstedt K, Forssman L, Giesecke J, Granath F. Risk factors for chlamydia trachomatis in 6810 young women attending family planning clinics. Int J STD AIDS. 1992;3:117–122.

62. Upchurch DM, Brady WE, Reichart CA, Hook EW III. Behavioral contributions to acquisition of gonorrhea in patients attending an inner-city sexually transmitted disease clinic. J Infect Dis. 1990;161:938–941.

63. Fennema JSA, van Ameijden EJC, Coutinho RA, van Den Hoek A. Clinical sexually transmitted diseases among human immunodeficiency virus-infected and noninfected drug-using prostitutes. Associated factors and interpretation of trends, 1986 to 1994. Sex Transm Dis. 1997;24:363–371.

64. Levine WC, Revollo R, Kaune V, et al. Decline in sexually transmitted disease prevalence in female Bolivian sex workers: impact of an HIV prevention project. AIDS. 1998;12:1899–1906.

65. Hooper RR, Reynolds GH, Jones OG, et al. Cohort study of venereal disease. I: the risk of gonorrhea transmission from infected women to men. Am J Epidemiol. 1978; 108:136–144.

66. Baeten JM, Nyange PM, Richardson BA, et al. Hormonal contraception and risk of sexually transmitted disease acquisition: results from a prospective study. Am J Obstet Gynecol. 2001;185:380–5.

67. Cates W Jr., Holmes KK. Re: condom efficacy against gonorrhea and nongonococcal urethritis. Am J Epidemiol. 1996;143:843–844.

68. Sanchez J, Gutuzzo E, Escamilla J. Sexually transmitted infections in female sex workers: reduced by condom use but not by a limited periodic examination program. Sex Transm Dis. 1998;25:82–89.

69. Schwartz MA, Lafferty WE, Hughes JP, Handsfield HH. Risk factors for urethritis in heterosexual men. Sex Transm Dis. 1997;24:449–455.

70. Hogewoning CJ, Bleeker MC, van den Brule AJ, et al. Condom use promotes regression of cervical intraepithelial neoplasia and clearance of human papillomavirus: a randomized clinical trial. Int J Cancer. 2003;107:811–6.

71. Bleeker MC, Hogewoning CJ, Voorhorst FJ, et al. Condom use promotes regression of human papillomavirus-associated penile lesions in male sexual partners of women with cervical intraepithelial neoplasia. Int J Cancer. 2003;107:804–10.

72. Alfonsi GA, Shlay J. The effectiveness of condoms for the prevention of sexually transmitted diseases. Current Women's Health Reviews. 2005;1:151–9.

73. Nielson CM, Harris RB, Nyitray AG, Dunne EF, Stone KM, Giuliano AR. Consistent condom use is associated with lower HPV prevalence in men. J Inf Dis. 2010;202:445–51.

74. Centers for Disease Control and Prevention. How to use a dental dam as a barrier for oral sex. Available from www.cdc.gov/condomeffectiveness/Dental-dam-use.html. Accessed October 26, 2017.

75. Halperin DT, Steiner MJ, Cassell MM, et al. The time has come for common ground on preventing sexual transmission of HIV. Lancet. 2004;364:1913–5.

76. American Academy of Pediatrics, Committee on Adolescence. Condom use by adolescents. Pediatrics. 2013;132:973–81.

77. Richens J, Imrie J, Copas A. Condoms and seat belts: the parallels and the lessons. Lancet. 2000;355:400–3.

78. Cassell MM, Halperin DT, Shelton JD, Stanton, D. Risk compensation: the Achilles' heel of innovations in HIV prevention? BMJ. 2006;332:605–7.

79. Kajubi P, Kamya MR, Kamya S, et al. Increasing condom use without reducing HIV risk: results of a controlled community trial in Uganda. J Acquir Immune Defic Syndr. 2005;40:77–82.

80. Imrie J, Stephenson JM, Cowan FM, et al. A cognitive behavioural intervention to reduce sexually transmitted infections among gay men: randomised trial. BMJ .2001; 322:1451–1456.

81. Anderson C, Gallo MF, Hylton-Kong T, et al. Randomized controlled trial on the effectiveness of counseling messages for avoiding unprotected sexual intercourse during sexually transmitted infection and reproductive tract infection treatment among female sexually transmitted infection clinic patients. Sex Transm Dis 2013;40:105–110.

82. Smoak ND, Scott-Sheldon LA, Johnson BT, Cary MP. Sexual risk reduction interventions do not inadvertently increase the overall frequency of sexual behavior: A meta-analysis of 174 studies with 116,735 participants. J Acquir Immune Defic Syndro. 2006;41:374–384.

83. Wilcox AJ, Dunson DB, Weinberg CR, Trussell J, Baird DD. Likelihood of conception with a single act of intercourse: providing benchmark rates for assessment of post-coital contraceptives. Contraception. 2001;63:211–5.

84. Cates W Jr., Steiner MJ. Dual protection against unintended pregnancy and sexually transmitted infections: What is the best contraceptive approach? Sex Transm Dis. 2002;29:168–174.

85. Centers for Disease Control and Prevention. Revised guidelines for HIV counseling, testing and referral. MMWR. 2001;50 (RR-19):1–58.

86. Grady WR, Klepinger DH, Nelson-Wally A. Contraceptive characteristics: the perceptions and priorities of men and women. Fam Plann Perspect. 1999;31:168–75.

87. Edwards JE, Oldman A, Smith L, et al. Women's knowledge of, and attitudes to, contraceptive effectiveness and adverse health effects. Br J Fam Plann.2000;26: 73–80.

88. Steiner MJ, Dalebout S, Condon S, et al. Understanding risk: a randomized controlled trial of communicating contraceptive effectiveness. Obstet Gynecol. 2003;102:709–17.

89. Steiner M, Piedrahita C, Glover L, Joanis C. Can condom users likely to experience condom failure be identified? Fam Plann Perspect. 1993;25:2820–223,226.

90. Steiner MJ, Hylton-Kong T, Figueroa JP, et al. Does a choice of condoms impact sexually transmitted infection incidence? A randomized, controlled trial. Sex Transm Dis. 2006;33:31–35.

91. Norris AE, Ford K. Associations between condom experiences and beliefs, intentions, and use in a sample of urban, low-income, African-American and Hispanic youth. AIDS Educ Prev. 1994;6:27–39.

92. Steiner MJ, Cates W Jr, Warner L. The real problem with male condoms is nonuse. Sex Transm Dis. 1999;26:459–62.

93. Warner L, Steiner MJ. Condom access does not ensure condom use: you've got to be putting me on. Sex Transm Inf. 2002;78:225.

94. Fishbein M, Pequegnat W. Evaluating AIDS prevention interventions using behavioral and biological outcome measures. Sex Transm Dis 2000;27:101–10.

95. Calzavara L, Burchell AN, Remis RS, et al. Delayed application of condoms is a risk factor for human immunodeficiency virus infection among homosexual and bisexual men. Am J Epidemiol. 2003;157:210–17.
96. Crosby RA, Sanders SA, Yarber WL, et al. Condom use errors and problems among college men. Sex Transm Dis. 2002;29:552–7.
97. Albert AE, Warner DL, Hatcher RA, Trussell J, Bennett C. Condom use among female commercial sex workers in Nevada's legal brothels. Am J Publ Health. 1995; 85:1514–1520.
98. Cook L, Nanda K, Taylor D. Randomized crossover trial comparing the eZ.on plastic condom and a latex condom. Contraception. 2001;63:25–31.
99. Valappil T, Kelaghan J, Macaluso M, et al. Female condom and male condom failure among women at high risk of sexually transmitted diseases. Sex Transm Dis 2005;32:35–43.
100. Macaluso M, Kelaghan J, Artz L, et al. Mechanical failure of the latex condom in a cohort of women at high STD risk. Sex Transm Dis. 1999;26:450–8.
101. Walsh TL, Frezieres RG, Peacock K, et al. Effectiveness of the male latex condom: combined results for three popular condom brands used as controls in randomized clinical trials. Contraception. 2004;70:407–13.
102. Mukenge-Tshibaka L, Alary M, Geraldo N, Lowndes CM. Incorrect condom use and frequent breakage among female sex workers and their clients. Int J STD AIDS. 2005;16:345–7.
103. Russell-Brown P, Piedrahita C, Foldesy R, et al. Comparison of condom breakage during human use with performance in laboratory testing. Contraception. 1992;45:429–37.
104. Silverman BG, Gross TP. Use and effectiveness of condoms during anal intercourse. A review. Sex Transm Dis. 1997;24:11–7.
105. Richters J, Kippax S. Condoms for anal sex. In: Mindel A, editor. Condoms. First ed. London: BMJ Publishing Group, 2000, 132–146.
106. McBride KR, Fortenberry JD. Heterosexual anal sexuality and anal sex behaviors: a review. J Sex Research. 2010;47:123–35.
107. Voeller B, Coulson AH, Bernstein GS, Nakamura RM. Mineral oil lubricants cause rapid deterioration of latex condoms. Contraception. 1989; 39:95–102.
108. Zaza S, Reeder JM, Charles LE, Jarvis WR. Latex sensitivity among perioperative nurses. AORN. 1994;60:806–812.
109. National Institute for Occupational Safety and Health. Preventing allergic reactions to natural rubber latex in the workplace [NIOSH alert]. National Institute for Occupational Safety and Health, June 1997 [DHHS (NIOSH) publication No. 97–135].
110. Food and Drug Administration. Allergic reactions to latex-containing medical devices [press release]. Rockville MD; Food and Drug Administration, March 29, 1991.
111. Food and Drug Administration. Don't be misled by "Latex Free" claims. Rockville MD; Food and Drug Administration, March 24, 2015 Available at: www.fda.gov/ForConsumers/ConsumerUpdates/ucm342641.html
112. Yassin MS, Lierl MB, Fischer TJ, et al. Latex allergy in hospital employees. Ann Allergy. 1994;72:245–249.
113. Hamann CP, Kick SA. Update: immediate and delayed hypersensitivity to natural rubber latex. Cutis. 1993;52:307–311.
114. Spencer B, Gerofi J. Can we tell them how to do it? In: Mindel A, editor. Condoms. First ed. London: BMJ Publishing Group, 2000, 207–219.
115. Glasser G, Hatcher RA. The effect on condom integrity of carrying a condom in a wallet for three months [abstract]. Proceedings of the American College of Obstetricians and Gynecologists District IV Conference. November 1992, San Juan, PR.

Coitus Interruptus (Withdrawal, Pulling Out)

15

Rachel K. Jones, PhD

- Sixty percent of all sexually active women report having used withdrawal at some point in their lives, and the proportion of couples currently relying on the method has increased in recent years.
- Withdrawal can be used alone, at the same time as other methods (dual use), or alternating with other methods (rotating use).
- Spermatozoa appear in the pre-ejaculatory fluid of some individuals, and there is a small chance this could cause pregnancy even if withdrawal occurs prior to ejaculation.

Coitus interruptus, more commonly referred to as withdrawal and pulling out, is the practice of withdrawing the penis from the vagina and away from the external genital organs of the woman before ejaculation, with the intention of avoiding pregnancy. Coitus interruptus was a natural response to the discovery that ejaculation into the vagina caused pregnancy. The method was probably widely practiced throughout history, playing a role in fertility declines that occurred prior to the advent of the pill.[1]

Over the last three decades, couples have increasingly relied on coitus interruptus. Some 60% of sexually experienced women report having *ever* practiced withdrawal according to the 2006-2010 National Survey of Family Growth (NSFG); comparable figures were 41% in 1995 and 25% in 1982.[2] Only pills and condoms were more often reported as methods ever used by the respondents.

Among women using contraception, 8% were currently relying on coitus interruptus in 2014, a significant increase from 5% in 2008.[3] But use of the method is likely more widespread. Most studies evaluate contraception based on the most effective method used. Using the 2002 NSFG, researchers found that reliance on withdrawal in the last month more than doubled when use of multiple methods were taken into account, from 5% to 11% among all women[4] and from 7% to 14% among adolescent females.[5]

Because it is perceived to be ineffective at preventing pregnancy, many individuals do not consider withdrawal to be a "real" method and may fail to report use unless they are specifically asked about it.[4,6–8]

MECHANISM OF ACTION

Withdrawal inhibits fertilization by preventing contact between spermatozoa and the ovum. The couple may have penile-vaginal intercourse until ejaculation is impending, at which time the penis is withdrawn from the vagina and away from the external genitalia of the partner. The individual must rely on his own sensations to determine when ejaculation is about to occur. The pre-ejaculate, which is usually released just prior to full ejaculation, generally goes unnoticed by both the partners during their course of sexual activity and so cannot be relied upon as a sign that ejaculation is about to occur.

EFFECTIVENESS

Withdrawal is in the bottom tier of contraceptive effectiveness (see Figure 3-1). The method has not been examined in clinical trials, but the perfect-use failure rate is estimated to be 4%. Data from the 2006-2010 NSFG suggest that 1 in 5 U.S. couples could expect to get pregnant over the course of a year if they relied solely on withdrawal (i.e., the typical-use failure rate is 20%).[9] The difference between the typical-use and perfect-use failure rates speak to the difficulty couples have in using withdrawal consistently and correctly.

When the penis becomes erect, pre-ejaculate, a lubricating secretion produced by the Littre or Cowper's glands, is emitted. Although two studies examining the pre-ejaculate for the presence of spermatozoa found none,[10,11] two other studies found spermatozoa, though in small numbers. In one of these studies, 8 of 23 samples contained clumps of a few hundred sperm, which could theoretically have posed a risk of fertilization.[12] In a study designed specifically to determine whether pre-ejaculate contained sperm potentially capable of fertilizing an egg, researchers examined the samples within 2 hours of production.[13] The pre-ejaculate of 37% of men (N=27) contained motile sperm, though the number of sperm in each sample was very low. Also worth noting is that this study found that subjects either consistently had sperm in their pre-ejaculate or consistently did not. The best available evidence suggests that the risk of pregnancy posed by pre-ejaculate is very low, though not zero.

As with other methods, withdrawal's efficacy in preventing pregnancy depends not only on characteristics of the method (whether the pre-ejaculate contains sperm) but also on characteristics of the user. Individuals who are less experienced with using the method or who have difficulty in foretelling when ejaculation will occur could have a greater risk of failure. Research also suggests that women reporting lower motivation to avoid pregnancy are more likely to use withdrawal,[5,14] and these attitudes may also result in inconsistent use of the method.

ADVANTAGES

As a method of contraception, withdrawal has several distinct advantages. It costs nothing, requires no devices, involves no chemicals, and is available in any situation. Some couples may select withdrawal as their method because it requires no physical examination or contact with a clinic or pharmacy.[15] Practicing coitus interruptus causes no medical side effects. It also enables both partners to take a responsible and active role in fertility regulation and may foster a dialogue on contraception and sexuality between the partners. It is also a back-up contraceptive that is always available and can enhance the effectiveness of other methods.

DISADVANTAGES AND CAUTIONS

Some pre-ejaculate fluid contains spermatozoa and could theoretically fertilize an egg.[12,13]

Because the method must be used every time a couple has sex, and complete withdrawal is required for it to be effective, the probability of pregnancy in typical users is substantially higher than that for hormonal methods or long-acting contraception. One reason for contraceptive failure may be that the male partner lacks the self-control demanded by the method for every act of intercourse.[16] For some couples, interruption of the excitement or plateau phase of the sexual response cycle may diminish pleasure. In addition, some men have difficulty foretelling when they will ejaculate, and some women may feel anxiety in relinquishing control over pregnancy prevention to men.

SPECIAL ISSUES

SEXUALLY TRANSMITTED INFECTIONS

Because not all pathogens are limited to seminal fluid, withdrawal does not completely protect couples from exposure to STIs presenting with actively infective surface lesions such as those from herpes genitalis or human papilloma virus.[17]

The seminal fluid that emerges from the penis prior to ejaculation may contain some human immunodeficiency virus (HIV).[12,17] However, coitus interruptus may decrease HIV exposure by reducing the amount of semen that enters the vagina. In stable discordant couples (the man was infected with HIV and the woman was not), coitus interruptus cut the HIV conversion rate of women by half in one study,[18] and by a larger percentage in another study.[19] Because these studies examined only stable heterosexual couples, the findings may not hold true for women with several HIV-infected partners.

Although coitus interruptus may be less likely than intercourse with ejaculation to transmit HIV, individuals have become infected while their partners consistently practiced withdrawal. Coitus interruptus has not been studied as a way to reduce HIV transmission from woman to man.

Use Patterns

Withdrawal is used in several different ways. One national study found that a majority of women using withdrawal in the last month also used another contraceptive, and only 35% of withdrawal users reported using this method alone.[14] Users of withdrawal were as likely to report that they used it with condoms as they were to report that they used it with a highly effective method such as the pill or the IUD. Similar patterns were observed among young adults in the NSFG.[5] (It is possible that some reports of dual use of condoms and withdrawal refer to situations where the penis was pulled out in order to put on a condom after insertive sex had begun.[20]) Some women reported using withdrawal and other methods at the same time (dual use), some reported switching between methods (rotating use), and still others reported adopting both strategies (dual and rotating use) over the one-month time period.[14] Other studies, both quantitative and qualitative, have also found that withdrawal is used in a variety of ways (dual and rotating use) and for a variety of reasons, including having no other method on hand, as "extra insurance" against pregnancy, enhancement of sexual pleasure, as well as others.[5–8,21]

Withdrawal is perceived to be used most frequently by adolescents, it presumably allows them to avoid acknowledging they are sexually active to health care providers or retail staff selling contraceptive methods. However, reliance on withdrawal is most common among individuals in their 20s.[22] Between 2008 and 2014, use of withdrawal as a primary method of contraception doubled, from 6% to 12%, among 25 to 29 year olds.[3] The shift toward greater reliance on withdrawal was most marked, and significant, for more advantaged populations, including white women (from 5% to 8%), those with family incomes >300% of poverty level (from 5% to 10%) and, interestingly, those with private insurance (from 5% to 9%). Levels of reliance on withdrawal were also higher than average among cohabiting women (13%) and women born outside the United States (13%). It is unclear what is responsible for the increase in reliance on withdrawal, but it suggests that information about withdrawal needs to be incorporated into educational and counseling materials. (See Chapter 2 for more complete discussion of patient-centered contraception counseling.)

PROVIDING THE METHOD

Many individuals, including those who rely on withdrawal, may not consider it to be a "real" method[4,6,8] and may fail to report that they use it when contraception is being discussed. Thus, health care providers may need to ask specifically about use of the method. Moreover, given that withdrawal can be part of several contraceptive strategies, providers should determine if dual, rotating, or both strategies are being used. Given increased reliance on the method in recent years, discussions of withdrawal are even more important. Indeed, it is possible that typical-use failure rates for the method would improve, approaching lower levels seen in other developed countries,[23] if couples had more information about it. Some users or potential users may have questions related to the fertile period, pre-ejaculate fluid, and the risk of any negative health effects, including exposure to STIs. Finally, inform the couple about emergency contraception, including intrauterine contraception, and provide a supply of emergency contraceptive pills and instruct them on their use to help decrease the risk of pregnancy. (See Chapter 10 on Emergency Contraception.)

USER INSTRUCTIONS FOR WITHDRAWAL*

1. To practice withdrawal, the man should withdraw his penis from his partner's vagina when he feels he is about to ejaculate, making sure that ejaculation occurs away from his partner's genitalia.
2. Withdrawal is not a good contraceptive method if the man cannot predictably withdraw prior to ejaculation.
3. Pre-ejaculate fluid can be released as soon as the penis becomes erect to as late as just before ejaculation. In some individuals, this pre-ejaculate fluid may contain small numbers of sperm, which could possibly cause a pregnancy. A man may not be aware that he has released pre-ejaculate fluid.

---

*These instructions are intended to guide providers in educating patients in how to use their method.

4. If more than one act of intercourse takes place within a relatively short period of time, the man should urinate and wipe off the tip of his penis before intercourse to remove any sperm remaining from a previous ejaculation.
5. Withdrawal does not effectively protect against sexually transmitted infections (STIs), including infection with the human immunodeficiency virus (HIV). Abstinence or use of latex or plastic condoms provide better protection.
6. Learn what options are available for postcoital protection should any ejaculate come in contact with the vagina. If you think you may have been exposed to a risk of pregnancy, contact your clinician about emergency contraception.

Emergency Contraceptives: Emergency contraceptive pills or placement of a copper intrauterine contraceptive after unprotected intercourse substantially reduces the risk of pregnancy.

Author Disclosures—none.

References

1. Santow G. Coitus interruptus and the control of natural fertility. Pop Stud 1995;49: 19–43.
2. Daniels K, Mosher W, and Jones J. Contraceptive methods women have ever used: United States, 1982–2010. 2013. Hyattsville, MD: National Center for Health Statistics.
3. Kavanaugh ML, Jerman J. Contraceptive method mix in the United States: Trends and characteristics with use between 2008 and 2014. Contraception 2017; 97:14–21.
4. Jones RK, Fennell J, Higgins JA, Blanchard K. Better than nothing or savvy risk-reduction practice? The importance of withdrawal. Contraception 2009;79:407–410.
5. Higgins JA, Wang Y. Which young adults are most likely to use withdrawal? The importance of pregnancy attitudes and sexual pleasure. Contraception 2015;91:320–327.
6. Arteaga S, Gomez AM. "Is that even a method of birth control?" A qualitative exploration of young women's use of withdrawal. J Sex Res 2015;626–632.
7. Frohwirth L, Blades N, Moore AM, Wurtz H. The complexity of multiple contraceptive method use and the anxiety the informs it: Implications for theory and practice. Arch Sex Behav 2016;45:2123–2135.
8. Whittaker PG, Merkh RD, Henry-Moss D, Hock-Long L. Withdrawal attitudes and experiences: a qualitative perspective among young urban adults. Perspect Sex Reprod H 2010;42:102–109.
9. Sundaram A, Vaughan B, Kost K et al. Contraceptive failure in the United States: Estimates from the 2006–2010 National Survey of Family Growth. Perspect Sex Reprod H 2017;49:7–16.
10. Ilaria G, Jacobs J, Polsky B et al. Detection of HIV-1 DNA sequences in pre-eajculatory fluid [letter]. Lancet 1992;340:1469.
11. Zukerman Z, Weiss D, Orvieto R. Does pre-ejaculatory penile secretion originating from Cowper's gland contain sperm? J Assist Reprod Gen 2003;20:157–159.

12. Pudney J, Oneta M, Mayer K, Seage G, Anderson D. Pre-ejaculatory fluid as potential vector for sexual transmission of HIV-1 [letter]. Lancet 1992;340:1470.
13. Killick S, Leary C, Trussell J, Guthrie K. Sperm content of pre-ejaculatory fluid. Hum Fertil 2011;14:48–52.
14. Jones RK, Lindberg LD, Higgins JA. Pull and pray or extra protection? Contraceptive strategies involving withdrawal among US adult women. Contraception 2014;90:416–420.
15. Rogow D, Horowitz S. Withdrawal: a review of the literature and an agenda for research. Stud Fam Plan 1995;26:140–153.
16. De Visser R. Delayed application of condoms, withdrawal and negotiation of safer sex among heterosexual young adults. AIDS Care 2004;16:315–322.
17. Howe J, Minkoff H, Duerr A. Contraceptives and HIV. AIDS 1993;8:861–871.
18. Musicco M, Saracco A, Lazzarin A. The role of contraceptive practices in HIV sexual transmisison from man to woman. In: Nicolosi A, ed. HIV methodology: models and methods. New York: Raven Press, Ltd; 1994.
19. DiVencenzi (for the European Study Group). A longitudinal study of human immunodeficiency virus transmission by heterosexual partners. New Engl J Med 2017; 331:341–346.
20. Crosby RA, Sanders SA, Yarber WL et al. Condom errors and problems among college men. Sex Transm Dis 2002;29:552–557
21. Sznitman SR, Romer D, Brown LK et al. Prevalence, correlates, and sexually transmitted infection risk related to coitus interruptus among African-American adolescents. Sex Transm Dis 2009;36:218–220.
22. Daniels K, Daugherty J, Jones J, and Mosher W. Current contraceptive use and variation by selected characteristics among women aged 15–44: United States 2011–2013. 2015. Hyattsville, MD: National Center for Health Statistics.
23. Moreau C, Trussell J, Rodriguez G et al. Contraceptive failure rates in France: results from a population-based survey. Hum Reprod 2007;22:2422–2427.

Permanent Contraception

16

Melody Y. Hou, MD, MPH
Danielle Roncari, MD, MPH

- Permanent contraception is one of the safest, most effective, and most cost-effective contraceptive methods.
- Permanent contraception is the most widely used method of family planning in the world in both developed and developing countries.
- Tubal surgery methods include transabdominal and transcervical approaches.
- Patients should be advised that these procedures should be considered permanent. Achieving pregnancy after permanent contraception is expensive, requiring either assisted reproductive technology (such as in vitro fertilization, or IVF) or highly technical surgery, and results cannot be guaranteed.
- Permanent contraception does not provide any protection against sexually transmitted infections (STIs), including human immunodeficiency virus (HIV).

Fallopian tube and vas deferens surgery are safe and effective permanent methods of contraception. Permanent contraception continues to be the most commonly used method in the United States: among individuals using a contraceptive method who were interviewed for the National Survey of Family Growth in 2011 to 2013, 25.1% relied on tubal surgery and 8.3% relied on vas surgery, totaling 12.5 million U.S. patients relying on permanent contraception.[1]

More than 30% of the world's couples use permanent contraception, but permanent contraception has its lowest prevalence in the least developed countries, with less than 10% of couples relying on this contraceptive method.[2]

A couple should consider both vas deferens and fallopian tube surgery as options for permanent contraception. Vas surgery carries fewer risks and greater efficacy than tubal surgery. There is no medical condition that would prohibit permanent contraception, although some conditions and circumstances may require certain surgical precautions.

FALLOPIAN TUBE SURGERY

In the United States, the most common approaches for fallopian tube surgery are laparotomy, if done at time of Cesarean delivery or immediately postpartum, and laparoscopy, if performed in the interval period (occurring at least 6 weeks postpartum). The Essure system, another method of interval surgery, uses a transcervical approach. Culdoscopy, which involves introducing a camera into the rectovaginal pouch through an incision in the posterior vaginal cul-de-sac, is not recommended due to its higher complication rate.[3] Although hysterectomy also confers permanent contraception, performing this major surgery solely for contraception is discouraged due to its risk of morbidity compared to other options for permanent contraception.

MECHANISM OF ACTION

Tubal surgery blocks fertilization by cutting, occluding, or removing the fallopian tubes to prevent the sperm and egg from uniting (Figure 16-1).

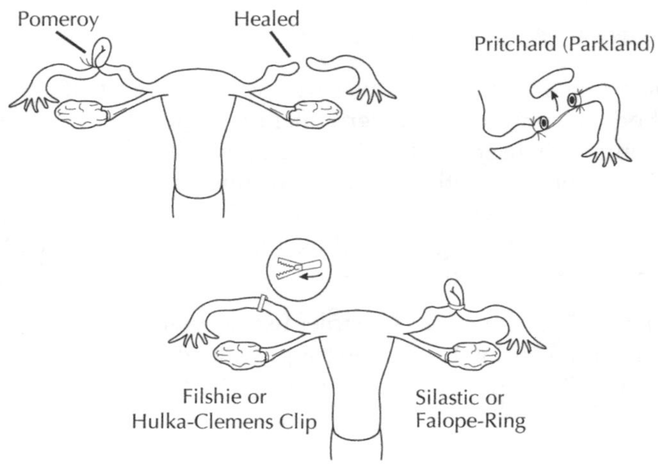

Figure 16-1 Possible tubal surgery techniques

EFFECTIVENESS

Following completion of childbearing, patients spend approximately 20 years using contraception. Tubal surgery is far more effective than short-term user-dependent reversible contraceptive methods, such as oral contraceptives, condoms, and injectable methods (See Figure 3-1 in Chapter 3). Failure rates of tubal surgery are roughly comparable to those of long-acting reversible methods, such as the contraceptive implants and intrauterine devices (IUDs), which are described in Chapters 4 and 5. The World Health Organization (WHO) and Centers for Disease Control and Prevention (CDC) place permanent contraception in the top tier of contraceptive effectiveness. The overall first-year typical-use failure rates are 0.5% for fallopian tube surgery and 0.15% for vas surgery (Table 27-1).

In 1996 the CDC conducted the Collaborative Review of Sterilization (CREST), a large, prospective, multicenter observational study of over 10,000 patients undergoing transabdominal tubal surgery in the U.S. who were followed for up to 14 years. The study demonstrated that transabdominal tubal surgery is highly effective.[4] Analysis of CREST data found that the 5-year cumulative probability of failure of aggregated surgical methods was 13 per 1,000 procedures.[4] The risk of failure persists for years after the procedure, and varies by several factors, including patient age at the time of surgery and surgical technique. Patients were more likely to have a contraceptive failure the younger they were at the time of surgery. Postpartum partial salpingectomy had the lowest 5-year and 10-year cumulative pregnancy rates (6.3 per 1,000 and 7.5 per 1,000 procedures, respectively). The highest 10-year cumulative pregnancy rates were found in patients younger than 28 years who had tubal occlusion with bipolar coagulation, at 54 pregnancies per 1,000 patients.[4] The results of the CREST study should be interpreted in context; the study included certain transabdominal occlusion methods whose surgical techniques were still evolving, and does not evaluate the titanium clip which was introduced in the United States in 1996 after the study was completed. According to the Royal College Working Party on Sterilization in 1999, efficacy of the titanium clip is comparable to other occlusion methods with a crude failure rate of 2 to 3 per 1,000 patients.[5]

Although complete salpingectomy has not yet been compared to other methods, we believe that the risk of pregnancy following complete salpingectomy would likely be the lowest of all methods. To date, there are only three case reports in the world literature of failure following salpingectomy.[6,7]

The Food and Drug Administration (FDA) has approved two transcervical permanent contraception systems: Essure and Adiana. Both rely on the placement of devices into the fallopian tubes that initiate a physiological response to cause tubal occlusion. Thus, successful bilateral device placement in the tubes is essential for effectiveness. Bilateral placement success rates for Essure are 81% to 98% among patients without tubal disease or adhesions, allowing for up to two separate attempts at placement. Among patients who have successful placement in clinical trials, 3.5% did not have occlusion by 3 months on hysterosalpingogram (HSG), but all had occlusion by 6 months.[8] An analysis using Markov modeling for any patient seeking permanent contraception via Essure in the office, Essure in the operating room setting, and laparoscopic approach in the operating room estimates the rate of successful occlusion in 1 year from the first attempt to be 87%, 88% and 99% respectively, assuming that 6% of patients who attempt a hysteroscopic approach will ultimately undergo laparoscopy.[9]

Some case reports of pregnancy following Essure have attributed procedure failure to patients or clinicians not adhering to manufacturer's instructions, but some pregnancies have occurred despite demonstrated adherence.[10–12] Markov modeling suggests that at 1 year, the expected pregnancy rates would be 57 in 1,000 patients who undergo hysteroscopic procedures, compared to 7 for laparoscopic silicone band and 3 for laparoscopic bipolar coagulation. In 10 years, using the same model, the cumulative pregnancy rate per 1,000 patients is estimated to be 96 for hysteroscopic occlusion, 24 for silicone band, and 30 for bipolar coagulation.[13]

Adiana retains FDA approval, although the manufacturer discontinued it in April 2012. Successful bilateral placement of Adiana was reported to be 94%, with a 36-month cumulative pregnancy rate of 16 in 1,000.[14] Long-term effectiveness has not been fully assessed for either hysteroscopic system.

Intrauterine Pregnancy

Intrauterine pregnancy following transabdominal tubal surgery carries no known added risk to the patient or the fetus. Pregnancy outcomes are unclear with Essure left in-situ. A portion of the coils trails into the uterine cavity, but trailing coils appear to shorten and become completely encapsulated in tissue on follow-up hysteroscopy. Clinical trials show that pregnancy rates are inferior when Essure is used to block hydrosalpinges prior to in vitro fertilization (IVF) than when laparoscopic salpingectomy is performed.[15–17] Although the extended follow-up of patients in the Phase III trial for Essure found no pregnancies among the 449 patients who completed all 5 years of follow up, unintended spontaneous intrauterine pregnancies have been reported in the literature or to the FDA following transcervical procedures, ending in miscarriage, ectopic pregnancy, abortion, and successful delivery.[10,11,18–20] These outcome data are from case reports and series, so more generalizable statements about transcervical procedures and safety in pregnancy cannot be made.

Ectopic Pregnancy

The overall risk of ectopic pregnancy in patients using permanent contraception is significantly lower than that of the general population, since the risk of becoming pregnant with permanent contraception is very low. However, if a patient becomes pregnant while using permanent contraception, the risk of that pregnancy being ectopic is high. An analysis of CREST data found that roughly 30% of pregnancies following permanent contraception were ectopic pregnancies.[21] The risk of ectopic pregnancy varies with the method of tubal surgery. The 10-year cumulative probability of ectopic pregnancy after transabdominal tubal occlusion by all methods was 7.3 per 1,000 procedures. For the titanium clip and silicone band, the 10-year cumulative probability was 8.5 and 7.3 per 1,000 procedures respectively. Postpartum partial salpingectomy had the lowest risk of ectopic pregnancy at 1.5 per 1,000 procedures. The risk of ectopic pregnancy did not diminish with the length of time since the tubal surgery, but did vary inversely with the age of the patient. The probability of ectopic pregnancy was greater for patients who initiated permanent contraception using these occlusion methods before age 30 than for patients 30 years or older. Young patients who had bipolar tubal coagulation had a 10-year cumulative probability of ectopic pregnancy of 31.9 per 1,000 procedures.[21] The rate of ectopic pregnancy following complete salpingectomy is unknown. However, since most ectopic pregnancies occur in the distal end of the fallopian tube, the rate of ectopic pregnancies following removal of the entire tube should be virtually zero. All three of the spontaneous pregnancies documented in case reports were intrauterine.[6,7]

There are no equivalent data on ectopic pregnancy risk for transcervical procedures, although there have been reports of ectopic pregnancies in Adiana trials and in postmarketing surveillance after Essure placement.[12,22]

Advantages and Indications

Tubal surgery is ideal for patients who are certain they wish to have no or no further children and need a reliable contraceptive method. Advantages include the following:

- Permanence
- High effectiveness
- High acceptability
- Safety
- Quick recovery
- Lack of significant long-term side effects

- Cost effectiveness
- No need to buy anything
- No need for partner compliance
- No need to interrupt coitus
- Privacy of choice

DISADVANTAGES AND CAUTIONS

Tubal surgery is not recommended for patients who are unsure of their desire for future fertility. Other disadvantages include the following:

- Restoring fertility after permanent contraception is difficult though possible. It is expensive, requires either costly assisted reproductive technology (such as IVF) or highly technical major surgery, and results cannot be guaranteed
- All surgical procedures carry some risk specific to the nature of the surgery and anesthetic used
- Regret for decision is high among some groups of patients
- Need for surgeon, procedure room (aseptic conditions), trained assistants, medications, and surgical equipment
- Expense at the time of the procedure
- Higher probability of pregnancy being ectopic if method fails
- No protection against sexually transmitted infections (STIs), including HIV

Patients with medical conditions or other special characteristics, such as a complicated history of abdominal surgeries or severe respiratory disease, may have surgical precautions for tubal surgery that differ from those of healthy patients.

SAFETY

Tubal surgery is a safe method of contraception. Death from transabdominal tubal surgery is extremely rare, and overall complication rates are low. Mortality rates in the United States have been estimated at 1 to 4 deaths per 100,000 procedures; most deaths in the U.S. have been associated with anesthetic complications[23–26] In the CREST study, no deaths were reported among 9,475 patients who underwent interval laparoscopic tubal surgery.[27]

Major complications from transabdominal tubal occlusion are also uncommon, with no difference in major morbidity between minilaparotomy and laparoscopy.[3] Complication rates for tubal occlusion, which include conversion to laparotomy, blood transfusion, febrile morbidity, and re-hospitalization, are estimated to be 0.9 to 1.6 per 100 procedures.[27] The types of complications vary by surgical procedure, anesthesia, and whether energy is used for tubal occlusion, but complications are overall extremely low.[28] Intraoperative complications include damage to bowel, bladder, or major vessels. Rarely, laparotomy and/or blood transfusion may be required to manage these events. Postoperative complications include wound infection and prolonged pelvic or abdominal pain. Risk factors for complications during transabdominal tubal occlusion include previous abdominal or pelvic surgery and obesity.[27]

Complete salpingectomy is a relatively new option for permanent contraception, so long-term safety data are unavailable. However, short-term safety data indicate that complete salpingectomy is a reasonable alternative to partial salpingectomy and other tubal occlusion methods as an interval method or following delivery.[29,30]

Based on published literature, major complications other than pregnancy from transcervical procedures have not been reported. Minor complications include tubal perforation, which was reported in 1% to 3% of Essure cases, with Essure devices found in the intraperitoneal cavity in 0.5% to 3% of patients. No perforations were reported during the Adiana trial.[31,32] In addition to infection, bleeding, and injury to surrounding organs, potential complications might include hypervolemia and possible hyponatremia from hysteroscopy.[31,32] No randomized trials compare safety outcomes of transcervical permanent contraception to transabdominal procedures.[28]

SPECIAL ISSUES

Ovarian Function

Several studies evaluated the vascular effects of tubal occlusion and subsequent ovarian function, as well as possible long-term outcomes such as menopausal symptoms. A prospective matched cohort evaluation of ovarian reserve and function in patients undergoing laparoscopic tubal occlusion using bipolar coagulation showed no functional impact after 5 years.[33] Another prospective study of minilaparotomy and laparoscopic tubal surgery found no difference in uterine or ovarian blood flow or ovarian hormone secretion after 6 months.[34] Likewise, complete salpingectomy had similar effect on ovarian reserve as tubal ligation at Cesarean delivery, with no differences in anti-Müllerian hormone levels before or after surgery.[35]

Despite relatively strong evidence that ovarian function is not affected by tubal occlusion, tubal occlusion may be associated with menopausal symptoms such as hot flushes, although age at menopause does not appear affected.[36–39]

Cancer Prevention

Transabdominal tubal surgery appears to have a protective effect against ovarian cancer that persists over many years.[40–42] A large case-control study showed tubal surgery was associated with a 39% reduction in the risk of ovarian cancer. The risk remained low up to 25 years after surgery and was irrespective of technique.[40] Results of a cohort study of more than 65,000 Danish patients not only showed an overall decrease in the risk of ovarian cancer, but also a reduced rate of endometrial cancer, although the association was not as strong.[41]

The protective effect of transabdominal tubal surgery on ovarian cancer risk extends to carriers of the BRCA1 mutation.[43,44] The risk reduction does not appear to include carriers of BRCA2, although this may be due to the small sample size.[44] Combined oral contraceptive (COC) use, especially long-term use, confers more protection in BRCA1 carriers, but the combination of COCs and tubal surgery offered greater protection than either method alone, conferring a risk reduction of 72%.[44]

The biological mechanism for ovarian cancer reduction in patients who have undergone transabdominal tubal surgery is unknown. However, increasing evidence indicates the distal end of the fallopian tube is the main site of origin of high grade serous ovarian carcinoma.[45] While occlusive techniques are estimated to lower a patient's lifetime risk of ovarian cancer by 24% to 36%, primarily by reducing the incidence of endometrioid and clear cell carcinoma, bilateral salpingectomy may create an overall 49% reduction in ovarian cancer that includes a decrease in serous carcinoma.[46,47] A number of organizations, including the American College of Obstetricians and Gynecologists in 2015, now recommends opportunistic complete salpingectomy during hysterectomy and tubal occlusion procedures.[48] An educational initiative promoting opportunistic salpingectomy for ovarian cancer reduction that took place in British Columbia, Canada was followed by an increase in salpingectomy for permanent contraception and with hysterectomy in that region.[49] The majority of surveyed obstetricians and gynecologists in the United States now perform salpingectomy at the time of hysterectomy and for permanent contraception for cancer reduction risk.[50]

Studies generally show no to mild protective association between tubal occlusion and breast cancer. One prospective cohort study of 619,199 patients suggested an inverse association between tubal surgery and breast cancer mortality (RR, 0.82), with a stronger benefit related to younger age at time of surgery (RR among women before age 35, 0.69).[51] However, data from the Nurses' Health Study, the Cancer and Steroid Hormone Study, and the Cancer Prevention Study II Nutrition Cohort yielded no overall association with breast cancer risk.[52,53]

The impact of transcervical procedures on these cancers has not been studied.

Menstrual Abnormalities

The long-term health effects of tubal surgery on menstrual pattern appear to be negligible. Menstrual disturbances following tubal surgery, known as post-tubal ligation syndrome, are likely due to inaccurate recall of previous menstrual patterns, weight changes, and pre-surgery use of hormonal contraceptives that can mask underlying menstrual dysfunction.[54–60] Although 2% to 4% of patients in the Essure and Adiana trials reported a disturbance in their menstrual patterns, the relationship of menstrual abnormalities to transcervical permanent contraception is unclear, with the same confounders as for other tubal occlusion procedures.[31,32]

Sexuality

Studies of female sexuality found no detrimental long-term effects from permanent contraception. The CREST study found that interval tubal surgery was not likely to change sexual interest or pleasure.[61] The majority of women who had changes in libido or sexual pleasure reported positive effects. Another study found an increase in coital frequency after 1 year among women who had permanent contraception as compared with women not using permanent contraception.[61,62]

Post-ablation Tubal Sterilization Syndrome (PATSS)

Post-ablation tubal sterilization syndrome (PATSS), in which menstrual blood trapped in the cornua or proximal tube causes painful distention, has an incidence of 8% to 33%.[63] Endometrial ablation has become an increasingly popular treatment for heavy or prolonged uterine bleeding. Although patients have reduced fertility after an ablation, they should still be advised not to undergo ablation unless they have completed childbearing due to the increased risk of abnormal placentation, spontaneous abortion, and preterm delivery in a subsequent pregnancy.[64] Permanent birth control is thus an appealing contraceptive option for these patients. However, after ablation, endometrial tissue can persist or regenerate in the cornual regions of the uterine cavity, even when the remaining cavity may be reduced in size or completely obliterated by the procedure.[65] Patients who have both endometrial ablation and tubal surgery may later develop retrograde bleeding from persistent endometrial tissue in the cornua and in isolated areas of the myometrium that can lead to PATSS.[63,66]

Performing transcervical procedures with ablation is not recommended for several reasons. Visualization of the tubal ostia for Essure placement following ablation can be challenging due to tissue destruction in the immediate period, and uterine synechiae in the delayed period.[67] Interpreting occlusion success by HSG may be difficult due to filling defects, so manufacturer instructions for Essure recommend confirming that the tubes are occluded prior to performing any planned ablations.[31] However, performing ablation after transcervical procedures also carries risk. The stainless steel core of in-situ Essure devices may conduct energy during global radiofrequency ablation, causing damage to surrounding organs.[10] The theoretical risk for global thermal methods and endometrial resection under direct visualization should be less than that of global radiofrequency ablation, but safety data are limited.[67,68] Although transcervical permanent birth control occludes the tubes more proximally than transabdominal procedures, PATSS can still occur following transcervical procedures and ablation.[63]

Chronic Pelvic Pain

Transabdominal tubal surgery does not seem to be associated with an increased risk of chronic pelvic pain if prior contraceptive use and previous menstrual patterns are considered.[54–56,58,60] Younger patients with pre-existing reports of menstrual dysfunction may be at increased risk following transabdominal surgery.[54]

Pelvic pain is the most common complaint after Essure placement.[69] In a retrospective study of 458 patients who underwent Essure placement, the incidence of acute pelvic pain after the procedure was 8.1%. By 3 months after the procedure, 4.2% of patients reported continued pain.[70] Most patients who experience pelvic pain after Essure will report pain within the first month after Essure placement, but an additional 19.2% reported the onset of pain between 1 and 12 months and 30.8% reported pain beginning 12 months or later.[71] The varying latency period documented in case reports and series about pain after Essure placement supports this finding, indicating that patients may still develop pain related to Essure placement months or years after the procedure.[72,73] Patients with a history of chronic pain, who had been excluded from the device approval trials, are more likely to report pain after hysteroscopic occlusion (OR 6.81; 95% CI 2.95-15.73).[70]

Following Adiana, 6% of the 635 patients who participated in the clinical trial reported cramping unrelated to menses; 5% reported dysmenorrhea, 3% reported pelvic pain and 1% reported dyspareunia.[32] There are no published data documenting incidence of chronic pelvic pain following Adiana, but some patients have reported chronic pelvic pain in the FDA device experience database.[74]

Hysterectomy

Although there is no known biological mechanism for tubal permanent contraception to increase the risk for hysterectomy, there is a strong association between transabdominal procedures and hysterectomy (RR, 1.6–4.4).[58,75,76] Patients who undergo tubal surgery appear to be 4.4 times more likely to undergo hysterectomy than those whose partners underwent vasectomy.[75] However, the majority of patients do not undergo subsequent hysterectomy; the cumulative probability of undergoing hysterectomy 14 years after tubal occlusion in the CREST study was 17%.[77] Increased risk was associated with a pre-surgery history of menstrual or other benign gynecologic disorders, such as endometriosis.[77] There are no data yet on the rate of hysterectomy following transcervical procedures, although case reports of hysterectomy due to pain or other complaints have been published.[78,79]

Regret

Most patients who choose tubal surgery as a contraceptive method never regret their decision. However, because of relationship changes and other life events, regret is always possible. Patients who undergo tubal surgery at age 30 or younger are at greater risk for regret.[80–82] The cumulative probability of regret over 14 years of follow-up in the CREST study was 12.7%.[80] However, the probability of regret was 20.3% for patients aged 30 years or younger at the time of surgery, compared with 5.9% for patients older than 30 years at the time of surgery. For all patients in the CREST study, the rate of regret following interval procedures within 1 year of delivery was 17.6%, compared to 17.8% following postpartum tubal ligation after vaginal delivery and 16.1% following Cesarean delivery. The cumulative probability of regret diminished steadily with the interval between delivery and surgery.[80] Immediate post-abortion procedures were not associated with increased regret when compared with interval procedures after abortion.[80,83,84]

Analysis of the data from the CREST study showed the 14-year cumulative probability of requesting reversal information was 14.3%, but in patients under the age of 24 years who underwent tubal surgery, the request for reversal information was as high as 40.4%.[82,84] The number of patients who requested information about IVF was not documented.

Risk factors for increased regret include having received less preoperative information about the procedure, having had less access to information about or support for other contraceptive methods, and having made the decision under pressure from a spouse or because of medical indications.[82,85,86] Younger patients are at greater risk for regret given the longevity of their future fertility and the opportunity for life events such as relationship changes or the death of a child.

Thorough and effective counseling is crucial in reducing the potential for regret in patients undergoing permanent contraception. Counseling should be in language the patient can easily understand. Both the patient and partner (when appropriate) should be counseled, and risk factors for regret should be addressed. However, the presence of strong risk factors for regret should not be used to uniformly restrict tubal surgery, but should indicate the need for more extensive counseling. Nulliparity and age should not be considered contraindications, and a nulliparous or young patient seeking permanent contraception should not be required to undergo a mental health evaluation due to a clinician's concern for patient regret.

Desire for Pregnancy Following Tubal Occlusion

Permanent contraception should be considered permanent, but some patients will have a change in personal circumstance and later desire to bear children. Assisted reproductive technologies such as IVF and microsurgical tubal reversal are options for a patient who desires pregnancy following tubal surgery, but success is not guaranteed. There are no randomized controlled trials comparing the success rates and costs of IVF with surgical reversal.

The choice between IVF and tubal surgery reversal for pregnancy is dependent on multiple factors, including the age of the patient at the time of treatment, severity of the tubal damage, remaining tubal length, and other fertility factors. With careful case selection and meticulous surgical technique, reasonable pregnancy rates of 42% to 69% can be achieved following microsurgical reversal of tubal occlusion.[88,89]

Patients should be aware that surgical reversal carries operative and anesthesia risks. Ectopic pregnancy is more common among pregnancies occurring after surgical reversal of tubal surgery than IVF. Published ectopic pregnancy rates following surgical reversal range from 4% to 8%.[89] Nonetheless, tubal occlusion reversal may be appealing for younger patients, couples who desire more than a single additional pregnancy, or those who are not comfortable with IVF. Both IVF and reversal surgery are costly and are often not covered by health insurance. Finally, patients undergoing tubal reversal surgery may have the need for future contraception.

In a large Canadian study, 23% of patients obtaining tubal reversal following tubal ligation went on to obtain a subsequent method of permanent contraception.[90]

There are limited data on outcomes after reversal of transcervical tubal occlusion. Issues with reversal of transcervical procedures include the location of the implants within the tubocornual junction rather than the tube itself, and the tissue ingrowth into the implants. One reversal technique that has resulted in successful pregnancies is removing the devices and reimplanting the tube into the uterus (tubouterine implantation).[91,92] IVF implantation and pregnancy outcomes are unknown with Essure left in situ, since a portion of the coils trail into the uterine cavity. Although there are case reports of successful IVF pregnancies following transcervical tubal occlusion, clinical trials show that using Essure to block hydrosalpinges prior to IVF is inferior to laparoscopic salpingectomy in ongoing pregnancy rates.[15–17] A successful pregnancy with IVF following device removal has been reported, but outcome data are still lacking.[93]

Tubal Occlusion Device Removal

Patients may request tubal occlusion device removal for reasons other than regret or desired fertility. Removal of transabdominal devices such as clips and rings can be done via laparoscopic salpingectomy. However, removal of transcervical devices, which lie at the tubocornual junction, is more challenging.[94] Patients are increasingly requesting Essure device removal for a variety of reasons, including unintended pregnancy, chronic pain, menstrual disorders, nickel hypersensitivity, or improper placement diagnosed after imaging.[94] In response to these complaints and FDA recommendations in November 2016, Essure now carries a black box warning and a patient-clinician discussion checklist for counseling.[95] Some patients may still request removal despite pre-procedural counseling, and clinicians should conduct careful history-taking, examination, imaging, and testing to eliminate other causes of the patient's complaints before attributing the symptoms to the devices. Treatment options for patients who request Essure device removal include leaving the devices in place with medical management of the presenting complaints, surgical removal of devices, or hysterectomy. Case reports and case series describe successful surgical removal of Essure devices using hysteroscopic removal, laparoscopic salpingectomy or salpingostomy, and wedge resection.[71,94,96–98] Outcomes after Essure device removal are generally favorable, with most patients reporting improvement in pelvic pain and nickel hypersensitivity reactions after Essure removal.[71] However, clinicians should caution patients that their specific complaints may not resolve after removal.[99]

There are no published case reports documenting removal for Adiana.

PROVIDING TUBAL SURGERY

COUNSELING GUIDELINES FOR TUBAL SURGERY

The goal of contraceptive counseling is to help patients select a method that they will use, will be effective, is most consistent with their reproductive intentions, and will not have adverse effects. The permanence of tubal surgery is a significant consideration for counseling. However, respect for a patient's autonomy, including a dialogue about the patient's reproductive desires and wishes, should be the primary concern during this discussion.[100]

The factors contributing to an individual's decision about permanent contraception vary. Each patient needs to weigh the risks, benefits, effectiveness, and side effects of the various contraceptive options available to them. Although racial disparities have been identified in tubal surgery rates, this association with race and ethnicity becomes no longer significant when adjusted for a history of unintended pregnancy.[87]

Counseling should address the following:

1. **Provide choices.** Present highly effective, long-acting, reversible methods as options, such as the contraceptive implant or IUD, as well as vas surgery.
2. **Assess the patient's understanding of the procedure.** Although awareness of tubal surgery for contraception is widespread in the United States, review the procedure, its effectiveness, and its risks with your patients to minimize misconceptions about the procedure.
3. **Facilitate the decision-making process.** Give the client sufficient time to make a thoughtful, informed decision about a permanent method of contraception, especially patients having immediate postpartum or post-abortion (spontaneous or induced) procedures. The patient should have decided she wants a permanent method well before delivery or a pregnancy-related event or procedure. (See Chapter 2 for more complete discussion of patient-centered contraception counseling.)
4. **Provide information about possible failure.** Inform patients that tubal surgery is not 100% successful and that failure can occur, even years after the procedure was performed. Additionally, there is a significant risk of ectopic pregnancy if the method fails.
5. **Discuss STI prevention.** Tubal surgery will not provide protection against STIs, including HIV. Thoroughly explain the risk to the patient and partner(s). Condom use will be necessary if the patient is at risk of such infections.

Components of Permanent Contraception Pre-Counseling 101

- Permanent nature of the procedure
- Alternative methods of contraception available including similar failure rates with long-acting reversible methods and vas surgery
- Details of the procedure, including risks and benefits of anesthesia
- The possibility of failure and risk of ectopic pregnancy
- The need to use condoms for protection against STIs, including HIV
- Need for post-procedure contraception following transcervical tubal surgery until occlusion is confirmed
- Federal and state Medicaid regulations about informed consent, including age of the patient, circumstances in which consent is obtained, and interval from time of consent to procedure
- Other state requirements beyond Medicaid

Informed Consent and Policy/Legal Issues. Informed consent is a process to ensure that a person can give consent, is fully informed about a surgical procedure and its consequences, and can make a voluntary decision. Provide information on tubal surgery in a language that the patient can understand. Patients must always sign or mark an informed consent form indicating that they understand the type of operation and intended permanence, possibility of failure, and risks and benefits, including the option to decline permanent contraception without loss of medical or financial benefits. The surgeon or authorized representative must also sign the form. Written informed consent should document, but not substitute for, the provider's active involvement in the patient's informed decision to have tubal surgery. Ensure that the patient has knowingly and freely requested the procedure. Understand that the federally mandated consent for permanent birth control does not replace surgical consent. If the patient elects Essure, the clinician must complete an FDA-required discussion checklist with the patient.[95]

Knowledge of federal, state and local, or institutional guidelines is important in the counseling and consent process. Some states have requirements about the consent process and its documentation, even if private funding is used.

- Strict adherence to informed consent procedures is mandatory prior to permanent contraception.[102]
- Partner or spousal consent in the United States is not legally required.[103]

- Patients using Medicaid funds for permanent birth control must be age 21 or older and mentally competent; they must wait 30 days after signing a valid consent document before receiving a permanent contraception procedure. In cases of premature delivery, patients must have signed their consent document 72 hours prior to delivery. Consent cannot be given when a patient is seeking or obtaining an abortion, is in active labor or childbirth, under the influence of alcohol or other drugs, or is institutionalized in a correctional facility, mental hospital, or other rehabilitative facility. Consent documents are invalid 180 days after signing.
- Patients whose procedures are funded by private insurance may not have the same restrictions as those using Medicaid funds, including age restrictions and waiting periods.

Federal guidelines that impose a waiting period for patients using Medicaid funds for permanent birth control, while initially developed to protect patients of vulnerable populations from involuntary procedures, have been called into question because they often unfairly restrict access for the very populations that they intend to protect. Particularly in the immediate postpartum period, timing of informed consent and availability of signed forms at the time of desired permanent tubal surgery can be a barrier to care. Approximately 24% to 44% of postpartum tubal surgery requests are not fulfilled because of Medicaid policy barriers.[104,105] Patients using private insurance do not face the same logistical hurdles to obtaining a permanent procedure.

Health care providers, policy makers, and the public should be aware of the ethical and legal issues involved in providing voluntary permanent contraception to those who may not be able to give informed consent.[106] When patients have limited mental capacity, the provider should consult with the patient's family, caregivers, and often institutional ethics committees to balance patient autonomy with what is understood to be in the best interests of the patient.[100] If an individual clinician or institution will not provide permanent contraception due to personal beliefs or institutional policy, the patient should be informed and referred elsewhere for care in a timely manner.[100]

Preoperative Screening. Take a preoperative history, perform a physical exam, and evaluate the general health condition of the patient. Order any standard pre-operative laboratory tests per the surgeon's or institution's policies, including tests pertinent to the patient's medical condition relevant to surgery, such as a blood type, complete blood count, or serum glucose level.

Timing

Tubal surgery can be performed postpartum (at the time of Cesarean delivery or shortly after vaginal delivery), after spontaneous or therapeutic abortion, or as an interval procedure (unrelated in time to a pregnancy).

The timing of the procedure influences both the surgical approach and the method of tubal surgery.

Postpartum Tubal Surgery. Approximately half of all permanent tubal procedures are performed in the postpartum period. Postpartum tubal surgery is performed after 10% of all hospital deliveries in the United States.[107] Tubal surgery may be done at the time of cesarean delivery or via minilaparotomy following vaginal delivery and should not extend the patient's hospital stay. Institutional barriers may create delays prevent fulfillment of postpartum tubal surgery requests. Since subsequent unintended pregnancy occurs in nearly 50% of patients not receiving their requested postpartum tubal surgery, hospital procedures should prioritize these procedures in the immediate postpartum period.[107]

Postpartum minilaparotomy should be done in a medically stable patient prior to the onset of significant uterine involution (within 1 to 2 days following delivery).[108] Fully assess maternal and neonatal well-being prior to the procedure. Consider postponing tubal surgery in the presence of medical or obstetric complications. Individualize the choice of anesthetic technique based on obstetrical outcomes and patient risk factors, but regional anesthesia is vastly preferred over general anesthesia.[109] Tubal surgery can be performed safely under local anesthesia.[108]

Postpartum tubal surgery requires counseling and informed consent before labor and delivery. Obtain the patient's consent during prenatal care, when the patient can make an informed decision, review the risks and benefits of the procedure, and consider alternative methods of contraception. For patients without private insurance who rely on federally-funded insurance programs, consider the regulations that address the timing of consent.[107]

Interval Tubal Surgery. In the United States, approximately one half of all tubal surgeries are performed as interval procedures.[108] Although transabdominal tubal surgery can be done at any time during the menstrual cycle, performing the procedure during the patient's follicular phase reduces the likelihood of concurrent (luteal phase) pregnancy, as does the patient's use of an effective method of contraception before the procedure. Highly-sensitive urine pregnancy tests can detect pregnancies as early as 1 week after fertilization.[110] For transcervical procedures with Essure devices, there may be a technical advantage to performing it in the early follicular phase for patients not using hormonal contraception, as the tubal ostia may be more easily seen due to a thinner endometrial lining.

Postabortion Tubal Surgery. Tubal surgery, either laparoscopically or via minilaparotomy, following uncomplicated first and second trimester abortions can be provided without added risk over interval procedures.[111] To avoid additional risk, use a single anesthetic for both the abortion and the tubal procedure. Transcervical procedures should not be performed immediately after an abortion procedure due to poor hysteroscopic visualization.

For patients using federal funds, tubal surgery cannot be performed simultaneously with an abortion.

Options For Approach

Laparoscopy. Laparoscopy is most commonly used for interval tubal surgery and is usually performed as an outpatient procedure. One advantage of laparoscopy over other surgical approaches is the opportunity to directly visualize the abdominal and pelvic organs. Laparoscopy results in small incision scars and allows a rapid return to full activity for the patient. The disadvantages of laparoscopy include the special training and equipment required, possible difficulty accessing the fallopian tubes due to adhesions or abnormal anatomy, and the risk of bowel, bladder, or major vessel injuries during surgery (Figure 16-2).

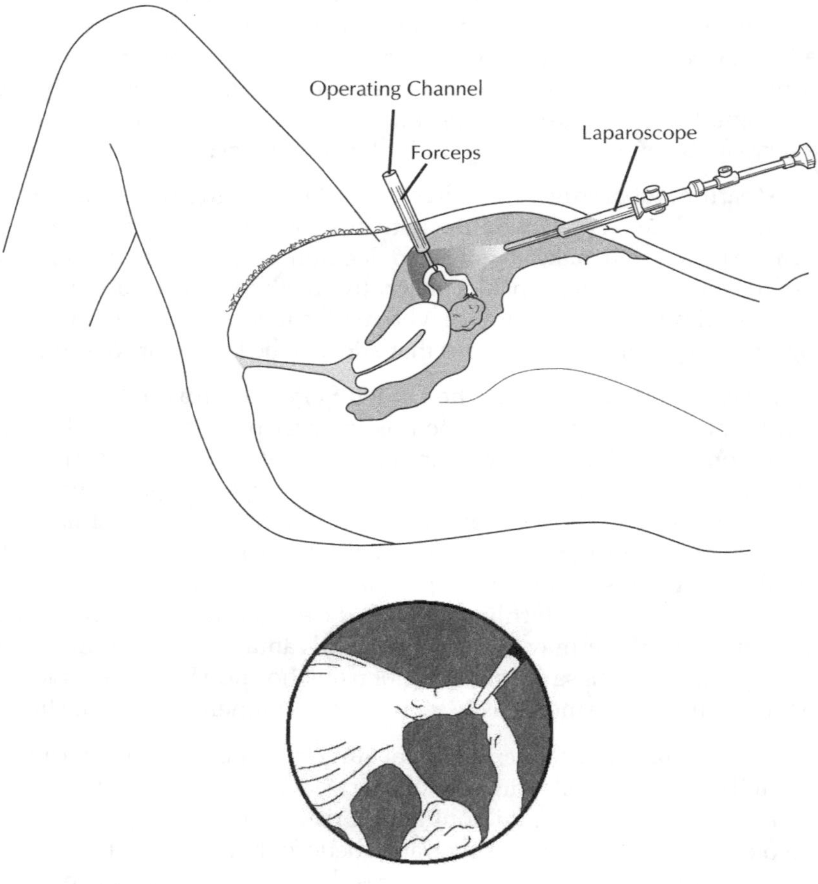

Figure 16-2 Laparoscopic tubal surgery approach

Choice of Laparoscopic Method

The choice of tubal surgery method depends on the provider's training and experience, the patient's medical history including prior abdominal or uterine surgery, and availability of supplies.

Electrocoagulation. Electrocoagulation for tubal occlusion is used exclusively with laparoscopic procedures.[101] Unipolar electrocoagulation is not recommended because of the increased risk of thermal bowel injury.[24] At least 3 cm of the isthmic portion of the tube must be coagulated using sufficient energy to achieve maximum efficacy.[112] Use of a current meter during bipolar coagulation is more accurate than visualizing tissue desiccation to indicate complete coagulation, and is associated with improved effectiveness.[112] Ectopic pregnancy rates are substantially higher with electrocoagulation methods than with other occlusion methods. In the CREST study, the risk of ectopic pregnancy for patients who underwent permanent birth control by bipolar coagulation before the age of 30 years was 27 times higher than for those patients who had a postpartum partial salpingectomy (31.9 vs. 1.2 ectopic pregnancies per 1,000 procedures).[21]

Mechanical Devices. Mechanical occlusion devices commonly used with laparoscopic procedures in the United States include the silicone band (Falope Ring), the spring clip (Hulka-Clemens clip), and the titanium clip (Filshie clip). All require special applicators and are most effective when used to occlude normal-appearing tubes. None of these methods involves risk of electrical injury.[113,114] While tubal occlusion by ring or clip should always be considered a permanent method, these devices typically destroy less of the fallopian tube than electrocoagulation methods, making future reversal efforts more likely to succeed.[101]

The silicone band was first developed in the 1970s in pursuit of a safer, non-thermal method. Two cm of tube is contained in a constricted loop following application. With this method, it is possible to lacerate the tube or surrounding vessels, and application may be more difficult when tubal abnormalities are present, such as adhesions or edema. The silicone band is one of the most commonly used tubal occlusion devices worldwide, with a cumulative 10-year failure rate in the CREST study at 33.2 per 1,000 procedures.[4] Postoperative pain was reported twice as often by patients receiving tubal rings than those receiving electrocoagulation.[28]

The spring clip was developed in the same time period as the silicone band, and was introduced in the United States in 1972. The hinged spring-loaded plastic clip with interlocking teeth is loaded in a special applicator and applied perpendicular to the tube across the isthmus, destroying less than 1 cm of tissue. The cumulative 10-year failure rate in the CREST study for the spring clip was 52.1 per 1,000 procedures.[4]

The titanium clip was approved in 1996. It is a hinged, locking clip made of titanium with a silicone rubber lining, which expands to keep the tube compressed as it flattens. It destroys 5 mm of tube and has a higher efficacy than the spring clip.[113,115] The titanium clip requires a special applicator for interval laparoscopic tubal surgery and for postpartum tubal occlusion.[115,116] The titanium clip has a similar safety and efficacy profile as other occlusion devices; data from the United Kingdom demonstrate a crude failure rate of 2 to 3 in 1,000 patients.[5] Studies do not support routine application of multiple clips per tube.[117,118] If a clip is misfired so that the tube is not occluded, a second one may be placed as close to the first as possible to reduce the risk of hydrosalpinx formation between the two clips.[118]

Salpingectomy. Laparoscopic salpingectomy is virtually 100% effective at preventing pregnancy.[119] Salpingectomy is gaining in popularity because of increasing evidence showing a reduction in ovarian cancer with this approach.[46,47] Limited available evidence suggests that laparoscopic salpingectomy takes approximately 6 minutes longer to complete than mechanical occlusion methods, with no increased risk of immediate or short-term complication rates.[29]

Minilaparotomy. In the United States, minilaparotomy is most commonly used for postpartum procedures prior to involution of the uterus. A small 2 to 3 cm incision is made just inferior to the umbilicus, allowing easy access to the fallopian tubes (Figure 16-3). Minilaparotomy requires only basic surgical instruments and training, although there is still a small

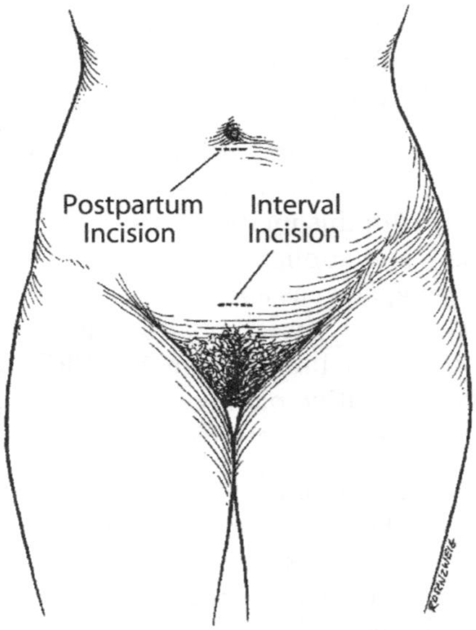

Figure 16-3 Postpartum and interval minilaparotomy incision site and size

risk of injury to the bowel, bladder, and other adjacent structures. In developing countries where laparoscopy is not available, suprapubic minilaparotomy is frequently used for non-postpartum tubal surgery.[108]

Choice of Minilaparotomy Method. The choice of tubal surgical method depends on the provider's training and experience and the patient's medical history including prior abdominal or uterine surgery.

Ligation and partial salpingectomy. Tubal surgery at the time of Cesarean delivery or postpartum or interval minilaparotomy is usually performed by ligation and resection of a portion of both fallopian tubes. A variety of partial salpingectomy techniques have been described, including the Pomeroy and Parkland methods.[108] The most common method used is a variation of the Pomeroy method using plain catgut, which degrades more rapidly than the original chromic suture type and thus decreases the risk of recannulization (Figure 16-4). The Irving and Uchida methods involve ligating and excising a segment of the tube and burying the proximal end either in the myometrium (Irving) or in the mesosalpinx (Uchida). Occasionally the distal end is also buried in the mesosalpinx, although it

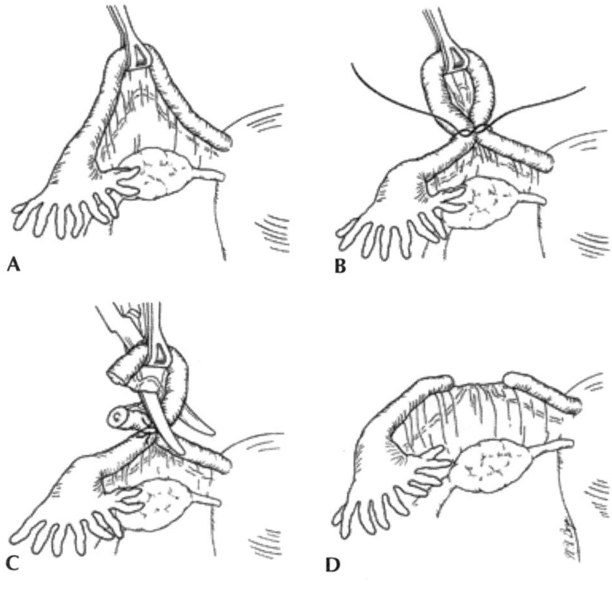

Figure 16-4 Pomeroy technique. A. A loop of the proximal portion of the tubal ampulla is elevated to reveal the vascular supply of the mesosalpinx. **B.** A strand of absorbable suture material is used to bilaterally ligate the tube and simultaneously provide hemostasis. **C.** A hemostat is placed on the suture strands immediately distal to the knot to prevent the tube from retracting into the abdomen. The open blade of the Metzenbaum scissors is used to pierce the mesosalpinx and approximately 1 cm of the tube is excised. **D.** The end result following dissolution of the absorbable suture material is return of the proximal and distal portions of the tube to their normal anatomic position.

is more frequently left exposed. The Irving and Uchida methods are seldom used in the United States, although failures with these methods are extremely rare.[108]

Salpingectomy. Salpingectomy can be safely performed at the time of cesarean delivery or via postpartum or interval minilaparotomy. Postpartum salpingectomy has a slightly longer operating time than postpartum partial salpingectomy (one study showed an increase of 11 minutes), but the procedures have similar blood loss and short-term complication rates.[30,120]

Hysteroscopy. The transcervical approach to tubal occlusion involves accessing the fallopian tubes via the cervix. Clinicians require special training to perform hysteroscopic procedures, which can be done only as an interval procedure. The procedure can be provided under local anesthesia, with or without sedation, in a properly equipped physician's office with appropriately dedicated resources for post-procedure recovery.

The Essure device, introduced in 2002, is currently the only FDA-approved method available in the United States. Essure is a soft, flexible device consisting of two concentric metal coils that is inserted into the proximal section of each fallopian tube using hysteroscopic guidance (Figure 16–5).[31] The nitinol (nickel-titanium) outer coil, which ends in platinum markers, anchors the device in the tubal lumen; the inner stainless steel coil anchors synthetic polyethylene terephthalate fibers which cause a benign inflammatory response. The inflammation stimulates growth of fibrous tissue, which occludes the tubes over the subsequent few weeks.

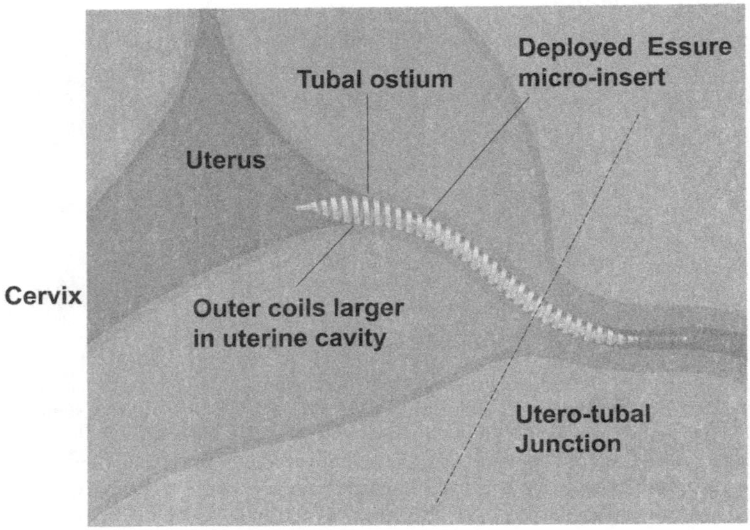

Figure 16-5 Hysteroscopic placement of Essure device within the tubal lumen

Patients must use an alternate method of reliable contraception for at least 3 months while tubal ingrowth is occurring. Confirmation of procedure success must be documented at least 3 months following procedure.[31]

Successful placement is not guaranteed and the procedure may be abandoned due to abnormal findings at the time of hysteroscopy or from failed attempts to place one or both devices.

Essure has relatively few contraindications, and is an acceptable alternative for patients with significant medical problems who desire permanent contraception. Patients with nickel sensitivity may have a reaction to the nickel component of the device. Use with caution in patients who are immunocompromised from HIV, immunosuppression medications, or chemotherapy, since the method relies on inflammation and scar tissue formation to cause tubal occlusion.[31]

Patients should undergo an Essure confirmation test (transvaginal ultrasound or modified HSG) to evaluate device retention and location. Providers should complete special training to identify proper placement of Essure devices post-procedure. HSG will confirm occlusion by the lack of free peritoneal dye spillage from the fallopian tubes. At least 6 radiographs must be performed to assess success: a scout film without contrast; minimal fill with a small amount of contrast; partial fill when nearly full of contrast; total fill of the cavity with the cornua distended with contrast; and magnifications of the distended cornua on each side.[31]

In cases where transvaginal ultrasonography will be used for confirmation, all of the following criteria must be met to conclude success:[31]

- No concern of possible perforation at the time of placement, including no use of excessive force
- No anatomical variations or technical difficulties making tubal ostia visualization challenging
- Provider is certain about adequate placement
- Procedure time $\leq$15 minutes (scope-in to scope-out)
- Placement with 1 to 8 trailing coils in the uterine cavity
- No unusual post-operative pain

Anesthesia And Pain Management

The most frequently used anesthesia approaches for tubal surgery in the United States are short acting general anesthesia for interval tubal procedures and regional anesthesia for postpartum procedures.[109] For patients undergoing transabdominal procedures under local anesthesia,

Table 16–1 Fallopian tube surgery approaches and available occlusion methods

Approach	Occlusion Method	Advantages	Disadvantages
Interval Tubal Occlusion			
Laparoscopy	• Complete salpingectomy • Silicone bands • Titanium clips • Bipolar electrocoagulation	• 2–3 small incisions • Less pain than from minilaparotomy • Low complication rate • Short recovery time	• Need for specialist with method-specific training necessary • Necessary equipment is often difficult to obtain and maintain • Need a fully equipped operating and recovery room with trained staff
Transcervical	Essure	• May be performed under local anesthesia • No incisions or scars • Can be safely performed in an outpatient setting	• Long-term effectiveness not known • Requires initial 3 months of backup contraception and confirmatory test
Suprapubic Minilaparotomy	• Complete salpingectomy • Pomery and Pritchard (Parkland) technique • Silicone bands • Titanium or spring clips	• Local or general anesthesia • Incision site usually not visible (below pubic hairline)	• Difficult technique if the patient is obese, the uterus immobile or the tubes have adhesions • Recovery can be more painful than with laparoscopy
Postpartum Tubal Occlusion			
Infraumbilical Minilaparotomy	• Complete salpingectomy • Pomeroy or Pritchard (Parkland) technique • Titanium clip	• Convenience • Lower costs • Ease of surgery • Does not necessarily extend hospital stay beyond that for a normal delivery	• Electrocoagulation not indicated • Titanium clip requires special postpartum applicator • Counseling must be prior to labor to reduce risk of regret
Cesarean Delivery	• Complete salpingectomy • Pomeroy or Pritchard (Parkland) technique • Titanium clip	• Convenience • Lower costs • Anatomy fully visible	• Cesareans should not be performed solely to occlude the tubes • Other disadvantages from infraumbilical minilapatoromy apply

(continued)

Table 16–1 Fallopian tube surgery approaches and available occlusion methods—*(continued)*

Approach	Occlusion Method	Advantages	Disadvantages
Postabortion Tubal Occlusion			
Laparoscopy	• Complete salpingectomy • Silicone bands • Titanium clips • Bipolar electrocoagulation	• Convenience • Patient motivation	• Need for careful counseling with consideration of risk of regret • If using general anesthesia, may increase the amount of blood loss with the abortion procedure
Suprapubic Minilaparotomy	• Complete salpingectomy • Pomeroy and Pritchard (Parkland) techniques	Same as above	Same as above

application of lidocaine 1% solution to the tubal surface may provide additional pain control.[121] Transcervical procedures may be provided using local anesthesia or minimal intravenous sedation, although paracervical block with lidocaine and/or conscious sedation significantly reduces pain.[122] Nonsteroidal anti-inflammatory medications may reduce pain and risk of tubal spasm during device placement, although studies on this have not been conducted.

All anesthetic methods need the attention of a trained professional who carefully monitors the patient and the drugs used. For more complete information on anesthetic techniques and regimens, go to www.engenderhealth.org.[123]

MANAGING PROBLEMS AND FOLLOW-UP

Major complications from tubal surgery are uncommon (1% to 3.5%), and vary by type of procedure and anesthesia used.[27,113,114] Risks include hemorrhage, infection, and the risk of death from anesthesia. These risks can be reduced by careful screening, use of local anesthesia or light sedation, close monitoring of vital signs, and careful aseptic surgical technique. The seriousness of complications can often be minimized by early recognition and aggressive management.

Intraoperative complications during any tubal occlusion approach can be minimized and addressed by an experienced surgeon and by adherence to standard protocols. No patient should leave the recovery room without both verbal and clear written instructions for follow-up, including

24-hour contact information for concerns or emergencies, immediate self-care, and a follow-up visit.

Patients who undergo transcervical permanent contraception (Essure) must return for an HSG or transvaginal ultrasonography for occlusion confirmation 3 months after the procedure.[31] In a successful placement, the HSG will demonstrate that the device is placed in both fallopian tubes and that there is no peritoneal spillage of contrast. On transvaginal ultrasonography, providers should look for appropriate positioning of the coils. Any equivocal or unsatisfactory ultrasound studies must be followed up with an HSG. The tubes may fail to occlude for idiopathic reasons or because the insert has been placed incorrectly, with possible myometrial perforation or loss of the insert intra-abdominally or externally. If perforation is suspected, obtain an ultrasound or a flat abdominal plain film to assess the position of the devices.[124] If occlusion has not been achieved and the devices are in the correct location, a repeat HSG may be performed 6 months postoperatively, with the patient continuing another method of contraception.[31] If correct placement is assured and occlusion is not achieved at 6 months, patients cannot rely on their transcervical procedure for contraception and must use another contraceptive method.[31] They may consider transabdominal procedures at this point as well as reversible methods, including long-acting methods such as IUDs or implants. As described above in the special consideration section, if a patient returns reporting of issues that are not clearly related to Essure, begin an appropriate workup of the presenting complaint. Attributing a complaint to Essure should be a diagnosis of exclusion before proceeding to removal.

PATIENT INSTRUCTIONS FOR TUBAL SURGERY*

Preoperative Instructions

1. Be completely sure of your decision to have a permanent contraception procedure. Know what it means to you and your family that this is a permanent procedure. You can change your mind at any time before the operation.

2. Before surgery while you are home, you may clip the hair around the top of your pubic bone. Do not shave. Wash the area to remove all loose hairs.

3. If you intend on having sedation or general anesthesia, do not eat or drink anything 6 to 8 hours prior to your procedure, and bring someone who can accompany you home after the procedure.

*These instructions are intended to guide providers in educating patients in pre- and post-care.

Postoperative Instructions

1. **Avoid intercourse or strenuous physical exercise for 1 week.** Strenuous exercise means hard physical exertion, lifting or straining that could bring pressure to the pelvis. When you resume having intercourse or strenuous activity, stop if it is uncomfortable.

2. Watch for the following symptoms:

Condition	Action
Temperature: >100.4 degrees Fahrenheit	Contact your provider immediately
Fainting: Fainting spells	Contact your provider immediately
Pain: Abdominal pain that is persistent, severe and/or increasing after 12 hours	Contact your provider immediately
Incision site issues (if transabdominal):	
Bleeding or spotting from incision sites	Put pressure and tape × 12 hrs If condition continues or worsens, contact provider
Pus or discharge from incision sites	Contact your provider immediately
Stitch in wound	Contact your provider – most stitches will dissolve and fall out, but any permanent suture must be removed by your provider

3. Take 1 or 2 analgesic tablets at 4- to 6-hour intervals if you need them for pain. (Note to provider: name and dose should be specified.) Do not use aspirin since it may promote bleeding.

4. If you think you are pregnant at any time in the future, return to the clinic immediately. Although pregnancy after tubal surgery is rare, chances are increased that it will be an ectopic pregnancy (outside the uterus) if it does occur. This can be a dangerous life-threatening condition and must be treated immediately.

5. You should know this method of birth control is permanent. Pregnancy is possible under certain conditions but reversal surgery and IVF results cannot be guaranteed.

Further instructions for **transabdominal** procedures:

6. **Return to the clinic for your postoperative visit** to make sure the healing process is normal.

7. You may bathe 24 hours after surgery but avoid putting tension on the incision and do not rub or irritate the incision for 1 week. Pat dry the incision site after bathing.

8. Stitches will dissolve and do not require removal. (Note to provider: this instruction must be modified if nonabsorbable sutures are used.)

Further instructions for **transcervical** procedures (Essure):

6. **Please return to your clinician for the confirmatory test** in 3 months so the success of the procedure can be assessed. Your provider will do either a hysterosalpingogram (HSG) or transvaginal ultrasound.
7. **Continue with your contraceptive method** until success of the tubal occlusion procedure has been confirmed. Until success is confirmed, you cannot rely on this method for contraception.

VAS SURGERY

Vas surgery is one of the safest and most effective family planning methods. The no-scalpel approach under local anesthesia is the most common method of vas surgery throughout the world, and is the most common non-diagnostic procedure performed by urologists in the United States. Vas surgery is the fifth most commonly used contraceptive method at 8.2% among patients aged 15 to 44 years in the National Survey of Family Growth, following oral contraceptive pills (25.9%), tubal surgery (25.1%), male condom (15.3%) and long-acting reversible contraception such as intrauterine devices and implants (11.6%).[1] The most common reasons that couples choose vas surgery are favorable reports from peers and recommendations by a clinician.[125] The most common sources of anxiety for patients who choose vas surgery are anticipated pain and fear of the unknown.[126]

Vas surgery is more effective than any tubal surgery method in preventing pregnancy. It is safer and faster in procedure and recovery time than tubal surgery, and costs one-fourth as much as tubal surgery.[127,128] Despite its cost-effectiveness, vas surgery lags far behind tubal surgery as the permanent contraceptive method of choice used in the United States; only a quarter of couples use vas surgery compared to tubal surgery for permanent contraception.[1]

MECHANISM OF ACTION

Permanent contraception via vas surgery blocks fertilization by cutting or occluding both vas deferens so that sperm cannot pass out of the body in the ejaculate (Figure 16-6).

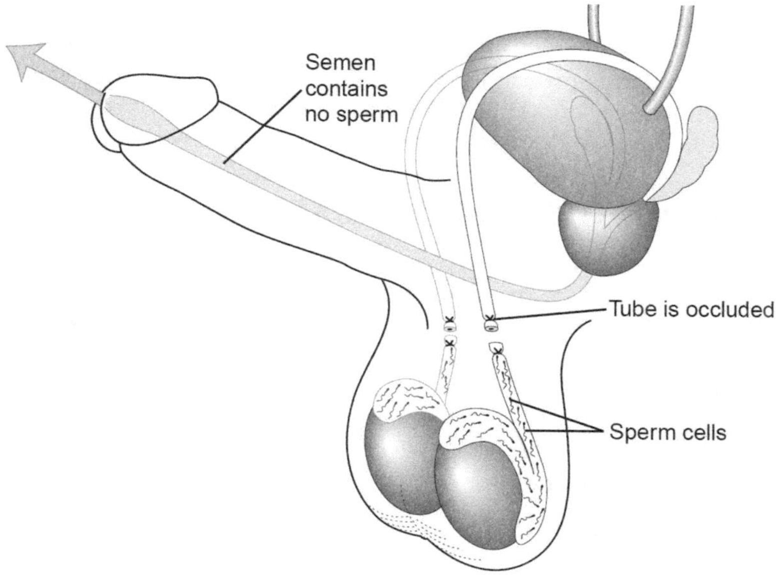

Source: Engenderhealth,[190] with permission

Figure 16-6 Anatomy following vas surgery

EFFECTIVENESS

Permanent contraception, along with intrauterine devices and implants, are in the WHO and CDC's top tier of contraceptive effectiveness. The overall first-year typical use failure rate for permanent contraception is 0.15% for vas surgery and 0.5% for tubal surgery (Table 27-1).

Vas surgery is not immediately effective. Once the vas is divided, time and ejaculations are needed to clear the sperm from the reproductive tract, and azoospermia or rare non-motile sperm (RNMS) must be confirmed before vas surgery can be deemed successful.[129–131] Approximately 25% to 50% of pregnancies after vas surgery occur during the period following surgery but before sperm are cleared.[132–134] True vas surgery failure occurs with technical failure, such as incorrect identification and division of structures at the time of surgery (such as occluding one vas twice without occluding the other), a rare unrecognized congenital duplication of the vas, or spontaneous recanalization of the divided vas.

The rate of pregnancy in partners of patients who have documented azoospermia after vas surgery is approximately 1 in 2,000.[129,135,136] The rate of failure to achieve azoospermia or RNMS after vas surgery, which then requires repeat surgery, is less than 1%. The CREST study by the CDC included 573 patients whose partners underwent vas surgery, and found that the cumulative probability of failure per 1,000 procedures was 7.4 at 1 year after surgery and 11.3 at 2, 3, and 5 years later.[133]

Advantages and Indications

Vas surgery is safer, less expensive, and as effective as tubal surgery. Vas surgery is ideal for those patients who are certain they wish to have no further children and need a reliable contraceptive method, and is preferred to tubal surgery if both are acceptable to patients and their partners. Advantages include the following:

- Permanence
- High effectiveness
- High acceptability
- Safety
- Quick recovery
- Lack of significant long-term side effects
- Cost-effectiveness (most cost-effective of all contraceptive methods)
- No need to buy anything
- No need for partner compliance
- No need to interrupt coitus
- Privacy of choice
- Removal of contraceptive burden from the partner
- Successful reversal rates higher than those following tubal surgery

Disadvantages and Cautions

Vas surgery is not recommended for patients who are not sure of their desire to end future fertility. Other disadvantages include the following:

- Restoring fertility after vas surgery is possible, though difficult. It can expensive, requires either costly assisted reproductive technology (such as IVF with intracytoplasmic sperm injection, or ICSI) or highly technical surgery, and results cannot be guaranteed.
- The effect of surgery is not immediate, and vas surgery cannot be depended on as a contraceptive method until sperm in the reproductive tract are cleared.

- All surgical procedures carry some risk specific to the nature of the surgery and anesthetic used.
- Regret for decision is high among some groups of patients
- Need for trained surgeon or other health professional, procedure room (aseptic conditions), trained assistants, medications, surgical equipment
- Expense at the time of the procedure
- Lack of protection against STIs, including infection with HIV

Patients with medical conditions or other special characteristics may have surgical precautions that differ from those of healthy patients. Since vas surgery is a non-abdominal surgery performed under local anesthesia, absolute surgical contraindications are rare. However, localized problems may make vas surgery more difficult to perform, such as inguinal hernia, large hydrocele or varicocele, and cryptorchidism.[137]

SAFETY

Vas surgery is a very safe method of contraception. Mortality due to the procedure itself is extremely rare, at 0.5 deaths per 100,000 patients undergoing the surgery worldwide. No deaths have been reported in the United States using contemporary surgical techniques.[138–141]

The rate of immediate post-operative complications is low. About 1% to 2% of patients experience hematoma formation and wound infection.[137,142–151] The relationship between surgical technique and complication rate is unclear, but higher-volume surgeons have less immediate post-operative complications than other clinicians.[144] Significant morbidity such as Fournier's gangrene is limited to very rare case reports.[152]

Extensive research has identified no significant long-term physical or mental health effects with vas surgery. Studies have consistently shown no adverse effects of vas surgery on cardiovascular disease, stroke, dementia, prostate or testicular cancer, and a variety of other conditions.[153] The American Urological Association states that clinicians do not need to routinely discuss these conditions during pre-surgical counseling because vas surgery is not a risk factor for these conditions.[141]

SPECIAL ISSUES

Chronic Scrotal Pain

Approximately 1% to 2% of patients undergoing vas surgery will develop severe chronic unilateral or bilateral scrotal pain or discomfort that interferes with quality of life and prompts patients to seek treatment.[154]

Also known as post-vasectomy pain syndrome, this diagnosis is defined as at least 3 months of chronic intermittent scrotal pain following vas surgery, in contrast to acute post-procedure pain which typically resolves 2 to 4 weeks post-procedure.[155] Chronic scrotal pain can have a delayed onset of months or years, unrelated to demographics or operative techniques.[156,157] Nearly 15% of patients have some scrotal discomfort following vas surgery, but only 1% to 2% report chronic pain causing regret or having a negative impact on their lives.[156,158] The pathophysiology of chronic scrotal pain after vas surgery is poorly understood, but may be related to epididymal or vas congestion, back pressure-induced epididymal blowout, sperm granuloma formation, or scrotal and spermatic cord nerve injury.[159–161] Conservative therapy such as scrotal support and rest, nonsteroidal anti-inflammatory drugs, tricyclic antidepressants, and/or gabapentin is sufficient treatment in most cases. If medical treatment fails, clinicians may consider spermatic cord nerve block, excision of site granulomas, epididymectomy or vasovasotomy, micro-denervation of the spermatic cord, or ultimately orchiectomy.[162] Very few men ever require surgical treatment for chronic scrotal pain following their vasectomy. According the American Urological Association, information about the low risk of severe, chronic scrotal pain is essential in pre-surgical counseling.[141]

Sexual Function

Many patients are concerned about erectile dysfunction, reduced orgasmic sensation, decreased semen volume, reduced libido, decreased genital sensation, or diminished sexual pleasure following vas surgery. Large numbers of studies consistently show that sexual function remains unaffected by vas surgery and surgery does not lead to impotence, other sexual difficulties, or reduction in the amount of semen ejaculated. Multiple studies have shown an increase in frequency or improvement in sexual satisfaction in half or more of patients and decrease in frequency of intercourse and sexual habits in only 5% of men.[163–165]

Anti-sperm Antibodies

Anti-sperm antibodies appear in 50% to 80% of men following vas surgery, compared to only 8% to 21% of men in the general population.[166,167] Multiple studies have shown no evidence of adverse health consequences, including immunological diseases, from anti-sperm antibodies.[168–170] The only possible clinical significance of anti-sperm antibodies is that very high levels may impair fertility after vas surgery reversal, which occurs infrequently.[171] The interpretation and clinical relevance of different types of anti-sperm antibody tests are controversial, and the presence of a specific antibody class may have more significance than titer level.[172,173] In any case, the presence of serum anti-sperm antibodies should not be considered a contraindication for vasectomy reversal.

Regret

Most patients who have vas surgery do not regret their decision; however, because of relationship changes and other life events, regret is always possible. The 1% to 2% risk of regret among patients after vas surgery is lower than the reported regret among patients after tubal surgery.[164,174] Partners of patients who have had vas surgery may have slightly higher rates of regret at 6% to 8% than those patients themselves, but this rate is similar to patients who had tubal surgery.[81,175] Regret following vas surgery is more common among patients who, at the time of the surgery, were less than 30 years old, were in an unstable marriage, had no or very young children, or made the decision for permanent contraception during a time of financial crisis or for reasons related to a pregnancy.[174,176] The most commonly reported reason for regret was the desire for more children, due to changing their mind, having a new partner, or losing a child.[177–179] Another reason for patient dissatisfaction or regret include feeling that a problem or complication following vas surgery was caused by the surgery itself. However, 80% to 100% of patients having vas surgery would recommend it to others.[141]

Thorough and effective counseling is crucial in reducing regret in patients choosing permanent contraception. Counseling should be in a language the patient can easily understand. Both the patient and partner (when appropriate) should be counseled, and risk factors for regret should be addressed. The presence of strong risk factors for regret should not be used to uniformly restrict vas surgery, but should indicate the need for more extensive counseling. Age and lack of children should not be considered contraindications, and patients seeking permanent contraception should not be required to undergo a mental health evaluation due to a clinician's concern for patient regret.

Desire for Pregnancy Following Vas Surgery

Permanent contraception should be considered permanent, but some patients will have a change in personal circumstance and later desire children. Assisted reproductive technologies and microsurgical vas surgery reversal are options for a patient who desires a pregnancy following vas surgery, but success is not guaranteed.[180]

The time elapsed between vas surgery and reversal is a major factor in the success of reversal; the longer the interval between vas surgery and reversal, the less likely the patient is to be fertile after the reversal.

Reversal is more successful when done within 10 years after surgery; pregnancy rates are less than 50% when reversal is performed more than 10 to 15 years after vas surgery.[179,181,182] Other factors that affect the success of vas surgery reversal include the skill of the surgeon, type of vas surgery originally performed, levels of anti-sperm antibodies, age of the partner, and partial obstruction of the vas after the reversal surgery that prevents movement of sperm through the vas.[183] After microsurgical reversal, the percentage of patients with sperm in the ejaculate is 75% to 100%.[179,184] However, presence of sperm in the ejaculate does not guarantee pregnancy. Reported pregnancy rates following microsurgical reversal range from 38% to 89%.[179,180,182,184] Finally, couples undergoing vas reversal surgery may have the need for future contraception.

Assisted reproductive technologies are a good option for patients who want children but do not want a vas surgery reversal or who already underwent unsuccessful reversal surgeries. Sperm can be retrieved from the epididymis or the testis and then used for intracytoplasmic sperm injection (ICSI) with IVF. Pregnancy rates per attempt following ICSI with IVF using epididymal or testicular sperm are reported to be 17% to 36%.[185] Data are conflicting on whether longer time elapsed between vas surgery and ICSI reduces the chance of pregnancy.[186–189]

Vas surgery reversal should be the first choice for patients who had vas surgery but now wish to have children, even for patients who have failed a previous reversal attempt.[181,187,190] Vas surgery reversal has the same if not better pregnancy rates and is less costly than ICSI using epididymal sperm.[187,188,191] However, both assisted reproductive technologies and reversal surgery are expensive and are often not covered by health insurance. Factors in deciding whether to have a reversal or ICSI with IVF should not only include cost but also the age and fertility of the partner and the number of children desired.

PROVIDING VAS SURGERY

COUNSELING GUIDELINES FOR VAS SURGERY

The goal of contraceptive counseling is to help patients select a method that they will use, will be effective, is most consistent with their reproductive intentions, and will not have adverse effects. The permanence of vas surgery is a significant consideration for counseling. However, respect for a patient's autonomy, including a dialogue regarding the patient's reproductive desires and wishes, should be the primary concern during this discussion.[100]

The factors contributing to an individual's decision about permanent contraception vary. Each patient needs to weigh the risks, benefits, effectiveness, and side effects of the various contraceptive options available to them.

Counseling should address the following:

1. **Provide choices.** Present highly effective, long-acting, reversible methods such as the contraceptive implant or IUDs as options available to the patient's partner.
2. **Assess the patient's understanding of the procedure.** Awareness of vas surgery is widespread in the United States, but patients often have misconceptions about the procedure. Review the procedure with patients so that they correctly understand it and clarify any misconceptions.
3. **Facilitate the decision-making process.** Give the patient sufficient time to make a thoughtful, informed decision about permanent contraception, especially when a patient's partner has just given birth or had an abortion, or when there are financial, marital, or sexual problems. (See Chapter 2 for more complete discussion of patient-centered contraception counseling.)
4. **Provide information about possible failure.** Inform the patient that vas surgery, although highly effective, is not immediately nor 100% successful. Failure can occur, even years after the procedure was performed.
5. **Discuss STI prevention.** Permanent contraception will not provide protection against STIs, including HIV. This should be thoroughly explained to patients or their partner(s). Condom use will be necessary if the patient is concerned about STI prevention.

Components of Pre-vasectomy Counseling[141]

- Permanent nature of the procedure
- Vas surgery is not immediately effective
- After vas surgery, another form of contraception is needed until occlusion is confirmed by post-vasectomy semen analysis (PVSA)
- The possibility of failure even after occlusion is confirmed
- Repeat surgery may be necessary in ≤1% of vas surgeries performed using a highly effective technique
- Patients must refrain from ejaculation for 1 week after the procedure
- Options for fertility after vas surgery may be expensive and may not be successful

- Rates of surgical complications are 1% to 2%, and vary with surgeon's experience
- Chronic scrotal pain that negatively affects quality of life occurs in 1% to 2% of patients, but rarely requires additional surgery
- Alternative methods of contraception available (including permanent and reversible methods for partners)

Other considerations for counseling include screening for risk indicators for regret, need for condoms to protect against STIs, and Federal and State Medicaid regulations about informed consent, including age of the patient, circumstances in which consent is obtained, and interval from time of consent to procedure.

Informed Consent and Policy/Legal Issues. See the Tubal Surgery section regarding informed consent, policy and legal issues.

Preoperative Screening. Take a preoperative history and perform a physical exam with attention to the inguinal area, scrotum, and testicles for factors that might affect the procedure such as an inguinal hernia, a large hydrocele or varicocele, or cryptorchidism. Evaluate the general health condition of the patient. Order any standard pre-operative laboratory tests per the surgeon or institution's policies, including tests pertinent to the patient's medical condition relevant to surgery, such as a blood type, complete blood count, or serum glucose level.

Options for Approach

The two key steps in vas surgery are to 1) isolate the vas and 2) occlude the vas. Immediate postoperative complications such as pain, bleeding, and infection are related to the method of isolation, whereas success and failure of vas surgery are related to occlusion method.

Vas Isolation

There are two methods for vas isolation: conventional vasectomy and minimally-invasive vasectomy (MIV), which includes no-scalpel vasectomy (NSV). Standard of care is MIV for vas isolation. Conventional vasectomy involves skin incisions 1.5 to 3 cm long that are made with a scalpel and then closed with suture. No special instruments are used to dissect and grasp the vas (Figure 16-7). MIV creates skin openings of <1 cm using special instruments, with minimal dissection around the vas. NSV was the first MIV technique, developed in 1974 in China by Dr. Li Shunqiang to make vasectomy a more acceptable method of contraception. In this method, the clinician places a vas ring clamp around the vas, perivasal tissue, and overlying skin before making the skin opening with

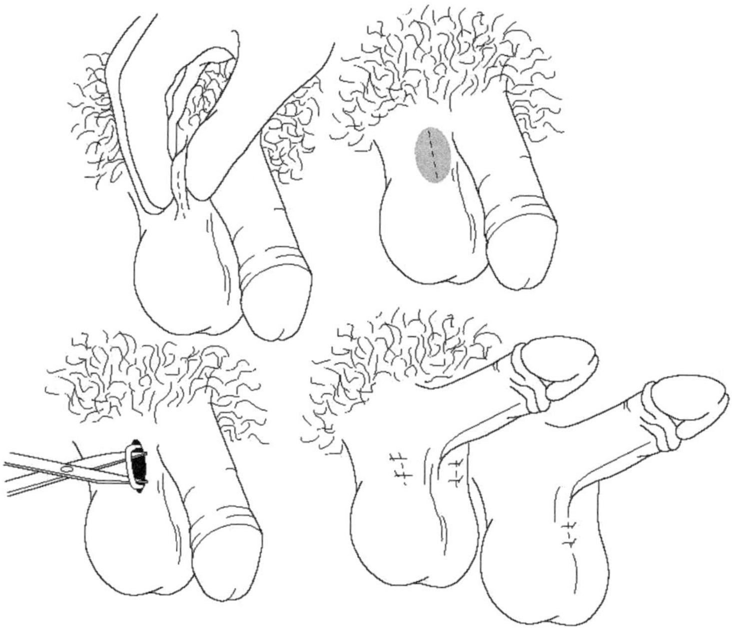

Figure 16-7 Conventional vasectomy

the vas dissector. The clinician will then use the vas ring clamp and dissector to isolate the vas before elevating, dividing, and occluding the ends of vas. The skin opening is left unsutured unless skin closure is necessary (Figure 16-8).[192] A detailed description can be found at www.engenderhealth.org (No-Scalpel Vasectomy: An Illustrated Guide For Surgeons).[193]

NSV has less bleeding, hematoma formation, infection, postoperative pain, and a shorter operation time compared to conventional vasectomy. If a single midline opening is used, the clinician must insure that both vas are occluded, rather than one vas occluded twice.[194] Several modifications to the NSV approach regarding finger placement, timing and placement of skin openings, and instrument design are published in the literature, although these variants should be referred to as MIV methods.[195–198]

Vas Occlusion

Once the vas is isolated, it is completely divided in nearly all occlusion techniques, with or without excision of a vas segment (division/excision) and with or without blockage of at least one end of the divided vas. Methods of blockage include ligation, application of clips, chemical occlusion, thermal or electrocautery, fascial interposition, or a combination of these.

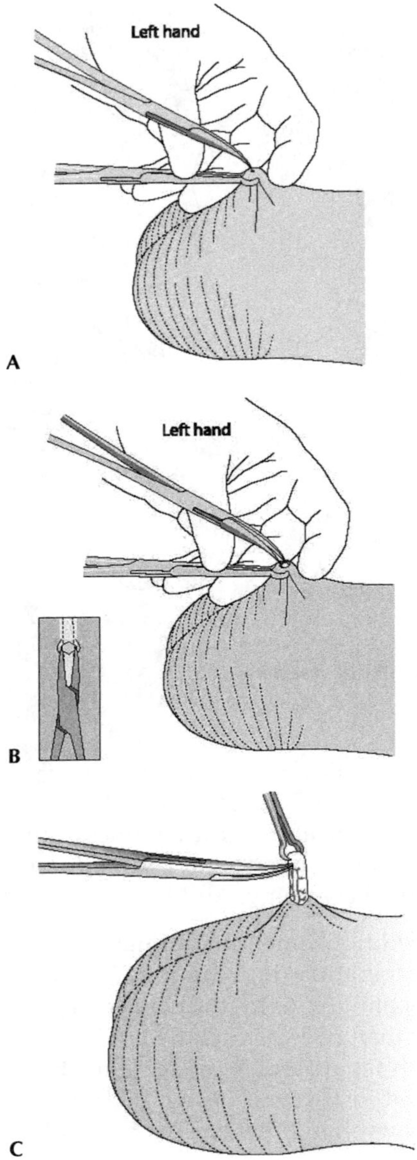

Source: Engenderhealth,[190]

Figure 16-8 No-scalpel vasectomy: A. Inserting both tips of the vas dissector into the puncture site; **B.** Spreading the tissues to make a skin opening twice the diameter of the vas **C.** Grasping a partial thickness of the elevated vas.

Ligation occludes the vas with ligatures, with division/excision of 1 cm length of vas between the sutures. The ligatures may be replaced with clips.[127] Mucosal cautery involves thermal or electrical cautery to the mucosa of the cut ends of the vas to destroy the luminal mucosa with minimal damage to the muscle layers. Cautery induces fibrosis to occlude the lumen; sparing the muscular layer decreases the risk of the cauterized portion sloughing off and the vas recanalizing.[137,199,200] Fascial interposition places a layer of internal spermatic fascia between the two divided ends, over the testicular or the abdominal end, and usually used with other techniques such as ligation and division/excision or mucosal cautery.[200,201] Folding and suturing each divided vas end on itself to prevent the cut ends from facing each other is not recommended.

Open-ended vasectomy involves division/excision followed by fascial interposition to cover the abdominal end of the divided vas. Theoretically, the open ends may minimize pressure and damage to the epididymis and increase success rates for vas surgery reversal.[202] Fascial interposition is necessary with this technique to prevent recanalization.

There are no well-designed randomized trials comparing these practices, except for one trial showing that simple ligation and division of the vas is more likely to fail compared to using fascial interposition.[127,201] One study investigating an intra-vas device of urethane filled with nylon thread showed lower success compared with no-scalpel vasectomy.[203]

The American Urological Association identified the following three division methods having data demonstrating excellent contraceptive and occlusive effectiveness, with failure rates consistently ≤1% in large numbers across different studies (Figure 16-9):[141]

1. Mucosal cautery with fascial interposition, without ligatures or clips
2. Mucosal cautery without fascial interposition and without ligatures or clips
3. Open-ended vasectomy, using mucosal cautery and fascial interposition on the abdominal end of the vas

Only one method, the Marie Stopes International technique, does not divide the vas but instead occludes it by using extended monopolar electrocautery to destroy 2.5 to 3 cm of the vas.[204] This method is not used in the United States but is considered a reasonable vas surgery technique by the American Urological Association.[141]

Data show no benefit of excising a short vas segment over no excision. If excision is performed, routine histological examination of the excised vas segments is not required, since a PVSA will confirm success.[141] However, if the surgeon suspects that the excised structure is not a section of vas, then histology may be helpful.

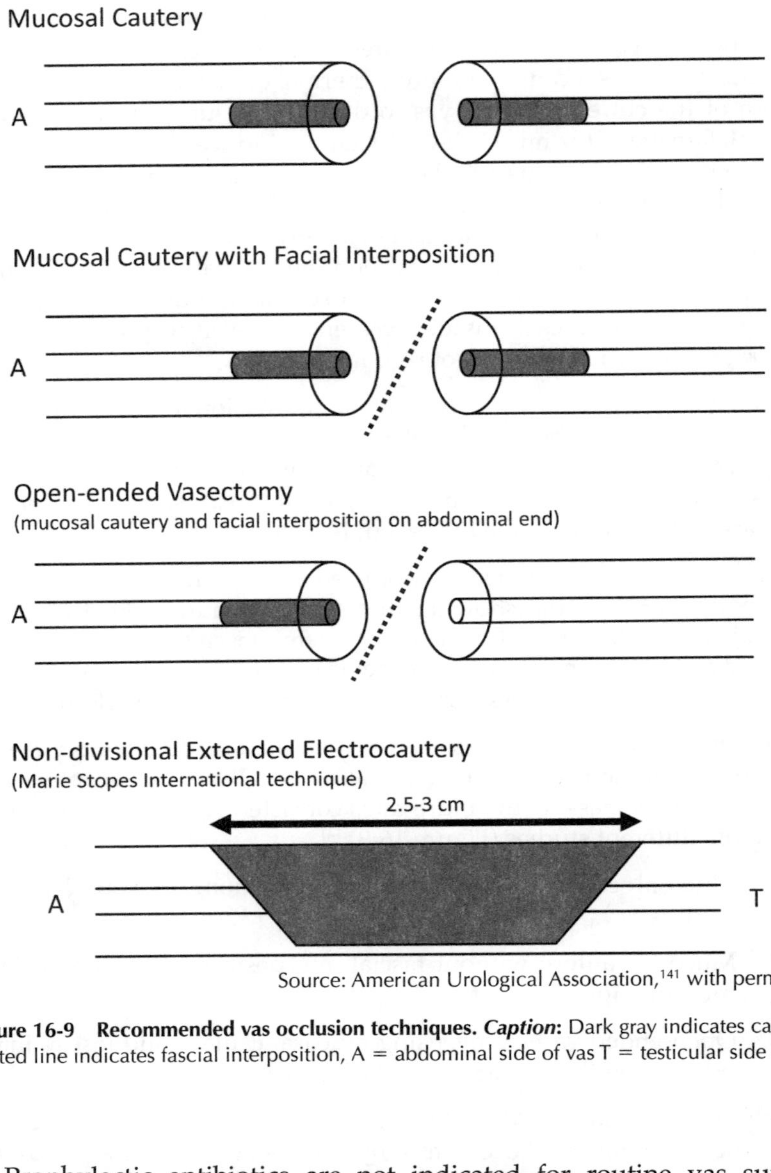

Source: American Urological Association,[141] with permission

Figure 16-9 Recommended vas occlusion techniques. ***Caption*:** Dark gray indicates cautery, dotted line indicates fascial interposition, A = abdominal side of vas T = testicular side of vas

Prophylactic antibiotics are not indicated for routine vas surgery unless the patient is at high risk of infection.[141] General risk factors for infection include advanced age, anatomic anomalies, poor nutritional status, smoking, chronic corticosteroid use, immunodeficiency, diabetes, and prolonged hospitalization.[205] However, the presence of one or more of these risk factors does not necessarily require the use of antimicrobial prophylaxis. The clinician should decide on a case-by-case basis whether prophylactic antibiotics are needed for vas surgery.

ANESTHESIA

Vas surgery is performed under local anesthesia alone in nearly all patients seeking vas surgery. Some patients whose anatomy may lead to a particularly difficult surgery or who are unable to tolerate the procedure under local anesthesia may benefit from oral or intravenous sedation or general anesthesia, although risks of anesthesia increase with deeper sedation. Topical anesthesia applied by the clinician to the surgical site is optional, but infiltration of local anesthesia into the skin and perivasal tissue should always be used.[141] Clinicians should administer local anesthetic using their smallest available needle, between 24 and 32 gauge, to minimize pain from the spermatic cord block.

All anesthetic methods need the attention of a trained professional who carefully monitors the patient and the drugs used.

MANAGING PROBLEMS AND FOLLOW-UP

Vas surgery is a minor surgical procedure. Fewer than 3% of cases require medical attention.[127] Intraoperative complications such as vasovagal reaction, lidocaine toxicity, and excessive bleeding, are unusual and can generally be prevented if appropriate guidelines and procedures are followed. Postoperative complications such as bleeding, infection, or vas surgery failure are infrequent. Most postoperative complications, including swelling of the scrotum, bruising, pain, and minor bleeding under the skin, are minor and subside within 1 or 2 weeks. Scrotal support, mild pain medication, and local application of cold therapy are usually sufficient for treatment. More significant complications such as heavy bleeding, hematoma, or infection are quite rare. Careful surgical technique, aseptic technique, early recognition of a problem, and proper postoperative care and follow-up greatly reduce the risks of both minor and major complications after vas surgery. A routine postoperative visit specifically to examine the scrotum is not necessary.

A patient's surgery is successful if the post-vasectomy semen analysis (PVSA) shows azoospermia or RNMS ($\leq$100,000 nonmotile sperm / mL).[206] All patients have motile and functional sperm in the ejaculate after surgery for some period of time, which can range from weeks to months based on factors such as frequency of ejaculation, patient age and anatomy, and surgical technique.[130,131,141,207] Patients should have a PVSA to confirm success, although instructions for when a patient should have the PVSA vary widely in terms of postoperative time or number of post-surgery ejaculations. The optimal time will minimize the number of PVSAs needed to establish success but still allow a patient to stop using other forms of contraception as soon as possible after surgery, and ranges from 1 week to 3 months. If motile sperm are still seen on PVSA at 6 months after vas surgery, the vas surgery should be considered a failure and repeat surgery considered.[141] In resource-poor settings, where semen analysis may not be available or practical, patients should use another form of contraception for at least 12 weeks after surgery.[201,208,209]

PATIENT INSTRUCTIONS FOR VAS SURGERY*

Preoperative Instructions

1. Be completely sure of your decision to have permanent contraception. You must be certain you understand and desire the permanence of vas surgery. You can change your mind at any time before the operation.
2. Before surgery while you are home, clip all the hair from around the penis and scrotum to about 1/4 inch long. Do not shave. Wash the penis and scrotum thoroughly to remove all loose hairs.
3. If possible, bring someone who can accompany you home after the procedure. Do not ride a bicycle; avoid walking long distances or using other transportation that may rub or put pressure on the scrotum.
4. Bring a pair of tight-fitting underwear or an athletic supporter to support the scrotum and minimize swelling.

Postoperative Instructions

1. **Use scrotal support for at least 2 days** (e.g., wearing brief-style underwear) to reduce pain. If possible, keep a cold pack on the scrotum for at least 4 hours to reduce the chances of swelling, bleeding, and discomfort. You may discontinue the scrotal support once you're comfortable without it.
2. If you don't have any bothersome discomfort, you may return to non-physical work the day of or the day after your surgery.
3. **Avoid ejaculation for 1 week after vas surgery** to allow the surgical sites to heal and to allow occlusion for methods that occlude the vas using mucosal cautery.[141]
4. **Avoid strenuous physical exercise for 1 week.** Strenuous exercise means hard physical exertion, lifting or straining that could bring pressure to the groin or scrotum. When you resume strenuous activity, stop if it is uncomfortable.
5. You will probably have some mild pain and swelling in the scrotal region, and the scrotum may be somewhat discolored. These conditions are normal and should not worry you.

---

*These instructions are intended to guide providers in educating patients in pre- and post-care.

6. You may notice blood in your ejaculate during the first month or 2 after surgery. This will resolve on its own and does not mean anything is wrong.

   Watch for the following symptoms:

Condition	Action
Temperature >100.4 Fahrenheit	Contact your provider immediately
Pain preventing sleep or work	If unrelieved by analgesic, contact your provider
Redness, discharge or inflammation at the incision site	Contact your provider
Bleeding from the incision site	Place pressure on the area for 10 minutes. If bleeding continues, contact your provider
Swelling greater than twice normal size	Contact your provider
Groin nodules larger than a nickel, painful and tender	Contact your provider
Stitches causing extreme pulling sensation	Contact your provider

7. Take 1 or 2 analgesic tablets at 4- to 6-hour intervals if you need them for pain. (Note to provider: name and dose should be specified.) Do not use aspirin since it may promote bleeding.
8. You may shower or bathe 24 hours after surgery but avoid putting tension on the incision and do not rub or irritate the incision for 1 week. Pat dry the incision site after showering or bathing.
9. Stitches will dissolve and do not require removal. (Note to provider: this instruction must be modified if nonabsorbable skin sutures or no sutures are used.)
10. **Please return to your clinician for the confirmatory test** in 3 months so the success of the procedure can be assessed.
11. **Use condoms or other contraceptive method** until you know that you are not releasing sperm in your ejaculate. For many patients, sperm will not be cleared from the body until after a minimum of 3 months. The best way of finding out if the surgery was successful is to have your semen looked at under a microscope about 3 months after the vas surgery. Until success is confirmed, you cannot rely on vas surgery as a contraceptive method.
12. **Remember, vas surgery is permanent.** Reversal surgery or assisted reproductive technologies are possible under certain conditions, but are expensive and require highly technical procedures. Results are not guaranteed.

Author Disclosures—Hou: none. Roncari: none.

REFERENCES

1. Daniels K, Daugherty J, Jones J, Mosher W. Current contraceptive use and variation by selected characteristics among women aged 15–44: United States, 2011–2013. Natl Health Stat Report 2015:1–14.
2. Department of Economic and Social Affairs. World contraceptive patterns. In: United Nations, ed. New York: United Nations; 2015.
3. Kulier R, Boulvain M, Walker D, Candolle G, Campana A. Minilaparotomy and endoscopic techniques for tubal sterilisation. Cochrane Database Syst Rev 2004:CD001328.
4. Peterson HB, Xia Z, Hughes JM, Wilcox LS, Tylor LR, Trussell J. The risk of pregnancy after tubal sterilization: findings from the U.S. Collaborative Review of Sterilization. Am J Obstet Gynecol 1996;174:1161–8; discussion 8–70.
5. Shaw R, Russell I, Settatree R, Templeton A, Filschie G, Argent V. Male and female sterilization: evidence based guidelines No. 4. London: Royal College of Obstetricians and Gynaecologists; 1999.
6. Bang A. [Pregnancy following bilateral salpingectomy]. Ugeskr Laeger 2008;170:1437–8.
7. Bollapragada SS, Bandyopadhyay S, Serle E, Baird C. Spontaneous pregnancy after bilateral salpingectomy. Fertil Steril 2005;83:767–8.
8. Hurskainen R, Hovi SL, Gissler M, et al. Hysteroscopic tubal sterilization: a systematic review of the Essure system. Fertil Steril 2010;94:16–9.
9. Gariepy AM, Creinin MD, Schwarz EB, Smith KJ. Reliability of laparoscopic compared with hysteroscopic sterilization at 1 year: a decision analysis. Obstet Gynecol 2011;118:273–9.
10. Smith RD. Contemporary hysteroscopic methods for female sterilization. Int J Gynaecol Obstet 2010;108:79–84.
11. Dhruva SS, Ross JS, Gariepy AM. Revisiting Essure- toward safe and effective sterilization. N Engl J Med 2015;373:e17.
12. Walter JR, Ghobadi CW, Hayman E, Xu S. Hysteroscopic sterilization with Essure: summary of the U.S. Food and Drug Administration actions and policy implications for postmarketing surveillance. Obstet Gynecol 2017;129:10–9.
13. Gariepy AM, Creinin MD, Smith KJ, Xu X. Probability of pregnancy after sterilization: a comparison of hysteroscopic versus laparoscopic sterilization. Contraception 2014;90:174–81.
14. la Chapelle CF, Veersema S, Brolmann HA, Jansen FW. Effectiveness and feasibility of hysteroscopic sterilization techniques: a systematic review and meta-analysis. Fertil Steril 2015;103:1516–25 e1-3.
15. Kerin JF, Munday D, Ritossa M, Rosen D. Tissue encapsulation of the proximal Essure micro-insert from the uterine cavity following hysteroscopic sterilization. J Minim Invasive Gynecol 2007;14:202–4.
16. Dreyer K, Lier MC, Emanuel MH, et al. Hysteroscopic proximal tubal occlusion versus laparoscopic salpingectomy as a treatment for hydrosalpinges prior to IVF or ICSI: an RCT. Hum Reprod 2016;31:2005–16.
17. Barbosa MW, Sotiriadis A, Papatheodorou SI, Mijatovic V, Nastri CO, Martins WP. High miscarriage rate in women treated with Essure(R) for hydrosalpinx before embryo transfer: a systematic review and meta-analysis. Ultrasound Obstet Gynecol 2016;48:556–65.
18. Munro MG, Nichols JE, Levy B, Vleugels MP, Veersema S. Hysteroscopic sterilization: 10-year retrospective analysis of worldwide pregnancy reports. J Minim Invasive Gynecol 2014;21:245–51.
19. Hitzerd E, Schreuder HW, Vleugels MP, Veersema S. Twelve-year retrospective review of unintended pregnancies after Essure sterilization in the Netherlands. Fertil Steril 2016;105:932–7.

20. Chudnoff SG, Nichols JE, Jr., Levie M. Hysteroscopic Essure inserts for permanent contraception: extended follow-up results of a phase III multicenter international study. J Minim Invasive Gynecol 2015;22:951–60.
21. Peterson HB, Xia Z, Hughes JM, Wilcox LS, Tylor LR, Trussell J. The risk of ectopic pregnancy after tubal sterilization. U.S. Collaborative Review of Sterilization Working Group. N Engl J Med 1997;336:762–7.
22. FDA approves new female sterlization device. FDA Talk Paper 2002;T02-41:1–2.
23. Escobedo LG, Peterson HB, Grubb GS, Franks AL. Case-fatality rates for tubal sterilization in U.S. hospitals, 1979 to 1980. Am J Obstet Gynecol 1989;160:147–50.
24. Peterson HB, Ory HW, Greenspan JR, Tyler CW, Jr. Deaths associated with laparoscopic sterilization by unipolar electrocoagulating devices, 1978 and 1979. Am J Obstet Gynecol 1981;139:141–3.
25. Hulka JF, Phillips JM, Peterson HB, Surrey MW. Laparoscopic sterilization: American Association of Gynecologic Laparoscopists' 1993 membership survey. J Am Assoc Gynecol Laparosc 1995;2:137–8.
26. Peterson HB, Hulka JF, Phillips JM, Surrey MW. Laparoscopic sterilization. American Association of Gynecologic Laparoscopists 1991 membership survey. J Reprod Med 1993;38:574–6.
27. Jamieson DJ, Hillis SD, Duerr A, Marchbanks PA, Costello C, Peterson HB. Complications of interval laparoscopic tubal sterilization: findings from the United States Collaborative Review of Sterilization. Obstet Gynecol 2000;96:997–1002.
28. Lawrie TA, Kulier R, Nardin JM. Techniques for the interruption of tubal patency for female sterilisation. Cochrane Database Syst Rev 2016:CD003034.
29. Westberg J, Scott F, Creinin MD. Safety outcomes of female sterilization by salpingectomy and tubal occlusion. Contraception 2017;95:505–8.
30. Shinar S, Blecher Y, Alpern S, et al. Total bilateral salpingectomy versus partial bilateral salpingectomy for permanent sterilization during cesarean delivery. Arch Gynecol Obstet 2017;295:1185–9.
31. Bayer HealthCare Pharmaceuticals I. Essure permanent birth control: instructions for use. Milpitas, CA: Bayer Healthcare LLC; 2002.
32. Hologic. Adiana permanent contraception: instructions for use. Hologic, Inc.; 2009.
33. Carmona F, Cristobal P, Casamitjana R, Balasch J. Effect of tubal sterilization on ovarian follicular reserve and function. Am J Obstet Gynecol 2003;189:447–52.
34. Cevrioglu AS, Degirmenci B, Acar M, et al. Examination of changes caused by tubal sterilization in ovarian hormone secretion and uterine and ovarian artery blood flow rates. Contraception 2004;70:467–73.
35. Ganer Herman H, Gluck O, Keidar R, et al. Ovarian reserve following Cesarean-delivery with salpingectomy versus tubal ligation - a randomized trial. Am J Obstet Gynecol 2017.
36. Whiteman MK, Miller KP, Tomic D, Langenberg P, Flaws JA. Tubal sterilization and hot flashes. Fertil Steril 2004;82:502–4.
37. Wyshak G. Menopausal symptoms and psychological distress in women with and without tubal sterilization. Psychosomatics 2004;45:403–13.
38. Ozkaya E, Gokmen O, Tosun A, et al. Unfavorable lipid profile and higher frequency of hot flashes during perimenopausal years after fallopian tube ligation. Gynecol Endocrinol 2013;29:559–62.
39. Nichols HB, Baird DD, DeRoo LA, Kissling GE, Sandler DP. Tubal ligation in relation to menopausal symptoms and breast cancer risk. Br J Cancer 2013;109:1291–5.
40. Green A, Purdie D, Bain C, et al. Tubal sterilisation, hysterectomy and decreased risk of ovarian cancer. Survey of Women's Health Study Group. Int J Cancer 1997;71:948–51.
41. Kjaer SK, Mellemkjaer L, Brinton LA, Johansen C, Gridley G, Olsen JH. Tubal sterilization and risk of ovarian, endometrial and cervical cancer. A Danish population-based follow-up study of more than 65 000 sterilized women. Int J Epidemiol 2004;33:596–602.
42. Irwin KL, Weiss NS, Lee NC, Peterson HB. Tubal sterilization, hysterectomy, and the subsequent occurrence of epithelial ovarian cancer. Am J Epidemiol 1991;134:362–9.

43. McGuire V, Felberg A, Mills M, et al. Relation of contraceptive and reproductive history to ovarian cancer risk in carriers and noncarriers of BRCA1 gene mutations. Am J Epidemiol 2004;160:613–8.
44. Narod SA, Sun P, Ghadirian P, et al. Tubal ligation and risk of ovarian cancer in carriers of BRCA1 or BRCA2 mutations: a case-control study. Lancet 2001;357:1467–70.
45. George SH, Garcia R, Slomovitz BM. Ovarian cancer: the fallopian tube as the site of origin and opportunities for prevention. Front Oncol 2016;6:108.
46. Cibula D, Widschwendter M, Zikan M, Dusek L. Underlying mechanisms of ovarian cancer risk reduction after tubal ligation. Acta Obstet Gynecol Scand 2011;90:559–63.
47. Yoon SH, Kim SN, Shim SH, Kang SB, Lee SJ. Bilateral salpingectomy can reduce the risk of ovarian cancer in the general population: a meta-analysis. Eur J Cancer 2016;55:38–46.
48. American College of Obstetricians and Gynecologists. Committee Opinion No. 620: Salpingectomy for ovarian cancer prevention. Obstet Gynecol 2015;125:279–81.
49. McAlpine JN, Hanley GE, Woo MM, et al. Opportunistic salpingectomy: uptake, risks, and complications of a regional initiative for ovarian cancer prevention. Am J Obstet Gynecol 2014;210:471 e1–11.
50. Jones NL, Schulkin J, Urban RR, et al. Physicians' perspectives and practice patterns toward opportunistic salpingectomy in high- and low-risk women. Cancer Invest 2017;35:51–61.
51. Calle EE, Rodriguez C, Walker KA, Wingo PA, Petrelli JM, Thun MJ. Tubal sterilization and risk of breast cancer mortality in US women. Cancer Causes Control 2001;12:127–35.
52. Eliassen AH, Colditz GA, Rosner B, Hankinson SE. Tubal sterilization in relation to breast cancer risk. Int J Cancer 2006;118:2026–30.
53. Gaudet MM, Patel AV, Sun J, Teras LR, Gapstur SM. Tubal sterilization and breast cancer incidence: results from the cancer prevention study II nutrition cohort and meta-analysis. Am J Epidemiol 2013;177:492–9.
54. Gentile GP, Kaufman SC, Helbig DW. Is there any evidence for a post-tubal sterilization syndrome? Fertil Steril 1998;69:179–86.
55. Bhiwandiwala PP, Mumford SD, Feldblum PJ. Menstrual pattern changes following laparoscopic sterilization with different occlusion techniques: a review of 10,004 cases. Am J Obstet Gynecol 1983;145:684–94.
56. DeStefano F, Perlman JA, Peterson HB, Diamond EL. Long-term risk of menstrual disturbances after tubal sterilization. Am J Obstet Gynecol 1985;152:835–41.
57. Rivera R, Gaitan JR, Ruiz R, et al. Menstrual patterns and progesterone circulating levels following different procedures of tubal occlusion. Contraception 1989;40:157–69.
58. Rulin MC, Davidson AR, Philliber SG, Graves WL, Cushman LF. Long-term effect of tubal sterilization on menstrual indices and pelvic pain. Obstet Gynecol 1993;82:118–21.
59. Sahwi S, Toppozada M, Kamel M, Anwar MY, Ismail AA. Changes in menstrual blood loss after four methods of female tubal sterilization. Contraception 1989;40:387–98.
60. Thranov I, Hertz JB, Kjer JJ, et al. Hormonal and menstrual changes after laparoscopic sterilization by Falope-rings or Filshie-clips. Fertil Steril 1992;57:751–5.
61. Costello C, Hillis SD, Marchbanks PA, Jamieson DJ, Peterson HB. The effect of interval tubal sterilization on sexual interest and pleasure. Obstet Gynecol 2002;100:511–7.
62. Shain RN, Miller WB, Holden AE, Rosenthal M. Impact of tubal sterilization and vasectomy on female marital sexuality: results of a controlled longitudinal study. Am J Obstet Gynecol 1991;164:763–71.
63. Tam T, Elgar C, Jirschele K, Lombard E. Post-ablation tubal sterilization syndrome (PATSS) following Novasure endometrial ablation: two case reports and a review of literature. J Minim Invas Gyn 2012:S71–122.
64. Lo JS, Pickersgill A. Pregnancy after endometrial ablation: English literature review and case report. J Minim Invas Gyn 2006;13:88–91.
65. McCausland AM, McCausland VM. Frequency of symptomatic cornual hematometra and postablation tubal sterilization syndrome after total rollerball endometrial ablation: a 10-year follow-up. Am J Obstet Gynecol 2002;186:1274–80; discussion 80–3.

66. Webb JC, Bush MR, Wood MD, Park GS. Hematosalpinx with pelvic pain after endometrial ablation confirms the postablation-tubal sterilization syndrome. J Am Assoc Gynecol Laparosc 1996;3:419–21.
67. Donnadieu AC, Fernandez H. The role of Essure sterilization performed simultaneously with endometrial ablation. Curr Opin Obstet Gynecol 2008;20:359–63.
68. Valle RF, Valdez J, Wright TC, Kenney M. Concomitant Essure tubal sterilization and Thermachoice endometrial ablation: feasibility and safety. Fertil Steril 2006;86:152–8.
69. Al-Safi ZA, Shavell VI, Hobson DT, Berman JM, Diamond MP. Analysis of adverse events with Essure hysteroscopic sterilization reported to the Manufacturer and User Facility Device Experience database. J Minim Invas Gyn 2013;20:825–9.
70. Yunker AC, Ritch JM, Robinson EF, Golish CT. Incidence and risk factors for chronic pelvic pain after hysteroscopic sterilization. J Minim Invas Gyn 2015;22:390–4.
71. Casey J, Aguirre F, Yunker A. Outcomes of laparoscopic removal of the Essure sterilization device for pelvic pain: a case series. Contraception 2016;94:190–2.
72. Jain P, Clark TJ. Removal of Essure(R) device 4 years post-procedure: a rare case. J Obstet Gynaecol 2011;31:271–2.
73. Mahmoud MS, Fridman D, Merhi ZO. Subserosal misplacement of Essure device manifested by late-onset acute pelvic pain. Fertil Steril 2009;92:2038 e1-3.
74. MAUDE - Manufacturer and User Facility Device Experience. Accessed 5/16/2017, at www.accessdata.fda.gov/scripts/cdrh/cfdocs/cfMAUDE/search.CFM.
75. Hillis SD, Marchbanks PA, Tylor LR, Peterson HB. Higher hysterectomy risk for sterilized than nonsterilized women: findings from the U.S. Collaborative Review of Sterilization. Obstet Gynecol 1998;91:241–6.
76. Goldhaber MK, Armstrong MA, Golditch IM, Sheehe PR, Petitti DB, Friedman GD. Long-term risk of hysterectomy among 80,007 sterilized and comparison women at Kaiser Permanente, 1971–1987. Am J Epidemiol 1993;138:508–21.
77. Hillis SD, Marchbanks PA, Tylor LR, Peterson HB. Tubal sterilization and long-term risk of hysterectomy: findings from the United States Collaborative Review of Sterilization. Obstet Gynecol 1997;89:609–14.
78. Sills ES, Dalton MM. Referrals for complications following hysteroscopic sterilisation: characteristics associated with symptomatic patients after the Essure procedure. Eur J Contracept Reprod Health Care 2016;21:227–33.
79. Hou MY. Discordant relationship between Essure microinsert position and tubal occlusion. BMJ Case Rep 2016;2016.
80. Hillis SD, Marchbanks PA, Tylor LR, Peterson HB. Poststerilization regret: findings from the United States Collaborative Review of Sterilization. Obstet Gynecol 1999;93:889–95.
81. Jamieson DJ, Kaufman SC, Costello C, Hillis SD, Marchbanks PA, Peterson HB. A comparison of women's regret after vasectomy versus tubal sterilization. Obstet Gynecol 2002;99:1073–9.
82. Schmidt JE, Hillis SD, Marchbanks PA, Jeng G, Peterson HB. Requesting information about and obtaining reversal after tubal sterilization: findings from the U.S. Collaborative Review of Sterilization. Fertil Steril 2000;74:892–8.
83. Wilcox LS, Chu SY, Eaker ED, Zeger SL, Peterson HB. Risk factors for regret after tubal sterilization: 5 years of follow-up in a prospective study. Fertil Steril 1991;55:927–33.
84. Wilcox LS, Chu SY, Peterson HB. Characteristics of women who considered or obtained tubal reanastomosis: results from a prospective study of tubal sterilization. Obstet Gynecol 1990;75:661–5.
85. Neuhaus W, Bolte A. Prognostic factors for preoperative consultation of women desiring sterilization: findings of a retrospective analysis. J Psychosom Obstet Gynaecol 1995;16:45–50.
86. Boring CC, Rochat RW, Becerra J. Sterilization regret among Puerto Rican women. Fertil Steril 1988;49:973–81.
87. Borrero S, Moore CG, Qin L, et al. Unintended pregnancy influences racial disparity in tubal sterilization rates. J Gen Intern Med 2010;25:122–8.

88. Lee DM, Patton PE. Tubal Surgery and Treatment of Infertility. In: Sciarra JJ, ed. Gynecology & Obstetrics. Philadelphia: Lippincott Williams & Wilkins; 2004.
89. van Seeters JA, Chua SJ, Mol BW, Koks CA. Tubal anastomosis after previous sterilization: a systematic review. Hum Reprod Update 2017:1–13.
90. Trussell J, Guilbert E, Hedley A. Sterilization failure, sterilization reversal, and pregnancy after sterilization reversal in Quebec. Obstet Gynecol 2003;101:677–84.
91. Monteith CW, Berger GS. Normal pregnancy after outpatient tubouterine implantation in patient with Adiana sterilization. Fertil Steril 2011;96:e45–6.
92. Monteith CW, Berger GS, Zerden ML. Pregnancy success after hysteroscopic sterilization reversal. Obstet Gynecol 2014;124:1183–9.
93. Salem SA, Peck AC, Salem RD, Sills ES. Can laparoscopic removal of Essure device before embryo transfer correct poor reproductive outcome pattern in IVF? A case report. Clin Exp Obstet Gynecol 2014;41:219–22.
94. Albright CM, Frishman GN, Bhagavath B. Surgical aspects of removal of Essure micro-insert. Contraception 2013;88:334–6.
95. Bayer HealthCare Pharmaceuticals I. Essure permanent birth control: patient information booklet. Milpitas, CA: Bayer Healthcare LLC; 2016.
96. Lannon BM, Lee SY. Techniques for removal of the Essure hysteroscopic tubal occlusion device. Fertil Steril 2007;88:497 e13–4.
97. Hur HC, Mansuria SM, Chen BA, Lee TT. Laparoscopic management of hysteroscopic Essure sterilization complications: report of 3 cases. J Minim Invas Gyn 2008;15:362–5.
98. Thiel J, Suchet I, Tyson N, Price P. Outcomes in the ultrasound follow-up of the Essure micro-insert: complications and proper placement. J Obstet Gynaecol Can 2011;33:134–8.
99. Brito LG, Cohen SL, Goggins ER, Wang KC, Einarsson JI. Essure surgical removal and subsequent symptom resolution: case series and follow-up survey. J Minim Invas Gyn 2015;22:910–3.
100. American College of Obstetricians and Gynecologists. Committee Opinion No. 695: Sterilization of women: ethical issues and considerations. Obstet Gynecol 2017;129:e109–e16.
101. American College of Obstetricians and Gynecologists. Practice Bulletin No. 133: Benefits and risks of sterilization. Obstet Gynecol 2013;121:392–404.
102. Soderstrom R. Clinical challenges: share warning information, court case teaches. Contraceptive Technology Update 1981;2:8–9.
103. Sterilization of persons in federally assisted family planning projects. 42 CFR 50 Subpart B2004.
104. Borrero S, Zite N, Potter JE, Trussell J, Smith K. Potential unintended pregnancies averted and cost savings associated with a revised Medicaid sterilization policy. Contraception 2013;88:691–6.
105. Wolfe KK, Wilson MD, Hou MY, Creinin MD. An updated assessment of postpartum sterilization fulfillment after vaginal delivery. Contraception 2017;96:41–6.
106. American College of Obstetricians and Gynecologists. Committee Opinion No. 371: Sterilization of women, including those with mental disabilities. Washington, D.C.: American College of Obstetricians and Gynecologists; 2007.
107. American College of Obstetricians and Gynecologists. Committee Opinion No. 530: Access to postpartum sterilization. Obstet Gynecol 2012;120:212–5.
108. Peterson H, Warshaw J, Pollack A, Levy B. Tubal sterilization. In: Jones HW, Rock JA, eds. Te Linde's operative gynecology. 10th ed. Philadelphia: Lippincott Williams & Wilkins; 2015.
109. Practice guidelines for obstetric anesthesia: an updated report by the American Society of Anesthesiologists Task Force on Obstetric Anesthesia. Anesthesiology 2007;106:843–63.
110. Kasliwal A, Farquharson RG. Pregnancy testing prior to sterilisation. BJOG 2000;107:1407–9.
111. Akhter HH, Flock ML, Rubin GL. Safety of abortion and tubal sterilization performed separately versus concurrently. Am J Obstet Gynecol 1985;152:619–23.

112. Peterson HB, Xia Z, Wilcox LS, Tylor LR, Trussell J. Pregnancy after tubal sterilization with bipolar electrocoagulation. U.S. Collaborative Review of Sterilization Working Group. Obstet Gynecol 1999;94:163–7.
113. Dominik R, Gates D, Sokal D, et al. Two randomized controlled trials comparing the Hulka and Filshie clips for tubal sterilization. Contraception 2000;62:169–75.
114. Sokal D, Gates D, Amatya R, Dominik R. Two randomized controlled trials comparing the tubal ring and Filshie clip for tubal sterilization. Fertil Steril 2000;74:525–33.
115. Sterilization device to offer ease of use. Contraceptive Technology Update 1996;17:53–64.
116. Update on female sterilization. The Contraception Report 1996;7:13–4.
117. Chi IC. Use of multiple clips for tubal occlusion in interval laparoscopic sterilization: circumstances and consequences. Contraception 1994;50:409–16.
118. Subair O, Uku A, Amu O. Hydrosalpinx complicating routine double clip sterilisation. J Obstet Gynaecol 2004;24:942–3.
119. Creinin MD, Zite N. Female tubal sterilization: the time has come to routinely consider removal. Obstet Gynecol 2014;124:596–9.
120. Danis RB, Della Badia CR, Richard SD. Postpartum permanent sterilization: could bilateral salpingectomy replace bilateral tubal ligation? J Minim Invas Gyn 2016;23:928–32.
121. Garwood S, Reeder M, Mackenzie IZ, Guillebaud J. Tubal surface lidocaine mediates pre-emptive analgesia in awake laparoscopic sterilization: a prospective, randomized clinical trial. Am J Obstet Gynecol 2002;186:383–8.
122. Kaneshiro B, Grimes DA, Lopez LM. Pain management for tubal sterilization by hysteroscopy. Cochrane Database Syst Rev 2012:CD009251.
123. EngenderHealth. Minilaparotomy for female sterilization: An illustrated guide for providers. New York: EngenderHealth; 2003.
124. Palmer SN, Greenberg JA. Transcervical sterilization: a comparison of Essure(r) permanent birth control system and Adiana(r) permanent contraception system. Rev Obstet Gynecol 2009;2:84–92.
125. Thompson B, MacGillivray I, Fraser C. Some factors in the choice of male or female sterilisation in Aberdeen. J Biosoc Sci 1991;23:359–63.
126. Sandlow JI, Westefeld JS, Maples MR, Scheel KR. Psychological correlates of vasectomy. Fertil Steril 2001;75:544–8.
127. Cook LA, Van Vliet HA, Lopez LM, Pun A, Gallo MF. Vasectomy occlusion techniques for male sterilization. Cochrane Database Syst Rev 2014:CD003991.
128. Trussell J, Lalla AM, Doan QV, Reyes E, Pinto L, Gricar J. Cost effectiveness of contraceptives in the United States. Contraception 2009;79:5–14.
129. Alderman PM. The lurking sperm. A review of failures in 8,879 vasectomies performed by one physician. JAMA 1988;259:3142–4.
130. Poddar AK, Roy S. Disappearance of spermatozoa from semen after vasectomy. J Popul Res 1976;3:61–70.
131. Richardson DW, Aitken RJ, Loudon NB. The functional competence of human spermatozoa recovered after vasectomy. J Reprod Fertil 1984;70:575–9.
132. Nazerali H, Thapa S, Hays M, Pathak LR, Pandey KR, Sokal DC. Vasectomy effectiveness in Nepal: a retrospective study. Contraception 2003;67:397–401.
133. Jamieson DJ, Costello C, Trussell J, Hillis SD, Marchbanks PA, Peterson HB. The risk of pregnancy after vasectomy. Obstet Gynecol 2004;103:848–50.
134. Deneux-Tharaux C, Kahn E, Nazerali H, Sokal DC. Pregnancy rates after vasectomy: a survey of US urologists. Contraception 2004;69:401–6.
135. Philp T, Guillebaud J, Budd D. Complications of vasectomy: review of 16,000 patients. Br J Urol 1984;56:745–8.
136. Davies AH, Sharp RJ, Cranston D, Mitchell RG. The long-term outcome following "special clearance" after vasectomy. Br J Urol 1990;66:211–2.
137. Labrecque M, Dufresne C, Barone MA, St-Hilaire K. Vasectomy surgical techniques: a systematic review. BMC Med 2004;2:21.

138. Grimes DA, Satterthwaite AP, Rochat RW, Akhter N. Deaths from contraceptive sterilization in Bangladesh: rates, causes, and prevention. Obstet Gynecol 1982;60:635–40.
139. Grimes DA, Peterson HB, Rosenberg MJ, et al. Sterilization-attributable deaths in Bangladesh. Int J Gynaecol Obstet 1982;20:149–54.
140. Khairullah Z, Huber DH, Gonzales B. Declining mortality in international sterilization services. Int J Gynaecol Obstet 1992;39:41–50.
141. Sharlip ID, Belker AM, Honig S, et al. Vasectomy: AUA guideline. Linthicum, MD2012.
142. Klapproth HJ, Young IS. Vasectomy, vas ligation and vas occlusion. Urology 1973;1:292–300.
143. Hieu DT, Luong TT, Anh PT, Ngoc DH, Duong LQ. The acceptability, efficacy and safety of quinacrine non-surgical sterilization (QS), tubectomy and vasectomy in 5 provinces in the Red River Delta, Vietnam: a follow-up of 15,190 cases. Int J Gynaecol Obstet 2003;83 Suppl 2:S77–85.
144. Kendrick JS, Gonzales B, Huber DH, Grubb GS, Rubin GL. Complications of vasectomies in the United States. J Fam Pract 1987;25:245–8.
145. Kjersgaard AG, Thranov I, Rasmussen OV, Hertz J. Male or female sterilization: a comparative study. Fertil Steril 1989;51:439–43.
146. Rees RW. Vasectomy: problems of follow up. Proc R Soc Med 1973;66:52–4.
147. Sobrero AJ, Kohli KL. Two years' experience of an outpatient vasectomy service. Am J Public Health 1975;65:1091–4.
148. Arellano Lara S, Gonzalez Barrera JL, Hernandez Ono A, Moreno Alcazar O, Espinosa Perez J. No-scalpel vasectomy: review of the first 1,000 cases in a family medicine unit. Arch Med Res 1997;28:517–22.
149. de los Rios Osorio J, Castro Alvarez EA. [Analysis of 5000 vasectomies at a family planning clinic in Medellin-Colombia]. Arch Esp Urol 2003;56:53–60.
150. Kumar V, Kaza RM, Singh I, Singhal S, Kumaran V. An evaluation of the no-scalpel vasectomy technique. BJU Int 1999;83:283–4.
151. Sokal D, McMullen S, Gates D, Dominik R. A comparative study of the no scalpel and standard incision approaches to vasectomy in 5 countries. J Urol 1999;162:1621–5.
152. Lema VM. Fournier's gangrene complicating vasectomy. East Afr Med J 2003;80:492–6.
153. EngenderHealth. Male sterilization. Contraceptive sterilization: global issues and trends. New York: EngenderHealth; 2002:161–77.
154. Valencic M. Re: Granitsiotis P, Kirk D. Chronic testicular pain: an overview. Eur Urol 2004;45:430-6 [letter]. Eur Urol 2005;47:720.
155. Tan WP, Levine LA. An overview of the management of post-vasectomy pain syndrome. Asian J Androl 2016;18:332–7.
156. Leslie TA, Illing RO, Cranston DW, Guillebaud J. The incidence of chronic scrotal pain after vasectomy: a prospective audit. BJU Int 2007;100:1330–3.
157. Nangia AK, Myles JL, Thomas AJ. Vasectomy reversal for the post-vasectomy pain syndrome: a clinical and histological evaluation. J Urol 2000;164:1939–42.
158. Manikandan R, Srirangam SJ, Pearson E, Collins GN. Early and late morbidity after vasectomy: a comparison of chronic scrotal pain at 1 and 10 years. BJU Int 2004;93:571–4.
159. Christiansen CG, Sandlow JI. Testicular pain following vasectomy: a review of postvasectomy pain syndrome. J Androl 2003;24:293–8.
160. Granitsiotis P, Kirk D. Chronic testicular pain: an overview. Eur Urol 2004;45:430–6.
161. Chen TF, Ball RY. Epididymectomy for post-vasectomy pain: histological review. Br J Urol 1991;68:407–13.
162. Levine LA, Hoeh MP. Evaluation and management of chronic scrotal content pain. Curr Urol Rep 2015;16:36.
163. Smith A, Lyons A, Ferris J, Richters J, Pitts M, Shelley J. Are sexual problems more common in men who have had a vasectomy? A population-based study of Australian men. J Sex Med 2010;7:736–42.
164. Shain RN. Psychosocial consequences of vasectomy in developed and developing countries. In: Goldsmith A, Spieler JM, Sciearra J, Zatuchni GI, eds. Male contraception: advances and future prospects. Philadelphia: Harper and Row; 1986:34–53.

165. Hofmeyr DG, Greeff AP. The influence of a vasectomy on the marital relationship and sexual satisfaction of the married man. J Sex Marital Ther 2002;28:339–51.
166. Ghazeeri GS, Kutteh WH. Autoimmune factors in reproductive failure. Curr Opin Obstet Gynecol 2001;13:287–91.
167. Gubin DA, Dmochowski R, Kutteh WH. Multivariant analysis of men from infertile couples with and without antisperm antibodies. Am J Reprod Immunol 1998;39:157–60.
168. Petitti DB, Klein R, Kipp H, Kahn W, Siegelaub AB, Friedman GD. A survey of personal habits, symptoms of illness, and histories of disease in man with and without vasectomies. Am J Public Health 1982;72:476–80.
169. Giovannucci E, Tosteson TD, Speizer FE, Vessey MP, Colditz GA. A long-term study of mortality in men who have undergone vasectomy. N Engl J Med 1992;326:1392–8.
170. Massey FJ, Jr., Bernstein GS, O'Fallon WM, et al. Vasectomy and health. Results from a large cohort study. JAMA 1984;252:1023–9.
171. Lea IA, Adoyo P, O'Rand MG. Autoimmunogenicity of the human sperm protein Sp17 in vasectomized men and identification of linear B cell epitopes. Fertil Steril 1997;67:355–61.
172. Helmerhorst FM, Finken MJ, Erwich JJ. Antisperm antibodies: detection assays for antisperm antibodies: what do they test? Hum Reprod 1999;14:1669–71.
173. Hjort T. Antisperm antibodies. Antisperm antibodies and infertility: an unsolvable question? Hum Reprod 1999;14:2423–6.
174. Holman CD, Wisniewski ZS, Semmens JB, Rouse IL, Bass AJ. Population-based outcomes after 28,246 in-hospital vasectomies and 1,902 vasovasostomies in Western Australia. BJU Int 2000;86:1043–9.
175. Pitaktepsombati P, Janowitz B. Sterilization acceptance and regret in Thailand. Contraception 1991;44:623–37.
176. Potts JM, Pasqualotto FF, Nelson D, Thomas AJ, Jr., Agarwal A. Patient characteristics associated with vasectomy reversal. J Urol 1999;161:1835–9.
177. Ehn BE, Liljestrand J. A long-term follow-up of 108 vasectomized men. Good counselling routines are important. Scand J Urol Nephrol 1995;29:477–81.
178. Miller WB, Shain RN, Pasta DJ. The pre- and poststerilization predictors of poststerilization regret in husbands and wives. J Nerv Ment Dis 1991;179:602–8.
179. Belker AM, Thomas AJ, Jr., Fuchs EF, Konnak JW, Sharlip ID. Results of 1,469 microsurgical vasectomy reversals by the Vasovasostomy Study Group. J Urol 1991;145:505–11.
180. Tanrikut C, Goldstein M. Obstructive azoospermia: a microsurgical success story. Semin Reprod Med 2009;27:159–64.
181. Donovan JF, Jr., DiBaise M, Sparks AE, Kessler J, Sandlow JI. Comparison of microscopic epididymal sperm aspiration and intracytoplasmic sperm injection/in-vitro fertilization with repeat microscopic reconstruction following vasectomy: Is second attempt vas reversal worth the effort? Hum Reprod 1998;13:387–93.
182. Practice Committee of the American Society for Reproductive Medicine. Vasectomy reversal. Fertil Steril 2004;82 Suppl 1:S194–8.
183. Nagler HM, Jung H. Factors predicting successful microsurgical vasectomy reversal. Urol Clin North Am 2009;36:383–90.
184. Lee HY. A 20-year experience with vasovasostomy. J Urol 1986;136:413–5.
185. Pollack AP, Barone MA. Reversing vasectomy. In: Sciarra JJ, ed. Gynecology & obstetrics. Philadelphia: Lippincot Williams & Wilkins; 2000.
186. Borges EJ, Rossi-Ferragut LM, Pasqualoto FF, Rocha CC, Iaconelli AJ. Different intervals between vasectomy and sperm retrieval interfere in the reproductive capacity from vasectomized men. J Assist Reprod Genet 2003;20:33–7.
187. Kolettis PN, Thomas AJ, Jr. Vasoepididymostomy for vasectomy reversal: a critical assessment in the era of intracytoplasmic sperm injection. J Urol 1997;158:467–70.
188. Fuchs EF, Burt RA. Vasectomy reversal performed 15 years or more after vasectomy: correlation of pregnancy outcome with partner age and with pregnancy results of in vitro fertilization with intracytoplasmic sperm injection. Fertil Steril 2002;77:516–9.

189. Sukcharoen N, Sithipravej T, Promviengchai S, Chinpilas V, Boonkasemsanti W. No differences in outcome of surgical sperm retrieval with intracytoplasmic sperm injection at different intervals after vasectomy. Fertil Steril 2000;74:174–5.

190. Pasqualotto FF, Lucon AM, Sobreiro BP, Pasqualotto EB, Arap S. The best infertility treatment for vasectomized men: assisted reproduction or vasectomy reversal? Rev Hosp Clin Fac Med Sao Paulo 2004;59:312–5.

191. Robb P, Sandlow JI. Cost-effectiveness of vasectomy reversal. Urol Clin North Am 2009;36:391–6.

192. Li SQ, Goldstein M, Zhu J, Huber D. The no-scalpel vasectomy. J Urol 1991;145:341–4.

193. EngenderHealth. No-scalpel vasectomy: an illustrated guide for surgeons. 3rd ed. New York: EngenderHealth; 2003.

194. Cook LA, Pun A, Gallo MF, Lopez LM, Van Vliet HA. Scalpel versus no-scalpel incision for vasectomy. Cochrane Database Syst Rev 2014:CD004112.

195. Chen KC. A novel instrument-independent no-scalpel vasectomy - a comparative study against the standard instrument-dependent no-scalpel vasectomy. Int J Androl 2004;27:222–7.

196. Jones JS. Percutaneous vasectomy: a simple modification eliminates the steep learning curve of no-scalpel vasectomy. J Urol 2003;169:1434–6.

197. Marmar JL, Kessler S, Hartanto VH. A minimally invasive vasectomy with the no suture, inline method for vas occlusion. Int J Fertil Womens Med 2001;46:257–64.

198. Moon HJ. Minimally invasive vas surgery using a newly designed double-ringed clamp. World J Urol 2010;28:205–8.

199. Barone MA, Irsula B, Chen-Mok M, Sokal DC. Effectiveness of vasectomy using cautery. BMC Urol 2004;4:10.

200. Sokal D, Irsula B, Chen-Mok M, Labrecque M, Barone MA. A comparison of vas occlusion techniques: cautery more effective than ligation and excision with fascial interposition. BMC Urol 2004;4:12.

201. Sokal D, Irsula B, Hays M, Chen-Mok M, Barone MA. Vasectomy by ligation and excision, with or without fascial interposition: a randomized controlled trial [ISRCTN77781689]. BMC Med 2004;2:6.

202. Shapiro EI, Silber SJ. Open-ended vasectomy, sperm granuloma, and postvasectomy orchialgia. Fertil Steril 1979;32:546–50.

203. Song L, Gu Y, Lu W, Liang X, Chen Z. A phase II randomized controlled trial of a novel male contraception, an intra-vas device. Int J Androl 2006;29:489–95.

204. Black T, Francome C. Comparison of Marie Stopes scalpel and electrocautery no-scalpel vasectomy techniques. J Fam Plann Reprod Health Care 2003;29:32–4.

205. Wolf JS, Jr., Bennett CJ, Dmochowski RR, et al. Best practice policy statement on urologic surgery antimicrobial prophylaxis. J Urol 2008;179:1379–90.

206. Lemack GE, Goldstein M. Presence of sperm in the pre-vasectomy reversal semen analysis: incidence and implications. J Urol 1996;155:167–9.

207. Labrecque M, St-Hilaire K, Turcot L. Delayed vasectomy success in men with a first postvasectomy semen analysis showing motile sperm. Fertil Steril 2005;83:1435–41.

208. Barone MA, Nazerali H, Cortes M, Chen-Mok M, Pollack AE, Sokal D. A prospective study of time and number of ejaculations to azoospermia after vasectomy by ligation and excision. J Urol 2003;170:892–6.

209. World Health Organization. Selected Practice Recommendations for Contraceptive Use. 3rd ed. Geneva: World Health Organization; 2016.

Contraception after Pregnancy

17

Kathy Irene Kennedy, DrPH, MA
Crystal Goldsmith, MD, MS

- Breast milk is the ideal source of nutrition for infants and confers immunological protection against many infections. It reduces the risk of some chronic diseases and includes factors that support growth. Family planning clinicians can play an important role in promoting breastfeeding.
- The Lactational Amenorrhea Method (LAM) can be an effective, *temporary* method of contraception. To maintain effective protection against pregnancy, another method of contraception must be used as soon as menstruation resumes, the frequency or duration of breastfeeds is reduced, bottle feeds or regular food supplements are introduced, or the baby reaches 6 months of age.
- Other good contraceptive options for breastfeeding women are (1) barrier methods, such as the male or female condom, which also confer protection against sexually transmitted infections; (2) the Copper T 380A intrauterine device (IUD); (3) *progestin-only* methods such as the progestin-only pill, Nexplanon or Depo-Provera, or one of the levonorgestrel IUDs; and (4) the permanent contraceptive methods of fallopian tube surgery and vasectomy for individuals or couples who do not want more children.
- The *combined hormonal methods*—pills, patches, injectables, or vaginal rings—are not good early contraceptive options for breastfeeding mothers because side effects include lowering milk supply.
- HIV can be transmitted through breastmilk. Therefore, in the United States, where safe alternatives to breastmilk are available, HIV-infected mothers are advised to avoid breastfeeding.

After childbirth, the recommended period before attempting the next pregnancy is at least 24 months.[1] However, and especially if not exclusively breastfeeding, a mother soon becomes capable of becoming pregnant again since the postpartum period of infertility may be brief and varies greatly across individuals. Although the breastfeeding mother will have a longer period of infertility than will the nonbreastfeeding one, fertility usually returns as the frequency of breastfeeds decreases. As the frequency of breastfeeds decreases, the mother should use a contraceptive method so as to breastfeed for as long as desired before becoming pregnant again. Fortunately, most family planning methods are compatible with breastfeeding, and the provider can play an important role in promoting both contraception and breastfeeding. In addition to helping to devise a postpartum plan for contraception, the provider can ensure that the mother has several breastfeeding sessions observed by an experienced lactation specialist before hospital discharge after delivery (see Figure 17-1[2]). Human milk is the ideal source

Clinical guidelines for the establishment of exclusive breastfeeding

1. Keep mothers and infants skin-to-skin until after the first breastfeeding.
2. Help mothers and infants achieve a comfortable position and an effective latch (attachment).
3. Keep the mother and infant together during the entire postpartum stay.
4. Teach mothers to recognize and respond to early infant feeding cues and confirm that their infants are being fed at least 8 times a day.
5. Confirm that mothers understand milk production, and the importance of milk removal.
6. Confirm that mothers are able to wake a sleepy infant.
7. Avoid using pacifiers (dummies) until breastfeeding is well established, unless medically indicated.
8. Avoid the use of artificial nipples (teats) and supplements unless medically indicated.
9. Observe and document at least one breastfeeding in each 8-hour period during the postpartum stay.
10. Assess mothers and infants for signs of effective breastfeeding, and intervene if milk transfer is inadequate.
11. Identify maternal and infant risk factors that may impact the ability to breastfeed effectively, and provide appropriate assistance, follow-up, and referral.
12. Identify any maternal and infant contraindications to breastfeeding.
13. If medically indicated, provide additional nutrition using a supplementation method that is least likely to compromise the transition to exclusive breastfeeding.
14. Confirm that infants have a scheduled appointment with a skilled health care provider within 5 to 7 days of age or 48-72 hours after discharge from the birthing facility. Provide mothers with contact information for breastfeeding resources in their community.
15. Provide appropriate education materials for mothers/families.
16. Support exclusive breastfeeding during any illness or hospitalization of mothers or infants.
17. Comply with the *International Code of Marketing of Breast-milk Substitutes* and subsequent resolutions.
18. Include family members or significant others in breastfeeding education.
19. Provide anticipatory guidance for common problems that can interfere with exclusive breastfeeding.
20. Confirm that mothers have realistic expectations regarding normal breastfed infant behaviors.
21. Discuss contraceptive options and their possible effect on milk production.

Source: International Lactation Consultant Association (2014).[2] Reprinted with permission.

Figure 17-1

of nutrition for infants and confers immunological protection against many infections. Health experts around the globe have declared that all mothers should be supported to breastfeed exclusively for 6 months, and to continue to breastfeed for a year or longer[3–11] and to have access to family planning information and services that allow them to sustain breastfeeding.[12]

POSTPARTUM INFERTILITY

During pregnancy, cyclic ovarian function is suspended. The corpus luteum, which arises from the ovulated follicle, secretes steroids, including estrogen and progesterone, that are essential in maintaining the early weeks of pregnancy. Later, steroids secreted by the placenta emerge to play a more dominant role in the hormonal support of the pregnancy. Luteal and placental steroids suppress the mother's circulating levels of follicle stimulating hormone (FSH) and luteinizing hormone (LH) but more importantly disrupt their pulsatile release from her pituitary.[13] When the placenta is delivered, the inhibiting effects of estrogen and progesterone are removed so that levels of FSH and LH gradually rise and the pituitary resumes the pulsatile release of FSH and LH.[14]

Most nonlactating women resume menses within 4 to 6 weeks of delivery, but about one third of first cycles are anovulatory, and a high proportion of first ovulatory cycles have a deficient corpus luteum that secretes subnormal amounts of steroids. In the second and third menstrual cycles, 15% are anovulatory and 25% of ovulatory cycles have luteal-phase defects. On average, the first ovulation occurs 45 days postpartum, although few first ovulations are followed by normal luteal phases.[15] The duration of postpartum infertility is variable and unpredictable.

LACTATIONAL INFERTILITY

Breastfeeding further extends the period of infertility and suppresses ovarian function.[16] Plasma levels of FSH return to normal follicular phase values by 4 to 8 weeks postpartum in breastfeeding women.[17] In contrast, LH pulsation is disorganized in terms of the frequency or the amplitude of the LH pulse in the majority of lactating women throughout most of the period of lactational amenorrhea.[18]

The mother's nipple and areola sensitivity increases at birth.[19] Infant suckling stimulates the nerve endings in the nipple and areola. Nerve impulses are passed to the hypothalamus, stimulating the release of various hormones, including prolactin. Prolactin controls the rate of milk production but is not believed to play a major role in suppressing ovarian function.[20] Instead, suckling appears to disrupt the pulsatile release of gonadotropin releasing hormone (GnRH) by the hypothalamus,[17] perhaps by increasing hypothalamic β-endorphin production.[21] The disruption of GnRH release in turn averts the normal pulsatility of LH, which is required for follicle stimulation in the ovary. Small amounts of secreted estrogen at this time are insufficient to trigger an LH surge necessary to induce ovulation.[17,22]

Ovulation can occur even though the breastfeeding mother has not yet resumed menstruation. Only about 60% of ovulations preceding first menses have an adequate luteal phase.[23] Lactational amenorrhea becomes increasingly unreliable as an indicator of infertility beyond 6 months postpartum. The probability that ovulation will precede the first menses increases over time:[23,24]

- 33% to 45% during the first 3 months postpartum
- 64% to 71% during months 4 through 12
- 87% to 100% after 12 months.

Full or nearly full (unsupplemented) breastfeeding is associated with longer periods of lactational amenorrhea and infertility than is combination feeding (formula and human milk). Frequent stimulation of the breast by suckling day and night helps maintain the cascade of neuroendocrine events that produces the contraceptive effect.[25] The breastfeeding characteristics that contribute significantly to delay the return of ovulation include a high frequency of breastfeeds, a long total duration of feedings, a short interval between breastfeeds, and the presence of night feeds.[24,26]

CONTRACEPTIVE BENEFITS OF LACTATION

In both traditional societies and developing countries, lactation plays a major role in prolonging birth intervals and thereby reducing fertility.[27] In developed countries, however, breastfeeding has a much smaller contraceptive effect because proportionately fewer infants are breastfed, and those who are breastfed are completely weaned at earlier ages. For example, in Indonesia, 96% of infants are breastfed, and those who are breastfed are not completely weaned until they are 2 years old on average.[28] In contrast, in the United States, only 81% of infants are ever breastfed with only 31% still breastfeeding at 1 year.[29] Work outside the home is a major barrier to breastfeeding in the United States and around the world. Although some protections for working mothers in the United States were created by the 2010 Patient Protection and Affordable Care Act, there is far from universal support for breastfeeding in the context of paid and unpaid work.[30]

The Lactational Amenorrhea Method (LAM) of Contraception

Women who breastfeed can learn to make use of breastfeeding's natural contraceptive effect. If the woman feeds her infant only from her breast and has not experienced her first postpartum menses (defined as any bleeding occurring after 56 days postpartum), then breastfeeding provides more than 98% protection from pregnancy in the first 6 months following a birth.[25,31,32] (See Figures 17-2 and 17-3.) The Lactational Amenorrhea Method (LAM) is the proactive application of exclusive breastfeeding during lactational amenorrhea for the first 6 months after delivery. Four prospective clinical studies of the contraceptive effect of LAM demonstrated a cumulative 6-month life-table perfect-use probability of pregnancy ranging from 0.5% to 1.5% among women who relied solely on LAM.[33–36] While pregnancy rates during the use of LAM compare favorably with those for many other methods of contraception

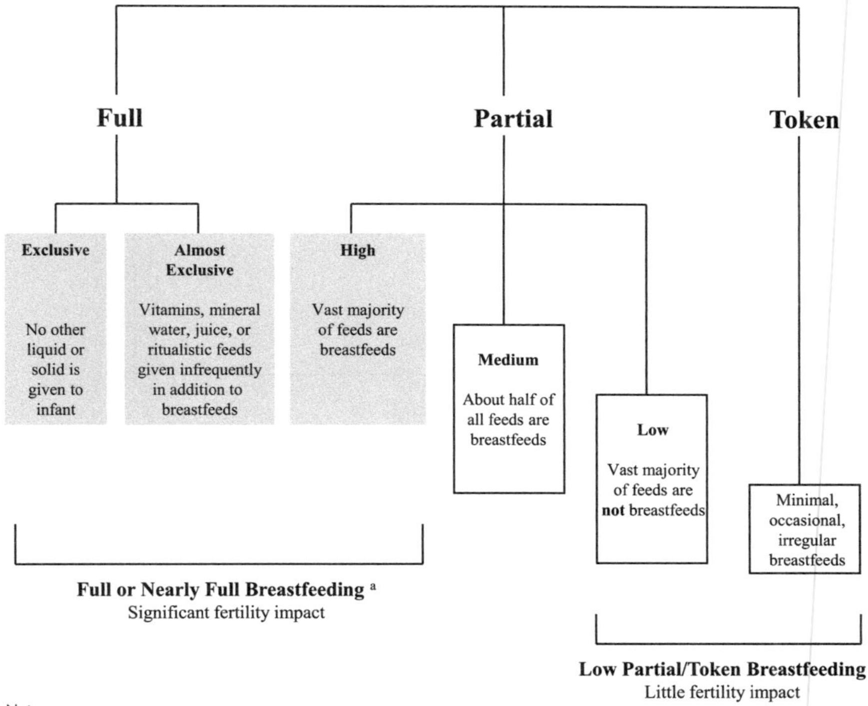

Notes:

[a]Intervals should not exceed 4 hours during the day and 6 hours at night; supplementation should not exceed 5 to 15% of all feeding episodes, preferably fewer. While the high-partial pattern is adequate for fertility suppression, counsel the mother that any supplementation or disruption of the breastfeeding pattern can increase the risk of fertility return.

Source: Labbok et al. (1994).[31]

Figure 17-2 Schema for breastfeeding definition

Ask the mother, or advise her to ask herself, these four questions:

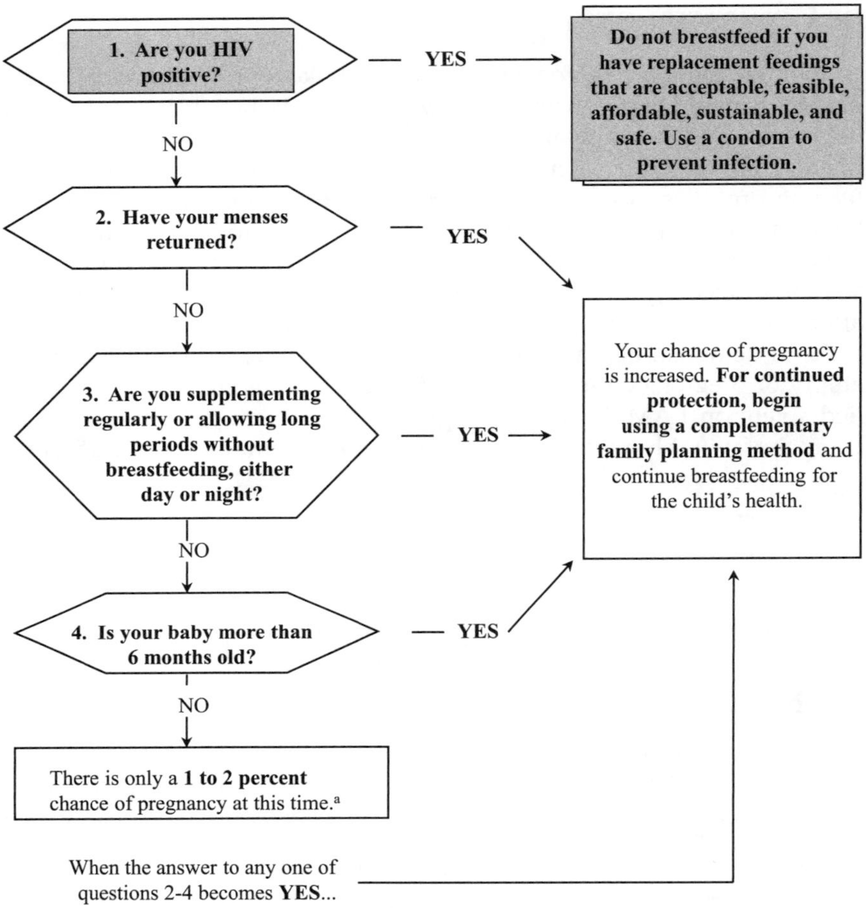

Notes:

[a]However, the mother may choose to use a complementary family planning method *at any time*.

Source: Adapted from Labbok et al. (1994).[31]

Figure 17-3 LAM: Lactational Amenorrhea Method

(see Chapter 26 on Contraceptive Efficacy), even greater efficacy could be achieved by a combination of breastfeeding and use of an additional method of contraception.

LAM requires "full or nearly full" breastfeeding because the infant who obtains nearly all nutritional requirements through breastfeeding is providing maximal suckling stimulation at the breast. As long as additional foods do not decrease this optimal amount of suckling, small amounts of supplementation should have little or no effect on the return of fertility. Thus, if LAM is to be used, supplements should be given only infrequently, in small amounts, and not by bottle. The only real challenge concerning the correct use of LAM is determining the allowable extent of supplementation to the infant's diet, if the mother wishes to supplement. Figure 17-2 defines different infant feeding patterns and can be helpful in determining whether the woman is fully or nearly fully breastfeeding.[31,37] *Milk expression, such as by hand or pump, is not a substitute for breastfeeding in terms of its fertility inhibiting effect.* A study of LAM used by working women reported an elevated 6-month probability of pregnancy (5.2%) indicating that frequent suckling, despite adequate milk production and full breastfeeding, is necessary to acquire the optimal benefits of LAM.[38]

Experience with LAM in the United States is limited. Nursing about every 3 hours is a key part of LAM; therefore, for many mothers needing to return to work—often within a few weeks postpartum—this makes LAM unrealistic. It is unknown whether more women would breastfeed if they appreciated the contraceptive effect of breastfeeding (or the other benefits of breastfeeding). Some U.S. women are already highly motivated to breastfeed, and they would be good candidates to use LAM as a temporary contraceptive option.[39] Women who choose to use LAM are basically choosing to fully or nearly fully breastfeed for at least some period (up to 6 months), so the choice to use LAM should be associated with the motivation to maintain frequent and exclusive breastfeeding. In the United States, LAM may be best promoted in the context of breastfeeding support (from the healthcare system, friends, employers), which facilitates full/nearly full breastfeeding and maximizes the duration of amenorrhea[40] and the duration for which women can use LAM.

If a woman wishes to avoid becoming pregnant when LAM protection ends, then she must begin to use another contraceptive method at that time.[41,42] Alternative contraception should be provided to women choosing LAM so that they are prepared when they need it.

POSTPARTUM SEXUALITY

A review of the return to sexual activity and intercourse postpartum indicates that many women resume sexual intercourse within several weeks of delivery.[43] In small samples of breastfeeding Western women, monthly coital frequency in the second month postpartum averaged 2.4, increasing to 3.2 to 4.9 in the third postpartum month.[44]

Contraception is only one counseling issue for postpartum women. Parents of newborns may experience reduced sexual feelings associated with bodily changes caused by pregnancy and delivery (even for the partner who had not been pregnant). Discussion of these bodily changes may help to alleviate a couple's anxiety:

- Tenderness in the perineum may make intercourse painful, especially if there has been an episiotomy.

- Reduced postpartum estrogen secretion may result in diminished vaginal lubrication and elasticity.
- Most women experience a heavy and bloody lochial discharge for about a month although it is not uncommon after 6 weeks postpartum.[45] This may interfere with sexual feeling.
- Couples may find that the exhaustion caused by the around-the-clock responsibilities of being a new parent temporarily decreases sexual drive.
- Lactation may diminish the erotic significance of the breasts. It is not uncommon for mothers to experience milk leakage during intimacy. Couples need to communicate feelings about whether sucking or touching the breasts is acceptable.
- Bonding between mother and child creates skills and commitment in the mother and trust and security in the infant but may interfere with the mother's emotional availability to her partner.
- Conversely, a birth (especially if planned) can be an exceedingly joyous experience that can enhance sexual intimacy. To some men and women, the shape or fullness of the lactating breast is particularly arousing.

INITIATING CONTRACEPTIVE USE POSTPARTUM

Counseling for postpartum contraception should begin in the prenatal period because many methods can be provided at the time of delivery or during the hospital stay, including progestin-only methods, intrauterine contraception, and female tubal surgery for permanent contraception. (See Chapter 2 for more complete discussion of patient-centered contraception counseling.) For these methods provided immediately upon delivery, it is important to plan in advance, preferably in the prenatal period, so informed choice is valid, and method choice and initiation are uncomplicated, convenient, and cost-effective. Insured and uninsured patients encounter several barriers in accessing postpartum contraception. Many women may not be able to attend a postpartum visit, either due to lack of healthcare coverage or challenges reaching the clinic. For those women who are able to attend postpartum visits, billing requirements, insurance approvals, and failure to stock contraceptive devices in clinics insure that many patients will need to return for multiple return visits in order to initiate longer-acting contraceptive methods. These hurdles illustrate the need for providers to be well educated regarding the safety and ease of initiating postpartum contraception.

Traditionally, a postpartum follow-up consultation occurred at 6 weeks because the uterus had mostly involuted and healed by this time, allowing for fitting of a diaphragm or cervical cap. However, a physical exam can reasonably occur at any time between 2 and 8 weeks postpartum.[46,47] In terms of contraceptive service delivery, routine adherence to the 6-week convention does not seem appropriate.[48] Therefore an individual approach to timing postpartum follow-up and contraceptive initiation is indicated. Although nearly all contraceptive methods can be used postpartum, the methods vary in terms of when in the postpartum period they should be initiated:[49,50]

- 6 weeks is too late to begin contraception for nonbreastfeeding mothers who wish to start using oral contraceptives, the patch, the vaginal ring, Nexplanon, or Depo-Provera.
- 2 weeks is too soon for fitting a diaphragm and may be earlier than patients desire IUD placement.
- If the couple has been unable to select a contraceptive method by the time of hospital discharge, they should plan a postpartum visit for 3 weeks.

When the couple's method of choice cannot be initiated during the hospital stay after delivery, they can choose temporary methods such as LAM, the brief interim use of condoms, or progestin-only pills and plan to initiate a longer-term method later. Schedule the first postpartum visit for the most logical time based on the specific woman's needs and plans for a longer-term method. For example, if a breastfeeding patient will be using the Copper T380A IUD (and did not receive one within 10 minutes of the delivery of the placenta), schedule a follow-up visit for 4 weeks postpartum, with the plan for using condoms, progestin-only pills or LAM until that time. Perhaps most important, contact the patient 1 to 4 weeks after delivery to check on postpartum recovery and breastfeeding success, and to confirm and support the success of the chosen contraception plan.

A systematic review of the research on the effectiveness of targeted postpartum counseling for contraception found that postpartum education results in more contraceptive use and fewer unplanned pregnancies compared to standard care.[51] As mentioned above, antenatal counseling is essential for informed choice for the immediate postpartum use of long-acting reversible and permanent methods. Individuals appear to be open and interested in family planning information at a variety of times, and their personal circumstances and opinions undoubtedly change over time as well. Thus, strategies for counseling before and after delivery, during the hospital stay, and after delivery, including with the infant's physician,[52] all have their place. We should not be limited to conventional approaches when considering the best time and place to reach couples regarding their needs for contraception.

The following considerations may prove useful when counseling and providing contraceptives to postpartum patients, whether or not they are breastfeeding:

- *Withdrawal* may be an acceptable method for couples in the postpartum period. Withdrawal is effective if used correctly and consistently. (See Chapter 15.)
- *Condoms* are an attractive option. They are readily available and do not require a medical practitioner for initiation. (See Chapter 14.)
- *Diaphragm and sponge* use may need to be delayed:
  - — The perineum may still be tender. Fitting a diaphragm may cause discomfort.
  - — Avoid the diaphragm and contraceptive sponge until 6 weeks after delivery. The diaphragm cannot be (re)fitted properly until that time. Moreover, the risk of toxic shock syndrome is increased when blood, including the postpartum lochia, is present.[53] (See Chapter 11.)
  - — The sponge (though not the diaphragm) has much higher failure rates among women who have delivered a child than among women who have not, *even during perfect use.* (See Chapter 11.) Inform women about this substantial decrease in efficacy for parous women so they can make an informed choice of a contraceptive method.
- *Postpartum abstinence,* if practiced properly, is 100% effective in preventing pregnancy. It can, however, be notoriously difficult to maintain. Counsel women about other contraceptive methods should they desire to resume intercourse. (See Chapter 13.)
- *Most progestin-only methods,* such as progestin-only pills, injectables, and contraceptive implants, have been deemed safe for immediate postpartum use. Progestin-only methods are not associated with increased risk for venous thromboembolism (VTE), as are estrogen-containing methods, and have been shown to have little impact on lactation.[49,54,55]
- *Intrauterine devices (IUDs)* are best inserted postpartum, either (1) immediately (within 10 minutes) after the expulsion of the placenta, or (2) after 4 weeks postpartum. It is less desirable to insert an IUD in the period between because of the high expulsion rate that occurs during uterine involution. However, more recent studies suggest the safety and acceptability of IUD insertion less than 4 weeks postpartum.[46,47] An IUD can be inserted during a cesarean delivery through the uterine incision prior to closure. IUD insertion should not be performed when chorioamnionitis

is present because of the elevated risk of infection.[56] Immediate postpartum insertion has not been associated with excessive bleeding or endometritis.[57] Expulsion rates following immediate postpartum insertion are higher than those following interval insertion 4 to 6 weeks postpartum or later. One small pilot study has examined expulsion rates in women receiving an immediate postplacental IUD after vaginal compared to cesarean birth and found that risk of expulsion was much greater following vaginal birth.[58] Subsequent studies report lower expulsion rates when an IUD is placed after cesarean birth when compared to placement after a vaginal birth.[59–61] Additionally, one study suggests that the LNG IUD demonstrates a greater risk of expulsion when placed immediately postpartum with compared to the Cu IUD. [62]

- *Permanent contraception* presents an option for appropriate candidates:
  - Vasectomy is an appropriate postpartum choice for couples who want a permanent method. As soon as the health of the mother and infant is determined to be sound, the vasectomy can be performed. If the woman is exclusively breastfeeding, a back-up method may not be needed while waiting for confirmation that the vasectomy has taken effect. As with tubal ligation, vasectomy requires counseling and reflection under nonstressful circumstances, preferably before delivery.
  - Tubal ligation (or salpingectomy) performed during the immediate postpartum period can be a more cost-effective and simpler technique than interval sterilization. While tubal ligation is a highly effective method of contraception, a small risk of sterilization failure persists for at least a decade. Partial salpingectomy performed postpartum, however, carries a very low 10-year pregnancy risk.[63] Discuss immediate postpartum contraceptive surgery well before the delivery to help ensure that consent is fully informed, since the decision to undergo permanent contraceptive surgery during the postpartum period is a risk factor for regret.[64,65] (See Chapter 16 on Permanent Contraception.) After a vaginal delivery, fallopian tube surgery should be performed by minilaparotomy within 48 hours or else delayed for 4 to 6 weeks. After 48 hours, access to the tubes is reduced and the risk of infection increased.[66] Tubal ligation can be performed through the abdominal incision after a cesarean delivery. As with minilaparotomy after vaginal delivery, cesarean sterilization may need to be delayed in the case of complications, such as severe pre-eclampsia, eclampsia, sepsis, severe hemorrhage, uterine rupture or perforation.[67] (If a vaginally-delivered woman who

intends to breastfeed chooses contraceptive fallopian tube surgery, then the procedure should be performed after the first hour of skin-to-skin contact with the neonate (known as the "golden hour"), including the first suckling episode, to prevent the disruption of breastfeeding.)[68]

Postpartum Contraception for the Nonbreastfeeding Woman

If she wishes to avoid becoming pregnant, the nonbreastfeeding woman should begin using a contraceptive method immediately postpartum or at least by the beginning of the fourth postpartum week.[48] Most nonbreastfeeding mothers have few restrictions placed on which method of contraceptive they can choose. Nonetheless, a few guidelines—in addition to those given above—are warranted:

- Combined oral contraceptives (COCs) and the combined patch, injectable, and vaginal ring (all of which contain estrogen and progesterone) may be *prescribed* immediately postpartum. However, caution women not to use them until at least 3 full weeks after delivery.[49,50] The risk of postpartum thrombophlebitis and thromboembolism in the postpartum period is 5 times the risk during pregnancy, and remains elevated through at least the 6th postpartum week.[69] Some leaders in the field advise postponing the initiation of COCs until 4 weeks[70] to 6.5 weeks postpartum,[50] and since COCs may increase the risk of venous thromboembolic disease 2 to 4 fold,[71] even up to 12 weeks postpartum.[72]
- Caution women that it is difficult to practice fertility awareness before their cycles are reestablished and cyclic signs of fertility return.
- Suggest that lubricated condoms are a good option at least for the short period before the woman becomes better suited to her preferred method.
- Nexplanon can be inserted and Depo-Provera injections can be safely initiated immediately postpartum. Discuss these options before delivery to ensure that consent is fully informed.

Initiating Contraceptive Use After Early Pregnancy Failure

Little research has been done in the area of contraceptive uptake following miscarriage. It is known that following miscarriage, fertility returns within 1 to 4 weeks.[73,74] The mean number of days to ovulation was 28, although patients may experience ovulation as early as 6 days after miscarriage. This does not appear to differ by gestational age at time of miscarriage.

The World Health Organization (WHO) recommends delaying subsequent pregnancy for 6 months following miscarriage, though this is guidance not based on studies of birth intervals following miscarriage. A recent cohort study compared patients conceiving in 0 to 3 months compared to >3 months after pregnancy loss of up to 20 weeks and found higher live birth rates among women conceiving within 3 months of pregnancy loss, with no difference in the incidence of repeat miscarriage.[75]

While one may assume that a patient experiencing miscarriage may not need contraception, there are many instances in which is it desirable. First, women who have had a miscarriage may not desire future pregnancy. Approximately one third of unintended pregnancies end in miscarriage.[76] Second, women experiencing miscarriage may need to grieve prior to conceiving again. This is particularly true among patients with multiple prior miscarriages and women at greater gestational age at the time of loss.[77] Contraception allows an opportunity to process the emotional burden of miscarriage prior to another pregnancy. Third, initiation and use of contraception after miscarriage provides an opportunity to medically optimize patients who have conditions associated with a high risk of miscarriage (such as diabetes, obesity, and hypertension.) Therefore, all individuals experiencing miscarriage should be counseled on contraceptive options following pregnancy loss. All contraceptive methods (including estrogen-containing methods) can safely be initiated immediately after first- or second-trimester miscarriage with the exception of standard contraindications (noted in Center for Disease Control and Prevention's 2016 Medical Eligibility Criteria for Contraceptive Use (MEC). (See the MEC summary chart insert in this book.) For example, an IUD placement should be delayed 3 months in the setting of septic abortion.[49]

Postpartum Contraception for the Breastfeeding Woman

Nonhormonal Methods

General comments regarding contraceptive use among postpartum women are given above. In addition, the following considerations are relevant for women who are breastfeeding. Breastfeeding is a condition for which there is no restriction on the use of nonhormonal methods.[49,50]

Tubal ligation can be performed immediately postpartum, although it can disrupt lactation if it requires general anesthesia or separation of mother and infant. Both problems can be minimized by performing the procedure with only regional or local anesthetic.[78] If tubal ligation does not occur while the mother is undergoing a cesarean delivery, it should be delayed until after the initial hour postpartum to allow for breastfeeding and family bonding. Breastfeeding should occur just before the mother leaves for the operating room for the procedure.[68] Regional anesthesia is preferred. Breastfeeding should be delayed immediately after the procedure until the mother is awake and alert to reduce the transfer of the anesthetic agent to the infant.[79] As soon as the mother is awake enough to hold her baby, it is safe for her to breastfeed.

The Copper T 380A IUD is also a good choice for breastfeeding women. The copper on the Copper T does not affect the quantity or quality of breastmilk.[80] (See the following section on Hormonal Methods for information on IUDs containing a progestin.) Some women experience mild uterine cramping when they breastfeed with an IUD in place, but the cramping does not usually interfere with lactation or with the effectiveness of the IUD. IUD placement is less painful, and pain and bleeding removal rates are lower, for the lactating mother. While uncommon, the risk of uterine perforation is higher among breastfeeding than nonbreastfeeding women (6.3/1,000 for LNG IUD and 3.7/1,000 for Cu IUD).[81] (See Chapter 5 on Intrauterine Devices.)

Spermicides and barrier methods have no effect on the ability to breastfeed. The lubricated condom is especially useful in the postpartum period because of increased vaginal dryness. Spermicides also may help offset dryness due to estrogen deficiency. In the United States, barrier methods are the most widely used contraceptive among lactating mothers in the first 6 months postpartum.[43] In animal studies, nonoxynol-9 is absorbed through the skin and secreted in breastmilk.[82] The question of whether nonoxynol-9 is secreted in breastmilk has not been completely evaluated in humans. (See Chapter 11 on Vaginal Barriers and Spermicides.)

Lactational Amenorrhea Method (LAM) provides effective protection against pregnancy for up to 6 months postpartum. If continued protection is desired, another method of contraception must be introduced when the LAM criteria indicate a return to the risk of pregnancy. It is useful and acceptable to many women to have a back-up method on hand to begin when any of the LAM criteria no longer apply. (See the detailed description of LAM earlier in this chapter.)

Fertility awareness methods can be difficult to use during the return of fertility, which can extend for many cycles during lactation.[83] The couple needs to abstain for 2 weeks in order to establish a "basic infertile pattern" of cervical mucus (and other) symptoms. Intercourse can then occur every other night unless/until there is some change in the basic infertile pattern, in which case more abstinence is necessary.[84] The changing fertility symptoms after the first postpartum menses may be especially difficult for new users to identify, and may lead to an increased risk for unplanned pregnancy.[85]

Basal body temperature cannot be ascertained unless a woman has at least 6 hours of uninterrupted sleep. Thus, the woman who gets up in the night to care for her infant is precluded from using the temperature symptom to help determine her fertility status.

The rules for using the symptothermal method during breastfeeding have been found to detect the onset of true fertility extremely well. However, these same rules often necessitate many days of abstinence when there is virtually no risk of pregnancy.[86] Recommend LAM to users of fertility awareness methods who are breastfeeding. LAM can eliminate the requirements for abstinence for up to 6 months with no apparent additional risk of unplanned pregnancy.[87] The transition from LAM use to the use of a fertility awareness method begins with the establishment of a basic infertile pattern.[85,87]

Hormonal Methods

Use of hormonal contraception in the postpartum period has been an area of intense research in an effort to balance the benefits of breastfeeding with the risks of unintended or short interval pregnancy. In 2016, the CDC revised the MEC to reflect the general safety of progestin-only methods in the immediate postpartum period, even among breastfeeding women.[49] These recommendations differ from the WHO MEC, (which are more conservative due to theoretical concerns about exposure of the neonate to exogenous steroids since all steroids pass through the breastmilk to the infant,)[50] and from the guidance of the Academy for Breastfeeding Medicine.[88]

It is important to consider not just epidemiologic data regarding the safety of hormonal contraception in the postpartum period, but also the individual characteristics of the patient when selecting a contraceptive method in the postpartum period. While is important to provide the full range of contraceptive methods available in the postpartum period, it is equally important to practice patient-centered counseling. This includes a complete discussion about the risks (including possible effects on breastmilk) and benefits.

Progestin-only contraceptives such as Nexplanon, the LNG IUD, Depo-Provera, and progestin-only pills do not have adverse effects on lactation, and some studies suggest they may even increase milk volume. They do not appear to have adverse effects on infant growth and development.[89,90] In addition, their contraceptive efficacy is high (see Chapter 26), and they are simple to use. Therefore, these methods are good options for breastfeeding women who wish to postpone a subsequent pregnancy. The U.S. CDC advises that progestin-only methods can be used in the first month postpartum as the advantages generally outweigh the risks during breastfeeding.[49]

The precipitous withdrawal of natural progesterone, usually 30 to 40 hours after birth, triggers the production of copious amounts of mature milk (although the mother may not perceive breast fullness for 50 to 73 hours), and the related changes in milk composition are largely completed by 72 hours.[91] Yet, most studies of the immediate postpartum use of progestin-only implants, pills, and IUDs suggest that these methods do not appear to interfere with the onset of lactogenesis, breastfeeding duration, or child growth or development. Perhaps the delivery of the placenta and the associated physiologic changes have more influence than just the drop in progesterone in propelling the development of mature milk. This argues for a better scientific understanding of the hormonal triggers at the onset of the second stage of lactogenesis.

Placement of the progestin-only contraceptive implant in the immediate postpartum period has been evaluated in a few small studies.[92–94] A randomized controlled trial assigned 69 women to contraceptive implant placement in the immediate postpartum period or at the postpartum visit. Of the 34 women randomized to placement at the postpartum visit, 20% did not attend a postpartum visit and therefore did not have an implant placed. All women in the immediate postpartum group had the implant placed. The 35 women receiving the contraceptive implant within 60 hours of delivery were compared to 34 women randomized to receive standard insertion 4 to 8 weeks postpartum. The duration of time until the onset of mature milk was not different between these groups (64 hours vs. 65 hours) and continuation of breastfeeding (both any and exclusive) did not differ at 6 months. No study has demonstrated a difference in breastmilk quality or infant growth or development save a single case report[95] among mothers utilizing an etonorgestrel contraceptive implant during breastfeeding.[92,96,97] Finally, use of postpartum implants is associated with a decrease in rapid repeat pregnancies and is highly cost effective.[98]

As with the Copper T 380A IUD, the CDC advises that the LNG IUD can be inserted at any time, including on the delivery table and during uterine involution. Until recently, data evaluating the effects of LNG IUD use in this immediate postpartum period on lactation included only a secondary analysis in which only 61% of the women enrolled even *initiated* breastfeeding.[99] Fortunately, a recent randomized controlled trial has evaluated time to lactogenesis and breastfeeding continuation in women assigned to post-placental versus standard insertion 4 to 8 weeks postpartum. No differences were noted in time to mature milk or in continuation of breastfeeding at 3 months.[100,101]

The use of progestin-only pills and progesterone rings is considered safe for use during lactation, though few studies have directly evaluated the use of these methods in the immediate postpartum period.[102–105] New mothers frequently are started on the progestin-only pill in the immediate postpartum period, with a plan to switch to combination hormonal methods when the risk for VTE has declined and lactation is better established. It is essential to counsel these women well regarding the differences in combination versus progestin-only pills. Specifically, the progestin-only pill is nearly entirely metabolized within 24 hours, requiring users take the pill at the same time daily. Additionally, patients need to be informed about the increased rates of breakthrough bleeding with the progestin-only pill. Finally patients should be given a clear timeline regarding when they may safely transition to a combination hormonal method.

The WHO's study of DMPA provided at 6 weeks postpartum demonstrated no impact on infant growth or development and small increases in the breastmilk production compared with nonhormonal methods of contraception.[105] Subsequently, focus turned toward provision of the progestin-only injectable in the immediate postpartum period. Two small studies have shown that a high dose of progestin (in DMPA) injected immediately postpartum has no impact on lactation.[94,106] It is important to note, however, that neither of these small studies had sufficient power to detect small but significant differences, and in at least one of the studies less than a quarter of the women in either group were exclusively breastfeeding at 6 weeks postpartum, suggesting that the immediate use of progestin methods may not influence breastfeeding duration among women who are not going to breastfeed much anyway. Ultimately, to date, the theoretical concern about administration of injectable progestin immediately upon delivery and before the onset of mature milk has not been supported. The U.S. MEC does not distinguish injectables from any other progestin-only method (although injectables result in faster, higher circulating levels of hormone than other delivery methods) and describes all progestin-only methods as having benefits that outweigh the risks of immediate postpartum use.[49]

Combined hormonal contraceptives (the combined pill, patch, injectable, and vaginal ring) used in the postpartum period have been the subject of multiple reviews.[54,107,108] The evidence is inconsistent regarding the effect of combined hormonal contraceptives on breastfeeding and insufficient regarding the impact on the infant when estrogen-containing methods were initiated less than 6 weeks postpartum. Older studies demonstrate a decrease in milk volume and breastfeeding, but they may reflect the use of COCs with higher doses of estrogen than are used today. Indeed, higher dose COCs were prescribed historically to suppress lactation.[109] Two newer studies suggest no impact on milk volume[110] or breastfeeding duration[111] but include only short-term data regarding breastfeeding.

Combined hormonal contraception is absolutely contraindicated <21 days postpartum due to safety concerns regarding the increased risk for VTE during the immediate postpartum period. The CDC then suggests the risks of CHC use outweigh the benefits in the first 30 to 42 days, depending on patient characteristics, which may increase VTE risk.[49] (However, the WHO considers the evidence regarding decreased breastmilk production to absolutely contraindicate the use of COCs in the first

6 weeks of breastfeeding and to relatively contraindicate it in the period from 6 weeks to 6 months.[50])

Counseling

When counseling women regarding both contraceptive methods and the timing of initiation, it is essential to consider the individual rather than the data alone. Breastfeeding provides significant health benefits to the mother-infant dyad and holds cultural importance for many women. While research to date suggests that the use of combined hormonal contraceptives is safe after 30 days, among women with breastfeeding challenges (preterm infants, poor milk production, etc.), it may be desired to avoid the introduction of estrogen-containing methods due to the possibility of decreased milk production. Likewise, while the CDC does not require a delay in administering Depo-Provera, as the WHO does, there may be ways in which the injection can be provided after mature milk comes in. This may be accomplished (a) by delaying hospital discharge (during which period breastfeeding support can be provided), or (b) by scheduling a nurse home visit after the 7th postpartum day, during which visit the injection can be given and continued breastfeeding support can be provided. (See Chapter 6 on Injectable Contraceptives.)

On the other hand, there are health risks with rapid repeat pregnancies. Women should be counseled regarding the full range of options available to them to best prevent pregnancy and meet their postpartum goals. Many women included in studies of postpartum contraception either failed to initiate breastfeeding or discontinued in the very early postpartum period for myriad reasons. Are there better ways to identify those women at risk for early discontinuation to provide better counseling and support? Are these women better served by providing the hormonal contraception immediately postpartum?

While many clinicians are deeply concerned about preventing early subsequent pregnancies in women described to be at high risk for not returning for postpartum care, it is equally important to recognize that these women simultaneously may be at high risk for early breastfeeding cessation, and we may be able to serve more than one of her needs by modifying the way we think about and deliver postpartum care.

Effects of Hormonal Contraception on the Breastfed Infant

Contraceptive steroids taken by the mother can be transferred to the nursing infant through breastmilk. The amounts, however, are small. While concern about the possible effects on the liver, sex organs, and other tissues of the neonate or premature infant is theoretical, it is prudent, when possible, to avoid exposing the neonate to exogenous steroids, which are not easily bound in plasma, conjugated by the liver, or excreted; additionally, the exogenous steroids may compete with natural hormones for receptor sites. Although studies are few and numbers are small, it appears that—

- The dose of contraceptive ethinyl estradiol reaching the infant of a mother taking combined pills is typically 1% or less of the maternal dose.[96]
- The quantity of progestin transferred to mother's milk varies with the type of progestin. The 17-hydroxy compounds (such as medroxyprogesterone acetate) enter the milk at approximately the same level as is found in the mother's blood, whereas the 19-nor compounds (such as norgestrel and norethindrone) enter the milk at only one-tenth the level in the blood.[112]

Hormonal contraceptive use during lactation is not the only possible source of estrogen and progestin exposure for the infant. When a mother becomes pregnant and continues to breastfeed a prior infant, that child is exposed to estrogen and progesterone in the mother's milk. Dairy cattle may also be pregnant at the time that they are milked, so that cow's milk and infant formula made from it may have relatively high levels of estrogen and progesterone.

Drug absorption, distribution, metabolism, and elimination are poorly understood in neonates. Although early studies of high-dose oral contraceptives did demonstrate some effect of hormones on nursing babies,[113] most of those reports were anecdotal and have not been corroborated in women using low-dose pills. One study of the male offspring of women who had used Depo-Provera found no effect on infant hormone regulation associated with breastfeeding exposure.[114]

Emergency Contraception and the Breastfeeding Woman

There is little, if any, published experience with emergency contraception during breastfeeding. Given what is known in general about breastfeeding and contraception, the U. K. Faculty of Family Planning and Reproductive Health Care Clinical Effectiveness Unit advises breastfeeding women that a contraceptive failure or unprotected sex before postpartum day 21 does not require the use of emergency contraception (EC), and that an IUD can be inserted as EC beginning in the fourth week[115] with the added benefit of providing subsequent ongoing contraception. The WHO and the CDC indicate that levonorgestrel EC can be used with no restriction by breastfeeding women.[49,50] Women should express and discard milk for 24 hours after taking ulipristal acetate since it is secreted into the breastmilk (with highest serum concentration in the first 3 hours after administration). Although levonorgestrel used for emergency contraception is also secreted into the milk (with highest concentrations in milk after 2-4 hours[116]) there appears to be no effect on lactation, and breastfeeding need not be withheld unless there is concern about infant exposure.[117]

The provision of a single packet of LNG EC during the postpartum LAM counseling has been shown to decrease the incidence of unplanned pregnancy during breastfeeding.[118]

BREASTFEEDING: ADVANTAGES TO THE INFANT

The practice of breastfeeding facilitates attachment—the psychological bond between mother and infant. Mother's milk has both nutritional and anti-infective advantages for the infant. The infant ingests substances that provide host-protection, humoral factors, and allergy prophylaxis. These are particularly concentrated in the colostrum, the high-protein, high-antioxidant fluid secreted in the first few days postpartum. The particular mixtures of protein, fat, carbohydrate, and trace elements in breastmilk change to meet the infant's evolving needs as breastfeeding proceeds from month to month.[119,120] There are both short-term and long-term health benefits of breastfeeding to the infant, and few, if any, liabilities. Even in developed country settings, breastfeeding reduces the risk of acute otitis media, nonspecific diarrheal disease, respiratory tract infections, atopic dermatitis, asthma, type 1 diabetes, childhood leukemia, sudden infant death syndrome, and necrotizing enterocolitis.[121] Later in life, having been breastfed is associated with significant positive effects in blood pressure, serum cholesterol, overweight and obesity, and risk of type 2 diabetes.[122]

Most medications taken by the breastfeeding mother are safe for the infant, and excellent references are available that list and describe those medications that may require an interruption of breastfeeding.[123,124] In the United States there are few contraindications to breastfeeding, with illicit drug use and maternal human immunodeficiency virus (HIV) infection as notable exceptions.[125]

BREASTFEEDING AND HIV

HIV, which causes acquired immune deficiency syndrome (AIDS), can be transmitted by an infected mother to her infant in utero, during childbirth, and through breastmilk. That HIV can be transmitted by breastfeeding has been conclusively demonstrated by case reports, laboratory data, and epidemiologic studies. Without effective anti-retroviral therapy, rates of vertical transmission during pregnancy and delivery are about 15% to 25%, and an additional 5% to 20% can become infected through breastfeeding.[126]

Thus, the majority of infants who are infected with HIV acquire the infection in utero or during childbirth, and the majority of infants who are breastfed by HIV-positive mothers do not become infected. Risk of transmission is greatest when maternal HIV viral load is high and immune function is poor. The risk of transmission is probably also affected by inflammatory breast conditions (such as mastitis), the mother's nutritional status, mode of feeding (exclusive breastfeeding is associated with less risk), and possibly HIV-specific anti-infective activities of the milk (such as inhibiting the binding of HIV glycoproteins to CD4 molecules).[127] It is also clear that breastmilk is normally protective (albeit to an unknown degree)[128] against enveloped viruses such as HIV and protects against childhood morbidity and mortality, so much so that research has shifted from studying the impact of infant feeding not only on HIV-free survival but also on overall infant survival.

However, there is a need to balance the risk of HIV transmission through breast milk with the risks of NOT breastfeeding. The decision to recommend breast or formula feeding depends on socioeconomic, cultural, and medical situations in each country. Specifically, the avoidance of breastfeeding should only be recommended when acceptable, feasible, affordable, sustainable and safe alternatives exist. In the United States, mothers living with HIV are instructed to avoid breastfeeding.[129]

In 2015, the WHO recommended lifelong antiretroviral (ARV) therapy for all individuals living with HIV upon diagnosis. The use of ARV therapy significantly decreases the risk of HIV transmission through breastmilk by suppressing the viral load. Among mothers using ARV therapy and breastfeeding exclusively for 6 months, risk of HIV transmission was 1.8% at 9 month compared to 1% among mothers choosing to formula feed in Rwanda.[130] The WHO recommendations now suggest that in locations where safe and exclusive use of formula is not possible, mothers should be encouraged to breastfeed exclusively for 12 months or longer. While exclusive breastfeeding is preferred, mixed feeding of formula and breastmilk is acceptable among mothers using ARV. There are currently no comparative data regarding mortality for infants with extended breastfeeding versus only 6 months of exclusive breastfeeding.

Women who are encouraged to breastfeed should do so exclusively while continuing ARV therapy. Within these guidelines, it is possible for HIV positive women to use LAM as a family planning method.

BREASTFEEDING: EFFECTS ON THE MOTHER

Breastfeeding has a major protective effect against premenopausal cancers of the ovary, endometrium, and breast and protects against type 2 diabetes, hypertension, cardiovascular disease, and stroke.[4,5,131–135]

Breastfeeding also promotes emotional bonding between mother and infant. Finally, the breastfeeding mother experiences a rapid return of uterine tone. Oxytocin, which induces uterine contraction, is released from the posterior pituitary when the nipple is stimulated by suckling.

During lactation, the body's estrogen levels are very low, and vaginal lubrication may be less than usual and begin later during sexual intercourse. Vaginal lubrication improves when cycling resumes or when the frequency of breastfeeding declines. Nursing mothers have added requirements for calories, protein, calcium, and iron, as well as several vitamins and other micronutrients. The increased needs for specific nutrients can be provided by a well-balanced diet, although U.S. women are often encouraged to continue their prenatal vitamins during breastfeeding. Supplements are generally unnecessary unless the diet is deficient in one or more of these nutrients.[136]

INSTRUCTIONS FOR AND INFORMATION ABOUT BREASTFEEDING*

1. Congratulations! Enjoy your baby, rest, and keep in touch with your clinician. Mother's milk is free and is always available at the right temperature, in contrast to infant formula.
2. Health experts concur that all women should be enabled to breastfeed, to breastfeed exclusively for 6 months, and to continue breastfeeding with complementary foods for 12 to 24 months or longer.
3. **If you are not breastfeeding, begin using a contraceptive method before or at your first sexual encounter**. You can become pregnant before your first menstrual period after childbirth because ovulation can begin before menstruation.
4. **If you are breastfeeding and providing bottle supplements, begin using a contraceptive method as soon as your clinician advises based on the method you have chosen.**
5. **If you are breastfeeding and using the Lactational Amenorrhea Method (LAM) as a temporary method of contraception, breastfeed your baby on demand (which usually means about every 3 hours), and avoid any bottle feeds**. Begin using another method of contraception when you resume menstruation (defined as any bleeding after 56 days postpartum), when you reduce the frequency or duration of breastfeeds, when you introduce bottle feeds or regular food supplements, or when your baby turns 6 months old. (See Figures 17-2 and 17-3.)

*These instructions are intended to guide providers in educating patients in how to use their method.

6. **You can become pregnant while breastfeeding your baby,** although the risk is greatly reduced before your first menstrual period. In the first 6 months of amenorrhea when you feed your baby on demand, avoid any bottle feeds, and provide minimal supplements by cup or spoon, your risk of pregnancy will be about 2%. This is equivalent to or lower than the risk associated with many other contraceptive methods. Most U.S. women do not follow breastfeeding patterns that confer maximum protection against pregnancy. However, women who choose LAM may adopt breastfeeding behaviors that maximize both milk production and the duration of amenorrhea.

7. **Breastfeeding is a convenient, inexpensive, and nutritious way to feed your baby, and it helps to protect the baby against infection, diarrhea, allergy, and sudden infant death syndrome. It also offers you protection against cancer of the breast, ovary, and uterus.**

8. **Neither intercourse nor menstruation affects the quality or quantity of your breastmilk. You do not need to stop breastfeeding because you start having intercourse again or start your period**. You can continue breastfeeding when you start using another contraceptive method.

9. **Lubricants, such as K-Y Jelly, spermicides, or saliva, may make intercourse easier after childbirth** because decreased estrogen production during breastfeeding diminishes vaginal lubrication.

10. **When you are nursing your child, your own nutrition is important.** Women can usually obtain all the calories and nutrients they need to breastfeed through their usual diet. There is no need to buy any special foods. Just eat a sensible, well-balanced diet, which is always a good idea.

11. **Avoid smoking**. Nursing women who smoke may transfer nicotine to their infant through their breastmilk. Nicotine is a poison that can harm the child. Inhaling smoke, including second-hand smoke, is also harmful to the baby. Smoking may also influence your ability to produce milk and decrease your supply.

12. **Alcohol that you drink enters your breastmilk**. Your baby will have more difficulty metabolizing alcohol than you do, especially in the first few weeks after delivery. Alcohol consumption inhibits milk ejection and temporarily reduces milk yield.[137] Thus it seems prudent to drink only modest amounts of alcohol and wait several hours after you have had a drink to nurse your baby, if possible, for example, wait 2 hours to breastfeed after drinking 4 ounces of alcohol.

13. **If you are using any medications while breastfeeding, be sure to tell your physician**. You can breastfeed while using virtually all common medications. However, for some medications you may need advice concerning the best timing for ingestion to decrease infant exposure. The InfantRisk Center (see Resource Materials) has a "warm line" that provides guidance regarding medication questions.
14. **If you are infected with HIV, be sure to get antiretroviral treatment. The virus that causes HIV/AIDS can be transmitted to your baby through breastmilk**. For this reason, most experts recommend that you not breastfeed your baby if you live in a country where replacement feedings are acceptable, feasible, affordable, sustainable and safe, as in the United States.
15. **It is indeed possible to combine work and breastfeeding successfully**, yet any separation of mother from infant for more than a few hours can create challenges to breastfeeding. Working women (or any breastfeeding woman!) should be sure to locate, preferably before delivery, a certified lactation consultant who can help in the event of any difficulty, from engorgement to declining milk supply. Lactation consultants are highly trained to give advice on a broad spectrum of breastfeeding issues, including the storage and transport of expressed milk, and can often help you rent an electric breast pump if you need one. The headquarters of the International Lactation Consultant Association can help you locate a certified lactation consultant near you (Website: www.ilca.org).

Resource Materials

- Academy of Breastfeeding Medicine: Clinical Protocols. (Guidelines for the care of breastfeeding mothers and infants) Available from: www.bfmed.org/Resources/Protocols.aspx. [Accessed May 13, 2017]
- App for the LactMed Drugs and Lactation database: https://toxnet.nlm.nih.gov/pda/lactmed.htm. [Accessed May 13, 2017]
- InfantRisk Center: (Counseling and data on the use of drugs and other substances in pregnant and breastfeeding mothers) www.infantrisk.com. [Accessed June 29, 2017]
- International Lactation Consultant Association: Resources to support breastfeeding are available at www.ilca.org/learning/resources. [Accessed May 13, 2017]

Disclosures—Kennedy: none. Goldsmith: none.

References

1. World Health Organization: Report of a WHO technical consultation on birth spacing. 2007 WHO Press, WHO/RHR/07.1 World Health Organization, Geneva, Switzerland. [Accessed May 13, 2017 at www.who.int/maternal_child_adolescent/documents/birth_spacing05/en/]
2. International Lactation Consultant Association (ILCA). Clinical guidelines for the establishment of exclusive breastfeeding. 3rd ed. ILCA, 2014:1–35.
3. World Health Assembly. Infant and young child nutrition. Fifty-fourth World Health Assembly Resolution WHA54.2. Geneva (Switzerland):WHO, 2001 May 18. [Accessed May 13, 2017 at: http://apps.who.int/gb/archive/pdf_files/WHA54/ea54r2.pdf]
4. American Academy of Pediatrics. Breastfeeding and the use of human milk. Pediatrics 2012:129(3): e827–841.
5. U.S. Department of Health and Human Services. The Surgeon General's call to action to support breastfeeding. Washington, DC: U.S. Department of Health and Human Services, Office of the Surgeon General; 2011. [Accessed May 13, 2017 at: www.ncbi.nlm.nih.gov/books/NBK52682]
6. World Health Organization. The optimal duration of exclusive breastfeeding: report of an expert consultation. Geneva (Switzerland): 2001 March 28–30. Geneva (Switzerland): WHO; 2002. [Accessed on May 13, 2017 at: www.who.int/nutrition/publications/infantfeeding/WHO_NHD_01.09/en]
7. Kramer MS, Kakuma R. The optimal duration of exclusive breastfeeding. Cochrane Database Syst Rev 2012;8:CD003517.
8. Academy of Nutrition and Dietetics. Position of the Academy of Nutrition and Dietetics: Promoting and supporting breastfeeding. J Acad Nutr Diet 2015:115:444–449.
9. Academy for Breastfeeding Medicine. ABM Position on breastfeeding—Revised 2015. Breastfeed Med 2015:10:407–411.
10. American College of Obstetrics and Gynecology. Optimizing support for breastfeeding as part of obstetric practice. ACOG Committee Opinion Number 658. Obstet Gynecol 2016;127:e86–92.
11. American Academy of Family Physicians. Breastfeeding (Policy Statement and Position Paper) 2014 [Accessed May 13, 2017 at: www.aafp.org/about/policies/all/breastfeeding.html]
12. UNICEF. Innocenti declaration on the protection, promotion and support of breastfeeding. New York: UNICEF; 1990. [Accessed May 13, 2017 at: www.unicef.org/programme/breastfeeding/innocenti.htm]
13. Hodgen GD, Itskovitz J. Recognition and maintenance of pregnancy. In: Knobil E, Neill JD, Ewing LL, Greenwald GS, Markert CL, Pfaff DW, (eds). The physiology of reproduction. New York: Raven Press; 1988. p. 1995–2021.
14. Willson JR. The puerperium. In: Willson JR, Carrington ER, Ledger WJ, Laros RK, Mattox JH, (eds). Obstetrics and gynecology. 8th ed. St. Louis (MO): CV Mosby Company; 1987. p. 598–607.
15. Gray RH, Campbell OM, Zacur H, Labbok MH, MacRae SL. Postpartum return of ovarian activity in non-breastfeeding women monitored by urinary assays. J Clin Endocrinol Metab 1987;64:645–50.
16. McNeilly AS. Lactational control of reproduction. Reprod Fertil Dev 2001;13:583–90.
17. McNeilly AS. Neuroendocrine changes and fertility in breastfeeding women. Prog Brain Res 2001;133:207–14.
18. Díaz S, Croxatto HB. Contraception in lactating women. Curr Opin Obstet Gynecol 1993;5:815–22.
19. Robinson JE, Short RV. Changes in breast sensitivity at puberty, during the menstrual cycle, and at parturition. Br Med J 1977;1(6070):1188–91.
20. Díaz S, Seron-Ferre M, Croxatto HB, Veldhuis J. Neuroendocrine mechanisms of lactational infertility in women. Biol Res 1995;28:155–63.

21. Gordon K, Renfree MB, Short RV, Clarke IJ. Hypothalamo-pituitary portal blood concentrations of β-endorphin during suckling in the ewe. J Reprod Fertil 1987;79:397–408.
22. McNeilly AS, Tay CCK, Glasier A. Physiological mechanisms underlying lactational amenorrhea. In: Campbell KL, Wood JW, (eds). Human reproductive ecology: interactions of environment, fertility and behavior. New York: Academy of Sciences; 1994. p. 145–55.
23. Lewis PR, Brown JB, Renfree MB, Short RV. The resumption of ovulation and menstruation in a well-nourished population of women breastfeeding for an extended period of time. Fertil Steril 1991;55:529–36.
24. Campbell OMR, Gray RH. Characteristics and determinants of postpartum ovarian function in women in the United States. Am J Obstet Gynecol 1993;169:55–60.
25. Kennedy KI, Rivera R, McNeilly AS. Consensus statement on the use of breastfeeding as a family planning method. Contraception 1989;39:477–96.
26. Gray RH, Campbell OM, Apelo R, et al. Risk of ovulation during lactation. Lancet 1990;335:25–9.
27. Becker S, Rutstein S, Labbok MH. Estimation of births averted due to breast-feeding and increases in levels of contraception needed to substitute for breast-feeding. J Bios Sci 2003;35:559–74.
28. Statistics Indonesia (Badan Pusat Statistik—BPS), National Population and Family Planning Board (BKKBN), and Kementerian Kesehatan (Kemenkes—MOH), and ICF International 2013. Indonesia Demographic and Health Survey 2012. Jakarta, Indonesia: BPS, BKKBN, Kemenkes, and ICF International. [Accessed on May 13, 2017 at: www.dhsprogram.com/PUBS/PDF/fr275/fr275.pdf]
29. Centers for Disease Control and Prevention. Breastfeeding Report Card, Progressing Toward National Breastfeeding Goals: United States, 2016 [Accessed on May 13, 2017 at: www.cdc.gov/breastfeeding/pdf/2016breastfeedingreportcard.pdf]
30. Murtagh L, Moulton AD. Working mothers, breastfeeding, and the law. Am J Public Health 2011:101:217–223.
31. Labbok M, Cooney K, Coly S. Guidelines: breastfeeding, family planning, and the Lactational Amenorrhea Method—LAM. Washington (DC): Institute for Reproductive Health, Georgetown University, 1994.
32. World Health Organization. The WHO multinational study of breastfeeding and lactational amenorrhea: III. Pregnancy during breastfeeding. Fertil Steril 1999;72:431–40.
33. Kazi A, Kennedy KI, Visness CM, Khan T. Effectiveness of the Lactational Amenorrhea Method in Pakistan. Fertil Steril 1995;64:717–23.
34. Labbok MH, Hight-Laukaran V, Peterson AE, Fletcher V, von Hertzen H, Van Look PFA. Multicenter study of the Lactational Amenorrhea Method (LAM): I. Efficacy, duration, and implications for clinical application. Contraception 1997;55:327–36.
35. Pérez A, Labbok MH, Queenan JT. Clinical study of the Lactational Amenorrhoea Method for family planning. Lancet 1992;339:968–70.
36. Ramos R, Kennedy KI, Visness CM. Effectiveness of lactational amenorrhea in prevention of pregnancy in Manila, the Philippines: non-comparative prospective trial. BMJ 1996;313:909–12.
37. Labbok M, Krasovec K. Toward consistency in breastfeeding definitions. Stud Fam Plann 1990;21:226–30.
38. Valdés V, Labbok MH, Pugin E, Pérez A. The efficacy of the lactational amernorrhea method (LAM) among working women. Contraception 2000;62:217–19.
39. Hight-Laukaran V, Labbok MH, Peterson AE, Fletcher V, von Hertzen H, Van Look PFA. Multicenter study of the Lactational Amenorrhea Method (LAM): II. Acceptability, utility, and policy implications. Contraception 1997;55:337–46.
40. Valdés V, Pérez A, Labbok M, Pugin E, Zambrano I, Catalan S. The impact of a hospital and clinic-based breastfeeding promotion programme in a middle class urban environment. J Trop Pediatr 1993;39:142–51.
41. Kennedy KI, Labbok MH, Van Look PFA. Consensus statement—Lactational Amenorrhea Method for family planning. Int J Gynaecol Obstet 1996;54:55–7.

42. Van Look PFA. Lactational Amenorrhoea Method for family planning. BMJ 1996:313: 893–4.
43. Labbok MH. Postpartum sexuality and the Lactational Amenorrhea Method for contraception. Clin Obstet Gynecol 2015:58:915–927.
44. Visness CM, Kennedy KI. The frequency of coitus during breastfeeding. Birth 1997;24:253–7.
45. Fletcher S, Grotegut CA and James AH. J Womens Health 2012;21:1290–1294.
46. Zerden ML, Stuart GS, Charm S, Bryant A, Garrett J, Morse J. Two-week postpartum intrauterine contraception insertion: a study of feasibility, patient acceptability and short-term outcomes. Contraception 2017;95:65–70.
47. Baldwin MK, Edelman AB, Lim JY, Nichols MD, Bednarek PH, Jensen JT. Intrauterine device placement at 3 versus 6 weeks postpartum: a randomized trial. Contraception 2016;93:356–63.
48. Speroff L and Mishell DR: The postpartum visit: it's time for a change in order to optimally initiate contraception. Contraception 2008; 78:90–98.
49. Curtis KM, Tepper NK, Jatlaoui TC, et al. U.S. Medical Eligibility Criteria for Contraceptive Use, 2016. MMWR Recomm Rep 2016;65:1–103.
50. World Health Organization. Medical eligibility criteria for contraceptive use, 5th ed. Geneva (Switzerland): World Health Organization; 2015, Department of Reproductive Health [Accessed May 13, 2017 at: www.who.int/reproductivehealth/publications/family_planning/MEC-5/en/]
51. Lopez LM, Hiller JE, Grimes DA. Education for contraceptive use by women after childbirth. Cochrane Database Syst Rev 2010;1:CD001863.
52. Fagan EB, Rodman E, Sorensen EA, Landis S, Colvin GF: A survey of mothers' comfort discussing contraception with infant providers at well-child visits. Southern Med J 2009;102:260–264.
53. Faich G, Pearson K, Fleming D, Sobel S, Anello C. Toxic shock syndrome and the vaginal contraceptive sponge. JAMA 1986;255:216–8.
54. Lopez LM, Grey TW, Stuebe AM, Chen M, Truitt ST, Gallo MF. Combined hormonal versus nonhormonal versus progestin-only contraception in lactation. Cochrane Database Syst Rev 2015;20:CD003988.
55. Bhardwaj NR, Espey E. Lactation and contraception. Curr Opin Obstet Gyn 2015;27: 496–503.
56. O'Hanley K, Huber DH. Postpartum IUDs: keys for success. Contraception 1992;45:351–61.
57. Welkovic S, Costa LOBF, Faúndes A, Ximenes RA, Costa CFF. Postpartum bleeding and infection after post-placental IUD insertion. Contraception 2001;63:155–8.
58. Letti Müller AL, Lopes Ramos JG, Martins-Costa SH, et al. Transvaginal ultrasonographic assessment of the expulsion rate of intrauterine devices inserted in the immediate postpartum period: a pilot study. Contraception 2005;72:192–5.
59. Levi E, Cantillo E, Ades V, Banks E, Murthy A. Immediate postplacental IUD insertion at cesarean delivery: a prospective cohort study. Contraception 2012;86:102–5.
60. Chen BA, Reeves MF, Creinin MD, Schwarz EB. Postplacental or delayed levonorgestrel intrauterine device insertion and breast-feeding duration. Contraception 2011;84:499–504.
61. Lester F, Kakaire O, Byamugisha J, et al. Intracesarean insertion of the Copper T380A versus 6 weeks postcesarean: a randomized clinical trial. Contraception 2015;91: 198–203.
62. Goldthwaite L, Hyer J, Sheeder J, Tocce K, Teal S. Postplacental levonorgestrel and copper intrauterine device insertion after vaginal delivery and expulsion by 12 weeks postpartum: a prospective cohort study. Contraception 2016;94:387.
63. Peterson HB: Sterilization. Obstet Gynecol 2008;111:189–203.
64. Wilcox LS, Chu SY, Eaker ED, Zeger SL, Peterson HB. Risk factors for regret after tubal sterilization: 5 years of follow-up in a prospective study. Fertil Steril 1991;55:927–33.
65. American College of Obstetricians and Gynecologists. Benefits and risks of sterilization. Obstet Gynecol 2003;102:647–58.

66. Association for Voluntary Surgical Contraception. Safe and voluntary surgical contraception. New York: AVSC International; 1995.
67. Chi IC, Thapa S. Postpartum tubal sterilization: an international perspective on some programmatic issues. J Biosoc Sci 1993;25:51–61.
68. Crenshaw JT. Healthy birth bractice #6: Keep mother and baby together—It's best for mother, baby, and breastfeeding. Perinatal Educ 2014;23:211–217.
69. Heit JA, Kobbervig CE, James AH, Petterson TM, Bailey KR and Melton LJ: Trends in the incidence of venous thromboembolism during pregnancy or postpartum: a 30-year population-based study. Ann Intern Med 2005;143:697–706.
70. American College of Obstetricians and Gynecologists. Use of hormonal contraception in women with coexisting medical conditions. Obstet Gynecol 2006:107:1453–72.
71. Sidney S, Petitti DB, Soff GA, Cundiff DL,Tolan KK and Qusenberry CP: Venous thromboembolic disease in users of low-estrogen combined estrogen-progestin oral contraceptives. Contraception 2004;70:3–10.
72. Tepper NK, Boulet SL, Whiteman MK, et al. Postpartum venous thromboembolism: incidence and risk factors. Obstet Gynecol 2014; 123:987.
73. Donnet ML, Howie PW, Marnie M, Cooper W, Lewis M. Return of ovarian function following spontaneous abortion. Clin Endocrinol 1990;33:13–20.
74. Lähteenmäki P. The disappearance of HCG and return of pituitary function after abortion. Clin Endocrinol 1978;9:101–12.
75. Finer LB, Zolna MR. Shifts in intended and unintended pregnancies in the United States, 2001–2008. Am J Public Health 2014;104(S1).
76. Schliep KC, Mitchell EM, Mumford SL, et al. Trying to conceive after an early pregnancy loss. Obstet Gynecol 2016;127:204–12.
77. Ockhuijsen HDL, Hoogen AVD, Boivin J, Macklon NS, Boer FD. Pregnancy after miscarriage: balancing between loss of control and searching for control. Res Nurs Health 2014;37:267–75.
78. Labbok MH. Contraception during lactation: considerations in advising the individual and in formulating programme guidelines. J Biosoc Sci 1985;9 Suppl:S55–66.
79. Burkman RT. Puerperium and breast-feeding. Curr Opin Obstet Gynecol 1993;5:683–7.
80. Wenof M, Aubert JM, Reyniak JV. Serum prolactin levels in short-term and long-term use of inert plastic and copper intrauterine devices. Contraception 1979;19:21–7.
81. Berry-Bibee EN, Tepper NK, Jatlaoui TC, Whiteman MK, Jamieson DJ, Curtis KM. The safety of intrauterine devices in breastfeeding women: a systematic review. Contraception 2017:94:725–738.
82. Chvapil M, Eskelson CD, Stiffel V, Owen JA, Droegemueller W. Studies on nonoxynol-9. II. Intravaginal absorption, distribution, metabolism and excretion in rats and rabbits. Contraception 1980;22:325–39.
83. Howie PW. Natural regulation of fertility. Br Med Bull 1993;49:182–99.
84. Parenteau-Carreau S, Cooney KA. Breastfeeding, Lactational Amenorrhea Method, and natural family planning interface: teaching guide. Washington (DC): Institute for Reproductive Health, Georgetown University; 1994.
85. Labbok MH, Stallings RY, Shah F, Pérez A, Klaus H, Jacobson M, Muruthi T. Ovulation method use during breastfeeding: is there increased risk of unplanned pregnancy? Am J Obstet Gynecol 1991;165:2031–6.
86. Kennedy KI, Gross BA, Parenteau-Carreau S, Flynn AM, Brown JB, Visness CM. Breastfeeding and the symptothermal method. Stud Fam Plann 1995;26:107–15.
87. Kennedy KI, Parenteau-Carreau S, Flynn A, Gross B, Brown JB, Visness C. The natural family planning - Lactational Amenorrhea Method interface: observations from a prospective study of breastfeeding users of natural family planning. Am J Obstet Gynecol 1991;165:2020–6.
88. Berens P,Labbok M and The Academy for Breastfeeding Medicine. Clinical Protocol #13 Contraception during breastfeeding. Breastfeeding Med 2015;10:3–12.
89. Phillips SJ, Tepper NK Kapp N, et al. Progestogen-only contraceptive use among breastfeeding women: a systematic review. Contraception 2016;94:226–52.

90. Kapp N, Curtis K and Nanda K: Progestogen-only contraceptive use among breastfeeding women: a systematic review. Contraception 2010;82:17–37.
91. Jones E and Spencer SA: The physiology of lactation. Ped Child Health 2007; 17: 244–248.
92. Gurtcheff SE, Turok DK, Stoddard G, Murphy PA, Gibson M, Jones KP. Lactogenesis after early postpartum use of the contraceptive implant. Obstet Gynecol 2011;117:1114–21.
93. Braga GC, Ferriolli E, Quintana SM, Ferriani RA, Pfrimer K, Vieira CS. Immediate post-partum initiation of etonogestrel-releasing implant. Obstet Gynecol Survey 2015;70:702–4.
94. Halderman LD, Nelson AL. Impact of early postpartum administration of progestin-only hormonal contraceptives compared with nonhormonal contraceptives on short-term breast-feeding patterns. Am J Obstet Gynecol 2002;186:1250–1256; discussion 1256–1258.
95. Stuebe AM, Bryant AG, Lewis R, Muddana A. Association of etonogestrel-releasing contraceptive implant with reduced weight gain in an exclusively breastfed infant: report and literature review. Breastfeeding Med 2016;11:203–6.
96. Brito MB, Ferriani RA, Quintana SM, Yazlle MEHD, Sá MFSD, Vieira CS. Safety of the etonogestrel-releasing implant during the immediate postpartum period: a pilot study. Contraception 2009;80:519–26.
97. Reinprayoon D, Taneepanichskul S, Bunyavejchevin S, et al. Effects of the etonogestrel-releasing contraceptive implant (Implanon®) on parameters of breastfeeding compared to those of an intrauterine device. Contraception 2000;62:239–46.
98. Han L, Teal SB, Sheeder J, Tocce K. Preventing repeat pregnancy in adolescents: is immediate postpartum insertion of the contraceptive implant cost effective? Am J Obstet Gynecol 2014;211:24e1–e7.
99. Chen BA, Creinin M, Reeves MS and Schwarz EB. Breastfeeding continuation among women using the levonorgestrel-releasing intrauterine device after vaginal delivery. Contraception 2009; 80:204–205.
100. Espey E, Turok D, Sanders J, Singh R, Thaxton L, Leeman L. Breastfeeding continuation in postplacental versus interval postpartum IUD insertion: the breastfeeding levonorgestrel IUD study (BLIS): a randomized controlled trial. Contraception 2016;94:407.
101. Turok D, Espey E, Sanders J, Eggebrotten J, Bullock H, Gawron L. The effect of postplacental versus interval postpartum IUD insertion on lactogenesis: the breastfeeding levonorgestrel IUD study (BLIS): a randomized controlled trial. Contraception 2016;94:390.
102. Moggia AV, Harris GS, Dunson TR, et al. A comparative study of a progestin-only oral contraceptive versus non-hormonal methods in lactating women in Buenos Aires, Argentina. Contraception 1991;44: 31–43.
103. Carr SL, Gaffield ME, Dragoman MV, Phillips S. Safety of the progesterone-releasing vaginal ring (PVR) among lactating women: A systematic review. Contraception 2016;94:253–61.
104. Bjarnadottir RI, Gottfredsdottir H, Sigurdardottir K, Geirsson RT, Dieben TOM. Comparative study of the effects of a progestogen-only pill containing desogestrel and an intrauterine contraceptive device in lactating women. BJOG 2001;108:1174–80.
105. Tankeyoon M, Dusitsin N, Chalapati S, et al. Effects of hormonal contraceptives on milk volume and infant growth. Contraception 1984;30:505–22.
106. Brownell EA, Fernandez ID, Fisher SG, et al. The effect of immediate postpartum depot medroxyprogesterone on early breastfeeding cessation. Contraception 2013;87:836–43.
107. Jackson E. Controversies in postpartum contraception: When is it safe to start oral contraceptives after childbirth? Thromb Res 2011;127.
108. Tepper NK, Phillips SJ, Kapp N, Gaffield ME, Curtis KM. Combined hormonal contraceptive use among breastfeeding women: an updated systematic review. Contraception 2016;94:262–74.
109. Anderson PO. Drugs that Suppress Lactation, Part 2. Breastfeed Med 2017;12:199–201

110. Bahamondes L, Bahamondes MV, Modesto W, et al. Effect of hormonal contraceptives during breastfeeding on infants milk ingestion and growth. Fertil Steril 2013;100: 445–50.
111. Espey E, Ogburn T, Leeman L, Singh R, Ostrom K, Schrader R. Effect of progestin compared with combined oral contraceptive pills on lactation. Obstet Gynecol 2012;119: 5–13.
112. Toddywalla VS, Mehta S, Virkar KD, Saxena BN. Release of 19-nor-testosterone type of contraceptive steroids through different drug delivery systems into serum and breast milk of lactating women. Contraception 1980;21:217–23.
113. Curtis EM. Oral-contraceptive feminization of a normal male infant. Obstet Gynecol 1964;23:295–96.
114. Virutamasen P, Leepipatpaiboon S, Kriengsinyot R, et al. Pharmacodynamic effects of depot-medroxyprogesterone acetate (DMPA) administered to lactating women on their male infants. Contraception 1996;54:153–7.
115. Faculty of Family Planning and Reproductive Health Care Clinical Effectiveness Unit. Contraceptive choices for breastfeeding women. J Fam Plann Reprod Health Care 2004;30:181–9.
116. Gainer E, Massai R, Lillo S, Reyes V, Forcelledo ML, et al: Levonorgestrel pharmacokinetics in plasma and milk of lactating women who take 1.5 mg for emergency contraception. Hum Reprod 2007;22:1578–1584.
117. Polakow-Farkash S, Gilad O, MerlobP, Stahl1 B, Yogev Y, Klinger G. Levonorgestrel used for emergency contraception during lactation-A prospective observational cohort study on maternal and infant safety. J Matern-Fetal Neo Med 2013:26:219–221.
118. Shaaban OM, Hassen SG, Nour SA, Kames MA, Yones EM. Emergency contraceptive pills as a backup for lactational amenorrhea method (LAM) of contraception: a randomized controlled trial. Contraception 2013:87:363–369.
119. Heinig MJ, Dewey KG. Health Advantages of breastfeeding for infants: a critical review. Nutrition Research Reviews 1996;9:89–110.
120. Riordan J and Wambach K (eds): Breastfeeding and human lactation (4th ed). Sudbury, MA: Jones and Bartlett, 2010.
121. Ip S, Chung M, Raman G, Chew P, Magula N, DeVine D, et al. Breastfeeding and maternal and infant health outcomes in developed countries. AHRQ Publication No. 07-E007. Rockville, MD: Agency for Healthcare Research and Quality. April 2007. [Accessed May 13, 2017 at: https://archive.ahrq.gov/downloads/pub/evidence/pdf/brfout/brfout.pdf]
122. World Health Organization. Horta BL, Bahl R, Martines JC, Victora CG. Evidence on the long-term effects of breastfeeding. Systematic reviews and meta-analyses 2007 WHO Press, World Health Organization, Geneva, Switzerland. [Accessed May 13, 2017 at: http://apps.who.int/iris/bitstream/10665/43623/1/9789241595230_eng.pdf]
123. American Academy of Pediatrics. Sachs HC and Committee on Drugs. The transfer of drugs and therapeutics into human breastmilk: An update on selected topics. Pediatrics 2013;132:e796–809.
124. National Institutes of Health, US National Library of Medicine. LactMed – A Toxnet Database. [Accessed May 13, 2017 at: https://toxnet.nlm.nih.gov/newtoxnet/lactmed.htm]
125. American Academy of Pediatrics. Human milk, breastfeeding and the transmission of Human Immunodeficiency Virus in the United States. Pediatrics 1995;96:977–9.
126. World Health Organization: HIV transmission through breastfeeding. A review of available evidence 2007. WHO Press. World Health Organization, Geneva Switzerland. Accessed on 5/31/2017 at www.who.int/maternal_child_adolescent/documents/9789241596596/en/
127. World Health Organization: Guideline: Updates on HIV and infant feeding 2016. WHO Press. World Health Organization, Geneva Switzerland. Accessed on 5/31/2017 at www.who.int/nutrition/publications/hivaids/guideline_hiv_infantfeeding_2016/en

128. World Health Organization: HIV transmission through breastfeeding: a review of available evidence: 2007 update. Geneva (Switzerland): World Health Organization; 2008. Available from: http://whqlibdoc.who.int/publications/2008/9789241596596_eng.pdf.
129. United States Department of Health and Human Services. AIDS info. Recommendations for use of antiretroviral drugs in pregnant hiv-1-infected women for maternal health and interventions to reduce perinatal HIV transmission in the United States. Accessed 5/31/2017 at https://aidsinfo.nih.gov/guidelines/html/3/perinatal-guidelines/0/#
130. Peltier CCAA, Ndayisaba GF, Lepage P, et al. Breastfeeding with maternal antiretroviral therapy or formula feeding to prevent HIV postnatal mother-to-child transmission in Rwanda. AIDS 2009;23:2415–23.
131. Collaborative Group on Hormonal Factors in Breast Cancer. Breast cancer and breastfeeding: collaborative reanalysis of individual data from 47 epidemiological studies in 30 countries, including 50302 women with breast cancer and 96973 women without the disease. Lancet 2002;360:187–195.
132. Rosenblatt KA, Thomas DB. Prolonged lactation and endometrial cancer: WHO Collaborative Study of Neoplasia and Steroid Contraceptives. Int J Epidemiol 1995;24:499–503.
133. Sung HK, Ma SH, Choi JY et al: The effect of breastfeeding duration and parity on the risk of epithelial ovarian cancer: a systematic review and meta-analysis. J Prev Med Public Health 2016:49:349–366.
134. Aune D, Norat T, Romundstad P et al. Breastfeeding and the maternal risk of type 2 diabetes: a systematic review and dose-response meta-analysis of cohort studies. Nutr Metab Cardiovasc Dis 2014 24:107–15.
135. Schwartz EB. Infant feeding in America: enough to break a mother's heart? Breastfeed Med 2013;8:454–7.
136. Institute of Medicine. Nutrition during lactation. Washington (DC): National Academy Press; 1991.
137. Haastrup MB, Pottegård A, Damkier P.Alcohol and breastfeeding. Basic Clin Pharmacol Toxicol 2014;14:168–73.

Contraception for Women with Medical Conditions

18

Rebecca H. Allen, MD, MPH
Carrie A. Cwiak, MD, MPH

- Individuals with chronic medical problems typically have an increased risk of health complications at baseline as a result of their condition(s).
- For patients with medical concerns, the risks associated with unintended pregnancy are often greater than the risks associated with contraceptive use.
- The United States Medical Eligibility Criteria for Contraceptive Use provides evidence-based guidelines, which facilitate the important task of helping patients with medical issues choose appropriate contraception.

Counseling individuals about contraception when they have co-existing medical conditions can be complicated and take more time. Nevertheless, most people with chronic medical conditions can safely use a variety of methods of contraception. Health care providers caring for individuals with medical conditions may be concerned about the effects of contraceptives on the medical condition, and therefore may avoid providing contraceptives or addressing family planning needs. However, adverse outcomes and disease progression are often greater during pregnancy than during contraceptive use. Unintended pregnancy itself can pose serious health risks to patients who have particular medical conditions (Table 18-1).[1] Given that the increase in maternal morbidity and mortality in the United States is due in part to chronic maternal conditions, providing appropriate contraceptive care is critical.[2]

Table 18-1 Conditions associated with increased risk for adverse health events as a result of pregnancy

- Breast cancer
- Complicated valvular heart disease
- Cystic fibrosis
- Diabetes: insulin dependent; with nephropathy, retinopathy, or neuropathy or other vascular disease; or of >20 years' duration
- Endometrial or ovarian cancer
- Epilepsy
- Hypertension (systolic ≥160 mm Hg or diastolic ≥100 mm Hg)
- History of bariatric surgery within the past 2 years
- HIV: not clinically well or not receiving antiretroviral therapy
- Ischemic heart disease
- Gestational trophoblastic disease
- Hepatocellular adenoma and malignant liver tumors (hepatoma)
- Peripartum cardiomyopathy
- Schistosomiasis with fibrosis of the liver
- Severe (decompensated) cirrhosis
- Sickle cell disease
- Solid organ transplantation within the past 2 years
- Stroke
- Systemic lupus erythematosus
- Thrombogenic mutations
- Tuberculosis

Adapted from: Curtis KM, et al. (2016).[1]

THE SAFETY OF CONTRACEPTIVE METHODS

UNDERSTANDING RISK ESTIMATES

Understanding the following fundamental statistical concepts will help in understanding the risks reported by studies and in interpreting those risks for our patients.

In contraceptive studies, the *relative risk* (RR) is the probability that an outcome will occur in users of a contraceptive method compared with the probability that that outcome will occur in nonusers of that method. Statistically, this is written as a ratio of users versus nonusers:

$$RR = \frac{\text{Probability of outcome X in } \textit{users} \text{ of method Y}}{\text{Probability of outcome X in } \textit{nonusers} \text{ of method Y}}$$

A relative risk of 1.0 means that use of a contraceptive method is not associated with the risk of an outcome either way: neither an increase nor a decrease. For example, because combined oral contraceptive (COC) use has no effect on eye color, the relative risk of having brown eyes with COC use compared with (for instance) condom use would be 1.0. However, if an outcome happens more often in users of that method, the relative risk will be greater than 1.0. Alternatively, if an outcome happens less often in users of the method, the relative risk will be less than 1.0. For example, the relative risk of developing ovarian cancer associated with COC use is 0.73, which means that, compared with women who have never used COC, COC users have a 27% reduction in the risk of developing ovarian cancer (1 − 0.73 = 0.27).[3] If there is only a slight increase in risk (RR = 1.10, or a 10% increase), the clinical importance of the increase in risk is generally small—unless the problem is very common or very serious. The "odds ratio" (OR) and the "hazard ratio" (HR) represent similar calculations and should be interpreted as you would a relative risk in clinical settings. The change in risk with use of a particular contraceptive method may be related to the method itself (causation) or to a common characteristic among users of that method (association).

The *absolute risk* of an outcome happening is also important to know. Even if the relative risk is very high, the absolute risk of an event may still be low, if the background risk in the population is low. For example, the relative risk of developing a benign liver tumor with COC use is 500. This risk appears to be quite high until you understand that this is such a rare occurrence that the chance that a COC user will develop a benign liver tumor (i.e., the absolute risk) is only 1 in 50,000 COC users.[30] A large multiple of a rare event is still a rare event.

The *attributable risk* reflects how much of the RR is associated with the use of the contraceptive method versus the background risk in the population of nonusers. For example, people frequently report having headaches. COC users also report having headaches. The attributable risk is typically what patients truly want to know: how much more or less often they are apt to have headaches because they are using COCs.

Finally, the *confidence interval* (CI) is another statistical principle that is useful. Studies will report both RR and its confidence interval. This is important because the RR calculated in a study is only an estimate. Because studies are based on *samples* of people, no one study ever reflects the experience of all individuals. So when researchers calculate the RR in a study, they also calculate (based on how many subjects were involved in the study and how similar the experiences of those subjects were) the probable limits within which the true answer would fall if all people were studied. The 95% confidence interval (95% CI) means that 95 times out of 100, the real answer lies between the 2 values quoted. For example, when a study of women with migraine with aura reports an increased risk of stroke with COC use with a RR = 3.0 (95% CI = 1.3, 11.3), the reader would know that the event occurred 3 times more often in COC users than in nonusers. However, the study also calculated with 95% confidence that the real risk lies somewhere between a 30% and an 11-fold increase.[4]

A crucial rule when interpreting the confidence interval is that a relative risk is statistically significant only if *both* confidence interval numbers reflect the same answer: either there is an increase or a decrease in risk.

A confidence interval that spans across the number 1 suggests that the answer is not clearly either an increased risk or a decreased risk, and therefore the relative risk is *not* statistically significant and should *not* change practice. For example, if a study of contraceptive patch users reports an increase in venous thromboembolism (VTE) with an RR = 2.0 (95% CI = 0.9, 4.1), the researchers are suggesting that patch users are 2 times more likely to experience the event compared to nonusers of the patch. However, the real answer is that the risk of the event could range widely, from 10% *less* often to 4.1 times *more* often.[5] Because the study could not determine whether the event actually increased or decreased among patch users, the outcome of the study is not statistically significant and should not alter clinical practice.

Permanent Contraception

Tubal sterilization for women and vasectomy for men are permanent, safe, and highly effective methods of contraception.[6] The risks of the procedures vary according to type of sterilization and anesthesia used. Vasectomy for men and hysteroscopic tubal occlusion for women can be performed under local anesthesia in the outpatient setting. In contrast, surgery on the fallopian tubes through laparotomy or laparoscopy is typically performed under regional or general anesthesia in a hospital. There are few medical conditions that represent a contraindication to the permanent contraceptive method itself. Examples include a known allergy to any components of the devices used to complete the procedure or extensive scarring due to previous surgeries or endometriosis that obscures the fallopian tubes. However, certain medical conditions place individuals at a higher risk for undergoing surgery, especially under general anesthesia. The risk of surgery must then be balanced against any acceptable alternative contraceptive methods that the person is eligible to use that are safer to administer and still effective at preventing pregnancy. (See Chapter 16 on Permanent Contraception.)

Intrauterine Contraception

Intrauterine contraception can be used by most individuals with chronic medical problems. Because the mechanism of action is local, intrauterine contraception has the advantage of no known drug-drug interactions. The main contraindications include pregnancy, active uterine or cervical infection, and a distorted uterine cavity unable to accommodate the device.[1] Other concerns include cancer in the genital tract (e.g., cervical cancer, endometrial cancer, gestational trophoblastic disease) and women with complicated solid organ transplantation (e.g., graft failure, rejection, or cardiac allograft vasculopathy). Due to its levonorgestrel (LNG) content, the hormonal intrauterine device (IUD) is contraindicated in patients with current breast cancer. Anecdotally, the LNG IUD is sometimes used by patients with a history of breast cancer if they also have abnormal uterine bleeding (AUB) and are not appropriate candidates for surgical management.[7] While the levonorgestrel acts directly on the uterus and cervix, there is a small amount of systemic absorption. A stable serum concentration of 150 to 200 pg/mL of levonorgestrel occurs after placement of the 52 mg LNG IUD.[8] This concentration is roughly 30-times lower than the 6.2 ng/mL from a 150 mcg levonorgestrel-containing oral contraceptive pill.[9] Due to the small amount of systemic absorption, there are theoretical concerns for the LNG IUD in individuals who have hepatocellular adenoma, hepatoma, and severe decompensated cirrhosis. The copper IUD is the only nonhormonal long-acting reversible contraceptive. For individuals with severe thrombocytopenia or severe anemia, there is concern that the copper IUD could increase menstrual blood loss. (See Chapter 5 on IUDs.)

Progestin-Only Contraceptives

Systemic progestin-only contraceptives have very few contraindications and can be used by most individuals with chronic medical problems. These methods include the etonogestrel subdermal implant (Nexplanon), depot medroxyprogesterone acetate (DMPA) injection, and progestin-only oral contraceptives (only available as norethindrone in the United States). Progestin-only contraceptives are effective options for patients who have cardiovascular risk factors or conditions because progestins do not increase the risk of cardiovascular complications: normotensive users of progestin-only methods do not have higher rates of venous thromboembolism (VTE), myocardial infarction (MI), or cerebrovascular accident (CVA) compared to normotensive nonusers.[10,11] Because DMPA is a high-dose contraceptive, there is theoretical concern that use of DMPA may be associated with slightly increased risk of cardiovascular complications compared to lower dose progestin-only methods. It is important to remind patients that their *absolute risk* of cardiovascular complications is not negligible, but that risk is primarily *attributable* to their chronic condition, and not to their contraceptive. In addition, progestin-only contraceptives may provide noncontraceptive benefits: inhibition of ovulatory cycling, decreased menstrual blood loss, and decreased anemia.[12] For patients with heavy menstrual bleeding, menstrual migraines, anticoagulant therapy, or sickle cell anemia, for example, the menstrual suppression provided by their contraceptive may actually improve their medical condition while providing effective protection from unintended pregnancy.

Progestin-only contraceptives are contraindicated in patients with current breast cancer. And progestins are metabolized in the liver via the microsomal P-450 system, so they must be used with caution in the setting of hepatocellular adenoma, hepatomas, and severe decompensated cirrhosis. Similarly, medication interactions are possible with low-dose progestin-only contraceptives (implant and POPs).[1] Although most medication interactions do not harm the contraceptive user per se, they may result in reducing the effectiveness of the contraceptive. Therefore, a back-up contraceptive may need to be added to preserve effectiveness, but the use of the primary method itself is not contraindicated. (See Chapter 4 on Contraceptive Implants, Chapter 6 on Injectable Contraceptives, and Chapter 9 on Progestin-only Pills.)

Combined Hormonal Contraceptives

For individuals with chronic medical conditions that increase their baseline risk of cardiovascular complications, the use of combined hormonal contraceptives (CHCs) is contraindicated. These methods include combined oral contraceptives (COCs), the transdermal patch, and the vaginal ring. Although the transdermal patch and the vaginal ring are non-oral, their estrogen component—ethinyl estradiol (EE)—nevertheless increases the risk of VTE compared to nonusers of CHCs. And although the risk of arterial thromboembolism (MI and CVA) associated with CHC use may be negligible in healthy users, individuals with hypertension, migraines with aura, or tobacco use age 35 and older will have further increases in risk that increase the risk of CHC use.[4,13,14] In individuals in whom CHCs are not contraindicated but should be used with caution (e.g. obesity), using the combined method with the lowest EE dose acceptable is still an option.

Use of the transdermal patch is associated with a 60% increase in EE exposure compared with a COC containing 30 mcg of EE. In contrast, use of the vaginal ring is associated with EE exposure 3 times lower than with the patch and 2 times lower than with COCs.[15] It is unclear whether this means use of the patch is associated with a comparatively increased risk, or use of the ring is associated with a comparatively decreased risk, of cardiovascular complications compared with use of COCs. Nevertheless, the relative EE exposure may be relevant when guiding a patient in choosing the CHC with the lowest EE dose acceptable to her.

Like progestin-only contraceptives, CHCs provide noncontraceptive benefits due to inhibition of ovulation, suppression of menstruation, and decrease in androgen levels.[12] For patients with menstrually-related disorders, AUB, or increased androgen levels, their contraceptive may add the benefit of improving their medical condition in addition to providing effective protection from unintended pregnancy.

As with all hormonal methods, CHCs are contraindicated in patients with current breast cancer. EE is metabolized in the liver to a greater extent than progestins, and so their use is contraindicated in the setting of hepatocellular adenoma, hepatomas, active hepatitis, and severe decompensated cirrhosis. Interactions can occur with medications that induce hepatic cytochrome P-450 metabolism.[1] A back-up contraceptive may need to be added to preserve effectiveness, but the use of the primary method itself is not contraindicated. (See Chapter 7 on Contraceptive Patch and Vaginal Contraceptive Ring and Chapter 8 on Combined Oral Contraceptives.)

Emergency Contraception

Oral emergency contraception includes the option of 1.5 mg of levonorgestrel or 30 mg of ulipristal acetate. Because the medications are a one-time dose, there is limited clinical impact and there are no contraindications.[1] All individuals with chronic medical problems should have access to emergency contraception. Placement of a copper IUD as an emergency contraceptive allows for ongoing contraception in this population. Women taking hepatic enzyme inducers should be warned that the efficacy of EC pills may be reduced, as enzyme inducers may increase metabolism of LNG and UPA. For these patients, the first-line option for EC is the copper IUD. For patients for whom the copper IUD is not acceptable or available, a double-dose of LNG (3 mg) may be used. This approach is safe, although the efficacy is not known. UPA is not recommended for patients taking enzyme inducers.[31]

RISKS OF UNINTENDED PREGNANCY

Unintended pregnancy is associated with small but real health risks; the risk of VTE is increased at least 22-fold in postpartum women compared to nonpregnant women of reproductive age.[16] For individuals with chronic medical conditions, risks of pregnancy complications such as VTE, uncontrolled blood pressure, or stroke are increased. In addition, pregnancy loss and congenital defects are more likely in patients with poorly controlled diabetes. Pregnancy in women taking teratogenic medications (e.g., antiepileptic drugs, isotretinoin) is associated with an elevated risk of birth defects. See Table 18-1 for the list of medical conditions associated with increased risk for adverse health events as a result of pregnancy. For these conditions, the known risks of unintended pregnancy are typically greater than any actual or theoretical risk associated with appropriate contraceptive use. When a pregnancy is planned, the risk-benefit ratio changes as the individual's goals for health (i.e., a healthy pregnancy) are thus changed. In this context, contraception may still be used to postpone pregnancy until therapy is completed (e.g., transplant, bariatric surgery, chemotherapy) or the medically condition is better controlled and therefore risks of pregnancy complications decreased.

CDC MEDICAL ELIGIBILITY CRITERIA FOR CONTRACEPTIVE USE

Development of the Guidelines

The Centers for Disease Control and Prevention (CDC) developed the United States Medical Eligibility Criteria for Contraceptive Use (U.S. MEC) as guidelines intended to assist health care providers in determining what methods are safe to use in the context of particular medical conditions.[1] (See the U.S. MEC color chart insert.) The World Health Organization (WHO) published the first MEC for global use in 1996. These guidelines were developed based on systematic reviews of the medical literature concerning the safety of contraceptive use in patients with chronic medical illnesses or other conditions. After review of the literature, an expert working group was convened to determine the final guidelines based on the literature. Therefore, where the literature was limited, expert opinion prevailed. The WHO MEC was designed as an overarching document as a starting point for countries to adapt their own guidelines for use. The CDC adapted the WHO guidance and published the first U.S. MEC in 2010. The United Kingdom published its MEC shortly before that. It is important to recognize that the CDC provided substantial technical support to the WHO in developing its MEC, and in turn relied on the same process for developing the U.S. MEC. Where the U.S. MEC appears to conflict from the WHO MEC, as in recommendations for breastfeeding women, for example, this reflects where the CDC adapted the MEC to be relevant to the U.S. population rather than a differing interpretation of the literature.

Using the Recommendations in Practice

The U.S. MEC will have the greatest benefit for women if it is used by health care providers in everyday practice in order to decrease unnecessary barriers to contraceptive access. The U.S. MEC app can be downloaded for free from the CDC for use in a smart phone. If a provider does not have access to a smart phone in their clinical setting, the guidelines can be downloaded to a desktop, or laminated charts can be used (apps, guidelines and charts are available for free from www.cdc.gov/reproductivehealth/contraception/mmwr/mec/summary.html).

The MEC uses a 4-tiered category system to denote level of risk associated with the use of a particular contraceptive among individuals with a particular condition, compared to the risk associated with unintended pregnancy.[1] Unintended pregnancy, rather than simply no risk, is the comparative condition because the great majority of sexually active patients (85%) will become pregnant within one year if using no contraceptive. (See Chapter 3 on Efficacy, Safety, Personal Considerations.) Category 1 conveys that benefits of use of the contraceptive outweigh the risks of use. Category 2 indicates that the benefits of use still outweigh the risks of use, but that additional follow up after initiation of the contraceptive may be warranted. Using category 1 and 2 contraceptive methods freely can eliminate barriers to contraceptive use that may be based on misperception of risk rather than actual evidence of risk. Use of category 1 and 2 contraceptives may be more easily incorporated into your clinical practice, more easily taught to trainees who may have limited family planning experience, or may provide assurance that additional referral before contraceptive initiation is not needed. Similarly,

Table 18-2 Conditions that are generally not a contraindication for contraceptives

Age	Benign breast cysts
Past ectopic pregnancy	Family history of cancer
Obesity	Ovarian cancer
Gestational hypertension	Dysmenorrhea
Gestational diabetes	Uterine fibroids
Varicose veins	Cervical dysplasia
Migraines without aura	HIV
Epilepsy	Thyroid disease
Depression	Cystic fibrosis
Abnormal uterine bleeding	Sickle cell anemia
Endometriosis	Iron deficiency anemia
Benign ovarian cysts	Antibiotic use

Adapted from: Curtis KM, et al. (2016).[1]

medical conditions for which all contraceptive methods are category 1 and 2 should be considered as conditions for which there are no significant contraceptive safety concerns due to the condition itself (see Table 18-2).

Categories Indicating Risk Potential

Category 3 indicates that the risks of using the contraceptive method outweigh the benefits, although the method may be used if nothing else is available or acceptable to the patient. This category most closely approximates the health care provider asking, "Are the risks from unintended pregnancy greater that the risks from this contraceptive method?" If yes, then clinical judgment guides us to use the contraceptive method. Health care providers may understandably require more family planning experience before they are comfortable prescribing category 3 methods to their patients. Within a group practice or clinic, category 3 methods may signal when referral to a more experienced health care provider is needed. Prescribing a category 3 contraceptive method typically requires more time within a clinical visit to explain to patients the risks and benefits of the method, as well as alternative methods. Follow up may be needed to assure that continued use is safe.

Category 4 conveys that an unacceptable risk is associated with use of that contraceptive in patients with that condition. Category 4 methods should be used only in rare circumstances and when there is no alternative method that is safe to use; for example, a patient with breast cancer using tamoxifen may benefit from protection of the endometrium conferred by the LNG IUD (the decision is best made in consultation with the medical oncologist).

The U.S. MEC allows for documentation of clinical decision-making to be more standardized, objective, recognizable, and feasible. For example, within an electronic medical record, a smart- or autotext can be used to concisely state, "Use of this contraceptive is category 1 (can use) in the CDC U.S. Medical Eligibility Criteria." Notes can be forwarded to other health care providers, such as the cardiologist caring for your patient with a history of peripartum cardiomyopathy, so that recommendations for care are well understood and communicated among the health care team. Finally, advocating for the highest quality care for our patients may require conversations with the other health care providers involved in their care. In these circumstances, the expertise of other health care providers should be respected. However, these providers might not have expertise in contraception and therefore may be uncomfortable due to their lack of knowledge or the myths they have heard. Their discomfort is understandable, but must be responded to with education and resources that provide accurate information about the risks of various contraceptive methods. The mutual goal is to provide safe care and minimize harm to the patient.

The U.S. MEC lists recommendations for contraceptive use in the presence of over 60 conditions. All contraceptive methods available in the United States are included; recommendations are listed separately for natural family planning, barrier methods, permanent contraception (the U.S. MEC lists this as 'sterilization'), and emergency contraception as they do not involve the prolonged provision of medication.

For Medical Conditions Not Listed in the U.S. MEC

Some medical conditions are not listed because there is not enough medical evidence on contraception use in that population of patients to inform recommendations. So how do health care providers manage the patient with a medical condition that is not listed in the U.S. MEC? In this case, the following options should be considered:

- Consider the risks inherent in the condition itself and review the recommendations for conditions that have similar risk. For example, cerebral aneurysm is not listed in the MEC but migraine with aura is, and so following the guidelines for migraine with aura might be prudent in order to avoid an increased risk of stroke with contraceptive use.
- Consider the themes of the U.S. MEC, including that—
  - Estrogen-containing contraceptives increase cardiovascular risk
  - Progestins generally do not
  - Nearly all women are eligible for at least one of the long-acting reversible contraceptive (LARC) methods
- Research other sources such as UpToDate, PubMed, etc. for guidance.
- Consult with the other health care providers involved in your patient's care.

Assessment of Medical Eligibility for Contraception

Screening for Medical Conditions

A comprehensive patient history, updated annually, will reveal the majority of contraindicating conditions. A pelvic examination will detect the majority of contraindications to IUD placement. The U.S. Selected Practice Recommendations for Contraceptive Use (SPR) provides guidelines to all health care providers as to how to prescribe contraception.[17] The SPR is included in the smart phone app that contains the U.S. MEC, and is also available at www.cdc.gov/reproductivehealth/contraception/mmwr/mec/summary.html. Specifically, the SPR reviews the screening tests that are needed before initiation of contraception. Blood pressure measurement before initiation of CHCs contributes to the safety of their use. COC users with unmeasured blood pressure were more likely to have complications after contraceptive initiation than users with measured blood pressure.[18] Documenting users' weight and body mass index (BMI) at initiation of all contraceptive methods may contribute to the effectiveness of follow up and future counseling as significant weight gain caused by contraceptive use is a common misconception and worry. Patients require a pelvic examination before IUD placement in order to decrease the risk of complications related to placement due to unrecognized infection, pregnancy, or cancer, but a pelvic examination is not required prior to initiating other contraceptive methods.[19] Screening for anemia, hyperlipidemia, or diabetes does not contribute to the safety of contraceptive use, so is it not required before initiating or continuing contraceptive use. Screening the general population for thrombogenic mutations before CHC use is not cost-effective, but it may be indicated in patients with a strong family history of thromboembolism.[20] The performance of STI testing, pap testing, and mammogram do not increase the safety of contraceptive use and should not be required before the provision of contraception unless an individual's history indicates the need for the test.[19]

Initiating a Method using MEC

Clinical Scenario 1

A 32-year-old patient with a known history of high blood pressure presents for contraception. She is not taking any medications, because she lost her health insurance. Her blood pressure is measuring consistently 160/100 mm Hg. Based on U.S. MEC recommendations (Table 18-3), estrogen-containing methods are considered contraindicated for this patient due to the higher risk of stroke, acute myocardial infarction, and peripheral arterial disease.[21,22] The patient is a candidate for an IUD, implant, or progestin-only pill. There are theoretical concerns about the effect of levonorgestrel on lipids and limited evidence suggests that among women with hypertension, those who used POPs or

Table 18-3 The U.S. MEC categories for clinical scenario 1

Hypertension	Cu-IUD	LNG-IUD	Implants	DMPA	POP	CHC
Adequately controlled hypertension	1	1	1	2	1	3
Elevated blood pressure levels Systolic 140–159 mm Hg or diastolic 90–99 mm Hg	1	1	1	2	1	3
Elevated blood pressure levels Systolic ≥160 mm Hg or diastolic ≥100 mm Hg	1	2	2	3	2	4
Vascular disease	1	2	2	3	2	4

Cu-IUD = copper intrauterine device, LNG-IUD = levonorgestrel intrauterine device, DMPA = depot medroxyprogesterone acetate, POP = progestin-only pill, CHC = combined hormonal contraception

DMPA had a small increased risk for cardiovascular events compared with women who did not use these methods.[23] However, because the absolute risk of cardiovascular events is quite small, the rating is only category 2 for POPs, LNG IUD, and the implant. For DMPA, there is further concern about its hypoestrogenic effects and reduced HDL levels which raises the rating to 3. Nevertheless, if no other methods are acceptable, DMPA is an option for this patient.

Clinical Scenario 2

When patients present with multiple medical conditions, the condition with the highest category number should determine the safety of the contraceptive choice for the patient. The U.S. MEC does have a category that helpfully provides recommendations for the patient with multiple conditions. The category is entitled *multiple risk factors for atherosclerotic cardiovascular disease,* and it takes into account older age, smoking, diabetes, hypertension, low HDL, high LDL, or high triglyceride levels.

A 25-year-old obese patient recently diagnosed with Type 2 diabetes mellitus presents for contraception (Table 18-4). She is currently taking metformin for diabetes. She also has a history of migraines with aura. Based on U.S. MEC recommendations, combined hormonal contraception is contraindicated in patients with migraines with aura due to the increased risk of stroke.[14] She is therefore a candidate for an IUD or a progestin-only method.

Table 18-4 The U.S. MEC categories for clinical scenario 2

	Cu-IUD	LNG-IUD	Implants	DMPA	POP	CHC
Migraine with aura	1	1	1	1	1	4
BMI ≥30 kg/m²	1	1	1	1	1	2
Non-insulin dependent diabetes mellitus	1	2	2	2	2	2

Cu-IUD = copper intrauterine device, LNG-IUD = levonorgestrel intrauterine device, DMPA = depot medroxyprogesterone acetate, POP = progestin-only pill, CHC = combined hormonal contraception

Table 18-5 The U.S. MEC categories for clinical scenario 3

	Cu-IUD	LNG-IUD	Implants	DMPA	POP	CHC
Inflammatory bowel disease (ulcerative colitis or Crohn's disease)	1	1	1	2	2	2/3

Cu-IUD = copper intrauterine device, LNG-IUD = levonorgestrel intrauterine device, DMPA = depot medroxyprogesterone acetate, POP = progestin-only pill, CHC = combined hormonal contraception

Clinical Scenario 3

Other U.S. MEC recommendations include two ratings for a single condition. In this case, it is the clinical circumstances or severity of the condition that will dictate which rating applies.

A 40-year-old patient with long-standing Crohn's disease presents for contraception (Table 18-5). In her case, use of combined hormonal contraception will depend on the severity of her disease. Women with inflammatory bowel disease are at baseline at a higher risk for VTE compared to unaffected women.[24] Nevertheless, for patients with mild inflammatory bowel disease and no other risk factors for VTE, the benefits of combined hormonal contraception generally outweigh the risks so a rating of 2 is given.[25] For those women with severe inflammatory bowel disease or other risk factors for VTE such as surgery or immobilization, the rating is increased to a 3 because the risks generally outweigh the benefits. She is a good candidate for IUDs or progestin-only methods.

Continuing a Method Based on the MEC

Certain U.S. MEC recommendations are subdivided into two subcategories: Initiation (I) of a new contraceptive method and Continuation (C) of a currently used contraceptive method. If an individual's condition changes or she develops a new medical condition while using a contraceptive, the category rating and risk-benefit profile may change.

Clinical Scenario 4

A 35-year-old patient with systemic lupus erythematosus presents for contraception (Table 18-6). She is negative for anti-phospholipid antibodies and is not taking immunosuppressants. She does have severe thrombocytopenia with platelets measuring 30,000. Both the copper IUD and DMPA are given a category 3 rating for initiation of the method in this setting. This is due to concerns for menstrual

Table 18-6 The U.S. MEC categories for clinical scenario 4

	Cu-IUD				DMPA			
	I	C	LNG-IUD	Implants	I	C	POP	CHC
Systemic lupus erythematosus with severe thrombocytopenia	3	2	2	2	3	2	2	2

I = initiation, C = continuation; Cu-IUD = copper intrauterine device, LNG-IUD = levonorgestrel intrauterine device, DMPA = depot medroxyprogesterone acetate, POP = progestin-only pill, CHC = combined hormonal contraception

Table 18-7 The U.S. MEC categories for clinical scenario 5

	Cu-IUD		LNG-IUD					
	I	C	I	C	Implants	DMPA	POP	CHC
Current PID	4	2	4	2	1	1	1	1

I = initiation, C = continuation; Cu-IUD = copper intrauterine device, LNG-IUD = levonorgestrel intrauterine device, DMPA = depot medroxyprogesterone acetate, POP = progestin-only pill, CHC = combined hormonal contraception

bleeding with severe thrombocytopenia that may be worsened by the copper IUD, and the potential for irregular bleeding with DMPA, a medication that cannot be reversed rapidly. However, if a patient already has a copper IUD in place or is on DMPA and develops severe thrombocytopenia, the recommendation changes to a category 2 rating. In this case, if the patient is already tolerating the method, one can consider continuing and observing for any signs of worsening bleeding.

Clinical Scenario 5

A 21-year-old patient desires an IUD for contraception. She presents with fever, pelvic pain, and foul-smelling vaginal discharge. She has cervical motion tenderness and uterine tenderness on exam. You diagnose her with pelvic inflammatory disease and treat her with antibiotics. In her case, placement of the IUD is contraindicated with current pelvic inflammatory disease (Table 18-7). She is eligible for all the other methods of contraception. However, if she had developed pelvic inflammatory disease with the IUD already in place, the recommendation for continuation is a category 2. The IUD can be continued while the infection is being treated provided the patient is clinically improving.[17]

Counseling Patients with Medical Conditions on Contraceptive Methods

Counseling medically complex patients will likely take additional time in order to address social determinants that likewise may be more complex in this population. If possible, allotting additional time for these patient visits will enable you to delve into the increased complexity of the medical decision-making that will be required. (See Chapter 2 for more on patient-centered counseling.)

Review All Medically Eligible Effective Methods

Once the patient has been screened for medical eligibility based on a review of the medical history and concomitant medications, review the available options. Individuals may have preconceived ideas regarding different methods of contraception, so dispel any misconceptions about efficacy or safety (see Chapter 3 on Efficacy, Safety, Personal Considerations). The effect of any particular method with the patient's disease process or the method's interaction with concomitant medication should be discussed. While you ideally should be able to provide the desired method that same day, the patient may need time to reflect and decide on a personal best option.

Discuss Future Pregnancy Plans

Individuals with chronic medical problems should be queried regarding their reproductive goals (see Chapter 2 for more on patient-centered counseling). If an individual is certain that future pregnancy is not desired, permanent contraception should be discussed. Individuals with chronic medical problems may want to time their pregnancy according to disease control or remission. If their medical condition would lead to serious pregnancy-related complications, then they may want to consider higher efficacy methods such as the IUD or implant. The IUD and contraceptive implant are highly cost-effective after just 1 year of use.[26,27] To minimize risks of birth defects and miscarriage, patients with diabetes mellitus should ideally have normal blood glucose levels prior to conception.[28] Similarly, patients with epilepsy should be evaluated for the possibility of discontinuing anti-epileptic medications or tapering to monotherapy with lower risk medication prior to conception to avoid the risk of birth defects.[29]

Consider Adherence Behaviors

Safety is not the only factor to address for patients with chronic medical conditions. Medication interactions can directly decrease their contraceptive hormonal levels and potentially decrease method effectiveness. In addition, they may face challenges in adhering to their contraceptive method. Consider your patient's existing medical regimen, requirements for therapy, or schedule of other health care visits. For example, patients with daily oral medication regimens might find it easy to incorporate a daily COC, but those with weekly dialysis will not be able to maintain adequate serum hormone levels with COCs, and individuals with frequent hospitalizations may not be able to return to your office or clinic on time for DMPA injections. The mental and physical capacity of the patient must be considered: e.g., has their history of stroke impaired their memory such that adherence to short-term contraceptives is impaired? Does their morbid obesity make vaginal ring insertion too difficult?

Individuals with chronic medical conditions may perceive they are not able to conceive; accordingly, adherence to contraception may not be a top priority for them. While it is true that these patients may have a lower absolute risk of unintended pregnancy than their healthy counterparts due to decreased fertility or decreased sexual activity as a result of their chronic disease, it is important to educate them that their overall risk from unintended pregnancy is still greater because the risk of pregnancy-related complications is greater. In this situation, reviewing the noncontraceptive benefits of various methods might motivate them to achieve other goals they have for their health.

Weigh Noncontraceptive Benefits and Bleeding Profiles

Individuals with chronic medical problems, depending on their condition, may benefit from the noncontraceptive effects of various methods. This may be an important part of their contraception decision-making process (see Chapter 3 on Efficacy, Safety, and Personal Considerations). For example, a hormonal method that reduces menstrual blood loss and dysmenorrhea may be of particular benefit for patients with severe anemia or women on anticoagulants. Long-term benefits such as protection against ovarian and endometrial cancer may be important to patients with a family history of ovarian cancer or with chronic anovulation, respectively.

Incorporate Contraceptive Choice

Compared to healthy individuals, those with medically complex conditions may have primary goals for their health that are more likely to be closely aligned with their major medical condition(s) rather than contraception itself. Even when the focus is contraception, individuals with chronic medical conditions will want to know: 1) how each of their contraceptive options will affect their chronic disease control or progression, 2) how each option might interact with their ongoing medication regimen, 3) how each option might increase the symptoms or side effects that currently challenge them. Whether healthy or medically complex, engaging in shared decision-making with the patient is key. As with other medications prescribed for a prolonged time, the process of informed consent before use of any contraceptive will require a review of the benefits and risks that are supported by evidence, with added clinical guidance when the evidence is lacking.

The additional social aspects that govern contraceptive choice cannot be ignored. For example, while a LARC method may be the safest method for your medically complex patients to use, they may feel hesitant choosing a contraceptive that they cannot stop on their own if they changed their mind. Listening to your patients' concerns and respecting their choices will foster a long-term provider-patient relationship that will be invaluable to successfully managing their health.

Author Disclosures—Allen: Nexplanon trainer (Merck). Cwiak: research support, advisory board (Medicines 360), research support (Contramed).

Acknowledgments—Kathryn M. Curtis, PhD, and Herbert B. Peterson, MD, for their work on the previous iteration of this chapter.

References

1. Curtis KM, Tepper NK, Jatlaoui TC, et al. U.S. medical eligibility criteria for contraceptive use, 2016. MMWR Recomm Rep 2016;65:1–104.
2. Creanga AA, Berg CJ, Syverson C, Seed K, Bruce FC, Callaghan WM. Pregnancy-related mortality in the United States, 2006-2010. Obstet Gynecol 2015;125:5–12.
3. Collaborative Group on Epidemiological Studies of Ovarian Cancer, Beral V, Doll R, Hermon C, Peto R, Reeves G. Ovarian cancer and oral contraceptives: collaborative reanalysis of data from 45 epidemiological studies including 23,257 women with ovarian cancer and 87,303 controls. Lancet 2008;371:303–14.
4. Chang CL, Donaghy M, Poulter N. Migraine and stroke in young women: case-control study. The World Health Organisation Collaborative Study of Cardiovascular Disease and Steroid Hormone Contraception. BMJ 1999;318:13–8.
5. Jick SS, Hagberg KW, Hernandez RK, Kaye JA. Postmarketing study of ORTHO EVRA and levonorgestrel oral contraceptives containing hormonal contraceptives with 30 mcg of ethinyl estradiol in relation to nonfatal venous thromboembolism. Contraception 2010;81:16–21.
6. American College of Obstetricians and Gynecologists. ACOG Practice bulletin no. 133: benefits and risks of sterilization. Obstet Gynecol 2013;121:392–404.
7. Chin J, Konje JC, Hickey M. Levonorgestrel intrauterine system for endometrial protection in women with breast cancer on adjuvant tamoxifen. Cochrane DB Syst Rev 2009:CD007245.
8. Mirena Prescribing Information 2008. (Accessed June 23, 2017, at www.accessdata.fda.gov/drugsatfda_docs/label/2008/021225s019lbl.pdf.)
9. Seasonique Prescribing Information 2010. (Accessed June 23, 2017, at www.accessdata.fda.gov/drugsatfda_docs/label/2010/021840s008lbl.pdf.)
10. Chakhtoura Z, Canonico M, Gompel A, Scarabin PY, Plu-Bureau G.Progestogen-only contraceptives and the risk of acute myocardial infarction: a meta-analysis. J Clin Endocrinol Metab 2011;96:1169–74.
11. Chakhtoura Z, Canonico M, Gompel A, Thalabard JC, Scarabin PY, Plu-Bureau G. Progestogen-only contraceptives and the risk of stroke: a meta-analysis. Stroke 2009;40:1059–62.
12. ACOG Practice Bulletin No. 110: noncontraceptive uses of hormonal contraceptives. Obstet Gynecol 2010;115:206–18.
13. World Health Organization. Ischaemic stroke and combined oral contraceptives: results of an international, multicentre, case-control study. WHO Collaborative Study of Cardiovascular Disease and Steroid Hormone Contraception. Lancet 1996;348:498–505.
14. Champaloux SW, Tepper NK, Monsour M, et al. Use of combined hormonal contraceptives among women with migraines and risk of ischemic stroke. Am J Obstet Gynecol 2017;216:489 e1–e7.
15. van den Heuvel MW, van Bragt AJ, Alnabawy AK, Kaptein MC. Comparison of ethinylestradiol pharmacokinetics in three hormonal contraceptive formulations: the vaginal ring, the transdermal patch and an oral contraceptive. Contraception 2005;72:168–74.
16. Jackson E, Curtis KM, Gaffield ME. Risk of venous thromboembolism during the postpartum period: a systematic review. Obstet Gynecol 2011;117:691–703.
17. Curtis KM, Jatlaoui TC, Tepper NK, et al. U.S. Selected Practice Recommendations for Contraceptive Use, 2016. MMWR Recomm Rep 2016;65:1–66.
18. Tepper NK, Curtis KM, Steenland MW, Marchbanks PA. Blood pressure measurement prior to initiating hormonal contraception: a systematic review. Contraception 2013;87:631–8.
19. Stewart FH, Harper CC, Ellertson CE, Grimes DA, Sawaya GF, Trussell J. Clinical breast and pelvic examination requirements for hormonal contraception: Current practice vs evidence. JAMA 2001;285:2232–9.
20. Vandenbroucke JP, van der Meer FJ, Helmerhorst FM, Rosendaal FR. Factor V Leiden: should we screen oral contraceptive users and pregnant women? BMJ 1996;313:1127–30.

21. Khader YS, Rice J, John L, Abueita O. Oral contraceptives use and the risk of myocardial infarction: a meta-analysis. Contraception 2003;68:11–7.
22. Gillum LA, Mamidipudi SK, Claiborne Johnston S. Ischemic stroke risk with oral contraceptives: a meta-analysis. JAMA 2000;284:72–8.
23. World Health Organization. Cardiovascular disease and use of oral and injectable progestogen-only contraceptives and combined injectable contraceptives. Results of an international, multicenter, case-control study. World Health Organization Collaborative Study of Cardiovascular Disease and Steroid Hormone Contraception. Contraception 1998;57:315–24.
24. Sridhar A, Cwiak CA, Kaunitz AM, Allen RH. Contraceptive considerations for women with gastrointestinal disorders. Digest Dis Sci 2017;62:54–63.
25. Zapata LB, Paulen ME, Cansino C, Marchbanks PA, Curtis KM. Contraceptive use among women with inflammatory bowel disease: A systematic review. Contraception 2010;82:72–85.
26. Mavranezouli I, Larc Guideline Development G. The cost-effectiveness of long-acting reversible contraceptive methods in the UK: analysis based on a decision-analytic model developed for a National Institute for Health and Clinical Excellence (NICE) clinical practice guideline. Hum Reprod 2008;23:1338–45.
27. Lipetz C, Phillips CJ, Fleming CF. The cost-effectiveness of a long-acting reversible contraceptive (Implanon) relative to oral contraception in a community setting. Contraception 2009;79:304–9.
28. Gabbe SG, Graves CR. Management of diabetes mellitus complicating pregnancy. Obstet Gynecol 2003;102:857–68.
29. Davis AR, Pack AM, Dennis A. Contraception for women with epilepsy. In: Allen RA, Cwiak C, eds. Contraception for the medically challenging patient. New York: Springer; 2014:135–46.
30. Kapp N, Curtis KM. Hormonal contraceptive use among women with liver tumors: a systematic review. Contraception. 2009 Oct;80:387-90.
31. Faculty of Sexual and Reproductive Healthcare. Clinical Guidance: Drug Interactions with Hormonal Contraception. 2018. Available at: www.fsrh.org/documents/ceu-clinical-guidance-drug-interactions-with-hormonal/

19

Contraception in the Later Reproductive Years

Amanda Black, MD
Anita L. Nelson, MD

- Although fertility and fecundity both decline with increasing age, contraception should still be used consistently by individuals in their later reproductive years when they wish to avoid unintended pregnancies.
- Pregnancies in this age group are associated with higher risks of poor fetal and maternal outcomes.
- No contraceptive methods are contraindicated on the basis of age alone. However, medical conditions tend to become more prevalent with increasing age and may limit choice of contraceptive methods.
- When counseling about contraceptive options for which the patient is medically eligible, discuss all the options in order of descending efficacy. Include a discussion of important noncontraceptive benefits that may help to improve quality of life during these years.
- The levonorgestrel-containing intrauterine devices and the etonogestrel implant provide effective contraception in the later reproductive years and then after, in an off-label use, as a progestin component of menopausal hormone therapy.

Menopause is a normal physiologic event defined as the final menstrual period; it indicates the cessation of ovarian follicular function and ovulation. However, menopause is a retrospective diagnosis that is made 1 year after the last natural menses. Perimenopause is the transitional period between the time when symptoms of hormonal changes first appear until menopause is diagnosed.[1] Due to the dwindling numbers of functional ovarian follicles, perimenopause is characterized by fluctuating hormone levels, irregular menstrual cycles, and the onset of vasomotor symptoms that generally increase in severity as menopause approaches.[2] The mean age of onset of perimenopause is 46 years, but the range is from

39 to 51 years. Perimenopause lasts an average of 5 years, but its duration varies from 2 to 8 years. Initially the follicular phase of the menstrual cycle shortens to 7 to 8 days, leading to a decrease in cycle length.[3] Menstrual cycle length becomes increasingly variable and unpredictable; later, episodes of amenorrhea occur.[4] However, even when cycles are longer than 50 to 60 days, ovulation will occur in 25% of them. Therefore, contraception is still required.[5]

Fluctuations in gonadotropins and estrogens seen during this time are so dramatic that they have been described as "hormonal chaos."[6] These vacillations in estrogen also lead to unpredictable bleeding; more than 75% of women experience abnormal uterine bleeding at some time during the perimenopause.[7] The Study of Women's Health Across the Nation (SWAN) study showed that anovulatory cycles without a bleeding episode represents relative hypoestrogenemia.[8] The increase in cycles with low estrogen levels can also explain other symptoms that are frequently experienced, such as moderate to severe vasomotor symptoms, vaginal dryness, dyspareunia, night sweats, sleep disturbances, reduced libido, mood swings, headaches, and bladder symptoms.[4,9–16] The prevalence of vasomotor symptoms in the perimenopause ranges from 42 to 79%.[14] In one large study, almost half (48.2%) of respondents aged 45 to 64 reported one or more personally distressing sexual concerns such as low sexual desire, low arousal, or orgasm difficulties.[16] The authors also reported a strong correlation between these concerns and other health issues. Disruptions of ovarian function have been linked to depression and increased cardiometabolic risk.[17–20] Other health issues occurring during this time include loss of bone mineral density and the emergence of cardiovascular disease, mental health problems, and gynecologic cancers.[18] The onset of menopause is not affected by the use of contraception, but different contraceptive methods may mask symptoms indicative of perimenopause or the start of menopause.

What is the probability of pregnancy in the years approaching menopause? The probability of becoming pregnant is dependent on the frequency of ovulation and the frequency of coitus, as well as male partner fertility and the consistency and efficacy of contraceptive use. The risk of pregnancy gradually declines with maternal age due to diminishing oocyte quality and ovarian reserve, an associated increase in anovulatory cycles and luteal insufficiency, and a decrease in coital frequency.[2,21] Evidence of luteal phase activity (ovulation) is seen in 87.9% of cycles up to 5 years before menopause and in 22.8% of cycles within 1 year of the final menstrual period.[2] The chance of naturally occurring pregnancy is approximately 30% per year at age 40 to 44 and decreases to 10% per year during age 45 to 49. Spontaneous pregnancy over the age of 50 is rare.[13] This contrasts with an 85% probability of pregnancy in 1 year for those in their 20s. If an individual is engaging in heterosexual sexual intercourse and does not desire pregnancy, an effective method of contraception should be used consistently until natural sterility is reached.

During the perimenopause, contraception appears to be used less consistently than earlier in life,[22] possibly due to a lower perceived risk of pregnancy. Very little data are collected about the contraceptives used by at risk people over 44 years of age.[23] A Massachusetts study of those at risk for pregnancy found nonuse of contraceptives varied by age from 9.3% of 18 to 24 year olds and 14.7% of 40 to 44 year olds, to 16.8% of 45 to 50 year olds.[24] However, the percentage of pregnancies that are unintended at this age is similar to or even higher than is found in younger age groups; almost half of unintended pregnancies during the perimenopause are terminated.[25]

What are the reproductive outcomes if pregnancy occurs after age 40? Reproductive outcomes are poorer for individuals over the age of 40, and the risks for serious maternal and neonatal complications are higher.[26] Age itself is an independent risk factor for these poor reproductive outcomes. However, these age-related risks may be magnified by medical comorbidities such as diabetes, hypertension, and obesity, which are all more prevalent among older reproductive age patients.[27,28] Although the absolute rate of maternal mortality is low, it is more than 5 times higher in this age group compared with those younger than 20.[26,29,30] Only 15% of births in the United States are to mothers who are age 35 or older, but over 27% of maternal deaths occur in this age group.[31] The risk of several maternal morbidities—including renal failure, shock, acute cardiac morbidity, amniotic fluid embolism and, as a measure of morbidity, ICU admission—increase dramatically with a maternal age over 39 years. Compared to mothers aged 20 to 24, the odds of severe maternal morbidity or mortality are 1.2 times higher for those aged 35 to 39, 2.2 times higher for those aged 45 to 49, and 5.2 times higher for those over age 50.[26]

With increasing age, there is also an increasing risk of spontaneous abortion and fetal aneuploidy. About half of pregnancies between the age of 40 to 44 years end in miscarriage; that rate increases to more than 90% over age 45.[32–34] The risk of chromosomal aneuploidy is reflected in both the increased risk of spontaneous abortion and the increased risk of having a child born with a chromosomal abnormality. The predicted odds of delivering a child at term with Trisomy 21 increases from 1 in 85 at age 40 to 1 in 35 at age 45.[34] The risks of ectopic pregnancy and stillbirth or perinatal death also increase with increasing maternal age.[32]

Other maternal complications also increase, including gestational diabetes, placenta previa, gestational hypertension, severe pre-eclampsia, and placental abruption.[27,29,30] The likelihood of Caesarean section is 2 to 3 times greater in those over the age of 35 years than in those younger than age 25. Neonatal complications, such as preterm delivery, low birthweight, intrauterine growth restriction, and perinatal mortality, also increase with increasing maternal age.[27–30]

It is important that the actual risks of pregnancy are addressed during any discussions about the risk of contraceptive options in the later reproductive years, particularly the risks of acute cardiovascular events and venous thromboembolism (VTE). For most patients, the health risks of pregnancy will generally far outweigh the risks with contraception.

CHANGING CONTRACEPTIVE NEEDS DURING THE LATER REPRODUCTIVE YEARS

Contraceptive needs change over the course of one's lifetime. The failure rate of every contraceptive method is lower in users over the age of 40 compared to younger individuals. Given this overall lower risk of pregnancy, methods offering less inherent efficacy may be suitable during these later reproductive years, but this decision must take into account the health risks posed by a pregnancy.

No contraceptive method is contraindicated on the basis of age alone.[35,36] For individuals in their later reproductive years, contraindications to contraceptive methods include all those that apply to younger users, such as VTE, malignancy, and certain medications. However, additional medical conditions frequently develop with increasing age that may raise contraceptive risks, particularly for estrogen-containing methods. Conditions to consider in this category include hypertension, obesity, tobacco use, diabetes, migraine, and cardiovascular disease (see Table 19-1 below).

In addition to the perimenopausal problems described above, symptomatic endometriosis is frequently found in this age group, as are heavy and prolonged bleeding episodes; these symptoms may improve with the use of some forms of contraception.[38] The goal of contraception should not only be to prevent pregnancy, but also to improve the user's quality of life and to provide protection against preventable adverse health conditions.

Table 19-1 Prevalence of health problems in women age 45-54 years

Hypertension	29.5%
Hyperlipidemia	31.2%
Cigarette smoking	21.2%
BMI > 30	35.3%
Heart disease	8.1%

Source: www.cdc.gov/nchs/hus/women.htm (2017)[37]

During individualized counseling, take into account baseline health risks for adverse clinical outcomes for both pregnancy and contraception, symptoms of the perimenopause, and the individual's life circumstances and goals. Present all the available contraceptive options for which the patient is eligible in descending order of efficacy. The relative appropriateness of each method should be assessed and discussed so that the best "contraceptive fit" can be determined for each individual. In fact, in many circumstances, methods may be used to achieve noncontraceptive benefits, even when there is no risk of pregnancy. Until menopause is confirmed, regularly review contraceptive use and available options, keeping in mind benefits, risks, and potential co-morbidities that may develop over time.

CONTRACEPTIVE OPTIONS DURING THE LATER REPRODUCTIVE YEARS

Other chapters provide detailed information about each of the individual methods. This chapter will summarize the features of each of the methods that are significant for people in the later reproductive years.

1. VOLUNTARY PERMANENT CONTRACEPTION

For those who have decided that their childbearing is complete, permanent birth control methods such as tubal ligation, salpingectomy, or partner vasectomy may be an option, although the benefit-to-risk ratios for performing these procedures decrease steeply with age. In the United States, rates of reliance upon voluntary permanent birth control methods are much higher than in many other countries; 50.6% of people who use contraception in the United States who are age 40 to 44 rely on tubal sterilization and 20% on vas sterilization.[39] As discussed in Chapter 16, tubal ligation and salpingectomy each have been shown to reduce the risk of all the major types of epithelial ovarian carcinoma.[40] However, if the procedure is provided late in reproductive years, it may not offer as great protection.

2. THE CONTRACEPTIVE IMPLANT

The single-rod subdermal contraceptive implant (Nexplanon) is the most effective contraceptive method and offers several features that are particularly relevant during the later reproductive years. Other 2-rod systems with levonorgestrel offered in other countries offer similar efficacy and safety. Nexplanon releases the progestin etonogestrel (ENG). Because the implant does not contain any estrogen, there are very few contraindications to its use. Even those who have serious medical comorbidities can usually safely use the implant.[35,36] (See Chapter 4 on Contraceptive Implant.) The implant is placed just beneath the skin in the upper arm during a 5-minute office procedure for which only minor training is needed. The progestin provides endometrial protection from the risks of unopposed estrogen associated with either anovulation or obesity, which are common problems in this age group. Extended use of the implant for up to 5 years' total duration is very appropriate in this age group.[41]

Changes in bleeding patterns are common with Nexplanon; 20% of users experience amenorrhea and more than 50% of younger users experience irregular bleeding (which is usually infrequent bleeding). How the implant impacts the abnormal bleeding patterns typically seen during these years is not well documented; perimenopausal hormonal fluctuations could theoretically increase the likelihood of abnormal bleeding patterns. Those abnormal bleeding patterns may raise concerns about the possibility of an underlying pathology. In this context, the question would be: "how should one interpret abnormal bleeding, especially for users who have risk factors for endometrial hyperplasia?" If bleeding changes coincide with implant initiation, then the new bleeding change should generally not raise concerns for endometrial pathology. However, if the bleeding is heavy or persists for more than 4 to 6 months or if new concerning bleeding changes develop after the implant has been used for a while, some evaluation may be prudent because the implant does not provide complete protection against all endometrial abnormalities.

Although ovulation is consistently inhibited by the ENG implant for the first few years of use, endogenous estradiol production continues; serum estradiol levels remain above the threshold needed to maintain normal bone mass. The evidence on the effect of implants on bone mineral density beyond 3 years is still limited but appears to be reassuring.[42,43]

Off-label, the implant provides adequate endometrial protection when estrogen therapies are being used to treat perimenopausal or postmenopausal symptoms.[5] There is no need to add extra progestin therapy in these settings.

3. Levonorgestrel Intrauterine Systems (LNG-IUS)

Levonorgestrel intrauterine systems (LNG-IUS) provide top-tier pregnancy protection and, depending upon the specific device, induce endometrial changes that address many uterine problems that tend to develop during perimenopause. The LNG-IUS 20 with 52 mg LNG (Mirena/Liletta) is the most effective medical treatment for heavy menstrual bleeding (HMB).[44] (See Chapter 5 on Intrauterine Devices.) HMB commonly develops during the perimenopausal years due to adenomyosis, anovulatory cycling, and other causes.[44] The LNG-IUS 20 is also the most effective medical therapy for endometrial hyperplasia. Although its use in this condition is off-label, comparative studies have demonstrated the significant superiority of intrauterine progestin therapy over oral therapies with medroxyprogesterone acetate (MPA) or mestranol for reversal of all categories of endometrial hyperplasia.[45,46] Because of these positive effects, the LNG-IUS 20 has been shown to reduce the risk of hysterectomy.[47] Bleeding from leiomyoma has been demonstrated to be reduced by high-dose LNG-IUS if the fibroids are not large (< 4 cm) and if they do not distort the uterine cavity. However, expulsion rates are higher when fibroids are present.[48] In younger users, lower-dose LNG-IUS options (LNG-IUS 12 Kyleena and LNG-IUS 8 Skyla/Jaydess) induce amenorrhea at much lower rates than seen with the LNG-IUS 20. The bleeding patterns with these lower-dose systems in older users are not well documented. However, the narrower diameter of the applicator for the lower-dose IUSs may make placement easier for older women.

Although the LNG-IUS 20 (Mirena/Liletta) is not currently approved by the U.S. FDA as a source of progestin for those with an intact uterus who use estrogen therapy to treat menopausal symptoms, it is approved for such use by medical agencies in over 100 other countries. Using the LNG-IUS 20 for contraception before menopause and later as the progestin component of post-menopausal hormone therapy for women with an intact uterus is an accepted strategy.[49]

Questions often arise about extending the length of time that the different hormonal IUDs can be used. Although there are not many clinical studies, those that exist support the off-label use of the LNG-IUS 20 for 7 years in women who are age 25 years or older at the time of LNG-IUS 20 placement.[50,51] (See Chapter 5 for a more detailed discussion.) Although each LNG-IUS provides *local* intrauterine concentrations of progestins, *serum* levels can reflect intrauterine LNG concentrations. Mean serum LNG levels after 7 years of use of the LNG-IUS 20 are 137 ± 12 pg/ml (range, 23-393),[50,52] which compares favorably with the mean serum LNG levels of 59 pg/ml reported at the end of the 3-year effective life of LNG-IUS 8.[53] Before advising off-label extended use of the LNG-IUS 20, consider the risks of removal and replacement and individual factors such as access to and the availability of replacement units.[50] In the advanced reproductive years with a low potential for pregnancy protection it is probably reasonable to allow continued use for contraception for at least 7 years. For off-label use as a source of endometrial protection from systemic estrogen therapy postmenopausally, even longer use may be considered; amenorrhea is a good sign of ongoing IUS function in this setting. Longer term use also allows for a smoother transition into menopause, avoiding the abnormal uterine bleeding patterns that affect many in this age group and disrupt their quality of life.

4. Copper Intrauterine Devices

The only copper IUD available at this time in the United States is ParaGard (TCu380A IUD). Many lower-dose copper IUDs are also available in other countries. As a group, copper IUDs are highly effective, long-acting, reversible contraceptives, but they are associated with increased menstrual blood loss. Therefore, they may not be suitable in the setting of abnormal or heavy uterine bleeding, which is fairly common during the late reproductive years. However, the copper IUD has some attractive features for users in this age group. It does not contain hormones, which is appealing if the patient has contraindications to hormone use or a strong desire to avoid use of any exogenous hormones. Copper IUD use is associated with a decreased risk of endometrial and, possibly, cervical cancer.[54–56] The copper IUD is also a very effective method of emergency contraception if placed within 5 days of an act of unprotected intercourse.[57]

The TCu380A IUD is a very cost-effective contraceptive method that can be used far beyond its 10-year on-label duration of use.[50,58] The potential for extended effectiveness is particularly important when a patient in the mid-to-late 40s presents after 10 years of using a CuIUD and asks for removal and placement of the device. In this instance, if the TCu380A IUD was placed at age 35 years or older, it is reasonable to leave the device in place until menopause.[50] IUD removal is advised if possible once menopause is diagnosed.

5. Injectable Progestins: Depo-Medoxyprogesterone Acetate

Depo-medroxyprogesterone acetate (DMPA; Depo-Provera) is an effective method of contraception that is associated with high amenorrhea rates.[59] Although successful treatment of heavy menstrual bleeding (HMB) is less likely with DMPA compared to the LNG-IUS,[60] DMPA can still be very useful for treating many types of HMB, including leiomyoma-related or adenomyosis-related HMB in poor surgical candidates and HMB in those with bleeding dyscrasia. (See Chapter 6 on Injectable Contraceptives.) Early unscheduled bleeding may discourage initiation of DMPA in this group, but practice suggests that pretreatment with GnRH agonists or other agents to establish amenorrhea may significantly reduce this transitional problem.

Lingering concerns about the adverse impact DMPA may have on bone mineral density have led to a proliferation of guidelines recommending stopping its use early in perimenopause to allow bone mineral density (BMD) to rebuild prior to the last menses. This ignores the fact that patients entering menopause on DMPA have already lost the bone density they would lose due to declining estradiol levels during the first 5 years of menopause. DMPA users will not experience that accelerated loss in bone density.[61,62] A systematic review of observational studies found that compared to never-users of DMPA, former users did not have higher rates of postmenopausal fractures, once those who had suffered prior fractures were excluded from the analysis.[63] Weight gain does occur in some users, but BMI >30 kg/m^2 is not a contraindication to use of DMPA. Just as in younger users, if early use is associated with a gain of 5% or more, further injections should be discouraged because continued weight gain is likely.[64,65]

DMPA is associated with a reduced risk of both endometrial hyperplasia and endometrial cancer, which is relevant in the later reproductive years when anovulatory cycles become more common and BMI is often increased.[66] DMPA use may be associated with hypoestrogenic symptoms due to the suppression of FSH-regulated ovarian estradiol production, but DMPA can be combined with menopausal estrogen therapy in appropriate candidates. DMPA alone has been shown to help reduce vasomotor symptoms in postmenopausal women.[67] Use of lubricants during intercourse may be recommended due to thinning of vaginal epithelium.

DMPA continuation beyond age 50 should be individualized; carefully consider whether the patient has other potential risk factors for osteoporosis that might increase liability risks. DMPA does not mask the menopausal rise in FSH levels.[68] Although DMPA use is less demanding of adherence than some other methods of reversible contraception, some users may still find it difficult to visit their clinicians every 3 months for repeat DMPA injections. This challenge may be overcome by using alternative health care providers or alternative sites for subsequent injections, such as pharmacist-administered injections or even self-injection when this is permitted by legislation.[69]

6. Combined Hormonal Contraception

Combined hormonal contraceptives (CHCs) raise the greatest number of clinical issues for patients in this age group, but may also provide the greatest numbers of noncontraceptive benefits. During the perimenopause, CHCs offer healthy candidates effective contraception as well as good cycle control (with the possibility of amenorrhea), decreased blood loss, treatment of vasomotor symptoms, at least partial protection against bone loss, and reduction in the risks of several cancers. (See Chapter 8 on Combined Oral Contraceptives and Chapter 7 on Contraceptive Patch and Vaginal Contraceptive Ring.) In particular, endometrial cancer rates can be reduced by about 50%, regardless of the age of the user.[70] Ovarian cancer risk reduction has been impressively demonstrated in younger users, but it is not clear how much the risk of ovarian cancer is reduced with CHC use in the later reproductive-age years.[71] More recently, the lifetime risk of colorectal cancer has been showed to be reduced by COC use, although the magnitude of the effect is not known when pills are used only during later reproductive years.[72,73]

Breast cancer risks alarm women, but the earlier studies that raised the concerns for increased breast cancer risk involved the use of high-dose formulations. Today, there does not appear to be an excess risk of breast cancer associated with long-term use of combined oral contraceptives, either during CHC use or later in life.[74,75] However, the risks of thrombotic stroke (TS) and myocardial infarction (MI) associated with combined hormonal contraceptives do increase with age.[5] In a Danish study, the risks of stroke and myocardial infarction increased by a factor of 20 and 100, respectively, in women age 45 to 49 compared to those age 15 to 19 after adjusting for CHC use. Higher estrogen dose formulations were associated with greater prevalence.[76]

Carefully monitor patients in this age group for development of category 4 conditions or combinations of category 3 conditions. (See the color insert of the U.S. Medical Eligibility Criteria.) Given the prevalence of obesity and underdiagnosed hypertension, diabetes, and cardiovascular risks, thorough periodic analysis of the health status of older CHC users must be done over time. Those found to be healthy without other contraindications to estrogen-containing methods can continue to use combined hormonal methods until menopause in the United States. However, the lack of evidence of the safety of CHCs in this population has prompted more conservative approaches in other countries. In Canada and in the United Kingdom, guidelines recommend considering changing at the age of 50 from CHC methods to a progestin-only method.[77]

Some companies have marketed lower-dose oral contraceptives specifically for this age group, but there is no consistent evidence that formulations with 10 or 20 mcg ethinyl estradiol are safer. Estrogen potency may be important; formulations with weaker estrogens may pose less thrombotic risk. In the late reproductive years, extended-cycle use of combined hormonal contraceptives (oral contraceptive pills and vaginal rings) may be particularly appealing, not only to achieve amenorrhea, but also to avoid development of vasomotor symptoms during hormone-free intervals. If the user wants scheduled bleeding, try to limit the number of hormone-free days with use of 24/4 formulations or 24/4 ring-use patterns. Some pill formulations have only 2 placebo pills and include low-dose estrogen-only pills during the rest of the scheduled bleeding days; this can reduce symptoms associated with estrogen withdrawal. Of note, the vaginal contraceptive ring increases vaginal lubrication and may help relieve symptoms of vaginal dryness and dyspareunia.

7. Progestin-Only Pills

With typical use, progestin-only pills (POPs) are as effective as CHCs containing estrogen. They can be used by virtually everyone; only current or recent (<5 years) breast cancer is listed as a category 4 condition.[35] (See the color insert of the U.S. Medical Eligibility Criteria.) They have not been shown to increase the risk of VTE or ATE, nor to adversely affect bone mineral density. POPs are excellent options to use when transitioning patients in the late reproductive years from longer acting methods that commonly induce amenorrhea (DMPA, LNG-IUS) or from those methods that cause cyclic bleeding (pills, patches, rings). If there is a question about an individual's menopausal status or whether she is still at risk for pregnancy when discontinuing one of the other contraceptive methods, switch the patient to POPs and look for absence of bleeding for at least 12 months to be sure that contraception is no longer needed.

Patient education requirements for POP use are minimal: take 1 pill every day at about the same time of day. The package contains only active pills; there are no placebos that can be taken out of order. Although globally there are several different progestins used in POPs (levonorgestrel, norethindrone, or desogestrel), only one formulation (norethindrone) is available in the United States and Canada at this time. POPs thicken the cervical mucus to prevent sperm ascent into the upper genital tract. The cervical mucus thins rapidly if there is a delay taking the norethindrone POP. So if administration is delayed more than 3 hours, a back-up method is needed for the next 2 days. Higher-dose POPs containing DSG available in other countries inhibit ovulation more reliably and are more forgiving of late pill ingestion. While POPs reduce blood loss and can help reduce vasomotor symptoms, they do not provide predictable scheduled bleeding. (See Chapter 9 on Progestin-only Pills.) Amenorrhea and unscheduled bleeding rates are generally higher with POPs than with combined hormonal contraceptives, but this does not seem to increase POP discontinuation rates in older users. POPs do not suppress the menopausal rise in FSH levels.[68]

8. Barrier and Behavioral Methods

As a group, barrier and behavioral methods have the highest contraceptive failure rates, but with their lower fertility potential, motivated users in their later reproductive years may find these methods attractive. These methods may pose specific challenges at this age. *Fertility awareness-based methods* that rely on knowledge of the timing of ovulation are not usually reliable in the perimenopause due to the difficulty interpreting markers of ovulation and the unpredictable nature of ovulation and cycle length. However, those techniques that monitor markers of ovulation on a daily basis (symptothermal technique or TwoDay method) may still be used during these years of transition. (See Chapter 12 on Fertility Awareness-Based Methods.)

Barrier methods, including male and female condoms, diaphragms, and cervical caps have lower failure rates during the perimenopause compared to younger age groups. Condoms have the additional advantage of protecting against sexually transmitted infections (STIs). Individuals in this age group may be re-entering the "dating scene" and initiating new relationships.[78] Reinforce the need for STI protection. Urogenital changes associated with estrogen deficiency, specifically vaginal dryness and mucosal thinning, can increase the risk of HIV acquisition.[79] However, those same physiologic changes may limit the acceptability of male condoms; lubricated condoms or use of water-based lubricants help ameliorate these problems during sexual intercourse. (See Chapter 14 on Male Condoms.) Male condom use may be more challenging if the partner is older or suffers from erectile dysfunction. In this case, female condoms may be an option. Female condoms may not be as readily available as they were in the past, because they now require a prescription in the United States. Users must also become familiar with their placement and removal.

Diaphragms (Caya) and, to some extent, the cervical cap (FemCap) rely on vaginal wall support to maintain their positioning. Patients with pelvic relaxation or significant urethral hypermobility may not be optimal candidates for these methods. Prescriptions are still needed to obtain these female barrier methods in the United States, but not in Canada or Europe. In general, clinician input is also helpful to ensure proper fit and to confirm the user's ability to correctly place and remove these devices. (See Chapter 11 on Vaginal Barriers and Spermicides.)

Spermicides may provide additional lubrication for coitus. However, failure rates with spermicides as a single agent are among the highest of any group of methods. The sponge has higher failure rates among parous compared to nulliparous users. All spermicides in the United States use nonoxynol-9 as their active ingredient, which has been associated with increased risk of HIV transmission. Those at higher risk of HIV acquisition should avoid the use of all nonoxynol-9 spermicides.

Coitus interruptus (withdrawal) also has higher typical-use failure rates. However, it may be appropriate in the perimenopause, especially if the couple is experienced using this method. (See Chapter 15 on Coitus Interruptus.)

9. Emergency Contraception

Individuals choosing a reversible contraceptive method other than implants or intrauterine devices should also be counseled about the availability, efficacy, and safety of emergency contraception (EC). Emphasize that EC should be used in the event of a method disruption or malfunction (e.g., condom slips or breaks, diaphragm is dislodged) or if unprotected intercourse occurs. Prescriptions for or packages of oral EC should be offered in advance of need to minimize the patient's out-of-pocket costs, but LNG EC is available over-the-counter if the user is willing to pay full cost. The choice of oral EC will depend upon body mass index (BMI) and the ongoing contraceptive method to be used after EC. The most effective method of EC is the copper IUD. (See Chapter 10 on Emergency Contraception).

WHEN CAN CONTRACEPTION BE RELIABLY STOPPED?

For any individual, it is not possible to know the precise age at which the risk of pregnancy disappears. No laboratory tests can reliably confirm when there is definitive loss of fertility. Single tests of FSH with or without estradiol are not reliable during the perimenopausal years.[6] In the face of the dramatic swings in hormone levels during the perimenopause, an elevation of FSH even with a low level of estrogen can incorrectly diagnose menopause; this can put the patient at risk for pregnancy if contraception were to be discontinued solely on the basis of these tests.

Contraception should be used until menopause is confirmed. Menopause may be confirmed in nonusers of hormonal contraception in the following instances:

- Amenorrhea for more than one year after age 50.
- Amenorrhea for 2 or more years if less than 50 years of age in those without functional hypothalamic amenorrhea.

Amenorrhea alone cannot be used to diagnose menopause in users of hormonal contraception. Some authorities endorse the concept that an elevated FSH (>30 IU/L) measured on 2 separate occasions 6 to 8 weeks apart while off combined hormonal contraception for at least 2 weeks can be diagnostic of menopause. Others recommend that the patient be switched to POPs or nonhormonal methods and observed for return of menses or amenorrhea.

Thus, recommendations for diagnosing menopause will vary depending on age, type of contraception used, clinical signs, and laboratory testing. Sterility is usually assumed at age 55, when 95% of individuals have reached menopause. It must be remembered standard menopausal hormone therapy is NOT a method of contraception.

Summary

- During the later reproductive years, one's contraceptive needs may change. New health problems or concerns may arise that require a method change or the use of a contraceptive method for its non-contraceptive benefits.
- Long-acting methods of reversible contraception are an excellent alternative to voluntary permanent birth control methods and may offer important non-contraceptive benefits for individuals in the later reproductive years.

- Reassess the need for and the safety of ongoing use of each individual's contraceptive method at each health care provider visit. Document the noncontraceptive benefits provided by the method.
- Do not hesitate to consider changing methods during the later reproductive years, particularly when new situations arise. In general, the implant and the progestin-only pills are the easiest "go-to" options given that they have very few medical contraindications. LNG-IUS 20 has additional benefits, including a substantial decrease in menstrual bleeding during perimenopause. Off-label, any of the LNG-containing intrauterine contraceptives and the ENG implant can be a source of progestin in postmenopausal hormonal therapy.
- In the absence of contraindications, combined hormonal contraceptives (CHC) may also provide relief from many perimenopausal symptoms.
- Male or female condoms can always be added for STI protection and should be considered when the need arises.
- Of course, emergency contraception should always be available in advance of need for those not using voluntary permanent contraception, IUDs or implants.
- Carefully counsel the patient about the need to continue using contraception until the diagnosis of menopause is confidently made.

Author Disclosure—Black: research grant from Mathra Pharma, consultant and speaker for Bayer and Pfizer. Nelson: research grants from Agile Pharma, ContraMed, Estetra SPRL, Evofem Inc., FHI360 (Mona Lisa), Mathra Pharma, Merck; speaker for Allergan, Bayer, Merck; advisory board member for Agile, Allergan, AMAG Pharma, Bayer, ContraMed, Merck, PharmaNest.

References

1. Shifren JL, Gass ML, Group NRfCCoMWW. The North American Menopause Society recommendations for clinical care of midlife women. Menopause 2014;21:1038–62.
2. Santoro N, Crawford SL, El Khoudary SR, et al. Menstrual cycle hormone changes in women traversing the menopause: Study of women's health across the nation. J Clin Endocrinol Metab 2017;102:2218–29.
3. Reid RL, BA M. Confronting the challenges of the menopausal transition. Women's Midlife Health 2015;1:1–9.
4. Santoro N. Perimenopause: From research to practice. J Womens Health (Larchmt) 2016;25:332–9.
5. Long ME, Faubion SS, MacLaughlin KL, Pruthi S, Casey PM. Contraception and hormonal management in the perimenopause. J Womens Health (Larchmt) 2015;24:3–10.
6. Santoro N, Brown JR, Adel T, Skurnick JH. Characterization of reproductive hormonal dynamics in the perimenopause. J Clin Endocrinol Metab 1996;81:1495–501.

7. Paramsothy P, Harlow SD, Greendale GA, et al. Bleeding patterns during the menopausal transition in the multi-ethnic study of Women's Health Across the Nation (SWAN): a prospective cohort study. BJOG 2014;121:1564–73.
8. Burger HG, Dudley EC, Robertson DM, Dennerstein L. Hormonal changes in the menopause transition. Recent Prog Horm Res 2002;57:257–75.
9. Hale GE, Robertson DM, Burger HG. The perimenopausal woman: endocrinology and management. J Steroid Biochem Mol Biol. 2014;142:121–31.
10. Martin VT, Pavlovic J, Fanning KM, Buse DC, Reed ML, Lipton RB. Perimenopause and menopause are associated with high frequency headache in women with migraine: results of the American Migraine Prevalence and Prevention Study. Headache 2016;56:292–305.
11. Jones HJ, Huang AJ, Subak LL, Brown JS, Lee KA. Bladder symptoms in the early menopausal transition. J Womens Health (Larchmt) 2016;25:457–63.
12. Avis NE, Crawford SL, Greendale G, et al. Duration of menopausal vasomotor symptoms over the menopause transition. JAMA Intern Med 2015;175:531–9.
13. Avis NE, Brockwell S, Randolph JF, et al. Longitudinal changes in sexual functioning as women transition through menopause: results from the Study of Women's Health Across the Nation. Menopause 2009;16:442–52.
14. Jackson EA, El Khoudary SR, Crawford SL, et al. Hot flash frequency and blood pressure: data from the Study of Women's Health Across the Nation. J Womens Health (Larchmt) 2016;25:1204–9.
15. Kravitz HM, Joffe H. Sleep during the perimenopause: a SWAN story. Obstet Gynecol Clin North Am 2011;38:567–86.
16. Shifren JL, Davis SR. Androgens in postmenopausal women: a review. Menopause 2017;24:970–79.
17. Bleil ME, Bromberger JT, Latham MD, et al. Disruptions in ovarian function are related to depression and cardiometabolic risk during premenopause. Menopause 2013;20:631–9.
18. Chang PY, Gold EB, Cauley JA, et al. Triglyceride levels and fracture risk in midlife Women: Study of Women's Health Across the Nation (SWAN). J Clin Endocrinol Metab 2016;101:3297–305.
19. El Khoudary SR, Santoro N, Chen HY, et al. Trajectories of estradiol and follicle-stimulating hormone over the menopause transition and early markers of atherosclerosis after menopause. Eur J Prev Cardiol 2016;23:694–703.
20. Joffe H, Crawford SL, Freeman MP, et al. Independent contributions of nocturnal hot flashes and sleep disturbance to depression in estrogen-deprived women. J Clin Endocrinol Metab 2016;101:3847–3855.
21. Steiner AZ, Jukic AM. Impact of female age and nulligravidity on fecundity in an older reproductive age cohort. Fertil Steril 2016;105:1584–8 e1.
22. Black A, Yang Q, Wen SW, Lalonde A, Guilbert E, Fisher W. Contraceptive use by Canadian women of reproductive age: Results of a national survey. J Obstet Gynaecol Can 2009;31:627–40.
23. Harlow SP, Dusendang JR, Hood MM, Wood NF. Contraceptive preferences and unmet need for contraception in midlife women: where are the data? Women's Midlife Health 2017;3:6–13.
24. Godfrey EM, Zapata LB, Cox CM, Curtis KM, Marchbanks PA. Unintended pregnancy risk and contraceptive use among women 45–50 years old: Massachusetts, 2006, 2008, and 2010. Am J Obstet Gynecol 2016;214:712.e1–8.
25. Finer LB, Zolna MR. Declines in unintended pregnancy in the United States, 2008–2011. N Engl J Med 2016;374:843–52.
26. Lisonkova S, Potts J, Muraca GM, et al. Maternal age and severe maternal morbidity: A population-based retrospective cohort study. PLoS Med 2017;14:e1002307.
27. Jacobsson B, Ladfors L, Milsom I. Advanced maternal age and adverse perinatal outcome. Obstet Gynecol 2004;104:727–33.

28. Klemetti R, Gissler M, Sainio S, Hemminki E. At what age does the risk for adverse maternal and infant outcomes increase? Nationwide register-based study on first births in Finland in 2005–2014. Acta Obstet Gynecol Scand 2016;95:1368–75.
29. Joseph KS, Allen AC, Dodds L, Turner LA, Scott H, Liston R. The perinatal effects of delayed childbearing. Obstet Gynecol 2005;105:1410–8.
30. Cleary-Goldman J, Malone FD, Vidaver J, et al. Impact of maternal age on obstetric outcome. Obstet Gynecol 2005;105:983–90.
31. Creanga AA, Berg CJ, Syverson C, Seed K, Bruce FC, Callaghan WM. Pregnancy-related mortality in the United States, 2006–2010. Obstet Gynecol 2015;125:5–12.
32. Nybo Andersen AM, Wohlfahrt J, Christens P, Olsen J, Melbye M. Maternal age and fetal loss: population based register linkage study. BMJ 2000;320:1708–12.
33. Heffner LJ. Advanced maternal age—how old is too old? N Engl J Med 2004;351:1927–9.
34. Morris J, Mutton D, Alberman E. Corrections to maternal age-specific live birth prevalence of Down's syndrome. J Med Screen 2005;12:202.
35. Centers for Disease Control and Prevention. U.S. Medical Eligibility Criteria for Contraceptive use, 2016. Morbidity and Mortality Weekly Report (MMWR) 2016;65:1–103.
36. World Health Organization. Medical eligibility criteria for contraceptive use. 5th Edition ed. Geneva, Switzerland 2015.
37. Centers for Disease Control and Prevention. Health, United States, 2015 - Women's Health 2016 Available from: www.cdc.gov/nchs/hus/women.htm.
38. Van Heertum K, Liu J. Contraception and conception in mid-life: a review of the current literature. Women's Midlife Health 2017;3:3.
39. Jones J, Mosher W, Daniels K. Current contraceptive use in the United States, 2006–2010, and changes in patterns of use since 1995. Natl Health Stat Report 2012:1–25.
40. Sieh W, Salvador S, McGuire V, et al. Tubal ligation and risk of ovarian cancer subtypes: a pooled analysis of case-control studies. Int J Epidemiol 2013;42:579–89.
41. Ali M, Akin A, Bahamondes L, et al. Extended use up to 5 years of the etonogestrel-releasing subdermal contraceptive implant: comparison to levonorgestrel-releasing subdermal implant. Hum Reprod 2016;31:2491–8.
42. Beerthuizen R, van Beek A, Massai R, Makarainen L, Hout J, Bennink HC. Bone mineral density during long-term use of the progestagen contraceptive implant Implanon compared to a non-hormonal method of contraception. Hum Reprod 2000;15:118–22.
43. Modesto W, Dal Ava N, Monteiro I, Bahamondes L. Body composition and bone mineral density in users of the etonogestrel-releasing contraceptive implant. Arch Gynecol Obstet 2015;292:1387–91.
44. Lethaby A, Hussain M, Rishworth JR, Rees MC. Progesterone or progestogen-releasing intrauterine systems for heavy menstrual bleeding. Cochrane Database Syst Rev 2015;4:CD002126.
45. Yuk JS, Song JY, Lee JH, Park WI, Ahn HS, Kim HJ. Levonorgestrel-releasing intrauterine systems versus oral cyclic medroxyprogesterone acetate in endometrial hyperplasia therapy: A meta-analysis. Ann Surg Oncol 2017;24:1322–29.
46. Gallos ID, Shehmar M, Thangaratinam S, Papapostolou TK, Coomarasamy A, Gupta JK. Oral progestogens vs levonorgestrel-releasing intrauterine system for endometrial hyperplasia: a systematic review and metaanalysis. Am J Obstet Gynecol 2010;203:547.e1–10.
47. Lahteenmaki P, Haukkamaa M, Puolakka J, et al. Open randomised study of use of levonorgestrel releasing intrauterine system as alternative to hysterectomy. BMJ 1998;316:1122–6
48. Youm J, Lee HJ, Kim SK, Kim H, Jee BC. Factors affecting the spontaneous expulsion of the levonorgestrel-releasing intrauterine system. Int J Gynaecol Obstet 2014;126:165–9.
49. Depypere HT, Hillard T, Erkkola R, et al. A 60-month non-comparative study on bleeding profiles with the levonorgestrel intrauterine system from the late transition period to estrogen supplemented menopause. Eur J Obstet Gynecol Reprod Biol 2010;153:176–80.

50. Wu JP, Pickle S. Extended use of the intrauterine device: a literature review and recommendations for clinical practice. Contraception 2014;89:495–503.
51. Ronnerdag M, Odlind V. Health effects of long-term use of the intrauterine levonorgestrel-releasing system. A follow-up study over 12 years of continuous use. Acta Obstetricia et Gynecologica Scandinavica 1999;78:716–21.
52. Hidalgo MM, Hidalgo-Regina C, Bahamondes MV, Monteiro I, Petta CA, Bahamondes L. Serum levonorgestrel levels and endometrial thickness during extended use of the levonorgestrel-releasing intrauterine system. Contraception 2009;80:84–9.
53. Bayer Inc. Jaydess Product Monograph November 21, 2014. At: www.bayer.ca/files/JAYDESS-PM-EN-174672-21NOV2014.pdf?.
54. Felix AS, Gaudet MM, La Vecchia C, et al. Intrauterine devices and endometrial cancer risk: a pooled analysis of the Epidemiology of Endometrial Cancer Consortium. Int J Cancer 2015;136:E410–22.
55. Castellsague X, Diaz M, Vaccarella S, et al. Intrauterine device use, cervical infection with human papillomavirus, and risk of cervical cancer: a pooled analysis of 26 epidemiological studies. Lancet Oncol 2011;12:1023–31.
56. Beining RM, Dennis LK, Smith EM, Dokras A. Meta-analysis of intrauterine device use and risk of endometrial cancer. Ann Epidemiol 2008;18:492–9.
57. Turok DK, Godfrey EM, Wojdyla D, Dermish A, Torres L, Wu SC. Copper T380 intrauterine device for emergency contraception: highly effective at any time in the menstrual cycle. Hum Reprod 2013;28:2672–6.
58. Sivin I, Stern J, Coutinho E, et al. Prolonged intrauterine contraception: a seven-year randomized study of the levonorgestrel 20 mcg/day (LNg 20) and the Copper T380 Ag IUDS. Contraception 1991;44:473–80.
59. Hubacher D, Lopez L, Steiner MJ, Dorflinger L. Menstrual pattern changes from levonorgestrel subdermal implants and DMPA: systematic review and evidence-based comparisons. Contraception 2009;80:113–8.
60. Kucuk T, Ertan K. Continuous oral or intramuscular medroxyprogesterone acetate versus the levonorgestrel releasing intrauterine system in the treatment of perimenopausal menorrhagia: a randomized, prospective, controlled clinical trial in female smokers. Clin Exp Obstet Gynecol 2008;35:57–60.
61. Cundy T, Cornish J, Roberts H, Reid IR. Menopausal bone loss in long-term users of depot medroxyprogesterone acetate contraception. Am J Obstet Gynecol 2002;186:978–83.
62. Beksinska ME, Smit JA, Kleinschmidt I, Farley TM, Mbatha F. Bone mineral density in women aged 40–49 years using depot-medroxyprogesterone acetate, norethisterone enanthate or combined oral contraceptives for contraception. Contraception 2005;71:170–5.
63. Lopez LM, Chen M, Mullins Long S, Curtis KM, Helmerhorst FM. Steroidal contraceptives and bone fractures in women: evidence from observational studies. Cochrane Database Syst Rev 2015;7:CD009849.
64. Lopez LM, Ramesh S, Chen M, et al. Progestin-only contraceptives: effects on weight. Cochrane Database Syst Rev 2016;CD008815.
65. Bonny AE, Secic M, Cromer B. Early weight gain related to later weight gain in adolescents on depot medroxyprogesterone acetate. Obstet Gynecol. 2011;117:793–7.
66. Kaunitz AM. Depot medroxyprogesterone acetate contraception and the risk of breast and gynecologic cancer. J Reprod Med 1996;41:419–27.
67. Bullock JL, Massey FM, Gambrell RD Jr. Use of medroxyprogesterone acetate to prevent menopausal symptoms. Obstet Gynecol 1975;46:165–8.
68. Beksinska ME, Smit JA, Kleinschmidt I, Farley TM. Assessing menopausal status in women aged 40–49 using depot-medroxyprogesterone acetate, norethisterone enanthate or combined oral contraception. S Afr Med J 2011;101:131–5.
69. Picardo C, Ferreri S. Pharmacist-administered subcutaneous depot medroxyprogesterone acetate: a pilot randomized controlled trial. Contraception 2010;82:160–7.

70. Iversen L, Sivasubramaniam S, Lee AJ, Fielding S, Hannaford PC. Lifetime cancer risk and combined oral contraceptives: the Royal College of General Practitioners' Oral Contraception Study. Am J Obstet Gynecol. 2017;216:580.e1–580.e9.
71. Braem MG, Onland-Moret NC, van den Brandt PA, et al. Reproductive and hormonal factors in association with ovarian cancer in the Netherlands cohort study. Am J Epidemiol. 2010;172:1181–9.
72. Gierisch JM, Coeytaux RR, Urrutia RP, et al. Oral contraceptive use and risk of breast, cervical, colorectal, and endometrial cancers: a systematic review. Cancer Epidemiol Biomarkers Prev. 2013;22:1931–43.
73. Bosetti C, Bravi F, Negri E, La Vecchia C. Oral contraceptives and colorectal cancer risk: a systematic review and meta-analysis. Hum Reprod Update. 2009;15:489–98.
74. Hannaford PC, Iversen L, Macfarlane TV, Elliott AM, Angus V, Lee AJ. Mortality among contraceptive pill users: cohort evidence from Royal College of General Practitioners' Oral Contraception Study. BMJ 2010;340:c927.
75. Thorbjarnardottir T, Olafsdottir EJ, Valdimarsdottir UA, Olafsson O, Tryggvadottir L. Oral contraceptives, hormone replacement therapy and breast cancer risk: a cohort study of 16,928 women 48 years and older. Acta Oncol 2014;53:752–8.
76. Lidegaard O, Lokkegaard E, Jensen A, Skovlund CW, Keiding N. Thrombotic stroke and myocardial infarction with hormonal contraception. N Engl J Med 2012;366:2257–66.
77. Faculty of Sexual & Reproductive Healthcare CEU. FSRH Guideline: Contraception for women aged over 40 years. 2017:1–66.
78. Copen CE, Daniels K, Vespa J, Mosher WD. First marriages in the United States: data from the 2006–2010 National Survey of Family Growth. Natl Health Stat Report 2012:1–21.
79. Senanayake P. Women and reproductive health in a graying world. Int J Gynaecol Obstet 2000;70:59–67.

20

Reproductive Tract Infections, Including HIV and Other Sexually Transmitted Infections

Jeanne M. Marrazzo, MD, MPH
Ina U. Park MD, MS

- Reproductive tract infections (RTIs) are frequently encountered by reproductive health professionals.
- RTIs include both sexually transmitted infections (STIs) and other common infections of the genital tract, such as bacterial vaginosis and vulvovaginal candidiasis. Important emerging infections, notably Zika virus, can also be sexually transmitted.
- RTIs can have serious health consequences:
  - Tubal occlusion leading to infertility and ectopic pregnancy
  - Pregnancy loss and neonatal morbidity caused by transmission of the infection to the infant during pregnancy and childbirth
  - Anogenital cancers
  - Enhanced transmission of human immunodeficiency virus (HIV)
- Assessing a client's risks for RTIs can help the client better select appropriate contraceptive methods and help the clinician provide better care. Ask each patient, "How do you protect yourself from infection with HIV and other sexually transmitted infections?"
- Preventing RTIs and their consequences requires sexually active persons to adopt safer sexual behaviors and clinicians to diagnose and treat existing infections effectively.
- Because reproductive-age patients constitute a major segment of the HIV epidemic in the United States, reproductive health care settings are a critical conduit to HIV testing and provision of

preventive services including HIV pre-exposure prophylaxis (PrEP). All patients should be offered counseling and voluntary HIV testing, and those at risk should be linked to services that provide HIV PrEP. A useful resource is the PrEP in Family Planning Tool Kit, available at www.hiveonline.org/prep4familyplanning.

- Routine HIV testing for all pregnant patients is the standard of care for prenatal services. Be certain that HIV-positive pregnant patients have access to antiretroviral treatment to improve health status, suppress viral load, and eliminate the likelihood of perinatal transmission.

In *Contraceptive Technology*, the generic term RTI covers three types of infections: (1) sexually transmitted infections (STIs), (2) vaginal infections including bacterial vaginosis and candidiasis, and (3) iatrogenic infections associated with the insertion of an intrauterine device (IUD) or induced abortion. Prevention of infection through risk reduction and screening/ treatment are the most effective ways to reduce the adverse consequences of RTIs, while recognition and correct management of RTIs that do occur can prevent complications in the individual and interrupt transmission in the community. This chapter provides general background about RTI management in the reproductive health care setting.

MAGNITUDE AND RISKS OF RTIs

The number of people infected with RTIs or affected by their consequences is a major problem for society.[1] For example, 2015 marked the highest number of sexually transmitted *Chlamydia trachomatis* cases (1,526,658 cases) ever reported to the Centers for Disease Control and Prevention (CDC).[2,3] Chlamydia is the most common condition reportable to the CDC. STIs are the most common cause of pelvic inflammatory disease (PID). Infertility caused by PID accounts for billions of dollars in healthcare costs as well as major emotional costs. STIs such as syphilis can cause neurologic sequelae such as blindness and devastating consequences in pregnancy including stillbirth. Lifetime costs associated with the morbidity and mortality due to the eight most common STIs contracted in a single year is 15.6 billion dollars.[4]

While the prevalence of RTIs by individual pathogen and across different geographic regions varies considerably, some general trends are notable. For example, individuals under 25 years of age account for a majority of RTI cases, with two-thirds of cases of gonorrhea and chlamydia reported in persons less than 25 years of age. Rates of chlamydia, gonorrhea, and PID are highest in adolescents and decline steadily with increasing age. RTIs are also concentrated in socio-geographic clusters, so-called "core populations," that generally reflect sexual networks, regional variation in disease prevalence and, possibly, access to care.

Finally, most RTIs exhibit a "biological sexism". Compared with men, women suffer more severe long-term consequences, including PID, infertility, ectopic pregnancy, chronic pelvic pain, and cervical cancer. Women may also be less likely to seek health care for assessment of RTI-related symptoms, because a higher proportion of their RTIs are asymptomatic or unrecognized as being serious. Women are also more likely than men to acquire RTIs, due to the transmission dynamics during an act of vaginal intercourse. The risk of acquisition increases when trauma occurs to the genital mucosa, as may be the case in sexual assault. For similar reasons, the risk increases from anal intercourse (a risk that also affects men who receive anal penetration). RTI acquisition is less likely during oral sex, digital penetration, or sex acts other than vaginal or anal intercourse.

TRANSMISSION OF RTIs

The probability that unprotected sexual intercourse will lead to RTIs or their consequences differs from the probability of unintended pregnancy. (See Table 20-1.) The risk of pregnancy varies according to the menstrual cycle. In contrast, while numerous complex factors probably modulate susceptibility to RTI, the risk of acquisition depends on (1) having sex with an infected person, (2) the gender of the infected person, (3) transmissibility of the particular RTI, and (4) use of barriers or other protective measures.[5,6] For example, the risk of acquiring gonorrhea from a single act of vaginal

Table 20-1 Comparative risk of adverse consequences from vaginal or anal intercourse: RTI and unintended pregnancy

Unintended pregnancy (per coital act)[10]	• 17%–30% midcycle <1% during menses
HIV transmission (per coital act)	• 0.08% receptive vaginal sex • 0.04% insertive vaginal sex • 1.3% receptive anal sex • 0.11% insertive anal sex
Gonococcal transmission (per coital act)[6]	• 50% receptive vaginal sex • 25% insertive vaginal sex
PID per woman infected with cervical chlamydia[11]	• 22% if not treated • 0% if promptly and adequately treated
Tubal infertility per PID episode[12]	• 8% after first episode • 20% after second episode • 40% after third or more episodes

intercourse (where one partner is infectious) is approximately 25% for men and 50% for women. The probability of suffering consequences from an RTI depends on whether or not proper diagnosis and treatment are affected. In the case of HIV, the quantity of serum (and presumably genital) HIV viral load directly influences risk of transmitting HIV to vulnerable partners. HIV viral load is extremely high in the context of early infection (the first several months after a person acquires the virus). Because sexual transmission of HIV frequently occurs during this early infection interval,[7] persons at risk need to consider HIV-prevention methods at all times.

There have been several breakthroughs related to preventing sexual transmission of HIV, including use of daily HIV antiretroviral medication (tenofovir-emtricitabine) for pre-exposure prophylaxis (PrEP).[8] Studies in Africa have also demonstrated that circumcision of male partners can significantly reduce the risk of these men acquiring HIV and other RTIs from their female partners.[9]

RTI RISK ASSESSMENT, PREVENTION AND RISK BEHAVIORS

Different individuals accept different levels of risk. Not everyone will follow every safer sex recommendation but, with the proper knowledge, each person can make his or her own informed choices about reducing risk. Some prevention messages are universal and should be reinforced (for example, barrier methods when appropriate). Additionally, client-centered counseling highlights the need to individualize risk assessment and tailor risk-reduction plans. The latter may include a discussion on selecting sex partners and building skills for negotiating safer sex.

Preventive measures for avoiding RTI transmission are generally consistent with guidelines for reducing risk of HIV infection. Risk-free options include having a mutually faithful relationship with an uninfected partner or completely abstaining from sexual activities that involve semen, blood or other body fluids, or skin-to-skin contact. Examining a partner for lesions, discussing each new partner's previous sexual history, and avoiding partners who have had many previous sex partners or known high-risk partners can augment other measures to prevent RTI transmission. Educating people about their bodies and teaching them to be active participants in their health care gives them more control over their reproductive health.

Contraceptive Choice

Choice of contraception directly affects the risk of RTI (Table 20-2). Condoms reduce the risks of both bacterial and viral RTIs; the evidence is

Table 20-2 Effects of contraceptives on bacterial and viral RTIs[21,22]

Contraceptive Method	Bacterial RTI	Viral RTI
Condoms	Protective	Protective
Spermicides	Not protective	Not protective
Diaphragm	Protective against cervical infection	Protective against cervical neoplasia
Hormonal contraception	Protective against symptomatic PID but not silent endometritis; Effect modified by estrogen vs. progesterone components	Not protective; DMPA associated with mildly elevated risk of HIV acquisition
IUD	Not protective; Associated with PID in first month after insertion	Not protective

See chapters on specific contraceptive methods for details.

strongest for condom effectiveness against HIV, trichomoniasis, genital herpes, and gonorrhea.[5] No recent data support spermicides' ability to prevent bacterial or viral infections, including HIV.[5] Diaphragms provide a barrier against cervical infection but have not demonstrated protection against HIV and most other RTIs.[13] In addition, diaphragms have been associated with changes in vaginal flora and urinary tract infections. Although oral contraceptives are usually associated with an increase in chlamydia detected in the cervix, they protect against symptomatic PID, but not asymptomatic endometritis.[14] Depot medroxyprogesterone acetate (DMPA) use has been associated with a modestly increased risk of HIV acquisition and of chlamydial infection in some studies.[15,16] Although older data suggested that copper IUD insertion was associated with a transient increased risk of PID in the first month after insertion, newer data indicates that RTI risk is both very low and not elevated after IUD insertion.[17] The overall risk of PID within 90 days of IUD insertion is less than 0.6%.[18,19] Routine antibiotic prophylaxis is not recommended before IUD placement. The IUD has a strong record of safety, even for HIV-positive patients.[20] At present, the data are insufficient to state whether the progesterone-releasing IUD has a differential effect on RTI acquisition or natural history.

Microbicides, defined as substances used topically that interrupt the ability of infectious agents to establish infection, continue to hold promise for prevention of both HIV and other STIs. The search for a nonspecific microbicide that offers protection against a wide variety of STIs, including HIV, has yielded disappointing results, and no available microbicide offers broad protection against RTIs. Furthermore, frequent use of certain topical agents such as nonoxynol-9 gel was associated with an increased risk of HIV acquisition.[23] Vaginal delivery of drugs such as tenofovir, with specific antiretroviral activity against HIV and herpes simplex virus (HSV), appears more promising. Use of tenofovir gel applied vaginally before and after sexual intercourse significantly reduced the rate of HIV acquisition (by 39%) in a study of South

African women and of HSV-2 acquisition by 50%.[24] Additional delivery systems in the form of subcutaneous implants or vaginal rings are under study.

Other Risk Behaviors

In addition to sexual behaviors, other practices have been linked to RTI risk. Routine douching for hygiene has been associated with an increased risk of PID and ectopic pregnancy. Douching is also a risk factor for bacterial vaginosis because it eradicates commensal hydrogen peroxide-producing vaginal *Lactobacillus* species.[25] Genital washing has been poorly studied but appear to have little effect, if any, on reducing the risk of acquiring an RTI. In some studies, these practices have been associated with an increased risk of HIV acquisition.

Drug use influences the transmission of RTIs. While hepatitis C is not typically considered an RTI, cases of sexual transmission have occurred, particularly among men who have sex with men.[26] Use of drugs such as methamphetamine and cocaine—through intravenous, intranasal, or other routes—has been associated with risky sexual behaviors. Outbreaks of syphilis, antibiotic-resistant gonorrhea, and chancroid have been linked to drug-related sexual behaviors and to sexual networks of drug users. Crystal methamphetamine has figured prominently in national outbreaks of syphilis in men who have sex with men, and the drug is especially harmful for its disinhibitory effects on sexual behavior. Abuse of alcohol, particularly binge drinking, has also been associated with risky sexual practices, including not using condoms.[27] Alcohol abuse is a notable concern for adolescents and young adults.

ASSESSMENT, DIAGNOSIS, AND TREATMENT OF RTIs

Comprehensive RTI-related care begins with routine risk assessment. Risk assessment should not be discarded due to common assumptions about either an individual patient (for example, a married patient) or "representative" types of patients (for example, patients who identify as lesbian).

At a minimum, ask clients about the following: (1) number of sex partners in the last 3 months; (2) anatomic sites exposed during sex (vagina, rectum, oropharynx), and (3) use of personal protective measures (e.g., condoms). Risk assessment also helps clinicians provide better contraceptive counseling and more cost-efficient RTI management. Balance the variety of demographic, behavioral, and clinical information (other than laboratory test results) to assess the likelihood that clients are infected with an RTI or are at high risk of future infection and to counsel clients in selecting appropriate contraceptive methods. For example, the RTI risk assessment scale can help identify patients who may be good candidates for barrier methods or inappropriate candidates for an IUD.[28]

Laboratory diagnosis of most RTIs can be performed in nearly every reproductive health care setting. Over the past decade, routine screening for chlamydia has been associated with a decreased prevalence of the infection among clients attending family planning clinics in several regions of the country, and with concomitant declines in PID and ectopic pregnancy.[29] In addition, some family planning clinics have extended their range of services to clients of all genders, including RTI diagnosis, treatment, and counseling. Many clinics provide *expedited partner management* (sometimes referred to as *expedited partner treatment*, or EPT), defined as provision of medications or a prescription for the partner of the index patient being treated, without a requirement for examination (see Partner Management in section on Counseling Patients About RTI Diagnosis And Treatment).

Routine screening for RTIs. Because most RTIs are asymptomatic and do not cause clinical signs such as cervicitis or PID, routine screening can provide early detection and prompt treatment, thus interrupting the progression to the sequelae of untreated disease. Counsel patients about the asymptomatic nature of most RTIs and that transmission typically occurs in the absence of symptoms. Chlamydial infections are the prototype, because up to 90% of these infections cause neither symptoms nor clinical signs (namely, cervicitis). The U.S. Preventive Services Task Force (USPSTF) recommends routine annual screening for target groups of patients, as delineated in Table 20-3.[30] The USPSTF also recommends routine screening for gonorrhea using similar criteria. Adults in the United States should be screened for HIV at least once, and more frequently if at ongoing risk of acquisition.[31] In contrast, the USPSTF recommends against routine screening for asymptomatic herpes simplex virus infection (genital

Table 20-3 Recommendations for screening of patients for genital infection with *Chlamydia trachomatis* and *Neisseria gonorrhoeae*

- All sexually active patients <25 years old
- Patients of any age at risk for infection, defined as having any of the following risk factors since their last negative test:
  - A new sex partner
  - More than 1 sex partner
  - A sex partner with concurrent partners or a sex partner who has an STI
  - Inconsistent condom use
  - Previous or coexisting STI
  - Exchanging sex for money or drugs

Screening should occur at least annually, or more frequently based on risk.

Source: U.S. Preventive Services Task Force[30]

herpes) using serology, citing the associated cost, imperfect performance of available screening assays, distress associated with receipt of a positive result, and lack of evidence that such an routine screening effects significant health benefit at the individual or population level.[32,33]

Counseling Patients About RTI Diagnosis and Treatment

Counseling patients with RTIs requires an approach different than that generally used in family planning settings. For couples trying to prevent unplanned pregnancies, counseling is typically nondirective to allow maximal opportunity for them to make an informed choice about the best contraceptive method. However, for patients who have RTIs, *directive* counseling is important to prevent new infections, increase adherence to treatment and follow-up, and offer guidance on talking to partners about their RTI exposure. Patients must be made aware of both the potential serious consequences of RTIs and the behaviors that increase the likelihood of reinfection.

Education about infection and treatment. Make sure patients understand what RTI they have, how it is transmitted, why it must be treated, and exactly when and how to take prescribed medication. Because unpleasant side effects from some medications may discourage patients from continuing treatment, discuss what to expect and ways to minimize side effects. For example, both azithromycin and doxycycline taken on an empty stomach may cause nausea that prompts the patient to stop taking the medication. Advise taking the medication with food unless directions specify otherwise.

Completion of treatment. Urge patients to finish their entire supply of medication even though symptoms, if present, may diminish or disappear in a few days. Discontinuing antibiotics before the infection is completely cured can lead to recurrent infection and increase the likelihood that hard-to-cure strains of the pathogen may flourish.

Abstinence during treatment. Advise patients to avoid sex until they complete the full course of therapy. For single-dose therapy like azithromycin, patients should abstain for the week following treatment.

Partner management. Failure to treat the partners of patients with RTIs is the most important risk factor influencing the high rates of chlamydia and gonorrhea recurrence in the months after initial treatment. An increasing number of family planning professionals are being trained in partner management skills. Confidentiality is crucial, just as it is in all aspects of family planning and RTI care. Notify and treat sex partner(s) to prevent both reinfection of the patient and spread of disease through the community. Assist patients in notifying their partners by coaching them in partner notification techniques (patient referral) and, if available, using trained STI public health program staff (provider referral) to help evaluate and treat partners. Another approach is asking patients to bring their partner with them for concurrent treatment (concurrent patient-partner therapy); this may be feasible for patients with one primary partner. *Expedited partner treatment (EPT)*, in which the patient is given either drugs or a prescription to give to partners without requiring that the partner be examined, is a highly effective way to increase the likelihood that partners are treated and to reduce the rate of recurrence in the index patient.[34–36] While legal regulations about the provision of expedited partner treatment vary by state, EPT is now legally permissible in 39 states, potentially legally permissible in 8, and not legal in only 3 states (www.cdc.gov/std/ept).

Comfort & support. Be attentive to patients' physical and psychosocial comfort to enhance adherence with treatment. Treat nausea, pain, itching, or other physiologic discomforts symptomatically, if possible. This is especially critical for patients who may be experiencing a first episode of symptomatic genital herpes, for example, or for patients with highly symptomatic vulvovaginal candidiasis. Overcoming the psychosocial component of genital discomfort is exceedingly important in RTI treatment. Patients may be afraid or ashamed to ask a partner to seek treatment, embarrassed to admit their sexual practices, or concerned about confidentiality. Reinforcing the messages that many RTIs are relatively common and can often be transmitted when people are experiencing no symptoms can help to minimize the stigma associated with these infections.

Concurrent infections. Managing RTIs requires that clinicians have a high index of suspicion for other infections. A patient may have two or more RTIs concurrently. Be alert for symptoms that differ from those normally associated with the primary RTI infection.

STI reporting. All states require that certain STIs, including chlamydia, gonorrhea, syphilis, be reported to public health officials. Reporting is not a breach of confidentiality; in fact, statutory protection of clients' names is a crucial part of control strategies. Accurate reporting helps identify trends in disease, gain resources for high prevalence communities, and evaluate RTI control efforts. Resources to assist with this process can be found online at state STD program websites, which are listed at the National Coalition of STD Directors website at https://npin.cdc.gov/featured-partner/national-coalition-std-directors-ncsd.

RTI During Pregnancy

Question pregnant patients and their sex partners about their risk of RTI; counsel them about the possibility of transmitting an infection to their infant. Because of the severe effects RTI may have on both the pregnancy and the developing fetus, all pregnant patients should be screened for infections with HIV, syphilis, and hepatitis B. Pregnant patients <25 years of age should also be screened for chlamydia and gonorrhea (see Tables 20-4 and 20-5). Cervical cancer screening should occur at the same intervals as for

Table 20-4 Risks of sexually transmitted bacteria and related syndromes in pregnancy and childbirth[37,38]

Organism/Syndrome	Infant Effects	Transmission Risk from Infected Mother	Prevention	Treatment of Mother, Neonate
Neisseria gonorrhoeae	Conjunctivitis, sepsis, meningitis	Approximately 30%	Screening: test mother; apply ocular prophylaxis	Ceftriaxone and Azithromycin
Chlamydia trachomatis	Conjunctivitis, pneumonia, bronchiolitis, otitis media	25%–50% conjunctivitis, 5%–15% pneumonia	Screening in third trimester: test mother, apply ocular prophylaxis	Azithromycin Amoxicillin Erythromycin
Treponema pallidum	Congenital syphilis, neonatal death	50%	Serologic screening in early and late pregnancy	Penicillin
Trichomonas vaginalis	Low birth-weight, preterm delivery	N/A	Diagnostic Testing	Metronidazole
Bacterial vaginosis	Low birth-weight, preterm delivery	N/A	Diagnostic Testing	Metronidazole Clindamycin

Source: Adapted from Cates (1995).[3]

[a]Percentage of pregnant patients with evidence of infection

Table 20-5 Risks of sexually transmitted viruses and related syndromes in pregnancy and childbirth[37,38]

Organism/Syndrome	Infant Effects	Transmission Risk from Infected Mother	Prevention	Treatment of Mother, Neonate
Hepatitis B Virus	Hepatitis, cirrhosis	10%–90%	Active HBV immunization	Post-exposure passive HBV immunization
Herpes Simplex Virus	Disseminated, central nervous system, localized lesions	Recurrent: 3% at delivery; primary: 30% at delivery	Cesarean delivery if lesions present at delivery	Acyclovir
Human Papillomavirus	Laryngeal papillomatosis	Rare	HPV immunization	Surgical
Human Immunodeficiency Virus	Pediatric HIV infection	27% without ART; <5% with ART	ART during pregnancy	Antiretrovirals (ART)

Source: Adapted from Cates (1995).[3]

[a]Percentage of pregnant women with evidence of infection

nonpregnant patients. Routine screening for human papillomavirus (HPV) infection is not recommended. Screening for herpes simplex virus type-2 (HSV-2) infection is not routinely recommended. Depending on the individual patient's concerns, HSV screening can be considered on a case-by-case basis. If serologic testing is obtained, it is critical to use a glycoprotein-G-based test, because this is the only type of assay that can reliably distinguish between antibody formed in response to HSV-2 infection from that formed in response to HSV-1 infection (a common cause of oral infection).

The management of some important RTI syndromes and related pathogens is discussed in more detail below. For more complete information, refer to the CDC STD Treatment Guidelines (www.cdc.gov/std/treatment) and for RTI in pregnant patients, refer to Guidelines for Perinatal Care, jointly published by the American College of Obstetricians and Gynecologists and the American Academy of Pediatrics.[37]

RTI and Sexual Assault

In cases of sexual assault and abuse, clinicians must attend not only to physical and psychological trauma but also to the possibility of pregnancy or RTI. Any of the sexually transmissible infections, including HIV, can be acquired during a sexual assault. Some RTIs, such as gonorrhea or syphilis, are almost exclusively sexually transmitted and are therefore useful markers of assault in persons who have not previously been sexually active. To reduce the risk of pregnancy, offer emergency contraception (see Chapter 10 on Emergency Contraception). To reduce risk of RTI, the CDC recommends the following approach:[38]

Adult evaluation. If possible, evaluate the survivor within 24 hours of the assault and take specimens for nucleic acid amplification testing (NAAT) of *N. gonorrhoeae* and *C. trachomatis*. Examine vaginal fluid microscopically for trichomoniasis and bacterial vaginosis (BV). Perform a pregnancy test, and keep a frozen serum sample for possible testing in the future. If treatment is not administered, schedule a repeat evaluation for 2 weeks later. Presumptive treatment may be provided at the survivor's request. Advise clients to use condoms until the test results are reported. While no regimen provides coverage against all potential pathogens, the following should be effective against the most frequent RTIs:

- Ceftriaxone 250 mg given intramuscularly (IM) PLUS
- Azithromycin 1 g given orally PLUS
- Metronidazole 2 grams (g) given orally (if vaginal penetration occurred)
- Hepatitis B vaccination, first dose (if survivor has not been vaccinated)

- HPV vaccination for female survivors between 9 and 26 years of age, and male survivors 9 to 21 years of age. Male survivors between 22 and 26 years of age should also be vaccinated.
- Postexposure prophylaxis against HIV, depending on risk assessment

Child evaluation. In general, the presence of an RTI in a child beyond the neonatal period suggests sexual abuse. However, unlike gonorrhea or syphilis, specific infections such as bacterial vaginosis (BV), genital mycoplasmas, and genital warts are not conclusive evidence of sexual abuse. Evaluation is essentially the same as described for adult victims (see previous section), except both culture and NAAT specimens should be collected from the pharynx and rectum as well as from the vagina or urethra because the child's report of assault may not be complete. Presumptive treatment may be given at the family's request. For more complete information regarding laboratory procedures, diagnosis, and treatment for child sexual assault and abuse victims, refer to the CDC 2015 Guidelines for Treatment of Sexually Transmitted Diseases (see www.cdc.gov/std/treatment).[38]

SPECIAL CONSIDERATIONS REGARDING RTI EVALUATION IN THE REPRODUCTIVE HEALTH SETTING

For many young people, reproductive health care clinics may be the only source of health care. Each patient should be asked "What do you do to protect yourself from infection with HIV and other sexually transmitted infections?" Providers may be able to determine readiness for behavior change by assessing this answer. The patient who answers, "I thought I would get some condoms while I'm here today," may be more receptive to behavioral change than the patient who answers, "Who, me?"

Although reproductive health providers are more likely than other primary care providers to ask about sex and drug behavior, many are reluctant to risk offending patients. It may be helpful to begin with, "I'm going to ask you some personal questions that I ask everyone, because I think it is so important to your health. Is that all right with you?"

Other Key Points. Avoid making assumptions about a patient's sexual and other behaviors based on appearances. In particular, avoid assumptions such as:

- Sexually experienced people know how to use safer sex techniques.
- People with stable jobs and families don't use drugs.

- Single people have lots of partners and risky sex practices.
- Older people have few partners and infrequent sex.
- Married people are heterosexual and don't have sex with partners of the same sex.

Remember that terminology can sometimes get in the way of clarity with this type of risk assessment. For example, teens may not know the word "monogamous." Some may think "sexually active" means vigorous sex, or many partners. Some people who engage in same-sex behavior do not think of themselves as "gay or lesbian," particularly in settings where acknowledging same-sex behavior or identity is stigmatized.

COUNSELING ABOUT SAFER SEX

Teach safer sex skills, including correct use of condoms and other latex and plastic barriers, to all at-risk patients (Table 20-6). Advise all patients

Table 20-6 Options for sexual intimacy and HIV and STI prevention

Safe	All unprotected sexual activities, when both partners are monogamous and known by testing to be free of HIV and other STIs; also mutual masturbation without contact with partner's semen, vaginal secretions, blood, or broken skin, as well as sexual fantasies, massage, hugging, body rubbing, dry kissing, erotic conversation, books, movies, videos, electronic images, erotic bathing, showering, non-penetrative behaviors that eroticize non-genital/non-oral/non-anal body parts, including feet, hands, hips, abdomen, ears
Low, but Potential Risk	All sexual activities, when both partners are monogamous but have not been tested; includes wet kissing with no broken skin, cracked lips, or damaged mouth tissue; hand-to-genital touching or mutual masturbation on healthy, intact skin or with a latex or plastic barrier; vaginal or anal intercourse using latex or plastic condom correctly with adequate lubrication; oral sex on a man wearing a latex or plastic condom; oral sex on a woman using a latex or plastic barrier such as a female condom, dental dam, or plastic wrap; hand-vaginal penetration with a glove
Unsafe in the absence of mutual monogamy and STI/HIV testing of both partners	Blood contact of any kind, including menstrual blood; any vaginal or anal intercourse without a latex or plastic condom; oral sex without a latex or plastic barrier (especially if there is any oral contact with menstrual blood, infected vaginal secretions, or semen); oral-anal contact; digital penetration of vagina or anus, shared sex toys or douching equipment; any sex that causes tissue damage or bleeding, such as rough vaginal or anal intercourse, rape, or fisting

that a crucial time for diligent safer sex practices is the first few months of a new relationship. Delaying intercourse may allow the couple the opportunity to get screened for common STIs, including HIV, together. Oral sex may also transmit gonorrhea, syphilis, HSV-1, and (to a much lower extent) HIV, especially with activities that expose the mouth to semen or blood.

Customize teaching methods for individual patients. Use audiovisual, print, and electronic teaching aids appropriate to the patient's age, language, culture, and learning style. Be sure to make your guidance specific to related to an individual's particular issues, rather than giving vague, global advice:

- "Starting today, put condoms on the night stand beside the bed," rather than "always use condoms."
- "You could reconsider whether to date this person, who is also dating other people," rather than "Have fewer, safer partners."
- "Next time you're out with friends and might have sex, avoid getting high on drugs or alcohol," rather than "Have safer sex."

Specific Concerns Related to HIV

Postexposure Prophylaxis, Sex, and Drugs

In cases of isolated high-risk exposures to HIV—unprotected vaginal or anal intercourse, rape, receptive oral sex with ejaculation, or sharing injection equipment when the partner is known or suspected to be infected—consider giving postexposure prophylaxis for HIV (HIV-PEP).[39] Although data on efficacy are limited, an increasing number of health care providers offer treatment to survivors of sexual assault as well. HIV-PEP should begin as soon as possible, and no later than 72 hours after the exposure. Treatment consists of a 28-day course of drugs combined from 2 or 3 antiretroviral drug groups, much like the combination therapy regimens used by persons with HIV. Discuss treatment protocol options with your local rape crisis center, or call the Postexposure Prophylaxis Hotline operated by the National HIV/AIDS Clinicians' Consultation Center for guidance on individual cases. The hotline is based at the University of California at San Francisco and can be reached toll-free 24 hours a day, 7 days a week at 1–888–448–4911.

Treatment may be costly, associated with side effects, and not always covered by health insurance. Thus, the decision to undertake HIV-PEP should be informed by a thorough discussion of all components of the risk-benefit assessment, including the risk associated with the exposure and the patient's individual concerns. Patients with ongoing risk for HIV exposure may consider transitioning from HIV-PEP to HIV-PrEP once their course of HIV-PEP is completed.

FACTORS AFFECTING SEXUAL TRANSMISSION

The likelihood of sexual HIV transmission is variable. The major determining factor is the HIV viral load in the infected partner's genital secretions (semen or vaginal fluid), which is directly proportional to the HIV viral load in their plasma.[40] Risk of sexual transmission may be increased under certain circumstances:

- During early HIV infection (the weeks after the infection is acquired), because HIV viral load, and thus infectivity, is very high
- During late or uncontrolled HIV infection, when viral multiplication is not suppressed by antiretroviral treatment
- When either partner, but especially the HIV-infected partner, has a concurrent STI including trichomoniasis, syphilis, gonorrhea, genital herpes, bacterial vaginosis, or chlamydia
- When blood or blood secretions are involved, or when tears in the exposed mucous membranes are present
- With anal sex (especially for the receptive partner), relative to vaginal or oral sex

The risk of sexual transmission from an infected partner may be decreased under the following circumstances:

- If the HIV-infected partner is being treated with antiretroviral medication and plasma HIV viral load is undetectable. While this does not guarantee that HIV is absent in genital secretions, the likelihood of sexual transmission is very low to negligible.
- If the partner's penis is circumcised, the risk of acquiring HIV is reduced by approximately half.

Advice for Patients Seeking Contraceptive Services

Until further data are available, it is prudent to advise all patients as follows:

- For vaginal or anal intercourse, use latex or plastic condoms each time you suspect any risk of exposure to HIV.
- For oral sex, use latex or plastic condoms for fellatio and latex or plastic vulvar barriers for cunnilingus any time you suspect any risk of HIV.
- Vaginal spermicides do not protect against HIV or other STIs.
- Any tissue damage to the vulva, vagina, anus, or penis could increase susceptibility to HIV. Avoid any intercourse until lesions are healed.

HIV Testing and Counseling

Reproductive health care providers represent the most important access point for patients to receive HIV testing. Thus, HIV testing should be a standard component of care.

When to Offer Testing

Offer routine HIV testing to *all adolescents and adults* between the ages 13 to 64 if they have never previously been tested. Routine HIV testing for all pregnant patients is already the standard of care in the United States.[41] Certain situations outside of the prenatal setting call for the care provider making a strong recommendation to seek testing and taking the extra effort to assure that patients have reasonable access to counseling and testing services:

- Known sexual exposure to an HIV-infected person
- Shared injection equipment with an HIV-infected person
- Possible recent occupational exposure
- Clinical settings with a ≥1% HIV seroprevalence
- Settings serving "populations at increased behavioral or clinical HIV risk," such as STI clinics, teen clinics with high rates of RTI, or correctional facilities, regardless of that setting's HIV seroprevalence
- Clinical signs or symptoms suggesting HIV infection (e.g., fever or illness of unknown origin, opportunistic infection without known reason for immune suppression)
- Diagnosis suggesting increased risk for HIV (such as another RTI or blood-borne infection)
- Patient's request

Prenatal testing. Many patients learn they have HIV when testing is done as part of routine prenatal care. Some prospective studies have indicated that pregnancy itself may also confer an increased risk of acquiring HIV infection.[42]

Counseling about pregnancy options is an especially important component of post-test counseling if the HIV diagnosis is made early in pregnancy; the patient may be overwhelmed by the news, and by the amount of information to absorb. Pregnant patients with HIV are faced with the same sorts of reproductive decisions as those without HIV, with similar percentages of terminated pregnancies and live births. For the HIV-positive patient who chooses to continue the pregnancy, consult appropriate guidelines for the use of antiretroviral therapy. Detailed guidelines are available at www.aidsinfo.nih.gov/guidelines.

Test Counseling

Reproductive health care providers should be prepared to explain how the test is done, what the routine screening procedure will and will not reveal, implications of anonymous vs. confidential testing, and instructions on how to obtain test results. A guide (Table 20-7) for providing this information and for giving negative and positive test results may be helpful.

Counseling and Testing Issues

Confidentiality. Confidential testing is name-linked, and information is protected to a degree determined by state law and, at the testing site, by formal policies and staff commitment to confidentiality.

Table 20-7 Components of counseling in the setting of HIV testing

Deciding whether to have the test
- Your right to decide whether to be tested
- Voluntary informed consent
- Who will see the results if test is done here; state law implications
- Other sites for testing; home test options

Benefits of being tested
- Peace of mind; knowing, one way or the other
- If infected:
  - — Options for HIV therapy, managing related problems
  - — Prevent transmission to others
  - — Make informed childbearing decisions
  - — Diagnose illness or symptoms
  - — Access assistance programs

Difficulties with being tested
- Learning you have a serious illness
- Disclosing results to sex or injecting-drug-equipment-sharing partners (public health departments can provide help with this task)

What results mean
- If antibody positive:
  - — You are infected
  - — You can pass the virus on to other people
  - — Need to establish care with knowledgeable provider and undergo further assessment for disease staging
- If antibody negative or indeterminate:
  - — You are not infected, or
  - — You are infected, but antibodies are not yet detectable

Reducing risk for HIV
- Develop a personalized risk-reduction plan today with counselor
- Offer condoms and other safer sex supplies
- Referral for drug, alcohol treatment
  - — Consider pre-exposure prophylaxis (PrEP)

Testing technology. Recommendations for laboratory-based HIV testing involve testing serum with a dual antigen / antibody enzyme immunoassay (EIA) followed by confirmation with an HIV1 / HIV2 differentiation assay, or in uncertain cases, an HIV nucleic acid test (Figure 20-1).[43] While both tests are very sensitive and specific, neither is perfect, so an HIV test is reported as positive only after obtaining positive results from at both the screening and confirmatory tests. As with any screening test, prevalence of the infection within the client's population is the major factor in determining a test's predictive value; the higher the prevalence, the greater the likelihood that a positive test result means that the person is truly infected. Always regard HIV test results in the context of the patient history and clinical picture, and re-evaluate when they are not in agreement.

Clinic-based point-of-care rapid testing, saliva testing, and home-based rapid testing are all FDA-approved and provide sensitivity and specificity comparable to those of traditional tests. Updated information on the types of tests available for HIV screening can be found at www.cdc.gov / hiv / testing / index.html.

Documentation of HIV Test Results. Recording HIV test results is important for ongoing medical care, although minimizing any risk to confidentiality should be prioritized. State and local professional associations may offer guidance for appropriate, lawful charting that does not compromise the patient, provider, or health care delivery. However, many states require reporting when HIV is detected; specific information is available at www.cdc.gov / hiv / guidelines / reporting.html.

SUMMARY OF MAJOR REPRODUCTIVE TRACT INFECTIONS, INCLUDING HIV, BY SYNDROME

VULVOVAGINAL SYNDROMES

Vulvovaginal complaints may be the most common reasons for seeking medical attention from reproductive health care providers. These complaints range from changes in normal vaginal discharge (increased amount, abnormal odor or color) to vulvar pruritus or pain. While the number of conditions that may be responsible is broad, a solid knowledge of the conditions discussed here is essential in the reproductive health care setting.

BACTERIAL VAGINOSIS (BV) is a clinical syndrome in which several species of vaginal bacteria (including *Gardnerella vaginalis* and other anaerobes) replace the normal hydrogen peroxide (H_2O_2)-producing *Lactobacillus* species. Bacterial vaginosis is a sexually associated condition,

Recommended Laboratory HIV Testing Algorithm for Serum or Plasma Specimens

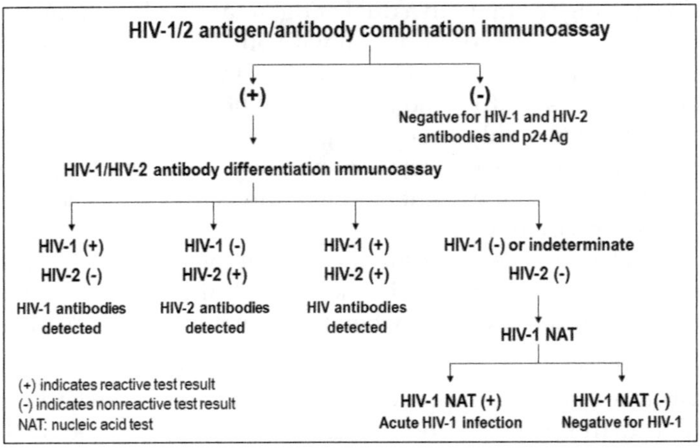

1. Laboratories should conduct initial testing for HIV with an FDA-approved antigen/antibody combination immunoassay* that detects HIV-1 and HIV-2 antibodies and HIV-1 p24 antigen to test for established HIV-1 or HIV-2 infection and for acute HIV-1 infection. No further testing is required for specimens that are nonreactive on the initial immunoassay.
2. Specimens with a reactive antigen/antibody combination immunoassay result (or repeatedly reactive, if repeat testing is recommended by the manufacturer or required by regulatory authorities) should be tested with an FDA-approved antibody immunoassay that differentiates HIV-1 antibodies from HIV-2 antibodies. Reactive results on the initial antigen/antibody combination immunoassay and the HIV-1/HIV-2 antibody differentiation immunoassay should be interpreted as positive for HIV-1 antibodies, HIV-2 antibodies, or HIV antibodies, undifferentiated.
3. Specimens that are reactive on the initial antigen/antibody combination immunoassay and nonreactive or indeterminate on the HIV-1/HIV-2 antibody differentiation immunoassay should be tested with an FDA-approved HIV-1 nucleic acid test (NAT).
    - A reactive HIV-1 NAT result and nonreactive HIV-1/HIV-2 antibody differentiation immunoassay result indicates laboratory evidence for acute HIV-1 infection.
    - A reactive HIV-1 NAT result and indeterminate HIV-1/HIV-2 antibody differentiation immunoassay result indicates the presence of HIV-1 infection confirmed by HIV-1 NAT.
    - A negative HIV-1 NAT result and nonreactive or indeterminate HIV-1/HIV-2 antibody differentiation immunoassay result indicates a false-positive result on the initial immunoassay.
4. Laboratories should use this same testing algorithm, beginning with an antigen/antibody combination immunoassay, with serum or plasma specimens submitted for testing after a reactive (preliminary positive) result from any rapid HIV test.

---

* *Exception: As of April 2014, data are insufficient to recommend use of the FDA-approved single-use rapid HIV-1/HIV-2 antigen/antibody combination immunoassay as the initial assay in the algorithm.*

Quick Reference Guide –
Laboratory Testing for the Diagnosis of HIV Infection: Updated Recommendations June 27, 2014
Source: Centers for Disease Control and Prevention, 2014[43]

Figure 20-1

Summary Chart of U.S. Medical Eligibility Criteria for Contraceptive Use

Condition	Sub-Condition	Cu-IUD	LNG-IUD	Implant	DMPA	POP	CHC
		I | C	I | C	I | C	I | C	I | C	I | C
Age		Menarche to <20 yrs:**2** ≥20 yrs:**1**	Menarche to <20 yrs:**2** ≥20 yrs:**1**	Menarche to <18 yrs:**1** 18-45 yrs:**1** >45 yrs:**1**	Menarche to <18 yrs:**2** 18-45 yrs:**1** >45 yrs:**2**	Menarche to <18 yrs:**1** 18-45 yrs:**1** >45 yrs:**1**	Menarche to <40 yrs:**1** ≥40 yrs:**2**
Anatomical abnormalities	a) Distorted uterine cavity	4	4				
	b) Other abnormalities	2	2				
Anemias	a) Thalassemia	2	1	1	1	1	1
	b) Sickle cell disease‡	2	1	1	1	1	2
	c) Iron-deficiency anemia	2	1	1	1	1	1
Benign ovarian tumors	*(including cysts)*	1	1	1	1	1	1
Breast disease	a) Undiagnosed mass	1	2	2*	2*	2*	2*
	b) Benign breast disease	1	1	1	1	1	1
	c) Family history of cancer	1	1	1	1	1	1
	d) Breast cancer‡						
	i) Current	1	4	4	4	4	4
	ii) Past and no evidence of current disease for 5 years	1	3	3	3	3	3
Breastfeeding	a) <21 days postpartum			2*	2*	2*	4*
	b) 21 to <30 days postpartum						
	i) With other risk factors for VTE			2*	2*	2*	3*
	ii) Without other risk factors for VTE			2*	2*	2*	3*
	c) 30-42 days postpartum						
	i) With other risk factors for VTE			1*	1*	1*	3*
	ii) Without other risk factors for VTE			1*	1*	1*	2*
	d) >42 days postpartum			1*	1*	1*	2*
Cervical cancer	Awaiting treatment	I: 4 | C: 2	I: 4 | C: 2	2	2	1	2
Cervical ectropion		1	1	1	1	1	1
Cervical intraepithelial neoplasia		1	2	2	2	1	2
Cirrhosis	a) Mild *(compensated)*	1	1	1	1	1	1
	b) Severe‡ *(decompensated)*	1	3	3	3	3	4
Cystic fibrosis‡		1*	1*	1*	2*	1*	1*
Deep venous thrombosis (DVT)/Pulmonary embolism (PE)	a) History of DVT/PE, not receiving anticoagulant therapy						
	i) Higher risk for recurrent DVT/PE	1	2	2	2	2	4
	ii) Lower risk for recurrent DVT/PE	1	2	2	2	2	3
	b) Acute DVT/PE	2	2	2	2	2	4
	c) DVT/PE and established anticoagulant therapy for at least 3 months						
	i) Higher risk for recurrent DVT/PE	2	2	2	2	2	4*
	ii) Lower risk for recurrent DVT/PE	2	2	2	2	2	3*
	d) Family history *(first-degree relatives)*	1	1	1	1	1	2
	e) Major surgery						
	i) With prolonged immobilization	1	2	2	2	2	4
	ii) Without prolonged immobilization	1	1	1	1	1	2
	f) Minor surgery without immobilization	1	1	1	1	1	1
Depressive disorders		1*	1*	1*	1*	1*	1*

Key:	
1 No restriction (method can be used)	3 Theoretical or proven risks usually outweigh the advantages
2 Advantages generally outweigh theoretical or proven risks	4 Unacceptable health risk (method not to be used)

Centers for Disease Control and Prevention
National Center for Chronic Disease Prevention and Health Promotion

Condition	Sub-Condition	Cu-IUD		LNG-IUD		Implant		DMPA		POP		CHC	
		I	C	I	C	I	C	I	C	I	C	I	C
Diabetes	a) History of gestational disease	1		1		1		1		1		1	
	b) Nonvascular disease												
	i) Non-insulin dependent	1		2		2		2		2		2	
	ii) Insulin dependent	1		2		2		2		2		2	
	c) Nephropathy/retinopathy/neuropathy‡	1		2		2		3		2		3/4*	
	d) Other vascular disease or diabetes of >20 years' duration‡	1		2		2		3		2		3/4*	
Dysmenorrhea	Severe	2		1		1		1		1		1	
Endometrial cancer‡		4	2	4	2	1		1		1		1	
Endometrial hyperplasia		1		1		1		1		1		1	
Endometriosis		2		1		1		1		1		1	
Epilepsy‡	(*see also Drug Interactions*)	1		1		1*		1*		1*		1*	
Gallbladder disease	a) Symptomatic												
	i) Treated by cholecystectomy	1		2		2		2		2		2	
	ii) Medically treated	1		2		2		2		2		3	
	iii) Current	1		2		2		2		2		3	
	b) Asymptomatic	1		2		2		2		2		2	
Gestational trophoblastic disease‡	a) Suspected GTD (immediate postevacuation)												
	i) Uterine size first trimester	1*		1*		1*		1*		1*		1*	
	ii) Uterine size second trimester	2*		2*		1*		1*		1*		1*	
	b) Confirmed GTD												
	i) Undetectable/non-pregnant ß-hCG levels	1*	1*	1*	1*	1*		1*		1*		1*	
	ii) Decreasing ß-hCG levels	2*	1*	2*	1*	1*		1*		1*		1*	
	iii) Persistently elevated ß-hCG levels or malignant disease, with no evidence or suspicion of intrauterine disease	2*	1*	2*	1*	1*		1*		1*		1*	
	iv) Persistently elevated ß-hCG levels or malignant disease, with evidence or suspicion of intrauterine disease	4*	2*	4*	2*	1*		1*		1*		1*	
Headaches	a) Nonmigraine (mild or severe)	1		1		1		1		1		1*	
	b) Migraine												
	i) Without aura (includes menstrual migraine)	1		1		1		1		1		2*	
	ii) With aura	1		1		1		1		1		4*	
History of bariatric surgery‡	a) Restrictive procedures	1		1		1		1		1		1	
	b) Malabsorptive procedures	1		1		1		1		3		COCs: 3 P/R: 1	
History of cholestasis	a) Pregnancy related	1		1		1		1		1		2	
	b) Past COC related	1		2		2		2		2		3	
History of high blood pressure during pregnancy		1		1		1		1		1		2	
History of Pelvic surgery		1		1		1		1		1		1	
HIV	a) High risk for HIV	2	2	2	2	1		2*		1		1	
	b) HIV infection					1*		1*		1*		1*	
	i) Clinically well receiving ARV therapy	1	1	1	1	If on treatment, see Drug Interactions							
	ii) Not clinically well or not receiving ARV therapy‡	2	1	2	1	If on treatment, see Drug Interactions							

Abbreviations: C=continuation of contraceptive method; CHC=combined hormonal contraception (pill, patch, and, ring); COC=combined oral contraceptive; Cu-IUD=copper-containing intrauterine device; DMPA = depot medroxyprogesterone acetate; I=initiation of contraceptive method; LNG-IUD=levonorgestrel-releasing intrauterine device; NA=not applicable; POP=progestin-only pill; P/R=patch/ring ‡ Condition that exposes a woman to increased risk as a result of pregnancy. *Please see the complete guidance for a clarification to this classification: www.cdc.gov/reproductivehealth/unintendedpregnancy/USMEC.htm.

Summary Chart of U.S. Medical Eligibility Criteria for Contraceptive Use

Condition	Sub-Condition	Cu-IUD I	Cu-IUD C	LNG-IUD I	LNG-IUD C	Implant I	Implant C	DMPA I	DMPA C	POP I	POP C	CHC I	CHC C
Hypertension	a) Adequately controlled hypertension	1*		1*		1*		2*		1*		3*	
	b) Elevated blood pressure levels (*properly taken measurements*)												
	i) Systolic 140-159 or diastolic 90-99	1*		1*		1*		2*		1*		3*	
	ii) Systolic ≥160 or diastolic ≥100‡	1*		2*		2*		3*		2*		4*	
	c) Vascular disease	1*		2*		2*		3*		2*		4*	
Inflammatory bowel disease	(*Ulcerative colitis, Crohn's disease*)	1		1		1		2		2		2/3*	
Ischemic heart disease‡	Current and history of	1		2	3	2	3	3		2	3	4	
Known thrombogenic mutations‡		1*		2*		2*		2*		2*		4*	
Liver tumors	a) Benign												
	i) Focal nodular hyperplasia	1		2		2		2		2		2	
	ii) Hepatocellular adenoma‡	1		3		3		3		3		4	
	b) Malignant‡ (hepatoma)	1		3		3		3		3		4	
Malaria		1		1		1		1		1		1	
Multiple risk factors for atherosclerotic cardiovascular disease	(e.g., older age, smoking, diabetes, hypertension, low HDL, high LDL, or high triglyceride levels)	1		2		2*		3*		2*		3/4*	
Multiple sclerosis	a) With prolonged immobility	1		1		1		2		1		3	
	b) Without prolonged immobility	1		1		1		2		1		1	
Obesity	a) Body mass index (BMI) ≥30 kg/m^2	1		1		1		1		1		2	
	b) Menarche to <18 years and BMI ≥ 30 kg/m^2	1		1		1		2		1		2	
Ovarian cancer‡		1		1		1		1		1		1	
Parity	a) Nulliparous	2		2		1		1		1		1	
	b) Parous	1		1		1		1		1		1	
Past ectopic pregnancy		1		1		1		1		2		1	
Pelvic inflammatory disease	a) Past												
	i) With subsequent pregnancy	1	1	1	1	1		1		1		1	
	ii) Without subsequent pregnancy	2	2	2	2	1		1		1		1	
	b) Current	4	2*	4	2*	1		1		1		1	
Peripartum cardiomyopathy‡	a) Normal or mildly impaired cardiac function												
	i) <6 months	2		2		1		1		1		4	
	ii) ≥6 months	2		2		1		1		1		3	
	b) Moderately or severely impaired cardiac function	2		2		2		2		2		4	
Postabortion	a) First trimester	1*		1*		1*		1*		1*		1*	
	b) Second trimester	2*		2*		1*		1*		1*		1*	
	c) Immediate postseptic abortion	4		4		1*		1*		1*		1*	
Postpartum (*nonbreastfeeding women*)	a) <21 days					1		1		1		4	
	b) 21 days to 42 days												
	i) With other risk factors for VTE					1		1		1		3*	
	ii) Without other risk factors for VTE					1		1		1		2	
	c) >42 days					1		1		1		1	
Postpartum (*in breastfeeding or non-breastfeeding women, including cesarean delivery*)	a) <10 minutes after delivery of the placenta												
	i) Breastfeeding	1*		2*									
	ii) Nonbreastfeeding	1*		1*									
	b) 10 minutes after delivery of the placenta to <4 weeks	2*		2*									
	c) ≥4 weeks	1*		1*									
	d) Postpartum sepsis	4		4									

Centers for Disease Control and Prevention
National Center for Chronic Disease Prevention and Health Promotion

<table>
<tr><th>Condition</th><th>Sub-Condition</th><th colspan="2">Cu-IUD</th><th colspan="2">LNG-IUD</th><th colspan="2">Implant</th><th colspan="2">DMPA</th><th colspan="2">POP</th><th colspan="2">CHC</th></tr>
<tr><td></td><td></td><td>I</td><td>C</td><td>I</td><td>C</td><td>I</td><td>C</td><td>I</td><td>C</td><td>I</td><td>C</td><td>I</td><td>C</td></tr>
<tr><td>Pregnancy</td><td></td><td colspan="2">4*</td><td colspan="2">4*</td><td colspan="2">NA*</td><td colspan="2">NA*</td><td colspan="2">NA*</td><td colspan="2">NA*</td></tr>
<tr><td>Rheumatoid arthritis</td><td>a) On immunosuppressive therapy</td><td>2</td><td>1</td><td>2</td><td>1</td><td colspan="2">1</td><td colspan="2">2/3*</td><td colspan="2">1</td><td colspan="2">2</td></tr>
<tr><td></td><td>b) Not on immunosuppressive therapy</td><td colspan="2">1</td><td colspan="2">1</td><td colspan="2">1</td><td colspan="2">2</td><td colspan="2">1</td><td colspan="2">2</td></tr>
<tr><td>Schistosomiasis</td><td>a) Uncomplicated</td><td colspan="2">1</td><td colspan="2">1</td><td colspan="2">1</td><td colspan="2">1</td><td colspan="2">1</td><td colspan="2">1</td></tr>
<tr><td></td><td>b) Fibrosis of the liver‡</td><td colspan="2">1</td><td colspan="2">1</td><td colspan="2">1</td><td colspan="2">1</td><td colspan="2">1</td><td colspan="2">1</td></tr>
<tr><td>Sexually transmitted diseases (STDs)</td><td>a) Current purulent cervicitis or chlamydial infection or gonococcal infection</td><td>4</td><td>2*</td><td>4</td><td>2*</td><td colspan="2">1</td><td colspan="2">1</td><td colspan="2">1</td><td colspan="2">1</td></tr>
<tr><td></td><td>b) Vaginitis (including trichomonas vaginalis and bacterial vaginosis)</td><td>2</td><td>2</td><td>2</td><td>2</td><td colspan="2">1</td><td colspan="2">1</td><td colspan="2">1</td><td colspan="2">1</td></tr>
<tr><td></td><td>c) Other factors relating to STDs</td><td>2*</td><td>2</td><td>2*</td><td>2</td><td colspan="2">1</td><td colspan="2">1</td><td colspan="2">1</td><td colspan="2">1</td></tr>
<tr><td>Smoking</td><td>a) Age <35</td><td colspan="2">1</td><td colspan="2">1</td><td colspan="2">1</td><td colspan="2">1</td><td colspan="2">1</td><td colspan="2">2</td></tr>
<tr><td></td><td>b) Age ≥35, <15 cigarettes/day</td><td colspan="2">1</td><td colspan="2">1</td><td colspan="2">1</td><td colspan="2">1</td><td colspan="2">1</td><td colspan="2">3</td></tr>
<tr><td></td><td>c) Age ≥35, ≥15 cigarettes/day</td><td colspan="2">1</td><td colspan="2">1</td><td colspan="2">1</td><td colspan="2">1</td><td colspan="2">1</td><td colspan="2">4</td></tr>
<tr><td>Solid organ transplantation‡</td><td>a) Complicated</td><td>3</td><td>2</td><td>3</td><td>2</td><td colspan="2">2</td><td colspan="2">2</td><td colspan="2">2</td><td colspan="2">4</td></tr>
<tr><td></td><td>b) Uncomplicated</td><td colspan="2">2</td><td colspan="2">2</td><td colspan="2">2</td><td colspan="2">2</td><td colspan="2">2</td><td colspan="2">2*</td></tr>
<tr><td>Stroke‡</td><td>History of cerebrovascular accident</td><td colspan="2">1</td><td colspan="2">2</td><td>2</td><td>3</td><td colspan="2">3</td><td>2</td><td>3</td><td colspan="2">4</td></tr>
<tr><td>Superficial venous disorders</td><td>a) Varicose veins</td><td colspan="2">1</td><td colspan="2">1</td><td colspan="2">1</td><td colspan="2">1</td><td colspan="2">1</td><td colspan="2">1</td></tr>
<tr><td></td><td>b) Superficial venous thrombosis (acute or history)</td><td colspan="2">1</td><td colspan="2">1</td><td colspan="2">1</td><td colspan="2">1</td><td colspan="2">1</td><td colspan="2">3*</td></tr>
<tr><td>Systemic lupus erythematosus‡</td><td>a) Positive (or unknown) antiphospholipid antibodies</td><td>1*</td><td>1*</td><td colspan="2">3*</td><td colspan="2">3*</td><td>3*</td><td>3*</td><td colspan="2">3*</td><td colspan="2">4*</td></tr>
<tr><td></td><td>b) Severe thrombocytopenia</td><td>3*</td><td>2*</td><td colspan="2">2*</td><td colspan="2">2*</td><td>3*</td><td>2*</td><td colspan="2">2*</td><td colspan="2">2*</td></tr>
<tr><td></td><td>c) Immunosuppressive therapy</td><td>2*</td><td>1*</td><td colspan="2">2*</td><td colspan="2">2*</td><td>2*</td><td>2*</td><td colspan="2">2*</td><td colspan="2">2*</td></tr>
<tr><td></td><td>d) None of the above</td><td>1*</td><td>1*</td><td colspan="2">2*</td><td colspan="2">2*</td><td>2*</td><td>2*</td><td colspan="2">2*</td><td colspan="2">2*</td></tr>
<tr><td>Thyroid disorders</td><td>Simple goiter/ hyperthyroid/hypothyroid</td><td colspan="2">1</td><td colspan="2">1</td><td colspan="2">1</td><td colspan="2">1</td><td colspan="2">1</td><td colspan="2">1</td></tr>
<tr><td>Tuberculosis‡</td><td>a) Nonpelvic</td><td>1</td><td>1</td><td>1</td><td>1</td><td colspan="2">1*</td><td colspan="2">1*</td><td colspan="2">1*</td><td colspan="2">1*</td></tr>
<tr><td>(see also Drug Interactions)</td><td>b) Pelvic</td><td>4</td><td>3</td><td>4</td><td>3</td><td colspan="2">1*</td><td colspan="2">1*</td><td colspan="2">1*</td><td colspan="2">1*</td></tr>
<tr><td>Unexplained vaginal bleeding</td><td>(suspicious for serious condition) before evaluation</td><td>4*</td><td>2*</td><td>4*</td><td>2*</td><td colspan="2">3*</td><td colspan="2">3*</td><td colspan="2">2*</td><td colspan="2">2*</td></tr>
<tr><td>Uterine fibroids</td><td></td><td colspan="2">2</td><td colspan="2">2</td><td colspan="2">1</td><td colspan="2">1</td><td colspan="2">1</td><td colspan="2">1</td></tr>
<tr><td>Valvular heart disease</td><td>a) Uncomplicated</td><td colspan="2">1</td><td colspan="2">1</td><td colspan="2">1</td><td colspan="2">1</td><td colspan="2">1</td><td colspan="2">2</td></tr>
<tr><td></td><td>b) Complicated‡</td><td colspan="2">1</td><td colspan="2">1</td><td colspan="2">1</td><td colspan="2">1</td><td colspan="2">1</td><td colspan="2">4</td></tr>
<tr><td>Vaginal bleeding patterns</td><td>a) Irregular pattern without heavy bleeding</td><td colspan="2">1</td><td>1</td><td>1</td><td colspan="2">2</td><td colspan="2">2</td><td colspan="2">2</td><td colspan="2">1</td></tr>
<tr><td></td><td>b) Heavy or prolonged bleeding</td><td colspan="2">2*</td><td>1*</td><td>2*</td><td colspan="2">2*</td><td colspan="2">2*</td><td colspan="2">2*</td><td colspan="2">1*</td></tr>
<tr><td>Viral hepatitis</td><td>a) Acute or flare</td><td colspan="2">1</td><td colspan="2">1</td><td colspan="2">1</td><td colspan="2">1</td><td colspan="2">1</td><td>3/4*</td><td>2</td></tr>
<tr><td></td><td>b) Carrier/Chronic</td><td colspan="2">1</td><td colspan="2">1</td><td colspan="2">1</td><td colspan="2">1</td><td colspan="2">1</td><td>1</td><td>1</td></tr>
<tr><td colspan="14">Drug Interactions</td></tr>
<tr><td>Antiretroviral therapy All other ARV's are 1 or 2 for all methods.</td><td>Fosamprenavir (FPV)</td><td>1/2*</td><td>1*</td><td>1/2*</td><td>1*</td><td colspan="2">2*</td><td colspan="2">2*</td><td colspan="2">2*</td><td colspan="2">3*</td></tr>
<tr><td>Anticonvulsant therapy</td><td>a) Certain anticonvulsants (phenytoin, carbamazepine, barbiturates, primidone, topiramate, oxcarbazepine)</td><td colspan="2">1</td><td colspan="2">1</td><td colspan="2">2*</td><td colspan="2">1*</td><td colspan="2">3*</td><td colspan="2">3*</td></tr>
<tr><td></td><td>b) Lamotrigine</td><td colspan="2">1</td><td colspan="2">1</td><td colspan="2">1</td><td colspan="2">1</td><td colspan="2">1</td><td colspan="2">3*</td></tr>
<tr><td>Antimicrobial therapy</td><td>a) Broad spectrum antibiotics</td><td colspan="2">1</td><td colspan="2">1</td><td colspan="2">1</td><td colspan="2">1</td><td colspan="2">1</td><td colspan="2">1</td></tr>
<tr><td></td><td>b) Antifungals</td><td colspan="2">1</td><td colspan="2">1</td><td colspan="2">1</td><td colspan="2">1</td><td colspan="2">1</td><td colspan="2">1</td></tr>
<tr><td></td><td>c) Antiparasitics</td><td colspan="2">1</td><td colspan="2">1</td><td colspan="2">1</td><td colspan="2">1</td><td colspan="2">1</td><td colspan="2">1</td></tr>
<tr><td></td><td>d) Rifampin or rifabutin therapy</td><td colspan="2">1</td><td colspan="2">1</td><td colspan="2">2*</td><td colspan="2">1*</td><td colspan="2">3*</td><td colspan="2">3*</td></tr>
<tr><td>SSRIs</td><td></td><td colspan="2">1</td><td colspan="2">1</td><td colspan="2">1</td><td colspan="2">1</td><td colspan="2">1</td><td colspan="2">1</td></tr>
<tr><td>St. John's wort</td><td></td><td colspan="2">1</td><td colspan="2">1</td><td colspan="2">2</td><td colspan="2">1</td><td colspan="2">2</td><td colspan="2">2</td></tr>
</table>

Updated in 2017. This summary sheet only contains a subset of the recommendations from the U.S. MEC. For complete guidance, see: http://www.cdc.gov/reproductivehealth/unintendedpregnancy/USMEC.htm. Most contraceptive methods do not protect against sexually transmitted diseases (STDs). Consistent and correct use of the male latex condom reduces the risk of STDs and HIV.

CS266008-A

but it is not usually considered a specific STI; however, it probably results at least initially from transfer of the associated bacteria from a sex partner who harbors them. For example, BV occurs frequently in women who regularly have sex with women, and BV-associated bacteria have been consistently detected on the scrotum and penis, especially underneath the foreskin. Although past studies did not find that treatment of the male partner was effective in enhancing cure of BV, this approach is currently under study. Because of the increased risk for postoperative infectious complications associated with BV, screening prior to pelvic surgery is recommended (for example, hysterectomy). Some specialists recommend that before performing surgical abortion, providers screen and treat BV in addition to providing routine antibiotic prophylaxis. Guidelines for BV screening prior to medical abortion are lacking, but there are no data to support this practice.

Symptoms. Excessive or malodorous discharge is a common finding. Erythema, edema, and pruritus of the external genitalia may be seen if vaginal discharge is profuse.

Diagnosis. The clinical diagnosis of BV is made if three of the following four (Amsel) criteria are present:

1. Increased amounts of homogenous discharge
2. Elevated vaginal pH (greater than 4.5)
3. Fishy odor after addition of 10% KOH
4. Identification of clue cells (small coccobacillary organisms associated with epithelial cells) on saline wet mount (>20% of vaginal epithelial cells)

Alternatively, rapid tests that detect high numbers of *Gardnerella vaginalis* bacteria, or byproducts of anaerobic metabolism such as sialidase, are also available. Primarily used in research, a Gram stain of the vaginal discharge reveals the relative absence of lactobacilli with replacement by other anaerobic organisms. Cultures and nucleic acid amplification assays (NAAT) such as polymerase chain reaction (PCR) for individual bacteria are not useful and should not be performed. NAATs that provide a result based on measuring the combination of bacteria present in vaginal fluid appear promising.

Treatment. Patients with symptomatic disease should be offered treatment. The three recommended regimens are:

1. Metronidazole, 500 mg orally twice daily for 7 days OR
2. Metronidazole gel, 0.75%, one full applicator (5 g) vaginally at bedtime for 5 days OR
3. Clindamycin cream, 2%, one full applicator (5 g) vaginally at bedtime for 7 days.

Other alternatives are oral clindamycin 300 mg two times a day for 7 days; clindamycin ovules 100 mg vaginally at bedtime for 3 days; tinidazole two grams orally once daily for 3 days; or tinidazole one gram orally once daily for 5 days. In pregnancy, oral regimens are generally preferred.

Potential complications. Recurrent infections are common. BV is associated with an increased risk of PID and may also cause cervicitis. BV is associated with an increased risk of adverse pregnancy outcomes, including preterm delivery and low birth weight. BV increases risk of acquiring chlamydia, gonorrhea, trichomoniasis, and HIV, and of transmitting HIV to male sex partners.

Behavioral messages to emphasize. The use of condoms by male partners has been associated with a reduced risk of recurrence of BV and may be a useful adjunct to antibiotic treatment, especially for patients with recurrent disease. Avoid douching, as this promotes loss of vaginal lactobacilli and likely exacerbates the problem. Avoid drinking alcohol until 24 hours after completing oral metronidazole therapy or 48 hours after completing tinidazole therapy. Exchange of vaginal fluid between sex partners should be minimized.

TRICHOMONIASIS is caused by *Trichomonas vaginalis,* a motile protozoan with an undulating membrane and four flagella.

Prevalence. Trichomoniasis is the most common curable STI in the United States and worldwide. Each year an estimated 3 million U.S. women become infected.

Symptoms. Excessive, frothy, diffuse, yellow-green vaginal discharge is common, although clinical presentation varies from no signs or symptoms to erythema, edema, and pruritus of the external genitalia. Dysuria and dyspareunia are also frequent. The type of symptoms or signs alone does not distinguish the microbial etiology. Sex partners may develop urethritis, balanitis, or cutaneous lesions on the penis; however, the majority are actually asymptomatic.

Diagnosis. Trichomoniasis is diagnosed when a vaginal culture, nucleic acid amplification test, or antigen test is positive for T. vaginalis OR typical motile trichomonads are identified in a saline wet mount of vaginal discharge. Trichomonads visualized on liquid-based cervical cytology (Pap smear) is specific (unlikely to be false positive), but Pap should not be used as a screening test for trichomoniasis.

Treatment. Metronidazole 2 g orally in a single dose. Alternative regimens are metronidazole 500 mg orally twice daily for 7 days or tinidazole 2 g orally at one time. Most treatment failures are due to failure to treat the index patient's sex partners; initial management should include retreatment of the patient and partners with single-dose metronidazole

(2 g). Metronidazole-resistant T. vaginalis, although uncommon, can occur. Most treatment failures respond to higher doses of metronidazole therapy or to a single dose of tinidazole (2 g). Additional regimens for persistent trichomonas are available from the CDC at www.cdc.gov/std/tg2015/trichomoniasis.htm. Sex partners should be simultaneously treated with the same regimen as the index client.

Potential complications. Secondary excoriation may occur. Recurrent infections are common. Trichomoniasis has been associated with an increased risk of salpingitis, low birthweight, prematurity, and acquisition of HIV.

Behavioral messages to emphasize. Make sure sex partner(s) are treated. Use condoms to prevent future infections. Avoid drinking alcohol until 24 hours after completing metronidazole therapy or 48 hours after tinidazole.

CANDIDIASIS (vulvovaginal candidiasis (VVC)) is caused by *Candida* species—usually *C. albicans*—that are dimorphic fungi that grow as oval, budding yeast cells and as chains of cells (hyphae). *Candida* are normal flora of the skin, mouth, and vagina. VVC is not considered an STI; however, sex partners do exchange orogenital strains of *Candida*. Risk factors for VVC are incompletely understood, but include immunosuppressed states, glucose intolerance, and (in some patients) antibiotic therapy.

Symptoms. Clinical presentation includes whitish vaginal discharge and erythema, edema, and pruritus of the external genitalia. Symptoms or signs alone do not distinguish the microbial etiology. Sex partners may develop balanitis or cutaneous lesions on the penis.

Diagnosis. The presumptive criteria are typical clinical symptoms of vulvovaginitis and microscopic identification of yeast forms (budding cells) or pseudohyphae in potassium hydroxide (KOH) wet-mount preparations of vaginal discharge. VVC is definitively diagnosed when a vaginal culture is positive for *C. albicans* or other *Candida* species in the presence of symptoms. Because up to 40% of patients are vaginally colonized with *Candida* species in the absence of VVC, cultures are not recommended unless chronic suppressive therapy is under consideration, in which case they are used to confirm the etiology and susceptibility to antifungal agents.

Treatment. Single-dose oral fluconazole, 150 mg, is a convenient therapy. In addition, many topical formulations provide effective candidiasis treatment. Examples include miconazole vaginal suppositories, 200 mg intravaginally at bedtime for 3 days; OR miconazole, 2%, vaginal cream, one full applicator (5 g) intravaginally at bedtime for 3 days (and applied externally for vulvitis); OR clotrimazole vaginal tablets, 100 mg intravaginally, daily for 3 days; OR butoconazole cream, 2%, 5 g intra-vaginally for 3 days. A variety of other effective treatment regimens exist. In general, more severe infections may need treatment of longer duration. Over-the-counter preparations for intravaginal administration of miconazole, clotrimazole, and butaconazole are available. Resistant VVC may respond to treatment with boric acid, provided as 600 mg in a type O gelatin capsule administered vaginally once daily for 2 weeks (avoid in pregnancy).

Potential complications. Secondary excoriation may occur. Recurrent infections are common, particularly with antibiotic use, immunosuppression, or diabetes.

Behavioral messages to emphasize. Wear a sanitary pad to protect clothing. Change pads frequently. To reduce moisture in the area, avoid panty hose, tight fitting clothing, and non-cotton panties. Store suppositories in a refrigerator. Continue taking medicine even during menses.

Other causes of vaginitis that reproductive health clinicians might encounter include:

Desquamative inflammatory vaginitis (DIV) is a relatively uncommon, but probably underdiagnosed, form of vaginitis characterized by copious, purulent vaginal discharge, typically accompanied by vaginal pain or burning and dyspareunia. DIV may be more common in older (peri- or postmenopausal) patients, though the epidemiology is poorly defined. Occasionally, frank vestibulitis or excoriations will occur. On examination of vaginal fluid, the characteristic findings are elevated vaginal pH (usually 5.5 to 7.4), few lactobacilli, and numerous Gram-positive cocci. Group B streptococcus may be involved in the pathogenesis of this condition. Treatment includes a relatively prolonged course of clindamycin 2% cream administered vaginally at bedtime, usually given for at least 14 days OR 10% hydrocortisone cream 5 g administered nightly at bedtime for at least 14 days. Longer courses of therapy are often required.

Irritant/chemical vaginitis occurs commonly, though few population-based data are available. Any substance that can elicit a mucosal inflammatory response, including douches, some spermicides, soaps or other cleansing agents, or other feminine-hygiene products, can be responsible if administered vaginally. This condition may result in vaginal discharge characterized by numerous white blood cells (WBCs). When evaluating a patient with vulvovaginal complaints take a careful history of use of any vaginal products or of products applied directly to the vulva.

Discrete Genital Lesions: Genital Ulcer Diseases (GUD), Including Genital Herpes, & Warts

Genital ulceration is often caused by STIs, especially herpes, which is the leading cause of this condition worldwide. The other main cause is syphilis. Chancroid is very uncommon in the United States, and should be suspected if herpes has been ruled out and there is a painful, single ulcer with inguinal lymphadenopathy, particularly if the patient reports transactional sex. Two other STIs that may involve GUD are lymphogranuloma venereum (LGV), discussed in the section on chlamydia, and granuloma inguinale. Granuloma inguinale is caused by a bacteria called *Klebsiella granulomatis* and is rare in the U.S. Initially, single or multiple subcutaneous nodules appear at the site of inoculation. Nodules erode to form granulomatous, heaped ulcers that are painless, bleed on contact, and enlarge slowly. The typical clinical presentation is sufficient to suggest the diagnosis.

GENITAL HERPES is caused by herpes simplex virus (HSV) types 1 and 2, DNA viruses that cannot be distinguished clinically; however, initial infection with HSV-1 is typically less severe and causes less frequent recurrences (sometimes none) relative to HSV-2. HSV-2 is more common in genital disease and is responsible for nearly all recurrent genital herpes.

Prevalence. Symptomatic primary (or initial) HSV infections affect an estimated 200,000 persons each year. Recurrent HSV infections are much more common. An estimated 45 million Americans are infected with genital HSV, though most infections are asymptomatic.[4] Persons without symptoms transmit most HSV infection.

Symptoms. Single or multiple vesicles, which are usually pruritic, can appear anywhere on the genitalia. Vesicles spontaneously rupture to form shallow ulcers that may be very painful. Lesions resolve spontaneously with minimal scarring. The first clinical occurrence is termed first episode infection (mean duration 12 days). Subsequent, usually milder, occurrences are termed recurrent infections (mean duration 4.5 days). The interval between clinical episodes is termed latency. Viral shedding from the cervix, vulva, or penile skin occurs intermittently without clinical symptoms during latency. HSV-2 genital infections are more likely to recur than are HSV-1 infections, thus identification of the type of infecting virus at initial infection has prognostic value.

Diagnosis. When typical genital lesions are present or a pattern of recurrence has developed, suspect herpes infection. An HSV tissue culture demonstrates the characteristic cytopathic effect following inoculation of a specimen from the cervix, the urethra, or the base of a genital lesion. HSV nucleic acid amplification tests can provide type-specific results from genital lesions. Several type-specific HSV serologic assays may help in the diagnosis of unrecognized infection, in management of sex partners of those with HSV, or in pregnant patients to diagnose HSV susceptibility or recent infection.

Treatment. No cure for HSV exists; however, antiviral drugs are helpful in reducing or suppressing symptoms. Oral administration is effective both in treating clinically symptomatic episodes and in suppressing or reducing recurrent outbreaks. Topical therapy is ineffective. Initial episodes can be treated with any of the following oral regimens, each given for 7 to 10 days. Treatment can be extended if healing is incomplete after 10 days of therapy

- Acyclovir
  - 400 mg three times a day OR
  - 200 mg capsules five times a day
- Famciclovir
  - 250 mg three times a day
- Valacyclovir
  - 1 g two times a day

Recurrent infections can be treated with any of the following oral regimens:

- Acyclovir
  - 400 mg three times a day for 5 days OR
  - 800 mg twice a day for 5 days OR
  - 800 mg three times a day for 2 days
- Famciclovir
  - 125 mg twice a day for 5 days
  - 1000 mg twice a day for 1 day
  - 500 mg PO × 1, then 250mg BID for 2 days
- Valacyclovir
  - 500 mg twice a day for 3 days OR
  - 1 g once a day for 5 days.

Daily prophylaxis with valacyclovir by HSV-infected persons reduces the risk of transmission to uninfected partners. Regimens given orally to prevent recurrences include the following (these regimens have been shown to be safe for long periods (years), so the duration of prophylaxis may be tailored to the individual patient's situation):

- Acyclovir 400 mg twice a day OR
- Famciclovir 250 mg twice a day OR
- Valacyclovir
  - 500 mg once a day OR
  - 1 gram once a day.

Famciclovir and valacyclovir offer more convenient dosing but are not more effective clinically at treating symptomatic disease than acyclovir;

however, famciclovir is less effective at suppressing subclinical shedding. For persons infected with HIV, increased dosages and/or extended duration of therapy is recommended.

Potential complications. HSV infection can cause neuralgia, meningitis, ascending myelitis, urinary retention, urethral strictures, and lymphatic suppuration. These outcomes are generally more common in the female genital tract. Pregnancy loss and preterm delivery have been associated with HSV infections, usually in primary infection occurring in the third trimester. *Neonates:* During vaginal delivery, virus from an active genital infection can cause neonatal herpes. This condition ranges in severity from clinically inapparent infections to local infections of the eyes, skin, or mucous membranes or to severely disseminated infection that may involve the central nervous system. Full-blown neonatal herpes has a high fatality rate, and survivors often have ocular or neurologic sequelae.

Behavioral messages to emphasize. Because both initial and recurrent lesions shed high concentrations of the virus, abstain from sexual activity while ulcers are present. However, most genital HSV transmission occurs during asymptomatic intervals. Condoms offer some protection from HSV acquisition. Prophylactic valacyclovir reduces HSV transmission risks. The risk of transmission to the neonate is highest with primary herpes infection (the first time they have been infected with either HSV-1 or HSV-2) during the third trimester, lower with non-primary first episodes of the disease, and lowest with recurrent herpes. At the onset of labor, describe any symptoms and examine for lesions. If no symptoms or signs are present, the infant may be delivered vaginally. Infants delivered through an infected birth canal should be cultured and followed carefully. Genital herpes (and other diseases causing genital ulcers) have been associated with an increased risk of acquiring HIV infections. Clinically evaluating asymptomatic partners has little value for preventing transmission of HSV.

SYPHILIS is caused by Treponema pallidum, a spirochete with 6 to 14 regular spirals and characteristic motility.

Prevalence. Primary and secondary syphilis currently are increasing in the United States. Congenital syphilis is also increasing in a limited number of counties. However, syphilis rates are increasing fastest among men who have sex with men, and it remains an important STI, with serious sequelae if not treated. In the United States, southeastern and western states have the highest rates of both syphilis and congenital syphilis.

Symptoms. *Primary:* The classical chancre is a painless, indurated ulcer, located at the site of exposure (e.g., genitals, rectum, oral cavity). The differential diagnosis for all genital lesions should include syphilis. *Secondary:* Patients may have a highly variable skin rash, mucous patches, condylomata lata (fleshy, moist tissue growths), lymphadenopathy, alopecia, or other signs. *Latent:* Patients are without clinical signs of infection.

Diagnosis. The 2015 CDC STD Treatment Guidelines discuss the types of serologic testing that are available. The clinical presentation by stage is as follows:

- *Primary:* Patients have typical lesion(s) and either a positive darkfield exam or a fluorescent antibody technique in material from a chancre, regional lymph node, or other lesion; or they have been exposed to syphilis within 90 days of lesion onset.
- *Secondary:* Patients have a typical clinical presentation and a strongly reactive serologic test; condyloma lata will be darkfield positive.
- *Latent:* Patients have serologic evidence of untreated syphilis without clinical signs.
- Primary and secondary syphilis are definitively diagnosed by demonstrating T. pallidum with darkfield microscopy or fluorescent antibody technique, but these can be presumptively diagnosed in the setting of a compatible clinical presentation and reactive serology. A definitive diagnosis of latent syphilis cannot be made under usual circumstances.

Treatment. *Primary, secondary, or early syphilis of less than 1 year duration:* benzathine penicillin G 2.4 million units IM in a single dose. Alternative regimens include ceftriaxone 1 gram IV or IM daily for 7 to 10 days.

Syphilis of indeterminate length or of more than 1 year duration: benzathine penicillin G 7.2 million units total; 2.4 million units IM, weekly, for 3 successive weeks.

Patients allergic to penicillin: Doxycycline 100 mg orally 2 times a day. [Note: Duration of therapy depends on the estimated duration of infection. If duration has been less than 1 year, treat the infection for 14 days; otherwise, treat for 28 days.]

Penicillin-allergic pregnant patients or for doxycycline-intolerant patients: Consult the 2015 CDC STD Treatment Guidelines.

Congenital syphilis or if the patient is simultaneously infected with syphilis and HIV: Refer to the 2015 CDC STD Treatment Guidelines.

Potential complications. Late syphilis and congenital syphilis, both complications of early syphilis, are preventable with prompt diagnosis and treatment. Sequelae of late syphilis include neurosyphilis (general paresis, tabes dorsalis, and focal neurologic signs), cardiovascular syphilis (thoracic aortic aneurism, aortic insufficiency), and localized gumma formation.

Behavioral messages to emphasize. Follow-up to monitor response to treatment is critical, and involves periodic testing. Timing of repeat testing depends on stage of disease and HIV status. Pregnant patients diagnosed with syphilis should be followed at least monthly. For early syphilis (primary, secondary, early latent), sex partner(s) from the prior 90 days should be evaluated and treated. Avoid sexual activity until treatment is completed, or at least 7 days if treated with benzathine penicillin injection.

HUMAN PAPILLOMAVIRUS (HPV) are common DNA viruses that include 170 types, with 40 types specific to the human genital tract, stratified as low or high-risk depending on oncogenic potential. Two major clinical syndromes arise from these infections: genital warts and epithelial (cervical, vulvar, vagina, anal) neoplasia. HPV vaccination should be a standard practice in reproductive health care. Genital warts are discussed below; cervical neoplasia is discussed in Chapter 21 on Reproductive Tract Cancers.

GENITAL WARTS (Condyloma accuminata) are caused by several low-risk types of human papillomavirus (HPV). Types 6 and 11 cause 90% of genital warts. ***Prevalence.*** Nearly every sexually active person will be exposed to HPV, and the CDC estimates that there are currently 79 million people infected. Genital warts account for more 350,000 physician office visits annually, making condyloma one of the most common symptomatic viral RTIs in the United States.[44] Risk for condyloma has been correlated with earlier onset of sexual activity, multiple sex partners, and a higher frequency of casual relationships compared with controls.

Symptoms. Single or multiple soft, fleshy, papillary or sessile, painless keratinized growths appear around the vulvovaginal area, penis, anus, urethra, or perineum. Condyloma may manifest as typical growths on the walls of the vagina or cervix, and patients may be unaware of their existence. Regular genital self-examinations may be helpful in detecting such growths on the external genitalia. From 60% to 90% of male partners of patients with condyloma have HPV infection on the penis, although infection is often not visible to the naked eye.

Diagnosis. No evidence supports the use of HPV DNA tests in the routine diagnosis or management of visible genital warts. A diagnosis is made from the typical clinical signs on the external genitalia. Colposcopy may be valuable for diagnosing flat warts, which are difficult to see. Exclude the possible diagnosis of condylomata lata by obtaining a serologic test for syphilis. A biopsy is usually unnecessary but can be done if the diagnosis is in question. When neoplasia is a possibility, take a biopsy of any atypical lesions or persistent warts before initiating therapy.

Treatment. Several different treatment regimens can be used, depending on client preference, available resources, and the experience of the health care provider. None of the currently available treatments is superior to others or ideal for all patients. The currently available treatments for visible genital warts consist of two types: (1) patient-applied therapies and (2) provider-administered therapies.

Patient-applied therapies:

- *Podofilox* 0.5% solution or gel. Patients apply podofilox solution with a cotton swab, or a podofilox gel with a finger, to visible genital warts twice daily for 3 days, followed by 4 days of no therapy. This process may be repeated up to a total of 4 times. Podofilox should not be used during pregnancy.
- *Imiquimod 3.75% or 5%* cream. Patients should apply imiquimod 3.75% cream with a finger, at bedtime nightly for up to 16 weeks. Imiquimod 5% cream is applied at bedtime, 3 times a week, for up to 16 weeks. For both formulations, patients should wash the area with mild soap and water after 6 to 10 hours. Imiquimod should not be used during pregnancy.
- *Sinecatechins* 15% ointment. Ointment should be applied to each wart 3 times daily, for up to 16 weeks. It should not be washed off after use.

Provider-administered therapies:

- *Cryotherapy* with liquid nitrogen or cryoprobe. Repeat applications every 1 to 2 weeks.
- *Trichloroacetic acid (TCA) or bichloroacetic acid (BCA)* 80% to 90%. Apply a small amount to only the warts and allow to dry, at which time a white "frosting" develops. Repeat weekly as needed.
- *Surgical removal*. Scissor or shaving excision, curette, or electrosurgery is possible.
- *Alternative regimen: Podophyllin resin* 10% to 25% in tincture of benzoin. A small amount of podophyllin should be applied to each wart and allowed to air dry. Avoid normal tissue. Wash off thoroughly in 1 to 4 hours to reduce local irritation. Podophyllin should not be used during pregnancy and is not recommended for vaginal use.

HPV is infectious even when asymptomatic. However, for most persons, it has a benign natural history, and some individuals may not be infectious for long periods of time. The effect of genital wart treatment on

HPV transmission and the natural history of HPV are unknown. Therefore, the goal of treatment is the temporary removal of visible genital warts and the amelioration of symptoms and signs, *not* the eradication of HPV.

Potential complications. Lesions may enlarge and destroy tissue. Giant condyloma, while histologically benign, may simulate carcinoma. In pregnancy, warts enlarge, are extremely vascular, and may obstruct the birth canal to necessitate a cesarean delivery. Neither routine HPV screening tests nor cesarean delivery for prevention of the transmission of HPV to the newborn is indicated. The perinatal transmission rate is unknown, although probably low. Persons with HIV disease can have rapidly growing genital warts. Patients infected with HIV have an increased risk of progressive HPV-related cervical disease.

Prevention. There is currently a nonavalent vaccine on the US market to prevent genital HPV infection that protects against acquisition of types 6, 11, 16, 18, 31, 33, 45, 52 and 58 (Gardasil9®). Large multicenter studies in young women and men indicate that both are nearly 100% effective in preventing HPV infection and associated disease outcomes including anogenital warts, cervical neoplasia, and anal neoplasia in men when given prior to HPV exposure. HPV vaccination should be routinely given to boys and girls 11 to 12 years of age, prior to the onset of sexual activity. Catch-up vaccination is recommended for females through 26 years of age and for males through 21 years of age. Males 22 to 26 may also be vaccinated. (See www.cdc.gov/mmwr/volumes/65/wr/mm6549a5.htm.)

Behavioral messages to emphasize. Return for regular treatment until lesions have resolved. Once warts have responded to therapy, no special follow-up is necessary. Because most partners are probably already infected, examination of sex partners is not necessary. Most new HPV infections are acquired from sex partners who have no symptoms or signs of the infection. To reduce risks of sequelae from cervical cancer, regular cervical cancer screening is crucial, regardless of whether a patient has received HPV vaccine. HPV testing is useful in triaging Pap smears showing ASCUS and co-testing for cervical neoplasia in patients 30 to 65 years of age. An assay for primary HPV screening has been approved by the U.S. FDA; national guidelines for primary HPV screening are in progress and may be found at the United States Preventive Services Task Force website: https://www.uspreventiveservicestaskforce.org/Page/Document/draft-recommendation-statement/cervical-cancer-screening2.

MOLLUSCUM CONTAGIOSUM is caused by the molluscum contagiosum virus, the largest DNA virus of the poxvirus group. This infection manifests as lesions that are 1 to 5 mm, smooth, rounded, firm, shiny flesh-colored to pearly-white papules with characteristically umbilicated centers. They are most commonly seen on the trunk and anogenital region and are generally asymptomatic. Exceptions occur in immunosuppressed patients (particularly HIV with low CD4 counts), in whom the lesions can be diffuse or become bulky.

Diagnosis. Infection is usually diagnosed on the basis of the typical clinical presentation. Microscopic examination of lesions or lesion material reveals the pathognomonic molluscum inclusion bodies.

Treatment. Lesions may resolve spontaneously without scarring. However, they may be removed by curettage after cryoanesthesia. Treatment with caustic chemicals (podophyllin, trichloroacetic acid, silver nitrate) and cryotherapy (liquid nitrogen) have been successful. If every lesion is not extirpated, the condition may recur.

Potential complications. Secondary infection, usually with staphylococcus, may occur. Lesions rarely attain a size greater than 10 mm in diameter.

Behavioral messages to emphasize. Return for reexamination 1 month after treatment so any new lesions can be removed. Sex partner(s) should be examined.

Chlamydia & Gonorrhea & Related Syndromes: Cervicitis, Urethritis & Pelvic Inflammatory Disease

Chlamydia & Gonorrhea

These two infections are often grouped together because they are often asymptomatic (especially in women), cause similar clinical syndromes, have similar adverse effects on reproductive health and risk of HIV transmission, and are targeted with national screening guidelines for women. They are discussed separately below.

CHLAMYDIA is the common name for infections caused by *Chlamydia trachomatis.* Genital chlamydial infection is the leading cause of preventable infertility and ectopic pregnancy. Chlamydia is the most commonly reported infectious disease in the United States. An estimated 3 million new cases occur annually. Because many chlamydial infections are asymptomatic and probably chronic, widespread screening is necessary to control this infection and its sequelae. CDC recommends that all sexually active women age younger than 25 years of age be screened annually for C. trachomatis (Table 20-3). For further information about the syndromes caused by *C. trachomatis,* see the sections on Cervicitis, Acute Urethral Syndrome, Nongonococcal Urethritis, and Pelvic Inflammatory Disease (PID) in this chapter.

The recommended regimens for all sites of uncomplicated chlamydial infection are azithromycin 1 g orally in a single dose OR doxycycline 100 mg orally twice a day for 7 days.

Alternatives are ofloxacin 300 mg orally two times a day for 7 days OR levofloxacin 500 mg orally for 7 days OR erythromycin base 500 mg orally four times a day for 7 days OR erythromycin ethylsuccinate 800 mg orally four times a day for 7 days.

During pregnancy, the recommended regimen is azithromycin 1 g orally in a single dose, and the alternative regimen is amoxicillin 500 mg orally three times daily for 7 days.

Alternatives are erythromycin base 500 mg orally four times daily for 7 days OR erythromycin base 250 mg orally four times daily for 14 days OR erythromycin ethylsuccinate 800 mg orally four times a day for 7 days OR erythromycin ethylsuccinate 400 mg orally four times a day for 14 days. In general, erythromycin-based regimens are inferior to the other drugs listed and should be viewed as second-line therapy. If alternative regimens are used, a test-of-use at 1 month after treatment is required.

Lymphogranuloma venereum (LGV) is caused by serovars L1, L2, or L3 of *Chlamydia trachomatis*. LGV infections are endemic in Asia and Africa and have been recently seen in the United States largely as outbreaks of rectal LGV (proctitis) among men who report unprotected receptive anal sex (most of whom are also HIV-positive). LGV should be suspected in any MSM with proctitis that does not respond to routine treatment for chlamydia and gonorrhea, or is especially severe. Such cases should be treated with 3 weeks of oral doxycycline and a specific diagnosis pursued, if possible.

GONORRHEA is caused by *Neisseria gonorrhoeae*, a Gram-negative bacterium seen as a diplococcus on Gram stain. The CDC estimates that 800,000 new cases of gonorrhea occur each year, making it the second most commonly reported infectious disease in the United States.

Symptoms. Cervical infections are most commonly asymptomatic, but patients may also present with abnormal vaginal discharge, abnormal vaginal bleeding, or dysuria. Infections of the penile urethra are often associated with dysuria, increased frequency of urination, and purulent discharge; an estimated one-fourth of these infections can be asymptomatic. Pharyngeal gonorrhea can occasionally produce symptoms of pharyngitis, but most infections are asymptomatic.

Diagnosis. Presumptive diagnosis relies on microscopically identifying typical gram-negative intracellular diplococci on smear of urethral exudates from the penis. Gram stain of endocervical secretions is positive only half the time in the presence of infection and is not commonly performed. Definitive diagnosis requires recovery of bacteria either by culture or molecular testing (NAAT). NAAT can be performed on urine or on self-collected vaginal swab. Although the use of culture allows for antimicrobial susceptibility testing, increasing use of NAAT has increased the number of patients tested and offers a noninvasive method for diagnosis. A definitive diagnosis by culture is required if important for medico-legal reasons (child abuse, sexual assault), or in cases of suspected treatment failure.

Treatment. Gonococcal antibiotic resistance is a growing concern, and treatment options are limited. Currently, dual antibiotic therapy is recommended for all anogenital and pharyngeal gonorrhea infections, regardless of the chlamydia test result. The recommended regimen for gonorrhea includes ceftriaxone 250 mg IM once plus azithromycin 1 g orally once. See the CDC's website on this topic for frequent updates (www.cdc.gov/std/treatment).

Potential complications. Up to 40% of untreated patients with cervical gonorrhea develop PID and are at risk for its sequelae (see the section on PID), including involuntary sterility and pelvic abscesses. Complications can also include epididymitis, urethral stricture, and sterility. Newborns are at risk for ophthalmia neonatorum, scalp abscess at the site of fetal monitors, rhinitis, or anorectal infection. All infected untreated persons are at risk for disseminated gonococcal infection.

Behavioral messages to emphasize. Anyone the index patient had sex with in the 60 days prior to diagnosis should be treated (see section on Expedited Partner Management). Avoid sex until completion of the prescribed course of medication and/or for 1 week after treatment was started. Understand how to take prescribed oral medications. Use condoms to prevent future infections, and understand potential consequences to future reproductive health if the infection is reacquired or not optimally treated.

CERVICITIS is a term used to refer to the syndrome of cervical inflammation that can accompany infection with some STIs, notably *Chlamydia trachomatis, Neisseria gonorrhoeae,* and *Mycoplasma genitalium,* and occasionally trichomoniasis and genital herpes. It is defined as the presence of endocervical mucopurulent discharge, easily induced bleeding, and/or edematous ectopy. Cervicitis can have noninfectious causes, including chemical trauma, and may also be promoted by progesterone-based hormonal therapy or bacterial vaginosis.

Prevalence. Based on extrapolation from local studies, cervicitis probably occurs more frequently than penile urethritis. Up to 3 million cases per year may occur annually.

Symptoms. Cervical mucopurulent discharge may be exuded from the cervix and may be perceived as abnormal vaginal discharge, and cervical bleeding may manifest as intermenstrual bleeding.

Diagnosis. Diagnosis is made by visualizing either mucopus on a swab of endocervical secretions or friability (bleeding) on gentle passage of a cotton-tipped swab. In most cases, a microbial organism cannot be identified. A definitive etiologic diagnosis is made when either chlamydia or gonorrhea (or less commonly, another STI) is isolated. NAAT is the preferred method of detection for M. genitalium, but no approved test is currently available.

Treatment. Presumptive treatment should be provided based on the individual patient's risk for chlamydial and/or gonococcal infections, and it should be directed at these organisms (particularly chlamydia). In patients at low risk for these STIs, the results of NAATs for *C. trachomatis* or *N. gonorrhoeae* should determine the need for treatment. Chlamydia is treated with azithromycin 1 g orally in a single dose OR doxycycline 100 mg orally twice a day for 7 days. The section on gonorrhea contains recommended treatment regimens for this infection. If treatment for these infections is ineffective, empiric treatment for *M. genitalium* may be considered, and is moxifloxacin 400 mg orally once daily (for 7 to 10 days).

Potential complications. PID (with subsequent infertility) may complicate infection. In addition, neonatal chlamydial infections, such as ophthalmia neonatorum or pneumonia, may be acquired during delivery if the cervix is infected. Postpartum endometritis may also occur.

Behavioral messages to emphasize. If infection involves *C. trachomatis* or *N. gonorrhoeae,* sex partner(s) should be treated for these bacteria. Anyone the index patient had sex with in the 60 days prior to diagnosis should be treated (see section on Expedited Partner Management). Avoid sex until completion of the prescribed course of medication and/or for 1 week after treatment was started. Understand how to take prescribed oral medications. Return early if symptoms persist or recur. Use condoms to prevent future infections, and understand potential consequences to future reproductive health if the infection is reacquired or not optimally treated.

PELVIC INFLAMMATORY DISEASE (PID) can be caused by varying combinations of *N. gonorrhoeae, C. trachomatis,* anaerobic bacteria, facultative gram-negative rods (such as *E. coli*), *Mycoplasma hominis,* and a variety of other microbial agents. Clinical PID is usually of polymicrobial etiology. *N. gonorrhoeae* and *C. trachomatis* may cause antecedent inflammation, which makes the tubes susceptible to invasion by anaerobic organisms.

Symptoms. Based on retrospective reports, many patients with PID have atypical or no symptoms. Symptoms can include pain and tenderness involving the lower abdomen, cervix, uterus, or adnexae, occasionally with fever, chills, and elevated white blood cell (WBC) count and erythrocyte sedimentation rate (ESR). The condition is more likely if the patient has multiple sex partners or a history of PID or is in the first 5 to 10 days of her menstrual cycle. More specific criteria, such as endometrial biopsy, magnetic resonance imaging, or diagnostic laparoscopy, are warranted only in selected instances.

Diagnosis. Patients with the typical clinical symptoms are presumed to have PID if other serious conditions, such as acute appendicitis or ectopic pregnancy, can be excluded. The diagnosis of PID is often based on imprecise clinical findings. Maintain a low threshold for diagnosing PID, because even mild or moderate PID has the potential for reproductive sequelae. Use objective criteria to monitor response to antibiotics, especially if ambulatory treatment is given. Direct visualization of inflamed (edema, hyperemia, or tubal exudate) fallopian tube(s) during laparoscopy or laparotomy confirms the diagnosis of PID. Cultures of tubal exudate may help establish the microbiologic etiology.

Treatment. Because the causative organism is usually unknown at the time of the initial therapy, use treatment regimens that are active against the broadest possible range of pathogens. Antimicrobial coverage should include *N. gonorrhoeae, C. trachomatis,* anaerobes, Gram-negative facultative bacteria, and streptococci.

Hospitalization and inpatient care: Since hospitalization is no longer synonymous with parenteral therapy, the decision to hospitalize is based on the clinician's discretion. Data show hospitalization did not improve short- or long-term outcomes in patients with symptomatic PID. Consider hospitalizing patients with acute PID when (1) surgical emergencies, such as appendicitis and ectopic pregnancy, are not definitely excluded; (2) severe illness precludes outpatient management; (3) the patient is unable to follow or tolerate an outpatient regimen; or (4) symptoms have not responded to outpatient therapy. Special consideration may be given to adolescents both to preserve their fertility and to improve their adherence.

Combined drug therapy is recommended in all cases since the full bacterial etiology of PID is not clear and is generally polymicrobial.

Parenteral treatment: Two parenteral regimens are recommended for both inpatient and outpatient care:

- *Regimen A:* Either cefotetan 2 g IV every 12 hours, OR cefoxitin 2 g IV every 6 hours for at least 24 hours after the patient clinically improves PLUS doxycycline 100 mg orally or IV every 12 hours. Continue doxycycline 100 mg orally twice daily after discharge to complete at least 14 days of therapy.
- *Regimen B:* Clindamycin 900 mg, IV three times a day, PLUS gentamicin 2 mg per kilogram (kg) IV loading dose and maintenance 1.5 mg/kg IV every 8 hours. Continue oral therapy as above.

Parenteral/Oral treatment: Either of two regimens is recommended:

- *Regimen B:* Ceftriaxone 250 mg IM in a single dose; OR
- Cefoxitin 2 g IM along with probenecid 1 g orally in a single dose PLUS doxycycline 100 mg taken orally twice daily for 14 days

Potential complications. Potentially life-threatening complications include ectopic pregnancy and pelvic abscess. Other sequelae are involuntary infertility, recurrent or chronic PID, chronic abdominal pain, pelvic adhesions, premature hysterectomy, and depression.

Behavioral messages to emphasize. For outpatient therapy, return for evaluation 2 to 3 days after initiation of therapy. Return for further evaluation 4 days after completing therapy. Refer sex partner(s) for evaluation and treatment (even if they are asymptomatic). Avoid sexual activity throughout the course of treatment. Understand how to take prescribed oral medications.

Urethritis, Including Nongonococcal Urethritis (NGU)

ACUTE URETHRAL SYNDROME (dysuria-pyuria syndrome) is a term reserved for the presentation of an acute urethral inflammation in patients that is distinct from bacterial cystitis and typically results from a direct urethral infection with the sexually transmitted pathogens *C. trachomatis* or *N. gonorrhoeae*. Bacterial cystitis itself is not sexually transmitted per se; however, it can be sexually associated. "Honeymoon" cystitis—that is, cystitis that occurs after frequent vaginal intercourse—is believed to be caused by friction against the urethra during sexual intercourse. In this case, the underlying etiology is mechanical, and coital movements help vaginal organisms ascend into the bladder. Use of the diaphragm with spermicides and spermicidally coated condoms have been associated with a higher risk of acute urethral syndrome.

Prevalence. Urinary tract infections are second in incidence only to upper respiratory infections. Depending on the population studied, as many as 10% to 25% of reproductive-age women report dysuria during the previous year. Among women with genital chlamydial infections, approximately 10% are infected at the urethra only.

Symptoms. Painful, urgent, and frequent urination as well as dyspareunia characterize this syndrome. Occasionally, hematuria is the precipitating event for seeking clinical evaluation. Consider pyelonephritis in the presence of fever, or if costovertebral angle pain or tenderness are present.

Diagnosis. Patients with >10 organisms (coliform bacteria or other uropathogens) per milliliter (ml) of urine have bacterial cystitis; however, a smaller number of organisms may also cause symptoms. Women with dysuria, frequency, pyuria (≥10 WBCs per 400× field on microscopic examination of urinary sediment), and lack of bacteriuria on standard urine culture, chlamydia should be strongly suspected. A definitive diagnosis of the etiologic organism requires cultures or nucleic acid amplification testing (for gonorrhea and chlamydia) of the urethra or urine. Dysuria may also be caused by vulvovaginitis or genital herpes simplex virus infection.

Treatment. Bacterial cystitis can be treated with a variety of antibiotics that achieve a high concentration in urine. Initial episodes of bacterial cystitis can be treated with appropriate single-dose therapy such as sulfamethoxazole 1.6 g plus trimethoprim 320 mg (Bactrim or Septra). Fluoroquinolones (e.g., ciprofloxacin 250 mg twice a day, OR ofloxacin 200 mg twice a day) can be effective. Three days is the usual course. If bacteriuria is absent in the presence of pyuria, consider presumptive treatment for chlamydial infection.

Potential complications. Left untreated, bacterial infections of the lower genitourinary tract can ascend to the upper tract, leading to pyelonephritis.

Behavioral messages to emphasize. Understand how to take any prescribed oral medications. Drink copious fluids to flush the genitourinary system. If *C. trachomatis* or *N. gonorrhoeae* organisms are isolated or strongly suspected, arrange for treatment of sex partner(s). (See the sections on these specific infections.)

URETHRITIS (Penile urethra) is caused by *C. trachomatis* or *N. gonorrhoeae* in less than half of cases. Other sexually transmissible agents, which may cause more than half of the cases, include *Trichomonas vaginalis, Mycoplasma genitalium,* herpes simplex virus, and *Ureaplasma urealyticum.* Among patients who engage in unprotected insertive anal sex, rectal coliform bacteria, such as E. coli, may contribute. The etiology of the remaining cases is unknown.

Symptoms. Dysuria, urinary frequency, and mucoid or mucopurulent urethral discharge are common.

Diagnosis. The syndrome of urethritis is defined by the sign of urethral discharge as noted above, and/or by the presence of at least 2 or more polymorphonuclear neutrophil (PMN) per high-power field (HPF) on Gram stain of urethral discharge. The latter test can also rule out gonorrhea if no Gram-negative intracellular diplococci are seen. However, urine NAAT for chlamydia and gonorrhea can test for both pathogens.

Treatment. When the etiology is *C. trachomatis,* or unknown, the following treatment is recommended: azithromycin 1 g orally in a single dose OR doxycycline 100 mg orally twice daily for 7 days. For patients who fail their first trial of antibiotics and whose partners have been treated, the persistent urethritis should be documented (either by visual examination of discharge or microscopy to quantify WBC).

For patients initially treated with doxycycline, azithromycin 1 g orally once should be given (with metronidazole 2 g orally for men who have sex with women). Patients initially treated with azithromycin should receive moxifloxacin 400 mg daily × 7 to 10 days (to cover *M. genitalium*) and men who have sex with women should also receive metronidazole 2 g orally as a single dose. For urethritis caused by genital herpes, see the relevant sections of this chapter.

Potential complications. Urethral strictures or epididymitis may occur. If C. trachomatis is transmitted to sex partners, the condition may result in mucopurulent cervicitis, PID, or proctitis. If *C. trachomatis* is acquired in pregnancy, complications may include neonatal infections such as conjunctivitis or pneumonia.

Behavioral messages to emphasize. If chlamydial infection or other STI is diagnosed, sex partner(s) with contact within the prior 60 days should be treated. Avoid sex until treatment is completed. Use condoms to prevent future infections.

VIRAL HEPATITIS

Hepatitis A, hepatitis B, and hepatitis C may all be sexually transmitted. Infections are clinically indistinguishable and are often asymptomatic. When symptoms occur, they may include fatigue, anorexia, nausea, vomiting, headache, fever, dark urine, jaundice, and moderate liver enlargement with tenderness. In all cases, diagnosis is made by serologic testing, sometimes in combination with measurement of plasma viral load by PCR testing. Specific features of each infection are described below.

HEPATITIS A is caused by hepatitis A virus (HAV), an RNA virus that is typically transmitted by the fecal-oral route. For this reason, HAV can be transmitted through oral-anal sexual contact.

Diagnosis. Serum IgM antiHAV is almost always detectable at the onset of symptoms, and IgG antiHAV levels rise soon thereafter. Measurement of serum IgM antiHAV is the diagnostic test of choice.

Treatment/Prevention. Therapy is supportive. Vaccination and postexposure prophylaxis strategies prevent the infection. Vaccinating all men who have sex with men, persons who use illicit drugs, and travelers to endemic areas against hepatitis A is currently recommended.

Potential complications. Long-term sequelae are rare. Rarely, acute fulminant hepatitis can occur, resulting in hepatic failure and death.

Behavioral messages to emphasize. HAV vaccination is strongly encouraged for target groups. Consult public health authorities regarding recommendations for postexposure prophylaxis of household contacts and sex partners.

HEPATITIS B is caused by hepatitis B virus (HBV), a DNA virus with multiple antigenic components. In the United States, about 5% of the general population show evidence of past HBV infections. An estimated 120,000 new cases of HBV infection are transmitted sexually each year. Heterosexual intercourse is now the predominant mode of HBV transmission.

Diagnosis. Diagnosis involves interpretation of several serologic tests as well as HBV serum PCR in some cases.

- Hepatitis B surface antigen (HBsAg): May indicate acute HBV infection a chronic active state (infectious in both)
- HBe antigen: Indicates active replication of the virus, and infectiousness
- AntiHBs (surface antibody): Indicates immunity conferred by past infection or successful immunization
- AntiHBc (core antibody): May indicate past or current infection; does not result from immunization

Guidance for interpretation of hepatitis B serology is available from the CDC at www.cdc.gov/hepatitis/hbv/pdfs/serologicchartv8.pdf

Treatment. Chronic active HBV can be treated with a variety of agents, including tenofovir, entecavir, and lamivudine, and should be initiated in consultation with a specialist. Guidelines can be found at www.aasld.org.

Potential complications. Long-term sequelae include chronic, persistent, active hepatitis, cirrhosis, hepatocellular carcinoma, hepatic failure, and death. Rarely, the course may be fulminant with hepatic failure.

Behavioral messages to emphasize. HBV vaccination is strongly encouraged for all young, sexually active clients. Specific vaccination and postexposure prophylaxis strategies are of proven efficacy in preventing hepatitis B. Vaccinating all newborn infants and adolescents against hepatitis B is currently recommended. In addition, the Advisory Committee on Immunization Practices recommends HBV vaccination for all men who have sex with men, persons seeking evaluation or treatment for an STI, and those who have a history of sexual activity with more than one partner in the previous 6 months. Subsidized HBV vaccine programs are available in many states.

HEPATITIS C is caused by hepatitis C virus (HCV), an RNA virus that is typically transmitted by the parenteral route (needle sharing or transfusion with contaminated blood). HCV has been detected in genital secretions, and sexual transmission has been documented, particularly in men who have sex with men. Transmission is more likely if sexual activity includes exchange of blood or bloody secretions.

Diagnosis. Serum IgM antiHCV is almost always detectable at the onset of symptoms, and IgG antiHCV levels rise soon thereafter.

Measurement of serum IgM antiHCV, possibly combined with HCV PCR, is the diagnostic approach of choice in the setting of acute hepatitis.

Treatment/Prevention. Direct-acting oral agents capable of curing hepatitis C virus (HCV) infection have been approved for use in the United States since 2011. Many more oral drugs are expected to be approved in the next few years. Existing guidelines for management can be found at www.hcvguidelines.org. No vaccine is available. Patients should be educated about ways to avoid transmission through contaminated needles or by sharing such items as razors with household or sexual contacts who are infected.

Potential complications. Long-term sequelae include chronic, persistent, active hepatitis, cirrhosis, hepatocellular carcinoma, hepatic failure, and death. Rarely, the course may be fulminant with hepatic failure.

Behavioral messages to emphasize. Sex partners already in an established relationship do not need to change their sexual practices if one partner is found to be HCV-infected; the partner of unknown status should be screened. If a person has HCV and is beginning a new sexual relationship, use safer sex precautions as applicable for routine STI protection (e.g., condoms).

ZIKA VIRUS. Sexual transmission of Zika virus has been documented for male-female, female-male, and male-male sex. The virus may be shed in semen for prolonged periods (as late as 188 days following the onset of illness), though in most cases will clear by 3 months. The main risk is for pregnant women, in whom high rates of congenital infection occur and may be manifested by a wide range of disorders, including microcephaly, macular scarring, and arthrogryposis (congenital contractures). The CDC recommends that before having unprotected sex, men should wait at least 6 months after symptom onset or last possible Zika virus exposure (if asymptomatic); women (symptomatic or not) are advised to wait at least 8 weeks after symptom onset or, if asymptomatic, after the last possible Zika virus exposure. More detailed information is available at www.cdc.gov/zika/index.html.

CONSULTATION FOR COMPLEX RTI

The National Network of Clinical STD Prevention Training Centers (NNPTC) has a national consultation service (STD Clinical Consultation Network) available for providers managing complex RTI cases who would like advice from a subject matter expert. Consults are answered in 1 to 5 business days depending on the urgency of the request. The STDCCN warm-line is staffed from Monday through Friday 8AM to 5PM, but consults can be entered anytime online at http://stdccn.org

Clinical Characteristics of HIV Infection

The current standard of care for HIV is highly active antiretroviral therapy (HAART), a combination of oral antiretroviral agents that inhibit different targets of the virus. HAART regimens can be composed of drugs from two, three, or more classes, including nucleoside analog reverse transcriptase inhibitors (NRTI), non-nucleoside reverse transcriptase inhibitors (NNRTIs), protease inhibitors (PIs), and integrase inhibitors; CCR-5 inhibitors and fusion inhibitors are used less commonly, largely in the setting of viral resistance. HAART should be initiated and managed by—or in close consultation with—an experienced HIV clinician in order to optimize care and a high likelihood of adherence, which is the main determinant of future success. HIV mutation and resistance can occur if the patient is not adherent with the regimen. While single daily dosing regimens and formulations that combine agents from several classes have emerged as the standard of care and have greatly simplified the approach to treatment, side effects still occur, and all regimens are expensive. Still, early initiation of therapy is beneficial for patients, regardless of their CD4 count at the time of diagnosis.[45] Viral load testing uses DNA or RNA detection assays to measure the actual amount of HIV in plasma, permitting an accurate determination of real-time viral activity and a rapid assessment of antiretroviral drug efficacy. For complete information on recommended regimens, see www.aidsinfo.nih.gov/guidelines/.

Reproductive health care would ideally be managed in the primary care/HIV care setting also, but in some cases these are two providers in two different sites, so careful attention to shared information, shared decision making, and collaboration is essential. Advice on medical management of patients with HIV is available from the National HIV/AIDS Clinicians' Consultation Center based at the University of California at San Francisco. This no-cost "warmline" is staffed Monday through Friday from 6:00 a.m. to 5:00 p.m. Pacific Time, and voicemail is available 24 hours a day, 7 days a week. Call 1–800–933–3413.

Gynecologic Management in HIV+ Patients

The keys to successful management of gynecologic infections among HIV-positive patients are a high index of suspicion, prompt diagnosis, aggressive treatment, and primary or secondary prophylaxis when appropriate. Table 20-8 outlines general stages of HIV infection and related concerns; a discussion of some specific conditions follows.

Vulvovaginal candidiasis (VVC). VVC is common in HIV-positive patients and may recur frequently if immune status deteriorates. Non-albicans species may be involved and may be less responsive to topical

Table 20-8 Stages of HIV infection and reproductive health concerns

	Primary HIV Infection/ Seroconversion	Symptom-Free	Early Symptoms	Discrete Illness/Cascade of Illness/Endstage
Duration	Average 1–8 weeks	Few months to many years	Few months to several years	Few months to several years
CD4 Cell Count × 106 /L Normal = 500–1600	Normal or slightly low	Typically >350	Typically <350	AIDS diagnosis at 200 or less
Viral Load copies/ml	High	Variable	Rising (without HAART)	High (without HAART)
Characteristics	Self-limited flu-like illness can occur; HIV antibody not detectable 6–12 weeks post-infection,* but serum viral assays positive.		Fevers, night sweats, zoster, vulvovaginal candidiasis, oral thrush, hairy leukoplakia, seborrheic dermatitis, weight loss, fatigue, loss of appetite	Mild or severe multiple opportunistic bacterial, viral, fungal, parasitic infections; cancers, including Kaposi's sarcoma, lymphoma, cervical cancer; Neurologic illness including dementia, peripheral neuropathy
Reproductive Health Concerns	Nonspecific presentation if primary infection is symptomatic; sex partner(s) and offspring may be at risk with ongoing risk behavior. Assess contraception, safer sex practices.	Usually asymptomatic, though risk of transmission less than with primary infection. Offer anticipatory guidance on future pregnancy planning. Appropriate Pap screening, aggressive management of abnormal findings. Assess contraception, safer sex practices.	Pregnancy likely to be normal except for transmission risk for offspring. Frequent Paps, aggressive management of abnormal findings. Assess contraception, safer sex practices.	Medications may interfere with hormonal contraception; assess drug interactions. Assist with short-range and long-range child care plans. Pregnancy may result in prematurity, low birthweight, premature rupture of membranes, other complications. Frequent Paps, aggressive management of abnormal findings. Assess contraception, safer sex practices.
Risk of Transmission to Offspring	Risk may increase above 25% baseline if primary infection occurs during pregnancy.	25% each pregnancy without treatment. Decreased to about 2% with effective HAART.	25% each pregnancy without treatment. Decreased to about 2% with effective HAART.	25% each pregnancy without treatment. Decreased to about 2% with effective HAART.

Source: Modified from Anderson (ed.) (2001).[46]

*Newer rapid tests may detect antibody to HIV earlier. See www.cdc.gov/hiv/topics/testing/rapid/index.htm for details and updated information.

imidazole or oral azole therapy. First-line treatment is a 7-day course of one of the topical imidazole antifungal agents. If topical treatment proves unsatisfactory, consider oral fluconazole (a single dose, 150 mg orally). Boric acid may be useful for infections with resistant *Candida* species.

Human papillomavirus and cervical disease. Genital warts caused by certain types of HPV (types 6 and 11) may progress more rapidly with immune compromise. Patients with HIV have significantly higher rates of Pap smear-detected abnormalities, dysplasia, and progression to cervical cancer relative to HIV-uninfected patients.

- HIV-positive patients <30 years of age should commence Pap screening within 1 year of the onset of sexual activity regardless of mode of HIV transmission (e.g., sexual activity, perinatal exposure) but no later than 21 years old.
- HIV-positive patients 21 to 29 years old should have a Pap test at the time of initial diagnosis with HIV. If the initial Pap test is normal, the next Pap test should be in 12 months. Some experts recommend a Pap test at 6 months after the baseline test. If the results of 3 consecutive Pap tests are normal, follow up Pap tests should be every 3 years. Co-testing (Pap test and HPV test) is not recommended for HIV-infected patients <30 years of age.
- HIV-positive patients 30 years of age and older can be screened with either Pap testing only or Pap testing and HPV co-testing. For screening with Pap tests alone, patients should have a Pap test at the time of HIV-diagnosis (baseline), then every 12 months. Some experts recommend a Pap test at 6 months after the baseline test. If the results of 3 consecutive Pap tests are normal, follow-up Pap tests should be every 3 years.

  If co-testing with Pap and HPV is available, then co-testing can be done at the time of diagnosis or age 30. Co-test negative patients (i.e., a normal Pap and negative HPV test) can have their next cervical cancer screening in 3 years. Those who are Pap-test normal but positive for HPV should have repeat co-testing in 1 year (unless genotype testing for 16 or 16/18 is positive). If either of the co-tests at 1 year is abnormal (i.e., abnormal cytology or positive HPV), referral to colposcopy is recommended.

  If the initial HPV results identify HPV16 or HPV16/18, then referral to colposcopy is recommended. If the HPV testing is positive, but the genotype specific testing for HPV16 or HPV 16/18 is negative, then repeat co-testing in 1 year is recommended. If either of the co-tests at 1 year is abnormal (i.e., abnormal cytology or positive HPV), referral to colposcopy is recommended.

Cervical cancer screening should continue throughout the patient's lifetime, and not stop at age 65 as in the general population.

Recommendations for management of abnormal cytology in HIV-positive patients are available at: https://aidsinfo.nih.gov/guidelines/html/4/adult-and-adolescent-oi-prevention-and-treatment-guidelines/343/hpv.

Finally, while the nonavalent HPV vaccine has not been extensively studied in HIV-positive patients, the vaccine is protein-based (no live virus) and is currently recommended for HIV-positive individuals between 9 to 26 years of age according to ACIP guidelines.

Pelvic inflammatory disease (PID). In general, PID does not require more aggressive treatment for HIV-positive patients, but the approach should be individualized. Depending on the severity of PID and immune status, providers should consider parenteral therapy and hospitalization, based on similar factors considerations for HIV-negative patients.

Genital herpes. In the presence of immune dysfunction, herpes lesions may be more extensive, more painful, atypical in location or appearance, and slower to heal. In a large study in Africa, suppressive therapy with twice daily oral acyclovir was associated with a reduction in plasma HIV viral load relative to placebo.[47] Benefits of suppressive therapy include reduction of symptomatic outbreaks, reduction in risk of HSV-2 transmission to sex partners (demonstrated in heterosexual couples), and possibly, a favorable effect on HIV itself due to direct activity against HIV. Treat symptomatic episodes of genital herpes should be accordance with standard guidelines for HIV-positive persons.

Psychological Care and Support for HIV+ Patients

Women with HIV often experience significant psychosocial stress, often related to the fact that they may be the primary caregivers for their families. They will often need guidance, support, and referral to assist with fundamental concerns including stable housing, economic stability, childcare, and addiction.

Reproductive Health Care for HIV+ Patients

For HIV-positive patients, the decision about whether to get pregnant is similar to that of HIV-negative patients, and their desire for a child is often profound. Counseling patients who are pregnant or contemplating pregnancy includes important medical issues:

- Impact of HIV on pregnancy
- Impact of pregnancy on HIV
- Effect of antiretroviral medication and other drugs on both the patient and developing fetus

- Risk of perinatal transmission and options for reducing risk
- Risk of breastfeeding for HIV transmission
- Course of HIV in perinatally infected infants
- Access to HIV-experienced obstetric and pediatric care
- Access to antiretroviral medications

Counseling for pregnancy optimally includes a full understanding of the patient's personal goals, support network, stressors in their life, and their overall physical and emotional status. Once this groundwork is in place, guide the patient through specific questions to help her predict how they would feel, how others would feel, and what might happen.

HIV-positive patients who do not wish to become pregnant are more likely to succeed with a contraceptive method they have chosen for themselves and feel comfortable using (Table 20-9). The goal is high contraceptive efficacy, low risk of HIV transmission to partners (if applicable), and low risk of STI acquisition. This goal is met by choices such as hormonal contraceptives or IUC, plus male condoms.

Thousands of patients with HIV give birth each year in the United States. Generally, HIV-positive patients with a competent immune system have uneventful pregnancies with normal labor and delivery. Just as with any patient with a serious systemic illness, HIV-positive patients may have complicated pregnancies, including prematurity, low birth weight, and premature rupture of membranes. However, the effects of HIV on pregnancy are hard to differentiate from the effects of poverty, poor health care, or addiction. Pregnancy itself does not appear to speed HIV progression.

Risks of HIV Transmission in the Perinatal Period

Without HAART, each offspring of an infected woman in the United States faces approximately a 25% risk of being infected in utero, during birth, or while breastfeeding. With HAART, the risk falls to 2% or less (see below).

Reducing perinatal transmission risk. Strategies to reduce perinatal HIV transmission continue to evolve rapidly. HAART is recommended for all pregnant patients with the goal of suppressing plasma HIV RNA to undetectable levels. Antiretroviral treatment is also recommended for HIV-exposed infants in their first weeks of life. HAART initiation for this purpose may be delayed until the second trimester.

Labor and delivery. In the absence of breastfeeding, an estimated 60% to 75% of perinatal HIV transmissions occur around the time of labor and

Table 20-9 Contraception for the HIV-positive patient[48]

Method	Possible Benefits	Possible Drawbacks
Oral Contraceptives	• Good effectiveness with consistent use • Less blood loss to avoid anemia	• Unclear interaction of steroids and immune function • Possible interaction with certain antibiotics, antiretrovirals, other drugs • No RTI protection • No HIV protection for partner
Depo-Provera	Good low-maintenance effectiveness	• Unclear interaction of steroids and immune function • No RTI protection • No HIV protection for partner
IUD	Good low-maintenance effectiveness	• Risk of infection during insertion interval • No RTI protection • No HIV protection for partner • Increased days of bleeding, possible anemia (copper IUD only)
Diaphragm	Some RTI protection for the cervix	• Increases vulnerability to UTIs for some users • Requires good technique
Male, Female Condom	Good RTI protection, HIV protection for partner	• Male condom requires partner cooperation; partner cooperation helpful with female condom • Requires good technique
Surgical Sterilization	Good low-maintenance efficacy for women who desire no more children	• No RTI protection • No HIV protection for partner

Sources: Adapted Cates W Jr. (2001)[3]

delivery, and a number of strategies can reduce exposure of the neonate to blood and secretions. In addition to intrapartum HAART, suggested approaches include vaginal disinfection, RTI treatment during pregnancy to lower viral shedding at term, avoidance of intrapartum invasive procedures, and cesarean delivery. Scheduled cesarean delivery before rupture of membranes is recommended for patients whose HIV viral load at 36 weeks or later is above 1,000 copies/mL. Avoid delays in delivery once membranes have ruptured. The risk of perinatal HIV transmission can double when fetal membranes rupture more than 4 hours before delivery.

Breastfeeding. Currently in the United States, bottle-feeding is recommended for infants to reduce the risk of postnatal HIV transmission via breast milk. The precise risk of HIV transmission via breast milk is difficult to quantify and may be influenced by the stage of the HIV disease (with high viral loads during primary infection and late stage disease), use of HAART, breastfeeding patterns, and other factors. Approximately

10% to 15% of all vertical transmissions are associated with breastfeeding. (See Chapter 17 on Contraception After Pregnancy.) Little is known about the impact of breastfeeding on the HIV-positive patient's nutritional status and overall health, or about the immunoprotective qualities of the breast milk produced by an immunocompromised patient.

Author Disclosures—Marrazzo: none. Park: none.

References

1. Eng TR, Butler WT. The hidden epidemic: confronting sexually transmitted diseases. Committee on Prevention and Control of Sexually Transmitted Diseases, IOM, U.S., Division of Health Promotion and Disease Prevention 1996.
2. Centers for Disease Control and Prevention. Sexually transmitted disease surveillance, 2015. Atlanta, GA: U.S. Department of Health and Human Services; November 2016.
3. Centers for Disease Control and Prevention, CDC Fact Sheet: Reported STDs in the United States. At www.cdc.gov/nchhstp/newsroom/docs/factsheets/STD-Trends-508.pdf. Accessed 9/14/2017.
4. Satterwhite CL, Torrone E, Meites E, et al. Sexually transmitted infections among US women and men: prevalence and incidence estimates, 2008. Sex Transm Dis 2013;40:187–93.
5. Cates W, Jr. Review of non-hormonal contraception (condoms, intrauterine devices, nonoxynol-9 and combos) on HIV acquisition. J Acq Imm Def 2005;38 Suppl 1:S8–10.
6. Garnett G. The transmission dynamics of sexually transmitted infections. In: Holmes KK, Sparling PF, Stamm WE, et al., eds. Sexually transmitted diseases. 4th ed. New York: McGraw-Hill; 2008:27–39.
7. Pilcher CD, Tien HC, Eron JJ, Jr., et al. Brief but efficient: acute HIV infection and the sexual transmission of HIV. J Infect Dis 2004;189:1785–92.
8. Baeten JM, Donnell D, Ndase P, et al. Antiretroviral prophylaxis for HIV prevention in heterosexual men and women. N Engl J Med 2012;367:399–410.
9. UNAIDS and WHO. New data on male circumcision and HIV prevention: policy and programme implications; WHO/UNAIDS technical consultation male circumcision and HIV prevention: research implications for policy and programming montreux. Geneva: Joint United Nations Programme on HIV/AIDS and World Health Organization, 2007.
10. Trussell J, Kost K. Contraceptive failure in the United States: a critical review of the literature. Stud Fam Plann 1987;18:237–83.
11. Herzog SA, Heijne JC, Althaus CL, Low N. Describing the progression from Chlamydia trachomatis and Neisseria gonorrhoeae to pelvic inflammatory disease: systematic review of mathematical modeling studies. Sex Transm Dis 2012;39:628–37.
12. Westrom L, Joesoef R, Reynolds G, Hagdu A, Thompson SE. Pelvic inflammatory disease and fertility. A cohort study of 1,844 women with laparoscopically verified disease and 657 control women with normal laparoscopic results. Sex Transm Dis 1992;19:185–92.
13. Padian NS, van der Straten A, Ramjee G, et al. Diaphragm and lubricant gel for prevention of HIV acquisition in southern African women: a randomised controlled trial. Lancet 2007;370:251–61.
14. Ness RB, Keder LM, Soper DE, et al. Oral contraception and the recognition of endometritis. Am J Obstet Gynecol 1997;176:580–5.
15. Polis CB, Phillips SJ, Curtis KM, et al. Hormonal contraceptive methods and risk of HIV acquisition in women: a systematic review of epidemiological evidence. Contraception 2014;90:360–90.

16. Morrison CS, Bright P, Wong EL, et al. Hormonal contraceptive use, cervical ectopy, and the acquisition of cervical infections. Sex Transm Dis 2004;31:561–7.
17. Steenland MW, Zapata LB, Brahmi D, Marchbanks PA, Curtis KM. Appropriate follow up to detect potential adverse events after initiation of select contraceptive methods: a systematic review. Contraception 2013;87:611–24.
18. Sufrin CB, Postlethwaite D, Armstrong MA, Merchant M, Wendt JM, Steinauer JE. Neisseria gonorrhea and Chlamydia trachomatis screening at intrauterine device insertion and pelvic inflammatory disease. Obstet Gynecol 2012;120:1314–21.
19. Turok DK, Eisenberg DL, Teal SB, Keder LM, Creinin MD. A prospective assessment of pelvic infection risk following same-day sexually transmitted infection testing and levonorgestrel intrauterine system placement. Am J Obstet Gynecol 2016;215:599 e1–e6.
20. Tepper NK, Curtis KM, Nanda K, Jamieson DJ. Safety of intrauterine devices among women with HIV: a systematic review. Contraception 2016;94:713–24.
21. Morrison CS, Turner AN, Jones LB. Highly effective contraception and acquisition of HIV and other sexually transmitted infections. Best Pract Res Clin Obstet Gynaecol 2009;23:263–84.
22. Polis CB, Curtis KM. Use of hormonal contraceptives and HIV acquisition in women: a systematic review of the epidemiological evidence. Lancet Infect Dis 2013;13:797–808.
23. Van Damme L, Ramjee G, Alary M, et al. Effectiveness of COL-1492, a nonoxynol-9 vaginal gel, on HIV-1 transmission in female sex workers: a randomised controlled trial. Lancet 2002;360:971–7.
24. Karim QA, Karim SS, Frohlich JA, et al. Effectiveness and safety of tenofovir gel, an antiretroviral microbicide, for the prevention of HIV infection in women. Science 2010;10:1126.
25. Klebanoff MA, Nansel TR, Brotman RM, et al. Personal hygienic behaviors and bacterial vaginosis. Sex Transm Dis 2010;37:94–9.
26. Jin F, Matthews GV, Grulich AE. Sexual transmission of hepatitis C virus among gay and bisexual men: a systematic review. Sex Health 2017;14:28–41.
27. Leigh BC. Alcohol and condom use: a meta-analysis of event-level studies. Sex Transm Dis 2002;29:476–82.
28. Cates W, Jr. A risk-assessment tool for integrated reproductive health services. Fam Plann Perspect 1997;29:41–3.
29. Zakher B, Cantor AG, Pappas M, Daeges M, Nelson HD. Screening for gonorrhea and Chlamydia: a systematic review for the U.S. Preventive Services Task Force. Ann Intern Med 2014;161:884–93.
30. LeFevre ML, USPSTF. Screening for Chlamydia and gonorrhea: u.s. Preventive services task force recommendation statement. Ann Intern Med 2014;161:902–10.
31. Screening for gonorrhea: recommendation statement. Ann Fam Med 2005;3:263–7.
32. Feltner C, Grodensky C, Ebel C, et al. Serologic screening for genital herpes: an updated evidence report and systematic review. for the US Preventive Services Task Force. JAMA 2016;316:2531–43.
33. USPSTF, Bibbins-Domingo K, Grossman DC, et al. Serologic Screening for Genital Herpes Infection: US Preventive Services Task Force Recommendation Statement. JAMA 2016;316:2525–30.
34. Golden MR, Whittington WL, Handsfield HH, et al. Effect of expedited treatment of sex partners on recurrent or persistent gonorrhea or chlamydial infection. N Engl J Med 2005;352:676–85.
35. Kissinger P, Mohammed H, Richardson-Alston G, et al. Patient-delivered partner treatment for male urethritis: a randomized, controlled trial. Clin Infect Dis : an official publication of the Infectious Diseases Society of America 2005;41:623–9.
36. Yu YY, Frasure-Williams JA, Dunne EF, Bolan G, Markowitz L, Bauer HM. Chlamydia partner services for females in California family planning clinics. Sex Transm Dis 2011;38:913–8.

37. American Academy of Pediatrics, American College of Obstetricians and Gynecologists. Guidelines for perinatal care. 7th ed. Elk Grove Village (IL): AAP; Washington, DC: American College of Obstetricians and Gynecologists; 2012. p. 109–110, 160, 12–194, 248.
38. Workowski K, Bolan G. Sexually Transmitted Disease Treatment Guidelines, 2015. MMWR 2015;64.
39. Centers for Disease Control and Prevention. Updated guidelines for antiretroviral post-exposure prophylaxis after sexual, injection-drug use, or other nonoccupational exposure to HIV—United States, 2016. www.cdc.gov/hiv/pdf/programresources/cdc-hiv-npep-guidelines.pdf.
40. Gray RH, Wawer MJ, Brookmeyer R, et al. Probability of HIV-1 transmission per coital act in monogamous, heterosexual, HIV-1-discordant couples in Rakai, Uganda. Lancet 2001;357:1149–53.
41. Centers for Disease Control and Prevention. Revised recommendations for HIV testing for adults, adolescents, and pregnant women in healthcare settings. MMWR 2006;55 (RR-14).
42. Gray RH, Li X, Kigozi G, et al. Increased risk of incident HIV during pregnancy in Rakai, Uganda: a prospective study. Lancet 2005;366:1182–8.
43. Centers for Disease Control and Prevention. Laboratory testing for the diagnosis of HIV infection: updated recommendations. 2014. http://dx.doi.org/10.15620/cdc.
44. Chesson HW, Ekwueme DU, Saraiya M, Watson M, Lowy DR, Markowitz LE. Estimates of the annual direct medical costs of the prevention and treatment of disease associated with human papillomavirus in the United States. Vaccine 2012;30:6016–9.
45. Group ISS, Lundgren JD, Babiker AG, et al. Initiation of antiretroviral therapy in early asymptomatic HIV infection. N Engl J Med 2015;373:795–807.
46. HIV/AIDS Bureau, Health Resources and Services Administration. A guide to the clinical care of women with HIV. In: Anderson RJe, ed. 1st ed. Rockville, MD: 2001.
47. Lingappa JR, Baeten JM, Wald A, et al. Daily aciclovir for HIV-1 disease progression in people dually infected with HIV-1 and herpes simplex virus type 2: a randomised placebo-controlled trial. Lancet 2010;375:824–33.
48. Curtis KM, Nanda K, Kapp N. Safety of hormonal and intrauterine methods of contraception for women with HIV/AIDS: a systematic review. AIDS 2009;23:S55–67.

Screening Women for Cervical, Ovarian, and Breast Cancer

21

Michael S. Policar, MD, MPH
George F. Sawaya, MD

- All current U.S. guidelines on cervical cancer screening state that for those at average risk, the following schedule applies:
  - — Begin at age 21
  - — Discontinue for individuals 65 years of age and older who in the prior 10 years have a history of 3 or more negative cervical cytology tests, or 2 negative co-tests. (A *co-test* combines a cervical cytology and a test for high-risk HPV DNA (hr-HPV).
- With the exception of women who are infected with HIV or who are otherwise immunocompromised, women younger than 21 years should not be screened regardless of the age of sexual initiation or the presence of other behavior-related risk factors.
- After total hysterectomy, individuals can discontinue screening if they have no prior history of a high-grade cervical pre-cancer or cancer.
- Women 21 to 29 years of age should have cervical cytology screening every 3 years. Women age 30 and older should receive *either* cervical cytology screening every 3 years or co-testing every 5 years.
- More variation exists in U.S. breast cancer screening guidelines, especially regarding the ages at which to start and stop mammograms, mammography intervals, and the use of screening clinical breast examination.
- Three U.S. guidelines differ in their recommendations for the inclusion of a screening pelvic exam at the time of a well-woman visit.
- For many asymptomatic individuals seen for a well-woman visit, a screening pelvic exam and screening breast exam will not be necessary. If indicated, a patient can collect a self-administered vaginal swab or urine sample for a NAAT testing screen for Chlamydia and gonorrhea, so there may be no need for a physical assessment beyond a blood pressure check.

A reproductive healthcare visit represents an ideal opportunity to offer periodic health screening services, including screening for genital tract cancers. As early as the 1920s, the prevalent philosophy of the American medical community was that individuals of all ages should receive an annual physical examination and a battery of routine screening tests to detect early, asymptomatic disease.[1] However, the wisdom of this practice has been challenged, and research studies and health policy discussions have focused upon the optimal content of periodic health screening: which tests should or should not be performed, how often each screening test should be done, and whether each test should be performed routinely or limited to persons with certain risk factors. While many approaches to periodic health screening have been proposed, the recommendations of the United States Preventive Services Task Force (USPSTF) are considered the blueprint for the screening guidelines developed by most state Departments of Health, professional specialty societies, and health plans. Using an evidence-based methodology, the USPSTF guidelines gauge the strength of each recommendation with a letter grade, which is assigned using a combination of the balance of net benefits and harms of the intervention and the level of certainty regarding net benefit, based upon the quality of the research studies used to develop the recommendation. In 2007, the USPSTF updated the definitions of the grades it assigns to recommendations and now includes "suggestions for practice" for each grade. In 2012, it further updated the definition of, and suggestions for practice, for the grade C recommendation.[2] (See Table 21-1.)

In the past, the concept of the "annual well-woman visit" included a screening breast exam, cervical cytology screening, and a screening pelvic exam in patients who had initiated sexual activity. Owing in part to the changes in cancer screening recommendations listed below, however, most people will no longer require yearly visits to receive screening tests, irrespective of their choice of contraceptive method. The USPSTF recommends that patients undergo a health screening visit once every 1 to 3 years, depending upon their underlying health status, sexual behaviors, the intervals of the recommended screening tests, and their own personal preferences. If the patient chooses not to receive this service, offer "opportunistic prevention" by providing prevention guidance and screening tests at the time of problem-oriented visits.

Another issue that may arise at a health-screening visit is whether to provide comprehensive preventive health services or only those related to sexual and reproductive health. As a result of health insurance coverage obtained through the Patient Protection and Affordable Care Act (ACA), most insured patients will have an established relationship with a primary care provider from whom they will receive some or all preventive health services. If so, it is important for the reproductive health care provider to avoid duplicating tests already completed, and ideally, with the permission of the patient, to transmit the record of the reproductive health

Table 21-1 Recommendation grades used by the U.S. Preventive Services Task Force, 2012

Grade	Definition	Suggestions for Practice
A	The USPSTF recommends the service. There is high certainty that the net benefit is substantial.	Offer or provide this service.
B	The USPSTF recommends the service. There is high certainty that the net benefit is moderate or there is moderate certainty that the net benefit is moderate to substantial.	Offer or provide this service.
C	The USPSTF recommends selectively offering or providing this service to individual patients based on professional judgment and patient preferences. There is at least moderate certainty that the net benefit is small.	Offer or provide this service for selected patients depending on individual circumstances.
D	The USPSTF recommends against the service. There is moderate or high certainty that the service has no net benefit or that the harms outweigh the benefits.	Discourage the use of this service.
I	The USPSTF concludes that the current evidence is insufficient to assess the balance of benefits and harms of the service. Evidence is lacking, of poor quality, or conflicting, and the balance of benefits and harms cannot be determined.	Read the clinical considerations section of USPSTF Recommendation Statement. If the service is offered, patients should understand the uncertainty about the balance of benefits and harms.

care visits to the primary care provider. In some cases, the only opportunity available to receive preventive health care services is during a patient's reproductive health care visit, so if you are adequately equipped in your practice, it is appropriate to offer the full range of recommended preventive interventions. Two helpful sources of age-specific disease prevention guidelines are the USPSTF (www.uspreventiveservicestaskforce.org) and "Preventing Cancer, Cardiovascular Disease, and Diabetes: A Common Agenda of the American Cancer Society, the American Diabetes Association, and the American Heart Association."[3] The USPSTF has a free app, the Electronic Preventive Services Selector, which facilitates point-of-care decisions about appropriate preventive services.

Over the years, health screening also has been linked with the provision of prescription hormonal contraceptives. In many cases, someone could get a prescription for combined hormonal contraceptives only if they underwent a well-woman visit. This attitude is now considered to be outdated, and only those medical conditions that could influence contraceptive choice, safety, or usage should be the subject of screening before writing a prescription for hormonal contraception. For example, the 2016 CDC Selected Practice Recommendations for Contraceptive Use (SPR) do not recommend breast or genital tract examination, cervical cancer screening, STI assessment, hemoglobin determination, or other routine lab tests as "contributing substantially to safe and effective use of a contraceptive method."[4] These guidelines also specify that, if available, it is desirable to measure blood pressure before initiating a patient on combined hormonal contraceptives, progestin-only pills, progestin-only injections, and implants. No other published domestic or international guidelines require screening for genital tract cancer or sexually transmitted infections prior to writing a prescription for contraceptives, based on the attitude that doing so is unnecessary for safe contraceptive use and that any unnecessary barriers to contraceptive services should be removed.[5] Furthermore, hormonal methods need not be restricted or withheld from a woman solely because she has an abnormal cervical cytology test. There is no reason to believe that the use of any contraceptive method will hasten the progression of an existing pre-invasive lesion to cervical cancer. All too often, the unfortunate result of withholding contraceptives from a woman with an abnormal cytology or biopsy result is unintended pregnancy, which makes diagnosis more difficult and often delays treatment.

CERVICAL CANCER

THE NATURAL HISTORY OF CERVICAL CANCER

The cause of pre-invasive cervical lesions and invasive cancer is an accumulation of DNA mutations in immature metaplastic cells in the cervix as a consequence of persistent high-risk human papilloma virus (hr-HPV) infection, in concert with other carcinogenic co-factors. A convenient and accurate analogy to describe the development of pre-invasive cervical lesions is the requirement for plant growth: a seed, receptive soil, and fertilizer to promote growth.

The Seed: Infection with high-risk HPV

Genital HPV infections are transmitted by skin-to-skin contact during sex. Although more than 100 DNA types of HPV have been identified, only a limited number are associated with premalignant and malignant epithelial lesions of the lower genital tract: HPV types 16 and 18 account for about 70% of high-grade squamous intraepithelial lesions (HSIL; also referred to as cervical intraepithelial neoplasia [CIN] 2 and 3 lesions) and cervical cancers. The remaining 30% are due to HPV types 31, 33, 35, 39, 45, 51, 52, 56, 58, 59, 66, and 68.[6] The high-risk HPV types exert their cancer-causing effects through a series of events leading to the degradation of the p53 tumor suppressor protein in infected cells, reducing the host's ability to reject cells with random DNA mutations. Infections due to HPV types 6 and 11, the cause of genital warts and most low-grade cervical lesions, exhibit no malignant potential.

The Soil: Squamous metaplasia within the transformation zone

The cervix consists of two types of epithelium:

- *Squamous epithelium*, covering the vagina and the vaginal portion of the cervix
- *Columnar epithelium*, covering the endocervical canal, and in some individuals, the area around the external cervical os

At menarche, the vaginal pH drops into an acidic range and causes the fragile columnar epithelial cells around the cervical os to be replaced by squamous epithelium, a process referred to as squamous metaplasia. As this process proceeds over decades, the advancing edge of the squamous epithelium (referred to as the squamocolumnar junction or SCJ) migrates centrally toward the cervical os and ultimately into the endocervical canal. The immature metaplastic cells found in younger women are particularly vulnerable to infection with HPV. Because squamous cell cancers and their precursors virtually always develop within the field of metaplasia (also called the transformation zone), both cytological and colposcopic evaluation focus upon this area.

The Fertilizer: An oncogenic cofactor

Since not all people who have persistent hr-HPV infection of their cervix develop a pre-invasive cervical lesion, it seems that persistent hr-HPV infection alone is insufficient to initiate the development of a pre-invasive cervical lesion. A facilitating agent, or oncogenic co-factor, appears to be necessary to act in concert with hr-HPV to initiate these premalignant changes. For example, cigarette smoking has been identified as a powerful cofactor,[7] doubling the risk of cervical cancer.

Risk Factors for Cervical Cancer

Epidemiological observations are consistent with the biological mechanism of cervical cancer. The following are primary epidemiological risk factors for the development of cervical cancer:

- Early onset of intercourse (defined as a sexual debut before 20 years old). Metaplasia is most active during adolescence, making a young woman more vulnerable to cell changes that result from hr-HPV infection.
- High number of sex partners. The greater the number of sex partners, the greater the risk of acquiring a high-risk type of HPV.

- A sex partner who has had other partners, especially if their previous partner had cervical cancer.
- Clinical history of condyloma acuminata. Infection with a low-risk type of HPV is a risk marker for co-infection with a high-risk type.[8]
- Infection with the human immunodeficiency virus (HIV) and other medical conditions associated with immunodeficiency. These illnesses decrease the ability of the immune system to recognize and reject abnormal cells. Women who use immunosuppressive drugs after major organ transplants also are at increased risk of cervical cancer.

Behavioral protective factors include no history of partnered sexual activity, long-term celibacy, life-long mutual monogamy, and long-term use of condoms. Factors that appear to have no effect on cervical cancer risk include a history of herpes simplex virus infection or the circumcision status of the partner. The effect of race and socioeconomic status are controversial. Studies show higher rates of cervical cancer among African American women and women of lower socio-economic status;[9,10] however, it is unclear whether the higher rates are related to poor access to medical care and, consequently, cervical cytology services, or other undetermined factors.[11] Cervical cancer incidence and mortality rates are higher in black and Hispanic women compared with white women among women living in rural areas, when compared with those living in urban areas.[10] It recently has been determined that African American women's risk of dying from cervical cancer is even higher than previously thought. The earlier risk estimate was based on population-based mortality statistics that had not been corrected for prior hysterectomy. The corrected cervical cancer mortality rate for African American women is 10.1 per 100,000, whereas the uncorrected rate is 5.7 per 100,000. The corrected rate for white women is 4.7 per 100,000, whereas the uncorrected rate is 3.2 per 100,000. Without the correction, the disparity in mortality was underestimated by 44%.[12]

HPV infections are widespread among sexually active adults, costly to characterize virologically through HPV DNA testing, and cannot be eradicated with antiviral drugs. HPV infections are transient in the vast majority of infected individuals; but persistent infection with high-risk HPV types is necessary for the development of high-grade lesions and cancer. Rather than to rely on a behavioral strategy that focuses on the sexual transmissibility of HPV, it makes more sense from a public health viewpoint to prevent cervical cancer and its precursors with primary prevention through HPV vaccination before sexual debut as well as secondary prevention through screening programs that will detect and permit treatment of high-grade pre-invasive lesions before life-threatening invasive cervical cancers have a chance to develop.

Prevention of Cervical Cancer With HPV Vaccination

Vaccination against high-risk HPV infection has been shown to be successful for primary prevention of cervical cancer precursors, as well as vaginal, vulvar and anal pre-cancer lesions due to HPV 16 and 18. The only product currently available in the U.S. is the nine-valent HPV (9vHPV) vaccine, Gardasil 9. The 4-valent and 2-valent HPV vaccines had been available since 2006 and 2009 respectively, but are no longer sold in the U.S.

The vaccine consists of genetically manufactured viral envelope proteins, rather than the live or attenuated virus, to stimulate the production of anti-HPV antibodies. When given to uninfected individuals, the vaccine has very high efficacy in preventing HSIL and cancers due to HPV types 16, 18, 31, 33, 45, 52, and 58. The 9vHPV vaccine also has high efficacy in protecting against genital warts, 90% of which are induced by HPV 6 and 11. The vaccine does not appear to cause any serious long-term adverse effects, but an important problem is that pain at the injection site can trigger a vasovagal fainting episode. For this reason, individuals receiving the vaccine should be monitored for at least 5 minutes after the injection to prevent an injury from an unwitnessed fall, and clinicians should be familiar with the recognition and treatment of vasovagal episodes. (For more, see Placement Technique in Chapter 5 on Intrauterine Devices.) Because 10% of HSIL lesions contain hr-HPV types not included in the vaccine, individuals who have been vaccinated are advised to receive routine cervical screening at currently recommended intervals. The 2016 CDC Advisory Committee on Immunization Practices (ACIP) has published guidelines regarding the use of HPV vaccine.[13]

- Routine vaccination of females and males aged 11 or 12 years is recommended. The vaccination series can be started beginning at age 9. Ideally, vaccine should be administered before potential exposure to HPV through sexual contact.
- Vaccination is recommended for females aged 13 through 26 years who have not been vaccinated previously or who have not completed the series. If a female reaches age 26 years before the vaccination series is complete, remaining doses can be administered after age 26 years.
- Males who are 13 to 21 years old should be vaccinated, although males 22 to 26 years may also be vaccinated. However, HPV vaccination is recommended through age 26 for men having sex with men and for immunocompromised persons (including those with HIV infection).[14]
- Initially, the CDC recommended HPV vaccination in a 3-dose schedule: first dose, second dose 1 to 2 months later, and third dose 6 months after the first. In 2016, the CDC added a 2-dose

schedule for 9 to 14 year olds (first dose, then second dose after 6 to 12 months), based on studies that showed that 2 doses were not inferior to 3 doses in this age group, as evidenced by seroconversion and antibody titers.

- The 9vHPV vaccine can be given at the same time as other vaccines, including TDaP, TD, and MCV4 vaccines. Lactating women can receive the HPV vaccine.
- HPV vaccination is not recommended in pregnant women. If a woman is found to be pregnant after initiating the vaccination series, the remainder of the 3-dose series should be delayed until completion of pregnancy. If a vaccine dose has been administered during pregnancy, no intervention is needed. Pregnancy registries for 4vHPV and 2vHPV vaccines have been closed because reports of problems in pregnant women or their newborns were no greater than in nonvaccinated women. A new pregnancy registry has been established for 9vHPV. Pregnancy testing is not indicated routinely before vaccination.
- Patients should be advised that vaccination has no therapeutic effect on an existing HPV infection, genital warts, or an abnormal cervical cytology.
- With increasing severity of prior abnormal cervical cytology findings, the likelihood of infection with HPV 16 or 18 increases, and benefits of vaccination decrease. Vaccination is still recommended for such patients, because vaccination can provide protection against infection with HPV vaccine types not already acquired.
- Pre-vaccination assessments (e.g., cervical cytology, screening for hr-HPV DNA, type-specific HPV tests, or HPV antibody) to establish the appropriateness of HPV vaccination are not recommended at any age.
- HPV vaccines are not live vaccines and can be administered to those who are immunosuppressed from disease or medications. However, the immune response and vaccine efficacy may be less than that in immunocompetent persons.

The American Cancer Society updated their HPV vaccination guideline in 2016.[15] It is similar to the ACIP guideline, but contains the caveat that late vaccination should be completed as soon as possible and that individuals should be informed that vaccination may not be effective at older ages.

Cervical Cancer Screening

Cervical cytology screening, more than any other screening test, has proven its cost-effectiveness over the years.[16] Based upon current screening patterns in the United States, early detection and treatment of pre-invasive cervical lesions prevents at least 70% of potential cervical cancers. In 2017, of the 12,820 Americans[17] who develop new cases of cervical cancer[18]—

- One half had not had a cervical cytology in the past 3 to 5 years.
- One half had received a cervical cytology within 3 to 5 years, but there was either a falsely negative result, the patient was not managed correctly, or there was inadequate follow-up of the patient.

False-negative results occur in about 25% of cervical cytology tests and occur either because the lesion exfoliated too few cells to be detected, there was a sampling error by the clinician, or there was an interpretive error in the cytopathology lab. In 1996, the U.S. FDA approved the technique of liquid-based cytology (LBC) with thin-layer preparation technique (Thin Prep, BD SurePath), which is intended to improve test quality by removing blood, mucus, and debris from the background of the sample. Early studies suggested that LBC improved screening accuracy over traditional practices;[19, 20] However, a large randomized clinical trial from the Netherlands[21] and a meta-analysis of eight studies[22] concluded that liquid-based cervical cytology is neither more sensitive nor more specific for detection of HSIL compared with the conventional cervical cytology test. Virtually all cytopathology labs in the United States have adopted this technology because it improves the efficiency of cytotechnicians, facilitates computerized screening or rescreening, and serves as a platform for evaluation of other pathogens in the cytology sample, specifically high-risk HPV, gonorrhea, and Chlamydia.

HPV Testing Used Alone or as an Adjunct to Cytological Screening

Hr-HPV DNA testing for 13 or 14 high-risk HPV types is used in one of four ways:

1. **Primary screening with cytology (co-testing)**, in which an hr-HPV DNA test and cervical cytology are performed simultaneously in those 30 years old and older.[23, 24]
2. **Primary hr-HPV screening,** using an hr-HPV test alone, in people 25 through 65 years of age who have not had a total hysterectomy.
3. **Triage** of an abnormal cervical cytology result. With this strategy, once the cytopathology laboratory reports an ASCUS result, a "reflex" hr-HPV DNA test is performed.[24]
4. **Co-testing** as follow-up of certain abnormal cytology results after colposcopy showing no high-grade precancerous lesion and for post-treatment surveillance.[24]

Primary cervical cancer screening with co-testing improves the sensitivity of screening for HSIL or cancer to at least 92% when compared with a sensitivity of about 75% for cytology alone.[23] Of equal importance is the negative predictive value of this approach, since people with negative results on both cytology and HPV tests have a less than 1% likelihood of developing HSIL or cancer within the next 10 years. Co-testing is not recommended for screening people under 30 years old due to the high prevalence of transient hr-HPV infections in younger individuals. Most important, people who are hr-HPV DNA negative and who have a normal cervical cytology result should not be rescreened before 5 years, because the risk of a new lesion is negligible and the likelihood of a false-positive test is substantial. The combination of a negative cervical cytology and a positive HPV test can be managed in one of two approaches. One option is to perform a co-test in 12 months. The second option, if it is available from your lab, is to test for HPV-16 or HPV-18 genotypes. If positive for HPV-16 or -18, refer the patient for colposcopy. If negative for both, recommend a 12-month follow-up with co-testing.[25] If you intend to perform cervical cancer screening with co-testing, it is critical to inform the patient in advance of sampling that they are being screened for HPV and will not need to have cervical rescreening earlier than 5 years if both tests are negative.

In April 2014, the FDA approved the cobas test for primary hr-HPV screening, based mainly on the results of a large U.S.-based study of HPV primary screening, known as ATHENA trial, which validated an effective triage algorithm. While primary hr-HPV screening detected approximately 50% more CIN 3+ compared with cytology, it also resulted in approximately double the number of colposcopies.[26] Interim clinical guidance has been published regarding the use of primary HPV testing for cervical cancer screening.[27] When HPV type 16 or 18 is identified, colposcopy is recommended. A positive test for one or more of the 12 other hr-HPV types should be followed with a cervical cytology, with the result used to triage the patient to colposcopy (if ASCUS or worse) or repeat testing in 1 year if negative. Re-screening after a negative primary hr-HPV screen should occur no sooner than every 3 years. In 2016, ACOG stated that if screening with primary HPV testing is used, it should be performed per the interim clinical guidance, which clarifies a number of important issues not specified in the product labeling. If primary screening is performed, it should be done with the approved test.[25]

The 2017 USPSTF Draft Recommendation Statement for cervical cancer screening includes two very significant modifications. They recommend first that hr-HPV testing alone replace the co-testing option for individuals aged 30 to 65, and second, that HPV-alone testing should be done every 5 years, rather than "not more often than every 3 years" as recommended by the interim clinical guidance. The rationale for this recommendation is that both clinical trial evidence and modeling suggest that co-testing increases the number of follow-up tests by as much as twofold and does not lead to increased detection of CIN 3 or cervical cancer compared with screening with hr-HPV testing alone. Therefore, the USPSTF did not include primary screening with co-testing in this recommendation statement.[28]

Technical Aspects of Cytological Screening

High accuracy in cytological screening depends on a good quality cervical sample, appropriately performed preparation, and competent cytopathologic interpretation.

- Cytological screening may be performed at any time of the cycle, because the presence of menstrual blood usually is not problematic in the interpretation of liquid-based cytology.
- Moisten the speculum with warm water or a small amount of lubricating gel applied away from the tip of the speculum. Samples most easily contaminated by blood should be taken early in the sampling sequence: nucleic acid amplification tests (NAATs) for Chlamydia and gonorrhea should be performed before the cervical cytology sample.
- Liquid-based cytology (LBC) sampling
  - — The cervix may be gently dabbed with a swab to wipe away mucus, discharge, or menstrual blood prior to collecting a LBC sample. However, do not wipe away material covering the cervix, as this practice may remove a significant amount of cellular material, resulting in a scanty sample.
  - — Use either a brush and spatula or a broom device that can be broken off and dropped into the solution, as instructed by the cytopathology lab used by your practice
  - — If using the brush, insert the brush into the cervix until only the bottom fibers are visible. Slowly rotate ¼ to ½ turn in one direction. Do not over-rotate as this may cause bleeding and loss of endocervical cells.
  - — Vigorously twirl the brush and spatula in the liquid at least 10 times. Push the brush against the side of the vial to remove any mucus. Use the spatula to mechanically remove mucus and cells from the brush.

Cervical Cytology Screening Intervals

The national recommendations for cervical cancer screening intervals include significant changes from earlier guidelines, often resulting in inconsistent, or even incorrect, practices among providers.[29] Between the 1940s and 2002, women in the United States were advised to have cervical cytology screening performed annually at the time of their well woman visit.[30] Currently, three major national organizations, the USPSTF,[31,32] the American Cancer Society, the American Society for Colposcopy and Cervical Pathology (ASCCP), and the American Society for Clinical Pathology[33]; and ACOG[25] have issued recommendations regarding the periodicity of cervical cancer screening. There is a great deal of overlap among the guidelines, and while minor differences exist among them, they constitute a single "national standard" regarding screening periodicity. Consequently, clinicians should be careful to explain the rationale in a woman's medical record if a decision is made to deviate from their content

Recommended routine cervical cancer screening intervals. The following recommendations apply to asymptomatic women who are being screened for cervical cancer, while those who are "under surveillance" for prior abnormal cytology results or who have undergone treatment for a pre-invasive cervical lesion are followed under other protocols.

- Age 21–29: every 3 years with cervical cytology alone
- Age 30–65: cervical cytology every 3 years or co-testing every 5 years
- Discontinue at age 65 after 3 consecutive negative cytology screening tests in the prior decade or two negative co-tests, with one in the last 5 years
- Discontinue routine screening after a hysterectomy with removal of the cervix (total hysterectomy) if the person has never had CIN 2 or higher. Once discontinued, routine cytology screening and hr-HPV testing should not be restarted for any reason. If there is a history of CIN 2 or higher, ACOG[25] guidelines state that screening with cytology alone every 3 years for 20 years after the initial post-treatment surveillance period "seems to be reasonable."
- The Panel on Opportunistic Infections in HIV-Infected Adults and Adolescents[34] recommends that women who are infected with HIV should have age-based cervical cancer screening:
  - HIV-positive individuals should begin screening with cytology alone within 1 year of onset of sexual activity or, if currently sexually active, within the first year after HIV diagnosis, but no later than 21 years of age. Repeat cytology in 6 to 12 months, but not HPV testing, is recommended for HIV-infected women younger than 21 years with ASCUS test results.
  - If the patient is younger than 30 years and the initial cytology screening result is normal, the next cytology screening should

be in 12 months. After 3 consecutive normal annual screenings, follow-up screening should be done every 3 years.

— Patients who are 30 years and older can be screened with cytology alone or co-testing. Once those screened with cytology alone have had 3 consecutive annual normal test results, or a single negative co-test result, follow-up screening can be every 3 years.

— Cervical cancer screening in HIV-positive patients should not stop at 65 years of age, but instead continue throughout their lifetime.[27]

- The 2016 ACOG guidelines state that it is reasonable to manage patients with non-HIV immunocompromise (for example, a solid organ transplant) in the same way as HIV-positive individuals, starting at 21 years of age. They also recommend that patients who were exposed to diethylstilbestrol (DES) in utero be screened annually.
- Patients 21 years of age and older who have never had genital sexual contact with another person should be advised that their risk of cervical cancer is extremely low, but not zero. Once counseled, either they may decline cervical cancer screening entirely or can opt to be screened routinely.
- Pregnant patients should be screened at the same intervals as those who are not pregnant. Unless the patient is due for screening at the time they enter antepartum care, "routine screening" is not needed if prior results are available and negative.

Studies show that performing cervical cancer screening more often than necessary can do more harm than good because the hazards of a false-positive test will exceed the negligible benefit of the shorter screening interval. For example, one study showed that in a cohort of 100,000 well-screened people between 45 to 59 years old, annual screening instead of every 3 years would require an additional 209,324 cervical cytologies and 11,502 colposcopies to prevent a single case of cervical cancer.[35]

A real problem for clinicians is that there has been no national consumer education campaign regarding the rationale for increased screening intervals, and many patients reject them as being financially motivated and not in the best interest of their health.[34] Some clinicians are reluctant to change their screening practices as well, and in one study, physicians felt that patients were uncomfortable with extended screening intervals and were concerned that patients would not come for annual exams without concurrent cytology screening.[36,37] Providers are fearful of encountering a patient with an interval cancer and being sued for a missed diagnosis. Despite these obstacles, clinicians should take the time to discuss with each patient the interval that applies to them and to counsel that being screened too often can be harmful to health. Over-screening minimally improves lesion detection rates, but it results in an excess risk of false-positive tests, which can lead to unnecessary colposcopy and biopsies, with attendant anxiety and inconvenience, as well as unnecessary financial costs to the patient[38] and the health delivery system. Health plans now recognize this as a patient safety issue. Going forward, expect quality metrics for cervical cancer screening to evaluate your practice, not only on the percentage of eligible patients who are screened for cervical cancer, but also for the average interval between tests in those who should be routinely screened every 3 to 5 years, which is intended to detect over-utilization of resources.

Management of Abnormal Cervical Cytology Results

The classification system recommended by the third Bethesda workshop (2014 Bethesda System for Reporting Cervical Cytology) contained a number of modifications to include new screening technologies, as well as to remedy points of confusion between pathologists and clinicians.[39]

Negative, but endocervical /transformation zone component absent or insufficient

The Bethesda System has eliminated the category of "satisfactory, but limited by . . .", but comments regarding suboptimal specimen quality still may be made. The finding that most often limits interpretation is a paucity of endocervical cells. Their presence confirms that in the process of sampling the transformation zone, the active squamocolumnar junction was included. Even with the best of sampling efforts, however, endocervical cells are absent in 10% to 20% of cervical cytology samples obtained from premenopausal patients and as many as 50% from those who are postmenopausal.[40] ASCCP guidelines recommend the following:[24]

- Age 21–29: Routine screening
- Age 30 or older: If HPV is negative, routine screening. If HPV is unknown, HPV testing is preferred, but repeat cytology in 3 years is acceptable. If the HPV test is positive, co-testing should be done in 1 year.

Unsatisfactory for evaluation

Inadequate sampling, obscuring inflammation and blood, or too much lubricant makes interpretation impossible. Because unsatisfactory smears have a greater likelihood of being abnormal,[41] repeat the test in 2 to 4 months,[24] preferably at mid-cycle and at least 24 hours after the most recent intercourse or use of vaginal products. If the repeat cytology again is unsatisfactory, perform a colposcopy. If it is negative, return to routine screening if the HPV result was negative or unknown, or co-test in 1 year if the HPV result was positive. If the proportion of unsatisfactory smears within a practice is greater than 5%, remedial action in consultation with the cytopathologist is recommended.

Negative for Intraepithelial Lesion or Malignancy: Organisms

Trichomonas vaginalis. While the cervical cytology is a relatively insensitive test for the detection of Trichomonas (it detects trichomonads in only about one-half of infected women), its specificity is as high as 98%.[42] Because the prevalence of trichomonas vaginal colonization in reproductive-aged women is about 5%, the positive predictive value of a cytological report of trichomonas is about 72%. When the report indicates presence of trichomonas, review the patient's medical record to determine whether the infection was recently treated. If it has been, no further action is required. If not, offer treatment to avoid horizontal transmission to a new sexual partner and to prevent conversion of asymptomatic trichomonas colonization into an uncomfortable case of symptomatic vaginal trichomoniasis. The practice of requiring microscopic saline suspension to confirm vaginal trichomonads is illogical because the sensitivity of this test is only 60%. Instead, if the saline suspension is negative and confirmation is desired, use a test with high sensitivity and specificity, such as the Aptima TMA test. Repeat the cytology test after the next routine screening interval, unless the narrative report mentions obscuring inflammation and indicates the need to repeat the cytology test after treatment.

Fungus morphologically consistent with Candida spp. In most cases, Candida detected on cervical cytology is due to normal vaginal colonization with low levels of Candida rather than frank vaginal candidiasis. Candida colonization is not dangerous to the patient or to sexual partner(s). Repeat the cytology test only if the inflammation due to the candidiasis is of sufficient severity that the cytopathologist recommends that the test be repeated after treatment is complete.

Shift in flora suggestive of bacterial vaginosis. This result refers to changes detected in the bacterial flora of the vagina in which the normal Lactobacillus are not abundant but coccobacilli are seen in numbers greater than normal. While this description was devised to suggest the possibility of bacterial vaginosis (BV), it is both an insensitive and nonspecific indicator of BV. The clinical diagnosis of BV is made solely on clinical findings (see Chapter 20 on Reproductive Tract Infections), and neither vaginal culture nor cervical cytology findings have any role in the diagnosis of this condition. Subsequent cervical cancer screening should be performed at the routine interval.

Bacteria morphologically consistent with Actinomyces spp. *Actinomyces israelii* is an anaerobic bacterium capable of causing a rare, but severe, pelvic infection called pelvic actinomycosis, especially in long-term IUD users over 35 years of age. The vast majority of IUD users with "Actinomyces-like organisms (ALO)" on cytology have an asymptomatic cervical colonization (not infection) that does not require either antibiotic therapy or removal of the IUD. However, IUD users with Actinomyces on their cytology report should have a bimanual pelvic examination to determine whether they have evidence of pelvic infection. If symptoms or physical findings suggest pelvic actinomycosis, remove the IUD and initiate intensive antibiotic therapy (see Chapter 5 on Intrauterine Devices). Advise the patient to use another method of contraception.

Cellular changes consistent with herpes simplex virus (HSV). Although an insensitive test of cervical herpes simplex shedding, cytology is a specific indicator. If the patient requests confirmation, a positive HSV-2 type-specific serology will confirm prior infection, but an HSV culture or PCR should be avoided, because viral shedding is intermittent and unpredictable. Unless inflammation interferes with the interpretation of the cytology sample, the next test should be performed at the routine interval.

Negative for Intraepithelial Lesion or Malignancy: Other Non-Neoplastic Findings

Reactive cellular changes associated with inflammation. Nonspecific reactive inflammatory changes may be associated with benign metaplasia, mechanical or chemical irritation, post-traumatic repair, chlamydial or gonococcal endocervicitis, trichomoniasis, viral infection, invasive cervical cancer, or other unknown factors. Of these possibilities, the only infectious conditions amenable to antibiotic therapy are gonococcal and chlamydial endocervicitis and vaginal trichomoniasis. Evaluate those who have not been screened recently by performing gonorrhea and chlamydia tests and treating patients who test positive. Rarely, the only cytological finding in a patient with an invasive cervical carcinoma is the persistent finding of inflammation. Some experts recommend that for those who have had consecutive cytology results with unexplained inflammation be evaluated by colposcopy, although the recommendation is not evidence-based.

Atrophy. Atrophy is most common in postmenopausal patients or those with estrogen-deficiency states. Treatment is indicated only if the patient has symptomatic genitourinary syndrome of menopause (GSM). Cervical cytology screening intervals do not need to be modified, and the patient does not need to be notified.

Endometrial cells, cytologically benign, in a woman 40 years of age or older. Endometrial cells found on cervical cytology are an insignificant finding in premenopausal women with normal ovulatory cycling.

However, because the postmenopausal endometrium normally is atrophic, the finding of endometrial cells may be the result of exfoliation from a focus of endometrial hyperplasia or adenocarcinoma. For this reason, consider the finding of endometrial cells in someone postmenopausal as a danger sign and evaluate the endometrium with either endometrial biopsy or pelvic ultrasound to measure endometrial stripe thickness. Because someone premenopausal with chronic anovulation also is at risk for endometrial hyperplasia, manage the finding of endometrial cells in the same way.

Epithelial Cell and Glandular Abnormalities

The management of atypical squamous cells of undetermined significance (ASCUS), low grade squamous intraepithelial lesion (LSIL), atypical squamous cells cannot exclude a high-grade squamous intraepithelial lesion (ASC-H), high grade squamous intraepithelial lesion (HSIL), and atypical glandular cells (AGC) results are detailed in the ASCCP 2012 updated consensus guidelines for the management of abnormal cervical cancer screening tests and cancer precursors.[24] Management algorithms are available online (www.asccp.org/asccp-guidelines). A useful management app for iPad, iPhone, and Android phones, called ASCCP Mobile, also is available.

Treatment of Histological Abnormalities

Since the early 1990s, management protocols have increasingly trended towards watchful waiting due to the recognition that most LSIL lesions will regress without treatment, rather than progress to higher-grade lesions or cancer. After completion of colposcopy, management is based on the correlation between cytology and cervical biopsy results, as well as colposcopic findings. Almost all patients will fall into one of three major management categories, based on the risk of having or developing a CIN 2 or worse lesion.[43]

- Low risk: Cytology plus HPV testing in 12 months (e.g., antecedent LSIL cytology, CIN 1 on biopsy)
- Moderate risk: Colposcopy and cytology in 6 months (e.g., CIN 2 on biopsy in a young woman)
- High risk: treatment with ablation (cryotherapy or laser) or excision (loop electrosurgical excision procedure [LEEP]) or cone biopsy (e.g., CIN 3 on biopsy).

Ovarian Cancer

In the United States in 2017, 22,440 patients were diagnosed with ovarian cancer, making this cancer the ninth most common among American women.[44] However, because of the low 5-year survival rates with this disease, especially in the later stages when it is more commonly diagnosed, it is the leading cause (53%) of gynecologic cancer deaths, accounting for 14,080 deaths in the United States in 2017. The average age at diagnosis is 63 years. It is more common in white women than in African-American women. The lifetime risk of ovarian cancer is about 1 in 75.

Although some risk factors for ovarian cancer are well known, a majority of people diagnosed with this condition have none.[45] Geographic differences are marked; rates in Sweden and the United States are 13 to 15 cases per 100,000 women per year, while the rate in Japan is 3 cases per 100,000 women per year. This difference in part may be related to dietary fat intake, which is higher in the United States and Scandinavia and lower in Japan. A long interval of ovulatory cycles also is associated with ovarian cancer; low parity, delayed childbearing, body mass index of 30 kg/m^2, and infertility are weak risk factors.[46]

Familial predisposition accounts for 5% to 10% of cases, and the risk of ovarian cancer is 5% if one first-degree relative had ovarian cancer and 7% if two or more first-degree relatives had the condition. A site-specific familial ovarian cancer syndrome has been described, which is mediated through a highly penetrant autosomal dominant gene; in these cases, the risk to a first-degree relative is up to 50%. In addition, women with BRCA mutations are at greater risk of ovarian cancer, about 35% to 70% for BRCA-1 and 10% to 30% for BRCA-2 by age 70.[46,47] Another genetic syndrome called hereditary non-polyposis colon cancer (Lynch syndrome) also is associated with increased risk of both ovarian and endometrial cancer. There is no accurate method to detect early ovarian cancer in these high-risk patients, and expert consensus guidelines recommend discussing prophylactic oophorectomy with patients who have completed childbearing and have either tested positive for one of the genetic syndromes or have two or more first-degree relatives with ovarian cancer.[44]

Other factors are known to protect against ovarian cancer. People who have had a term pregnancy before age 26 have a lower risk of ovarian cancer than those who have not, and risk goes down with each full-term pregnancy.[47] Oral contraceptive use reduces the risk of ovarian cancer by as much as 80% in people age 40 to 59 years. Not only does longer duration of use provide more protection, but the effect lasts for as long as 15 years after oral contraceptives are discontinued.[48] The same effect is seen with DMPA; a case control study in Thailand[49] showed a 83% risk reduction for epithelial ovarian cancer when the duration of DMPA use was longer than 3 years. There is a decreased risk of ovarian cancer in women who have chronic anovulation (i.e., polycystic ovary syndrome); protection also is seen with greater duration of lactation. Tubal surgery for permanent contraception is associated with a 40% to 50% reduction in the risk of ovarian cancer, and hysterectomy (without oophorectomy) with a 35% reduction.

This may be explained by growing evidence that most ovarian cancers originate in the fallopian tube epithelium, both in those that are high-risk and in the general population.[50] As a result, prophylactic salpingectomy with conservation of the ovaries until menopause has become a more common practice for premenopausal patients undergoing risk-reducing surgery,[50,51,52] as well as offering bilateral salpingectomy as an option for an elective contraceptive sterilization instead of a tubal occlusion procedure.[53] (For more, see Chapter 16 on Permanent Contraception.)

Ovarian Cancer Screening

Ovarian cancer usually is diagnosed during an evaluation of someone who is symptomatic, but it may be detected as a mass found incidentally during pelvic examination or ultrasound. While early ovarian cancer has been long considered a "silent cancer," 70% of patients recall having symptoms for 3 months or longer before their diagnosis. Ovarian cancer can be associated with pelvic pain, abdominal discomfort and distention, bloating after meals, feeling full quickly, constipation, nausea, urinary frequency, and rarely, irregular vaginal bleeding. In advanced stages, ovarian cancer is often accompanied by fatigue, nonspecific gastrointestinal symptoms, poor appetite and weight loss, increased abdominal girth, or shortness of breath due to pleural effusion. Women who experience such symptoms daily for more than a few weeks should be evaluated. The best way to promptly diagnose ovarian cancer is for both the patient and their clinician to have a high index of suspicion when characteristic symptoms occur.[54]

Three techniques have been suggested to screen for the early stages of asymptomatic ovarian cancer: periodic bimanual pelvic examination, serum CA-125 measurement, and transvaginal ultrasound. The USPSTF recommends against routine screening for ovarian cancer with any of these modalities (D Statement), because the potential harms outweigh the potential benefits.[55] However, guidelines from the U.S. National Institutes of Health state that these tests should be offered annually to women who have familial risk factors for ovarian cancer, starting at 25 to 30 years of age.[46]

For decades, conducting a screening pelvic exam (SPE) as part of a well-woman visit has been justified as being a screening test for ovarian cancer, but it is insensitive and has poor specificity.[56] Recent national guidelines contain inconsistent recommendations.

- The USPSTF issued a statement in March 2017 that "current evidence is insufficient to assess the balance of benefits and harms of performing SPE in asymptomatic, non-pregnant adult women" . . . an [I] statement.[57]

- ACOG recommends an annual screening pelvic exam in women 21 years of age and older, despite acknowledging that no evidence supports or refutes routine exam in low-risk individuals.[58,59] However, they qualify this recommendation by stating that the inclusion of speculum exam, bimanual exam, or both, in an otherwise healthy woman should be a shared, informed decision between patient and provider.
- The American College of Physicians (ACP) recommends against routine screening bimanual pelvic examination.[60] Their rationale is that the accuracy of SPE for detecting ovarian cancer is low and that no studies have assessed the benefit of SPE for other conditions, such as PID, benign conditions, or other gynecologic cancers. They emphasize that SPE rarely detects non-cervical cancer or other treatable conditions, and of note, that outcomes are not improved. However, the harms of SPE include falsely positive findings that lead to unnecessary laparoscopies or laparotomies; fear, anxiety, embarrassment, pain, and discomfort for the patient; and unnecessary costs to the health care system.

Consequently, a dilemma for clinicians is deciding what to advise asymptomatic people about the need for a screening pelvic exam at the time of a well-woman visit. An example of an "active" approach is to state that "there are three national guidelines; each one says something different. All three agree that there is no evidence that the SPE is beneficial. There is evidence of harms, including false alarms."[61] A "passive" approach is to say nothing about the SPE and only respond to questions or to a request for an exam.

Screening with the serum tumor marker CA-125 will detect up to 80% of advanced non-mucinous ovarian cancers, but the test is only 50% to 70% sensitive for early-stage cancers and has poor specificity (many false-positive results), which may lead to unnecessary invasive and costly workups. Screening those at average risk with this test is not recommended because of the low prevalence of ovarian cancer and the test's moderate sensitivity and poor specificity. Vaginal-probe pelvic ultrasound also has been suggested as a screening test because of its high sensitivity (98%), but it has poor specificity and the highest cost of any of the screening modalities.

The utility of screening asymptomatic average risk people for ovarian cancer was evaluated in the Prostate, Lung, Colorectal and Ovarian (PLCO) Cancer Screening Randomized Controlled Trial.[62] This clinical trial was conducted between 1993 and 2001 and enrolled 78,216 women who were 55 to 74 years of age. Each was assigned to annual screening or usual care; the screened women had a CA-125 for 6 years and transvaginal ultrasound for 4 years. The cohorts were followed on average 12.4 years [range, 10.9 to 13.0 years] with a cancer diagnosis and death as outcomes. Simultaneous screening with CA-125 and transvaginal ultrasound compared with usual care did not reduce ovarian cancer mortality. However, diagnostic evaluation following a false-positive screening test result was associated with complications. Of 3,285 women with false-positive results, 1,080 underwent surgery as part of the diagnostic workup. Of these women, 15% experienced distinct major complications, resulting in a rate of 20.6 complications per 100 surgical procedures. This large RCT is consistent with others in showing that screening for ovarian cancer, at least with these modalities, has no benefit for those at average risk, but it does have substantial risk of falsely positive results that can lead to complications during diagnostic evaluation.

BREAST CANCER

Breast cancer was the second leading cause of female cancer deaths in the United States, accounting for 28% of all cancer cases and 15% of cancer deaths in women (about 40,600 deaths in 2017).[63] Incidence rates of breast cancer increased 1% per year since the 1970s, but from 1999 to 2006 the rates decreased by 2% per year. Mortality also has been falling since 1990, as a result of earlier diagnosis and improved treatments. A woman's lifetime risk of breast cancer, assuming she lives to old age, is about 1 in 8. The chance that a woman will die from breast cancer is about 1 in 37 (about 2.7%).

Risk factors are helpful indicators of risk but do not predict the development of breast cancer in the majority of cases. Of women with breast cancer, 21% of those age 30 to 54 years have risk factor(s), as do 29% of those between 55 and 84 years old.[64] (See Table 21-2.)

Recent studies have focused on the role of breast density as a risk factor for breast cancer. Breast density normally decreases with advancing age, menopause, heavier body weight, and earlier childbearing, while in general there is increased breast density in those using hormone therapies. Patients with dense breasts have a modestly increased risk of breast cancer and experience a 10% to 20% reduction in the sensitivity of mammography to detect breast cancer. In postmenopausal patients, an increase in mammographic breast density score over time (when it should be stable or decreasing) is an important risk factor for breast cancer.[65] A four-category scoring system for mammographic breast density is now used with all screening mammograms.[66] (See Table 21-3.) Numerous states have passed legislation that requires health care providers to inform women with dense breasts of the modest increased risk of breast cancer and reduced sensitivity of mammography, and several states require practitioners to discuss supplemental tests to screening mammography, despite the lack of evidence regarding which additional tests should be done and the degree to

Table 21-2 Risk characteristics of breast cancer

Factor	High-Risk Group	Low-Risk Group
Relative risk >4.0		
Age	Old	Young
Country of birth	North America, Northern Europe	Asia, Africa
Two first-degree relatives with breast cancer diagnosed at an early age	Yes	No
History of cancer in one breast	Yes	No
Relative risk = 2.1–4.0		
Nodular densities on mammogram (postmenopausal)	Densities occupy >75% of breast volume	Parenchyma composed entirely of fat
One first-degree relative with breast cancer	Yes	No
Biopsy-confirmed atypical hyperplasia	Yes	No
High-dose radiation to chest	Yes	No
Oophorectomy before age 35	No	Yes
Relative risk = 1.1–2.0		
Socioeconomic status	High	Low
Place of residence	Urban	Rural
Race/ethnicity		
—Breast cancer at ≥40 years	Caucasian	Asian
—Breast cancer at <40 years	Black	Asian
Religion	Jewish	Adventist, Mormon
Age at first full-term pregnancy	≥30 years	<20 years
Age at menarche	<12 years	>14 years
Age at menopause	>55 years	<45 years
Obesity (postmenopausal)	Obese	Slender
Breastfeeding	None	Several years
—Breast cancer <45 year		
Hormone replacement therapy >10 years	Yes	No
Height	Tall	Short
History of primary cancer in endometrium, ovary, or colon	Yes	No
Alcohol consumption	Yes	No

Source: Adapted from Hulka BS, et al.[60] with updates

which they improve screening outcomes and that insurance often does not cover these additional tests. In their 2015 guideline, ACOG does not recommend routine use of alternative or adjunctive tests to screening mammography for those with dense breasts who are asymptomatic and have no additional risk factors, based on the fact that published evidence does

Table 21-3 **BI-RADS breast density categories, demographics, sensitivity of cancer detection, and breast cancer risk**[62]

Category	Description	Percentage of Population*	Sensitivity (%)	Relative Risk of Breast Cancer‡
1	Almost entirely fat	10	88	—
2	Scattered fibroglandular densities	43	82	—
3	Heterogeneously dense	39	69	1.2 (compared with average breast density)
4	Extremely dense	8	62	2.1 (compared with average breast density)

not demonstrate meaningful outcome benefits with supplemental tests, such as ultrasonography, MRI, breast tomosynthesis, or thermography.[66] The recommendations for screening mammography intervals are the same for individuals with dense breasts as for others.

Given the multiplicity of breast cancer risk factors, and their relative contribution to breast cancer risk, it is challenging for a clinician to forecast an individual patient's likelihood of acquiring breast cancer. Three free internet-based programs are available to quickly calculate a patient's breast cancer risk

- *The Breast Cancer Risk Assessment Tool,* sponsored by the National Cancer Institute, projects a person's individualized of risk for invasive breast cancer over a 5-year period and over a lifetime. It can be found at www.cancer.gov/bcrisktool.
- Breast Cancer Surveillance Consortium Risk Calculator. This tool integrates mammographic breast density: https://tools.bcsc-scc.org/bc5yearrisk/calculator.htm.
- *The Detailed Breast Cancer Risk Calculator* produces estimates using each of the Gail Model 1 and NSABP model-2. It is located at www.halls.md/breast/risk.htm.

Breast Cancer Screening

Breast self-examination (BSE). The longstanding recommendation that all adult women practice monthly BSE has been abandoned.[67] Although BSE may provide those who perform them with a sense of empowerment and occasionally may result in earlier detection of a breast mass than might occur by coincidence, two very large randomized clinical trials have shown that breast cancer mortality and survival is no greater in those who are taught BSE than in those who are not. The larger study, involving 266,000 women in Shanghai, China, concluded that BSE actually might cause more hazard than benefit, owing to the many false positives that result from BSE.[68] From a public health standpoint, these studies suggest that financial and educational resources should not be used to implement population-based BSE programs. For individuals, the message in these studies is that a formal, timed regimen of BSE is no more effective in preventing death from breast cancer than the incidental discovery of unusual breast changes. Nonetheless, patients still should be counseled to take note of changes in their breasts, and when they occur, and bring the finding to the attention of their clinician, a concept that ACOG refers to as "breast awareness."[69]

For women who continue to practice BSE, the optimal time for performing BSE is 1 to 7 days after the end of the menses. Performing the exam after a shower, while the skin still is wet, may improve accuracy. After inspecting their breasts while sitting or standing in front of a mirror, they should palpate each breast in turn, with the hand on the side of the breast being examined placed behind the head. The objective of BSE is to detect a significant change in the breasts from one month to the next, not necessarily the finding of a dominant nodule.

Screening Clinical Breast Examination (CBE). CBE is not a highly accurate screening test, having a sensitivity of only 54% and a false positive rate of 6%. However, one benefit of CBE is that about 2% to 6% of breast cancers missed on mammography can be palpated on CBE, the combination thereby slightly improving detection rates. As with screening pelvic exams, three national guidelines differ regarding the benefits and harms of screening clinical breast examination.

- In 2013, the USPSTF concluded that the current evidence is insufficient (I statement) to assess the additional benefits and harms of screening CBE beyond screening mammography in women 40 years or older.[67] No comment was made regarding CBE in the 2016 update.[70,71]
- ACOG recommends that screening CBE may be offered to asymptomatic, average-risk women in the context of an informed, shared decision-making approach that recognizes the uncertainty of additional benefits and the possibility of adverse consequences of CBE beyond mammography. Screening intervals of every 1 to 3 years for women aged 25–39 and annually for women 40 and older are reasonable.[69]
- The American Cancer Society does not recommend CBE for breast cancer screening among average-risk women at any age, because there is no evidence of any benefit of a CBE alone or in conjunction with screening mammography.[72] However, there is

moderate-quality evidence that adding CBE to mammography increases the false-positive rate, resulting in harms that are not balanced by improved outcomes.

When performing CBE for screening or diagnostic purposes, having good technique is important for optimal detection of abnormalities.[73] Examine the breasts while the patient is sitting with hands on hips or behind the head. Repeat the exam while the patient is lying down. Examine each breast in vertical stripes. Palpate with flat portion of your fingers rather than your fingertips. If a patient has very pendulous breasts, place your hand between the breast and chest wall, then palpate the tissue between your hands. Be sure to include the axillary tail of the breast in the examination. Lymph node examination of the supraclavicular and axillary nodes is an integral component of the examination. Draw a diagram in the medical record indicating the position and size of abnormalities, noting that dominant nodules have measurable dimensions, while fibrocystic change does not.

MAMMOGRAPHY

When used as a screening test, the purpose of mammography is to detect preclinical breast cancer before a mass can be palpated clinically. Large-scale studies show that in women who receive at least biennial mammograms over a 10-year period, breast cancer mortality is reduced by an average of 24%, with the largest reduction in women 50 to 69 years old. The accuracy of mammography as a screening test has improved over the last two decades, resulting in a false-negative rate of 5% to 15% and a false-positive rate of 3% to 6%.

Digital screening mammography has almost completely replaced film mammography in the United States. An even newer version of digital breast imaging called digital breast tomosynthesis (DBT), also known as 3D mammography, uses a computer algorithm to reconstruct multiple low-dose digital images of the breast into thin "slices" to include the entire breast. Tomosynthesis is typically performed as a supplement to standard two-view digital screening mammography, which more than doubles the total radiation exposure compared to a standard digital mammography screening examination. DBT reduces follow-up for additional imaging or testing (lower recall rates) and increase cancer detection rates compared with conventional digital mammography alone.[71] However, these studies did not evaluate whether there is an incremental clinical benefit to detecting these cancers earlier than with conventional digital mammography. In addition, no studies of DBT looked at clinical outcomes, such as breast cancer morbidity or mortality or quality of life.[71]

The three national guidelines differ regarding the benefits and harms of screening mammograms, as reflected in the age ranges for when to start and stop screening mammograms, as well as how often they should be performed.

- The USPSTF 2016 updated guidelines for breast cancer screening recommend every-other-year (biennial) screening mammograms for women between the ages of 50 and 74 years (B statement).[70,71] For women 40 and older, the decision to start regular, biennial screening mammography before the age of 50 years should be an individual one and "women who place a higher value on the potential benefits than the potential harms may choose to begin biennial screening between the ages of 40 and 49 years" (C Statement). These guidelines should not be interpreted to mean that mammograms should not be performed in the younger age group. Clinicians should *routinely counsel* women regarding the pros and cons of mammography and leave the decision to the client.

  The USPSTF also concluded that current evidence is insufficient to assess the benefits and harms of DBT as a primary screening method for breast cancer. For women identified as having dense breasts on an otherwise negative screening mammogram, evidence also is insufficient to recommend breast ultrasonography, magnetic resonance imaging (MRI), DBT, or other methods as additional screening modalities (I statement).

- ACOG guidelines recommend that women at average risk of breast cancer should be offered screening mammography starting at age 40 years.[69] If they have not initiated screening in their 40s, they should begin screening mammography by no later than age 50 years. The decision about the age to begin mammography screening should be made through a shared decision-making process, which includes information about the potential benefits and harms. Women at average risk of breast cancer should have screening mammography every 1 or 2 years. Biennial screening mammography, particularly after age 55 years, is a reasonable option to reduce the frequency of harms, as long as patient counseling includes a discussion that with decreased screening comes some reduction in benefits.

- The American Cancer Society guidelines made a qualified recommendation that women should have the opportunity to begin screening at age 40 years and a strong recommendation that women should undergo regular screening mammography starting at age 45 years.[72] Women aged 45 to 54 should be screened every year and biennially starting at 55 years of age.

Patients with an increased risk of breast cancer should initiate mammographic screening before age 40. According to the guidelines of the American College of Radiology,[74] younger people should start mammograms at the following times:

- 10 years before the age of diagnosis of a first-degree relative with breast cancer, but not before the age of 30
- After the diagnosis of breast cancer
- Age 25 to 30 years if known or suspected carrier of the BRCA-2 breast cancer gene
- Age 20 to 25 years if known or suspected carrier of BRCA-1 breast cancer gene
- 6 to 12 months after radiation therapy if breast tissue is conserved, then every 6 to 12 months for 1 to 2 years, then annually
- A breast biopsy result of lobular carcinoma in situ (LCIS) or atypical ductal hyperplasia
- 8 years after radiation therapy to the chest or mediastinum, or by age 25, whichever occurs last

An international reporting system for mammogram results, developed by the American College of Radiologists and adopted internationally, is entitled BI-RADS (Breast Imaging Reporting and Data System).[75] The seven categories of assessment and management of each are contained in Table 21-4. Patients with assessments of BI-RADS 4 or 5 should be referred immediately for breast biopsy. Also pay special attention to patients with category "zero" results, as they will need to receive additional imaging studies. Pay special attention to those with category 3 results, because they will need further follow-up imaging studies at an interval specified by the radiologist. Patients

Table 21-4 BI-RADS mammogram, breast ultrasound, and breast MRI reporting system

Category	Assessment	Cancer risk	Recommendation
0	Incomplete		Further studies needed until a final category can be assigned
1	Negative	0	Routine screening interval
2	Benign finding	0	Routine screening interval
3	Probably benign	>0% to <2%	Short-interval (6 month) follow-up
4	Suspicious	50%	Biopsy
4A	Low suspicion	2% to ≤10%	"
4B	Moderate suspicion	>10% to ≤50%	"
4C	High suspicion	>50% to <95%	"
5	Highly suspicious	>95%	"
6	Known biopsy-proven malignancy	N/A	Surgical excision

with BI-RADS category 3 results who are at increased risk of breast cancer should be referred to a breast specialist. When used as a diagnostic test in someone with a breast abnormality, diagnostic mammography paired with ultrasound can suggest malignancy at the location of the finding and exclude malignancy elsewhere in the same or opposite breast. In the presence of a dominant breast nodule, a negative diagnostic mammogram does not exclude the diagnosis of breast cancer. In this case, tissue sampling, either by core needle biopsy, fine-needle aspiration cytology, or excisional biopsy, is the only definitive procedure to exclude cancer.

Useful algorithms describing the management of women with abnormal mammograms and other breast complaints or clinical findings have been developed by the California Department of Health Services[76] and can be found at https://qap.sdsu.edu/screening/breastcancer/bda/index.html.

Author Disclosures—Policar: none; Sawaya: none

References

1. American Medical Association. Periodic health examination: a manual for physicians. Chicago: American Medical Association, 1940.
2. U.S. Preventive Services Task Force Grade Definitions. Grade definitions after July 2012. At www.uspreventiveservicestaskforce.org/Page/Name/grade-definitions.
3. Eyre H, Kahn R, Robertson RM et.al. Preventing cancer, cardiovascular disease, and diabetes: a common agenda for the American Cancer Society, the American Diabetes Association, and the American Heart Association. CA Cancer J Clin 2004;54:190–207.
4. Curtis KM, Jatlaoui TC, Tepper NK, et al. U.S. Selected Practice Recommendations for Contraceptive Use, 2016. MMWR Recomm Rep 2016 Jul 29;65:1–66.
5. Stewart FH, Harper CC, Ellertson CE, Grimes DA, Sawaya GF, Trussell J. Clinical breast and pelvic examination requirements for hormonal contraception: Current practice vs. evidence. JAMA 2001;285:2232–9.
6. Munoz N, Bosch FX, de Sanjose S, et al. Epidemiologic classification of human papillomavirus types associated with cervical cancer. N Eng J Med 2003;348:518–27.
7. Winkelstein W, Jr. Smoking and cervical cancer—current status: a review. Am J Epidemiol 1990;131:945–57.
8. Workowski KA, Bolan GA; Centers for Disease Control and Prevention. Sexually transmitted diseases treatment guidelines, 2015. MMWR Recomm Rep 2015;64:1–137.
9. Centers for Disease Control. Black-white differences in cervical cancer mortality—United States, 1980–1987. MMWR 1990;39:245–8.
10. Musselwhite LW, Oliveira CM, Kwaramba T, et al. Racial/ethnic disparities in cervical cancer screening and outcomes. Acta Cytol 2016;60(6):518–526. Epub 2016 Nov 9.
11. Singh GK, Williams SD, Siahpush M, Mulhollen A. Socioeconomic, rural-urban, and racial inequalities in US cancer mortality: Part I - all cancers and lung cancer and Part II - colorectal, prostate, breast, and cervical cancers. J Cancer Epidemiol 2011;2011:107497.
12. Beavis AL, Gravitt PE, Rositch AF. Hysterectomy-corrected cervical cancer mortality rates reveal a larger racial disparity in the United States. Cancer 2017 May 15;123:1044–50.
13. Petrosky E, Bocchini JA Jr, Hariri S, et al.; Centers for Disease Control and Prevention (CDC). Use of 9-valent human papillomavirus (HPV) vaccine: updated HPV vaccination recommendations of the advisory committee on immunization practices. MMWR 2015 Mar 27;64:300–4.

14. Centers for Disease Control and Prevention (CDC). Recommendations on the use of quadrivalent human papillomavirus vaccine in males—Advisory Committee on Immunization Practices (ACIP), 2011. MMWR 2011 Dec 23;60:1705–8.
15. Saslow D, Andrews KS, Manassaram-Baptiste D, et al.; American Cancer Society Guideline Development Group. Human papillomavirus vaccination guideline update: American Cancer Society guideline endorsement. CA Cancer J Clin 2016;66:375–85.
16. Koss LG. The Papanicolaou test for cervical cancer detection. A triumph and a tragedy. JAMA 1989;261:737–43.
17. American Cancer Society. Cancer Facts & Figures 2016. Atlanta: American Cancer Society; 2016. At www.cancer.org/content/dam/cancer-org/research/cancer-facts-and-statistics/annual-cancer-facts-and-figures/2016/cancer-facts-and-figures-2016.pdf. Accessed Aug 19, 2017.
18. Kristensen GB, Skyggebjerg KD, Holund B, et al. Analysis of cervical smears obtained within 3 years of the diagnosis of invasive cervical cancer. Acta Cytol 1991;35:47–50.
19. Hessling JJ, et al. Effectiveness of thin-layer preparations vs. conventional Cervical cytology in a blinded split-sample study. Extended cytologic evaluation. J Repro Med 2001;46:880–6.
20. Wertlake P. Results of AutoPap system-assisted and manual cytologic screen comparison. J Reprod Med 1999;44:11–7.
21. Siebers AG, Klinkhamer PJ, Grefte JM, et al. Comparison of liquid-based cytology with conventional cytology for detection of cervical cancer precursors: a randomized controlled trial. JAMA 2009;302:1757–64.
22. Arbyn M, Bergeron C, Klinkhamer P, et al. Liquid compared with conventional cervical cytology: a systematic review and meta-analysis. Obstet Gynecol 2008;111:167–77.
23. Wright TC Jr, Schiffman M, Solomon D, et al. Interim guidance for the use of human papillomavirus DNA testing as an adjunct to cervical cytology for screening. Obstet Gynecol 2004;103:304–9.
24. Massad LS, Einstein MH, Huh WK, et al. 2012 ASCCP Consensus Guidelines Conference. 2012 updated consensus guidelines for the management of abnormal cervical cancer screening tests and cancer precursors. Obstet Gynecol 2013;121:829–46.
25. ACOG. Practice Bulletin No. 168 Summary: Cervical cancer screening and prevention . Obstet Gynecol 2016;128:e112–e130.
26. Wright TC, Stoler MH, Behrens CM, et al. Primary cervical cancer screening with human papillomavirus: end of study results from the ATHENA study using HPV as the first-line screening test. Gynecol Oncol 2015;136:189–97.
27. Huh WK, Ault KA, Chelmow D, et al. Use of primary high-risk human papillomavirus testing for cervical cancer screening: interim clinical guidance. Obstet Gynecol 2015;125:330–7.
28. USPSTF Draft Recommendation Statement Cervical Cancer: Screening. September 2017. At www.uspreventiveservicestaskforce.org/Page/Document/UpdateSummary Draft/cervical-cancer-screening2. Accessed October 5, 2017
29. Yabroff KR, Saraiya M, Meissner HI, et al. Specialty differences in primary care physician reports of Papanicolaou test screening practices: a national survey, 2006 to 2007. Ann Intern Med 2009;151:602–11.
30. Chelmow D, Waxman A, Cain JM, Lawrence HC. The evolution of cervical screening and the specialty of obstetrics and gynecology. Obstet Gynecol 2012;119:695–699.
31. U.S. Preventive Services Task Force, Screening for Cervical Cancer, March 2012. www.uspreventiveservicestaskforce.org/Page/Document/UpdateSummaryFinal/cervical-cancer-screening. Accessed October 5, 2017.
32. Moyer VA; U.S. Preventive Services Task Force. Screening for cervical cancer: U.S. Preventive Services Task Force recommendation statement. Ann Intern Med 2012;156:880–91.
33. Saslow D, Solomon D, Lawson HW, et al. American Cancer Society, American Society for Colposcopy and Cervical Pathology, and American Society for Clinical Pathology screening guidelines for the prevention and early detection of cervical cancer. J Low Genit Tract Dis 2012;16:175–204.

34. Panel on Opportunistic Infections in HIV-Infected Adults and Adolescents. Guidelines for the prevention and treatment of opportunistic infections in HIV-infected adults and adolescents: recommendations from the Centers for Disease Control and Prevention, the National Institutes of Health, and the HIV Medicine Association of the Infectious Diseases Society of America. Available at: http://aidsinfo.nih.gov/contentfiles/lvguidelines/adult_oi.pdf.
35. Sawaya GF, McConnell KJ, Kulasingam SL, et al. Risk of cervical cancer associated with extending the interval between cervical-cancer screenings. N Engl J Med 2003;349:1501–9.
36. Meissner HI, Tiro JA, Yabroff KR, Haggstrom DA, Coughlin SS. Too much of a good thing? Physician practices and patient willingness for less frequent pap test screening intervals. Med Care 2010;48:249–59.
37. Perkins RB, Anderson BL, Gorin SS, Schulkin JA. Challenges in cervical cancer prevention: a survey of U.S. obstetrician-gynecologists. Am J Prev Med 2013;45:175–81.
38. Bettigole C. The thousand-dollar Pap smear. N Engl J Med 2013;369:1486–7.
39. Nayar R, Wilbur DC. The Bethesda System for reporting cervical cytology: a historical perspective. Acta Cytol 2017;61(4–5):359–372.
40. Kivlahan C, Ingram E. Papanicolaou smears without endocervical cells. Are they inadequate? Acta Cytol 1986;30:258–260.
41. Ransdell JS, Davey DD, Zalesky S. Clinicopathologic correlation of the unsatisfactory Papanicolaou smear. Cancer 1997;81:139–43.
42. Krieger JN, Tam MR, Stevens CE, et al. Diagnosis of trichomoniasis: comparison of conventional wet mount examination with cytologic studies, cultures, and monoclonal antibody staining of direct specimens. JAMA 1988;259:1223–7.
43. Sawaya GF, Smith-McCune K. Clinical Expert Series. Cervical Cancer Screening. Obstet Gynecol 2016;127:459–67.
44. American Cancer Society. Key statistics for ovarian cancer. https://www.cancer.org/cancer/ovarian-cancer/about/key-statistics.html. Accessed October 5, 2017.
45. Whittemore AS, Harris R, Itnyre J. Characteristics relating to ovarian cancer risk. Collaborative analysis of 12 US case-control studies. II. Invasive epithelial ovarian cancers in white women. Am J Epidemiol 1992;136:1184–1203.
46. National Institute of Health Consensus Development Panel on Ovarian Cancer, NIH consensus conference. Ovarian cancer. Screening, treatment, and follow up. JAMA 1995;273:491–7.
47. American Cancer Society. What are the risk factors for ovarian cancer? https://www.cancer.org/cancer/ovarian-cancer/causes-risks-prevention/risk-factors.html Accessed Sept 2, 2017.
48. Rosenberg L, Palmer JR, Zauber AG. A case control study of oral contraceptive use and invasive epithelial ovarian cancer. Am J Epidemiol 1994;139:654–61.
49. Wilailak S, Vipupinyo C, Suraseranivong V et al. Depot medroxyprogesterone acetate and epithelial ovarian cancer: a multicentre case-control study. BJOG 2012;119:672–7.
50. Corzo C, Iniesta MD, Patrono MG, Lu KH, Ramirez PT. Role of fallopian tubes in the development of ovarian cancer. J Minim Invasive Gynecol 2017;24:230–234.
51. Hartmann LC, Lindor NM The role of risk-reducing surgery in hereditary breast and ovarian cancer. N Engl J Med 2016;374:454–68.
52. Long Roche KC, Abu-Rustum NR, et.al. Risk-reducing salpingectomy: Let us be opportunistic. Cancer 2017;123:1714–1720.
53. Creinin MD, Zite N. Female tubal sterilization: the time has come to routinely consider removal. Obstet Gynecol 2014;124:596–9.
54. American College of Obstetricians and Gynecologists Committee on Gynecologic Practice. Committee Opinion No. 477: the role of the obstetrician-gynecologist in the early detection of epithelial ovarian cancer. Obstet Gynecol 2011;117:742–6.
55. Moyer VA; U.S. Preventive Services Task Force. Screening for ovarian cancer: U.S. Preventive Services Task Force reaffirmation recommendation statement. Ann Intern Med 2012;157:900–4.
56. Doroudi M, Kramer BS, Pinsky PF. The bimanual ovarian palpation examination in the Prostate, Lung, Colorectal and Ovarian cancer screening trial: Performance and complications. J Med Screen 2017;24:220–222.

57. US Preventive Services Task Force, Bibbins-Domingo K, Grossman DC, et al. Screening for Gynecologic Conditions with Pelvic Examination: US Preventive Services Task Force Recommendation Statement. JAMA 2017;317:947–953.
58. ACOG Committee on Gynecologic Practice Committee opinion No. 534: Well-woman visit. Obstet Gynecol 2012;120(2 Pt 1):421–4.
59. Conry JA, Brown H. Well-Woman Task Force: Components of the well-woman visit. Obstet Gynecol 2015;126:697–701.
60. Qaseem A, Humphrey LL, Harris R, Starkey M, Denberg TD; Clinical Guidelines Committee of the American College of Physicians. Screening pelvic examination in adult women: a clinical practice guideline from the American College of Physicians. Ann Intern Med 2014;161:67–72.
61. Sawaya GF. Screening pelvic examinations: the emperor's new clothes, now in 3 sizes? JAMA Intern Med 2017;177:467–46.
62. Buys SS, Partridge E. et.al. Effect of screening on ovarian cancer mortality: the Prostate, Lung, Colorectal and Ovarian (PLCO) Cancer Screening Randomized Controlled Trial. JAMA 20118;305:2295–303.
63. American Cancer Society. How common is breast cancer? https://www.cancer.org/cancer/breast-cancer/about/how-common-is-breast-cancer.html. Accessed August 20, 2017.
64. Hulka, BS, Stark AT. Breast cancer: cause and prevention. Lancet 1995;346:883–7.
65. Kerlikowske K. Longitudinal measurement of clinical mammographic breast density. JNCI 2007;99:386.
66. ACOG Committee Opinion #625 Management of Women with Dense Breasts Diagnosed by Mammography. Obstet Gynecol 2015;125:750–1.
67. USPSTF Archived final recommendation statement breast cancer: screening. Originally published on: December 30, 2013. At www.uspreventiveservicestaskforce.org/Page/Document/RecommendationStatementFinal/breast-cancer-screening#clinical-considerations. Accessed on August 20, 2017.
68. Thomas DB. et.al. Randomized trial of breast self-examination in Shanghai: final results. J Natl Cancer Inst 2002;94:1445–57.
69. ACOG Committee on Practice Bulletins—Gynecology. Practice Bulletin Number 179: breast cancer risk assessment and screening in average-risk women. Obstet Gynecol 2017;130:e1–e16.
70. USPSTF breast cancer: screening. Release Date: January 2016. At www.uspreventiveservicestaskforce.org/Page/Document/UpdateSummaryFinal/breast-cancer-screening1. Accessed on August 20, 2017.
71. Siu AL on behalf of the U.S. Preventive Services Task Force. Screening for Breast Cancer: U.S. Preventive Services Task Force Recommendation Statement. Ann Intern Med 2016;164:279–296.
72. Oeffinger KC, Fontham ET, Etzioni R, et.al. Breast cancer screening for women at average risk: 2015 guideline update from the American Cancer Society. JAMA 2015;314: 1599–614.
73. Barton MB, Harris R, Fletcher S. Does this patient have breast cancer? The screening clinical breast exam: should it be done? How? JAMA 1999;282:1270.
74. Lee CH, Dershaw DD, Kopans D. Breast cancer screening with imaging: recommendations from the Society of Breast Imaging and the ACR on the use of mammography, breast MRI, breast ultrasound, and other technologies for the detection of clinically occult breast cancer. J Am Coll Radiol 2010;7:18–27.
75. Liberman L, Abramson AF Squires FB, et al. The breast imaging reporting and data system: positive predictive value of mammographic features and final assessment categories. Am Jour Radiol 1998;171:35–40.
76. Cancer Clinical Services Quality Assurance Project. Breast diagnostic algorithms for primary care clinicians, 2011.(Last updated: July 9, 2013). At http://qap.sdsu.edu/screening/breastcancer/bda/index.html. Accessed August 30, 2017.

Sexuality & Contraception

22

Jenny A. Higgins, PhD, MPH
Patty Cason MS, FNP

- While natural, sexuality is also cultural. Physiologic aspects of sexuality (for example, libido and arousal) are strongly linked with social and psychological factors.
- There is a wide variety of sexual preferences and behaviors.
- The majority of people, including adolescents, have sexual experiences, which may or may not include penile-vaginal intercourse.
- The way our society thinks about gender influences sexual behaviors and attitudes, including how sexual problems are defined and treated within the sexual and reproductive health field.
- Contraceptive research has often overlooked the sexual aspects of contraceptive methods that are designed for female bodies. However, a few studies have explored how methods (including combined oral contraceptives [COCs], intrauterine devices [IUDs], and contraceptive implants) influence sexual experiences.
- Findings from these studies show that some people experience a decreased interest in sex during COC use; however, the causal mechanism remains unclear. Other people experience increases in sexual desire and well-being while using COCs or other methods, including IUDs and implants.
- Clients want practitioners to be more open with them about sexuality.
- The relationship between sexuality and contraception is complex and is a highly variable experience.

The reproductive health field would be non-existent without sex; yet many providers and researchers remain under-informed about the biopsychosocial elements of sex and sexual functioning, including contraception's impact on sex and, in turn, sex's impact on contraception. Sexually graphic images may saturate the media in the United States, but conversations about sexuality remain taboo and are often omitted from clinical encounters. Few of us feel sexually fluent; able to speak with our clients and colleagues about sex in a respectful but comfortable way.[1,2] Barriers to such conversations include time, provider skills or knowledge, and both provider and patient comfort.[3,4] Continuing medical education offers few tools to improve clinicians' sexual fluency.[2] Even practitioners well versed in sexuality research may be uncomfortable speaking with clients about sex; we eagerly assume that people prefer privacy.

As individuals, many people tend to focus on how sex can benefit relationships, inform identities, and bring intimacy, pleasure, satisfaction, passion, relaxation, and stress reduction. But as professionals, clinicians may feel as if they have to focus on the negative consequences of sex: the risk and threat of exposure to undesired conception, disease, or violence.[5–7] While many health care providers feel comfortable asking patients about sexual behaviors as they relate to the potential risk of pregnancy and sexually transmitted infections, far fewer speak with patients about sexual knowledge, pleasure, or satisfaction.[1,7] Clients report that practitioners rarely ask them about sex, despite the evidence suggesting that discussions about positive sexual experiences and satisfaction (and not merely sexual risk) yield significant benefits for patient health as well as the quality of the provider-patient relationship.[8,9] The perceived dangers of sexuality (versus the benefits and pleasures) become even more pronounced in our work with adolescents.[10] This *pleasure deficit*[11] characterizes contraceptive research and development, acceptability studies, and marketing.[12]

There are three clear reasons why a positive and proactive approach to sexuality should matter to family planning practitioners and researchers. First, in a practical way, understanding the sexual context informs clinical conversations that help couples choose and use suitable contraceptive methods. Addressing the notion that *the way sex feels matters to patients* could have extraordinarily positive, even revolutionary, impact on contraceptive practices; it would also acknowledge patients as sexual agents with unique experiences and priorities rather than merely as targets of contraceptive programs.

Second, clients *want* us to care about sexuality. Most patients wish to discuss sexual concerns, but many are uncomfortable initiating such topics,[4] and many report that providers neither inquire about nor follow up on sexual issues.[13] In one study of 1,500 routine gynecologic patients, 78% said they wanted to discuss their sexual concerns, but 70% of these women reported feeling too embarrassed to bring up the topic with their physician. The overwhelming majority (89%) said they would have discussed sexual concerns had their physician initiated the topic.[14]

And third, promoting positive sexuality has the potential to directly influence rates of unintended pregnancy and sexually transmitted infections (STIs). Cross-cultural comparisons with the United States indicate that Western Europeans' greater candidness about sexuality fosters an improved overall sexual experience,[15] which may contribute to increased contraceptive use, reduced STI acquisition, and lower rates of unintended pregnancy.[16–18] For the last century family planning practitioners, have had the opportunity to be pioneers of greater sexual openness and improved sexual and reproductive health at the national and international level.

In this chapter, we first provide some basic definitions and concepts related to gender, sexuality and desire. We review epidemiological and theoretical highlights from the sexuality field. Then, method by method, we describe burgeoning research that examines connections between people's sexual experiences and contraceptive acceptability and practices. We conclude with resources and recommendations to assist practitioners in addressing sexuality during clinical encounters.

Please note several important caveats to this chapter. We do not include a comprehensive discussion of the sexual response cycle or sexual dysfunction, as authoritative guides on those topics can be found elsewhere.[19] Second, we refer you to Chapter 13 for a discussion of sexual abstinence. In the current chapter we focus on vaginal intercourse, since this sexual behavior is most pertinent to contraception. That said, we make no assumptions about the sexual or gender identities of people who have penile-vaginal intercourse or who use contraception. Though the term "women" sometimes appears in this chapter, we recognize that not all contraceptive users identify as women. We encourage the development of contraceptive programs and services that are inclusive of transgender and genderqueer individuals. Additionally, we may use language that refers to female-based and male-based methods for ease of communication. However, we encourage practitioners to move away from this contraceptive binary, given that decisions about contraceptive use are often made within a relationship (versus individual) context. Finally, although the term "sex" can refer to many activities (both with and without a partner),[20] here we generally use this term to mean penile-vaginal intercourse.

SEXUALITY 101: SEXUAL BEHAVIOR IN SOCIAL CONTEXTS

Although sex appears to be a biological and physical activity, it is deeply set in our social and cultural context, and it becomes symbolic of the various attitudes and values to which our culture subscribes.[21] Behaviors that we may consider second nature are also *social* in nature. Even practices such as kissing, primal to sexual expression in the West, are not uniformly practiced across cultures. Sexuality varies greatly, not only across the globe but also across socio-demographic groups within our society. In this section, we first review some key terms and concepts pertaining to sex, gender, and sexual identity. We then review some typical sexual behavior patterns, but we remind readers that any single sexual behavior is ensconced in multiple layers of social meaning.

Sex, Gender, And Beyond: Some Basic Definitions

It is helpful for family planning clinicians to understand and be sensitive to the definitions of terms related to gender, sexual preference, and orientation. Gender, in particular, is nuanced and complicated and may be confusing for clinicians attempting to be sensitive toward gender non-conforming patients. The following definitions are intended to broaden clinicians' understanding of these terms.

Gender and biologic sex: Often, the terms "gender" and "sex" are used interchangeably; however, they are not synonymous. At birth we are assigned a *biologic sex* based on physical attributes, such as external genitalia, internal reproductive structures, or if tested, sex chromosomes. This assignment is done for the purpose of identifying an individual as male, female, or intersex. In the case of an individual with unambiguous, XX or, XY chromosomes and without an endocrine or other disorder that alters the development of the reproductive tract, that person's biologic sex describes the individual's inherent chromosomal sex assignment. When both phenotype and sense of self match genotype, as they do in the vast majority of people, this sex assignment causes no dissonance. Sex assignment is a label that a person typically carries for life. *Intersex* is a general term used for a variety of conditions in which a person is born with a chromosomal configuration or reproductive or sexual anatomy that doesn't seem to fit the typical definitions of female or male.[22] Examples of intersex variations include androgen insensitivity syndrome and congenital adrenal hyperplasia. Not all intersex people have mixed or indeterminate genitalia. Those who do, however, have historically been surgically intervened upon as infants and children to make the genitalia appear more typically male or (usually) female. This practice is strongly opposed by intersex activists and most health care providers.[23] These groups emphasize that intersex variations are both healthy and normal, though rare.

Gender differs from biologic sex in that gender is neither inherently nor solely connected to an individual's physical anatomy or genetic sexual assignment. Gender is the intersection of a person's internal sense of self (gender identity), gender expression, and biologic sex. A person's gender is also strongly influenced by how others perceive it. Regardless of what kind of chromosomes or body individuals are born with (that is, their biologic sex), they may choose to identify with a gender identity that best aligns with their own self-perception.

Gender is a core aspect of self that society often views as a binary concept, with two options—boy/man or girl/woman—that are firmly fixed at birth. While this binary framework is entrenched in most societies, this duality does not allow for an accurate description or a sensitive understanding of the spectrum of gender that exists and that clinicians are exposed to. This spectrum includes a variety of anatomical presentations, from those that are in the range that is considered biologically normal to those triggered by chromosomal or endocrine differences. Gender concepts and the spectrum of gender reach beyond anatomy and physiology and are often independent of physical considerations.

Compared to sex, which is a biologic concept based on chromosomes and physiologic structures, gender is a purely social construct. An expression that captures this idea is, "Sex is what you're born with; gender is what you choose." Gender may also be what one chooses later in life. Gendered interactions between parent and child begin at birth and often earlier. Expectations of gendered roles inform all aspects of upbringing, media, religion, relationships, and culture. From a feminist perspective, it is important to question the rigidity of gender roles and their expectations and understand who is served by the consistent reinforcement of these expectations.

Gender identity can be defined as one's internal concept of one's gender and sense of self as a boy/man, a girl/woman, both, or neither or other (e.g., genderqueer). Gender identity also includes what one calls oneself: he, she, they, ze, shim, or another description.

Most people's gender identity matches the sex assignment they received at birth (for example, a baby assigned female at birth who grows up to identify as a woman). These folks are sometimes referred to as *cisgender* or *cis*. Cisgender refers to people whose biologic sex, gender identity, and gender expression are aligned. Cisgendered individuals experience gender privilege as being part of the dominant social norm. Yet they may be unlikely to perceive or acknowledge this social privilege unless they have had personal experiences that allow them to appreciate the experience of a gender-expansive or transgendered person clashing with societal norms when, for instance, filling out forms, using public restrooms, or shopping for clothing.

For some, gender identity differs from their biologic or assigned sex (for example, a baby assigned male at birth who grows up to identify as a woman or as genderqueer). These folks are often referred to as *transgender* or *trans*. Transgender can refer to behavior or identity that is not contained within stereotypical gender norms. In its narrow definition, a trans person is someone whose gender identity does not match the assigned birth gender. Trans people may seek to match their gender expression with their gender identity, rather than their birth-assigned sex. Very importantly, being transgender does not imply any particular sexual orientation. Some people choose to socially, hormonally, or surgically change their sex to match more fully their gender identity. But not all people who identify as trans will modify their body or even their appearance.

Transman or FTM (female to male) is a person with a typically masculine gender identity who was not assigned a male sex at birth. A transman may use the pronoun he, she, or some other choice. A transman may or may not use androgens and may or may not have had breast, genital, facial, or neck surgery. It is important not to make assumptions about the gender of a transman's partners. These individuals still need reproductive services, and may need contraception.

Transwoman or MTF (male to female) is a person with a typically feminine gender identity who was not assigned a female sex at birth. A transwoman may use the pronoun she, he, or some other choice. A transwoman may or may not use estrogens and may or may not have had breast, genital, facial, neck, or other surgery.

Gender fluidity describes a range of gender expression that may change at any time. A gender-fluid person may move in and out of specific genders.

Gender roles are the set of expectations and behaviors assigned to girls / women and boys / men by society.

Gender expression is one's outward presentations and behaviors related to one's gender identity, including one's gender role. The masculine role has the qualities attributed to men, and the feminine role has the qualities attributed to women. The communication of gender expression can be through appearance, hairstyle, mannerisms, clothing, or voice. Gender expression incorporates the way in which people assign gender to others based on their gendered characteristics. Gender expression is not an indication of sexual orientation.

Gender-expansive refers to people who in one or another aspect of their lives or behavior function outside of commonly held definitions of gender expression, gender identity, or gender norms. Perhaps they do not identify with being on the gender binary as either men or women, or perhaps they identify as a blend of both. Additionally, an individual may identify with a particular gender but express gender in non-stereotypical ways. Given that gender is contextual within a social construct, gender-expansive expression in one time period or culture can be gender normative in another. Men or women wearing tattoos, earrings, or brightly colored clothing are all examples of the malleability of societal expectations about gender expression.

Why Gender Matters For Sexuality And Contraception

Gender identity has an enormous impact on sexuality and sexual and reproductive behavior. It is critical that health care providers not make assumptions regarding the gender of partners based on the patient's gender identity. These individuals still need appropriate sexual and reproductive health services including contraceptive services. Yet there are often significant barriers for gender non-conforming individuals to access appropriate services. The less providers make assumptions and the more open and accepting providers are to these individuals, the better we will be at providing equitable reproductive healthcare for our patients. Perhaps less malleable than societal expectations about gender expression is the power and privilege surrounding gender roles, and the sometimes painful experiences of those in non-dominant roles. In their groundbreaking work, "A New View of Women's Sexual Problems," Ellen Kaschak and colleagues describe a non-medicalized feminist classification system that provides a framework for understanding issues related to female sexuality.[24] Framed with this perspective, a person's perceived inability to meet cultural norms regarding gender creates potential for sexual avoidance, distress, anxiety, and shame about one's body, fantasies, or desires.

Along those lines, gender influences virtually all aspects of sexual attitudes and experiences.[25] And gender stereotypes surrounding sex continue to be reinforced by society and culture. Social movements in the 20th century, including the sexual revolution and the feminist movement, transitioned women and men into more egalitarian relationships and roles in virtually all spheres of our society. Women now enjoy more sexual autonomy and, arguably, more sexual satisfaction than at any other moment in U.S. history. But many women still cannot capitalize on their right to enjoyable sex.[26] Girls are socialized to protect and preserve their sexuality; by contrast, boys learn that they have the right to pleasurable sex.[27,28] Some young women report that unprotected intercourse "just happened"; preparing for sex would mean acknowledging they are sexual.[29] In order to justify their sexual interests, women may also feel the need to be swept away by passionate, romantic feelings,[30] a phenomenon that can also undermine successful contraceptive use. More concerning, women's risks of sexual harm—which include harm from STIs and unintended pregnancy as well as damage to one's reputation—sexual manipulation and coercion, and outright assault and incest, far outweigh the risks faced by men (see Table 22-1). Men may also sabotage women's contraceptive attempts.[31] These gender inequalities dramatically shape women's sexual interest, enjoyment, and motivations to use contraception.

Despite these discouraging gender disparities regarding sexual violence and coercion, we need to remember that all people, including women and other marginalized people, deserve to have healthy, happy, life-enhancing sex. We would be remiss to ignore how gender inequality and sexual violence drastically undermine patients' ability

Table 22-1 Statistics on lifetime prevalence of intimate partner violence, sexual violence, coercion, and stalking in the United States[32]

	Men	Women
Severely physically assaulted by intimate partner	14.0%	22.3%
Raped*	1.7%	19.3%
Experienced other forms of sexual violence, including sexual coercion, unwanted sexual contact, and being made to penetrate	23.4%	43.9%
Stalked	5.7%	15.2%
Proportion of homicide victims killed by an intimate partner[33]	5.0%	45.0%

*Rape was defined as completed or attempted forced penetration.

to achieve this. However, we would be equally remiss to ignore the positive aspects of gender differences in patients' sexual experiences and factors contributing to optimal sexual functioning. (For example, some female-assigned individuals may experience multiple orgasms during sexual activity—a phenomenon not generally experienced by male-bodied individuals.)

Furthermore, as practitioners, we have the opportunity to promote sexual well-being not only as a desirable outcome in itself but also for its connection to better overall physical, emotional and relationship health[34]—including more effective contraceptive use. Current data support the premise that engaging in consistent, non-coercive, wanted, pleasurable, partnered or solo[35] sex confers a variety of health benefits.[36] Young women who masturbate, for example, are more likely to report consistent contraceptive use and positive communication with their partners than are those who haven't masturbated.[37] In a recent nationally representative internet-based survey, women who used vibrators currently or in the past were significantly more likely to have had a gynecological exam during the past year than women who had never used vibrators.[38]

In addition to a positive relationship between sexuality and use of health care, patients may be pleased to know that physically satisfying sex and frequent orgasm[39] is associated with cardiovascular health[40,41] and longevity.[42] Reported high levels of sexual satisfaction correlate with lower levels of stress,[43] higher levels of general well-being,[44] life satisfaction,[45] happiness,[46] and overall quality of life.[43] Satisfying coupled sex is highly correlated with relationship satisfaction[47,48] and is causally associated with healthier relationships that are more likely to remain intact.[49]

In other words, there are good clinical reasons to invest in patients' pleasure and to encourage conversations and openness about sex during clinical encounters.

"NORMAL" SEXUAL BEHAVIORS

Unfortunately, research on sexuality remains limited and underfunded. Few nationally representative, population-based surveys inform our knowledge of sexual behavior, and research on sexuality can be even more socially biased than other types of behavioral research. The last such U.S. study, the National Survey of Sexual Health and Behavior (NSSHB), was conducted in 2010 among 5,865 individuals between the ages of 14 and 94.[50–55] Investigators found that penile-vaginal intercourse, both within the last month and last year, was the most common sex act reported by women and men regardless of age.

We should remind readers that penile-vaginal intercourse is *much* more strongly associated with satisfying orgasm for the person with the penis than the person with the vagina.[56] Female-assigned people are more likely to experience orgasms through direct stimulation of the clitoris and surrounding structures (see image of clitoral anatomy in Figure 22-3) by way of a hand, mouth, vibrator, or other object.

However, penile-vaginal intercourse is hardly the only sexual behavior in which people engage. Investigators of the NSSHB found that beginning with the 30-and-older age groups, an increasing proportion of women reported no vaginal intercourse within the past year. Investigators also found a greater proportion of people reporting oral and anal sexual activity and experience compared with former sexuality studies. For example, more than 40% of women between the ages of 20 and 49 had experienced receptive anal intercourse. Masturbation activities are also common. In the last year alone, 40% of all women (except women over 70) had masturbated, and 20% had masturbated within the last month.

Studies about sexual activities and behavior rely on self-report and may be significantly biased by gender role expectations. Studies of sexual behavior traditionally find, for example, that men report more sexual experiences and more sexual partners than women.[57] In a series of experiments with college students, participants were asked a series of questions about both non-sexual and sexual behaviors such as number of lifetime sexual partners. They were then asked the same questions when they believed that their responses were being monitored by a lie detector,[58] which was in fact fake. As could be predicted, when participants did not believe their responses were being monitored, the male participants reported more sexual partners and were more likely to report having engaged in sexual intercourse than the female participants. When participants believed their responses were being monitored by a lie detector, women were more likely than men to report having engaged in sexual intercourse and to report having more lifetime sexual partners. Importantly, when participants were asked questions not related to sexual behaviors there was no difference in the reports with or without use of the (fake) lie detector. It appears from these studies that individuals' self-reported responses are based on discomfort about defying gender norms, calling into question the validity of much of what we believe we know about incidence, direction and extent of sexual differences and gender.

Sexual frequency. Clients sometimes worry about whether their personal sexual frequency is normal. To normalize variability of sexual frequency, a good statistic for clinicians to keep in their white-coat pocket is that roughly equal proportions of North Americans reported sex with a partner at least twice a week, a few times a month, or only a few times a year, if at all.[50,59] In other words, there is wide variation in sexual frequency, and frequent activity is as common as little or no sexual activity. Age can also influence sexual frequency, with sexual frequency generally declining with age. Some clients may take their sexual frequency into account when exploring their contraceptive preferences.

Onset of sexual activity. Adolescence, the period between puberty and adulthood, brings sexual desires and experiences for most young people. The vast majority of U.S. adolescents are involved in dating relationships with at least some physical component: 85% have had a boyfriend or girlfriend, 85% to 90% have kissed someone, and 79% have engaged in "deep kissing."[60,61] The median age at first vaginal intercourse is 17.3 years for young men and 17.5 years for young women (remarkably similar to those in other industrialized countries),[62] and 7 in 10 U.S. adolescents have had vaginal intercourse by age 19.[63] This age has not shifted considerably over the last few decades.

Policy makers and health care providers often apply their own moral values to adolescent sexual activity. This phenomenon can be observed in certain policies, including sex education legislation, and among providers, who may counsel their young patients regarding health behaviors. Adolescents themselves, however, assign great meaning, importance, and positivity to their sexual experiences.[64–66] Moreover, most sexually active adolescents are using contraception. In 2002, 83% of teen girls and 91% of teen boys reported using contraceptives at most recent sex.[63] These proportions represent a marked increase; in 1995, only 71% of girls and 82% of boys reported having used a contraceptive method at last sex.[63]

That said, compared to adults, adolescents engage in shorter-term relationships that can make effective contraceptive use more challenging. This is because people of all ages often frame their decisions about contraception around their current relationship(s) rather than their own goals, desires, and attitudes about reproduction. Chapter 2 presents strategies to help patients clarify what they want regarding reproduction and contraception and how best to help them achieve those goals. Some patients will discontinue their hormonal method after a breakup, for example, when they do not anticipate being reunited with their partner. Patients who prioritize effectiveness and for whom prevention of pregnancy is very important may prefer highly effective methods such as implants or intrauterine contraception regardless of their sexual frequency or current partnership status.[67] Male condoms in particular are overwhelmingly the method of choice for first vaginal intercourse experiences (66% of young women and 71% of young men reported condom use at first vaginal intercourse),[63] so always speak with young people about condoms—for both STI and pregnancy prevention. It is critical to include condoms in comprehensive contraception counseling. Conversations about condom negotiation skills, including language your patients can use with their partner to initiate condom use, are also very important.

Same-gender sexual behavior. The term *sexual minority* refers to people whose sexual identity, orientation, or practices differ from the majority of society—for example, gay and queer people. Sexual minorities are an important consideration for sexual and reproductive health care providers. A sizable minority of people in our society either label themselves with non-heterosexual identity or engage in non-heterosexual sexual behaviors. (Of course, these rates vary by age group, geographic location, and other factors.) For example, almost 20% of U.S. youth claim a sexual minority identity such as "mostly heterosexual," "bisexual," or "gay/lesbian."[68] National estimates of same-gender behavior are elusive, due in part to variability in which questions and which persons are asked. In the dated (1999) but nationally-representative National Health and Social Life Survey (NHSLS),[69] 9% of men and 4% of women said they had a same-gender sexual partner at least once since puberty, but a greater proportion of women (6%) said they found the thought of having sex with a same-gender partner very appealing or appealing.[69] In a more recent (2010) national study of sexual behavior, estimates of same-sex sex behaviors were much higher. Among 18 to 59 year-olds, 9% to 15% of men and 8% to 17% of women reported receiving oral sex from a same-sex partner in their lifetime.[50]

The sexuality field has increasingly embraced Lisa Diamond's notion of *sexual fluidity.* In this model, emotional connection, rather than gender, drives relationships; women in particular may flow in and out of sexual relationships with both men and women.[70] Young women may engage in sexual activity with other women at one point in their lives but choose men as their primary sexual partners at another life stage. Being receptive to hearing from your patients how they identify regarding sexual orientation can build rapport and trust. But beware of making any contraceptive assumptions based on someone's sexual orientation. You will serve clients' contraceptive needs best by asking about the potential of clients' current sexual partner(s) to get pregnant or cause pregnancy rather than about their sexual orientation. Alternately, given that some people have fluid gender identification, practitioners may wish to ask questions pertaining to specific anatomical parts rather than gender. For example, "Do you have sex with anyone with sperm?"

A growing body of research documents that, compared to their heterosexual peers, sexual minority youth are at increased risk of unintended pregnancy. Specifically, bisexual- and lesbian-identified girls as well as girls who behave bisexually report unintended pregnancy rates that are significantly greater than heterosexuals.[71–75] Although few studies have examined sexual orientation disparities in unintended pregnancy among "older" (non-adolescent) women, evidence that suggests that sexual minority women's elevated risk for unintended pregnancy extends into adulthood.[76] While most sexual minority women engage in penile-vaginal intercourse at least occasionally,[77,78] they are less likely than heterosexual women to seek contraception or to think of themselves as contraceptive consumers. More research is needed to develop appropriate counseling, clinical, and social marketing interventions to decrease unintended pregnancy among sexual minority women. In the meantime, you may wish to remember three things: not all your clients will identify as heterosexual, even those clients seeking contraception; many people's sexual identity will shift over time; and your sexual minority clients may be at particular risk for unintended pregnancy and deserve compassionate and sensitive contraceptive care.

REASONS FOR WANTING—AND *NOT* WANTING—TO HAVE SEX

Sexual researchers have documented an enormous array of sexual motivations, including (but not limited to) a shared experience of significance and intimacy with another person, relationship maintenance, stress relief, and identity building.[79] In their analysis of college students, Meston and Buss ranked the strength and intensity of 50 different sexual motivations (e.g., "I wanted to show my affection to the person," "I realized I was in love," "The person really desired me").[80] The top three reasons were "I was attracted to the person," "I wanted to experience physical pleasure," and "It feels good". Of course, these motivations are likely to change over one's relationship and life course. For example, adolescents may be more motivated than adults to learn how to be sexual and to gain self-knowledge. Another study tried to document some of the different varieties of sexual pleasures that people seek in sex, such as the pleasures of physical-erotic sensation, pleasing one's partner, spontaneity, and close, skin-on-skin contact.[81] In both studies, gender significantly shaped people's sexual motivations and types of pleasure-seeking. For example, particularly within heterosexual relationships, cisgender women may be more focused on their *partners'* pleasure as a goal, while cisgender men may be comparatively more focused on their own orgasm.

Research must continue to explore how sexual motivations and pleasures influence contraceptive practices. For example, women who are highly focused on men's pleasure are less likely to promote male condom use.[81] At the very least, practitioners should recognize that clients have a range of motivations for engaging in sexual behaviors, which may be very different from those the provider personally experiences or endorses. For example, a provider may insist that patients and their partners will not notice an IUD string during intercourse, but a patient may insist that the string is bothersome and request a change in method because of this discomfort. When you acknowledge the variety of potential sexual experiences, you can help validate patients concerns, maintain a good patient-provider relationship, and support positive health behaviors.

There are also many reasons—social, cultural, or religious—why people *don't* want to have sex. Fear of pregnancy often sexually inhibits patients, and sometimes their partners as well.[82,83] For this reason, with *all* clients, practitioners are advised to proactively discuss the potential for contraception to provide a sexual benefit by alleviating anxiety about risk of pregnancy. Protection from pregnancy could be promoted as a way to enhance a couple's enjoyment of sex, especially among those whose arousal is diminished by pregnancy risk. Indeed, some people report enjoying sex more after menopause, when the threat of pregnancy is no longer a concern.

That said, some people may be sexually turned on by the idea of conceiving a baby with one's partner, even if a child isn't fully desired.[84] Others may be afraid that they can't get pregnant and so take deliberate risks of becoming pregnant even though they don't currently want a child. A nationally representative report from the National Campaign to Prevent Teen and Unplanned Pregnancy (now called Power to Decide) found that an astonishing percentage of 18 to 30 year-olds expressed concern about infertility: 59% of women and 47% of men reported at least some concern, and 19% of women and 14% of men reported *extreme* concerns.[85] Thus, while some might not be able to enjoy sex unless completely protected against unintended pregnancy, others may take deliberate procreative risks related to their confusion and anxiety about infertility. Chapter 2 presents patient-centered approaches to help providers discuss these and other seemingly contradictory concerns that patients have about fertility, contraception, and reproduction. As a provider, you can acknowledge these concerns and normalize the variety of preferences and experiences that exist.

SEXUAL PROBLEMS

Despite our interest in promoting positive sexuality, we recognize that many clients, if they bring up sexuality at all, are most likely to bring up sexual concerns or problems. In a national probability sample of 987 U.S. women between the ages of 20 and 65, Bancroft et al. found that one in four (24%) women reported marked distress about their sexual relationship or their own sexuality.[86] The strongest predictors of distress were lower levels of general emotional well-being and quality of the emotional relationship with the partner. These predictors of distress did not correlate well with the diagnostic criteria that are used to diagnose sexual dysfunction in the *Diagnostic and Statistical Manual of Mental Disorders, 5th Edition*, or *DSM-5*.[87] In the DSM-5, diagnoses of sexual problems (for example, erectile difficulties, lubrication difficulties) tend to be based primarily on physiologic indicators. That said, the DSM-5 stipulates that to make the diagnosis, "sexual dysfunction" must include both a disturbance in functioning *and* personal distress.

Health care providers need to respond sensitively when patients report distressing sexual problems, and sexual complaints need to be considered within their social and cultural context. What we think of as sexually ideal for women and men has shifted over time, and it will continue to shift. For example, climaxing too early is considered a problem for men, but rarely for women; this may not have been a problem at all 150 years ago in our country, nor is it a problem in all other societies. Similarly, women's lack of orgasm or "low" sexual desire have not always been considered dysfunctional.[88,89] Negative attitudes, messages, and values regarding sex strongly influence desire and function.

Table 22-2 includes prevalence estimates of several sexual problems from two different U.S. studies. Unfortunately, there is a scarcity of epidemiologic studies of sexual dysfunction,[90] and the most recent estimates available focus on 40 to 80 year-old adults.[91] Plus, the figures presented here are from relatively dated publications (1999, 2008), and they may not be perfectly relevant for individuals of reproductive age. Estimates from the nationally-representative National Health and Social Life Survey (NHSLS),[69] presented in *JAMA* in 1999, were striking: 43% of women and 31% of men reported at least one sexual problem in the previous year.[92] The sexual problems measured included lack of interest in sex, inability to achieve orgasm, reports of sex not being pleasurable, anxiety about performance, trouble lubricating (women only), pain during sex

Table 22-2 Prevalence estimates of common sexual problems in the United States

	NHSLS*		Shifren et al. study**	
	Men	Women	Women	Women Distressed by Problem
Lack of Interest in sex/low desire	16%	33%	39%	10%
Low arousal or arousal problems			26%	5%
Unable to achieve orgasm	8%	24%	21%	5%
Experienced pain during sex	3%	14%		
Sex not pleasurable	8%	21%		
Anxious about performance	18%	12%		
Climax too early	28%	10%		
Trouble lubricating		19%		
Unable to keep an erection	11%			
Premature ejaculation	29%			

*National Health and Social Life Survey (1994)[69,92,97]

**Shifren et al. (2008)[93]

(women only), climaxing too early (men only), and trouble achieving or maintaining an erection (men only). Sexual problems were most common among young women, older men, and nonmarried and poorly educated respondents. Importantly, respondents did not indicate whether these problems were persistent or distressing for them. Thus, NHSLS figures may dramatically overstate the prevalence of sexual "problems" in the United States. Many NHSLS respondents rated their relationships positively: nearly half of respondents described their relationships as "extremely" emotionally and physically satisfying.[69]

In their 2008 nationally representative study of sexual problems, Shifren et al. found much lower rates of persistent sexual problems among women, particularly since investigators explored whether women themselves were *distressed* by sexual problems.[93] Using a panel study of 31,640 women, aged 18 to 102 (mean age of 49 years), researchers assessed measures related to desire, arousal, and ability to reach orgasm; they also used the Female Sexual Distress Scale (FSDS) to determine women's comfort or discomfort with their sexual functioning. The age-adjusted sexual problem prevalence was 42%, almost identical to the previously cited study in *JAMA*.[92] But approximately half of those women (22% overall) reported sexually related personal distress. Those most likely to report distressing sexual problems were poorly educated, ranked poorly on self-assessed health, and were more likely to have depression, anxiety, thyroid conditions, and urinary incontinence. A separate analysis of women in this study who reported "low sexual desire," fewer than 1 in 3 (27.5%), or 10% of the entire sample, reported sexual distress.[94] These sizeable gaps between the prevalence of sexual problems and the prevalence of any distress associated with those problems are important reminders of how the nature of a sexual problem depends on whom you ask, when, and in what context.[95,96]

SEXUAL DESIRE

As noted above, insufficient sexual desire is a very common sexual complaint among cisgender women. However, there is disagreement about how patients conceptualize these difficulties[98] and even about the meaning of the term sexual desire.[99] Desire is variably described as a "spontaneous" drive, low-level arousal, or a sexual eagerness or wanting. Simply defined, it is the motivation to engage in sexual acts.[100] Often, the term sexual desire refers to "spontaneous" desire rather than desire that is experienced in "response" to arousing sexual stimuli.[99,101] However, a body of evidence supports the concept that "spontaneous desire" does not exist and even desire that seems spontaneous is actually in response to sexual stimuli.[102]

When queried, individuals report motivation to engage in sexual acts for a range of reasons, including sexual release, orgasm, pleasing their partner, desire for intimacy, emotional closeness, love, and feeling sexually desirable. Clearly, what is meant by sexual desire and what individuals in fact "desire" is complicated and highly influenced by biology, psychology, and society.[100]

An individual's perception and interpretation of their sexual desire and their sexual self in general is shaped by their personal psychosexual history and thus influenced both positively and negatively by conditioning.[103,104] The alarming statistics shown in Table 22-1 on sexual violence underline the possibility that for a given individual, there is a statistically reasonable chance that sexual difficulties are the consequence of sexual trauma. For this reason, clinicians addressing sexual complaints must consider the possibility that sexual trauma is a contributing factor. Another likely contributing factor is familial, societal, religious, and cultural rules about what is acceptable or taboo regarding sexuality.[105,106]

Interestingly, the current emphasis on female desire is relatively new.[107] Following the introduction of the oral contraceptive pill in 1960 and the following evolution of sexual mores in the 1960s and 1970s, women in the United States were increasingly acknowledged to be sexual beings. The subsequent introduction in 1998 of sildenafil, a medication used to treat erectile difficulties, followed by other medications in the same class (PDE 5 inhibitors), created a market for blockbuster medications to treat sexual dysfunctions. There is heated controversy[101] among feminists, researchers, authors, sexual medicine specialists, and pharmaceutical companies over sexual desire and desire difficulties:[108] how it is described, defined in the DSM, represented in the media, and most importantly, how to address or treat it.

Thankfully, a simple and very welcome fact that all parties agree on is that that a person does not have to experience "spontaneous desire" in order to have pleasurable, satisfying sex.[102] Sexual experiences are equally satisfying in the absence of "spontaneous desire" because human beings easily respond to arousing sexual stimuli with "responsive desire".

As of this writing, there are several medications under development aimed at increasing sexual desire in female-assigned people. One FDA-approved medication, flibanserin, is indicated for "the treatment of premenopausal women with acquired, generalized hypoactive sexual desire disorder (HSDD) as characterized by low sexual desire that causes marked distress or interpersonal difficulty".[109] Of note for clinicians caring for reproductive-age women is flibanserin's potential for drug interactions with alcohol and with medications that are CYP3A4 inhibitors. Strong and moderate CYP3A4 inhibitors such as ketoconazole, miconazole, fluconazole, and ciprofloxacin are contraindicated and weak inhibitors such as oral contraceptives must be used with caution.

The current DSM-5 amalgamated female disorders of desire and arousal into a single diagnosis called "female sexual interest/arousal disorder" replacing hypoactive sexual desire disorder (HSDD). Clinicians who interact with women who have concerns about levels of desire may be helped by an understanding of the changing perception and meaning of sexual desire, and the changing landscape within which sexual desire complaints have developed. In addition to considering a diagnosis of "female sexual interest/arousal disorder" as defined by the DSM-5, clinicians can embrace a more complex and holistic view of sexual desire to help patients explore how familial, religious, cultural, or societal expectations or in many cases, sexual trauma, may be influencing their concerns or limiting their own experience of desire. Reassure patients that spontaneous desire may not exist, as such, and is not necessary for sexual arousal or pleasurable, satisfying sex; this knowledge can help normalize and validate an individuals' experiences and support them as agents of their own sexuality.

Clinicians who are not experts in sexual medicine *can* help patients who experience sexual difficulties.[110] The last section of this chapter contains tools and resources that are useful for clinicians engaging in sensitive conversations about sexuality and sexual complaints.

THE SEXUAL ACCEPTABILITY OF CONTRACEPTIVE METHODS

Most people wish to have only one or two children in their lifetime. People who have sex with partners with whom they could procreate will need to use contraception for well over 25 years of their sexual lives.

Therefore, the majority of sexual activity during the reproductive years occurs during times when patients wish to avoid pregnancy. A central but overlooked aspect of the acceptability of contraceptive products is *sexual acceptability,* or how contraceptive methods influence sexual experiences, which has subsequent, direct implications for contraceptive use patterns.[111–113] Contraceptive methods are only effective if used, and they must be designed to fit patients' sexual lives rather than vice versa.

Although contraception is expressly designed for nonprocreative sexual activity, we know little about how contraceptives affect the sexuality of individuals at risk of pregnancy. This gap is striking when compared to research on male condoms[114,115] or male-based hormonal methods that are being researched.[116–118] Researchers have recognized that male-assigned individuals are less likely to use these methods if they hinder sexual experiences. In comparison, female-based contraceptives are de-sexualized in both research and our culture at large.[11]

A growing body of data also indicates that the potential impact on the user's sexual experience is important if not critical to female patients as they select which contraceptive method(s) to use.[119–121] In one U.S. study of 382 participants, the most frequently desired contraceptive feature was "does not interfere with the pleasure of sex," which was selected by proportionally more respondents than the response saying a method "is 99% effective without having to do anything" (87% versus 74%, respectively).[122] Similar findings emerged from a study of 189 patients seeking a new contraceptive method at family planning clinics. When asking about what factors the patients valued in choosing a new method, investigators listed two sexual acceptability factors alongside more common characteristics

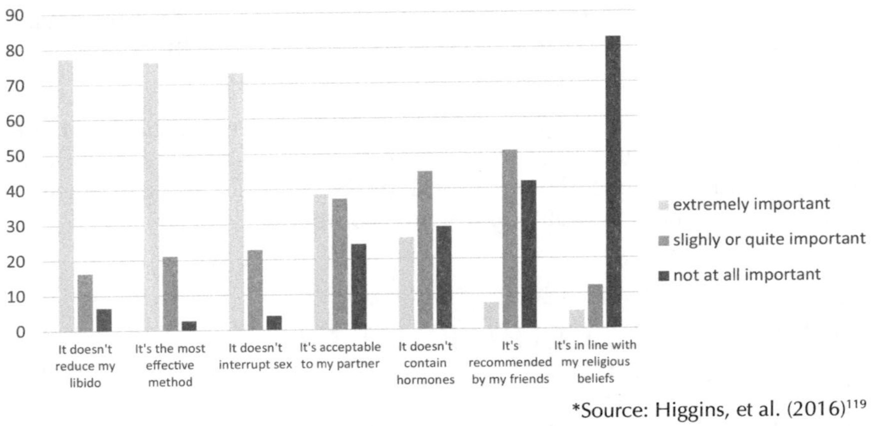

Figure 22-1 Percent of family planning clients evaluating criteria in their selection of a new method

such as efficacy and partner acceptability. As seen in Figure 22-1, patients ranked factors of "doesn't reduce my libido" and "doesn't interrupt sex" just as highly as efficacy and more highly than all other criteria.[119]

Encouragingly, in recent years, researchers have shown progressive interest in how contraception affects female-bodied patients' sexuality and how sexuality may influence people's contraceptive choices and practices. Scholars have published several reviews on this topic, particularly in terms of hormonal contraception and sexual functioning.[123–126] This growing body of research suggests significant associations between contraceptives' sexual acceptability—particularly with regards to the domain of sexual function—and how consistently and continuously women use these methods.

However, the majority of studies use a relatively narrow approach to sexual acceptability—sometimes with only a single question.[127,128] Researchers most frequently use measures of classic sexual functioning such as arousal, desire (libido), lubrication, orgasm, satisfaction, and pain. The most common assessment tool is the Female Sexual Function Index (FSFI),[129] but researchers use a variety of scales and measures. Most of these sexuality measures were originally developed to identify sexual dysfunction, usually in mid-life patients experiencing sexual or other health problems. As a result, they may not be particularly useful in identifying contraceptive-related sexual outcomes in younger, healthy patients.

Some professionals have advocated for a broader approach to contraception's sexual acceptability. After all, sexuality encompasses many factors, including physiological function and sensation, partner- and relationship aspects, and broader psychological well-being. Contraception could affect all these sexual domains. Contraceptive side effects such as bleeding, cramping, mood changes, or breast tenderness could all have sexual repercussions. Individual sexual preferences for disinhibition, inhibition, or spontaneity could also contribute to how acceptable or unacceptable a patient finds a particular method. Moreover, the broader socio-cultural context influences virtually *all* of the ways in which contraception potentially influences sexuality.

Based on a review of the literature, Higgins and Smith[12] proposed a conceptual model of contraceptive sexual acceptability that incorporates a wider range of sexual aspects (Figure 22-2). On the outer-most layer of the model, macro-level factors serve as the context in which individuals and couples experience contraceptives in their lives. The middle layer of the model—relationship factors—acknowledges that sexual activity takes place in dyads. These relationship dynamics and partner factors can connect directly to contraceptive practices and contraception's sexual acceptability. They work interactively with an individual's particular sexual experiences and preferences, which are at the core of the model.

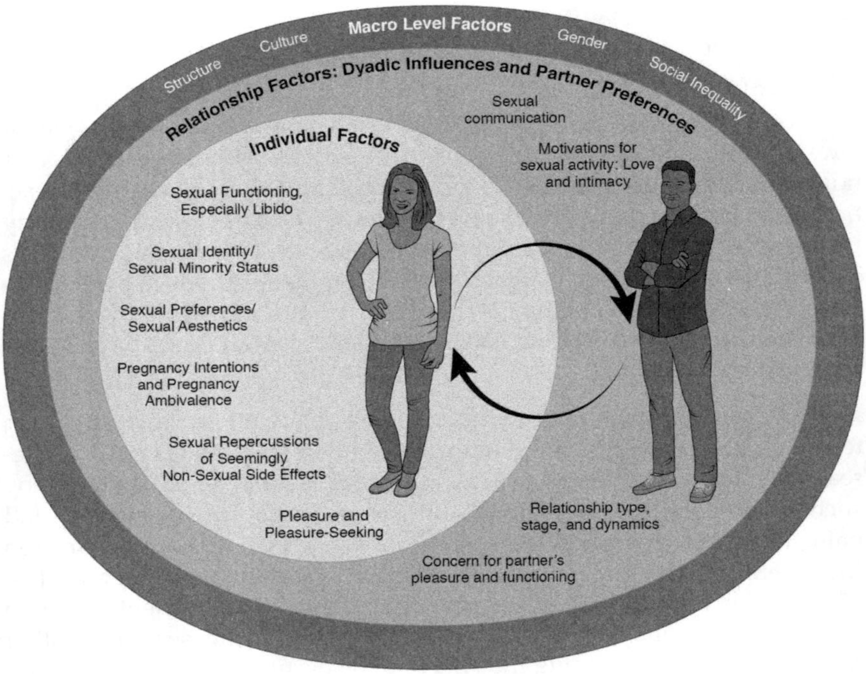

+Source: Higgins and Smith (2016),[12] with permission.

Figure 22-2 Higgins and Smith's Conceptual Model of the Sexual Acceptability of Contraception+

Few studies of contraceptive methods' sexual outcomes address all aspects of the above model. The majority of studies focus primarily on individual-level factors, particularly sexual functioning. Nonetheless, readers and practitioners may want to keep this broader approach to sexuality in mind as they review method-by-method sections.*

Male Condoms

Though male condoms help prevent STIs, they also play an enormous role in pregnancy prevention. At least 1 in 3 penile-vaginal sex acts among 15–44 year-old adults in the U.S. involves the use of male condoms.[130] Prior studies have examined the sexual acceptability of male condoms, with findings that condoms can reduce pleasure and sensation on the penis. Moreover, the people who report these condom-related sexual detractions are less likely to use them than those who do not report them as strongly.[131,132] Research has also documented males' experiences

*Much of the material in the following section comes directly from Higgins and Smith's 2016 review of this topic.[12]

of sexual condom-use problems, including condom-associated erection loss.[133–135]

Research has been slower to document female-assigned people's sexual experiences with condoms.[136] However, the winds may be shifting: more than 20 articles from the last 10 years have dealt in some way with women's sexual experiences of condoms.[12] Taken cumulatively, these studies confirm prior findings that some women perceive condoms as a barrier to intimacy and trust, which can lead to a waning of condom use as a relationship develops,[137–140] and that sexual motivations pertaining to love (versus, say, pleasure or fun) can undercut the likelihood of condom use.[141]

These studies also convincingly demonstrate that female-assigned people can also experience reductions of both pleasure and sensation with condom use.[131,142] For example, especially when used in the absence of exogenous lubricants, condoms may reduce vaginal lubrication, which can cause some women discomfort or pain.[143,144] There is also the potential for latex sensitivity or allergy, which have an adverse impact on comfort and pleasure. In fact, findings exhibit far more gender similarities than differences, with reporting of condom "turn-offs" similar for women and men.[131,142] (Exceptions include the following: people with penises can be more likely to report "fit and feel" issues with male condoms,[142] and female-assigned people can be more likely to report pain associated with condom use.[143]) Most notably, though men were proportionally more likely than women in these studies to say that condoms diminish their physical pleasure,[115,145–147] the associations between such pleasure attitudes and actual condom practices may be just as strong if not stronger for women.[148]

Contraceptive researchers and clinicians should start with the assumption that at least some female-assigned people may experience reductions in pleasure and sensation when using male condoms. Compared to male-assigned people, female-assigned people may also uniquely experience condom-related pain and reductions in vaginal lubrication. We should take care to assess contraceptive users' beliefs about and experiences with condom-related pleasure reduction. Failure to do so could mean overlooking one of the largest predictors of condom non-use. Sexual health professionals might also wish to share ideas on how to better integrate condoms into the sexual experience with all clients, regardless of gender or body parts. People with penises may struggle with condoms' fit and feel, whereas people with vaginas might dislike texture or lubrication attributes. Clients should be encouraged to try a variety of condom types, sizes, and lubricants. Water- or glycerin-based lubricants, either with or without condoms, may help overcome sexual discomfort and lackluster sexual satisfaction.[149]

That said, as with any contraceptive method, condoms offer both minuses and plusses in terms of sexual acceptability, and some female-assigned people love condoms. Positive sexual aspects of condoms include (if desired) prolonged intercourse, less mess and easier cleanup after sexual activity, and of course, the ability to have intercourse with greatly reduced worry about STIs.

Combined Oral Contraceptives (COCs)

Variable study methodology and quality as well as confusion regarding the pathways of action make it hard to definitively answer the question of if and how COCs affect sexual desire, enjoyment, and functioning.[150,151] For example, sexual effects could result from hormonally mediated physiological changes in female bodies (vaginal dryness or lower androgens), psychological changes (e.g., feeling more protected against pregnancy and thus less sexually inhibited), potential placebo or nocebo effects (feeling sure that the pill will lower one's sex drive), or a combination of physiological and psychological effects.[151] Furthermore, the majority of studies on pill use and sexuality have been cross-sectional in nature, an inherent limitation if one wants to understand the effects of the pill on sexual functioning and enjoyment over time.

Most research on COCs and sexuality examines libido. Several reviews of this topic have found reports of both increased and decreased libido with COC use.[124,150,152] These reviews also noted the lack of high-quality studies of this topic. Few studies are randomized and placebo-controlled, and fewer meet every single standard for high quality reporting of randomized clinical trials (CONSORT guidelines[153]). A well-conducted trial demonstrated a decrease in libido in COC users compared to placebo in a sample of women in Scotland (higher baseline libido) but not in a sample of women in the Philippines (lower baseline libido).[154] A prospective study in the U.S. followed 100 new COC users for 1 year.[155] Among those 47% of patients who stopped using their pills over the course of the study, decreased sexual thoughts and decreased psychosexual arousability were the strongest predictors of discontinuation. While this study, like other observational studies, could not establish if COCs definitely *caused* the lower libido, it nonetheless highlights the importance of lowered libido in this sample of patients and its effect on discontinuation.

The standard, albeit controversial, explanation for how COCs influence sexual functioning, including desire, primarily involves the role of androgens. Given that COCs inhibit luteinizing hormone (LH) and prevent ovulation, they also decrease ovarian production of testosterone. COC-related increases in estrogen levels also raise the amount of sex hormone binding globulin (SHBG), which also contributes to declines in levels of free testosterone.[156] While most studies do show an increase in SHBG as well as a decrease in total and free testosterone in COC users, the majority of those studies do not demonstrate a negative impact on libido.[157] Some researchers however, have concluded that lower levels of free testosterone contribute to lowered libido in COC users, particularly given that non-contraception-focused trials suggest that addition of exogenous testosterone may improve libido significantly more than placebo.[158] As a result, some researchers have been studying the effects of "androgen-restored contraception," which supplements combined oral contraceptives with testosterone.[159]

Significant debate surrounds these pathways, including which hormones (estrogen, progesterone, testosterone, or oxytocin)[160] exert the greatest influence on sexual functioning, and how,[125] or even if hormonal changes are really that important relative to women's subjective experiences of their sexuality. And though testosterone decreases are perhaps the most popular explanation for how COCs affect women's sexual functioning, testosterone research itself may be marred by possible confounders that bias the interpretation of findings.[161] In those not taking hormonal contraception, different levels of endogenous androgens among individuals do not correlate with differences in sexual functioning or libido. No particular androgen level is predictive of "low" female sexual function,[162] and patients vary in the degree to which they are sensitive to these hormonal changes[163] or the degree to which lowered testosterone has any clear effect on sexual interest.[164] Moreover, the context of sexual activity matters just as much if not more than the relative amount of hormones present in the body. Additionally, emerging scientific inquiry is beginning to investigate the role of genetics in sexual well-being,[165] particularly in relation to androgen-sensitivity and sexual desire.[166] Our understanding of how our genetics may predispose susceptibility to sexual dysfunction and how COCs may confound these effects is in its infancy. However, future research shows exciting promise in this regard. In sum, we urge readers to use caution in assuming that androgens always contribute directly to increased sexual desire in women—or that COCs thus result in universal changes to sexual libido. Encouragingly, preliminary findings suggest that COC users who experience issues with libido or arousal may find relief when switching to a different hormonal formulation.[167–169]

Many people using COCs experience no negative sexual functioning outcomes.[170–173] Birth control pills also relieve dysmenorrhea and lighten menstrual bleeding,[173,174] two potential sexual benefits for many individuals and couples. COCs can mitigate negative effects of health conditions such as endometriosis and polycystic ovarian syndrome (PCOS) that adversely affect sexuality. For example, COCs have been associated with reductions in endometriosis-related pelvic pain[175] and unwanted aesthetic aspects of PCOS such as hirsutism (increased facial and body hair)[176] and acne.[173,176] COCs can treat acne in the non-PCOS patient as well. Other positive sexual outcomes associated with COCs in the literature include improvements in sexual function and libido, reductions in benign breast disease and improvements in skin problems.[177–179] However, other aspects of COC use such as breakthrough bleeding, breast tenderness,[180,181] and vaginal dryness[182] are likely to detract from sexual acceptability.

Combined Hormonal Vaginal Ring

The vaginal ring provides a powerful and unique glimpse into the sexual acceptability of contraception. Routine use calls for placing the pliable ring into the vagina for 3 to 4 weeks and then removing it for a ring-free (hormone free) interval every month. The ring can also be used continuously without any hormone free interval. The largest studies of this method strongly suggested that women who associated the method with positive sexual attributes were more likely to continue using it over time.[183] More specifically, studies document several pathways through which the ring may affect sexual functioning. The ring requires touching one's genitals, which necessitates an element of sexual self-comfort. In one U.S. study of adolescent women, those participants most willing to try the ring also expressed more comfort with their genitals.[184] Women less apt to try the method were concerned that the ring could get lost inside or easily fall out of the vagina. To address concerns among those less comfortable touching their genitals, providers may wish to give patients additional information about the vagina as well as alternative strategies for placement such as placing the ring while showering, using an applicator,[184] or enlisting a partner's assistance to place and remove the ring.

The *mechanics* of the ring also affect its sexual acceptability, for both users and their partners. In one review comparing the ring to COCs, women reported that the ring was more likely to interfere with sex, and a significantly larger proportion of women reported that their sex partners preferred the pill.[185] Ring-related events, such as feeling the ring inside the vagina, interference with sex, and expulsion, were associated with higher rates of discontinuation.[185] On the other hand, the overwhelmingly majority of male partners reported that they never felt the ring during sex, expressed no change in sexual sensations, reported that being able to feel the ring did not bother them nor reported that the ring disrupted sex.

As with any hormonal method, *hormonal influences* affect the ring's sexual acceptability in both negative (mostly) and positive ways. Mild adverse hormone-related outcomes include bleeding, nausea, headache, breast tenderness, and vaginal discomfort.[185,186] However, compared to COC users, ring users experienced comparatively fewer issues with vaginal dryness in one study.[185] Extended cycle use has been associated with improvements in Italian women's dyspareunia, sexual function, sexual distress, and quality of life.[186] Highly satisfied ring users in one U.S. study reported fewer side effects than with pills, no detection of the ring during normal use, and either no change or an increase in sexual pleasure and/or sexual frequency; these satisfied women were more likely to continue ring use.[187]

Intrauterine Device (IUD)

A 2014 systematic review of women's sexual experiences with IUDs located only 10 studies published in the past 30 years.[188] Use of the IUD was more commonly associated with positive or neutral sexual effects than negative ones; however, the review identified mixed results, a lack of U.S. studies, and potential methodologic limitations. A 2016 U.S. study found copper IUD users significantly less likely than depot medroxyprogesterone acetate users to report lack of sexual desire in the previous 6 months;[189] however, it did not include baseline sexuality measures, which could have affected study results. A prospective, 2016 U.S. study addressed these gaps by documenting sexual acceptability using a variety of sexuality measures among women initiating an IUD or implant method.[119] Investigators controlled for baseline sexual functioning, relationship length, general health and well-being, and other factors that can influence sexuality. Measured after both 1 and 3 months of use, the total Female Sexual Function Index scores or New Sexual Satisfaction Scale scores of new IUD and implant users did not differ from baseline. However, participants *were* significantly more likely to report perceived improvements (versus detractions) to their sexual lives.[119] For example, at 1 month, 38% of women indicated their new method had improved their sex life in the last 4 weeks, compared to 15% reporting their method had made their sex life worse. By 3 months, 40% of women still reported improvements. Among those reporting sexual detractions due to their contraceptive method, 88% said they had experienced an increase in vaginal bleeding. Perceived sexual improvements were strongly associated with the ability to "let go" in sex and with one's sense of control over pregnancy prevention, suggesting that many women may be able to enjoy sexual activity more when the threat of pregnancy is reduced.

While the above studies document objective sexual outcomes in relationship to IUD use, other studies have assessed more subjective aspects of this method. A recent U.S. qualitative study of the sexual acceptability of IUDs revealed mostly positive themes such as increased sexual disinhibition due to the method's high contraceptive efficacy, greater allowance for sexual spontaneity compared to condoms, and psycho-sexual benefits of no or fewer synthetic hormones compared to other hormonal methods.[190] These sexual themes connected to users' method satisfaction and non-users' openness to the method. In the U.S. qualitative study mentioned earlier, non-users' most frequently cited sexual concern about IUDs was the potential for their partner to feel or be "poked" by the string.[190] Familiarity with the data regarding potential sexual effects from IUDs helps clinicians respond more effectively to sexual concerns.

Individuals' preferences for and responses to menstrual bleeding patterns (and changes) with IUD use will affect sexual acceptability. For patients preferring little to no menstrual bleeding, a levonorgestrel (LNG) IUD may be particularly enticing as blood flow decreases significantly in the vast majority of users. The bleeding patterns seen with each of the IUDs is discussed in more detail in Chapter 5 on Intrauterine Devices (IUDs). The bleeding profile associated with LNG IUD use is likely to increase sexual acceptability of this method, though it is important to note that some women prefer monthly periods.[191] Since copper IUD users have no hormonal change to their menstrual cycles, their menstrual cycles will come at the same time each month as they would if they were using no contraception. The ovary is not affected in any way and the user continues to ovulate in precisely the same way as if not using contraception. Many patients prefer to feel themselves cycle and ovulate naturally. During ovulation, people are more likely to masturbate and more likely to initiate sexual activity with a partner,[192,193] so use of a method that does not suppress ovulation can have a sexual benefit. On the other hand, the sexual acceptability of copper IUDs may be thwarted for patients who experience increases in amount of blood, unscheduled bleeding, or cramping with the device.[119]

In sum, while studies demonstrate mostly positive effects of IUDs on patients' sexuality, this method's sexual acceptability will vary according to individual user characteristics, including bleeding preferences, comfort with an object inside the body, and tolerance for hormone-related side effects for people using hormone-containing devices. Individuals who desire a hormone-free method may find the copper IUD particularly appealing. IUDs may also be extremely desirable methods for those who have trouble "letting go" in sex unless securely protected against pregnancy. On the other hand, they may be less appealing to people who want more hands-on, day-to-day control over their contraception.

Progestin-Only Transdermal Implant

Although its extremely high efficacy is likely to enhance sexual disinhibition in many users, the progestin-only transdermal implant may also decrease sexual acceptability through its associated unpredictable and potential irregular bleeding profile.[194–197] Studies suggest that 20% to 25% of implant users report frequent or prolonged bleeding within the first year of use.[195,197] However, at least a third (32% to 42%) of users experience amenorrhea,[195,196] and an additional 20% experience minimal bleeding.

This is highly desired by many women but concerning or undesirable to others.[198] A variety of other possible implant side effects may indirectly decrease sexual acceptability, including headaches, acne,[195,196] or mood changes.[195]

Implant use has also been associated with positive sexual outcomes. One study reported significantly higher Female Sexual Function Index scores measuring arousal, orgasm, satisfaction, and pain after 3 months of Nexplanon use compared to baseline assessments, and these higher scores persisted at 6 months.[174] Though 2% to 9% of new implant users across several studies reported libido loss,[194–196] these figures are smaller than those seen in studies of oral contraceptives and other hormonal methods.

Progestin-Only Injectable Contraceptive

Sexual acceptability of the injectable contraceptive DMPA will in part be based on an individual's response to high-dose progestin. Many people using DMPA will have a decrease in their endogenous estrogen levels due to the impact of this high dose of progestin on the ovarian production of estradiol. Several studies have documented decreased libido with DMPA use,[199–201] with one study reporting that up to 21% of women reported reductions in sexual desire (compared to only 8% reporting increases).[202] The latter study also found that 20% of women using DMPA reported breast tenderness and 9% experienced sexual pain, perhaps due to the hypoestrogenic effect on vaginal tissue.[200] DMPA has also been associated with negative changes in mood and is highly correlated with weight gain, with a subset of users experiencing large increases in weight.[199,201] Both of these factors could shape DMPA users' sexual well-being. In an attempt to better understand the "lived experiences" of DMPA use, Gubrium's qualitative interview findings from 34 U.S. women highlighted that side effects are not experienced in isolation, but rather as a constellation of factors including weight gain, changes in body image, unpredictable bleeding, and emotionality. Taken together, these factors can enact changes in sexual desire or libido, thus contributing in important and understudied ways to the sexual acceptability of this contraceptive method.[201]

Permanent Contraception

Fallopian Tube Surgery

Fallopian tube surgery for permanent contraception was the most commonly used contraceptive method in the U.S. for decades, only recently surpassed in popularity by oral contraceptives (in 2014, 15.5% versus 16.0%, respectively).[203] Despite the widespread prevalence of this method, few recent studies assess its sexual acceptability. However, the literature suggests that, for most people, there is no negative impact and a potentially positive impact[204] on patients' sexual function after the procedure.

Before undergoing tubal surgery, some individuals report concerns about losing their femininity or their desire for or ability to enjoy sex, though few may actually experience these outcomes after the procedure.[205] Though not documented in the literature, subsequent "sexual disinhibition" due to high contraceptive efficacy may counteract potential negative psychological impacts that potentially affect sexuality. Especially after a reproductive lifetime of trying to prevent unintended pregnancy, many patients may enjoy the psychological and sexual freedoms of no longer having to actively "practice" contraception. Celebrating the high sexual acceptability of permanent contraception (such as tubal surgery), particularly if done in tandem with in-depth counseling for sexual concerns, may prove beneficial for clients seeking permanent contraception.

Vas Surgery

Besides the male condom and withdrawal, vas surgery is the only contraceptive option currently available for male-assigned people in the US. This method is highly effective and safe; it is also extremely underutilized in part due to a reluctance to suggest it by health care providers and counseling staff. A common misconception is that male-assigned people will not want permanent contraception. Compared to tubal surgery, vas surgery is cheaper, more cost-effective, and associated with fewer post-operative complications; however, the ratio of vas surgeries to tubal surgeries in the United States is 1:3.[203] In a large number of countries, from Bangladesh to Morocco to Zimbabwe, vas surgery is rarely if ever carried out.[206] This underutilization of vas surgery pertains at least in part to widespread concerns, documented in the United States and abroad, related to "loss of manhood" and potential interference with erection and ejaculation.[207,208] Dispelling these misconceptions and highlighting the rapid return to sexual function after the procedure may result in increased use among individuals and couples seeking permanent contraception. Moreover, vasectomy is associated with few sexual side effects and may even promote better couple-level sexual outcomes. In a study of Austrian couples, while men reported no changes in sexual function after 6 months, their female *partners* reported improved sexual functioning.[209] Findings from this study underscore the psychosexual benefits that many people feel when protected against pregnancy.

Withdrawal (Coitus Interruptus)

The family planning community sometimes overlooks withdrawal as a method of contraception. However, withdrawal is commonly practiced the world over, both as a sole or extra method. As Chapter 15 on Coitus Interruptus describes, estimates from the 2006–2010 National Survey of Family Growth show that the majority of sexually-experienced women in the U.S. have *ever* used withdrawal, and 8% currently rely on withdrawal as their contraceptive method.[210,211] While these rates present increases from prior years,[211] they still may be underestimates, particularly when multiple methods are taken into account. In a 2014 study of 4,634 adult women in the U.S., Jones et al. found that 33% reported any use of withdrawal in the last 30 days, and 13% reported withdrawal exclusively.[212] For a variety of cultural reasons, certain countries such as Turkey have particularly large rates of withdrawal use, with estimates of one quarter to one third of all Turkish couples reporting some recent use of withdrawal, with rates holding steady since the 1990s.[213,214]

The few studies available suggest several sexual implications of the method. Although withdrawal interrupts the moment, requires climax awareness and control for effective use,[215] and can interfere with pleasure for both partners, it may still be sexually preferable to male condoms for some individuals and couples.[216–219] In one nationally representative study of U.S. young adults, both women and men who reported that condoms can reduce their pleasure had significantly greater odds of having used withdrawal at their last penile-vaginal episode.[216] A similar finding emerged from studies of withdrawal in both Turkey[217] and Uganda.[220] Particularly if couples want to engage in additional pregnancy prevention (that is, dual or even triple method use), withdrawal may provide a more sexually acceptable "double-up option" than condoms if STI risk is not present. Other couples may prefer extra-vaginal ejaculation versus ejaculation inside the vagina.

The Female Condom and Other Barrier Methods

Other than male condoms, female condoms are the only currently available contraceptive method that helps prevent both pregnancy and STIs, including human immunodeficiency virus (HIV). Though used less commonly than male condoms, they provide vital dual-prevention prophylaxis[221,222]—especially for sex workers, among whom their use has been the most promoted by public health officials and policy makers.[223] Studies suggest that female condoms can be sexually acceptable to many female-assigned people by way of enhanced level of lubrication,[221,224] greater pleasure and sensation than the male condom,[221] clitoral stimulation through the outer ring,[221] capacity to comfortably accommodate all penis sizes,[224] ability to place it prior to penetrative sexual activity[221] (since the female condom does not rely on a penile erection, it can be placed at any time), and may have a better smell than male condoms.[224] Indeed, women's experiences of greater pleasure and sexual sensations helped predict long-term use of female condoms among 255 women in Brazil.[225] However, not all people's sexual experiences with this device are positive, and—just as with male condoms—a barrier to more widespread female condom use is the perception that it interferes with sexual satisfaction and pleasure for both partners.[226,227]

At least two articles have assessed the sexual acceptability of the diaphragm—a method that has received increased research attention in recent years as a potential for use with spermicide/microbicide combinations that aim to provide dual prevention against both pregnancy and STIs, including HIV. There are no spermicide/microbicide combination products currently on the market. Available data on use of the diaphragm studied prior versions of the diaphragm, which had a variety of sizes. The current diaphragm has only one size and no data concerning sexual acceptability for this particular product. Using a diaphragm may promote sexual autonomy for users as it can be used covertly when placed before sex.[228] Contraceptive users report liking the notion that the diaphragm can be placed up to six hours before sexual activity, thereby being less sexually disruptive.[228] Others feel confident they could use a diaphragm while sexually excited without breaking the mood.[229] Women in one clinical trial studying use of a novel microbicidal/spermicidal gel described the importance of having partner support when using the diaphragm, which some obtained by erotizing safety and highlighting the pleasurable, lubricating aspects associated with using microbicidal/spermicidal gel along with the diaphragm.[228] All currently available spermicidal products, including spermicidal gel or cream for use with a diaphragm or cervical cap as well as the sponge, vaginal contraceptive film, gel and foam, contain nonoxynol 9. Nonoxynol 9 is a surfactant/detergent and can denude the vaginal epithelium.[230,231] This effect may not be evident in some individuals, and may become more bothersome with repeated or frequent use.

Barrier methods such as the female condom, diaphragm, sponge, and cervical cap require comfort with putting something inside the vagina. Thorburn et al. (2006) found that almost 20% of U.S. college-based women preferred a method that does not require genital touching, so these methods may not be well-suited for everyone.[229,232] Prolonging sexual activity prior to intercourse or enlisting a partner's help with placement could increase intimacy and encourage both partners' active engagement in family planning. More research is needed on how couples erotically incorporate barrier methods, including technologies such as dental dams and microbicides and spermicides into their sexual routine.

Fertility Awareness Based Methods

Recent research has paid scant attention to fertility awareness based methods in the contraceptive literature, despite the United Nations' estimate that 41 million couples worldwide used some form of these methods.[215] Only three articles in the last 15 years reference sexual outcomes associated with fertility awareness based methods,[233,234] one of which is a systematic review.[215] This latter review highlighted increased bodily awareness and self-control as common positive experiences among users of fertility awareness based methods.[215] Particularly given the necessity of *couple* participation with these methods, couple factors are likely to influence uptake and sexual acceptability. Many couples may choose fertility awareness based methods due to their "naturalness," facilitation of skin-to-skin contact, or lack of hormonal influences. However, unless people use a barrier method during the fertile window, these methods do not allow for spontaneous sexual activity during periods of peak fertility—a phenomenon that could serve as a sexual turn-off for many potential users. Another turn-off could be these methods' relatively high typical-use failure rates, which could stymie sexual disinhibition. On the other hand, couples who do not feel like pregnancy prevention is a priority or who want a pregnancy to "just happen" could deliberately select a fertility awareness based method for the positive attributes listed above. Further, changing technology related to fertility awareness based methods, including mobile phone apps, may increase these methods' effectiveness and user appeal. (See Chapter 12 on Fertility Awareness-Based Methods.)

Summary

Contraceptives affect family planning patients' sexuality in both positive and negative ways. These influences include, but are not limited to, direct hormonal effects on sexual functioning, indirect psychosexual impacts of efficacy or side effects, and more subjective user assessments of contraceptive-related pleasure and satisfaction. Though a few findings are unidirectional across studies (e.g., no study participants reported that condoms enhance sensation or that breast tenderness improves one's sex life), many other themes show strong variability—with the very contraceptive feature sexually desired by one person disdained by another (e.g., timing or method of application, effect on menstrual bleeding). We strongly encourage practitioners to familiarize themselves with existing literature and help clients find a good fit between their sexual preferences and contraceptive method.

We would applaud more research on the sexual acceptability of contraceptive methods, but we also hope for a more innovative approach that taps into the sexual-improvement potential in contraceptive marketing and counseling. What if clinicians and contraceptive marketers were to tout the potential sexual benefits of methods? For example, practitioners may wish to inform contraceptive users about the potentially sexuality-enhancing aspects of IUDs—that is, that a greater proportion of IUD users will perceive positive compared with negative sexual effects as a result of their method, and the overwhelming majority will experience either no sexual change or a positive sexual change.[119,235] This information could help address patient concerns about use of an IUD and result in increased patient satisfaction. Existing contraceptive advertisements often portray women as empowered medical consumers but not as sexual agents. Ads promote convenience, efficacy, and noncontraceptive benefits (e.g., menstrual timing and regulation, acne improvement) but not their potential ability to facilitate pleasurable, worry-free sex. Sexual and reproductive health clients could be well served by investigations of the feasibility and benefits of eroticizing of contraceptives.[236] This trend can be seen globally in pleasure-centered sexual health promotion efforts, including the eroticization of safer-sex campaigns[237,238] (see also www.thepleasureproject.org). The contraceptive field should follow suit.

TOOLS & FURTHER RESOURCES

HOW CLINICIANS CAN PROMOTE SEXUAL HEALTH AND HELP THEIR CLIENTS LEAD SATISFYING SEX LIVES

Be familiar with sexual anatomy. Clitoral anatomy in particular is poorly understood.[243]

Most people think of the clitoris as the small nub beneath the clitoral hood. It is surprising to many people that in addition to this small tip of the clitoris (called the glans), the clitoris is made up of a neck and body (shaft), legs (crura) and large bulbs of erectile tissue (clitoral bulbs or vestibular bulbs). Figure 22-3 depicts the entire clitoris and labels the various parts. All parts of the clitoris are capable of being highly responsive to arousal and touch.

Include sexuality in discussions about contraception.

- Consider and address possible sexual effects, both positive and negative, when providing information about contraceptive methods.
- Identify sexual problems that may have been attributed to use of a contraceptive method.
- Explore whether sexual side effects led to discontinuation of methods in the past.
- Ask questions that clarify what, if any, specific sexual effects are of concern or important to an individual.

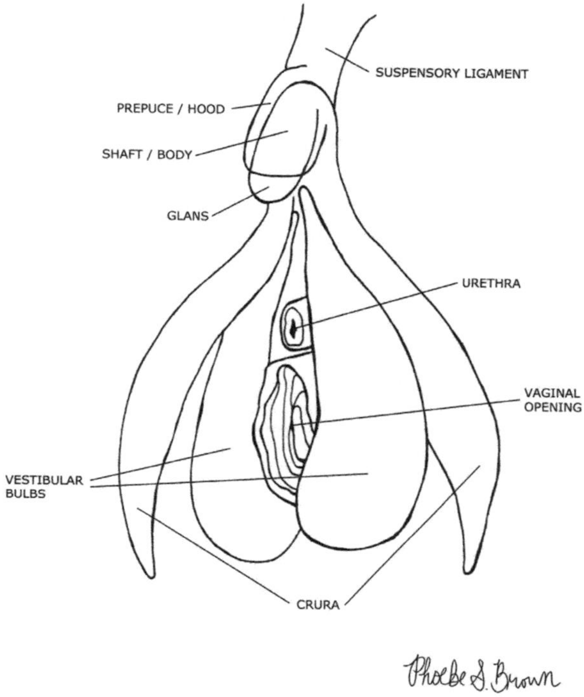

Figure 22-3 Anatomy of the clitoris

Some clinicians may be reluctant to bring up sexual health if they feel unprepared to adequately handle patient concerns. An open conversation to identify problems may in itself naturally provide education and simple suggestions that help. Simply being asked respectful but direct questions may encourage patients to think more openly about sex and sexuality and may support sexual self-comfort. Table 22-3 contains some helpful questions to get you started.

We want to emphasize that treatment begins with an open, nonjudgmental conversation. One way to be responsive to a patient's sexual issues is called PLISSIT: permission, limited information, specific suggestions, and intensive therapy (explored more below).[239] The PLISSIT model is used by many nontherapist clinicians. It gives patients permission to discuss the problem, validates their concerns as legitimate, and provides limited information and suggestions.

- **Permission**: (1) For health care provider to discuss sex with the patient; (2) for patient to discuss sexual concerns now or in the future.

Table 22-3 Suggested questions clinicians can ask to offer a conversation about sexuality*

1. Sexual health is important to overall health; therefore, I always ask patients about it. Is it okay with you if I ask you a few questions about sexual matters now?

   or

2. At this point in the exam, I generally ask some questions regarding your sexual life. Will that be okay?
3. How are things going sexually?
4. Are there any sexual problems or worries that you would like to discuss?
   - *Normalize issues. For example, "It's not uncommon for people ________ (who have diabetes, as they get older, who have a new baby/young children, around menopause, etc.) to have that problem."*
   - *"For many people, ________ (orgasm, pain, decreased interest in sex, etc.) can be a problem. I would be happy to discuss these or other issues with you. If I can't answer your question, I'll find someone who can."*

*Some of these questions taken from Nusbaum and Hamilton (2002).[8]

- **Limited Information**: Clarify misinformation, dispel myths, and provide factual information in a limited manner.
- **Specific Suggestions**: Provide specific suggestions directly related to the particular problem.
- **Intensive Treatment**: Provide (or give referrals for) highly individualized therapy for more complex issues.

The following simple educational interventions also may be helpful: normalizing sexual frequency, understanding a mismatch between partners' libidos, suggesting use of lubricants, and explaining anatomy and relevant sexual responses.

RESOURCES *to learn more about responding to people with sexual complaints*

Patients who need more in-depth counseling for treatment can be referred to a qualified sex therapist; such therapists can be located via the American Association of Sexuality Educators (www.aasect.org) or the International Society for the Study of Women's Sexual Health (www.isswsh.org). The American Physical Therapy Association (APTA)'s section specializing in women's health is an excellent source of referrals for women with dyspareunia and a variety of vulvar and vaginal pain issues (www.womenshealthapta.org).

Clinicians who would like more information on diagnosis and treatment of sexual problems and concerns can refer to the following:

- The leading clinical reference and text in the field, originally developed by the late Sandra Leiblum: *Principles and Practice of Sex Therapy*.[110]

- Volume 10, issue 1 of the Journal of Sexual Medicine (2013) contains a variety of standard operating procedures for diagnosing and treatment of sexual dysfunctions including desire disorder,[240] arousal disorder,[241] genital pain,[242] as well as guidelines for taking a sexual history.[243]

The Association of Reproductive Health Professionals (ARHP) has created:

- A fact sheet for talking with patients about sexuality and sexual health: www.arhp.org/uploadDocs/sexandsexfactsheet.pdf
- A clinical competency document in sexuality: www.arhp.org/uploadDocs/SHF_Competencies.pdf. This document has excellent guidance yet is somewhat dated. For example, it cites the DSM-4 versus the more updated DSM-5.
- A guide on "Sex Therapy for non-Therapists": www.arhp.org/Publications-and-Resources/Clinical-Fact-Sheets/SHF-Therapy.

Sex-Positive Educational Resources for Patients and Providers

Books

Comprehensive information about sex

- Joannides, P., Gross, D. (2015). *Guide to Getting It On: A Book About the Wonders of Sex* (8th ed.). Waldport, OR: Goody Foot Press.
  A dictionary/encyclopedia format using informal language, quotations from interviewing a diverse demographic, and illustrations in order to provide accurate, approachable, and memorable information about sex and anatomy.
- Joannides, P., Gross, D., & Johnson, T. (2017). *Guide to Getting It On: Unzipped!* Oregon: Goofy Foot Press.
  Streamlined version of *Guide to Getting it On*.
- Winston S. (2010) *Women's Anatomy of Arousal*. Kingston, NY: Mango Garden Press, (English and Spanish *in press*)
  A book with beautiful anatomy illustrations.

Desire

- Hall, K. (2004). *Reclaiming Your Sexual Self: How You Can Bring Desire Back into Your Life*. Hoboken, NJ: John Wiley & Sons, Inc.
  This book explores sexual desire, or lack thereof. A sex therapist discusses how to assert control of your health and sexual life.

- Nagoski, E. (2015). *Come as You Are: The Surprising New Science That Will Transform Your Sex Life*. New York: Simon & Schuster Paperbacks.
  This book presents science about desire in layperson's language with a focus on female sexuality.

Orgasm

- Cass, V. (2007). *The Elusive Orgasm: A Woman's Guide to Why She Can't and How She Can Orgasm.* Cambridge, MA: Da Capo Press.
  Clinical psychologist and sex therapist Vivianne Cass explores the causes of women's orgasm difficulties and how to remedy them. This book provides a full overview of women's sexual pleasure, covering sexual triggers, stages of arousal, the power of mind, and how women differ from men.

Comic book

- Gonick, L., & DeVault, C. (1999). *The Cartoon Guide to Sex.* New York, NY: HarperCollins Publishers.
  This book explores the spectrum of human sexuality, sexual arousal and response, sexual communication, love, marriage and other arrangements, contraception, and sexual health through approachable and scientifically accurate comics.

Disabilities and sex

- Kaufman, M., Silverberg, C., & Odette, F. (2007). *The Ultimate Guide to Sex and Disability: For All of Us Who Live with Disabilities, Chronic Pain & Illness.* San Francisco, CA: Cleis Press, Inc.
  This book, written by a medical doctor, a sex educator, and a disability activist, is the first complete sex guide for people who live with disabilities, pain, illness, or chronic conditions (although it is useful for anyone). This book provides readers with encouragement, support, and all the information they need to create a sex life that works for them.

Sexual pleasure: techniques

- Kerner, I. (2010). *She Comes First: the Thinking Man's Guide to Pleasuring a Woman*. New York, NY: William Morrow, an imprint of HarperCollins. (English)
  This book provides a step by step guide to oral sex techniques.

  Kerner, I. (2007). *Ellas Llegan Primero: el Libro para los Hombres Que Quieren Complacer a las Mujeres*. Madrid: Punto de Lectura. (Spanish)
  This book provides a step by step guide to oral sex techniques.

- Moon, A., & Diamond, K. (2015). *Girl Sex 101.* Oregon: Lunatic Ink. This book offers information about sex for women and women lovers of all genders and identities through playful and informative illustrations and voices.

Parenting, children's sexual development

- Roffman, D. (2012). *Talk to Me First: Everything You Need to Know to Become Your Kids' "Go To" Person About Sex.* Boston, MA: Da Capo Press. This book is a teaching tool for parents in a time when children are exposed to sex and sexuality at an early age. It prepares parents to be the most credible and influential resource about sexuality in their children's lives.
- Silverberg, C., & Smyth, F. (2015). *Sex Is a Funny Word: A Book About Bodies, Feelings, and YOU.* Seven Stories Press.
  This kid-friendly comic book is a resource about bodies, gender and sexuality. It opens up conversations between young people and the adults in their lives.

Pregnancy and postpartum

- Young, M. (2016). *The Ultimate Guide to Sex Through Pregnancy and Motherhood: Passionate, Practical Advice for Moms.* Jersey City, NJ: Cleis Press.
  The author uses her own personal experiences to discuss sex and sexuality throughout pregnancy and motherhood so that women are encouraged to embrace themselves, their feelings and their desires.

Websites and Online Media for Sex Education

- A Woman's Touch Sexuality Resource Center: www.sexuality resources.com
- www.ashasexualhealth.org
- www.sexsmartfilms.com
- NPR sexual health podcast
- www.thepleasureproject.org

Websites that sell sex toys:

- www.goodvibrations.com
- www.evesgarden.com
- www.sexualityresources.com

Tips for Toys

Sex toys enable exploration and self-satisfaction. Counselors and providers may wish to emphasize the following points when talking to patients about sex toys:

- Use of lubrication is important. A variety of lubricants can be bought at most drugstores.
- Patients should avoid toys that are made of toxic materials that contain phthalates; they should seek out toys that do not have a chemical or plastic smell. Safe options include:
  - — non-porous materials
  - — 100% silicone
  - — glass
  - — surgical steel
  - — sealed ceramics
  - — medical-grade plastics
- A helpful experiment: trying vibrations on different parts of the body. People should try a range of speeds and types of vibrations to see what they like.
- Patients should be encouraged to relax and have fun! There is no right or wrong way to use a vibrator; it's about pleasure.
- People will not become addicted to vibrators or unable to orgasm without them. Vibrators may help someone orgasm more quickly, but they will not create desensitization to the stimulation that leads to orgasms.
- Some people like to use vibrators on the clitoris directly (intense); others use them on the lips of the vulva; others use them on the inside of the vagina. Some like to move the vibration around to all three places. Patients won't know unless they try.
- For most people, arousal that can lead to orgasm occurs when the clitoris, lips of the vulva, and first 1 to 3 inches of the vagina (closest to the outside of the body) are stimulated.
- Many people enjoy partnered vibrator play. People may want to try using their vibrator with a partner.

Author Disclosures—Higgins: none. Cason: advisory board member or consultant to Teva, Medicines 360, Allergan, Merck, Bayer, ContraMed, Evofem; trainer/speaker for Merck, Medicines360, Teva, ContraMed.

References

1. Sobecki JN, Curlin FA, Rasinski KA, Lindau ST. What we don't talk about when we don't talk about sex: results of a national survey of U.S. obstetrician/gynecologists. J Sex Med 2012;9:1285–1294.
2. Parish SJ, Rubio-Aurioles E. Education in sexual medicine: proceedings from the international consultation in sexual medicine, 2009. J Sex Med 2010;7:3305–3314.
3. Akers AY, Gold MA, Borrero S, Santucci A, Schwarz EB. Providers' perspectives on challenges to contraceptive counseling in primary care settings. J Women Health 2010;19:1163–1170.
4. Berman L, Berman J, Felder S, et al. Seeking help for sexual function complaints: what gynecologists need to know about the female patient's experience. Fertil Steril 2003;79:572–576.
5. Moore K, Helzner JF. 'What's sex got to do with it?': challenges for incorporating sexuality into family planning programs. New York: The Population Council; 1996.
6. Dixon-Mueller R. The sexuality connection in reproductive health. Stud Fam Plann 1993;24:269–282.
7. Wimberly YH, Hogben M, Moore-Ruffin J, Moore SE, Fry-Johnson Y. Sexual history-taking among primary care physicians. J Natl Med Assoc 2006;98:1924–1929.
8. Nusbaum MR, Hamilton CD. The proactive sexual health history. Am Fam Physician 2002;66:1705–1712.
9. Nusbaum MRH, Gamble GR, Pathman DE. Seeking medical help for sexual concerns: Frequency, carriers, and missed opportunities. J Fam Practice 2002;51:1–5.
10. Lerum K, Dworkin SL. "Bad girls rule": an interdisciplinary feminist commentary on the report of the APA Task Force on the Sexualization of Girls. J Sex Res 2009;46:250–263.
11. Higgins JA, Hirsch JS. The pleasure deficit: revisiting the "sexuality connection" in reproductive health. Perspect Sex Reprod Health 2007;39:240–247.
12. Higgins JA, Smith NK. The sexual acceptability of contraception: reviewing the literature and building a new concept. J Sex Res 2016;53:417–456.
13. Maurice WL, Bowman MA. Sexual medicine in primary care. St. Louis: Mosby Year Book; 1999.
14. Nusbaum MR, Gamble G, Skinner B, Heiman J. The high prevalence of sexual concerns among women seeking routine gynecological care. J Fam Pract 2000;49:229–232.
15. Schwartz IM. Affective reactions of American and Swedish women to their 1st premarital coitus: a cross-cultural comparison. J Sex Res 1993;30:18–26.
16. Schalet A. Adolescent sexuality viewed through two cultural lenses. In: Kuriansky J, Tepper MS, Owens AF, eds. Sex, love, and psychology: Sex Health (Vol. 3). Westport, CT: Praeger; 2007.
17. Schalet A. Raging hormones, regulated love: adolescent sexuality and the constitution of the modern individual in the United States and the Netherlands. Body & Society 2000;6:75–105.
18. Dodge B, Sandfort TG, Yarber WL, de Wit J. Sexual health among male college students in the United States and the Netherlands. Am J Health Behav 2005;29:172–182.
19. Bancroft J. Human sexuality and its problems. 3rd ed. Edinburgh ; New York: Churchill Livingstone/Elsevier; 2009.
20. Wynn LL, Foster AM, Trussell J. Would you say you had unprotected sex if . . . ? Sexual health language in emails to a reproductive health website. Cult Health Sex. 2010;21:499–514.
21. Millett K. Sexual politics. [1st ed. Garden City, N.Y.,: Doubleday; 1970.
22. Intersex Society of North America. What is intersex? Available at: www.isna.org/faq/what_is_intersex 2017. Accessed March 29, 2017.
23. Intersex Society of North America (ISNA). Our Mission. Available at: www.isna.org 2017. Accessed July 2, 2017.
24. Kaschak E, Tiefer L. A new view of womens sexual problems. New York: Haworth Press; 2001.

25. Schwartz P, Rutter V. The gender of sexuality. Thousand Oaks, CA: Pine Forge Press; 1998.
26. Reiss IL, Reiss HM. An end to shame: shaping our next sexual revolution. Buffalo, N.Y.: Prometheus Books; 1990.
27. Fields J. Risky lessons: sex education and social inequality. New Brunswick, NJ: Rutgers University Press; 2008.
28. Fine M. Sexuality, schooling, and adolescent females: the missing discourse of desire. Harvard Educational Review 1988;58:29–53.
29. Tolman DL. Dilemmas of desire: teenage girls talk about sexuality. Cambridge, MA: Harvard University Press; 2002.
30. Cassell C. Swept away: why women fear their own sexuality. New York: Simon & Schuster; 1984.
31. Moore AM, Frohwirth L, Miller E. Male reproductive control of women who have experienced intimate partner violence in the United States. Soc Sci Med.70:1737–1744.
32. Breiding MJ, Smith SG, Basile KC, Walters ML, Chen J, Merrick MT. Prevalence and characteristics of sexual violence, stalking, and intimate partner violence victimization—national intimate partner and sexual violence survey, United States, 2011. MMWR Surveill Summ 2014;63:1–18.
33. Catalano S, Smith E, Snyder H, Rand M. Female victims of violence. Available at: www.bjs.gov/content/pub/pdf/fvv.pdf. U.S. Department of Justice 2009.
34. Jannini EA, Fisher WA, Bitzer J, McMahon CG. Is sex just fun? How sexual activity improves health. J Sex Med 2009;6:2640–2648.
35. Levin RJ. Sexual activity, health and well-being: The beneficial roles of coitus and masturbation. Sexual and Relationship Therapy 2007;22:135–148.
36. Liu H, Waite LJ, Shen S, Wang DH. Is sex good for your health? A national study on partnered sexuality and cardiovascular risk among older men and women. J Health Soc Behav 2016;57:276–296.
37. Hogarth H, Ingham R. Masturbation among young women and associations with sexual health: an exploratory study. J Sex Res 2009;46:558–567.
38. Herbenick D, Reece M, Sanders S, Dodge B, Ghassemi A, Fortenberry JD. Prevalence and characteristics of vibrator use by women in the United States: results from a nationally representative study. J Sex Med 2009;6:1857–1866.
39. Seldin DR, H.S. F, Martin LR. Sexual activity as a predictor of life-span mortality risk. Pers Indiv Differ 2002;33:409–425.
40. Drory Y. Sexual activity and cardiovascular risk. Eur Heart J Supplements 2002;4: H13–H18.
41. Ebrahim S, May M, Ben Shlomo Y, et al. Sexual intercourse and risk of ischaemic stroke and coronary heart disease: the Caerphilly study. J Epidemiol Community Health 2002;56:99–102.
42. Buettner D. The Blue Zones: 9 lessons for living longer from the people who have lived the longest. Washington, DC: National Geographic Society;2008.
43. Flynn KE, Lin L, Bruner DW, et al. Sexual satisfaction and the importance of sexual health to quality of life throughout the life course of U.S. adults. J Sex Med 2016;13:1642–1650.
44. Lee DM, Vanhoutte B, Nazroo J, Pendleton N. Sexual health and positive subjective well-being in partnered older men and women. J Gerontol Series B, Psychological sciences and social sciences 2016;71:698–710.
45. Davison SL, Bell RJ, LaChina M, Holden SL, Davis SR. The relationship between self-reported sexual satisfaction and general well-being in women. J Sex Med 2009;6:2690–2697.
46. Lowenstein G, Krishnamurti T, Kopsic J, McDonald D. Does increased sexual frequency enhance happiness? J Econ Behav Organ 2015;116:206–218.
47. Muise A, Giang E, Impett EA. Post sex affectionate exchanges promote sexual and relationship satisfaction. Arch Sex Behav 2014;43:1391–1402.

48. Heiman JR, Long JS, Smith SN, Fisher WA, Sand MS, Rosen RC. Sexual satisfaction and relationship happiness in midlife and older couples in five countries. Arch Sex Behav 2011;40:741–753.
49. Yeh HC, Lorenz FO, Wickrama KA, Conger RD, Elder GH, Jr. Relationships among sexual satisfaction, marital quality, and marital instability at midlife. J Fam Psychol 2006;20:339–343.
50. Herbenick D, Reece M, Schick V, Sanders SA, Dodge B, Fortenberry JD. Sexual behavior in the United States: results from a national probability sample of men and women ages 14–94. J Sex Med 2010;7 Suppl 5:255–265.
51. Reece M, Herbenick D, Schick V, Sanders SA, Dodge B, Fortenberry JD. Background and considerations on the National Survey of Sexual Health and Behavior (NSSHB) from the investigators. J Sex Med 2010;7 Suppl 5:243–245.
52. Schick V, Herbenick D, Reece M, et al. Sexual behaviors, condom use, and sexual health of Americans over 50: implications for sexual health promotion for older adults. J Sex Med 2010;7 Suppl 5:315–329.
53. Fortenberry JD, Schick V, Herbenick D, Sanders SA, Dodge B, Reece M. Sexual behaviors and condom use at last vaginal intercourse: a national sample of adolescents ages 14 to 17 years. J Sex Med 2010;7 Suppl 5:305–314.
54. Reece M, Herbenick D, Schick V, Sanders SA, Dodge B, Fortenberry JD. Sexual behaviors, relationships, and perceived health among adult men in the United States: results from a national probability sample. J Sex Med 2010;7 Suppl 5:291–304.
55. Herbenick D, Reece M, Schick V, Sanders SA, Dodge B, Fortenberry JD. Sexual behaviors, relationships, and perceived health status among adult women in the United States: results from a national probability sample. J Sex Med 2010;7 Suppl 5:277–290.
56. Blair KL, Cappell J, Pukall CF. Not all orgasms were created equal: differences in frequency and satisfaction of orgasm experiences by sexual activity in same-sex versus mixed-sex relationships. J Sex Res 2017:1–15.
57. Baumeister RF, Catanese KR, Vohs KD. Is there a gender difference in strength of sex drive? theoretical views, conceptual distinctions, and a review of relevant evidence. Pers Soc Psychol Rev 2001;5:242–273.
58. Fisher TD. Gender roles and pressure to be truthful: the bogus pipeline modifies gender differences in sexual but not non-sexual behavior. Sex Roles 2013;68:401–414.
59. Laumann EO. The social organization of sexuality: sexual practices in the United States. Chicago: University of Chicago Press; 1994.
60. Coles R, Stokes F. Sex and the American teenager. New York: Harper and Row; 1995.
61. Haffner DW, Stayton WR. Sexuality and reproductive health. In: Hatcher RA, ed. Contraceptive technology 17th rev. ed. New York: Ardent Media; 1998:13–41.
62. Wellings K, Collumbien M, Slaymaker E, et al. Sexual behaviour in context: a global perspective. Lancet 2006;368:1706–1728.
63. Abma JC. Teenagers in the United States: sexual activity, contraceptive use, and childbearing, 2002. Vital Health Stat 2004;24:1–48.
64. Hawes ZC, Wellings K, Stephenson J. First Heterosexual Intercourse in the United Kingdom: A Review of the Literature. J Sex Res 2010;47:137–152.
65. Carpenter LM. Gender and the meaning and experience of virginity loss in the contemporary United States. Gender & Society 2002;16:345–365.
66. Carpenter LM. Virginity lost: an intimate portrait of first sexual experiences. New York: New York University; 2005.
67. Trussell J, Schwarz EB, Guthrie K. Research priorities for preventing unintended pregnancy: moving beyond emergency contraceptive pills. Perspect Sex Reprod Health.42:8–9.
68. Savin-Williams RC, Ream GL. Prevalence and stability of sexual orientation components during adolescence and young adulthood. Arch Sex Behav 2007;36:385–394.
69. Laumann EO. The social organization of sexuality: sexual practices in the United States. Chicago: University of Chicago Press; 1994.

70. Diamond LM. Sexual fluidity: understanding women's love and desire. Cambridge, MA: Harvard University Press; 2008.
71. Goldberg SK, Reese BM, Halpern CT. Teen pregnancy among sexual minority women: results from the national longitudinal study of adolescent to adult health. J Adolesc Health 2016;59:429–437.
72. Tornello SL, Riskind RG, Patterson CJ. Sexual orientation and sexual and reproductive health among adolescent young women in the United States. J Adolesc Health 2014;54:160–168.
73. Saewyc EM. Adolescent pregnancy among lesbian, gay, and bisexual teens. In: Cherry A, Dillon M, eds. International Handbook of Adolescent Pregnancy: Springer; 2014:159–169.
74. Charlton BM, Corliss HL, Missmer SA, Rosario M, Spiegelman D, Austin SB. Sexual orientation differences in teen pregnancy and hormonal contraceptive use: an examination across 2 generations. Am J Obstet Gynecol 2013;209:204 e201–208.
75. Lindley LL, Walsemann KM. Sexual orientation and risk of pregnancy among New York City high-school students. Am J Public Health 2015;105:1379–1386.
76. Everett BG, McCabe KF, Hughes TL. Unintended pregnancy, depression, and hazardous drinking in a community-based sample of sexual minority women. J Womens Health 2016;25:904–911.
77. Morrow KM, Allsworth JE. Sexual risk in lesbians and bisexual women. J Gay Lesbian Med Assoc 2000;4:159–165.
78. Diamond LM. Female bisexuality from adolescence to adulthood: results from a 10-year longitudinal study. Dev Psychol 2008;44:5–14.
79. Meston CM, Buss DM. Why women have sex: understanding sexual motivations, from adventure to revenge (and everything in between) 1st ed. New York: Times Books; 2009.
80. Meston CM, Buss DM. Why humans have sex. Arch Sex Behav 2007;36:477–507.
81. Higgins JA, Hirsch JS. Pleasure, power, and inequality: incorporating sexuality into research on contraceptive use. Am J Public Health 2008;98:1803–1813.
82. Graham CA, Sanders SA, Milhausen RR, McBride KR. Turning on and turning off: a focus group study of the factors that affect women's sexual arousal. Arch Sex Behav 2004;33:527–538.
83. Higgins JA, Tanner AE, Janssen E. Arousal loss related to safer sex and risk of pregnancy: implications for women's and men's sexual health. Perspect Sex Reprod Health 2009;41:150–157.
84. Higgins JA, Hirsch JS, Trussell J. Pleasure, prophylaxis and procreation: a qualitative analysis of intermittent contraceptive use and unintended pregnancy. Perspect Sex Reprod Health 2008;40:130–137.
85. Kaye K, Suellentrop K, Sloup C. The fog zone: how misperceptions, magical thinking, and ambivalence put young adults at risk for unplanned pregnancy. Washington, DC: The National Campaign to Prevent Teen and Unplanned Pregnancy, 2009.
86. Bancroft J, Loftus J, Long JS. Distress about sex: A national survey of women in heterosexual relationships. Arch Sex Behav 2003;32:193–208.
87. American Psychiatric Association. Diagnostic and statistical manual of mental disorders: DSM-5. Washington, DC: American Pychiatric Association; 2013.
88. Heiman J. Orgasmic disorders in women. In: Leiblum SR, ed. Principles and practice of sex therapy. 4th edition. ed. New York, NY: The Guilford Press; 2007:84–123.
89. Jutel A. Framing disease: the example of female hypoactive sexual desire disorder. Soc Sci Med 2010;70:1084–1090.
90. Derogatis LR, Burnett AL. The epidemiology of sexual dysfunctions. J Sex Med 2008;5:289–300.
91. Laumann EO, Glasser DB, Neves RC, Moreira ED, Jr., Group GI. A population-based survey of sexual activity, sexual problems and associated help-seeking behavior patterns in mature adults in the United States of America. Int J Impot Res 2009;21:171–178.
92. Laumann EO, Paik A, Rosen RC. Sexual dysfunction in the United States: prevalence and predictors. JAMA 1999;281:537–544.

93. Shifren JL, Monz BU, Russo PA, Segreti A, Johannes CB. Sexual problems and distress in United States women: prevalence and correlates. Obstet Gynecol 2008;112:970–978.
94. Rosen RC, Shifren JL, Monz BU, Odom DM, Russo PA, Johannes CB. Correlates of sexually related personal distress in women with low sexual desire. J Sex Med 2009;6:1549–1560.
95. Brotto LA. The DSM diagnostic criteria for hypoactive sexual desire disorder in women. Arch Sex Behav 2010;39:221–239.
96. Carvalheira AA, Brotto LA, Leal I. Women's motivations for sex: exploring the diagnostic and statistical manual, fourth edition, text revision criteria for hypoactive sexual desire and female sexual arousal disorders. J Sex Med 2010;7:1454–1463.
97. Michael RT, Gagnon JH, Laumann EO, Kolata G. Sex in America: A definitive survey. New York, NY: Warner Books; 1994.
98. McCabe MP, Goldhammer DL. Prevalence of women's sexual desire problems: what criteria do we use? Arch Sex Behav 2013;42:1073–1078.
99. Brotto LA. The DSM diagnostic criteria for hypoactive sexual desire disorder in women. Arch Sex Behav 2010;39:221–239.
100. Mark K, Herbenick D, Fortenberry D, Sanders S, Reece M. The object of sexual desire: examining the "what" in "what do you desire?" J Sex Med 2014;11:2709–2719.
101. Driscoll M, Basson R, Brotto L, et al. Empirically supported incentive model of sexual response ignored. J Sex Med 2017;14:758–759.
102. Laan E, Both S. What makes women experience desire? Fem Psychol 2008;18:505–514.
103. Brotto LA, Petkau AJ, Labrie F, Basson R. Predictors of sexual desire disorders in women. J Sex Med 2011;8:742–753.
104. Pfaus JG, Kippin TE, Coria-Avila GA, et al. Who, what, where, when (and maybe even why)? How the experience of sexual reward connects sexual desire, preference, and performance. Arch Sex Behav 2012;41:31–62.
105. Ringa V, Diter K, Laborde C, Bajos N. Women's sexuality: from aging to social representations. J Sex Med 2013;10:2399–2408.
106. Peixoto MM, Nobre P. Dysfunctional sexual beliefs: a comparative study of heterosexual men and women, gay men, and lesbian women with and without sexual problems. J Sex Med 2014;11:2690–2700.
107. Kingsberg SA, Rezaee RL. Hypoactive sexual desire in women. Menopause 2013;20:1284–1300.
108. Tiefer L. Apples and oranges: "sexual medicine" and the effort to deny that counting and classifying are political acts. J Sex Marital Ther 2017;43:246–249.
109. Thurston RC, Ewing LJ, Low CA, Christie AJ, Levine MD. Behavioral weight loss for the management of menopausal hot flashes: a pilot study. Menopause 2015;22:59–65.
110. Binik YM, Hall KSK. Principles and practice of sex therapy. Fifth edition/ed. New York: The Guilford Press; 2014.
111. Severy LJ, Newcomer S. Critical issues in contraceptive and STI acceptability research. J Soc Iss 2005;61:45–65.
112. Higgins JA, Davis AR. Sexuality and contraception (chapter 1). In: Hatcher RA, et al., eds. Contraceptive technology 20th ed. New York, NY: Ardent Media; 2011:1–28.
113. Higgins JA, Davis AR. Contraceptive sex acceptability: a commentary, synopsis and agenda for future research. Contraception 2014;90:4–10.
114. Hensel DJ, Stupiansky NW, Herbenick D, Dodge B, Reece M. When condom use is not condom use: an event-level analysis of condom use behaviors during vaginal intercourse. J Sex Med 2011;8:28–34.
115. Randolph ME, Pinkerton SD, Bogart LM, Cecil H, Abramson PR. Sexual pleasure and condom use. Arch Sex Behav 2007;36:844–848.
116. Oudshoorn N. The male pill: a biography of a technology in the making. Durham, NC: Duke University Press; 2003.
117. Solomon H, Yount KM, Mbizvo MT. 'A shot of his own': the acceptability of a male hormonal contraceptive in Indonesia. Cult Health Sex 2007;9:1–14.

118. WHO. Hormonal contraception for men: acceptability and effects on sexuality. World Health Organization Task Force on Psychosocial Research in Family Planning, Special Programme of Research, Development and Research Training in Human Reproduction. Stud Family Plann 1982;13:328–342.
119. Higgins JA, Sanders JN, Palta M, Turok DK. Women's sexual function, satisfaction, and perceptions after starting long-acting reversible contraceptives. Obstet Gynecol 2016;128:1143–1151.
120. Grady WR, Klepinger DH, Nelson-Wally A. Contraceptive characteristics: the perceptions and priorities of men and women. Fam Plann Perspect 1999;31:168–175.
121. Lessard LN, Karasek D, Ma S, et al. Contraceptive features preferred by women at high risk of unintended pregnancy. Perspect Sex Repro Health 2012;44:194–200.
122. Gomez AM, Clark JB. The relationship between contraceptive features preferred by young women and interest in IUDs: an exploratory analysis. Perpect Sex Repro Health 2014;46:157–163.
123. Burrows LJ, Basha M, Goldstein AT. The effects of hormonal contraceptives on female sexuality: a review. J Sex Med 2012;9:2213–2223.
124. Schaffir J. Hormonal contraception and sexual desire: a critical review. J Sex Marital Ther 2006;32:305–314.
125. Stuckey BGA. Female sexual function and dysfunction in the reproductive years: the influence of endogenous and exogenous sex hormones. J Sex Med 2008;5:2282–2290.
126. Welling LL. Psychobehavioral effects of hormonal contraceptive use. Evolutionary Psychology 2013;11:718–742.
127. Wiebe E. Capturing the sexual side effects of hormonal contraception. Contraception 2009 Dec;80:540–54. Contraception 2010;82:581–581.
128. Graesslin O, Barjot P, Hoffet M, Cohen D, Vaillant P, Clerson P. The EVAPIL scale, a new tool to assess tolerance of oral contraceptives. Contraception 2009;80:540–554.
129. Rosen R, Brown C, Heiman J, et al. The Female Sexual Function Index (FSFI): a multidimensional self-report instrument for the assessment of female sexual function. J Sex Marital Ther 2000;26:191–208.
130. Higgins JA, Smith NK, Sanders SA, et al. Dual method use at last sexual encounter: a nationally representative, episode-level analysis of US men and women. Contraception 2014;90:399–406.
131. Crosby R, Milhausen R, Yarber WL, Sanders SA, Graham CA. Condom 'turn offs' among adults: an exploratory study. Int J STD AIDS 2008;19:590–594.
132. Hensel DJ, Stupiansky NW, Herbenick D, Dodge B, Reece M. Sexual pleasure during condom-protected vaginal sex among heterosexual men. J Sex Med 2012;9:1272–1276.
133. Sanders SA, Yarber WL, Kaufman EL, Crosby RA, Graham CA, Milhausen RR. Condom use errors and problems: a global view. Sex Health (14485028) 2012;9:81–95.
134. Crosby R, Sanders S, Yarber WL, Graham CA. Condom-use errors and problems: a neglected aspect of studies assessing condom effectiveness. Am J Prevent Med 2003;24:367–370.
135. Sanders SA, Hill BJ, Crosby RA, Janssen E. Correlates of condom-associated erection problems in young, heterosexual men: condom fit, self-efficacy, perceptions, and motivations. AIDS Behavior 2014;18:128–134.
136. Higgins JA, Fennell JL. Providing for women's pleasure in the next generation of condoms. J Sex Med 2013;10:3151–3153.
137. Bolton M, McKay A, Schneider M. Relational influences on condom use discontinuation: a qualitative study of young adult women in dating relationships. Canadian Journal of Human Sexuality 2010;19:91–104.
138. Sanders SA, Reece M, Herbenick D, Schick V, Dodge B, Fortenberry JD. Condom use during most recent vaginal intercourse event among a probability sample of adults in the United States. J Sex Med 2010;7:362–373.
139. Versteeg M, Murray M. Condom use as part of the wider HIV prevention strategy: experiences from communities in the North West Province, South Africa. SAHARA J : journal of Social Aspects of HIV/AIDS Research Alliance/SAHARA, Human Sciences Research Council 2008;5:83–93.

140. Wang X. The role of attitude functions, efficacy, anticipated emotions, and relationship status on college students' condom use intentions. J Sex Res 2013;50:704–714.
141. Gebhardt WA, Kuyper L, Dusseldorp E. Condom use at first intercourse with a new partner in female adolescents and young adults: the role of cognitive planning and motives for having sex. Arch Sex Behav 2006;35:217–223.
142. Crosby RA, Milhausen RR, Mark KP, Yarber WL, Sanders SA, Graham CA. Understanding problems with condom fit and feel: an important opportunity for improving clinic-based safer sex programs. J Prim Prev 2013;34(1–2):109–115.
143. Fennell J. "And isn't that the point?": pleasure and contraceptive decisions. Contraception 2014;89:264–270.
144. Higgins JA, Hirsch JS. Pleasure, power, and inequality: incorporating sexuality into research on contraceptive use. Am J Public Health 2008;98:1803–1813.
145. Kaneko N. Association between condom use and perceived barriers to and self-efficacy of safe sex among young women in Japan. Nurs Health Sci 2007;9:284–289.
146. Træen B, Gravningen K. The use of protection for sexually transmitted infections (STIs) and unwanted pregnancy among Norwegian heterosexual young adults 2009. Sex Cult 2011;15:195–212.
147. Widdice LE, Cornell JL, Liang W, Halpern-Felsher BL. Having sex and condom use: potential risks and benefits reported by young, sexually inexperienced adolescents. J Adol Health 2006;39:588–595.
148. Higgins JA, Wang Y. The role of young adults' pleasure attitudes in shaping condom use. Am J Public Health 2015;105:1329–1332.
149. Higgins JA, Trussell J, Moore NB, Davidson JK. Virginity lost, satisfaction gained? Physiological and psychological sexual satisfaction at heterosexual debut. J Sex Res 2010:1–11.
150. Davis AR, Castano PM. Oral contraceptives and libido in women. Annu Rev Sex Res 2004;15:297–320.
151. Schaffir J. Hormonal contraception and sexual desire: a critical review. J Sex Marital Ther 2006;32:305–314.
152. Burrows LJ, Basha M, Goldstein AT. The effects of hormonal contraceptives on female sexuality: a review. J Sex Med 2012;9:2213–2223.
153. Moher D, Schulz KF, Altman DG. The CONSORT statement: revised recommendations for improving the quality of reports of parallel-group randomised trials. Lancet 2001;357(9263):1191–1194.
154. Graham CA, Ramos R, Bancroft J, Maglaya C, Farley TM. The effects of steroidal contraceptives on the well-being and sexuality of women: a double-blind, placebo-controlled, two-centre study of combined and progestogen-only methods. Contraception 1995;52:363–369.
155. Sanders SA, Graham CA, Bass JL, Bancroft J. A prospective study of the effects of oral contraceptives on sexuality and well-being and their relationship to discontinuation. Contraception 2001;64:51–58.
156. Devineni D, Skee D, Vaccaro N, et al. Pharmacokinetics and pharmacodynamics of a transdermal contraceptive patch and an oral contraceptive. J Clin Pharmacol 2007;47:497–509.
157. Pastor Z, Holla K, Chmel R. The influence of combined oral contraceptives on female sexual desire: a systematic review. Euro J Contracep Repro 2013;18:27–43.
158. Braunstein GD. Androgen insufficiency in women. Growth Horm IGF Res 2006;16: S109–S117.
159. Zimmerman Y, Foidart JM, Pintiaux A, et al. Restoring testosterone levels by adding dehydroepiandrosterone to a drospirenone containing combined oral contraceptive: II. Clinical effects. Contraception 2015;91:134–142.
160. Salonia A, Nappi RE, Pontillo M, et al. Menstrual cycle-related changes in plasma oxytocin are relevant to normal sexual function in healthy women. Horm Behav 2005;47:164–169.
161. van Anders SM, Goldey KL, Bell SN. Measurement of Testosterone in Human Sexuality Research: Methodological Considerations. Arch Sex Behav 2014;43:231–250.
162. Davis SR, Davison SL, Donath S, Bell RJ. Circulating androgen levels and self-reported sexual function in women. JAMA 2005;294:91–96.

163. Warnock JK, Clayton A, Croft H, Segraves R, Biggs FC. Comparison of androgens in women with hypoactive sexual desire disorder: those on combined oral contraceptives (COCs) vs those not on COCs. J Sex Med 2006;3:878–882.
164. Graham CA, Bancroft J, Doll HA, Greco T, Tanner A. Does oral contraceptive-induced reduction in free testosterone adversely affect the sexuality or mood of women? Psychoneuroendocrino 2007;32:246–255.
165. Bishop JR, Ellingrod VL, Akroush M, Moline J. The association of serotonin transporter genotypes and selective serotonin reuptake inhibitor (SSRI)-associated sexual side effects: Possible relationship to oral contraceptives. Hum Psychopharm Clin 2009;24:207–215.
166. Elaut E, Buysse A, De Sutter P, et al. Relation of androgen receptor sensitivity and mood to sexual desire in hormonal contraception users. Contraception 2012;85:470–479.
167. Bednarczyk RA, Davis R, Ault K, Orenstein W, Omer SB. Sexual activity-related outcomes after human papillomavirus vaccination of 11-to 12-year-olds. Pediatrics 2012;130:798–805.
168. Strufaldi R, Pompei LM, Steiner ML, et al. Effects of two combined hormonal contraceptives with the same composition and different doses on female sexual function and plasma androgen levels. Contraception 2010;82:147–154.
169. Shahnazi M, Bayatipayan S, Khalili AF, et al. Comparing the effects of the second-and third-generation oral contraceptives on sexual functioning. Iran J Nurs Midwif Res 2015;20:47–55.
170. Witting K, Santtila P, Jern P, et al. Evaluation of the female sexual function index in a population based sample from Finland. Arch Sex Behav 2008;37:912–924.
171. Machado RB, de Melo NR, Prota FE, Lopes GP, Megale A. Women's knowledge of health effects of oral contraceptives in five Brazilian cities. Contraception 2012;86:698–703.
172. Hoga LAK, Rodolpho JRC, Penteado PED, Borges ALV, Alvarez REC. Religiosity and sexuality: Counseling provided by Brazilian Protestant pastors. Sex Reprod Health 2013;4:57–63.
173. Wonglikhitpanya N, Taneepanichskul S. Effects of biphasic oral contraceptives containing desogestrel (Oilezz) on cycle control facial acne and seborrhea in healthy Thai women. J Med Assoc Thailand 2006;89:755–760.
174. Di Carlo C, Gargano V, De Rosa N, Tommaselli GA, Sparice S, Nappi C. Effects of estradiol valerate and dienogest on quality of life and sexual function according to age. Gynecol Endocrinol 2014;30:925–8.
175. Guzick DS, Huang LS, Broadman BA, Nealon M, Hornstein MD. Randomized trial of leuprolide versus continuous oral contraceptives in the treatment of endometriosis-associated pelvic pain. Fertil Steril 2011;95:1568–1573.
176. Caruso S, Rugolo S, Agnello C, Romano M, Cianci A. Quality of sexual life in hyperandrogenic women treated with an oral contraceptive containing chlormadinone acetate. J Sex Med 2009;6:3376–3384.
177. Caruso S, Agnello C, Romano M, et al. Preliminary study on the effect of four-phasic estradiol valerate and dienogest (E2V/DNG) oral contraceptive on the quality of sexual life. J Sex Med 2011;8:2841–2850.
178. Caruso S, Malandrino C, Cicero C, Ciancio F, Cariola M, Cianci A. Quality of sexual life of women on oral contraceptive continued-regimen: pilot study. J Sex Med 2013;10:460–466.
179. Goretzlehner G, Waldmann-Rex S, Schramm GA. Extended cycles with the combined oral contraceptive chlormadinone acetate 2 mg/ethinylestradiol 0.03 mg: pooled analysis of data from three large-scale, non-interventional, observational studies. Clin Drug invest 2011;31:269–277.
180. Mabrouk M, Montanari G, Di Donato N, et al. What is the impact on sexual function of laparoscopic treatment and subsequent combined oral contraceptive therapy in women with deep infiltrating endometriosis? J Sex Med 2012;9:770–778.
181. Roumen F. The contraceptive vaginal ring compared with the combined oral contraceptive pill: a comprehensive review of randomized controlled trials. Contraception 2007;75:420–429.

182. Sabatini R, Cagiano R. Comparison profiles of cycle control, side effects and sexual satisfaction of three hormonal contraceptives. Contraception 2006;74:220–223.
183. Merkatz RB, Plagianos M, Hoskin E, Cooney M, Hewett PC, Mensch BS. Acceptability of the Nestorone(R)/ethinyl estradiol contraceptive vaginal ring: development of a model; implications for introduction. Contraception 2014;90:514–521.
184. Terrell LR, Tanner AE, Hensel DJ, Blythe MJ, Fortenberry JD. Acceptability of the vaginal contraceptive ring among adolescent women. J Ped Adol Gynecol 2011;24:204–210.
185. Roumen FJ. Review of the combined contraceptive vaginal ring, NuvaRing. Ther Clin Risk Manag 2008;4:441–451.
186. Caruso S, Cianci S, Malandrino C, Cicero C, Lo Presti L, Cianci A. Quality of sexual life of women using the contraceptive vaginal ring in extended cycles: preliminary report. Euro J Contracept Repro Health 2014;19:307–314.
187. Huang Y, Merkatz R, Zhu H, Roberts K, Sitruk-Ware R, Cheng L. The free perinatal/postpartum contraceptive services project for migrant women in Shanghai: effects on the incidence of unintended pregnancy. Contraception 2014;89:521–527.
188. Sanders JN, Smith NK, Higgins JA. The intimate link: a systematic review of highly effective reversible contraception and women's sexual experience. Clin Obstet Gynecol 2014;57:777–789.
189. Boozalis A, Tutlam NT, Chrisman Robbins C, Peipert JF. Sexual desire and hormonal contraception. Obstet Gynecol 2016;127:563–572.
190. Higgins JA, Ryder K, Skarda G, Koepsel E, Bennett EA. The sexual acceptability of intrauterine contraception: A qualitative study of young adult women. Perspect Sex Repro Health 2015;47:115–122.
191. Bastianelli C, Farris M, Benagiano G. Use of the levonorgestrel-releasing intrauterine system, quality of life and sexuality. Experience in an Italian family planning center. Contraception 2011;84:402–408.
192. Roney JR, Simmons ZL. Hormonal predictors of sexual motivation in natural menstrual cycles. Horm Behav 2013;63:636–645.
193. Caruso S, Agnello C, Malandrino C, Lo Presti L, Cicero C, Cianci S. Do hormones influence women's sex? Sexual activity over the menstrual cycle. J Sex Med 2014;11:211–221.
194. Aisien AO, Enosolease ME. Safety, efficacy and acceptability of implanon a single rod implantable contraceptive (etonogestrel) in University of Benin Teaching Hospital. Nigerian Journal Of Clinical Practice 2010;13:331–335.
195. Duvan CI, Gözdemir E, Kaygusuz I, Kamalak Z, Turhan N. Etonogestrel contraceptive implant (Implanon): analysis of patient compliance and adverse effects in the breastfeeding period. Journal of the Turkish-German Gynecological Association 2010;11:141–144.
196. Gezginc K, Balci O, Karatayli R, Colakoglu MC. Contraceptive efficacy and side effects of Implanon®. Euro J Contracep Repro Health 2007;12:362–365.
197. Visconti F, Zullo F, Marra ML, et al. A new long-term reversible contraception method: sexual and metabolic impact. Translational medicine @ UniSa 2012;4:86–89.
198. Gezginc K, Balci O, Karatayli R, Colakoglu MC. Contraceptive efficacy and side effects of Implanon. Euro J Contracep Repro Health 2007;12:362–365.
199. Wanyonyi SZ, Stones WR, Sequeira E. Health-related quality of life changes among users of depot medroxyprogesterone acetate for contraception. Contraception 2011;84:e17–22.
200. Sedigheh E, Maryam GT, Ali B, Mehdi P. Comparison of complications and marital satisfaction in women taking contraceptive ampoules of cyclofem and Id contraceptive pills. Healthmed 2012;6:2689–2693.
201. Gubrium A. 'I've lost my mojo, baby': A narrative perspective on the effect of Depo-Provera on libido. Sex Res Soc Pol 2011;8:321–334.
202. Tabari MG, Moslemi L, Esmaelzadeh S, Bijani A. Comparison of side effects and marital satisfaction between the women taking cyclofem and depo-medroxyprogesterone contraceptive ampoules. Afr J Pharm Pharmaco 2012;6:1933–1937.
203. Daniels K, Daugherty J, Jones J. Current contraceptive status among women aged 15–44: United States, 2011–2013. Hyattsville, MD: National Council for Health Statistics;2014.

204. ACOG. Treatment of menorrhagia and sexual function. ACOG Clinical Review 2008;13:7–7.
205. Schaffir J, Fleming M, Waddell V. Patient perceptions regarding effect of gynecological surgery on sexuality. J Sex Med 2010;7:826–831.
206. EngenderHealth. Contraceptive Sterlization: Global Issues and Trends. New York: EngenderHealth;2002.
207. Shih G, Dube K, Sheinbein M, Borrero S, Dehlendorf C. He's a real man: a qualitative study of the social context of couples' vasectomy decisions among a racially diverse population. Am J Mens Health 2013;7:206–213.
208. Bunce A, Guest G, Searing H, et al. Factors affecting vasectomy acceptability in Tanzania. Intl Fam Plann Perspect 2007;33:13–21.
209. Al-Ali BM, Shamloul R, Ramsauer J, et al. The Effect of Vasectomy on the Sexual Life of Couples. J Sex Med 2014;11:2239–2242.
210. Daniels K, Mosher WD, Jones J, Division of Vital Statistics. Contraceptive methods women have ever used: United States, 1982–2010. Hyattsville, MD: National Council for Health Statistics;2013.
211. Jones J, Mosher WD, Daniels K, Division of Vital Statistics. Current contraceptive use in the United States, 2006–2010, and changes in patterns of use since 1995. Hyattsville, MD: National Council for Health Statistics;2012.
212. Jones RK, Lindberg LD, Higgins JA. Pull and pray or extra protection? Contraceptive strategies involving withdrawal among US adult women. Contraception 2014;90: 416–21.
213. Ciftcioglu S, Erci B. Coitus interruptus as a contraceptive method: Turkish women's perceptions and experiences. J Adv Nurs 2009;65:1686–1694.
214. Cindoglu D, Sirkeci I, Sirkeci RF. Determinants of choosing withdrawal over modern contraceptive methods in Turkey. Euro J Contracep Repro Health 2008;13:412–421.
215. Freundl G, Sivin I, Batar I. State-of-the-art of non-hormonal methods of contraception: IV. Natural family planning. Euro J Contracep Repro Health 2010;15:113–123.
216. Higgins JA, Wang Y. Which young adults are most likely to use withdrawal? The importance of pregnancy attitudes and sexual pleasure. Contraception 2015;91:320–327.
217. Ortayli N, Bulut A, Ozugurlu M, Cokar M. Why withdrawal? Why not withdrawal? Men's perspectives. Reprod Health Matter 2005;13(25):164–173.
218. Rahnama P, Hidarnia A, Amin Shokravi F, Kazemnejad A, Ghazanfari Z, Montazeri A. Withdrawal users' experiences of and attitudes to contraceptive methods: a study from Eastern district of Tehran, Iran. BMC Public Health 2010;10:779.
219. Whittaker PG, Merkh RD, Henry-Moss D, Hock-Long L. Withdrawal attitudes and experiences: a qualitative perspective among young urban adults. Perspect Sex Reprod Health 2010;42:102–109.
220. Higgins JA, Gregor L, Mathur S, Nakyanjo N, Nalugoda F, Santelli JS. Use of withdrawal (coitus interruptus) for both pregnancy and HIV prevention among young adults in Rakai, Uganda. J Sex Med 2014;11:2421–2427.
221. Mathenjwa T, Maharaj P. 'Female condoms give women greater control': A qualitative assessment of the experiences of commercial sex workers in Swaziland. Euro J Contracep Repro Health 2012;17:383–392.
222. Naidu M. Perceptions around second generation female condoms: Reporting on women's experiences. Anthropol Noteb 2013;19:25–34.
223. Peters AJ, van Driel FT, Jansen WH. Silencing women's sexuality: global AIDS policies and the case of the female condom. J Int AIDS Soc 2013;16:18452.
224. Mack N, Grey TG, Amsterdam A, Williamson N, Matta CI. Introducing female condoms to female sex workers in Central America. International Perpect Sex Repro Health 2010;36:149–155.
225. Telles Dias PR, Souto K, Page-Shafer K. Long-term female condom use among vulnerable populations in Brazil. AIDS Behav 2006;10:S67–75.

226. Okunlola MA, Morhason-Bello IO, Owonikoko KM, Adekunle AO. Female condom awareness, use and concerns among Nigerian female undergraduates. J Obstet Gynecol 2006;26:353–356.

227. Sobze Sanou M, Fokam J, Guetiya Wadoum R, et al. Condom perception and prevention of HIV/AIDS infection in Cameroon: appraisal of knowledge, attitudes and practices among level one students of the University of Dschang. Igiene e sanita pubblica 2013;69:183–194.

228. Sahin-Hodoglugil NN, Montgomery E, Kacanek D, et al. User experiences and acceptability attributes of the diaphragm and lubricant gel in an HIV prevention trial in Southern Africa. AIDS Care 2011;23:1026–1034.

229. Kraft JM, Harvey SM, Thorburn S, Henderson JT, Posner SF, Galavotti C. Intervening with couples: assessing contraceptive outcomes in a randomized pregnancy and HIV/STD risk reduction intervention trial. Women Health Iss 2007;17:52–60.

230. World Health Organization. WHO/CONRAD technical consultation on nonoxynol-9: WHO, Geneva, 9–10 Octover 2001 summary report. Geneva: World Health Organization 2003.

231. Grimes DA, Lopez LM, Raymond EG, Halpern V, Nanda K, Schulz KF. Spermicide used alone for contraception. Cochrane Database Syst Rev 2013:CD005218.

232. Thorburn S, Harvey SM, Tipton J. Diaphragm acceptability among young women at risk for HIV. Women Health 2006;44:21–39.

233. Badcock PB, Smith AMA, Richters J, et al. Characteristics of heterosexual regular relationships among a representative sample of adults: the Second Australian Study of Health and Relationships. Sex Health 2014;11:427–438.

234. Fataneh G, Marjan MH, Nasrin R, Taraneh T. Sexual function in Iranian women using different methods of contraception. J Clin Nurs 2013;22:3016–3023.

235. Sanders JN, Smith NK, Higgins JA. The intimate link: a systematic review of highly effective reversible contraception and women's sexual experience. Clinical Obstet Gynecol 2014;57:777–789.

236. Severy LJ, Spieler J. New methods of family planning: Implications for intimate behavior. J Sex Res 2000;37:258–265.

237. Scott-Sheldon LA, Johnson BT. Eroticizing creates safer sex: a research synthesis. J Primary Prevent 2006;27:619–640.

238. Philpott A, Knerr W, Boydell V. Pleasure and prevention: when good sex is safer sex. Reprod Health Matters 2006;14:23–31.

239. Annon J. The PLISSIT model: a proposed conceptual scheme for the behavioral treatment of sexuality problems. J Sex Educ Ther 1976;2:1–15.

240. Bitzer J, Giraldi A, Pfaus J. Sexual desire and hypoactive sexual desire disorder in women. Introduction and overview. Standard operating procedure (SOP Part 1). J Sex Med 2013;10:36–49.

241. Laan E, Rellini AH, Barnes T, International Society for Sexual M. Standard operating procedures for female orgasmic disorder: consensus of the International Society for Sexual Medicine. J Sex Med 2013;10:74–82.

242. Fugl-Meyer KS, Bohm-Starke N, Damsted Petersen C, Fugl-Meyer A, Parish S, Giraldi A. Standard operating procedures for female genital sexual pain. J Sex Med 2013;10:83–93.

243. Althof SE, Rosen RC, Perelman MA, Rubio-Aurioles E. Standard operating procedures for taking a sexual history. J Sex Med 2013;10:26–35.

244. Caruso S, Agnello C, Intelisano G, Farina M, Di Mari L, Sparacino L, Cianci, A. Prospective study on sexual behavior of women using 30 microg ethinylestradiol and 3 mg drospirenone oral contraceptive. Contraception 2005;72:19–23.

Mental Health and Contraception

23

Kelli Stidham Hall, PhD, MS, FNP
Julia R. Steinberg, PhD, MA

- Contraception should be situated in the broader context of patients' mental, physical, and reproductive health and wellbeing.
- Education and counseling for patients with mental health considerations should emphasize that modern contraceptives do not appear to *cause* clinically significant mood symptoms or mental health conditions, and in fact, combined oral contraceptives may improve mood symptoms for many patients.
- The majority of patients with depression and related disorders are eligible for all available contraceptive methods. Drug interactions between hormonal contraceptives and commonly used antidepressants, including selective serotonin reuptake inhibitors, are rare.
- Ethical issues surrounding reproductive autonomy and contraceptive decision-making in light of potential cognitive, emotional, and motivational impairments of patients with mental health conditions, especially serious mental illnesses, require careful consideration

Among the leading causes of disability worldwide, depression is commonly experienced by patients in their reproductive years.[1-9] Compared to men, women in the United States are approximately 1.5 to 3 times more likely to experience depression.[9] One-fifth of adult women in the United States will experience a depressive disorder in their lifetime; one in ten will experience one each year; one in nine will experience postpartum depression.[8] Figure 23-1 highlights depression prevalence rates among U.S. women over the life course – with notably steady inclines across adolescence and young adulthood, a peak in mid-adulthood, and the onset of decline in older adulthood.[10] Among younger groups of women, the prevalence of depressive disorders has been increasing over

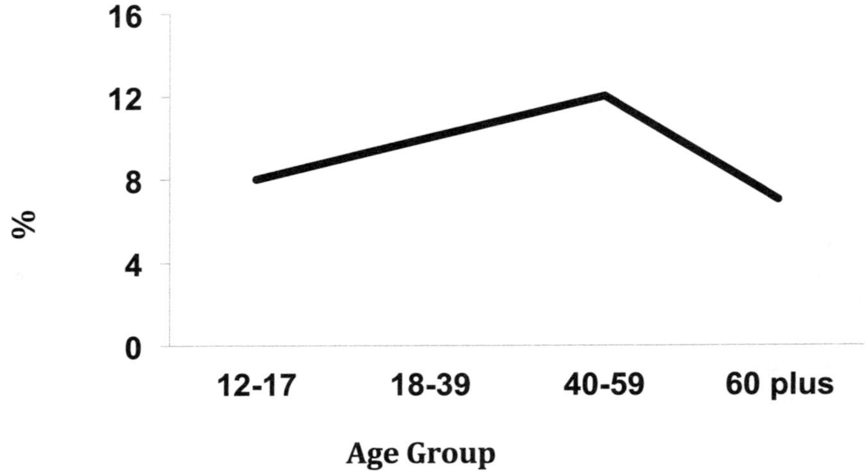

Figure 23-1 Depression prevalence rates among U.S. women, by age group[10]

the last decade.[10-14] Poor, unemployed, and less educated women experience disproportionately high rates of depressive disorders compared to socially advantaged women.[14-17] Mood disorders are highly co-morbid with other mental health conditions including anxiety, substance use, and eating disorders.[1-4]

Detection and treatment rates for depression are low among reproductive-aged women,[22,23,26-30] as are rates of mental health service use.[18,19,21] Recent population- and clinic-based studies have suggested that less than half of pregnant and non-pregnant reproductive-aged U.S. women with a major depressive episode or those meeting criteria for clinical depression receive a mental health diagnosis or treatment, even though the majority (e.g. >70%) have had contact with a health provider in the last year.[26,28,30] Compared to white women, black and Hispanic women are even less likely to receive a mental health diagnosis or treatment.[24-26] Collectively, the same groups of socially disadvantaged women who are at risk for unmet mental health needs are the very same groups of women who experience the highest rates of unintended pregnancy.[31,32]

Most people in the United States have their first depressive episode in their 20s.[7,9] Usually a depressive episode does not occur at only one single time point in a person's life, and the majority of those experiencing depression have more than one episode over their lifetime.[4] Risk factors for recurrence include severity of past depressive episode(s), being younger at time of most recent episode, and having had more than one episode already.[33,34]

Collectively, the epidemiologic trends and risk factors for depression and related disorders among reproductive-aged women have implications for the body of research linking mental and reproductive health outcomes—literature which we cover in detail later in this chapter.[35-53]

ETIOLOGY OF MOOD DISORDERS

The causes of mood disorders are not fully understood. Clinical studies of depression and anxiety suggest that deficiencies in neurotransmitters that affect mood, including serotonin, norepinephrine, dopamine, gamma-aminobutyric acid (GABA), and peptides, are likely involved.[1-4] Genetic predisposition appears to be an important precursor to such neurotransmitter deficiencies.[4] While specific "depression genes" remain unknown, there is scientific evidence of a genetic component, as women and men who have first degree relatives with depression experience a 1.5- to 3-fold risk of experiencing the condition themselves.[1-4] Additionally, psychosocial stressors may further contribute to or exacerbate the onset and symptomatology of a mood disorder. Indeed, adverse life experiences, including physical and sexual violence or trauma, poverty or economic hardship, racial/ethnic discrimination, chronic medical illnesses such as cancer, stroke or HIV/AIDs, and other social stressors are known risk factors for depression among both women and men.[1-4] Gene-environmental interactions exacerbate these risks, as biological dysfunction associated with the stress process is believed to result in altered neuronal size, functioning, repair capabilities, production of new neurons, and reduced hippocampus volume and neurocircuitry changes as a result of elevated cortisol—all of which may contribute to depression.[1-4]

THE POTENTIAL IMPACT OF HORMONAL CONTRACEPTION ON MOOD

Early contraceptive researchers in the 1960s hypothesized that synthetic estrogens and progestins in combined oral contraceptives (COCs) could potentially interact with mood-related neurotransmitters.[54-58] Articles published in the 1970s and 1980s suggested that the large steroid dosages in COCs (e.g. Enovid: 5mg norethynodrel, 75mcg mestranol) could interfere with serotonin, noradrenaline, tryptophan (an amino acid precursor to serotonin), and vitamin and endocrine metabolism.[54-58] Pyridoxine deficiency was thought to result from estrogen-related reductions in noradrenaline and serotonin in the hypothalamus,[54,55,57] while enzymatic breakdown of neurotransmitters could result from progestin-related cerebral monoamine oxidase activity.[58]

These dose-related mechanistic theories may no longer be relevant, as modern formulations of hormonal contraceptives have significantly lower steroid dosages.[58] While methodological limitations in research designs have made comparisons of findings across studies difficult and have likely contributed to conflicting results,[58-61] the majority of the most rigorous and recent studies, including placebo-controlled trials, prospective cohorts, and comprehensive reviews, has largely disputed the claims that modern hormonal contraceptives "cause" depression or mood symptoms. In fact, some have found lower rates of depression or mood symptoms in women who use COCs compared to those who do not.[64-70] Collectively, this body of scientific evidence suggests that the steroidal activity of modern methods do not have a clinically relevant physiological impact on women's mood or mood-related neuroendocrine functioning. A 2016 critical analysis of studies published over the last 30 years focusing on combined hormonal contraception and its effects on mood had four major conclusions:

- Most women using combined hormonal contraceptives reported no effect or a beneficial effect on mood, with a low incidence of adverse effects.
- Contraceptives containing less androgenic progestins may have fewer adverse effects on mood.
- Continuous and perhaps non-oral dosing of combined hormonal contraceptives have the fewest mood effects.
- Women with underlying mood disorders may be predisposed to mood symptoms, but this may reflect factors related to mood disorder itself rather than hormonal contraception.[59]

The Medical Eligibility Criteria for Contraceptive Use (MEC) report recently updated in 2016 by the U.S. Centers for Disease Control and Prevention (CDC) concluded there are no contraindications to hormonal contraception for patients with depression, basing their recommendation on evidence that does not support a causal relationship.[62] Few studies if any have used brain imaging and hormonal bioassays to assess hormonal contraception's potential impact on mood-related neuroendocrine processes. Such techniques could be useful in further clarifying these relationships.

Beyond COCs, other clinical research studies have examined whether mental health symptoms occur at higher rates among women initiating other hormonal contraceptive methods. This work is less comprehensive but has explored methods such as the depot medroxyprogesterone acetate (DMPA) injectable, the transdermal patch, vaginal ring, and long-acting reversible contraceptives (LARC) including the subdermal implant, levonorgestrel-releasing intrauterine devices (IUDs), and the copper-containing IUD.[71-78] Collectively, these studies have also found no adverse effects of these contraceptive methods on depression, anxiety, or mood symptoms.[71-78]

The Impact of Mental Health on Family Planning Outcomes

A growing body of literature documents the impact of mental health symptoms on family planning outcomes.[79-96] Women with depression and anxiety are at greater risk of experiencing an unintended pregnancy, compared to women without depression and anxiety.[83-85,93] Patients experiencing elevated mental health symptoms, like depression, anxiety and stress, are likely at higher risk of unintended pregnancies because these symptoms influence their sexual and contraceptive behaviors. Sexual behaviors that have been examined include increased numbers of sexual partners, earlier sexual debut, and more frequent sexual activity.[86-89] Contraceptive behaviors that have been examined include contraceptive choice, continuation, and consistency of use.[90-92,95-97] With respect to contraceptive choice and use, some studies find more depressive, anxiety, or stress symptoms are associated with choosing or using less effective methods,[26,91] while in contrast a few other studies with specific populations (e.g., veterans, post-abortion patients) have found more depressive, anxiety, or stress symptoms are associated with using or choosing more effective methods[79,80,96] or found no association between mental health symptoms and contraceptive behaviors at all.[81]

With respect to other contraceptive behaviors such as time to discontinuation or consistency of method use, studies have usually found that elevated depressive, anxiety, or stress symptoms are associated with early discontinuation or inconsistent method use.[71,74,82,91,92,95,97] These findings have been most widely noted for condoms and COCs and for samples of adolescent and young adult women, but have also been demonstrated for the DMPA injectable, IUDs, and implants and among cohorts spanning all reproductive ages.

In order to shed light on the direction of the relationship between mental health and contraceptive behaviors, it may be necessary to concurrently study the underlying mechanisms linking mood disorders to contraceptive behaviors. Several interesting hypotheses exist regarding behavioral and biological pathways, though they have not been investigated. First, depression and related disorders like anxiety may affect cognitive and behavioral processes around contraception use, including risk assessment, planning, social learning, and cost-benefit analysis of using contraception, perceptions of susceptibility to pregnancy, and interactions with providers.[98-110] Depressed patients may pay particular attention to negative side effects and risk-related information about hormonal contraceptives because they are attuned to negative cues in their environment.[101-103] Indeed, one study found that women experiencing elevated depressive symptoms were more likely to perceive negative mood side effects they attributed to their COC and they were also more likely to discontinue the method compared to women without depressive symptoms.[97] Excessive worry that can accompany mood disorders could potentially contribute to irrational concerns about contraceptive side effects or safety. Decreased motivation and desire for self-care could influence women's abilities to use certain user-dependent methods, like daily COCs.[99,105,108,109] Alternatively, in the provider-patient interaction, a depressed woman who lacks self-efficacy and agency may be more likely to rely on the provider's method recommendations. Collectively, these cognitive and behavioral processes may have implications for initiation and effective and continued use of contraceptive methods by patients with mental health considerations.

Second, from a biological perspective, neuroendocrine pathology associated with mood disorders could potentially amplify perceived physical symptomatology attributed to COCs. Perceived mood symptoms continue to be a primary reason why women report not using, misusing, or discontinuing hormonal contraceptives (e.g., discontinuation rates ranging from 14% to 21%),[111,112] even despite literature refuting a causal relationship between contraception and mood symptoms. Some research has suggested that women with depression, anxiety, and stress conditions are more likely to *perceive* negative mood symptoms than those without those symptoms.[97] It is possible that sensory, rather than pathophysiological, processes related to physical symptoms may be altered in COC users with mental health conditions. Rubino-Watkins et al. found that COC users with psychological stress had higher self-reported negative cognitive patterns and emotions over time than stressed women not using COCs; greater negative affect was attributed to more daily stressors among OC users versus nonusers.[101] Somatization (recurrent and frequently changing physical symptoms which cannot be explained by any known medical condition) and hypochondriasis (excessive worry about illness and the belief that one has an undiagnosed physical disease) are associated with higher rates of reported side effects of active and placebo medications among general samples.[102,103] These conditions reflect symptomatologies commonly occurring with mood disorders and thus have potential implications for patients with depression or anxiety who use hormonal contraception.

Overall, these hypotheses linking mental health and family planning, while interesting, have not been rigorously evaluated and require further study in order to inform our understanding of and clinical approaches for managing contraception in the context of depression and related conditions.

CLINICAL MANAGEMENT OF DEPRESSION IN REPRODUCTIVE HEALTH CARE SETTINGS

Patients' mental health status can have an impact on their contraceptive behaviors. Thus, detecting and diagnosing of depression and related disorders is not only important in its own right but may help patients to achieve their sexual and reproductive health goals. The following section presents a brief overview of clinical management of common mood disorders for reproductive health professionals. It should be noted, however, that scientific evidence examining what clinical practices help patients who are experiencing elevated depressive, anxiety, and stress symptoms to engage in their preferred sexual and reproductive behaviors is lacking.

Assessment of personal or family risk factors for new, recurring, or chronic mental health conditions begins with the past and family medical histories, including prior psychiatric diagnoses, cognitive behavioral and/or pharmacologic treatments, hospitalizations, suicide attempts, and social history for co-occurring issues like substance use and violence.[113-118] Suspicions of an undiagnosed or diagnosed mental health issue may arise as early during the interview as the history of present illness. Clinical presentations of mood disorders in reproductive health settings may be directly related to depression symptomatology (e.g., sad or depressed mood) but may also include more indirect presentations. An underlying problem may present with multiple and vague complaints; non-specific symptoms or pain-related syndromes, such as non-specific vulva, pelvic, vaginal, coital, or menstrual-related pain, headaches; or gastrointestinal disturbances.[118] If so, the history of present illness provides a moment to assess co-occurring mental health symptoms, including their onset, severity, and degree of functional impairment.

Other considerations for the patient interview and patient-provider communication, which are appropriate for all clinical encounters but may be given particular attention when seeing patients with diagnosed or suspected mood disorders, are listed in Table 23-1. Many patients with undiagnosed symptomatology may lack awareness and insight into their mental health status and may not recognize they are depressed. Even when they do, the stigma surrounding mental health disorders may render disclosure of depression symptoms difficult.[113-118]

Table 23-1 Patient interview techniques that are mental health sensitive

- Disclosure
- Reflective listening
- Actively engage patient
- Cultural competence
- Patience
- Non-judgmental tone
- Introduce mental health with educational statements and not questions
- Empathy
- Knowledge of mental health resources
- Reflect on your own reactions

Reproductive health providers, whose focus is often on patients' health promotion and disease prevention, are uniquely well-suited to broach holistic discussions about patients' overall health and psychological well-being as it influences sexual and reproductive health. Patients are likely to feel more comfortable and open to discussion with providers who exude patience, empathy, and a non-judgmental tone.[103-108] Reflective listening, use of open-ended questions, and simple educational statements can normalize the experience, reduce stigma, and foster trust. For example, a statement like, "Depression is one of the most common issues affecting reproductive-aged patients, and so I like to check in with all my patients about their own mental health status," may be an effective approach to initiate a conversation, whereas directive, confrontational questions should be avoided. Subtle cues of an underlying mood or anxiety disorder may be detected through careful observation of a sad voice, anxious expressions, or lethargic posture. Health providers should be attuned to transference (i.e., feeling down, sad, or upset after seeing a patient with depression or anxiety) and take the opportunity to reflect on their own feelings, emotions, and mood during and after the clinical encounter.[113,114] Helping a patient to understand that her mental health is as important as her reproductive health and that the two are interrelated may facilitate honesty, trust, and effective communication.

Standardized mental health screening instruments are effective, efficient methods to screen patients for mood disorders and should be routinely and systematically conducted in reproductive-health settings, most readily with well-woman exams or new patient visits or during any encounter in which the patient appears to have ongoing or suspected mental health symptoms.[119-131] Screening instruments elicit self-reported information about recent (e.g., over the past two weeks or month) symptoms that can be diagnostic of major depressive episode, persistent depressive disorder, or other specified or unspecified depressive disorder, as defined by a standard source such as the Diagnostic and Statistical Manual of Mental Health Disorders (DSM) or the International Statistical Classification of Disease. Commonly used instruments are noted in Table 23-2.

Table 23-2 Common depression screens

Instrument Name	Abbreviation	# of Items
PRIME-MD Patient Health Questionnaire	PHQ	2–15
Beck Depression Inventory	BDI-I or BDI-II	7–21
Center for Epidemiologic Studies Depression Scale	CES-D	4–20
Edinburgh Postnatal Depression Scale	EPDS	10
Inventory of Depressive Symptomatology – Self Rated	QIDS-SR	16

Abbreviated screens are the most feasible options for busy clinical practices where large volumes of patients are seen and time per patient is limited. The two-item Patient Health Questionnaire (PHQ-2), which is a validated shortened version of the PHQ-9 used to assess "little interest or pleasure in doing things" or "feeling down, depressed or hopeless" has documented high sensitivity (83%) and specificity (92%) rates or detecting major depressive disorder.[123] Similarly, commonly used mnemonics offer easy-to-remember guides for assessing diagnostic symptoms. For instance, with the mnemonic "*SIG E CAPS,*" a positive screen would entail reports of at least five of the following symptoms present for at least 2 weeks, all of which represent DSM-5 criteria:

Sleep – increased or decreased (if decreased, often early morning awakening)

Interest – decreased

Guilt/worthlessness

Energy – decreased or fatigued

Concentration/difficulty making decisions

Appetite and/or weight increase or decrease

Psychomotor activity – increased or decreased

Suicidal ideation

For a clinical diagnosis of a mood or anxiety disorder, typically a more comprehensive, formal structured psychiatric interview, such as the Composite International Diagnostic Interview or the Structured Clinical Interview for DSM, is required and should be conducted by a trained mental health professional.[4,10] Having readily available materials and information on local social work counselors, psychology or psychiatric services, and insurance or medication assistance programs can help providers further address patients' mental health needs. Any patient exhibiting suicidal ideation or other severe symptoms should be assessed with a suicide screening instrument and immediately referred to specialized or emergency care.[131]

Differential diagnoses of patients presenting with new onset mental health symptoms in reproductive health contexts may include pregnancy, reproductive endocrine conditions that cause estrogen deficiency, and chronic diseases like hypothyroidism, diabetes mellitus, anemia, cancer, and multiple sclerosis. These differential diagnoses are not uncommon among reproductive-aged women and can cause mood-related symptoms that mimic depression.[113,115-118] Moreover, medications such as beta-blockers or calcium channel blockers, glucocorticoids, and GnRH analogues can cause mood symptoms.[113,115-118] Laboratory evaluation to help rule out such alternative diagnoses may include serum testing for complete blood counts, basic metabolic panel, fasting glucose, fasting lipid profile, prolactin, and thyroid stimulating hormone, as well as urine testing for pregnancy.

The role of the reproductive health provider should, at a minimum, entail screening for common mood disorders, differentiating sub-clinical symptomatology from a diagnosable disorder, ruling out differential diagnoses, and providing or referring for further psychiatric evaluation and treatment when indicated. However, many such providers and settings are also equipped with the relevant knowledge, training, services, and resources to initiate and maintain a simple treatment regimen for common mental health conditions. Depression treatment options generally depend upon the severity of symptoms. Evidence-based psychological therapies, most commonly cognitive behavioral therapy or interpersonal psychotherapy, are often considered the first-line treatment for mild symptoms.[115-118, 125-127] On the other hand, pharmacologic therapy may represent the best, preferred, or most feasible and accessible treatment option for many patients. Pharmacotherapy is more effective when used in conjunction with psychotherapy.[115-118] For patients with moderate or severe symptoms, a combination of pharmacologic and psychological therapies is recommended, and in the cases of severe symptoms, primary management by a mental health specialist is advised.[115-118]

Table 23-3 summarizes the treatment goals, length, and approaches for the 3 phases of depression treatment: acute, continuation and maintenance.[113,117] Selective serotonin reuptake inhibitors (SSRIs), which work on mood-related neurotransmitters in the brain, are the most commonly used class of antidepressants and are generally a preferred treatment option because they are accompanied by fewer side effects than are other psychiatric drug classes.[113,128] The closely related serotonin-norepinephrine reuptake inhibitors (SNRIs) (e.g., duloxetine venlafaxine, and desvenlafaxime) work on both serotonin and norepinephrine. Counseling for patients initiating SSRIs and SNRIs should emphasize that mild side effects may

Table 23-3 Phases of depression treatment

Phase	Goal	Length	Treatment
Acute	Induce remission	6–8 weeks	Psychotherapy, pharmacotherapy, or both
Continuation	Preserve remission; prevent relapse	16–20 weeks	Continue treatment from acute phase
Maintenance	Protect against reoccurrence and relapse	Varies by frequency/ severity of previous episode	Continue treatment if episode was severe, risk of reoccurrence, comorbid conditions or patient preference

occur initially but generally improve with time: loss of interest, nausea, drowsiness, headache, dizziness, appetite/weight changes, decreased libido, restlessness, sweating, tremors, and dreams.[113,128] Adverse events, such as fractures and liver/renal impairment, are less common but should be monitored. Additionally, SSRIs inhibit the hepatic P450 cytochrome system (see contraceptive management section below), and older generation SSRIs like paroxetine and fluoxetine have the highest rates of drug interactions, followed by sertraline and, finally, citalopram and escitalopram, with the fewest interactions.[113,128] It may be necessary to check therapeutic blood levels and to monitor for an increase in the side effects when SSRIs are initiated in patients taking beta blockers, calcium channel blockers, digoxin, tegretol, or dilantin.[113,128] For patients with concerns about libido or weight or who have concurrent needs such as for smoking cessation or sleep aides, atypical antidepressants such as bupropion (a psychostimulant which inhibits dopamine and norepinephrine), mirtazapine (a noradrenergic and specific serotonergic antidepressant), and trazodone (a serotonin agonist and reuptake inhibitor) may offer alternatives to SSRIs and SNRIs.[113,128] Table 23-4 summarizes starting and standard dosages of the most commonly used safe and effective antidepressants that may be appropriate and feasible to initiate and manage in reproductive health settings.[113]

Several older generation classes of antidepressants still used for cases of chronic, severe or refractory depression include tricyclics (e.g., amitriptyline, imipramine, nortryptyline) and monoamine oxidase inhibitors (e.g., phenelzine, isocarboxazid). Both classes come with greater side effect profiles, are more likely to be lethal with overdose, and have higher levels of interaction with other drugs and foods.[113,116,117,128] St. John's wort (hypericum perforatum), a widely used and studied over-the-counter herbal therapy has mild antidepressant, sedative, and anxiolytic properties, but it is a cytochrome P450 (CYP450) inhibitor and thus has high levels of interactions with other medications.[136,137] Other alternative or adjunct therapies,

Table 23-4 Dosing of commonly used antidepressants[113]

Agent	Class	Starting Dose mg/day	Standard Dose mg/day
Fluoxetine (Prozac)	SSRI	20	20–40
Paroxetine (Paxil)	SSRI	20	20–40
Sertraline (Zoloft)	SSRI	50	50–150
Citalopram (Celexa)	SSRI	20	20–40
Escitalopram (Lexapro)	SSRI	10	10–20
Venlafaxine (Effexor)	SNRI	37–75	75–225
Bupropion (Wellbutrin)	NDRI	150	150–300
Duloxetine (Cymbalta)	SNRI	30	30–90

including exercise, phototherapy, sleep, acupuncture, and omega 3 fatty acid supplements, may be used as complementary or self-initiated treatments by some patients but are not to be considered first-line treatment options because the evidence regarding their effectiveness for depression remains conflicting or insufficient.[113,116,117]

In summary, there is a range of roles that reproductive health providers can play in meeting patients' mental health needs. While understudied, promoting mental health and wellbeing is not only an end in and of itself, but it may also support contraceptive management to improve patients' family planning outcomes.

Contraceptive Initiation and Management in the Context of Mental Health

Contraceptive Method Eligibility, Drug Interactions, and Safety Considerations

An overview of contraceptive method options and considerations for patients with depression and related specific mental health issues is presented in Table 23-5.[138,139] For the most part, a patient-provider shared decision-making process should inform contraceptive method selection based upon the patient's individual health circumstances, contraceptive preferences, and family planning needs, rather than a mental health diagnosis or treatment. Depression is considered a category 1 by the CDC MEC, which cites no evidence for restrictions of hormonal contraception use for patients with the mood disorder.[62] Drug interactions between modern pharmacologic antidepressant agents and hormonal contraceptives are relatively rare, and the best available scientific evidence suggests SSRIs and SNRIs do not interact with hepatic metabolism of synthetic steroids in COCs or other locally acting hormonal contraceptives.[140,141] Additionally, many patients with depression and anxiety are treated with non-pharmacologic therapies including cognitive behavioral therapy, interpersonal psychotherapy, and adjunct therapies like exercise, sleep, and healthy diet. These treatments should also not interfere with contraception or preclude use of any methods. Providers can encourage patients to participate in these treatment modalities since the principles and self-care techniques learned (e.g., problem-solving and coping skills) may also benefit patients' reproductive health decision-making and behaviors. Overall, the full range of available contraceptive methods is appropriate for the majority of patients with depression and related conditions, including those taking SSRIs or SNRIs or using adjunct therapies.

Table 23-5 Contraceptive initiation and management considerations for specific mental health issues[138,139]

	Contraceptive Method				
Mental Health Issues	**Long-acting reversible contraception (LARC)** (copper-containing intrauterine device (IUD), levonorgestrel-releasing IUD, subdermal implants)	**Progestin-only contraception** (depot medroxyprogesterone acetate injectable (DMPA), progestin-only pills (POP))	**Other hormonal contraceptive methods** (vaginal ring, transdermal patch)	**Combined oral contraceptives (COCs)**	**Condoms**
1. Adherence concerns	Highly effective and reversible with low user-maintenance; Should be considered first line	DMPA acceptable option, POPs not optimal because less tolerant of missed or late pill dosages	Less ideal than LARC and DMPA because requires monthly (ring) or weekly (patch) replacement, but acceptable; counseling on appropriate use and regular assessment for adherence necessary; emergency contraceptive provision as back-up	Not optimal; requires counseling and education on appropriate use and frequent assessment of daily adherence, missed pills; emergency contraceptive provision as back-up	Dual use of condoms plus another more effective method should be routinely encouraged to prevent sexually transmitted infections; not an optimal option for primary contraceptive method in most cases due to higher typical use failure rates than other effective methods, adherence concerns considerable user effort, and necessary partner cooperation; acceptable when all other effective options are not feasible

(continued)

Table 23-5 Contraceptive initiation and management considerations for specific mental health issues[138,139]—*(continued)*

	Contraceptive Method				
Mental Health Issues	**Long-acting reversible contraception (LARC)** (copper-containing intrauterine device (IUD), levonorgestrel-releasing IUD, subdermal implants)	**Progestin-only contraception** (depot medroxyprogesterone acetate injectable (DMPA), progestin-only pills (POP))	**Other hormonal contraceptive methods** (vaginal ring, transdermal patch)	**Combined oral contraceptives (COCs)**	**Condoms**
2. Mood side effect concerns	Copper-containing IUD optimal option for patients who prefer not to take hormones, other LARC methods also acceptable; no evidence to support LARC causes mood symptoms	Acceptable; no evidence to support DMPA or POPs cause mood symptoms	Acceptable; no evidence to support ring or patch cause mood symptoms; assess regularly for adherence issues	No evidence to support COCs cause mood symptoms; may consider lower dosage and monophasic formulations, extended cycle regimens or continuous dosing; assess regularly for adherence issues	
3. Concerns about menstrual irregularities	Acceptable; irregular bleeding patterns possible	Acceptable; irregular bleeding patterns possible with DMPA; irregular bleeding may occur with missed dosages of POPs	Acceptable	Optimal option for menstrual control; may be optimal option for patients who prefer to be in "regular" control of using contraception	
4. Postpartum depression and breast feeding	Acceptable	Acceptable	CDC MEC category 3 for patients <1 month postpartum due to potential estrogen transmission in breast milk	CDC MEC category 3 for patients <1 month postpartum due to potential estrogen transmission in breast milk	

(continued)

Table 23-5 Contraceptive initiation and management considerations for specific mental health issues[138,139]—*(continued)*

	Contraceptive Method				
Mental Health Issues	**Long-acting reversible contraception (LARC)** (copper-containing intrauterine device (IUD), levonorgestrel-releasing IUD, subdermal implants)	**Progestin-only contraception** (depot medroxyprogesterone acetate injectable (DMPA), progestin-only pills (POP))	**Other hormonal contraceptive methods** (vaginal ring, transdermal patch)	**Combined oral contraceptives (COCs)**	**Condoms**
5. Peri-menopausal depression	Acceptable	Acceptable	Acceptable; assess for contraindications to estrogen	Optimal option; has therapeutic benefit for peri-menopausal symptoms; assess for contraindications to estrogen	
6. Premenstrual dysphoric disorder (PMDD)	Acceptable	Acceptable	Acceptable	Drospirenone-containing COCs have FDA approval for PMDD	
7. Medical comorbidities including cardiovascular risks, over age 35 years and a smoker, and other estrogen contraindications	Acceptable	DMPA not optimal since may contribute to weight gain, truncal fat deposit and peripheral glucose intolerance	CDC MEC categories 3–4; contraindicated due to increased risk of VTE	CDC MEC categories 3–4; contraindicated due to increased risk of VTE	
8. Taking modern antidepressants including SSRIs or SNRIs	Acceptable	Acceptable	Acceptable	Acceptable	
9. Taking older generation antidepressants including TCAs, MAOIs or St. John's wort	Acceptable	Acceptable	Acceptable	Drug interaction concerns; not recommended	

(continued)

Table 23-5 Contraceptive initiation and management considerations for specific mental health issues[138,139]—*(continued)*

	Contraceptive Method				
Mental Health Issues	**Long-acting reversible contraception (LARC)** (copper-containing intrauterine device (IUD), levonorgestrel-releasing IUD, subdermal implants)	**Progestin-only contraception** (depot medroxyprogesterone acetate injectable (DMPA), progestin-only pills (POP))	**Other hormonal contraceptive methods** (vaginal ring, transdermal patch)	**Combined oral contraceptives (COCs)**	**Condoms**
10. Taking mood stabilizers and/or anti-epileptics	Acceptable	Acceptable	Acceptable	Drug interaction concerns; monitor drug levels, adjust dosages as necessary if other methods not feasible	
11. Taking atypical antipsychotics	Acceptable	Acceptable	Acceptable	Acceptable, may have therapeutic benefit for hyperprolactinemia	
12. Intimate partner violence	May be optimal option due to inconspicuous nature and infrequent health service visit requirements	DMPA optimal option due to inconspicuous nature but requires more frequent health service visits	Not optimal option for patients with unsupportive partner due to conspicuous nature	Not optimal option for patients with unsupportive partner due to conspicuous nature	
13. Impaired decision-making capacity	Ethical considerations due to long-term nature and informed consent for medical procedures, but reversible	DMPA optimal option because less invasive, highly effective and reversible	Not optimal since requires intact cognitive functioning	Not optimal since requires intact cognitive functioning	

Adapted with permission from Hall KS, Steinberg J, Marcus S. Contraception for Women with Mental Health Conditions. In C. A. Cwiak & R. H. Allen (Eds.), Contraception for the Medically Challenging Patient. 2014. Springer Science: New York.

Notes: LARC = long acting reversible contraception; IUD = intrauterine device; DMPA = depot medroxyprogesterone acetate; POPs = progestin-only pills; COCs = combined oral contraceptives; TCAs = tricyclic antidepressants; MAOIs = monoamine oxidase inhibitors; CDC MEC = Center for Disease Control and Prevention Medical Eligibility Criteria 2010; VTE = venous thrombotic event; SSRI = selective serotonin reuptake inhibitors; SNRI = serotonin norepinephrine reuptake inhibitors

The older generation antidepressants can interact with contraceptive steroid metabolism in the liver through inhibition of cytochrome P450 (CYP450), potentially leading to decreased contraceptive efficacy; additionally, reduced hepatic metabolism can also lead to antidepressant side effects or toxicity.[113-118,141] St. John's wort may induce the cytochrome P450 system and subsequently reduce contraceptive steroid availability, by 13% to15% one study found.[136,137] So while systemic hormonal contraceptive methods are not unsafe or contraindicated for patients taking these more intensive psychiatric treatments, and decreased hormonal serum hormonal levels do not appear to translate to clinically relevant increased pregnancy rates, back-up methods should be advised. Other safe alternatives for patients on tricyclic antidepressants, monoamine oxidase inhibitors, and St. John's wort include DMPA and locally-acting hormonal contraceptive methods, such as the levonorgestrel-releasing IUD, as well as non-hormonal methods such as the copper-containing IUD. Contraceptive contraindications for other psychiatric medication classes that may be used among patients with serious mental illnesses are discussed later in this chapter.

Another consideration in method selection for patients with mental health considerations is reproductive autonomy. Patients with depression may be more likely to lack agency and thus may be more likely to defer to the provider to make the contraceptive decision than would patients without depression who may be more assertive and active in the decision-making process. Generally, providers have a responsibility to provide patients with information about all available contraceptive methods—including their strengths and limitations in the context of mental and physical health status—and empower them with confidence to make an informed decision that is best for their health status and needs.

Hormonal Formulation Considerations

Most patients with depression and related disorders will do well on most types of COCs, and in fact research has suggested that the experiences of women generally with perceived side effects are similar across the many different available formulations of COCs (there are more than 90 different Food and Drug Administration (FDA)-approved COCs in the U.S. alone).[143-145] Contraceptive counseling should emphasize this point. However, several theoretical considerations may be useful in helping patients select the most suitable formulation, particularly for those patients who may have difficulty finding a satisfactory pill. Of note, these considerations have been given little to no attention in research, but they may have physiologic and mechanistic relevance and thus may be useful in guiding clinical management of hormonal contraception for patients with mood disorders.

A primary consideration is dosage, given the dose-response relationship with COCs and side effects noted with the earliest pills. Thus, formulations with the lowest possible dosages (i.e., 20 mcg versus >20 mcg) may potentially minimize the risk of mood side effects.[146]

Progestin type, phasic dosing, and extended or continuous regimens are other considerations for COC selection among patients with depression and related conditions. A recent comprehensive review found that COCs containing less androgenic progestins may be less likely to contribute to mood symptoms compared to pills with higher androgenic properties.[59] Fourth-generation drospirenone-containing COCs have an FDA-approved indication for treatment of premenstrual dysphoric disorder (PMDD)-related mood symptoms and thus may be beneficial for some patients with depression and anxiety disorders (see more on PMDD later in this chapter).[145] Levonorgestrel- and norgestrel-containing COCs (second generation) are not known to contribute to mood symptoms, and given their widespread use, also offer suitable options.[147-149] Many of these progestins are available in various phasic dosages, which could have relevance for cyclic mood symptoms due to variable circulating estrogen levels during ovulation and menses. For patients with cyclic mood concerns, monophasic formulations offer a steady dose (versus triphasic or 4-phasic formulations) to better stabilize hormone levels and minimize the risk of mood symptoms.[149,150] Patients who report mood symptoms during their placebo week (i.e., estrogen withdrawal) may benefit from COCs with extended cycle regimens (e.g., 24/4) or continuous dosing (i.e. skipping inactive pills), which would reduce or eliminate the estrogen withdrawal period.[150]

Other Method Considerations

As noted, patients with mood or anxiety disorders are potentially eligible for the full range of contraceptive methods. In the context of mood disorders, however, other factors beyond safety should be considered in a shared patient-provider contraceptive decision-making process. Most notably, adherence issues should be addressed in initiation and management of contraceptive methods given that some research finds patients with depression, anxiety and psychological stress are at increased risk for contraceptive nonuse, misuse and discontinuation; the most compelling body of evidence presented earlier in this chapter is for user-dependent methods including condoms and COCs. In addition, given that some research has found more depressive symptoms are associated with choosing or using more effective methods, providers should make sure patients are exercising their desires rather than those of the provider. As hypothesized in previous sections, cognitive difficulty with memory, distraction, disinterest, lack of energy, and emotional lability that accompany depression and anxiety may make taking a daily COC difficult for some patients. Similarly, lack of autonomy may make condom negotiation challenging. Long-acting reversible contraceptive methods (LARCs), including IUDs and the subdermal implant, have the greatest contraceptive efficacy, are cost-effective, require little user burden, induce less worry and hassle, and may offer the ideal method choices for patients with mental health considerations who wish to avoid an unintended pregnancy.[145,151-154] For others who may not prefer LARCs or who desire more hands-on control of using their method or worry about menstrual irregularity, the vaginal ring, transdermal patch, or COCs are alternative options.

Contraceptive Counseling Considerations

Education and counseling are a critical components of contraceptive initiation and management for patients with mental health considerations. The scope of counseling needs among patients with mood disorders may be broad, and counseling should ultimately be tailored to individual patient's specific needs and circumstances. Contraceptive counseling should occur within a larger discussion of sexuality, reproductive health promotion, risk reduction and disease prevention, pregnancy intentions and readiness for pregnancy (emphasizing the value of stable social conditions and interpersonal relationships), and individual contraceptive expectations and preferences.[142] Several key education and counseling strategies which may be universally applicable are summarized in Table 23-6. At a minimum, contraceptive counseling should dispel myths about side effects, reinforce the benefits of modern methods for pregnancy prevention and non-contraceptive effects (e.g., improved mood and acne, protection from ovarian and uterine cancer), address sexual risk behaviors

Table 23-6 Contraceptive counseling strategies in consideration of mental health

- Employ universal mental health screening to identify patients with elevated symptoms who are potentially at risk of contraceptive nonuse, misuse, and discontinuation.
- Assess for reduced reproductive autonomy.
- Emphasize method efficacy and effectiveness in context of mental health symptoms.
- Educate about the mood benefits of most available modern hormonal formulations.
- Dispel myths about mood side effects.
- Discuss benefits of long-acting methods.
- Assess for non-adherence with antidepressants, which may raise a red flag for non-adherence with contraception.
- Facilitate informed and shared patient-provider decision-making, tailoring method selection to patients' preferences and needs.
- Address dual protection and risk for sexually transmitted infections.

and condom use given an increased risk for sexually transmitted infections experienced among patients with depression and anxiety, and evaluate concurrent treatment adherence issues among patients who are taking antidepressants and contraception.[155-164] (See Chapter 2 for more complete discussion of patient-centered contraception counseling.)

Providers should also be aware that the patient-provider interaction may be affected by patients' mental health symptoms. Those with more depressive, anxiety, or stress symptoms may feel less control of their lives and so be more accepting of a provider's recommendation for a contraceptive method. Thus, ensuring patients are comfortable with and own their choice of the method may be critical to their using it correctly and consistently.

Knowledge of contraceptive methods is low among reproductive-aged women generally,[156] and for patients with mental health conditions, provision of repeated and specific educational information on user-related method characteristics including effectiveness rates may be useful. Contraceptive information presented should be accurate, simple, clear, and provided at a time when patients are most receptive.[142] Evidence-based counseling techniques like motivational interviewing can be used to focus attention on specific behaviors that may need to change (e.g., frequent missed pills, condom nonuse), to evoke motivation for change by increasing confidence and readiness, and to plan practical steps to improve contraceptive behaviors.[118,157,165] Equipping patients with strategies to improve accuracy and consistency of medication use in the context of daily life, such as setting a cell phone reminder or taking pills when brushing teeth before bedtime may increase the likelihood of contraceptive method continuation and satisfaction.[145] Simple written educational materials can supplement verbal communication. (See Chapter 8 on Combined Oral Contraceptives.)

SPECIAL CASES OF MENTAL HEALTH AND CONTRACEPTIVE MANAGEMENT

Beyond common mood disorders, there are several other special cases of mental health or related conditions that may be encountered in reproductive health settings.

Premenstrual Dysphoric Disorder (PMDD)

PMDD is a severe, chronic, and disabling form of premenstrual syndrome (PMS) that follows a predictable cyclic pattern with symptoms beginning in the late luteal phase of the menstrual cycle after ovulation and then ending shortly after menses begins.[166,167] Both PMS and PMDD both have associated physical and emotional symptoms that may include moodiness, abdominal cramps, headache, bloating, breast tenderness, fatigue, or changes in sleep and eating habits.[166,167] However, PMDD can cause extreme moodiness or similar behavioral symptoms, including sadness or hopelessness, anxiety or tension, or marked irritability or anger. Underlying depressive or anxiety disorders commonly co-occur in women with PMDD or PMS, and cyclic hormonal changes can worsen mood symptomatology.[166,167] The goal of treatment for PMDD is to help alleviate the patient's one or two most troubling symptoms, which should be identified through counseling and shared decision-making. Patients can be educated on the symptom-reducing benefits of lifestyle modifications, including diet, exercise, and sleep. COCs may be therapeutic to control or reduce symptoms, particularly if taken as an extended cycle or continuous dosing regimen with no hormone-free period (i.e., placebo period) or a shortened hormone-free period.[166,167] The fourth-generation drospirenone/ethinyl estradiol pill has an FDA indication for psychiatric treatment of PMDD. Commonly used antidepressants, particularly SSRIs, may also be recommended as the first-line treatment for many patients with PMDD.[166,167] The management of SSRIs for PMDD is generally similar to their management for major depressive disorder, such that for the most part they are taken as standard dosing all month long.[166,167] However, they may also be prescribed only in the interval between ovulation and onset of menses (days 14-28). Finally, there is equivocal evidence on the effectiveness of alternative therapies for treatment of PMDD, but for some women helpful stress reduction techniques include yoga, acupuncture, massage, and nutritional supplements including calcium (1200 mg/day), vitamin B6, magnesium, and L-tryptophan.[166,167] (See Chapter 1 on menstrual cycle issues.)

Postpartum and Perimenopausal Depression

Rates of postpartum and perimenopausal depression among U.S. women are estimated at 10% to 20%.[4, 168-170] These reproductive-specific cases of depression have diagnostic criteria similar to major depressive disorder except when onset occurs following pregnancy or during perimenopause.[4,168,169, 171-175] First-line treatment recommendations for postpartum and perimenopausal depression are the same as those for major depressive disorder—psychotherapy and SSRIs, which should not interfere with modern hormonal contraceptive methods. For breastfeeding postpartum patients, it is believed that possible reductions in breast milk production and venous thromboembolism (VTE) risk may occur with the estrogen in many hormonal methods, and thus, progestin-only methods including the levonorgestrel-releasing IUD, subdermal implant, DMPA injectable, or progestin-only pills are safer alternatives for those with depressive symptoms.[62,145] For perimenopausal patients who may experience hormonal fluctuations and mood, menstrual and hot flash symptoms, COCs, the patch, or ring can help stabilize hormone levels while also preventing pregnancy.[170-175] However, other contraindications to estrogen use should be evaluated prior to initiation and throughout treatment for perimenopausal patients with cardiovascular risk factors and tobacco use.[62] Notably, given that postpartum and perimenopausal patients may not be aware of their risks for unintended pregnancy, explicit discussions of contraception should occur during education and counseling sessions in these periods.

Intimate Partner Violence

Intimate partner violence is an issue closely related to mental and reproductive health with important implications for reproductive autonomy that should be addressed within contraceptive counseling and management. Intimate partner violence—rape, physical violence, or stalking by a sexual partner—is estimated to affect more than 1 in 3 women in their lifetimes.[176,177] Rates of depression and anxiety are higher among women who have experienced violence compared to those who have not, and women with mental health disorders may be particularly susceptible to being victims of intimate partner violence.[176-178] Women in violent relationships may experience reproductive coercion, contraceptive sabotage, intentional exposure to sexually transmitted infections, unintended pregnancy, and lack of control over contraceptive use, their pregnancy outcomes, and access to health services.[34,176,179,180] Routine screening for intimate partner violence with simple questions such as, "Has your partner ever hit, slapped, kicked, bitten, pushed, choked, shoved, or physically hurt you?" can identify patients who may have special contraceptive considerations.[176] Providers can work with patients to select methods that minimize the likelihood of exacerbating partner resistance or violence and maximize contraceptive control and reproductive autonomy. IUDs or the sub-dermal implant may offer other subtle, highly effective options that require less frequent health service visits, while the DMPA injectable is an effective, inconspicuous contraceptive method that is controlled by the woman.

Serious Mental Illness (SMI)

While psychotic disorders like schizophrenia, bipolar disorder, and borderline personality disorder occur less commonly among reproductive-aged women than do mood and anxiety disorders,[181,182] these serious mental illnesses (SMIs) have important implications for patients' family planning.[183] Patients with SMI may experience cognitive impairments, impulsivity, self-destructive behaviors, poor judgment, deficits in reality testing (objective evaluation of an emotion or thought in context of real life), and co-occurring substance misuse that can affect contraceptive decision-making and behaviors.[142,183-193] Patients taking atypical antipsychotics may believe they are not at risk for pregnancy because of menstrual irregularities or they may believe that their antipsychotic medication offers contraceptive protection, neither of which is correct. While understudied, patients with SMI may be at greater risk of sex-associated adverse consequences than are patients without SMI. Patients with SMI tend to lack basic knowledge of sexuality and reproduction, have misperceptions about contraception, have limited access to contraceptive methods, and experience higher rates of non-adherence to contraceptive regimens, unintended pregnancy, sexually transmitted infections, and non-consensual and transactional sex.[142,183-193] Thus, reproductive health providers can play an important role in health promotion and unintended pregnancy prevention for this vulnerable group.

Reproductive autonomy and coercion are concerns when providing contraceptive care for patients with SMI, whose dynamic individual reproductive desires and values should be weighed with their risk of unintended pregnancy. Reproductive health providers have an ethical responsibility to try to help these patients understand, to the extent possible, the adverse health and social consequences that unintended pregnancy can have for themselves and their offspring.[183,185,186] A comprehensive contraceptive education, counseling, and shared decision-making process can help patients with SMI optimize choices, taking into account co-occurring medical conditions, individual preferences, and the likelihood of method success. Routine mental status exams will ensure they are able to attend to, absorb, retain, and recall information disclosed in contraceptive counseling sessions, appreciate the information and its significance for their lives, evaluate the consequences, express both cognitive and evaluative understanding, and communicate a decision based upon that understanding.[189,190] When shared decision-making and informed consent is not fully possible, providers should rely upon highly effective reversible contraceptive methods so that family planning needs in the context of a patient's mental health status can be regularly re-evaluated.

The majority of patients with SMI are eligible for the wide range of available contraceptive methods. Permanent sterilization may not be ethically appropriate for many patients with SMI given their reduced decision-making and informed consent capacity, but LARC methods are highly effective and reversible alternatives. In most cases, levonorgestrel-releasing and copper-containing IUDs and the subdermal implant should be considered as first line methods for patients with SMI desiring contraception. Given high occurrence of SMI with other chronic disease comorbidities including diabetes, obesity, breast cancer, or hypertension, and smoking over 35 years of age, non-estrogen containing methods like LARCs also offer the safest options, and are highly effective, have few adherence issues, and little cardiovascular risk.[62,188,191-194]

On the other hand, LARCs require provider-controlled insertion and removal procedures, which may also present a dilemma for informed consent. Other progestin-only methods like the DMPA injectable and progestin-only pills (POPs) are intermediate or shorter-acting, effective methods that offer strong alternatives to LARCs for patients with SMI who have contraindications to estrogen. However, DMPA requires the patient to come back for a shot every 3 months, which may be hard for someone with an SMI. Patients using neuroleptics who have medical morbidities and are using DMPA may be at risk for weight gain, truncal fat deposit, and peripheral glucose intolerance, so monitoring is indicated.[195-197]

For patients with SMI who are eligible for estrogen-containing contraceptives and who do not want or have access to LARC, reasonable options include combined hormonal methods, including the vaginal ring, transdermal patch, and COCs.[145] The effectiveness of these methods relies heavily on correct use. This is even more true for patients on POPs, which must be taken within a 3-hour time-frame daily for effectiveness and have irregular bleeding profiles with missed or late dosages.[145] Highly user-dependent barrier methods like condoms and diaphragms should be considered low priority options for patients with SMIs. Although, given the elevated HIV/STI risk among this population, dual method use (i.e., condoms plus another effective contraceptive) should be encouraged.[198-201] Emergency contraception offers a back-up strategy for unplanned, unprotected sex. (See Chapter 10 on Emergency Contraception.)

Another major consideration for contraceptive method selection for patients with SMIs is safety and drug interactions with medications used to treat schizophrenia and bipolar disorder. Mood stabilizers, including lamotrigine, carbamazepine, and topiramate, can induce CYP450 3A4 causing enhanced hepatic metabolism of contraceptive steroids, particularly those found in oral formulations, and potentially decreased contraceptive efficacy.[196,197, 202-208] Antipsychotic medications, including clozapine and chlorpromazine, are metabolized by the liver, and contraceptive steroids can cause a significant increase in antipsychotic levels resulting in severe side effects such as hypotension, sedation, and tremor.[209-211] Serum circulating levels of anti-epileptics, such as valproate and lamotrigine, can be reduced by contraceptive steroids, rendering them less effective.[208-211] Providers should monitor psychiatric drug levels and adjust dosages as needed for oral hormonal contraceptive users.[208-211] For patients with SMIs and the potential for drug interactions, the local action of the IUDs or the high dose of the DMPA injectable offer effective alternative contraceptive options; both methods have comparable continuation rates and low rates of psychiatric complications and hospitalization.[193,212,213]

A final drug consideration for patients with SMI is hyperprolactinemia and suppression of the hypothalamic-pituitary-gonadal axis resulting from use of older atypical antipsychotics (risperidone>aripiprazole>ziprasidone). This suppression can cause menstrual irregularities, amenorrhoea, sexual dysfunction, infertility issues, and galactorrhoea.[214,215] For these patients, estradiol supplementation for neuroendocrine regulation is recommended, and some research has shown that estrogen, in the form of COCs, may be therapeutic in modulating the expression of psychotic symptoms.[215-219] Hypothalamic-pituitary-gonadal axis suppression is less of a concern for patients taking newer antipsychotics.[214,216,219] Should COCs be used as primary contraception for patients on atypical antipsychotics, education and counseling should emphasize the importance of correct and continued use of the daily pill, along with the benefits of dual protection with condoms.

Conclusions

Helping patients plan healthy pregnancies and prevent unintended pregnancies should be a clinical priority for all everyone, but especially for those with depression and related disorders. Contraception should be situated in the holistic context of patients' mental, physical, and reproductive health and wellbeing. Family planning providers, who are often the sole source of healthcare for reproductive-aged women, are uniquely well-suited to address interrelated mental and reproductive health needs. In this chapter, we have attempted to highlight an integrated approach to family planning care—one that prioritizes mental health screening and basic treatment in reproductive health settings, and vice versa—the value of contraceptive initiation and management strategies tailored to mental health considerations. While these suggestions for the management of contraception in the context of depression and related disorders are based upon the best available scientific evidence and clinical practices to date, many questions regarding the interrelationships between mental health and contraception remain unanswered. There are several notable areas for future research. First, the specific cognitive, behavioral, and biological mechanisms linking depression, anxiety and related conditions to risky sexual and contraceptive behaviors, as well as perceived mood side effects, warrants attention. A more nuanced understanding of the dynamic and longitudinal interrelationships between mental and reproductive health across patients' lifespans could provide insight into potentially vulnerable periods that may benefit from targeted psychiatric screening and treatment strategies, as well as tailored family planning education and counseling interventions. It is unknown whether treatment of depression and related disorders may also directly or indirectly improve patients' contraceptive behaviors and outcomes. The impact of mental health morbidity on reproductive autonomy and decision-making has received little research attention but is a timely consideration in efforts around improving patient-centered models of reproductive healthcare. Finally, the potentially unique family planning needs of patients with SMIs have been understudied. Future work in these areas may ultimately inform more holistic, rigorous, evidence-based approaches to contraceptive care in the broader realm of patients' mental and physical health.

Author Disclosures—Hall: None. Steinberg: None.

References

1. U.S. Department of Health and Human Services' Office on Women's Health; Substance Abuse and Mental Health Services Administration. Action steps for improving women's mental health. 2009: 1–64. www.store.samhsa.gov/shin/content/OWH09-PROFESSIONAL/OWH09-PROFESSIONAL.pdf. Accessed August 17, 2017.
2. U.S. Department of Health and Human Services. Mental Health. Healthy people 2020. Accessed September 27, 2013. http://www.healthypeople.gov/2020/LHI/mentalHealth.aspx
3. World Health Organization. The World Health Report 2001, Mental Health: new understanding, new hope. 2001: 1–169. www.who.int/whr/2001/en/whr01_en.pdf?ua=1. Accessed August 17, 2017.
4. American Psychiatric Association. Diagnostic and statistical manual of mental disorders, 5th edition. Text revised. Washington, DC: APA. 2013.
5. Gore FM, Bloem PJN, Patton GC, Ferguson J, et al. Global burden of disease in young people aged 10–24 years: a systematic analysis. Lancet 2011;377;2093–2102.
6. World Health Organization. The Global burden of disease: 2004 update. Geneva, Switzerland: WHO.
7. Kessler RC. Epidemiology of women and depression. J Affect Dis 2003;74:5–13.
8. Harvard Medical School. National Comorbidity Survey. 2009. www.hcp.med.harvard.edu/ncs/index.php. Accessed September 27, 2013.
9. Kessler RC, Berglund P, Demler O, Jin R, Koretz D, Merikangas KR, et al. The epidemiology of major depressive disorder: Results from the National Comorbidity Survey Replication (NCS-R). JAMA 2003;289:3095–3105.
10. Centers for Disease Control and Prevention. Prevalence of current depression among persons aged ≥12 years, by age group and sex—United States, National Health and Nutrition Examination Survey, 2007–2010. MMWR 2012;60:1747.
11. Cross-National Collaborative Group. The changing rate of major depression. Cross-national comparisons. JAMA 1992;268:3098–3105.
12. Compton WM, Conway KP, Stinson FS, Grant BF. Changes in the prevalence of major depression and substance use disorders in the United States between 1991–1992 and 2001–2002. Am J Psychiatry 2006;163:2141–2147.
13. Wittchen Hu, Zhao S, Kessler RC, Eaton WW. DSM-III-R generalized anxiety disorder in the National Comorbidity Survey. Arch Gen Psychiatry 1994;51:355–64.
14. American Psychological Association. Women and depression. www.apa.org/about/gr/issues/women/depression.aspx. Accessed October 24, 2012.
15. Mcleod JD, Kessler RC. Socioeconomic status differences in vulnerability to undesired life events. J Health Soc Behav 1990;31:162–72.
16. Office of the Surgeon General, Center for Mental Health Services, National Institute of Mental Health. Mental health: culture, race, and ethnicity: a supplement to mental health: a report of the Surgeon General 2001. Rockville (MD): Substance Abuse and Mental Health Services Administration.

17. Lorant V, Deliege D, Eaton W, Robert A, Philippot P, & Ansseau M. Socioeconomic inequalities in depression: A meta-analysis. Am J Epidemiol 2003;157:98–112.
18. National Institute of Mental Health. Use of mental health services and treatment among adults. www.nimh.nih.gov/statistics/3USwE_MT_ADULT.shtml. Accessed October 24, 2012.
19. National Institute of Mental Health. Use of mental health services and treatment among children. www.nimh.nih.gov/statistics/1NHANES.shtml. Accessed October 24, 2012.
20. Higgins ES. A review of unrecognized mental illness in primary care; prevalence, natural history and efforts to change the course. Arch Fam Med 1994:3:3908–917.
21. Wang PS, Lane M, Olfson M, Pincus HA, Wells KB, Kessler RC. Twelve month use of mental health services in the United States. Arch Gen Psychiatry 2005;62:629–640.
22. Barrio L, Burt V. Depression in pregnancy: Strategies for primary care management. Dealing with under-diagnosed and undertreated problem. Women's Health Prim Care 2000;3:490.
23. Miranda J, Chung JY, Green BL, Krupnick J, Siddique J, Revicki DA, Belin T. Treating depression in predominantly low-income young minority women: a randomized controlled trial. JAMA 2003;290:57–65.
24. Carrington CH. Clinical depression in African American women: Diagnosis, treatment and research. J Clin Psychol 2006;62:779–91.
25. Das AK, Ofson M, McCurtis HL, Weissman MM. Depression in African Americans: breaking barriers to detection and treatment. J Fam Pract 2006;55:30–9.
26. Farr SL, Dietz PM, Williams JR, Gibbs FA, Tregear S. Depression screening and treatment among non-pregnant women of reproductive age in the United States, 1990–2010. Prev Chron Dis 2011;8:A122.
27. Lee Li-Ching, Casanueva CE, Martin SL. Depression among female family planning patients: prevalence, risk factors and use of mental health services. J Women's Health 2005;14:225–232.
28. Ko JY, Farr SL, Dietz PM, Robbins CL. Depression and treatment among US pregnant and non-pregnant women of reproductive age, 2005-2009. J Women's Health 2012;21:830–6.
29. Dennis CL, Ross LE, Grigoriadis S. Psychosocial and psychological interventions for treating antenatal depression. Cochrane Database Syst Rev 2007;3.
30. Farr SL, Bitsko RH, Hayes DK, Dietz PM. Mental health and access to services among US women of reproductive aged. Am J Obstet Gynecol 2010;203:e1–9.
31. Finer LB, Henshaw SK. Disparities in rates of unintended pregnancy in the United States, 1994 and 2001. Persp Sex Reprod Health 2006;38:90–6.
32. Frost JJ, Singh S, Finer LB. Factors associated with contraceptive use and nonuse, United States, 2004. Perspect Sex Reprod Health 2007; 39:48–55.
33. Coryell W, Endicott J, Keller MB. Predictors of relapse into major depressive disorder in a nonclinical population. Am J Psychiat 1991;148:1353–1358.
34. Eaton WW, Anthony JC, Gallo J, et al. Natural history of diagnostic interview schedule/DSM-IV major depression. The Baltimore Epidemiologic Catchment Area follow-up. Arch Gen Psychiat 1997; 54:993–999.
35. Grote NK, Bridge JA, Gavin AR, Melville JL, Iyengar S, Katon WJ. A meta-analysis of depression during pregnancy and the risk of pre-term birth, low birth weight and intrauterine growth restriction. Arch Gen Psychiatry 2010;67:1012–1024.
36. Flynn HA, Walton MA, Chermack ST, Cunningham RM, Marcus SM. Brief detection and co-occurrence of violence, depression and alcohol risk in prenatal care settings. Arch Women's Ment Health 2007;10:155–161.
37. Alder J, Fink N, Bitzer J, Hosli I, Holzgreve W. Depression and anxiety during pregnancy: A risk factor the obstetric, fetal and neonatal outcome? A critical review of the literature. J Maternal-Fetal Neonatal Med 2007;20:189–209.
38. Kelly RH, Russo J, Holt V, et al. Psychiatric and substance use disorders as risk factors for low birth weight and preterm delivery. Obstet Gynecol 2002;100:297–304.

39. Vesga-Lopez O, Blanco C, Keyes K, Olfson M, Grant BF, Hasin DS. Psychiatric disorders in pregnant and postpartum women in the United States. Arch Gen Psychiatr 2008;65:805–815.
40. Williams KE, Marsh WK, Rasgon NL. Mood disorders and fertility in women: a critical review of the literature and implications for future research. Hum Reprod Update 2007;13:607–616.
41. Bennett I M, Culhane JF, McColuum KF, Elo IT. Unintended rapid repeat pregnancy and low education status: Any role for depression and contraceptive use? Obstet Gynecol 2006;194:749–54.
42. Steinberg JR, Trussell J, Hall KS, Guthrie K. Fatal flaws in a recent meta-analysis on abortion and mental health. Contraception 2012;86:4307.
43. Takahashi S, Tsuchiya KJ, Matsumoto K, Suzuki K, Mori N, Takei N. Psychosocial determinants of mistimed and unwanted pregnancy: the Hamamatsu birth cohort study. J Matern Child Health 2012;16:947–955.
44. Steinberg JR, Becker D, Henderson JT. Does the outcome of a first pregnancy predict depression, suicidal ideation, or lower self-esteem? Data from the National Comorbidity Survey. Am J Orthopsychiatry 2011;81:193–201.
45. Steinberg JR, Finer LB. Examining the association of abortion history and current mental health: A reanalysis of the National Comorbidity Survey using a common-risk-factors model. Soc Sci Med 2011;72:72–82.
46. Kessler RC, Berglund PA, Foster CL, Saunders WB, Stang PE, Walters EE Social consequences of psychiatric disorders, II: Teenage parenthood. Am J Psychiatry 1997;154:1405–1411.
47. Lancaster CA, Gold KJ, Flynn HA, Yoo H, Marcus SM, Davis MM. Risk factors for depressive symptoms during pregnancy: A systematic review. Am J Obstet Gynecol 2010;205:5–14.
48. Gavin NI, Gaynes BN, Lohr KN, Meltzer-Brody S, Gartlehner G, Swinson T. Perinatal depression: a systematic review of prevalence and incidence. Obstet Gynecol 2005;106:1071–83.
49. Marcus S, Flynn H, Blow F, Barry K. Depressive symptoms among pregnant women screening in obstetrics settings. J Women's Health 2003;12:373–380.
50. Milgrom J, Gemmill AW, Bilszta JL, et al. Antenatal risk factors for postnatal depression: a large prospective study. J Affect Dis 2008;108(1-2):147–57.
51. Beck CT. Predictors of postpartum depression: An update. Nursing Research 2001; 50:278–285.
52. Marcus SM, Flynn HA, Young E, Ghaziuddin N, Mudd S. Recurrent depression in women through the lifespan. In American Psychiatric Press Review of Psychiatry, M. Riba and J Oldham (eds.). American Psychiatric Press, Inc., Washington DC, 2:19–50.
53. Silverman JG, Raj A, Mucci LA, Hathaway JE. Dating violence against adolescent girls and associated substance use, unhealthy weight control, sexual risk behavior, pregnancy, and suicidality. JAMA 2001;286:572–579.
54. Moller SE. Effect of oral contraceptives on tryptophan and tyrosine availability: Evidence for a possible contribution to mental depression. Neuropsychobio 1981;7: 192–200.
55. Parry BL, Rush AJ. Oral contraceptives and depressive symptomatology: Biologic mechanisms. Compar Psychiatr 1979:20:347–58.
56. Sheenan DV, Sheenan KH. Psychiatric aspects of oral contraceptive use. Psychiatr Ann 1976;6:500–8.
57. Winston F. Oral contraceptives, pyridoxine and depression. Am J Psychiatr 1973;130:1217–21.
58. Robinson SA, Dowell M, Pedulla D, McCauley L. Do the emotional side-effects of hormonal contraceptives come from pharmacologic or psychological mechanisms? Med Hypotheses 2004;63:268–73.
59. Schaffir J, Worly BL, Gur T. Combined hormonal contraception and its effects on mood: a critical review. Eur J Contraception Reprod Health Care 2016;21:347–355.

60. Zethraeus N, Dreber A, Ranehill E, Blomberg L, Labrie F, Schoultz B, Johannesson M, Hirschberg AL. A first-choice combined oral contraceptive influences general well-being in healthy women: a double-blind randomized placebo-controlled trial. Fert Steril 2017;107:128–1245.
61. Skovlund CW, Morch LS, Kessing LV, et al. Association of hormonal contraception with depression. JAMA Psychiat 2016;73:1154–1162.
62. Centers for Disease Control and Prevention. U.S. Medical Eligibility Criteria for Contraceptive Use, 2016. MMWR 2016;65:1–104.
63. Vessey MP, McPherson K, Lawless M, Yeates D. Oral contraception and serious psychiatric illness: absence of an association. Br J Psychiatr 1985;146:45–49.
64. Duke JM, Sibbritt DW, Young AF. Is there an association between the use of oral contraception and depressive symptoms in young Australian women? Contraception 2007;75:27–31.
65. Walker A, Bancroft J. Relationship between premenstrual symptoms and oral contraceptive use: a controlled study. Psychosom Med 1990;52:86–96.
66. O'Connell K, Davis AR, Kerns J. Oral contraceptives: side effects and depression in adolescent girls. Contraception 2007;75:299–304.
67. Deijen JB, Duyn KJ, Jansen WA, Klittsie JW. Use of a monophasic low-dose oral contraceptive in relation to mental functioning. Contraception 1992;46:359–67.
68. Almagor M, Ben-Porath MS. Mood changes during the menstrual cycle and their relation to the use of oral contraceptives. J Psychosom Res 1991;35:721–8.
69. Sanders SA, Graham CA, Bass JL, Bancroft J. A prospective study of the effects of oral contraceptives on sexuality and wellbeing and their relationship to discontinuation. Contraception 2001;64:51–8.
70. Segebladh B, Borgstrom A, Odlind V, Bixo M, Sundstrom-Poromaa I. Prevalence of psychiatric disorders and premenstrual dysphoric symptoms in patients with experience of adverse mood during treatment with combined oral contraceptives. Contraception 2009; 79:50–5.
71. Westhoff C, Truman C, Kalmuss D, et al. Depressive symptoms and Depo-Provera. Contraception 1998;57:237–40.
72. Gupta N, O'Brien R, Jacobsen LJ, et al. Mood changes in adolescents using depo-medroxyprogesterone acetate for contraception. J Ped Adolesc Gynecol 2001;14:71–76.
73. Tsai, S. Effect of depot medroxyprogesterone acetate on postpartum depression. Contraception 2010;82:174–77.
74. Westhoff C, Truman C, Kalmuss D et al. Depressive symptoms and Norplant contraceptive implants. Contraception 1998;57:241–245.
75. Lopez LM, Grimes DA, Gallo MF, Schulz KF. Skin patch and vaginal ring versus combined oral contraceptives for contraception. Cochrane Database Syst Rev 2010;17(3)pub3.
76. Sucato GS, Land SR, Murray PJ, Cecchini R, Gold MA. Adolescents experiences using the contraceptive patch versus pills. J Pediatr Adolesc Gynecol 2011;24:197–203.
77. Mansour D, Korver T, Marintcheva-Petrova M, Fraser IS. The effects of Implanon on menstrual bleeding patterns. Eur J Contracept Reprod Health Care 2008;13:13–28.
78. Elovainio M, Teperi J, Aalto AM, et al. Depressive symptoms as a predictor of discontinuation of treatment of menorrhagia by levonorgesterol releasing intrauterine system. Int J Behav Med 2007;14:70–5
79. Callegari LS, Zhao X, Nelson KM, Lehavot K, Bradley KA, Borrero S. Associations of mental illness and substance use disorders with prescription contraception use among women veterans. Contraception 2014;90:97–103.
80. Francis J, Presser L, Malbon K, Braun-Courville D, Linares LO. An exploratory analysis of contraceptive method choice and symptoms of depression in adolescent females initiating prescription contraception. Contraception 2015;91:336–343.
81. Faisal-Cury A, Menezes PR, Huang H. The relationship between perinatal psychiatric disorders and contraception use among postpartum women. Contraception 2013;88:498–502.

82. Walsemann K, Perez A. Anxiety's relationship to inconsistent use of oral contraceptives. Health Ed Behav 2006;33:197–214.
83. Steinberg JR, McCulloch CE, Adler NE. Abortion and mental health: Findings from the National Comorbidity Survey-Replication. Obstet Gynecol 2014;123:263–270.
84. Steinberg JR, Russo NF. Abortion and anxiety: What's the relationship? Soc Sci Med 2008;67:238–252.
85. Hall KS, Kusunoki Y, Gatny H, Barber J. Unintended pregnancy risk among young women with psychological stress and depression symptoms. Soc Sci Med 2014;100:62–71.
86. Hall KS, Kusunoki Y, Gatny H, Barber J. Stress and the frequency of sexual intercourse among young women. J Sex Med 2014;11:1982–90.
87. Lehrer JA, Shrier LA, Gortmaker S, Buka S. Depressive symptoms as longitudinal predictors of sexual risk behaviors among US middle and high school students. Pediatrics 2006;118:189–200.
88. Shrier LA, Harris SK, Sternberg M, Beardslee WR. Associations of depression, self-esteem, and substance use with sexual risk among adolescents. Prev Med 2001;33:179–189.
89. Chen YW, Stiffman AR, Cheng LC, Dore P. Mental health, social environment and sexual risk behaviors of adolescent service users: a gender comparison. J Child Fam Stud 1997;6:9–25.
90. Garbers S, Correa N, Tobier N, Blust S, Chiasson MA. Associations between symptoms of depression and contraceptive method choices among low-income women at urban reproductive health centers. Mat Child Health 2010;14:102–109.
91. Hall K, Moreau C, Trussell J, Barber J. Role of young women's depression and stress symptoms in their weekly use and nonuse of contraceptive methods. J Adolesc Health 2013;53:241–248.
92. Hall K, Moreau C, Trussell J, Barber J. Young women's consistency of contraceptive use – do depression and stress matter? Contraception 2013;88:641–649.
93. Brooks TL, Harris SK, Thrall JS, Woods ER Association of adolescent risk behaviors with mental health symptoms in high school students. J Adolesc Health 2002;31:240–46.
94. Lee Li-Ching, Casanueva CE, Martin SL. Depression among female family planning patients: prevalence, risk factors and use of mental health services. J Women's Health 2005;14:225–232.
95. Zink TM, Shireman TI, Ho M, Buchanan T. High-risk teen compliance with prescription contraception: An analysis of Ohio Medicaid Claims. J Ped Adolesc Gynecol 2002;15: 15–21.
96. Steinberg JR, Tschann JM, Henderson JT, Drey E A, Steinauer JE, Harper CC. Psychological distress and post-abortion contraceptive choice at an urban clinic. Contraception 2013;88:717–724.
97. Hall K, Reame N, O'Connell K, Rickert V, Weshoff C. Influence of depressed mood and psychological stress symptoms on perceived oral contraceptive side effects and discontinuation in young minority women. Contraception 2012;86:518–25.
98. Alvy LM, McKirnan DJ, Mansergh G, Koblin B, Colfax GN, Flores SA, Hudson S. Project MIX Study Group. Depression is associated with sexual risk among men who have sex with men, but is mediated by cognitive escape and self-efficacy. AIDS Behavior 2011;15:1171–1179.
99. Clery-Melin ML, Schmidt L, Lafargue G, Baup N, Fossati P, Pessiglione M. Why don't you try harder? An investigation of effort production in major depression. PLoS One 2011;6:1–8.
100. Hartley CA, Phelps EA. Anxiety and decision-making. Biol Psychiatr 2012;72:113–118.
101. Rubino-Watkins MF, Doster JA, Franks S, et al. Oral contraceptive use: implications for cognitive and emotional functioning. J Nerv Mental Dis 1999;187:275–80.
102. Barsky AJ, Saintfort R, Rogers MP, Borus JF. Nonspecific medication side effects and the Nocebo phenomenon. JAMA 2002;287,:22–7.
103. Katon W, Lin E, Von Korff M, et al. Somatization: A spectrum of severity. Am J Psych 1991;148:34–40.

104. Mathews A, MacLeod C. Cognitive vulnerability to emotional disorders. Ann Rev Clin Psychology 2005;1:167–195.
105. Beck AT, Cognitive models of depression. J Cognitive Psychotherapy 1987;1:5–37.
106. Maner JK, Schmidt NB. The role of risk avoidance in anxiety. Behav Ther 2006;37:181–189.
107. Yuen KSL, Lee TMC. Could mood state affect risk-taking decisions? J Affect Disorders, 2003;75:11–18.
108. Ruscher S, de Wit R. Mazimanian D. Psychiatric patients' attitudes about medication and factors affecting noncompliance. Psych Services 1997;48:82–5.
109. Patel MS, David AS. Medication adherence: predictive factors and enhancement strategies. Psychiatry 2004;3:41–4.
110. Calev A. Assessment of neuropsychological functions in psychiatric disorders. Washington DC: American Psychiatric Press, 1999.
111. Westhoff C, Heartwell S, Edwards S, et al. Oral contraceptive discontinuation: do side effects matter? Am J Obstet Gynecol 2007;196:412e1–412e7.
112. Rosenberg MJ, Waugh MS, Long S. Unintended pregnancies and use, misuse and discontinuation of oral contraceptives. J Reprod Med 1995,40:355–60.
113. Mann JJ. The medical management of depression. NEJM 2005;353:1819–34.
114. Roter DL, Frankel RM, Hall JA, Sluyter D. The expression of emotion through nonverbal behavior in medical visits. Mechanisms and outcomes. J Gen Intern Med 2006;21:s28–34.
115. Hackley B, Sharma, C, Kedzior A, Sreenivasan S. Managing mental health conditions in primary care settings. J Midwifery Women's Health 2010;55:9–19.
116. National Institute for Health and Clinical Excellence Clinical guidelines CG90, TMAP Guidelines, The MacArthur Initiative on Depression and Primary Care 2009.
117. University of Michigan Depression Center Toolkit. www.depressiontoolkit.org/treatmentoptions/Psychotherapy/dbt.asp. Accessed December 20, 2012.
118. ARHP's Clinical Advisory Committee for The Reproductive Health Implications of Depression. September 2011. www.arhp.org/core. Accessed February 1, 2013.
119. American Psychological Association. Assessment tools. www.apa.org/pi/about/publications/caregivers/practice-settings/assessment/tools/index.aspx. Accessed February 1, 2013.
120. Bohannon RW, Maljanian R, Goethe J. Screening for depression in clinical practice: reliability and validity of a five-item subset of the CES-Depression. Percept Motiv Skills 2003;97:855–61.
121. Cohen S, Kamarck T, Mermelstein R. A global measure of perceived stress. J Health Soc Behav 1993;24:385–96.
122. Radloff, L.S. The CES-D scale: A self-report depression scale for research in the general population. Applied Psych Meas 1977;1:385–401.
123. Kroenke K, Spitzer RL, Williams JB. The patient health questionnaire-2: validity of a two-item depression screener. Med Care 2003;41:1284–92.
124. Andresen EM, Malmgren JA, Carter WB, Patrick DL. Screening for depression in well older adults: evaluation of a short form of the CES-D (Center for Epidemiologic Studies Depression Scale). Am J Preven Med 1994; 10:77–84.
125. Spitzer RL, Kroenke K, Williams JBW, and the Patient Health Questionnaire Primary Care Study Group. Validation and utility of a self-report version of PRIME-MD: The PHQ Primary Care Study. JAMA 1999;282:1737–1744.
126. Richter P, Werner J, Heerlein A, Kraus A, Sauer H. On the validity of the Beck Depression Inventory: a review. Psychopathology 1998;31:160–168.
127. Lovibond PF & Lovibond SH. The structure of negative emotional states: Comparison of the Depression Anxiety Stress Scales (DASS) with The Beck Depression and Anxiety Inventories. Behav Res Ther 1995;33:335–343.
128. Fydrich T, Dowdall D, Chambless DL. Reliability and validity of the Beck Anxiety Inventory. J Anxiety Dis 1992;6:55–61.
129. Beck AT, Steer RA. Manual for the Beck Anxiety Inventory. San Antonio, TX: Psychological Corporation, 1990.

130. Spielberger CD, Gorsuch RL, Lushene R, Vagg PR, Jacobs GA. State-trait anxiety inventory for adults: Manual, Test Booklet and Scoring Key. Palo Alto, CA: Consulting Psychologist Press, Inc., 1983.
131. McDowell AK, Lineberry TW, Bostwick JM. Practical suicide-risk management for the busy primary care physician. Mayo Clin Proc 2011;86:792–800.
132. Hunot VM, Caldwell D, Jones DP, Furukawa TA, Lewis G, Churchhill R. Cognitive behavioural therapies versus treatment as usual for depression. Cochrane Database Syst Rev 2010:CD008699.
133. Hunot V, Churchill R, Teixeira V, Silva de Lima M. Psychological therapies for generalised anxiety disorder. Cochrane Database Syst Rev 2007;1:CD0001848.
134. Churchill R, Davies P, Caldwell D, Moore THM, Jones H, Lewis G, Hunot V. Interpersonal, cognitive analytic and other integrative therapies versus treatment as usual for depression. Cochrane Database Syst Rev 2010;9:CD008703.
135. Anderson IM, Edwards JG. Guidelines for choice of selective serotonin reuptake inhibitor in depressive illness. Adv Psychiatr Treat 2001:170–180
136. Will-Shahab L, Bauer S, Kunter U, Roots I, Brattstrom A. St John's wort extract (Ze 117) does not alter the pharmacokinetics of a low dose oral contraceptive. Eur J Clin Pharmacol 2009;65:287–94.
137. Murphy PA, Kern SE, Stanczyk FZ, Westhoff CL. Interaction of St. John's wort with oral contraceptives; effects on the pharmacokinetics of norethindrone and ethinyl estradiol, ovarian activity and breakthrough bleeding. Contraception 2005; 71:402–8.
138. Hall KS, Steinberg J, Marcus S. Contraception for Women with Mental Health Conditions. In C. A. Cwiak & R. H. Allen (Eds.), Contraception for the medically challenging patient. Springer Science: New York, 2014.
139. Hall, KS, Steinberg JR, Cwiak C, Allen, R, Marcus, SM. Contraception for women with depression and anxiety: a commentary on the evidence and principles for practice. Am J Obstet Gynecol 2015;212:740–46.
140. Koke SC, Brown EB, Miner CM. Safety and efficacy of fluoxetine in patients who receive oral contraceptive therapy. Am J Obstet Gynecol 2002;187;551–5.
141. D'Arcy PF. Drug interactions with oral contraceptives. Drug Intell Clin Pharm 1986;20:353–62.
142. Buckley P (Ed.) Sexuality and serious mental illness. Netherlands: Harwood Academic Publishers, 2013.
143. Moreau C, Trussell J, Gilbert F, Bajos N, Bouyer J. Oral contraceptive tolerance: does the type of pill matter? Obstet Gynecol 2007;109:1277–85.
144. Hall KS, Trussell J. Types of combined oral contraceptives used by US women. Contraception 2012;86:659–65.
145. Hatcher RA, Trussell J, Stewart F, et al. Contraceptive technology, 20th revised edition. New York, Ardent Media, 2004.
146. Gallo MF, Grimes NK, Lopez LM, Schulz KF. 20ug versus >20ug estrogen combined oral contraceptives for contraception. Cochrane Database Syst Rev 2011; 8:CD003989.
147. Maitra NN, Kulier R, Bloemenkamp K, Helmerhorst FM, Gulmezogul AM. Progestogens in combined oral contraceptives for contraception. Cochrane Database Syst Rev 2004;3:CD004861.
148. Lawrie TA, Helmerhorst FM, Maitra NN, Kulier R, Bloemenkamp K, Gulmezoglu AM. Types of progestogens in combined oral contraception: effectiveness and side-effects Cochrane Database Syst Rev 2011;5:CD004861.
149. Van Vliet HAAM, Grimes DA, Lopez LM, Schulz KF, Helmerhorst FM. Triphasic versus monophasic oral contraceptives for contraception. Cochrane Database Syst Rev 2011;11:CD003553.
150. Edelman A, Gallo MF, Jensen JT, Nichols MD, Grimes DA. Continuous or extended cycle vs. cyclic use of combined hormonal contraceptives for contraception. Cochrane Database Syst Rev 2014;7:CD004695.

151. World Health Organization (WHO) Department of Reproductive Health and Research, Johns Hopkins Bloomberg School of Public Health/Center for Communication Programs (CCP). Knowledge for health project. Family planning: a global handbook for providers (2011 update). Baltimore, MD; Geneva, Switzerland: CCP and WHO.
152. Trussell J, Vaughn B. Contraceptive failure, method-related discontinuation and resumption of use: results from the 1995 NSFG. Fam Plann Persp 1999;31:64–72,93.
153. Mosher WD, Jones J. Use of contraception in the United States: 1982-2008. Vital Health Stat 2010;23:1–43.
154. Kost K, Singh S, Vaughan B, Trussell J, Bankole A. Estimates of contraceptive failure from the 2002 National Survey of Family Growth. Contraception 2008;77:10–21.
155. Frost JJ, Lindberg LD, Finer LB. Young adults' contraceptive knowledge, norms and attitudes: associations with risk of unintended pregnancy. Persp Sex Reprod Health 2012,44:2:107–116.
156. Hall KS, Castano P, Stone P, Westhoff C. Measuring oral contraceptive knowledge: a review of research findings and limitations. Pat Ed Couns 2010;81:388–94.
157. Akers AY, Gold MA, Borrero S, et al. Structured contraceptive counseling—a randomized controlled trial. J Women's Health 2010;19:1163–70.
158. Hall K. The Health Belief Model can guide modern contraceptive research. J Midwif Women's Health 2011;57,74–81.
159. Lopez LM, Tolley EE, Grimes DA and Mario CM. Theory-based strategies for improving contraceptive use: a systematic review. Contraception 2009; 79:411–1
160. Tessler SL, Peipert JF. Perceptions of contraceptive effectiveness and health effects of oral contraception. Women's Health Issues 1997;7:400–6.
161. Rickert VI, Berenson AB, Williamson AJ et al. Immediate recall of oral contraceptive instructions: implications for providers. Am J Obstet Gynecol 1999;180:1399–1406.
162. Grimes DA, Schulz KF. Nonspecific side effects of oral contraceptives: nocebo or noise? Contraception 2011;83:5–9.
163. DiMatteo MR, Lepper HS, Croghan TW. Depression is a risk factor for noncompliance with medical treatment: meta-analysis of the effects of anxiety and depression on patient adherence. Arch Intern Med 2000;160:2101–7.
164. Osterberg L, BlasckeT. Adherence to medication. N Engl J Med 2005;353:487–97.
165. O'Mahen HA, Himle JA, Fedock G, Henshaw E, Flynn HA. A pilot randomized controlled trial of cognitive behavioral therapy for perinatal depression adapted for women with low incomes. Depression Anxiety 2013;30:679–687.
166. Johns Hopkins Medicine. Premenstrual dysphoric disorder (PMDD). Health Library. www.hopkinsmedicine.org/healthlibrary/conditions/gynecological_health/premenstrual_dysphoric_disorder_pmdd_85,P00580/. Accessed 24 June 2017.
167. Mayo Clinic. Premenstrual syndrome (PMS): What's the difference between premenstrual dysphoric disorder (PMDD) and premenstrual syndrome (PMS)? Diseases and Conditions. www.mayoclinic.org/diseases-conditions/premenstrual-syndrome/expert-answers/pmdd/faq-20058315. Accessed 24 June 2017.
168. Centers for Disease Control and Prevention. Depression Among Women. www.cdc.gov/reproductivehealth/depression. Accessed May 31, 2017.
169. O'Hara MW, McCabe JE. Postpartum depression: Current status and future directions. Ann Rev Clin Psychol 2013;9:379–407.
170. Steinberg EM, Rubinow DR, Bartko JJ, et al. A cross-sectional evaluation of perimenopausal depression. J Clin Psychiatry 2008;69:973–980.
171. Ward RK, Zamorski MA. Benefits and risks of psychiatric medication during pregnancy. AAFP 2002;66:629–36.
172. Flynn HA, O'Mahen HA, Massey L, Marcus S. The impact of a brief obstetrics clinic-based intervention on treatment use for perinatal depression. J Women's Health 2006;15:1195–204.
173. Marcus SM, Barry KL, Flynn HA, Tandon R, Greden JF. Treatment guidelines for depression in pregnancy. Int J Obstet Gynecol 2001;72:61–70.

174. Freeman EW, Samuel MD, Lin H, Nelson DB. Associations of hormones and menopausal status with depressed mood in women with no history of depression. Arch Gen Psychiatry 2006;63:375–382.
175. Parry BL. Optimal management of perimenopausal depression. Int J Womens Health 2010;2:143–151.
176. ACOG. Intimate partner violence. Committee Opinion No. 518. American College of Obstetricians and Gynecologists. Obstet Gynecol 2012;119:412–7.
177. Black MC, Basile KC, Breidig MJ, Smith SG, Walters ML, Merrick MT, et al. The National Intimate Partner and Sexual Violence Survey (NISVS): 2010 summary report. Atlanta (GA): National Center for Injury Prevention and Control, Centers for Disease Control and Prevention, 2011.
178. Lehrer JA, Buka B, Gortmaker, Shrier LA. Depressive symptomatology as a predictor of exposure to intimate partner violence among US female adolescents and young adults. Arch Ped Adolesc Med 2006;160:270–276.
179. Gee RE, Mitra N, Wan F, Chavkin DE, Long JA. Power over parity: intimate partner violence and issues of fertility control. AJOG 2009:201:e1–e7.
180. Miller E, Decker MR, McCauley HL, Tancredi DJ, Levenson RR, Waldman J, Schooenwald P, Silverman JG. Pregnancy coercion, intimate partner violence and unintended pregnancy. Contraception 2010;81:316–322.
181. National Alliance on Mental Illness. About mental illness. www.nami.org/template.cfm?section=about_mental_illness. Accessed June 2, 2013.
182. National Institute of Mental Health Prevalence of serious mental illness among U.S. Adults by age, sex and race. www.nimh.nih.gov/statistics/SMI_AASR.shtml. Accessed August 20, 2013.
183. Matevosyan NR. Reproductive health in women with serious mental illnesses: a review. Sexuality Disab 2009;27:109–18.
184. Miller LJ. Sexuality, reproduction, and family planning in women with schizophrenia. Schizoprhenia Bulletin 1997;23:623–35.
185. Miller LJ, Finnerty M. Family planning knowledge, attitudes and practices in women with schizophrenic spectrum disorders. J Psychsom Obstet Gynecol 1998;19:210–217.
186. Krumm S, Killan R, Becker T. Mentally ill women's subjective views on social context of desire for children. A qualitative approach. Psychiatr Prax 2011;38:23–30
187. Guedes TG, Moura ERF, Almeida PC. Particularities of family planning in women with mental disorders. Rev Latino-am Enfermagem 2009;17:639–44.
188. Seeman MV, Ross R. Prescribing contraceptives for women with schizophrenia. J Psychiatr Prac 2011;17:258–269.
189. McCullough LB, Coverdale J, Bayer T, Chernenak FA. Ethically justified guidelines for family planning interventions to prevent pregnancy in female patients with chronic mental illness. Am J Obstet Gynecol 1992;167:19–25.
190. Coverdale JH, Bayer TL, McCullough LB, Chervenak FA. Respecting the autonomy of chronic mentally ill women in decisions about contraception. Hosp Comm Psychiatr 1993;44:671–674.
191. Magalhaes PVS, Kapczinkski F, Kauer-Sant'Anna M. Use of contraceptive methods among women treated for bipolar disorder. Arch Women's Ment Health 2009;12:183–185.
192. Lang DL, Sales JM, Salazar LR, et al. Determinants of multi-method contraceptive use in a sample of adolescent women diagnosed with psychological disorders. Infectious Dis Obstet Gynecol 2011:1–8.
193. Berenson AB, Asem H, Tan A, Wilkinson GS. Continuation rates and complications of intrauterine contraception in women diagnosed with bipolar disorder. Obstet Gynecol 2011;118:1331–1336.
194. Whitmore EA, Mikulich SK, Ehlers KM, Crowley TJ. One-year outcome of adolescent females referred for conduct disorder and substance abuse/dependence. Drug Alcohol Depend 2000;59:131–141.

195. Verhaeghe J. Hormonal contraception in women with the metabolic syndrome: a narrative review. Eur J Contracept Reprod Health Care 2010;15:305–13.
196. Crawford P. Interactions between antiepileptic drugs and hormonal contraception. CNS Drugs 2002;16:263–272.
197. Dutton C, Foldvary-Schaefer N. Contraception in women with epilepsy: pharmacokinetic interactions, contraceptive options, and management. Int Rev Neurobiol 2008; 83:113–134.
198. Smith MD. HIV risk in adolescents with severe mental illness: literature review. J Adolesc Health, 2001;29:320–329.
199. Auslander WF, McMillen JC, Elze D, Thompson R, Jonson-Reid M, Stiffman A. Mental health problems and sexual abuse among adolescents in foster care: relationship to HIV risk behaviors and intentions. AIDS Behav 2002;6:351–359.
200. Tubman JG, Gil AG, Wagner EF, Artigues H. Patterns of sexual risk behaviors and psychiatric disorders in a community sample of young adults. J Behav Med 2003;26:473–500.
201. DiClemente RJ, Ponton LE. HIV-related risk behaviors among psychiatrically hospitalized adolescents and school- based adolescents. Am J Psychiatr 1993;150:324–325.
202. Gaffield ME, Culwell KR, Lee CR. The use of hormonal contraception among women taking anticonvulsant therapy. Contraception 2011;83:16–29.
203. Spina E, Pisani F, Perucca E. Clinically significant pharmacokinetic drug interactions with carbamazepine. An update. Clin Pharmacokinet 1996;31:198–214.
204. Herzog AG, Blum AS, Farina EL, et al. Valproate and lamotrigine level variation with menstrual cycle phase and oral contraceptive use. Neurology 2009;72:911–4.
205. Wegner I, Edelbroek PM, Bulk S, et al. Lamotrigine kinetics within the menstrual cycle, after menopause, and with oral contraceptives. Neurology 2009;73:1388–93.
206. Bialer M, Doose DR, Murthy B, et al. Pharmacokinetic interactions of topiramate. Clin Pharmacokinet 2004;43:763–80.
207. Johannessen Landmark C, Patsalos PN. Drug interactions involving the new second- and third-generation antiepileptic drugs. Expert Rev Neurother 2010;10: 119–40.
208. Reddy DS. Clinical pharmacokinetic interactions between antiepileptic drugs and hormonal contraceptives. Expert Rev Clin Pharmacol 2010;3:183–92.
209. Gabbay V, O'Dowd MA, Mamamtavrishvili M, et al. Clozapine and oral contraceptives: A possible drug inter- action. J Clin Psychopharmacol 2002;22:621–2.
210. Brown D, Goosen TC, Chetty M, et al. Effect of oral contraceptives on the transport of chlorpromazine across the CACO-2 intestinal epithelial cell line. Eur J Pharm Biopharm 2003;56:159–65.
211. Chetty M, Miller R. Oral contraceptives increase the plasma concentrations of chlorpromazine. Ther Drug Monit 2001;23:556–8.
212. Abel K, Rees S. Reproductive and sexual health of women service users: What's the fuss? Adv Psychiatr Treat 2010;16:279–80.
213. Cropsey KL, Matthews C, Campbel S, et al. Long-term, reversible contraception use among high-risk women treated in a university-based gynecology clinic: comparison between IUD and Depo-Provera. J Women's Health 2010;19:349–53.
214. Seeman MV. Antipsychotic-induced amenorrhea. J Ment Health 2011;20:484–91.
215. Richer-Rossler A, Schmid C, Bleuer S, Birkhauser M. Antipsychotics and hyperprolactinaemia: pathophysiology, clinical relevance, diagnosis and therapy. Neuropsychiatr 2009;23:71–83.
216. Riecher-Rössler A. Oestrogen effects in schizophrenia and their potential therapeutic implications—review. Arch Women's Ment Health 2002;5:111–118
217. Kulkarni J, de Castella A, Fitzgerald PB, et al. Estrogen in severe mental illness: A potential new treatment approach. Arch Gen Psychiatr 2008;65:955–60.
218. Riecher-Rössler A, de Geyter C. The forthcoming role of treatment with oestrogens in mental health. Swiss Med Wkly 2007;137:565–72.
219. Currier GW, Simpson GM. Psychopharmacology: Antipsychotic medications and fertility. Psychiatr Serv 1998;49:175–6.

Pregnancy Testing and Assessment of Early Normal and Abnormal Pregnancy

24

Maureen K. Baldwin, MD, MPH
Alison B. Edelman, MD, MPH

- Early pregnancy confirmation is an essential family planning service.
- Early pregnancy diagnosis allows consideration of all options for pregnancy care: parenthood, abortion, and adoption.
- Once a pregnancy is visualized on ultrasound examination, then human chorionic gonadotropin hormone (hCG) testing is rarely useful.
- A negative pregnant test permits rapid initiation of effective contraception.

ESSENTIAL PREGNANCY INFORMATION FOR EVERYONE

Certain situations provide key opportunities to educate women regarding the prevention or planning of a pregnancy. For example, clinician visits to screen for sexually transmitted infection (STI) are a common and an under-utilized opportunity for intervention. As many as one-quarter of all adolescent girls with a positive pregnancy test have previously had one or more visits for pregnancy screening, representing a missed opportunity for education and intervention.[3]

Once an unintended pregnancy occurs, the opportunity to prevent or prepare is lost. Integration of pregnancy prevention and preconception care into primary care is cost-effective and strongly recommended.[5] These

Box 24-1 Pregnancy screening visit goals

1. Determine if patient is pregnant.
2. Educate the patient about options and implement a plan for the pregnancy.
3. Identify other issues that might require further evaluation or urgent intervention.
4. Review use of medications (over-the-counter, prescription), herbs/vitamins, illegal or recreational substance use.
5. Assess gestational dating.
6. Screen for sexually transmitted infections.
7. Document Rh status and obtain relevant laboratory tests.

visits allow for a review of the medical history and medication list, timely completion of recommended screening tests and immunizations, and planning and preparing for pregnancy, including initiation of folic acid.[6]

Although confirmation of a healthy pregnancy is a pressing issue for most patients, a general history, review of the medication list and, if possible, a physical exam should also be performed, as this may reveal additional items that need to be addressed (Box 24-1).

EDUCATION AND COUNSELING

Family planning is a complex issue influenced by social, familial, biologic and psychological factors. Because nearly half of pregnancies are unintended,[8] a pregnancy diagnosis visit is an important time to clarify a patient's feelings about pregnancy and pregnancy intent. (See Chapter 2 on patient-centered counseling.) Before conducting the pregnancy test, find out how the patient feels about the possibility of pregnancy. Realize that ambivalence is common. When presenting the test result, elicit the patient's reaction and allow time to express feelings. Assess the patient's support system. Provide referrals if a patient feels counseling would be helpful, or if the patient is unsupported or alone with this decision. Emphasize that a decision regarding the outcome of this pregnancy does not need to be made that day. Encourage the patient to talk with a partner, family, or friends. Outline all the options available whether or not the test is positive including:

Pregnant and plans to continue the pregnancy:

- Provide education about healthy antenatal practices and resources for prenatal care.
- Review the pregnancy warning signs (severe pain, bleeding, faint or dizzy, fever).

Pregnant and plans to continue the pregnancy, but does not want to parent:

- In addition to the above initial prenatal care education and resources, provide resources for adoption services.
- Provide resources for an unbiased counselor.

Pregnant and does not plan to continue the pregnancy:

- Provide a referral for abortion services.
- Provide a general overview of what can be expected with the process to obtain an abortion based on state laws, access to services, and gestational dating. (See Chapter 25 on Abortion.)

Not pregnant but wants to be pregnant:

- Provide age-based fertility counseling (such as from www.reproductivefacts.org).
- If appropriate, provide a referral for fertility evaluation.
- Provide preconception education, including advice to take a daily vitamin that includes folic acid (400 mcg daily) before and during the first trimester of pregnancy.[9]
- Provide assessment to optimize medical conditions and medications.
- Review if up to date on vaccinations.
- Update travel warnings (Zika exposure, see www.cdc.gov).

Not pregnant and does not want or unsure about pregnancy:

- Provide counseling about contraceptive options, including relative effectiveness. (See Chapter 26 on Contraceptive Efficacy.)
- Initiate effective contraception (including QuickStart).
- Provide risk-based STI screening.
- Provide age-based fertility counseling.

Pregnancy Care Referral

If the patient is pregnant and plans to continue the pregnancy, encourage early entry into pregnancy care so gestational dating can be confirmed and baseline vital signs can be documented. If the patient selects to continue the pregnancy, perform screening tests in the first trimester, which also include prenatal diagnosis for genetic abnormalities (if desired).

If the patient is pregnant and selects pregnancy termination, expedient care is important as earlier procedures are associated with less morbidity.[10]

If prenatal or abortion care is not provided on-site, then facilitate the patient's access to care. In making a referral, consider factors such as the patient's insurance coverage, primary language, indications for high-risk perinatal care, accessibility of the clinic/hospital logistically and financially and any special delivery needs (e.g., need for cesarean section) or desires (e.g., epidural or water-birth delivery, access to permanent contraception, availability of immediate postpartum or postabortion contraception). Many insurance plans require a referral in order for the patient to be seen for abortion care.

There is often a delay of several weeks until the patient will have a first pregnancy care appointment, so review the signs and symptoms (i.e., severe pain or bleeding, faint or dizzy, fever) that may signal problems during early pregnancy. Provide instructions to the patient, including whom to contact if a problem or emergency arises in the interim. Patients who have medical conditions such as diabetes, heart disease, or hypertension may need an urgent referral to a high-risk obstetrician.

PREGNANCY EVALUATION: GESTATIONAL DATING, HISTORY, SYMPTOMS, PHYSICAL EXAM, LABORATORY EVALUATION, ADDITIONAL SCREENING

Estimate Gestational Dating

Confirm a pregnancy with a urine pregnancy test and estimate the gestational dating by reviewing the timing of pregnancy signs and symptoms, obtaining the last menstrual period (LMP), and performing a pelvic exam. LMP dating is the first day of full flow of menstrual bleeding. Be mindful that not all bleeding episodes represent a true menses. For instance, if the bleeding is light or mistimed, if the periods are irregular, if hormonal contraception is misused, or if there is lactation—then the LMP may not be accurate. Document these issues as well as how sure or unsure the patient is about the LMP date. Ultrasound dating can be used to confirm LMP dating or in some cases used instead of LMP dating.

A pelvic exam correlates uterine enlargement with the estimated gestational dating based on the LMP. For example, an 8-week intrauterine gestation enlarges the uterus to the size of a softball or large orange.[11] The pelvic exam may also help to screen for an abnormal pregnancy (e.g., ectopic pregnancy) or uterine abnormalities (e.g., fibroids). If performed, a speculum exam can aid in the diagnosis of sexually transmitted infections (e.g., chlamydia). If the uterine size by bimanual examination does not

Table 24-1 Possible reasons for uterine size and dates discrepancy

Uterus Smaller Than Expected	Uterus Larger Than Expected
Fertilization later than dates suggest	Fertilization earlier than dates suggest
Ectopic pregnancy	Uterine fibroids
Miscarriage	Twin gestation
Error in pregnancy test	Hydatidiform mole*
Normal variation	Normal variation

*Molar pregnancy: 28% are larger than expected and 14% are smaller than expected.[2]

correspond to the estimated gestational dating based on LMP, consider the possible reasons for the discrepancy (Table 24-1). Ultrasound evaluation can both document pregnancy location and confirm gestational dating. Ultrasound confirmation is limited before 6 weeks gestation and should be interpreted with caution (see Ultrasound section).

Gestational Dating Definitions

The term *gestational age* is used interchangeably with *menstrual age (LMP)*, but they are different.[12] If the *menstrual age (LMP)* is used for dating a pregnancy then this is based on the first day of the LMP and normal pregnancy duration is 40 weeks. When the actual date of conception is known (e.g., as in assisted fertility), then the date of conception or *gestational age* can be used instead. Assuming a person ovulates mid-cycle, the duration of a full-term pregnancy is 38 weeks. This chapter will refer to gestational dating based on the *menstrual age (LMP)*.

Normal Early Pregnancy Symptoms

As early as 2 weeks after conception, even before the first missed menstrual period, hormonal changes may make breasts tender, sore, fuller, or heavier. Fatigue, nausea, and urinary frequency may be noted at 4 weeks following the LMP. Women may also report irregular light bleeding or spotting. This is common in a normal early pregnancy and is due to the trophoblastic tissue of the early pregnancy (blastocyst) invading into the endometrium.[13,14] However, heavy bleeding, particularly when accompanied by lower abdominal pain, may signal a threatened spontaneous abortion or ectopic pregnancy.[15] An ectopic pregnancy may be completely asymptomatic, but the presence of pain accompanied by spotting or moderate to severe bleeding should alert the clinician to the possibility of ectopic pregnancy[16] (discussed later in the chapter). Any time a pregnant patient mentions bleeding or spotting, Rh status should be reviewed.

Rh Screening

Rh typing is a standard screening test for any pregnant person. Patients whose blood is typed as Rh D negative are typically administered anti-D immune globulin under the following circumstances:

a. When undergoing spontaneous or induced abortion

b. When experiencing vaginal bleeding or trauma

c. Routinely at 28 weeks gestation

d. After delivery, if the infant is Rh positive

Administering anti-D immune globulin under these circumstances prevents the risk of Rh sensitization. However, the majority of Rh sensitization is caused from a fetal-maternal hemorrhage at the time of delivery. Rh sensitization from first-trimester events is rare.[17] The recommendation to give anti-D immune globulin for first-trimester bleeding, miscarriage, or abortion varies between countries;[18,19] however, the American Congress of Obstetricians and Gynecologists (ACOG) recommends 50 mcg of anti-D immune globulin in the above situations.[17] After the first trimester, whether pregnancy ends by spontaneous or induced abortion, ACOG recommends the standard 300 mcg dose.

Other Early Pregnancy Screening

Screening for a few medical conditions at a pregnancy test visit can improve pregnancy outcomes considerably. Review a baseline blood pressure measurement, the medication list, risk for intimate partner violence and smoking cessation. A hemoglobin or hematocrit can be helpful at the time of initial evaluation to assess the need for iron or nutritional supplementation, to perform additional screening for thalassemia, to assess the cumulative extent of any bleeding, and to provide an important baseline for later comparison. If a patient has a known history of diabetes or is obese, a baseline hemoglobin A1C or fasting glucose level can be helpful to determine current and recent glycemic control. Document a resting blood pressure. Screen for chlamydia, HIV, and syphilis as part of routine prenatal testing. Even if the patient is considering abortion, screen for STIs to minimize the risk of postabortion infection.[20] Additional routine tests for prenatal care include a urine culture, Rubella antibody to determine immune status, and Hepatitis B surface antigen.

Possible Early Pregnancy Exposure to Teratogens

At the time of a positive pregnancy test, briefly review and discuss use of prescription drugs, over-the-counter (OTC) medications or herbs, and illegal substances.[21,22] Some of these products may be teratogenic. Cessation of the use of potential teratogenic drugs could prevent abnormalities, and awareness of the risks associated with their use could influence decisions regarding pregnancy continuation. Classic examples include warfarin or lithium. In some cases, the benefit of the medication may outweigh risks, so urgent consultation may be necessary to evaluate possible alternatives. The Organization of Teratology Information Services (www.otispregnancy.org) provides up-to-date resources and fact sheets about both maternal and paternal exposures to medications, herbal products, infectious agents, vaccines, medical conditions, illicit substances, and alcohol dependency.

Intimate Partner Violence Screening and Referral

The prevalence of intimate partner violence in pregnancy is as high as 23%.[23] Homicide and suicide remain the two leading causes of maternal mortality in the United States (2008), and half of these cases are directly related to intimate partner violence.[24–26] **Because of the prevalence of domestic violence, particularly among women in the prenatal and postpartum period, clinicians providing gynecologic care, pregnancy screening, and prenatal care are in a unique position to screen, recognize, and intervene.** Women who have experienced intimate partner violence often report that a question by a health care worker was the first step in disclosure and recognition.[27]

Clinicians should be aware of community-based resources such as local domestic violence hotlines, shelters, advocacy organizations, and support groups for victims of intimate partner violence. National resources include the National Domestic Violence Hotline (1–800–799-SAFE) and the National Sexual Violence Resource Center (1–877–739–3895). Internet sites include the National Domestic Violence Hotline (www.ndvh.org), the Family Violence Prevention Fund (http://endabuse.org), the National Coalition against Domestic Violence (www.ncadv.org), and local domestic violence hotlines (www.usdoj.gov/ovw/).

Pregnant with an Intrauterine Device (IUD)

Perform an exam to confirm that the IUD strings are visible. If the strings are present, any available provider should remove the IUD immediately, whether there is a plan to continue the pregnancy or to have an abortion. Patients considering an abortion may ultimately decide to continue the pregnancy or they may choose medication abortion—in both instances, it is important to have removed the IUD. The passage of time (even a couple of days) may lead to retraction of the strings as the uterus increases in size. An IUD left in place increases the risk of septic abortion and other complications such as late miscarriage, preterm delivery, and placental abruption.[28] Counsel the patient that the risk of miscarriage with immediate removal is less than the risk with keeping it in place. Beyond the risk associated with removing the IUD or leaving it in place, miscarriage is a risk for *all* pregnancies.[29] (See Chapter 5 on Intrauterine Devices.)

If the strings are not visible and the patient desires to continue the pregnancy, then provide urgent referral to a specialized family planning service. The patient could potentially be offered hysteroscopic removal. Always, earlier is better. For a patient who chooses to have an abortion, an IUD without visualized strings can be removed simultaneously during a vacuum aspiration. While the number of pregnancies that occur with an IUD in place is extremely low, the proportion of these pregnancies that are ectopic is higher than for patients not using an IUD. Therefore, localize the site of the pregnancy by ultrasound as soon as possible.

HUMAN CHORIONIC GONADOTROPIN HORMONE (hCG) LEVELS IN PREGNANCY, PREGNANCY TESTING, PITFALLS OF PREGNANCY TESTS

It is rarely necessary to obtain serum hCG in early pregnancy. Asymptomatic patients without risk factors for ectopic pregnancy can undergo confirmation of pregnancy with qualitative urine hCG testing. For symptomatic patients, serum hCG may be necessary:

- To identify or rule out an ectopic pregnancy
- To confirm that an ongoing pregnancy is not present following an abortion in a patient with a pregnancy of unknown location

Timing Early Pregnancy Events

Following ovulation, fertilization of the ovum by sperm occurs within the fimbria of the fallopian tube and the fertilized ovum remains in the tube until it is a ball of cells (the morula or embryo) when it then enters the uterine cavity. By 6 days after ovulation, the *embryo* implants into the *decidua*, which is the modified endometrium specialized for implantation and support of a pregnancy. Cells from the embryo form early placental tissue that produces hCG. The hCG maintains the corpus luteum of the ovary, which continues to secrete progesterone until the placental tissue produces increasing quantities of progesterone by 6 to

7 weeks after fertilization. The hCG is the molecule that is detected by a pregnancy test.[30]

hCG Detection in Pregnancy

Pregnancy tests detect the hCG in a pregnant person's urine, blood, or serum. Serum or urine pregnancy tests today detect four independent molecules.[31]

- Intact hCG
- Hyperglycosylated hCG (H-hCG)
- Free β-subunit
- Pituitary hCG

hCG is the term used in this text to denote the types of hCG tested in pregnancy and replaces the formerly used term βhCG.

Highly Sensitive Urine Pregnancy Tests

The OTC pregnancy tests sold for home use and those used in clinics are essentially the same. Cross-reactions with other hormones are not a problem for highly sensitive urine pregnancy tests. Most have a stated sensitivity of 25 mIU/mL.[32]

Home Pregnancy Tests

Home pregnancy test kits offer the advantages of privacy, anonymity, and convenience. Because home pregnancy tests are easily accessible, patients may identify pregnancies early and thus be more able to be active managers of their own health care. Most home pregnancy tests available are sensitive to 25 to 50 mIU/mL hCG. Even tests commonly available at "dollar store" pricing are accurate and sensitive to 100 mIU/mL hCG.

Test accuracy can be affected by the technique and experience of the user, and by the user's ability to follow the test instructions precisely.[32] The most common error with home pregnancy tests is a negative result because the test was performed too early in pregnancy. In addition, a person using a home pregnancy test may have difficulty understanding the directions packaged in the test kit. In an evaluation of instructions from thirteen OTC urine pregnancy tests, the reading level required to understand the instructions ranged from a 7th to a 14th grade reading level.[33] A false-positive test can occur if the test is not read within the designated number of minutes. This phenomenon occurs because a negative test appears faintly positive due to evaporation of the urine sample, which gives rise to an evaporation line.

Sensitivity and Specificity

Highly sensitive urine pregnancy tests, including home pregnancy tests, are intended to provide accurate qualitative (positive/negative) results with hCG levels as low as 5 to 100 mIU/mL. Tests can be positive as early as the day of the first missed menses, depending on the sensitivity of the test. One study reported that 98% of women have a positive pregnancy test within 28 days LMP.[34] On the other hand, another study reported that, even using an extremely sensitive test (0.13 mIU/mL), among 142 women with self-reported onset of LMP, 10% of clinical pregnancies were undetectable on the first day of missed menses. This is due to the variable timing of implantation, which can even occur after the first day of the next expected menses.[35]

Early pregnancies produce quite a variable range of hCG levels, and the time at which a pregnancy is detected accurately by different pregnancy tests varies widely. Moreover, few clinic pregnancy tests or home tests have been calibrated against the three critical forms of hCG: intact hCG, H-hCG, and free β-subunit.[30]

Accuracy

A study of 18 different OTC home urine pregnancy tests demonstrated hCG levels from 23 to 2,438 mIU/mL in well-dated pregnancies 28 to 30 days LMP.[32] This study found that most tests were consistently accurate at a urine hCG of 100 mIU/mL and that some brands had technical or design problems.[32] Thus, for a test to detect 95% of pregnancies at the time of missed menses, it would need to consistently detect hCG of at least 12.4 mIU/mL. Manufacturers' claims that a pregnancy test can detect pregnancy "as early as the day of the missed menstrual period" are based on data that are almost 30 years old that assumed that urine hCG concentrations were the same as serum hCG concentrations. In fact, the average urine hCG concentration is generally less than half of the corresponding serum hCG concentration, depending on the duration of pregnancy and specificity of the test.[30]

Less-Sensitive Urine Pregnancy Tests

Less-sensitive urine pregnancy tests can detect hCG from 200 to 2,000 mIU/mL. These tests are not currently available outside research settings. They have a fairly narrow range of use. They are not appropriate to "rule out" pregnancy, because early pregnancy, ectopic pregnancy, impending spontaneous abortion and, in rare cases, even later pregnancies (16 to 20 weeks) may be missed due to their low hCG levels. Less-sensitive tests can be used to confirm pregnancy ≥6 weeks LMP or to document the decline of hCG after abortion. However, even for this use, a less-sensitive test (sensitivity 1,500 to 2,000 mIU/mL) had a 60.8% false-positive rate 2 weeks after successful medication abortion.[36] A negative less-sensitive pregnancy test after medication abortion is reassuring, but a positive test may not mean much.

Quantitative Serum hCG Tests

A quantitative serum hCG test is designed to provide a *level* or number of hCG mIU/ml; thus, the rise or fall of the hCG level may provide important information about the status of the pregnancy. Use of a serum *quantitative* hCG test only to confirm early pregnancy does not have any advantages over *qualitative* (yes/no) highly sensitive urine tests. Highly sensitive urine pregnancy kits are equally specific for hCG and provide immediate results at much lower cost. Only certain clinical situations justify the additional expense of serum hCG testing.

Serum quantitative hCG tests provide accurate results with levels as low as 5 mIU/ml. Thus they reliably detect pregnancy sooner after implantation around 21 days LMP. Tests are usually "batched" because of expense; test processing requires 1 to 2 hours. Be sure to specify *quantitative* hCG when ordering this test. In addition, it is optimal but not essential to use the same laboratory for serial hCG tests to limit inter-assay variation between laboratories.[37] Given that some patients often have to travel significant distances for repeat hCG tests, it may be difficult to have all samples sent to the same laboratory.

Uses for Serum hCG

Repetitive or serial testing of serum hCG can be used to check the increasing or decreasing trend of hCG levels. **A single serum hCG result alone is rarely meaningful**[38] and, as mentioned earlier, if you just need a yes/no answer (pregnant or not pregnant) then a qualitative highly sensitive urine test works just as well. Rather, the pattern of hCG in conjunction with other diagnostic tests, such as ultrasound examination, clinical evaluation of the patient, and consideration of risk factors can help to differentiate between a normal or abnormal intrauterine pregnancy or ectopic pregnancy.[38] Very high levels of hCG (>100,000 prior to 10 weeks) can be associated with molar pregnancy or multiple pregnancies, such as twins.

Pitfalls of Pregnancy Tests

Any test result can be wrong. Laboratory errors do occur, including specimen mix-up and incorrectly performed test procedures. Consider repeating the test when an unexpected result occurs.

False-Negative Pregnancy Tests

False-negative results can occur either when the test is performed too early or when there are extremely high hCG levels. Urine that is too diluted can also be responsible for false-negative results. It is rare but known in the literature that urine and serum pregnancy tests may yield false-negative results when hCG is present at extreme concentrations. Known as the *high-dose hook effect*, the *secondary* antibody binding sites become saturated with free hCG so that the *primary* antibody complex is unable to bind, preventing detection of the antigen.[39] In one case of molar pregnancy, only after multiple dilutions of the serum was hCG of 1.5 million mIU/ml detected.[40] In another case of complete molar pregnancy, the hCG level was 3,704,085 mIU/ml.[41] If you suspect a molar pregnancy, notify the laboratory so that they can perform dilutions, if necessary. The important thing to remember is that laboratory test results should be questioned if they are discordant with clinical findings.

False-Positive Pregnancy Tests

In very rare cases, urine pregnancy test results are positive even when the patient is not pregnant. This occurs when hCG is present and originating from a source other than pregnancy. A false-positive result could occur if the person has had treatment involving an hCG injection within the preceding 14 days. hCG injections are used in fertility treatments to stimulate ovulation. Faint false-positive results have also been reported with urine samples contaminated by blood or recent use of Chinese herbal medication and with the fad hCG diet.[42] If you suspect a false-positive result, obtain a serum quantitative hCG.

A pregnancy test may also be positive if hCG is present due to incomplete resolution of a previous pregnancy, including gestational trophoblastic disease, or due to an hCG-secreting tumor. Low levels of hCG (5 to 30 mIU) may be associated with tumors of the pancreas, ovaries, breast, and many other sites.[43] Some normal postmenopausal women also have low levels of circulating hCG-like substance of pituitary origin.[44–46] In addition, patients with end-stage renal disease may produce hCG, which registers as a false-positive pregnancy test, due to decreased urinary clearance.[47]

Phantom hCG or heterophilic antibodies can cause a *serum* hCG to be positive (typically at low levels) but urine tests to be negative. These antibodies are present only in the blood and at high enough levels to interfere with serum hCG radioimmunoassay in a small number of women (1/3,300).[41,48,49] In these cases, hCG is falsely detected due to interfering antibodies found in human serum. While uncommon, false-positive or phantom hCG tests have led to the misdiagnosis of ectopic pregnancy, or to the erroneous assumption of post-gestational choriocarcinoma. Since these interfering antibodies are present only in blood, perform a urine pregnancy test as a confirmatory hCG measurement when clinically indicated to rule out the false-positive serum hCG results due to heterophilic antibodies.[30] For confirmation, the laboratory should be notified to perform serial dilutions.

Biochemical Pregnancy

Very early pregnancy loss, or a *biochemical* pregnancy, refers to a pregnancy that fails to implant and grow in the uterus successfully. Serum hCG levels appear approximately 1 week after conception, peak at approximately 10 to 100 mIU/ml, then drop. A normal or heavier than usual menstrual period follows, which may or may not be delayed. Women may have a positive pregnancy test in the last week of their menstrual cycle, but if the test is repeated later, the test is negative; transient hCG may extend to 5 days after the time of the missed menses.[32]

SERUM hCG LEVELS IN EARLY PREGNANCY

Elevated hCG can be detected in serum at low levels as early as 21 days LMP, very soon after implantation occurs.[51] In general, serum levels of hCG reach 50 to 250 mIU/ml by the time of the first missed menstrual period; hCG reaches a peak of >100,000 mIU/ml at approximately 10 to 12 weeks LMP and then declines to a plateau that is maintained until delivery (See Figure 24-1).[52] Low levels of hCG may simply indicate that a normal pregnancy is earlier in gestation than menstrual dates suggest. These values can also vary significantly between individuals. During the first 10 weeks of pregnancy, an hCG rise of 66% over 2 days or 48 hours is generally considered acceptable evidence of a viable intrauterine pregnancy.[53] However, hCG increase over 48 hours can be as high as 228% and as low as 33% for a viable pregnancy, though values are dependent on

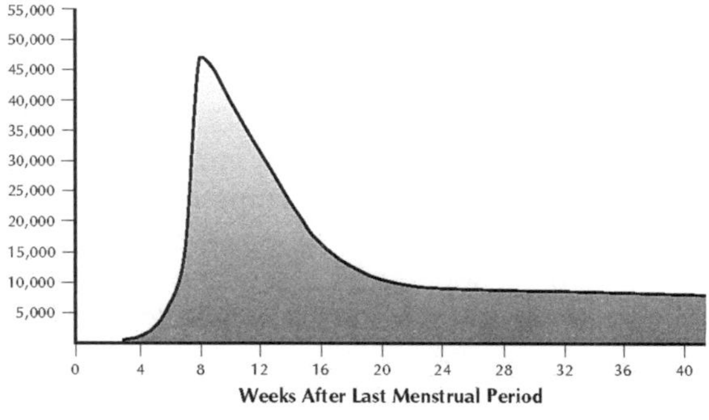

Source: Braunstein (1976) with permission.[50]

Figure 24-1 hCG levels during normal pregnancy

initial hCG levels.[54,92] With an hCG trend that is less than expected, consider obtaining a third value for confirmation. Elevated levels of hCG are seen with a multiple gestation, reflecting the increased placental mass, as well as in the setting of gestational trophoblastic disease.[52]

A single hCG value tells you if a person is pregnant, but it does not determine the pregnancy's location or whether it is growing normally. More information can be obtained from serial assessment of hCG change over time, usually over 24 or 48 hours. An hCG level of 2,000 to 3,000 mIU/ml or higher correlates with the ability to visualize a pregnancy via transvaginal ultrasound, also called the "discriminatory zone" (See Ultrasound section, below).[55,56] If an intrauterine pregnancy can be visualized on ultrasound examination, the appearance of anatomic landmarks and growth of the embryo over time on ultrasound should be the primary method of assessing viability. If there is a question about viability of an intrauterine pregnancy, the ultrasound is generally repeated in 7 days if an embryonic pole was seen, or in up to 10 days if only a gestational sac with or without a yolk sac was seen.

Typically, the pattern of hCG rise, fall, or plateau, in combination with the clinical picture, ultrasound examination (if performed), and risk factors for ectopic pregnancy is more important than a single hCG value in determining the location and status of the pregnancy (See Box 24-3 Risk Factors for Ectopic Pregnancy).

hCG Trends in Abnormal Pregnancy

Regardless of its location, an abnormal pregnancy could have already stopped growing, could be growing abnormally, or currently could be growing normally. Subsequently, in abnormal pregnancies, hCG levels often increase abnormally, plateau, or decrease, but can also have a normal trend initially. One study demonstrated that almost 30% of women with ectopic pregnancies had initial patterns of hCG change that mimicked either an intrauterine pregnancy or a complete miscarriage.[57] The rate of rise of hCG in ectopic pregnancy generally is lower than for intrauterine pregnancies, but the curves overlap.[4]

Extremely high hCG production, with hCG levels as high as 2 million mIU/ml, can occur with a molar pregnancy, such as hydatidiform mole or gestational trophoblastic disease, though some molar gestations have normal hCG levels.[52] Abnormally low hCG levels often occur with an abnormal pregnancy, such as before a spontaneous abortion or with an ectopic pregnancy, but they can also represent a normal pregnancy earlier than expected.

If an abnormal hCG trend occurs but the pregnancy is desired, obtain an ultrasound as soon as the hCG level reaches the discriminatory zone. Consider following an abnormally low rise of serum hCG with a third serial hCG value for confirmation.

Table 24-2 Rise or decline in sequential quantitative hCG values in early viable intrauterine pregnancy, complete spontaneous abortion, and ectopic pregnancy

Type of Pregnancy	%
Early viable intrauterine pregnancy	
Mean rise in hCG in 2 days, % increase	124
Minimum expected rise in hCG in 2 days, % increase[a]	53
Complete spontaneous abortion	
Range of minimum expected decline in hCG, % decrease[b]	21–35
Ectopic pregnancy[c]	
% of women who experienced a **rise** in hCG (Group A)	60
• % of pregnancies in Group A whose first two hCG values were consistent with intrauterine pregnancy	35
• Median rise in hCG in 2 days, % increase	75
% of women who experienced a **decline** in hCG (Group B)	40
• % of pregnancies in Group B whose first two hCG values were consistent with complete spontaneous abortion	20
• Median decline in hCG in 2 days, % decrease	27
Group A and Group B combined	
• % of pregnancies with first two hCG values out of range for normal intrauterine pregnancy or complete spontaneous abortion	71
• % of pregnancies with first two hCG values consistent with range for normal intrauterine pregnancy	21
• % of pregnancies with first two hCG values consistent with range for complete spontaneous abortion	8

Sources: Barnhart et al (2004), Seeber and Barnhart (2006), Silva et al (2006) with permission.

[a] hCG will increase at this rate or faster in 99% of early viable intrauterine pregnancies.

[b] The rate of decrease depends on the initial hCG value.

[c] 287 women presented to ER with pain or bleeding; initial hCG was <5,000, pregnancy not visualized with transvaginal ultrasound. The first two hCG tests were taken at least 24 hours but no more than 7 days apart.

hCG Trends After Pregnancy Completion or Termination

After a pregnancy ends and the placenta has separated from the uterus, hCG levels decrease, first quickly and then more slowly. Figure 24-2 represents the hCG disappearance curve following uterine aspiration abortion at 7 to 13 weeks (upper curve), miscarriage at 6 to 15 weeks (middle curve), and surgical treatment of ectopic pregnancy (bottom curve).[58] Following complete evacuation of a pregnancy of any gestation, hCG becomes undetectable by 3 to 4 weeks in most patients.

If a medication abortion or a first-trimester vacuum aspiration successfully ended the pregnancy, the hCG level initially declines steadily, halving by 48 hours.[59–61]

The outcome of medication abortion can be followed by quantitative hCG instead of ultrasound, making a return to the clinic for an in-person

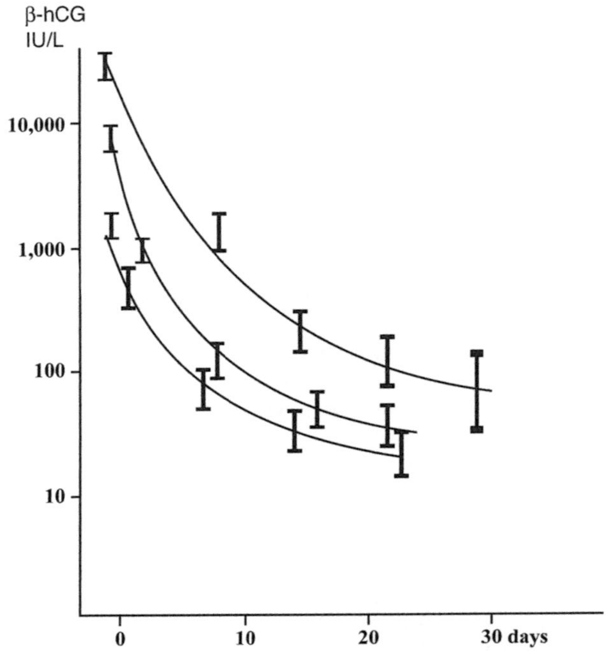

Disappearance curves of serum hCG in three groups of women. Semilogarithmic scale. Upper curve represents women (n = 36) who had elective vacuum aspiration abortion at 7–13 weeks LMP. Middle curve represents women (n = 35) with spontaneous abortion at 6–15 weeks LMP treated with uterine aspiration. Lower curve represents women (n = 35) with ectopic pregnancies diagnosed 2.5–11.0 weeks after LMP and removed surgically.

Source: Steier et al. (1984)[58] with permission.

Figure 24-2 Disappearance curve of hCG after abortion, surgical evacuation of miscarriage and surgical treatment of ectopic pregnancy

examination unnecessary. This is especially helpful for those who must travel a great distance to obtain mifepristone and misoprostol and for those who have received the medication by mail for self-administration. For patients undergoing a medication abortion, hCG continues to increase following mifepristone but then declines precipitously after expulsion of the pregnancy.[62] By 6 to 18 days after taking mifepristone, the hCG level can be expected to drop by 80% from the initial value (measured on the day of mifepristone) in 98.5% of successful medication abortions.[63]

When an hCG level is used to confirm completed vacuum aspiration abortion, a 50% decline in hCG by 48 hours is considered successful uterine evacuation based on trends after medication abortion.[60–66] Often, hCG will drop 50% in 24 hours, allowing for a faster confirmation. Likewise, if hCG is used to confirm complete uterine evacuation in the setting of pregnancy of unknown location or uterine aspiration without identification of gestational tissue, a 50% decline is considered to confirm completed pregnancy and is suggestive of intrauterine location. (See Chapter 25 on Abortion for further discussion.)

Follow-Up After Spontaneous Abortion

Serum hCG is not recommended following a spontaneous abortion if a prior ultrasound documented an intrauterine pregnancy or if the gestational sac and placental tissue were confirmed by direct visualization after uterine evacuation. Ultrasound examination can be used to identify whether the gestational sac has completely expelled. If intrauterine pregnancy has not been confirmed by one of these methods, then serial hCG testing should demonstrate a rapid decline if complete expulsion has occurred. Without prior evidence of intrauterine pregnancy, these cases should be treated as pregnancy of unknown location (See Pregnancy of Unknown Location section below). In some cases, weekly serial hCG followed to nonpregnant levels might be necessary to ensure completion of the pregnancy.

ULTRASOUND IN VERY EARLY PREGNANCY

Targeted ultrasound examination in the outpatient setting at the time of a positive pregnancy test has the primary goal of dating and localizing the pregnancy. Trained providers will also want to assess pregnancy viability for patients with desired pregnancy. Transvaginal ultrasound allows for visualization of the entire pelvis: identification of the uterus, ovaries, presence or absence of ovarian cysts, and presence or absence of fluid in the cul-de-sac.[56]

PREGNANCY LOCALIZATION

Identifying the location of a pregnancy with a very early ultrasound, such as prior to 6 weeks gestation, is important in the setting of a symptomatic patient or a patient planning to undergo abortion. Patients with pain or bleeding could have an ectopic pregnancy or be undergoing a miscarriage. However, very early ultrasound can have confusing results. Performing ultrasound examination for an asymptomatic desired pregnancy should ideally be done after 6 to 7 weeks gestation.

Earliest Ultrasound Visualization of Pregnancy

The landmarks for timing of findings by transvaginal ultrasound are as follows:

Table 24-3 Timing of landmarks in early pregnancy (with transvaginal ultrasound based on 28-day cycle)[67]

20–32 days gestation from LMP	positive highly-sensitive urine pregnancy test
35 days LMP (5 weeks)	gestational sac can usually be visualized
40 days LMP (5½ weeks)	yolk sac virtually always is seen
48 days LMP (6½ weeks)	embryonic pole with cardiac motion is seen

Visualization of the uterus with transvaginal ultrasound should be performed in a systematic fashion and include evaluation both in the longitudinal and transverse views. Avoid the temptation of focusing only on the gestational sac, because other important findings can be missed with this approach (e.g., twins, ectopic pregnancy, uterine anomalies, fluid in the cul-de-sac, ovarian mass). The longitudinal view captures the uterus on its long axis, making it possible to visualize the cervix and endometrial cavity up to the fundus and to orient the viewer in the pelvis.

Visualization of the Gestational Sac

A true gestational sac can be challenging to distinguish from a *pseudosac,* which can be present with an ectopic pregnancy. A pseudosac is the sloughing of decidua that produces a fluid collection in the endometrial cavity.[68] Approximately 10% of patients with ectopic pregnancy have a pseudosac visualized on ultrasound.[69]

The following are characteristics of a normal gestational sac:

1. A three-dimensional round or oval structure, implanted off-center to the midline, that normally grows about 1 mm/day.[70] (See Figures 24-3A and B.)
2. Completely surrounded by a multi-layered echogenic choriodecidual reaction, known as the double decidual reaction. The appearance is of a multi-layered fluffy white cloud surrounding the

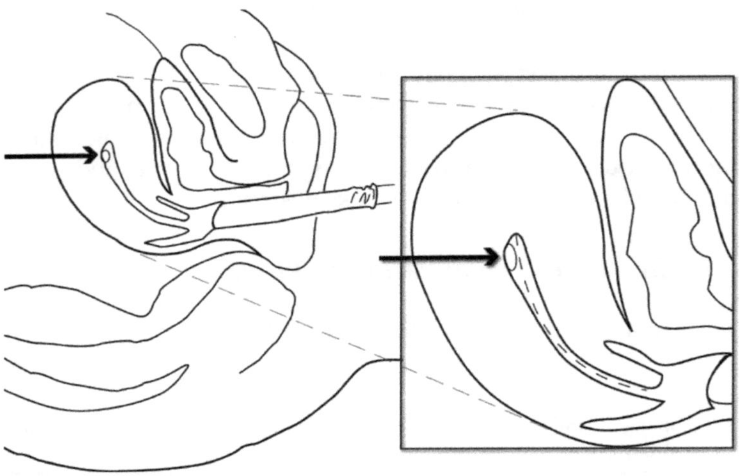

Figure 24-3A Illustration of eccentric implantation. The pregnancy implants into the thickened endometrium or decidua. In effect, it burrows into the endometrial lining; it does not float in the endometrial cavity. That's why the gestational sac is off-center to the midline of the endometrial cavity (arrow). (Courtesy of Mary Fjerstad, NP).

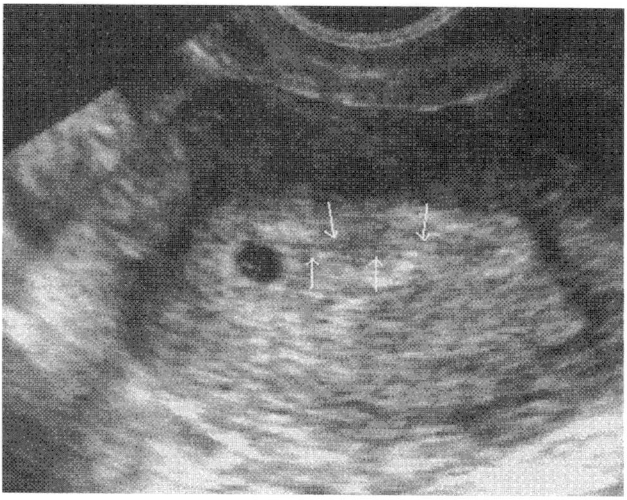

Figure 24-3B Longitudinal view of an intrauterine gestational sac, choriodecidual reaction and endometrial cavity line. Note the thin black line that extends longitudinally through the endometrial cavity, sometimes referred to as the endometrial cavity line (arrows). The gestational sac is adjacent to, but does not displace, the endometrial cavity line, thereby demonstrating an eccentric implantation.[72] In addition, the double decidual reaction (multi-layered echogenicity) surrounding the gestational sac is seen. (Courtesy of Mary Andrews, NP)

gestational sac, whiter near the sac and at the outer edge of the reaction. Another description of the appearance of the choriodecidual reaction is that of an orange rind or halo (see Figure 24-4A and B).[71,72]

In contrast, the illustration (Figure 24-5A) and ultrasound images (Figure 24-5B) demonstrate pseudosacs.

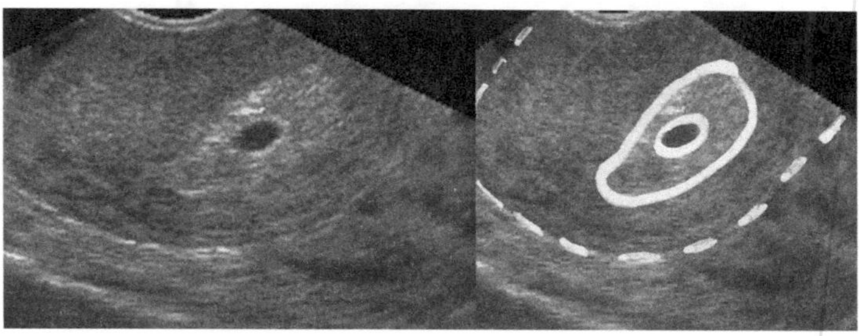

Figure 24-4A and Figure 24-4B Intrauterine gestational sac with choriodecidual reaction. The double decidual reaction is seen in which the ring closest to the sac is bright white (echogenic), somewhat faded in the middle of the reaction, and then brighter again at the edge of the choriodecidual reaction. In view B, the inner and outer rings of the reaction are outlined with solid white lines and the uterus is outlined with a broken white line. (Courtesy of Mary Fjerstad, NP)

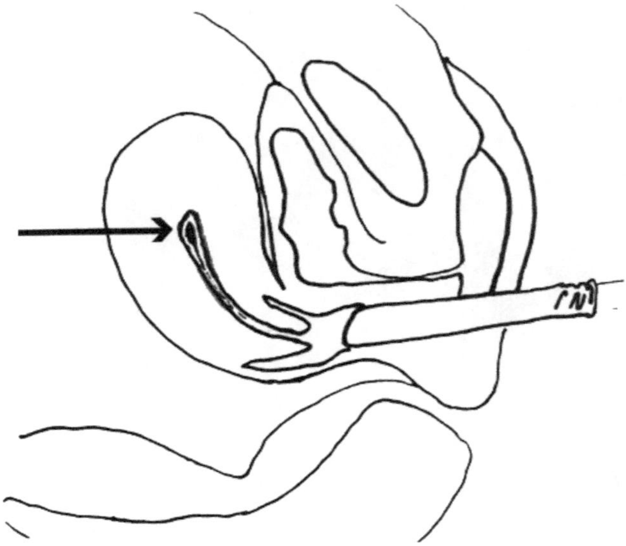

Figure 24-5A Illustration of a pseudosac. This is a fluid collection within the endometrium; the fluid collection can be large or small, irregular shaped or round (at least when viewed in one plane), but it is not implanted in the decidual lining; it is midline in the cavity, not eccentric to the midline. (Courtesy of Mary Fjerstad, NP)

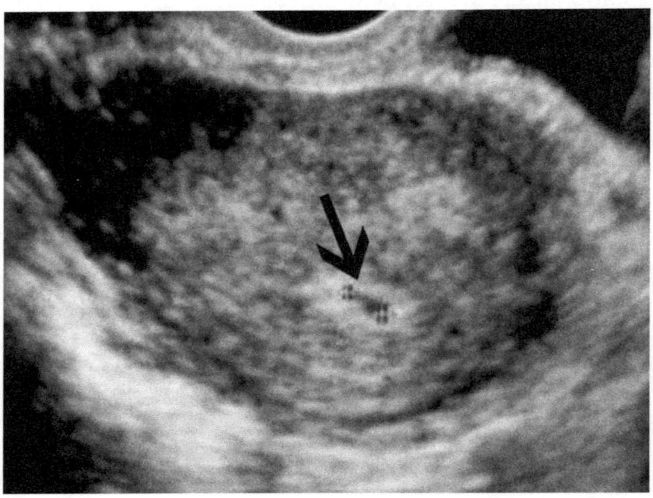

Figure 24-5B Pseudosac. Note that the choriodecidual reaction is not multi-layered; it is a thin, homogenous echogenic rim. Note also that the fluid-filled sac (arrow) is mid-line in the uterine cavity, not eccentrically implanted as would be a true gestational sac. Also note that the fluid-filled sac is irregularly shaped. Another view taken at the same session demonstrates that the sac lost all semblance of roundness when it was viewed in a different plane (Figure 24–11). (Courtesy of Mary Fjerstad, NP)

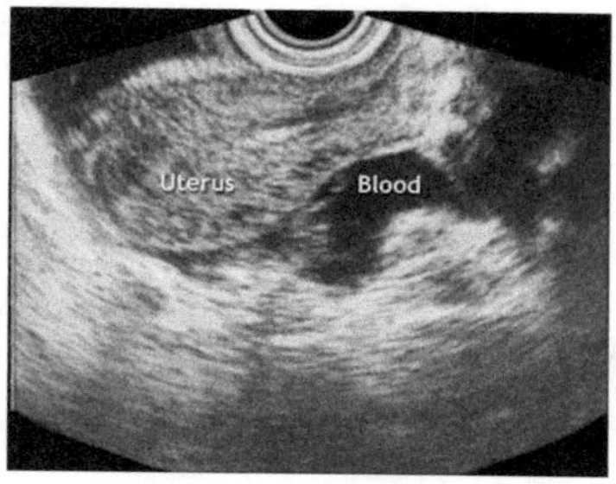

Figure 24-6 Free fluid in the cul-de-sac. (Courtesy of Matthew Reeves, MD)

Small amounts of free pelvic fluid can be seen in intrauterine pregnancies, as well as in ectopic pregnancies. The presence of a moderate to large amount of fluid in the cul-de-sac has 96% specificity for diagnosing ectopic pregnancy. In 15% of confirmed ectopic pregnancies, sonolucent fluid in the cul-de-sac was the *only* extrauterine finding.[73] One study found that visualization of any free fluid had 63% sensitivity and 80% specificity in diagnosing ectopic pregnancy in patients presenting to the emergency department.[74] In other words, ectopic pregnancy itself was not visualized directly in the adnexa, but fluid in the cul-de-sac was the only visual sonographic clue of ectopic pregnancy, along with absence of intrauterine gestational sac. In the ultrasound image (Figure 24-6), free fluid in the cul-de-sac is seen.

Visualization of the Yolk Sac

The yolk sac is derived from embryonic tissue; therefore a pseudosac will not produce a yolk sac. When a yolk sac is seen within an intrauterine sac, it confirms that it is a true intrauterine gestational sac (See Figure 24-7). The sensitivity for diagnosing intrauterine gestations greater than 5.5 weeks approaches 100%.[75]

Ultrasound Measurements

Transvaginal ultrasound will be necessary for appropriate visualization and measurements prior to about 10 week size. Prior to when an embryo can be visualized at about 6½ week size, measure the gestational sac in 3 dimensions to obtain a mean sac diameter in mm. Use the following formulas to estimate gestational dating (by menstrual age) in days:

- Embryo pole (mm) + 42
- Mean sac diameter (mm) + 30

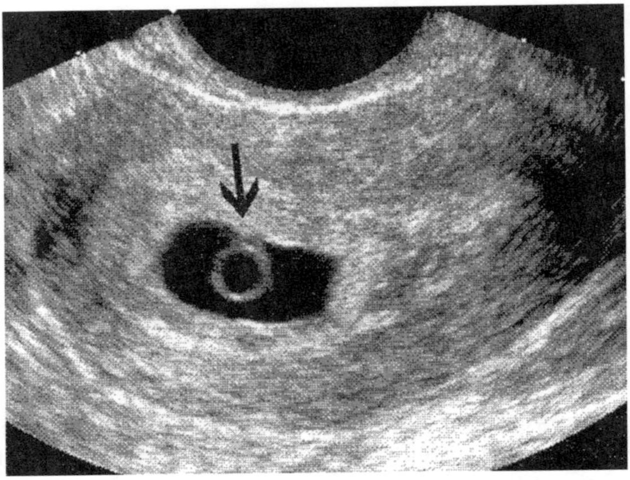

Figure 24-7 Yolk sac appears within the intrauterine gestational sac (arrow).

Correlation of hCG, Ultrasound Findings and Clinical Picture

When pregnancy cannot be visualized by transvaginal ultrasound, the clinician must evaluate the expected gestational dating, ultrasound findings, the pregnancy test results, knowledge of expected hCG values, and the patient's clinical picture in conjunction with risk factors of ectopic pregnancy. The most likely scenario is that a pregnancy is intrauterine, since approximately only 2% of pregnancies are reported to be ectopic in the general population.[76]

When a patient's highly sensitive urine pregnancy test is positive but no gestational sac is visualized by transvaginal sonography, there are several possible explanations:

- Very early intrauterine pregnancy; too early for a gestational sac to be visualized (<4.5 weeks)
- Abnormal pregnancy—intrauterine pregnancy not growing normally
- Ectopic pregnancy
- Elevated hCG due to reasons other than pregnancy

In addition, certain things can delay the visualization of a normal gestational sac including body habitus (i.e., obesity), fibroids, uterine anomalies, or an acutely retroverted uterus. Abnormal or delayed growth of a pregnancy can also prevent visualization at the expected time. For example, a multiple gestation pregnancy will have higher hCG levels than a singleton pregnancy before it can be visualized.

hCG Discriminatory Zone

The amount of hCG in early pregnancy directly correlates with the quantity of pregnancy tissue growing. The hCG level at which a gestational sac *should* be seen on transvaginal ultrasound is called the "discriminatory zone." The current accepted discriminatory zone of hCG is 2,000 to 3,000 mIU / mL with transvaginal ultrasonography.[38]

ABNORMAL PREGNANCY ASSESSMENT

EARLY PREGNANCY LOSS

Miscarriage occurs in approximately 15% of all clinically recognized pregnancies.[29,77]

The terminology to describe miscarriage includes:

- **Missed abortion or early pregnancy failure (EPF):** a nonviable pregnancy without bleeding or cervical dilation. EPF can be further categorized based on ultrasound findings:
    1. **Anembryonic gestation ("blighted ovum"):** mean sac diameter of ≥25 mm without an embryo on *transvaginal* ultrasound *or* no growth of gestational sac size over 5 to 7 days.
    2. **Embryonic/fetal demise:** presence of embryo ≥7mm in length without cardiac motion. Note: If the embryo is smaller than 7mm with no cardiac motion, this is NOT diagnostic of demise. In the situation of a wanted pregnancy, ultrasound should be repeated in about 1 week to evaluate viability.
- **Incomplete abortion:** clinical and ultrasound findings of an open cervix and passage of some but not all of the products of conception (POCs).
- **Threatened abortion:** uterine bleeding, closed cervix, and no passage of POCs.
- **Inevitable abortion:** cervical dilation, with / without bleeding or cramping, and where passage of tissue will eventually occur.

The diagnosis of spontaneous abortion may be made on the basis of a pelvic examination, abnormal bleeding, or ultrasound findings. If ectopic pregnancy has been excluded and bleeding is not heavy, women have a choice of several options for management, including expectant management, medical treatment (misoprostol), or vacuum aspiration.[78] Expectant and medical management should be followed with evaluation to confirm that the gestational sac has successfully expulsed. Approximately 15% of

Table 24-4 Guidelines for transvaginal ultrasonographic diagnosis of pregnancy failure in a woman with an intrauterine pregnancy of uncertain viability (Doubilet 2013)[38]

Findings Diagnostic of Pregnancy Failure	Findings Suspicious For, But Not Diagnostic of, Pregnancy Failure
Crown-rump length of ≥7mm and no heartbeat	Crown-rump length of <7 mm and no heartbeat
Mean sac diameter of ≥25 mm and no embryo	Mean sac diameter of 16–24 mm and no embryo
Absence of embryo with heartbeat ≥2 wks after a scan that showed a gestational sac without a yolk sac	Absence of embryo with heartbeat 7–13 days after a scan that showed a gestational sac without a yolk sac
Absence of embryo with heartbeat ≥11 days after a scan that showed a gestational sac with a yolk sac	• Absence of embryo with heartbeat 7–10 days after a scan that showed a gestational sac with a yolk sac • Absence of embryo ≥6 wks after last menstrual period • Empty amnion (amnion seen adjacent to yolk sac, with no visible embryo) • Enlarged yolk sac (>7 mm) • Small gestational sac in relation to the size of the embryo (<5 mm difference between the mean sac diameter and crown rump length)

patients do not experience expulsion even after misoprostol and may require uterine aspiration. Women should be offered all options and may decide on management based on appointment availability, desire to avoid a procedure, or need for predictable timing.

Anembryonic Pregnancy

Anembryonic pregnancy, formerly known as *blighted ovum,* refers to a pregnancy in which the gestational sac developed normally but the embryo never materialized, or an embryo developed but was then reabsorbed. Trophoblastic tissue continues to function, causing continued growth of the gestational sac, although at a slower than normal rate. An anembryonic pregnancy is diagnosed when a transvaginal ultrasound reveals a mean sac diameter (MSD) exceeding 25 mm with no detectable embryo.[38]

Pregnancy of Unknown Location (PUL)

Evaluation of the location of very early pregnancies can be challenging. A small proportion (estimated 2%) of these pregnancies may be ectopic pregnancies, which are important to identify and monitor or treat.[79] About half of women presenting with very early pregnancy of unknown location have an undesired pregnancy and it is acceptable to proceed with abortion

Box 24-2 Clinical steps for pregnancy of unknown location

1. Perform urine pregnancy test.
2. Document whether the patient plans to continue or terminate the pregnancy.
3. Assess symptoms (bleeding, pain, etc.).
4. Document the last menstrual period.
5. Conduct pelvic exam with attention to adnexal exam and uterine size.
6. Obtain a transvaginal ultrasound.
7. Draw serum for hCG measurement if no visible intrauterine pregnancy.
8. Determine Rh status (If bleeding/spotting, administer Rhogam if Rh negative and obtain CBC).

(medical or surgical) prior to localization of the pregnancy in certain circumstances. In stable patients with desired pregnancy, serial hCG should be obtained to determine if the pregnancy is abnormal prior to any intervention. All patients with pregnancy of unknown location need follow-up to ensure resolution of the pregnancy, but the length of the follow-up may vary.

First, determine whether the patient is stable and symptomatic (bleeding, pain, etc.). Determine if the pregnancy is desired or whether the patient would like to proceed with an abortion.

Initial Evaluation of Pregnancy of Unknown Location

Symptomatic Patients. The following symptoms may require further evaluation or management: abdominal or pelvic pain, vaginal bleeding, and free fluid noted in the pelvis on ultrasound examination. Obtain a detailed medical and surgical history, including risk factors for ectopic pregnancy (assisted reproductive technologies, prior tubal occlusive surgery, intrauterine contraception, prior ectopic, history of pelvic infections, prior pelvic surgery, and smoking). Symptomatic patients can undergo initial triage evaluation in an outpatient clinic setting unless they demonstrate severe pain, unstable vital signs, ongoing heavy bleeding, or other symptoms concerning for ruptured ectopic pregnancy.

Asymptomatic Patients. Asymptomatic patients who have an undesired pregnancy can proceed with medical or surgical abortion regardless of pregnancy localization and without waiting. The probability of ectopic pregnancy in this setting is estimated to be 0.4% if they are asymptomatic and have expected gestational dating based on menstrual age of less than 35 days.[80]

Asymptomatic patients who have a positive urine pregnancy test with a desired pregnancy, no risk factors for ectopic pregnancy, and normal exam findings can be scheduled for routine prenatal care. An ultrasound can be performed at the first prenatal visit to aid in accurate gestational

Table 24-5 hCG levels in pregnancies of unknown origin

If hCG <2,000–3,000 mIU/mL and the pregnancy is desired

- Obtain another serum hCG level in 48 hours.

Normal rise (>53%)[54]:

- A rise of greater than 53% over 48 hours is suggestive of intrauterine pregnancy. No further hCG testing is necessary.
- Multiple gestations will have a higher hCG level before being detectable by ultrasound.

Abnormal rise (≤40% to 53%):[92]

- Consider a third hCG value for confirmation.
- A lower rise over 48 hours is suggestive of an abnormal intrauterine pregnancy or an ectopic pregnancy.
- Consider uterine aspiration. Abrupt hCG decline >50% within 24 to 48 after aspiration is suggestive of intrauterine pregnancy. No further evaluation is necessary in the setting of abrupt decline after aspiration. (See Chapter 25 on Abortion for further discussion.)

Plateau (±15%):

- Consider uterine aspiration as above.

Decline (>15%):

- If the hCG levels are low (<200) and are declining spontaneously by more than 15% weekly, the patient can be monitored with weekly hCG levels until the hCG level is 2 or less (non-pregnant).

If hCG >3,000 mIU/mL and the pregnancy is desired

- Refer for formal ultrasound.
- If the ultrasound is unable to confirm the location of the pregnancy, or if it suggests ectopic pregnancy, the next step is urgent referral to a site where ectopic pregnancy can be managed.

dating as well as pregnancy localization. Waiting until after 6 weeks gestation to perform this visit is less likely to lead to additional testing or confusion and anxiety about the results. A clinical dilemma arises when a serum hCG level or an ultrasound is obtained in asymptomatic patient and is non-diagnostic, either for pregnancy viability or localization.

Uterine Aspiration for Pregnancy Localization. Uterine aspiration with serial hCG assessment can be used for pregnancy location and is particularly helpful in the following scenarios:

- A patient with undesired pregnancy who desires termination
- A patient with a desired pregnancy and abnormal hCG rise (≤40%), plateau, or decline

Gross pathologic or histologic examination of the uterine tissue should be performed either by the clinician and/or a pathologist. The sensitivity of visualization of chorionic villi is similar between clinicians and pathologists at around 60%.[66,81–83] Since not seeing villi might result in an over-diagnosis of ectopic pregnancy, serial hCG should be obtained for correlation. Additionally, false-positive visualization of villi can occur resulting in over-reassurance.

Ongoing serum hCG monitoring should be performed after the uterine aspiration. A repeat serum hCG between the day of the procedure and 48 hours later, but as soon as 12 hours later, documenting decline of >50% demonstrates a completed pregnancy and suggests that the pregnancy was intrauterine. No further follow-up is necessary.[60,84] If the serum hCG does not decline, either the uterine evacuation was not complete or the pregnancy may be ectopic. The next step in this scenario is to repeat an ultrasound.

Abortion in the Setting of Pregnancy of Unknown Location. In an asymptomatic patient with an undesired pregnancy who wants an abortion and has a pregnancy of unknown location, in most cases it is reasonable to proceed with medical or surgical abortion. In these instances, obtain an hCG prior to the abortion and then 24 to 48 hours after the surgical abortion or after the patient thinks the products of pregnancy passed following a medication abortion. The initial hCG results may not be received prior to the patient initiating or completing the abortion. If the initial hCG is above the discriminatory zone of 2,000 to 3,000 (see hCG Discriminatory Zone section above), then the concern for ectopic pregnancy is increased and formal ultrasound examination is the next step along with obtaining a serial hCG trend and referral to a facility where ectopic pregnancy could be managed.

Further evaluation may also be warranted if the estimated menstrual age is more than 35 days LMP because those patients are much more likely to have an ectopic pregnancy. In this case, the potential risk of ectopic pregnancy should be discussed with the patient and uterine aspiration could be considered over medication abortion. Additionally, consider consultation or referral for ultrasound that could identify pelvic free fluid and adnexal masses prior to an intervention if those radiologic characteristics cannot be adequately evaluated by the abortion clinic.

Ectopic Pregnancy

Assess the risk factors for ectopic pregnancy through the patient's history (see Box 24-3 Risk factors for ectopic pregnancy). However, more than half of identified ectopic pregnancies occur in women without known risk factors.[85]

Box 24-3 Risk factors for ectopic pregnancy

- Previous ectopic pregnancy[1]
- History of tubal surgery (female sterilization or tubal reconstruction)
- Intrauterine contraceptive in place[4]
- Pelvic inflammatory disease[7]

Heterotopic pregnancy is the simultaneous occurrence of two or more implantation sites, most commonly a concomitant intrauterine pregnancy and an ectopic pregnancy.[86] The incidence of heterotopic pregnancy in the general population is reported as 1 in 4,000.[87] The risk of heterotopic pregnancy in women undergoing assisted reproductive techniques is as high as 1%.[88]

Molar Pregnancy

Hydatidiform mole (molar pregnancy) is an abnormal conception with excessive trophoblastic proliferation. Molar pregnancies are classified as either complete (genetic material exclusively of paternal origin, no embryo present) or partial (one maternal and two paternal contributions—usually two sperm fertilize a normal oocyte, and an embryo is often present).[89] Patients with molar pregnancies typically present in the first trimester with abnormal bleeding and very high levels of hCG[90] (see Pitfalls of Pregnancy Testing). With a complete mole, uterine size is often greater than expected due to hydropic trophoblastic tissue. Although molar pregnancies are initially benign, their high hCG levels can cause medical sequelae including hyperemesis gravidarum, hyperthyroidism, hypertension, or large ovarian theca lutein cysts.

Trophoblastic tissue of molar pregnancies may become invasive, which can lead to malignant conditions such as gestational trophoblastic neoplasia (GTN) and choriocarcinoma. GTN is highly curable if detected early; occasionally, however, patients with metastatic disease still die.[91] These conditions

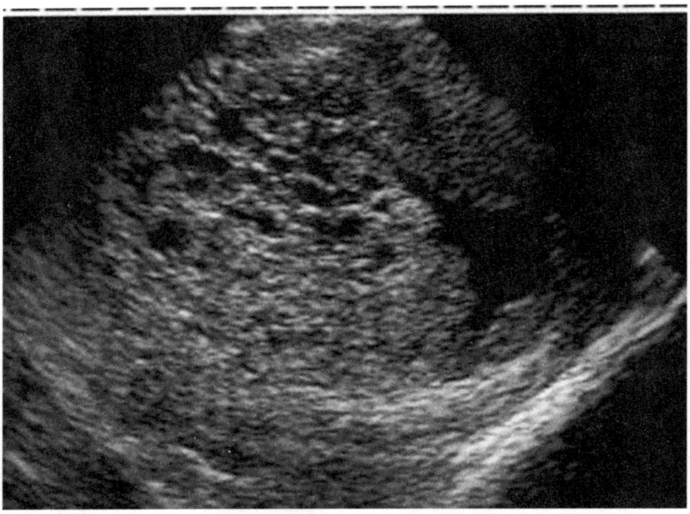

Figure 24-8 Molar pregnancy. The "snow storm" appearance of a molar pregnancy is the result of multiple small cystic spaces. The larger cysts are visible as sonolucent spaces while the smaller cysts create echogenic areas due to the multiple interfaces between the cysts. (Courtesy Matthew Reeves, MD).

are more likely with complete (20%) than partial (<5%) moles.[90] The standard of care for treatment is uterine evacuation with close surveillance of post-evacuation serum hCG for 6 to 12 months. Evacuation can usually be performed in the same setting as surgical management of a miscarriage or abortion of the same uterine size. Tissue should be sent for formal pathologic evaluation. Because the occurrence of a new pregnancy during the monitoring phase can mask malignancy or confuse the clinical picture, we strongly recommend use of effective contraception during this time-period.

Author Disclosures—Baldwin: Nexplanon trainer for Merck. Edelman: none.

REFERENCES

1. Ankum WM, Mol BW, Van der Veen F, Bossuyt PM. Risk factors for ectopic pregnancy: a meta-analysis. Fertil Steril 1996;65:1093–9.
2. Soto-Wright V, Bernstein M, Goldstein DP, Berkowitz RS. The changing clinical presentation of complete molar pregnancy. Obstet Gynecol 1995;86:775–9.
3. Zabin LS, Emerson MR, Ringers PA, Sedivy V. Adolescents with negative pregnancy test results. An accessible at-risk group. JAMA 1996;275:113–7.
4. Barnhart KT. Clinical practice. Ectopic pregnancy. N Eng J Med 2009;361:379–87.
5. Wilkes J. AAFP Releases Position Paper on Preconception care. Am Fam Physician 2016;94:508–10.
6. ACOG technical bulletin. Preconceptional care. Number 205—May 1995. American College of Obstetricians and Gynecologists. Int J Gynaecol Obstet 1995;50:201–7.
7. Hillis SD, Owens LM, Marchbanks PA, Amsterdam LF, Mac Kenzie WR. Recurrent chlamydial infections increase the risks of hospitalization for ectopic pregnancy and pelvic inflammatory disease. Am J Obstet Gynecol 1997;176:103–7.
8. Finer LB, Zolna MR. Shifts in intended and unintended pregnancies in the United States, 2001–2008. Am J Public Health 2014;104 Suppl 1:S43–8.
9. Erickson JD. Folic acid and prevention of spina bifida and anencephaly. 10 years after the U.S. Public Health Service recommendation. MMWR Recomm Rep 2002;51:1–3.
10. Kapp N, Whyte P, Tang J, Jackson E, Brahmi D. A review of evidence for safe abortion care. Contraception 2013;88:350–63.
11. Fox GN. Teaching first trimester uterine sizing. J Fam Pract 1985;21:400–1.
12. Fielding JR, Brown DL, Thurmond AS. Gynecologic imaging. Philadelphia, PA: Elsevier/Saunders; 2011.
13. Hasan R, Baird DD, Herring AH, Olshan AF, Jonsson Funk ML, Hartmann KE. Patterns and predictors of vaginal bleeding in the first trimester of pregnancy. Ann Epidemiol 2010;20:524–31.
14. Promes SB, Nobay F. Pitfalls in first-trimester bleeding. Emerg Med Clin North Am 2010;28:219–34.
15. Hasan R, Baird DD, Herring AH, Olshan AF, Jonsson Funk ML, Hartmann KE. Association between first-trimester vaginal bleeding and miscarriage. Obstet Gynecol 2009;114:860–7.
16. Barnhart KT, Sammel MD, Gracia CR, Chittams J, Hummel AC, Shaunik A. Risk factors for ectopic pregnancy in women with symptomatic first-trimester pregnancies. Fertil Steril 2006;86:36–43.
17. ACOG practice bulletin. Prevention of Rh D alloimmunization. Number 4, May 1999 (replaces educational bulletin Number 147, October 1990). Clinical management guidelines for obstetrician-gynecologists. American College of Obstetricians and Gynecologists. Int J Gynaecol Obstet 1999;66:63–70.

18. Van Look PF, Cottingham J. The World Health Organization's safe abortion guidance document. Am J Public Health 2013;103:593–6.
19. Qureshi H, Massey E, Kirwan D, et al. BCSH guideline for the use of anti-D immunoglobulin for the prevention of haemolytic disease of the fetus and newborn. Transfus Med 2014;24:8–20.
20. Sawaya GF, Grady D, Kerlikowske K, Grimes DA. Antibiotics at the time of induced abortion: the case for universal prophylaxis based on a meta-analysis. Obstet Gynecol 1996;87:884–90.
21. Werler MM, Mitchell AA, Hernandez-Diaz S, Honein MA. Use of over-the-counter medications during pregnancy. Am J Obstet Gynecol 2005;193:771–7.
22. Schwarz EB, Maselli J, Norton M, Gonzales R. Prescription of teratogenic medications in United States ambulatory practices. Am J Med 2005;118:1240–9.
23. Chambliss LR. Intimate partner violence and its implication for pregnancy. Clin Obstet Gynecol 2008;51:385–97.
24. Plichta SB. Intimate partner violence and physical health consequences: policy and practice implications. J Interpers Violence 2004;19:1296–323.
25. Palladino CL, Singh V, Campbell J, Flynn H, Gold KJ. Homicide and suicide during the perinatal period: findings from the National Violent Death Reporting System. Obstet Gynecol 2011;118:1056–63.
26. Berg CJ, Callaghan WM, Henderson Z, Syverson C. Pregnancy-related mortality in the United States, 1998 to 2005. Obstet Gynecol 2011;117:1230.
27. Rodriguez MA, Quiroga SS, Bauer HM. Breaking the silence. Battered women's perspectives on medical care. Arch Fam Med 1996;5:153–8.
28. Kim SK, Romero R, Kusanovic JP, et al. The prognosis of pregnancy conceived despite the presence of an intrauterine device (IUD). J Perinat Med 2010;38:45–53.
29. Rai R, Regan L. Recurrent miscarriage. Lancet 2006;368:601–11.
30. Davies S, Byrn F, Cole LA. Human chorionic gonadotropin testing for early pregnancy viability and complications. Clin Lab Med 2003;23:257–64, vii.
31. Cole LA. Human chorionic gonadotropin and associated molecules. Expert Rev Mol Diagn 2009;9:51–73.
32. Cole LA, Khanlian SA, Sutton JM, Davies S, Rayburn WF. Accuracy of home pregnancy tests at the time of missed menses. Am J Obstet Gynecol 2004;190:100–5.
33. Wallace LS, Zite NB, Homewood VJ. Making sense of home pregnancy test instructions. J Womens Health 2009;18:363–8.
34. Chard T. Pregnancy tests: a review. Hum Reprod 1992;7:701–10.
35. Wilcox AJ, Baird DD, Dunson D, McChesney R, Weinberg CR. Natural limits of pregnancy testing in relation to the expected menstrual period. JAMA 2001;286: 1759–61.
36. Godfrey EM, Anderson A, Fielding SL, Meyn L, Creinin MD. Clinical utility of urine pregnancy assays to determine medical abortion outcome is limited. Contraception 2007;75:378–82.
37. Desai D, Lu J, Wyness SP, et al. Human chorionic gonadotropin discriminatory zone in ectopic pregnancy: does assay harmonization matter? Fertil Steril 2014;101:1671–4.
38. Doubilet PM, Benson CB, Bourne T, Blaivas M. Diagnostic criteria for nonviable pregnancy early in the first trimester. N Eng J Med 2013;369:1443–51.
39. Kazemi MR, Vargas JE, Lo JC. Hyperthyroidism and a negative urine hCG test in molar pregnancy. Am J Med 2004;117:889–90.
40. Tabas JA, Strehlow M, Isaacs E. A false negative pregnancy test in a patient with a hydatidiform molar pregnancy. N Engl J Med 2003;349:2172–3.
41. Cole LA. Human chorionic gonadotropin tests. Expert Rev Mol Diagn 2009;9:721–47.
42. Butler SA, Cole LA. Evidence for, and associated risks with, the human chorionic gonadotropin supplemented diet. J Diet Suppl 2016;13:694–9.
43. Bandi ZL, Schoen I, Waters M. An algorithm for testing and reporting serum choriogonadotropin at clinically significant decision levels with use of "pregnancy test" reagents. Clin Chem 1989;35:545–51.

44. Cole LA, Khanlian SA, Muller CY. Normal production of human chorionic gonadotropin in perimenopausal and menopausal women and after oophorectomy. Int J Gynecol Cancer 2009;19:1556–9.
45. Cole LA, Khanlian SA, Muller CY. Detection of perimenopause or postmenopause human chorionic gonadotropin: an unnecessary source of alarm. Am J Obstet Gynecol 2008;198:275 e1–7.
46. Cole LA, Ladner DG. Background hCG in non-pregnant individuals: need for more sensitive point-of-care and over-the-counter pregnancy tests. Clin Biochem 2009;42:168–75.
47. Fahy BG, Gouzd VA, Atallah JN. Pregnancy tests with end-stage renal disease. J Clin Anesth 2008;20:609–13.
48. Knight AK, Bingemann T, Cole L, Cunningham-Rundles C. Frequent false positive beta human chorionic gonadotropin tests in immunoglobulin A deficiency. Clin Exp Immunol 2005;141:333–7.
49. Rotmensch S, Cole LA. False diagnosis and needless therapy of presumed malignant disease in women with false-positive human chorionic gonadotropin concentrations. Lancet 2000;355:712–5.
50. Braunstein GD, Rasor J, Danzer H, Adler D, Wade ME. Serum human chorionic gonadotropin levels throughout normal pregnancy. Am J Obstet Gynecol 1976;126:678–81.
51. Lohstroh PN, Overstreet JW, Stewart DR, et al. Hourly human chorionic gonadotropin secretion profiles during the peri-implantation period of successful pregnancies. Fertil Steril 2007;87:1413–8.
52. Cole LA, Laidler LL, Muller CY. USA hCG reference service, 10-year report. Clin Biochem 2010;43:1013–22.
53. Kadar N, Caldwell BV, Romero R. A method of screening for ectopic pregnancy and its indications. Obstet Gynecol 1981;58:162–6.
54. Barnhart KT, Sammel MD, Rinaudo PF, Zhou L, Hummel AC, Guo W. Symptomatic patients with an early viable intrauterine pregnancy: hCG curves redefined. Obstet Gynecol 2004;104:50–5.
55. Timor-Tritsch IE, Rottem S. Transvaginal sonography. 2nd ed. New York: Elsevier; 1991.
56. Doubilet PM. Ultrasound evaluation of the first trimester. Radiol Clin North Am 2014;52:1191–9.
57. Dart RG, Mitterando J, Dart LM. Rate of change of serial beta-human chorionic gonadotropin values as a predictor of ectopic pregnancy in patients with indeterminate transvaginal ultrasound findings. Ann Emerg Med 1999;34:703–10.
58. Steier JA, Bergsjo P, Myking OL. Human chorionic gonadotropin in maternal plasma after induced abortion, spontaneous abortion, and removed ectopic pregnancy. Obstet Gynecol 1984;64:391–4.
59. Aral K, Gurkan Zorlu C, Gokmen O. Plasma human chorionic gonadotropin levels after induced abortion. Adv Contracept 1996;12:11–4.
60. Schaff EA, Fielding SL, Eisinger S, Stadalius L. Mifepristone and misoprostol for early abortion when no gestational sac is present. Contraception 2001;63:251–4.
61. Walker K, Schaff E, Fielding S, Fuller L. Monitoring serum chorionic gonadotropin levels after mifepristone abortion. Contraception 2001;64:271–3.
62. Rorbye C, Norgaard M, Nilas L. Prediction of late failure after medical abortion from serial beta-hCG measurements and ultrasonography. Hum Reprod 2004;19:85–9.
63. Fiala C, Safar P, Bygdeman M, Gemzell-Danielsson K. Verifying the effectiveness of medical abortion; ultrasound versus hCG testing. Eur J Obstet Gynecol Reprod Biol 2003;109:190–5.
64. Creinin MD. Methotrexate and misoprostol for abortion at 57–63 days gestation. Contraception 1994;50:511–5.
65. Pocius KD, Bartz D, Maurer R, Stenquist A, Fortin J, Goldberg AB. Serum human chorionic gonadotropin (hCG) trend within the first few days after medical abortion: a prospective study. Contraception 2017;95:263–8.
66. Edwards J, Carson SA. New technologies permit safe abortion at less than six weeks' gestation and provide timely detection of ectopic gestation. Am J Obstet Gynecol 1997;176:1101–6.

67. Norton ME, Scoutt LM, Feldstein VA. Callen's ultrasonography in Obstet Gynecol. Sixth edition. ed. Philadelphia, PA: Elsevier; 2017.
68. Paul M. Management of unintended and abnormal pregnancy : comprehensive abortion care. West Sussex, England: Wiley-Blackwell; 2009.
69. Bhatt S, Ghazale H, Dogra VS. Sonographic evaluation of ectopic pregnancy. Radiol Clin North Am 2007;45:549–60.
70. Timor-Tritsch IE, Rottem S. Transvaginal sonography. New York, N.Y.: Elsevier; 1988.
71. Doubilet PM, Benson CB. Double sac sign and intradecidual sign in early pregnancy: interobserver reliability and frequency of occurrence. J Ultrasound Med 2013;32:1207–14.
72. Yeh HC. Efficacy of the intradecidual sign and fallacy of the double decidual sac sign in the diagnosis of early intrauterine pregnancy. Radiology 1999;210:579–82.
73. Della-Giustina D, Denny M. Ectopic pregnancy. Emerg Med Clin North Am 2003;21: 565–84.
74. Mahony BS, Filly RA, Nyberg DA, Callen PW. Sonographic evaluation of ectopic pregnancy. J Ultrasound Med 1985;4:221–8.
75. Gracia CR, Barnhart KT. Diagnosing ectopic pregnancy: decision analysis comparing six strategies. Obstet Gynecol 2001;97:464–70.
76. Centers for Disease C, Prevention. Ectopic pregnancy—United States, 1990–1992. MMWR 1995;44:46–8.
77. Sotiriadis A, Makrydimas G, Papatheodorou S, Ioannidis JP. Expectant, medical, or surgical management of first-trimester miscarriage: a meta-analysis. Obstet Gynecol 2005;105:1104–13.
78. Pauleta JR, Clode N, Graca LM. Expectant management of incomplete abortion in the first trimester. Int J Gynaecol Obstet 2009;106:35–8.
79. American College of Obstetricians and Gynecologists. ACOG Practice Bulletin No. 94: Medical management of ectopic pregnancy. Obstet Gynecol 2008;111:1479–85.
80. Li CL, Song LP, Tang SY, et al. Efficacy, safety, and acceptability of low-dose mifepristone and self-administered misoprostol for ultra-early medical abortion: a randomized controlled trial. Reprod Sci 2017;24:731–7.
81. Lindahl B, Ahlgren M. Identification of chorion villi in abortion specimens. Obstet Gynecol 1986;67:79–81.
82. Dean G. Accuracy of POC detection after early abortion with MVA vs EVA: a randomized trial. The Forum; 2012 Oct 27, 2012; Denver, CO.
83. Paul M, Lackie E, Mitchell C, Rogers A, Fox M. Is pathology examination useful after early surgical abortion? Obstet Gynecol 2002;99:567–71.
84. Pocius KD, Maurer R, Fortin J, Goldberg AB, Bartz D. Early serum human chorionic gonadotropin (hCG) trends after medication abortion. Contraception 2015;91:503–6.
85. Murray H, Baakdah H, Bardell T, Tulandi T. Diagnosis and treatment of ectopic pregnancy. CMAJ 2005;173:905–12.
86. Kulp JL, Barnhart KT. Ectopic pregnancy: diagnosis and management. Womens Health 2008;4:79–87.
87. Seeber BE, Barnhart KT. Suspected ectopic pregnancy. Obstet Gynecol 2006;107:399–413.
88. Dumesic DA, Damario MA, Session DR. Interstitial heterotopic pregnancy in a woman conceiving by in vitro fertilization after bilateral salpingectomy. Mayo Clin Proc 2001;76:90–2.
89. Sebire NJ. Histopathological diagnosis of hydatidiform mole: contemporary features and clinical implications. Fetal Pediatr Pathol 2010;29:1–16.
90. Soper JT, Mutch DG, Schink JC, American College of Obstetricians and Gynecologists. Diagnosis and treatment of gestational trophoblastic disease: ACOG Practice Bulletin No. 53. Gynecol Oncol 2004;93:575–85.
91. El-Helw LM, Hancock BW. Treatment of metastatic gestational trophoblastic neoplasia. Lancet Oncol 2007;8:715–24.
92. Barnhart KT, Guo W, Cary M, et al. Differences in serum human chorionic gonadotropin rise in early pregnancy by race and values at presentation. Obtstet Gynecol 2016;128:503-11.

Abortion

25

Siripanth Nippita, MD, MS
Maureen Paul, MD, MPH

- Access to legal, safe abortion is a critical part of primary reproductive health care.
- Approximately 90% of all abortions in the United States occur during the first trimester; two-thirds take place at or before 8 weeks following the onset of the individual's last normal menstrual period.
- Medication methods (most commonly mifepristone followed by misoprostol) are effective and safe options for individuals seeking abortion during the early weeks of pregnancy.
- Resources are available for facilitating abortion referrals, and for providing financial and logistical assistance to those in need of these services.
- Clinicians should address expeditiously any individual's request for pregnancy confirmation and provide information on all options, including prompt services or referral for abortion if the individual so desires.

Individuals have abortions for many reasons. In large U.S. surveys,[1,2] respondents most frequently cited financial concerns, relationship problems, or work, school, or family responsibilities as reasons for their decision to have an abortion. Approximately 12% of individuals reported concerns about their own health or that of the embryo or fetus as reasons for the abortion, and 1% reported that they were ending a pregnancy that resulted from coerced sex. In other studies, women who presented for second-trimester abortions were more likely to have had a delayed diagnosis of pregnancy and to have encountered logistical difficulties in accessing services, such as finding a provider, obtaining public insurance, or arranging transportation.[3–5] The decision to terminate a pregnancy is based on an individual's unique situation, and it often involves complex considerations regarding responsibilities to self and others.

Each individual deserves to feel respected and supported when making this decision.

This chapter provides an overview for clinicians who evaluate and refer patients for abortion services, as well as those who offer early medication or aspiration abortion in their practices. In the past, many clinicians delayed scheduling an abortion until 7 weeks following the onset of the last menstrual period (LMP) because pregnancy tests lacked the sensitivity to confirm early pregnancy. Today, highly sensitive pregnancy tests, ultrasonography, and improved abortion methods allow clinicians to diagnose pregnancy and offer safe and effective abortion options during the earliest weeks of pregnancy. Several excellent reviews describe the various clinical abortion techniques in more detail.[6,7]

LEGAL STATUS OF ABORTION

On January 22, 1973, the U.S. Supreme Court decided *Roe v. Wade* [410 U.S. 113 (1973)], the landmark case that legalized abortion nationwide. The *Roe* Court recognized the decision to continue or end a pregnancy as part of a fundamental constitutional right to privacy, thereby affording it high protection. Holding that the government could not interfere with an individual's choice to have an abortion unless it had a "compelling" reason to do so, the Justices attempted to balance the interests involved by establishing a "trimester framework":[8]

1. In the first trimester, the abortion decision and procedure must be left to the judgment of the pregnant patient and the physician, largely unimpeded by governmental regulations.
2. In the second trimester, each state may choose to regulate abortion procedures in ways that are reasonably related to the pregnant patient's health.
3. In the third trimester, if and when a fetus reaches viability, the state may elect to promote its interest in potential human life by prohibiting abortion, as long as it provides an exception for abortions necessary to protect the patient's life or health.

As demand for legal abortion services grew in the United States, abortion opponents introduced legislation at the local, state, and national levels to reduce access to abortion services. Passage of the Hyde Amendment in 1976 restricted federal funding for abortion, thereby curtailing access for the poor,[9,10] and numerous states regulated minors' access to abortion through provisions for parental involvement. Under *Roe*, the Supreme Court upheld such limitations on poor and young individuals' access to abortion, but it generally struck down other kinds of abortion restrictions.[8]

The Supreme Court's 1992 landmark decision in *Planned Parenthood of Southeastern Pennsylvania v. Casey* [505 U.S. 833 (1992)] greatly encouraged additional regulation of abortion by replacing *Roe's* trimester framework with a standard that allowed state restrictions on abortion as long as they did not impose an "undue burden" on an individual's ability to seek abortion. Under this less protective standard, the Supreme Court has upheld mandatory waiting periods, biased counseling provisions, and burdensome design requirements for facilities that provide abortion services; such laws have proliferated in recent years. Although the *Casey* Court weakened considerably the legal standard used to test the constitutionality of abortion restrictions, it affirmed individuals' fundamental right to choose abortion before fetal viability and upheld the requirement that any ban on abortion at a point when the fetus is viable must provide an exception to safeguard a patient's life or health.[8]

In the 1990s, after the *Casey* decision failed to overturn *Roe*, abortion opponents launched a concerted campaign to restrict methods of abortion. These efforts remained largely unsuccessful until 2007 when the U.S. Supreme Court, made increasingly conservative by two George W. Bush appointees, considered the federal Partial-Birth Abortion Ban Act of 2003 [18 U.S.C. 1531 (2003)]. In a sweeping 5 to 4 ruling, the Court upheld this federal abortion ban, which criminalizes certain safe second-trimester abortion procedures even when a physician believes that such a procedure is necessary to preserve a patient's health. This decision invited further abortion restrictions by crediting an asserted state interest in promoting respect for "embryonic and fetal life" [Gonzales v. Carhart, 550 U.S. 124, 163 (2007)], while dismissing decades of Supreme Court precedent that held women's health paramount.[11,12]

Election of the pro-choice President, Barack Obama in 2008 represented a positive shift for reproductive rights. Early in his administration, President Obama helped to restore critical health services worldwide by rescinding the "global gag rule," a regulation that had prohibited U.S. support for foreign nongovernmental organizations that provided information, counseling, or referrals for abortion, or that engaged in any kind of abortion advocacy work.[13] Following the murder of Kansas abortion provider Dr. George Tiller, in May 2009, the Department of Justice revitalized the National Task Force on Violence Against Reproductive Health Care Providers that had remained largely dormant under the preceding Bush administration. This Task Force aims to uphold the 1993 Freedom of Access to Clinic Entrances (FACE) Act [18 U.S.C. 248 (1994)] and other laws by coordinating efforts to prevent, investigate, and prosecute acts of violence and harassment against abortion providers.[8]

Notwithstanding these efforts and others, however, the struggle against the long-standing erosion of reproductive rights remains a formidable challenge. Lawmakers who oppose abortion won a number of seats in state legislatures following midterm elections in 2010. From 2011 to 2016, lawmakers passed 30% of the anti-abortion legislation enacted since *Roe*.[14] Examples of such legislation include ultrasound requirements, mandated counseling provisions, abortion bans after 20 to 22 weeks' gestation or under particular circumstances, and restrictions related to the facilities where abortions may be performed. Many restrictions are not based on sound scientific evidence.[15] Also worrisome are existing life-long appointments of conservative judges to some state and federal courts and to the Supreme Court,[16] as well as an anti-abortion movement that is determined to overturn *Roe* altogether.

Advocates for reproductive rights have won important victories, however. In 2013, Texas lawmakers passed House Bill 2, which mandated that abortion providers maintain local hospital admitting privileges and that clinics adhere to standards for ambulatory surgical centers. These regulations shuttered more than half of the state's abortion clinics, severely curtailing individuals' access to abortion. In 2016, the Supreme Court ruled in *Whole Woman's Health vs. Hellerstedt* that these two provisions posed an undue burden to obtaining an abortion without any apparent benefit.[17] Thus, they violate the Fourteenth Amendment, which guarantees an individual's right to privacy and protects the right to terminate a pregnancy before fetal viability.

The election of Donald Trump to the United States presidency in 2016 has brought with it an aggressive conservative agenda that includes accelerated infringement on abortion access, reinstatement and expansion of the global gag rule, and threats to the family planning safety net in the United States. In addition, undermining access to contraception without cost-sharing may reverse the current U.S. trends of lower rates of unintended pregnancy and abortion[18] and increasing rates of use of effective contraceptive methods.[19] At the same time, however, activism to protect women's health and rights is on the rise, and many states are enacting legislation to preserve or extend access to family planning services.[14]

THE PUBLIC HEALTH IMPACT OF LEGAL ABORTION

The *Roe v. Wade* decision ushered in a new era in reproductive health, producing immediate public health benefits. Abortion-related morbidity and mortality plummeted because abortion was more readily available closer to home, earlier in pregnancy, and at lower cost.[20] Abortion practices became safer after studies in the 1970s revealed that vacuum aspiration carried less morbidity than sharp curettage, local anesthesia was safer than general anesthesia, abortions performed in freestanding clinics were safer than those performed in hospitals, and dilation and evacuation (D&E) was safer than the second-trimester labor induction methods used at the time.

According to the Guttmacher Institute, the annual number of legal induced abortions rose dramatically following the *Roe* decision to reach 1.5 million in 1980. The number remained stable throughout the 1980s, peaking at 1.6 million in 1990 and falling to a historic low of 926,200 in 2014.[21] The abortion rate (number of abortions per 1,000 women aged 15 to 44 years) also fell to 14.6 per 1,000 in 2014, from a peak of 27.4 per 1,000 in 1980.[21] (See Figure 25-1.[22]) This change in the abortion rate is due primarily to a decline in the rate of unintended pregnancy, which decreased to 54 per 1,000 women in 2011, from 45 per 1,000 in 2008.[18] Both increased contraceptive use overall and use of highly effective contraception, including long-acting reversible methods, likely have contributed to

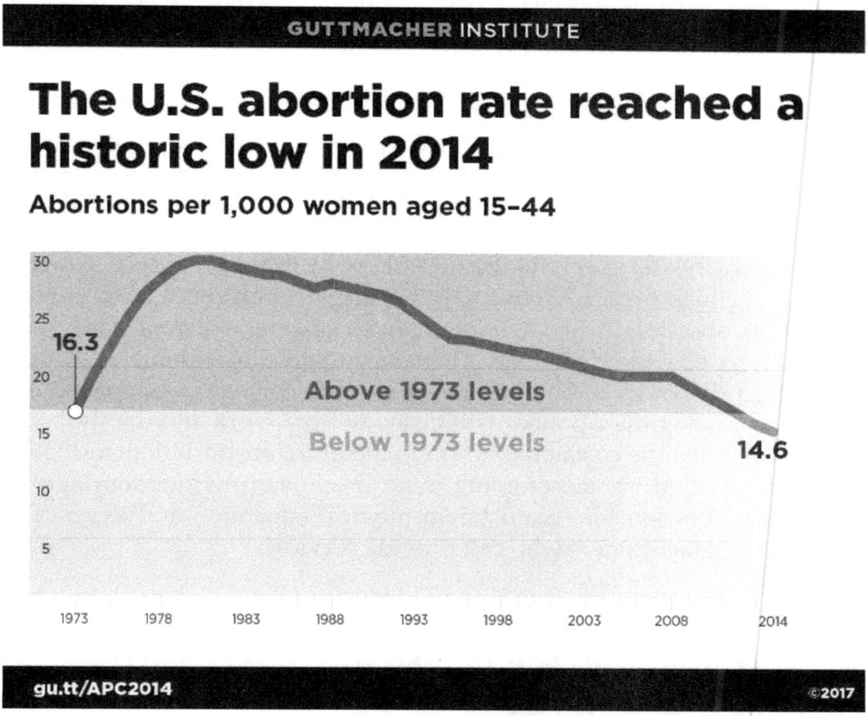

Source: Guttmacher Institute (2017)[22]

Figure 25-1 Abortion rates in the United States, 1973–2014

the decline. The Affordable Care Act has increased access to contraception by providing full coverage without cost-sharing for all Food and Drug Administration-approved contraceptive methods.

About 92% of abortions take place in the first trimester, a figure that has remained fairly stable over time; however, the proportion of abortions occurring at 8 weeks or less has increased from 38% in 1973 to 66% in 2013.[23] Moreover, very early abortions (6 weeks' gestation or less) have become more common, accounting for 38% of abortions performed at ≤13 weeks' gestation in 2013.[23] In contrast, the small percentage of abortions (about 5%) performed at or after 16 weeks' gestation has remained largely unchanged.[23]

To maintain the important public health benefits brought by the *Roe v. Wade* decision, abortion must remain not only safe and legal, but also available to individuals who need them. In the groundbreaking Turnaway study,[24] researchers followed individuals who obtained wanted abortions and those who were denied abortions because they exceeded the facilities' gestational age limits. Compared with individuals who obtained abortions, those who were denied abortions were less likely to rise out of poverty or have aspirational one-year life plans and more likely to remain in abusive relationships and experience pregnancy-related complications.[25] They were also more likely to experience anxiety and depressive symptoms shortly after being denied an abortion.[26]

In addition to increasing restrictions on abortion, the shortage of trained providers limits access to services.[27] According to a survey of National Abortion Federation members collected in 2002, more than 60% of U.S. abortion doctors were at least 50 years old,[28] and many had begun to retire. Between 2011 and 2014 the number of facilities providing abortion services declined from 1,720 to 1,671, leaving 90% percent of U.S. counties without an abortion provider.[29] Some physicians travel across states lines regularly to provide abortions. However, many individuals still must travel long distances to obtain their abortion.[30–32] This travel burden not only adds to the time a patient will be away from work and family, but it also compounds the costs of abortion to include transportation and lodging. Important efforts are ongoing to address this provider shortage by integrating abortion into mainstream medical education and expanding the range of practitioners who can provide services.

CHARACTERISTICS OF INDIVIDUALS WHO OBTAIN ABORTIONS

Not surprisingly, most individuals who have abortions are young and unmarried. In 2014, women in their twenties had more than half of all

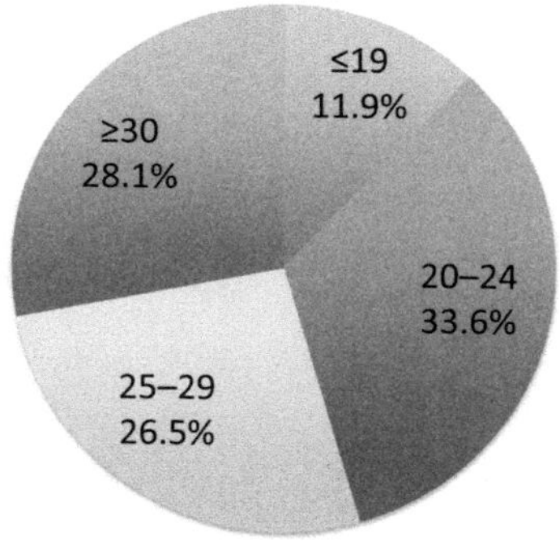

Data source: Jerman J, et al. (2016)[33]

Figure 25-2 Age distribution of abortion patients, 2014

reported abortions in the United States (Figure 25-2).[33] Teenagers obtained 12% of abortions that year, a dramatic decrease from nearly 33% in 1973. The racial and ethnic composition of individuals having abortions was similar in 2014 (Figure 25-3) and 2008, with black and Hispanic women overrepresented compared with white women.[33] Eighty-five percent of individuals who obtained abortions in 2014 were unmarried (Figure 25-4). In addition, the majority (60% in 2014) already had at least one child (Figure 25-5).[29,33]

Reflecting growing health disparities, poor and low-income individuals bear a disproportionate share of the burden of unintended pregnancy and its consequences. Although the unintended pregnancy rate fell between 2008 and 2011, rates among individuals below the poverty level were two to three times the national average.[18] In 2014, three-quarters of abortion patients were poor or low-income.[33] Paying for abortion services

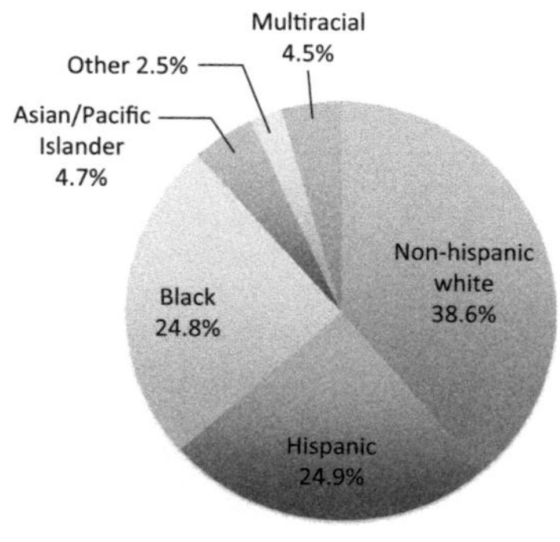

Data source: Jerman J, et al. (2016)[33]

Figure 25-3 Self-reported race of abortion patients, 2014

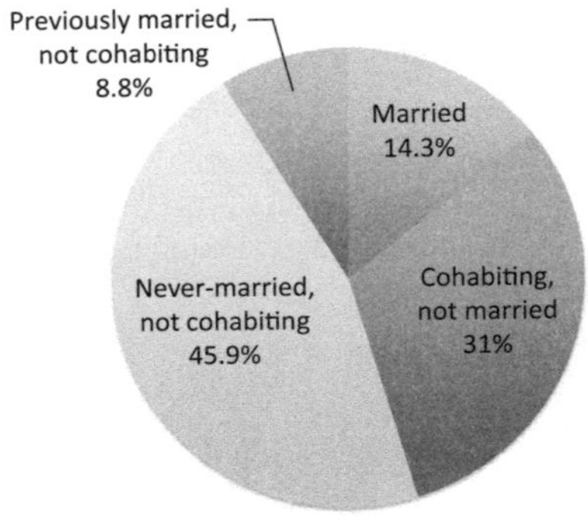

Data source: Jerman J, et al. (2016)[33]

Figure 25-4 Abortion patients' relationship status at the time of conception, 2014

poses a particular hardship for them, especially if they live in states where public insurance does not cover this care. Indeed, three-quarters of individuals obtaining abortion who lived in these states reported paying for the procedure themselves in 2014.[33]

An individual's ability to manage fertility depends on many factors, including access to affordable and effective contraception. About half of the unintended pregnancies in the United States occur in contraceptive non-users.[34] Common reasons for non-use among those having abortions include a perceived low risk of pregnancy, concerns or ambivalence about contraception, and problems accessing contraception. Although 51% of individuals obtaining abortions report that they used contraception during the month that they became pregnant, they may rely on less-effective

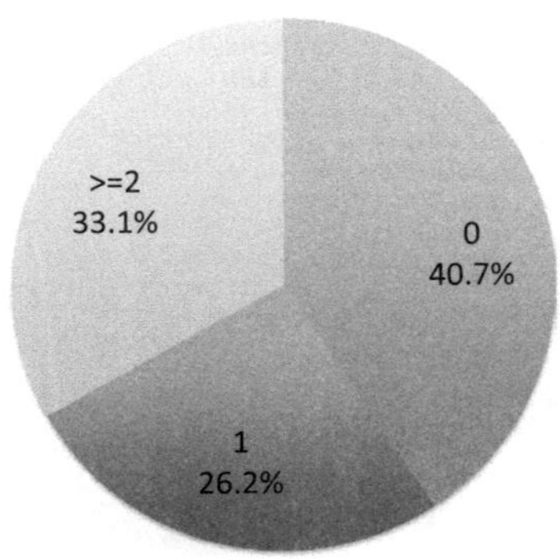

Data source: Jerman J, et al. (2016)[33]

Figure 25-5 Prior births reported by abortion patients, 2014

methods or use methods inconsistently or incorrectly.[35] Providers of abortion care can help address this situation by informing patients about contraceptive options, offering them the method of their choice, and helping them overcome any barriers to effective use.

EVALUATION AND PREPARATION OF PATIENTS FOR ABORTION

DECIDING WHETHER TO CONTINUE A PREGNANCY

The process of deciding whether to continue a pregnancy commonly begins as soon as an individual suspects pregnancy. Some will have made a firm decision by the time they seek pregnancy confirmation; others may need to explore their options further. Providing prompt and convenient pregnancy confirmation services has important benefits, including the following:

- Allows the patient ample time to consider options
- Facilitates the initiation of prenatal care
- Increases the likelihood that an individual will be eligible for the full range of early abortion options
- Decreases the risks of adverse events and morbidity
- Expedites the diagnosis of pregnancy abnormalities, such as ectopic pregnancy

Clinicians can facilitate patients' decision-making by providing accurate and unbiased information about the pregnancy and helping them explore their feelings in a supportive and nonjudgmental setting. This is especially important given that many individuals experience stigma or may internalize stigma so deeply that they feel judged even when others are supportive.[36] The aim of the discussion is to allow patients to evaluate how continuing this pregnancy or deciding to have an abortion would affect their lives, future plans, and significant others. Some individuals experience ambivalence or find the decision complicated.[37] Basic factual information and discussion will meet the needs of most individuals; some patients may desire more extensive education, evaluation, or counseling to ensure that they are making an informed decision. Depending on the scope of services that your practice provides, you may need to refer patients for financial assistance, further counseling, first- or second-trimester abortions, prenatal care, adoption services, or other necessary care. Helpful resources for abortion referrals and funding assistance are listed in Table 25-1.

Table 25-1 Resources for abortion services and funding

Resource	Contact Information	Services
Planned Parenthood	www.plannedparenthood.org 1-800-230-PLAN	Directs women to nearest Planned Parenthood clinic
National Abortion Federation	https://prochoice.org/think-youre-pregnant/naf-hotline/ Abortion referrals: 1-800-257-0012 Funding support: 1-800-772-9100	Refers to nearest NAF member clinic
National Network of Abortion Funds	https://abortionfunds.org/need-abortion/	Financial assistance through 70 member funds
Patient Navigation Program	1-617-616-1636 patientnavigation@pplm.org	Based in New England; assists patients regardless of geographic location. General information about referrals and funding; judicial bypass coordination for Massachusetts minors; application counseling for Massachusetts health insurance

Pre-Abortion Evaluation

Because most individuals who request abortion are young and healthy, the pre-abortion medical evaluation is usually straightforward. The main goals of the evaluation include the following:

- Confirm pregnancy and estimate gestational age
- Identify possible problems that require further evaluation or intervention, such as ectopic pregnancy
- Identify medical or gynecologic conditions that might influence the choice of abortion methods or necessitate a hospital-based abortion

History-Taking

Ask the patient about recent menstrual history, including the regularity of menstrual cycles and the onset of the last normal menstrual period. Recording a contraceptive history, including recent use of hormonal methods, helps establish the accuracy of gestational dating based on LMP. Inquire as well about future contraceptive plans, so that the patient can start a contraceptive method immediately after abortion if desired.

The medical history should include the following:

- Any relevant obstetric and gynecologic history, including outcomes of prior pregnancies, adverse events or morbidity with previous abortions, history of uterine abnormalities (e.g., large leiomyomata [fibroids], bicornuate uterus), and any surgery involving the cervix or uterus (e.g., conization of the cervix, cesarean delivery)

- Acute or chronic illnesses that may require additional evaluation or adjunctive therapy
- Allergies to latex, local anesthetics, antiseptic solutions, analgesics, antibiotics, antiprogestins, prostaglandins, or other medications
- Use of tobacco, alcohol, or street drugs
- Current medications including asthma medications, anticoagulants, or systemic corticosteroids

This history may affect the provider's recommendations for abortion method, pre-abortion testing, pain control, or follow-up. Rarely, with medically complicated patients, it may be appropriate to perform the abortion in a hospital setting where staff and resources are readily available to manage any serious problems that may arise.

Clinical Examination

Perform a targeted physical assessment that includes vital signs. Some freestanding clinics are not able to accommodate patients with certain medical conditions or a body mass index above a specific cutoff, and referring providers should be aware of any such restrictions when coordinating care. Perform a pelvic examination to determine uterine size and position before aspiration abortion and to confirm gestational age based on LMP if the patient has not had an ultrasound. Note any findings, such as large uterine fibroids or cervical stenosis, which may indicate the need for further evaluation or influence the selection of an abortion method. If a pregnant patient has an intrauterine contraceptive device in place, remove it expeditiously to prevent the risk of septic abortion. If the patient chooses medication abortion, the clinician should remove the device at the time of mifepristone ingestion. Clinicians may perform a surgical abortion and remove intrauterine contraception concurrently if the interval between pregnancy confirmation and the procedure is reasonably brief.

Ultrasonography

Although many abortion providers in the United States use ultrasound routinely for gestational dating,[28] the National Abortion Federation guidelines do not require it before first-trimester abortion as long as the gestational age estimate by LMP and uterine size reasonably concur.[38] In many cases, clinical assessment of gestational age by history of LMP and pelvic examination, combined with a protocol for ultrasound as needed, suffices for provision of safe early abortion.[39] Consider ultrasound evaluation if the patient has an uncertain LMP, if you suspect pregnancy beyond 9 weeks, if you detect an adnexal mass or suspect ectopic pregnancy, or to evaluate other pelvic findings further. Ultrasound dating is the standard of care for second-trimester abortion in the United States.[38]

Laboratory Tests

Routine laboratory evaluation prior to abortion is minimal and includes a urine pregnancy test (unless ultrasound is performed to confirm the pregnancy and gestational age) and Rh typing. Additional testing may be necessary as determined by the patient's history or physical examination findings. These tests may include:

- Hemoglobin or hematocrit
- Screening for reproductive tract infection (The U.S. Preventive Services Task Force recommends routine screening for gonorrhea and chlamydia in sexually active women under age 25. Some U.S. providers routinely screen for chlamydia at the abortion visit, whereas others prefer to treat all patients prophylactically without screening.[28] If gonorrhea, chlamydia, or bacterial vaginosis is suspected or identified, initiate treatment prior to or at the time of the abortion.)
- Serial serum quantitative hCG levels to monitor a possible ectopic pregnancy or evaluate a missed or incomplete spontaneous abortion. (In addition, some clinicians may choose to follow serial hCG levels to confirm successful completion of a medication abortion in lieu of performing an ultrasound.[39])

Patient Education and Informed Consent

An individual seeking abortion will need information about available methods: how they are done; their safety, success rates, risks, costs, time required; and follow-up care. Although the patient may want a partner or other supportive persons involved in the information session, provide the opportunity to talk privately with you in case there are any confidential concerns, as well as to screen for intimate partner violence or coercion. Providers must follow any state regulations regarding the information given to patients, as well as those governing parental notification or consent for minors seeking abortion.[40] Once the patient has the information needed to make a decision and has all questions answered, ask for a signature on the appropriate consent forms before the abortion.

More than any other factor, the gestational age of the pregnancy determines which abortion method the individual may choose (Figure 25-6).

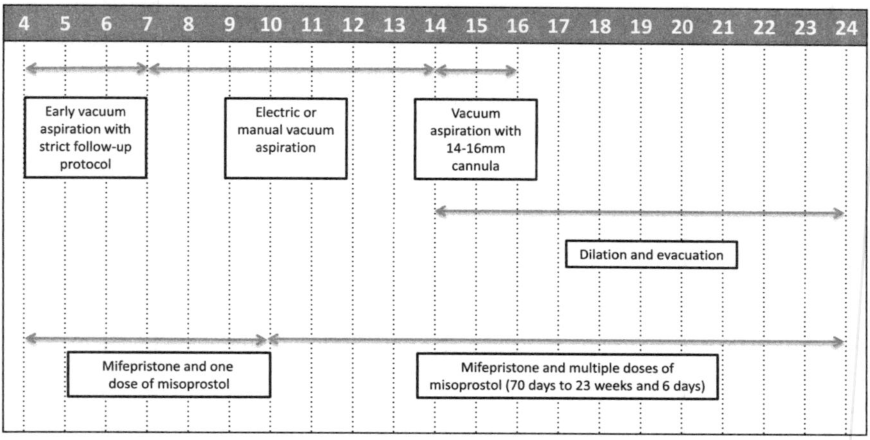

Adapted from: Royal College of Obstetricians and Gynaecologists. The Care of Women Requesting Induced Abortion. RCOG Evidence-based Clinical Guideline No. 7. London: RCOG; 2011, with the permission of the Royal College of Obstetricians and Gynaecologists.

Figure 25-6 Options for terminating pregnancy, by duration of pregnancy

A patient may opt for a vacuum aspiration abortion throughout the first trimester or an early medication abortion during the first 70 days (10 weeks) of pregnancy. After the first trimester, abortion methods include dilation and evacuation (D&E) or medical induction. A patient's options may be limited by other factors, such as cost or lack of skilled D&E providers in the community.[21] In addition, some medical conditions or problems, such as severe anemia or abnormal uterine anatomy, may affect which abortion method or clinical setting would be safest for the individual.

The choice between a medication or aspiration abortion mostly depends on the patient's preferences. In helping the patient decide between medication abortion and aspiration, explain the important features of each method (Table 25-2), emphasizing that both methods are highly effective. Most individuals will express a clear preference and be highly satisfied with the method they choose.

The main advantages of vacuum aspiration are its speed and predictability, and the option for oral analgesia or anxiolytics, sedation, or general anesthesia. The drawbacks are the procedure's invasiveness and the small risk of uterine perforation. Reasons commonly cited for choosing medication abortion include that it is non-invasive and more "natural" and that it affords individuals greater privacy and control over the abortion process.[41] Some individuals may consider a medication abortion similar to a miscarriage, and for them the experience may carry less stigma. Disadvantages of medication methods include the length of time required to complete the abortion process and the longer period of bleeding and cramping that commonly accompanies passage of the pregnancy.

Table 25-2 Characteristics of early abortion methods

Vacuum Aspiration Abortion	Medication Abortion
Highly effective	Highly effective
Procedure brief	Abortion process usually takes several hours to a few days, depending on regimen
Involves invasive procedure	Avoids invasive procedure (aspiration) if successful
Usually done with cervical anesthesia; allows option of oral analgesia/anxiolytics, sedation, or general anesthesia	Avoids anesthesia
Usually requires only 1 visit	May involve 2 visits or more
Lighter perceived bleeding	Heavier perceived bleeding
Requires clinical setting	May occur in privacy of home

CLINICAL PROVISION OF ABORTION METHODS

FIRST-TRIMESTER MEDICATION ABORTION

Since the introduction of mifepristone in Europe more than two decades ago, its use for abortion has risen worldwide. The U.S. Food and Drug Administration (FDA) approved mifepristone for abortion in September of 2000, and by 2014 medication abortion in the United States accounted for 32% of all abortions and 45% of those occurring before 9 weeks LMP.[21] Planned Parenthood affiliates and most members of the National Abortion Federation currently offer early medication abortion services, and many private doctors, including obstetrician-gynecologists and family practice physicians, provide abortion care within their primary care offices. In several states, advanced practice clinicians (nurse practitioners, certified nurse midwives and physician assistants) provide some or all aspects of early medication abortion care in accordance with state laws.[42] Efforts are ongoing to expand access to medication abortion by diverse types of practitioners.

Substantial research supports the effectiveness of medication abortion during the first 7 to 10 weeks of pregnancy, depending on the regimen used. These regimens include mifepristone-misoprostol, methotrexate-misoprostol, and misoprostol alone. Use of mifepristone-misoprostol predominates in the United States, but the other regimens represent critical alternatives where mifepristone is unaffordable or unavailable.

Medications Used in Early Abortion

Mifepristone. Mifepristone is sold in the United States under the brand name Mifeprex. Mifepristone is a 19-norsteroid with a high affinity for progesterone receptors; it also binds to glucocorticoid receptors and, to a lesser extent, androgen receptors. The drug blocks the action of progesterone, which is necessary to establish and maintain placental attachment. Mifepristone also softens the cervix and stimulates synthesis of prostaglandins by cells of the early decidua.[7]

Millions of women worldwide have used the combination of mifepristone and misoprostol for early abortion with an impressive safety record, and in 2016 the FDA approved its use through 70 days (10 weeks).[43] However, some limitations apply to the use of mifepristone for abortion. It should not be used in women with known or suspected ectopic pregnancy because it is ineffectual in eliminating a conceptus outside the uterine cavity. In addition, the FDA drug label for mifepristone-misoprostol abortion advises against its use in the following circumstances:

- Intrauterine contraception in place (must be removed before treatment)
- Chronic adrenal failure
- Current long-term systemic corticosteroid therapy
- History of allergy to mifepristone, misoprostol, or other prostaglandin
- Hemorrhagic disorders or concurrent anti-coagulant therapy
- Inherited porphyrias

Misoprostol. Misoprostol is a prostaglandin E1 analogue that softens the cervix and stimulates uterine contractions, thereby facilitating expulsion of the pregnancy. Although misoprostol alone can induce abortion, protocols that combine it with mifepristone are more effective.[44] Sold in the United States as a generic drug, as well as under the brand name Cytotec, misoprostol is a widely available, inexpensive medication marketed for prevention of gastrointestinal ulcer disease. The FDA has approved an early abortion regimen using mifepristone in combination with misoprostol.

Misoprostol can cause mild, short-term systemic prostaglandin effects, including nausea, vomiting, diarrhea, and temporary elevation of body temperature—side effects that patients commonly report with all medication abortion regimens. It can be administered orally (swallowed), vaginally, buccally (tucked between cheek and gum), or sublingually (placed under the tongue) for abortion, and the pharmacokinetics of the drug differ by route of administration. An oral dose of misoprostol results in rapid, high peak blood levels with relatively weak stimulation of the uterus, while a vaginal, buccal, or sublingual dose produces overall lower blood levels but a more sustained uterine effect.[45] Prenatal exposure to misoprostol has been associated with major congenital anomalies, primarily of the skull and limbs, but the absolute risk is low (less than 1%).[45,46]

Methotrexate. Methotrexate is a folic acid analogue that competitively inhibits dihydrofolate reductase, an enzyme necessary for DNA synthesis. Methotrexate causes abortion by its action on the rapidly dividing cells of the early placenta; when combined with misoprostol, it is effective in inducing abortion through 49 days (7 weeks) of gestation.[47] Methotrexate is FDA approved for treatment of choriocarcinoma and certain other types of cancer, severe psoriasis, and rheumatoid arthritis. Use of methotrexate for treatment of ectopic pregnancy or early medication abortion is not included in the FDA drug label, but these uses are supported by published evidence accumulated over many years.

Before mifepristone became available in the United States, clinicians commonly employed a regimen of methotrexate and vaginal misoprostol for early medication abortion. The efficacy of methotrexate-misoprostol through 7 weeks of gestation compares favorably to mifepristone regimens, but it is associated with a longer duration until complete abortion.[48] Single-dose methotrexate therapy for medication abortion or ectopic pregnancy has little, if any, systemic toxicity, but it should not be administered to individuals with chronic renal or hepatic disease. Methotrexate is a known teratogen when used in high, multiple doses; the teratogenic risk associated with single-dose methotrexate is unknown but warrants caution.[7]

Facility and Staffing Considerations

Medication abortion is well-suited to the scope of practice of primary care providers, including nurse practitioners, nurse midwives, and physician assistants. The FDA stipulates that medication abortion providers must be able to assess the duration of pregnancy, diagnose ectopic pregnancy, and provide or refer for vacuum aspiration or emergency treatment when necessary (e.g., hemorrhage or signs of sepsis); personal expertise in ultrasound or aspiration is not required. These capabilities do not differ from those needed by any clinician caring for reproductive-aged patients who may present for diagnosis or evaluation of early pregnancy. Laws in many states, however, restrict the extent to which clinicians other than physicians can practice medication abortion,[40] so checking state-specific requirements before initiating the service is important.

Providing medication abortion does not require specialized facilities, and services via telemedicine are also available.[49] For in-office visits, a typical medical office with space for private consultation, physical examination if indicated, equipment and medication for handling an allergic reaction suffices along with a capacity to arrange for a urine pregnancy test and Rh typing. In addition, the office must have a protocol for backup or referral, 24-hour emergency telephone service, and trained staff. Other practical issues to consider include state laws or regulations specific to facilities that provide abortion services (if any), as well as any requirements for information provision, waiting periods, or parental consent or notification for minors seeking abortion care. Several organizations can provide additional information about these issues, including the National Abortion Federation.

In the United States, mifepristone is not available through pharmacies; rather, it is sold directly to licensed healthcare providers who meet the aforementioned FDA qualifications after they sign and return a Prescriber's Agreement provided by the drug's distributor. Prescribers agree to report adverse events and to give each patient a Medication Guide to read and a Patient Agreement to read and sign. Information and forms necessary to enroll as a mifepristone provider are available at http://www.earlyoptionpill.com.

Information Provision

An individual undergoing medication abortion needs detailed information about the medications, when and how to take them, what to expect during the process, possible side effects and problems, and what to do if questions or concerns arise (Table 25-3).

Mifepristone-Misoprostol Regimens

Although use of mifepristone alone results in abortion in some cases, the addition of misoprostol increases efficacy substantially. Researchers have studied different doses, routes of administration, and timing of misoprostol following mifepristone ingestion; the FDA revised labeling in 2016 to reflect an evidence-based regimen.

The early abortion regimen approved by the FDA in 2000 was based on studies that used 600 mg of mifepristone orally at the first visit, followed 2 days later by 400 mcg of misoprostol orally at the second visit. The patients then returned in approximately 2 weeks for a follow-up visit to assess whether the pregnancy had passed. The success rate (complete abortion without the need for aspiration) of this regimen ranged from 92% to 96% in women with pregnancies of 49 days' duration or less but fell significantly thereafter.[50,51]

Subsequent studies conducted in the United States and internationally led to the development of improved evidence-based mifepristone regimens that were more effective and convenient with fewer side

Table 25-3 Patient education for early medication abortion

1. Discuss the patient's decision to have an abortion and confirm that the decision is certain and voluntary.
2. Discuss the treatment alternatives (medication abortion or vacuum aspiration) and explain the benefits and risks of each method.
3. Describe the medication regimen that will be followed.
4. Explain what to expect in regard to bleeding and cramping. These symptoms typically intensify during expulsion of the pregnancy (usually 2 to 4 hours) and then gradually subside. Passage of clots is common during expulsion. Lighter bleeding or spotting typically can last for up to 2 weeks, but may be longer.
5. Explain that the patient is unlikely to see products of conception unless the pregnancy is close to 9 weeks' gestation or more, in which case the embryo will be very small and often obscured by blood clots.
6. Discuss known side effects of the medication abortion regimen including mild gastrointestinal symptoms; short-term fever, warmth or chills; or oral ulcers (methotrexate only).
7. Explain that the drugs used for medication abortion may increase the risk of birth defects if the pregnancy were to continue. **Emphasize that aspiration abortion is advised if the medication abortion method fails.**
8. Discuss possible morbidity including failed abortion (continuing pregnancy), incomplete abortion, hemorrhage, or infection. Emphasize that atypical infections have occurred rarely after use of mifepristone combined with misoprostol, and review how to take antibiotics if prescribed (see text).
9. Provide instructions about how to administer the misoprostol. Depending on the regimen used, routes of administration can include oral (swallowed), buccal (tucked between cheek and gum), sublingual (under the tongue), or vaginal (inserted deep into the vagina after washing hands). A drawing or picture of buccal or sublingual placement may be helpful, because these terms are unfamiliar to most individuals. Also explain how to use pain medications.
10. Explain the time commitment and expected number of visits.
11. Provide 24-hour emergency contact information and emphasize warning signs that may require evaluation, including the following:
    a. Prolonged or heavy bleeding (≥2 soaked maxi-pads for 2 consecutive hours);
    b. Fever (≥100.4° F) lasting more than 4 hours or beginning in the days after misoprostol administration;
    c. Abdominal pain or discomfort or 'feeling sick' (including weakness, nausea, vomiting or diarrhea, with or without fever) more than 24 hours after using misoprostol.
12. Provide information about available contraceptive methods and when to initiate the chosen method, if any.
13. Address any concerns about confidentiality.
14. Review all required consent forms, which must be signed before administration of the medication regimen.

effects (Table 25-4). In brief, key research findings underpinning these new protocols included the following:

- Mifepristone, 200 mg, is as effective as a 600 mg dose when combined with misoprostol in various regimens.[52,53]
- Self-administration of misoprostol at home is safe, effective, and highly acceptable to women.[54–57]

Table 25-4 Selected clinical protocols for early medication abortion

Visit*	Mifepristone and misoprostol regimens† (≤70 days)	Misoprostol-only regimens (≤13 weeks)
One	*Day 1* Give 200 mg mifepristone to take orally, in the clinic or at home	*Day 1*
	Provide four 200 mcg misoprostol tablets (800 mcg total) to take home,‡ with instructions for administration: • Vaginally§ in 6–48 hrs, <u>OR</u> • Buccally‖ in 24–48 hours, <u>OR</u> • Sublingually¶ in 24–48 hours	Provide a sufficient number of 200 mcg misoprostol tablets with instructions for use as follows: • Four tablets (800 mcg) sublingually every 3 hours for 2-3 doses • Four tablets (800 mcg) vaginally or buccally every 3-12 hours for 2–3 doses
	Offer contraceptive counseling • May initiate medroxyprogesterone acetate or etonogestrel implant on Day 1 if desired • May initiate combined oral contraceptive pill or patch on the day of misoprostol administration	Offer contraceptive counseling
	Administer Rh_o(D)-immune globulin 50-mcg to Rh_o(D)-negative women. Provide analgesics and instructions for their use.	
Two	*Day 3–14 (at least 24 hrs after misoprostol administration)* Assess outcome • If abortion complete, offer contraceptive counseling; may place IUD at this visit. If abortion has not occurred, offer repeat dose of misoprostol (800 mcg) unless patient prefers aspiration • If ongoing viable pregnancy, follow up in about 1 week • If persistent non-viable pregnancy, follow-up may occur in about 4 weeks	*Day 4–9 (at least 24 hrs after misoprostol insertion)* Assess outcome • If abortion complete, offer contraceptive counseling • If abortion has not occurred, provide repeat doses of misoprostol (800 mcg) unless patient prefers aspiration • If ongoing viable pregnancy, follow up at about Day 14 • If persistent nonviable pregnancy, follow up in about 4 weeks
Three	*Day 14–21 (only needed if viable pregnancy on previous visit)* Schedule aspiration abortion if viable pregnancy persists	*Day 14 (only needed if viable pregnancy on previous visit)* Schedule aspiration abortion if viable pregnancy persists
Four	*Approximately 4–5 weeks after initiation of treatment for patients who are awaiting resolution of a non-viable pregnancy.* Offer aspiration if nonviable pregnancy persists.	

*Routine visits subsequent to day 1 may not be necessary if providers are using hCG testing rather than ultrasound to confirm complete abortion.

†Efficacy decreases with increasing gestational age as follows for mifepristone 200 mg and misoprostol 800 mcg given buccally: ≤49 days, 98%; 50–56 days, 97%; 57–63 days, 95%; 64–70 days, 93%.[69] Sublingual and vaginal misoprostol have similar efficacy through 63 days.[62,70–72]

‡Simultaneous administration of mifepristone and misoprostol has been found to have acceptable efficacy through 63 days LMP.[67]

§Vaginal administration has fewer side effects compared with buccal or sublingual administration.

‖Instruct the patient to swallow any residual pill fragments after 30 minutes.

¶The revised FDA-approved regimen specifies buccal administration. The patient should swallow any residual pill fragments after 30 minutes.

- Compared with the oral route of misoprostol used in the original FDA-approved regimen, administration of misoprostol 800 mcg vaginally, buccally, or sublingually following mifepristone extends acceptable efficacy through 70 days of gestation,[58–61] and most studies report a lower incidence of side effects as well. Sublingual misoprostol 800 mcg produces more side effects compared with the vaginal route.[62–64]

- Shorter dosing intervals between mifepristone and misoprostol (24 hours for buccal or sublingual administration and 6 to 24 hours for vaginal administration) do not decrease efficacy significantly.[61,65,66] Simultaneous administration of mifepristone and vaginal misoprostol also has acceptable efficacy through 63 days LMP.[67]

During the first few years following FDA approval of mifepristone, the evidence-based regimen of mifepristone 200 mg followed by 800 mcg vaginal misoprostol was common practice in the United States. Reports of serious infections in a small number of women using this regimen, including a few deaths from clostridial infections,[68] prompted many U.S. clinicians to adopt protocols using alternative routes of misoprostol administration. However, an association between these infections and the vaginal route of misoprostol administration was never confirmed, and the absolute rate of serious infection is extremely low. A regimen of mifepristone 200 mg followed by buccal misoprostol 800 mcg predominates in the United States; vaginal or sublingual misoprostol administration is also safe and effective. The current American College of Obstetricians and Gynecologists guideline does not recommend routine antibiotic administration during medication abortion,[7] although some providers prefer to continue this practice.

Misoprostol-only regimens

Although misoprostol alone is not as effective as combined mifepristone regimens,[44,73] it remains an important alternative in countries where mifepristone is not available or abortion is illegal or inaccessible.[74] Researchers have studied a variety of early-abortion regimens using misoprostol alone; most involve multiple doses and therefore higher rates of side effects than occur with mifepristone regimens (Table 25-4).[73,75] In a study involving more than 2,000 women, success rates of 83% to 85% were achieved with use of 800 mcg misoprostol vaginally every 3 or 12 hours or sublingually every 3 hours; sublingual doses taken at 12-hour intervals were less effective. Side effects (primarily fever) are increased with sublingual administration compared with the vaginal route.[76]

Anecdotal evidence suggests that some populations in the United States are using misoprostol to self-induce abortion.[77] Some individuals prefer to self-manage abortion, and this practice may grow if access continues to decrease. Online resources are available to provide information to women in these circumstances (e.g., https://abortionpillinfo.org/en/sass, https://plancpills.org/). Individuals occasionally may present for follow-up or management of problems, such as heavy bleeding or incomplete abortion. In addition to following guidelines for problem management and referral used for other medication abortion patients (see below), (1) strongly advise aspiration abortion if the pregnancy is viable to avoid the potential teratogenic effects of misoprostol; and (2) help the patient obtain information, family planning care, and other needed health services.

Methotrexate-misoprostol regimens

Prior to the availability of mifepristone in the United States, U.S. researchers developed other regimens for early medication abortion using methotrexate and misoprostol. Because these drugs are widely available and inexpensive, they offer an important alternative when mifepristone is unaffordable or unavailable. Used in combination with vaginal misoprostol 800 mcg, methotrexate is 92% to 96% successful in terminating pregnancy through 49 days of gestation.[47,48,78] However, 15% to 25% of patients may need to wait up to a month for expulsion of the gestational sac to occur.[47,48,79] During this delay, they will no longer feel pregnant if the pregnancy has stopped growing.

Most protocols use intramuscular methotrexate at a dose of 50 mg per square meter of body surface, but a 50 mg dose taken orally (dissolved in orange juice to disguise the taste) is comparably effective.[79,80] Three to 7 days after methotrexate treatment, the patient inserts misoprostol 800 mcg vaginally. The misoprostol dose can be repeated if bleeding does not occur after 24 hours or if abortion has not occurred by the time of the 1-week follow-up visit. Most patients will abort successfully by 4 weeks following initiation of treatment.

Follow-up After Medication Abortion

No matter which drug combination or regimen they use, individuals undergoing medication abortion are likely to experience cramping and bleeding. In most cases, pain can be managed with nonsteroidal anti-inflammatory drugs (NSAIDs), such as ibuprofen, or acetaminophen with codeine phosphate (300 mg/30 mg). NSAIDs do not interfere with the effectiveness of misoprostol.[81] Although bleeding may seem abundant to those experiencing it, the amount of bleeding is rarely clinically significant. One study that used mifepristone with oral or vaginal misoprostol through 63 days' gestation found median blood losses ranging from 83 ml to 89 ml,[82] compared with the 50 ml typically lost during menses or the nearly 500 ml typically given in a blood donation. Although the range of bleeding varies widely among women, meaningful changes in hemoglobin seldom occur.[82] Bleeding is usually heaviest during expulsion of the pregnancy; lighter flow or spotting lasts about 2 weeks on average, but may be longer.[83] Use of combined oral contraceptives does not alter bleeding patterns after medication abortion.[83,84]

Providing patients with parameters for excessive bleeding enhances safety. Advise the patient to call if the bleeding soaks 2 or more large pads per hour for 2 consecutive hours. If the patient feels otherwise well, monitoring periodically by telephone for another 2 hours is acceptable. Patients whose bleeding does not slow after this interval warrant prompt in-person evaluation. Some providers treat excessive bleeding with another dose of misoprostol or an ergot alkaloid such as methylergonovine maleate (Methergine) before resorting to aspiration. Heavy bleeding that prompts a patient to contact the clinician may occur in the several days following misoprostol administration or it may be delayed for 3 to 5 weeks.[85] Bleeding heavy enough to require aspiration occurs in less than 1% of patients, and less than 1 in 1,000 women will need a blood transfusion for excessive bleeding.[7,86]

Side effects common with all medication abortion regimens include nausea, headache, vomiting, diarrhea, dizziness, fever, and chills.[7] These side effects typically subside within a few hours and seldom require treatment. Temperature elevation (100.4° F or more) that lasts more than 4 hours or that begins in the days after misoprostol administration, however, warrants clinical assessment.

A disadvantage of medication abortion is that it often involves at least two office visits (Table 25-4), depending on the regimen used. With the evidence-based mifepristone-misoprostol regimens used in the United States, two office visits are common: the first to evaluate the patient and provide the medications, and a second visit to assess whether the pregnancy has ended. Data suggest that the second office visit may be replaced by telephone follow-up combined with a urine pregnancy test at home.[87–91] Patients may also opt to have a baseline serum quantitative hCG level drawn at the initial clinic visit and a second serum hCG test at a more convenient laboratory or facility instead of returning for a follow-up visit.

Additional office visits may be necessary if state regulations require a separate counseling visit before the patient has an abortion, or if the medication abortion fails. If a growing pregnancy persists for 2 to 3 weeks after treatment, aspiration abortion is strongly recommended because of the potential risk of birth defects following exposure to misoprostol. If the pregnancy has stopped growing but has not completely passed from the uterus, the patient may choose to have another course of misoprostol, an aspiration procedure, or simply wait for expulsion to occur.

Clinical methods used to confirm abortion include a history of bleeding with evidence of uterine involution on follow-up examination, serum or urine hCG testing, or ultrasonography. Although most medication abortion researchers in the United States relied on ultrasonography to assess gestational age and clinical outcomes, many providers offer safe medication abortion services without routine use of ultrasound.[39,92,93] Whichever method you choose to follow patients, remember these important guidelines:

- If a patient has a gestational sac on initial ultrasound examination and no sac on follow-up, then the abortion is complete. Aspiration for a thickened endometrial stripe or "debris" in the uterus is not indicated unless the patient is bleeding heavily or has symptoms or signs of infection.[94]
- If the patient has a gestational sac on initial ultrasound and you are following serum hCGs in lieu of sonography to determine treatment success, draw an initial quantitative hCG test on the day of mifepristone administration and a second test 3 to 5 days after misoprostol. It should drop by at least 50% within that timeframe.[95] (See Chapter 24 on Pregnancy Testing and Early Assessment of Normal and Abnormal Pregnancy.)
- If the patient does not have a gestational sac on initial ultrasound and is asymptomatic, mifepristone may be given with appropriate counseling including ectopic pregnancy warnings. Draw an initial quantitative serum hCG test on the day of mifepristone administration and a second test 24 to 48 hours after misoprostol administration.
- If the hCG values fall by at least 50% after 24 hours, then the abortion is most likely complete.[96] Patients need further follow-up if hCG levels do not drop by at least 50% within 24 to 48 hours. Rapidly rising hCG values typically signal a continuing pregnancy, while a slow rise, plateau, or slow fall may indicate ectopic pregnancy or incomplete abortion.[97]
- Absent or minimal bleeding after taking misoprostol may indicate treatment failure.
- hCG may not clear from the body for a month or more after complete abortion, and pregnancy testing during this time may yield misleading results. Although a negative urine pregnancy test result 1 to 2 weeks following treatment is reassuring, a positive test does not necessarily mean that the pregnancy is continuing.[98]

First-Trimester Vacuum Aspiration Abortion

Introduced in the United States in 1967, vacuum aspiration (suction curettage) is used for virtually all first-trimester instrumental abortions in the United States.[23] Aspiration is a safe and simple way to empty the uterus completely and quickly using modest cervical dilation and a hand-held syringe (manual vacuum aspiration) or an electric vacuum pump. Most states limit abortion provision to physicians; however, in a few states without such restrictions, advanced practice clinicians have provided aspiration abortions for years with an impressive safety record.[99]

Vacuum aspiration using local cervical anesthesia with or without oral NSAIDs and/or anxiolytics or, alternatively, intravenous moderate sedation can be provided safely and appropriately in a medical office setting. The office should be equipped with the same emergency back-up equipment and supplies needed to provide injectable medications (drugs and resuscitation equipment to manage an allergic reaction, seizure, respiratory depression, or cardiac arrest). In addition, clinicians should have available the medications needed to treat uterine bleeding and a plan in place for transferring a patient to a surgical facility in the rare event that an evaluation may be needed for uterine perforation or severe hemorrhage. The availability of portable and inexpensive manual vacuum aspirators has facilitated abortion provision in primary care settings that do not have electric pumps, as well as resource-poor settings worldwide. Research indicates that manual vacuum aspiration (MVA) is as effective and safe as electric vacuum aspiration (EVA);[100,101] although pain is comparable,[102,103] women prefer the quietness of the MVA device.[103] The ability of providers to identify products of conception in the tissue aspirate after very early abortion (less than 6 weeks) does not differ significantly with use of MVA or EVA.[104]

1. As the first step in an aspiration procedure, perform a bimanual examination to determine the size and position of the uterus. Insert a short-bladed speculum, such as a Moore Graves design or a customized weighted speculum, to draw the cervix close to the perineum for adequate visualization and to straighten a flexed uterus. Vaginal cleansing with an antiseptic solution is common practice but does not reduce the incidence of post-procedure infection.[105] Many clinicians use a *no-touch technique,* i.e., not touching the parts of instruments, including the tips of dilators or cannulae, that will enter the sterile uterine cavity.[106]

2. Administer a local anesthetic such as lidocaine amide to the cervix to reduce pain. The total amount of lidocaine administered should not exceed 200 mg (20 cc of 1% lidocaine or 40 cc of 0.5% lidocaine). Inject 2 to 3 cc of the anesthetic into the lip of the cervix before placing a tenaculum to keep the cervix stabilized, and

then administer the remaining solution at two to four sites either directly into the cervical stroma or paracervically. Consistent strong evidence documents the superior efficacy of deep injections (2 to 3 cm) compared with superficial injections.[107]

3. Using tapered, graduated metal or plastic dilators, stretch the cervix gently and incrementally as needed to accommodate an aspiration cannula of appropriate size for the gestation. Typically, the diameter of the cannula in millimeters corresponds to the duration of the pregnancy in weeks. For example, a clinician may choose a 7 mm cannula to evacuate a pregnancy at 7 weeks. On occasion, smaller cannulas may be necessary due to difficult cervical dilation, or they may simply be equally effective. Insert a cannula connected to either a manual vacuum syringe or an electric vacuum pump through the dilated cervix and remove the products of conception by a combination of rotary and back-and-forth motions. Detection of a "gritty" sensation as the cannula moves across the endometrial surface typically indicates that the uterus is empty.

4. Examining the removed tissue helps to confirm complete evacuation. If the products of conception are not readily apparent, suspending the tissue in water, saline, or white vinegar and checking with backlighting may facilitate the evaluation.[106] If pregnancy tissue still is not identified, a post-procedure ultrasound may confirm retained products or assist in the diagnosis of uncommon

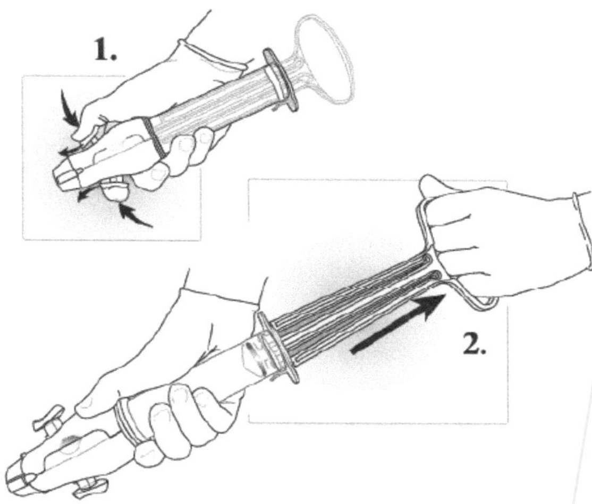

Prepare the manual vacuum aspirator (MVA) by pushing the valve buttons down and forward until they lock into place (1). Pull the plunger back until the arms snap outward and catch on the cylinder base (2).

Figure 25-7A Charging the manual vacuum aspirator

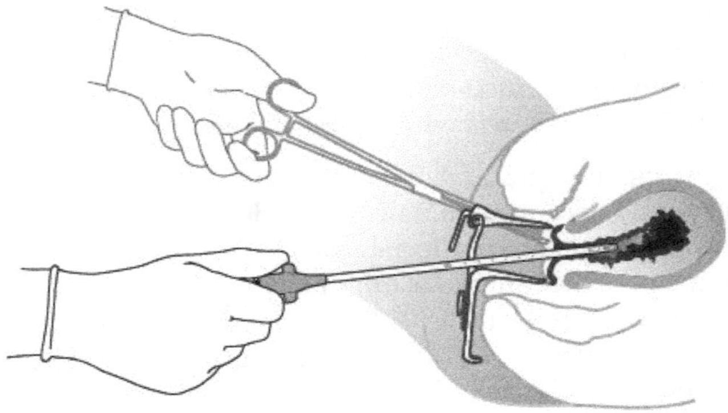

After administering paracervical anesthesia and applying a tenaculum, open the cervix as needed with mechanical dilators to allow for insertion of an appropriately sized cannula. In general, the diameter of the cannula should approximate the gestational age in weeks (e.g., use a 7-mm cannula to evacuate a 7-week pregnancy).

Figure 25-7B Inserting the cannula

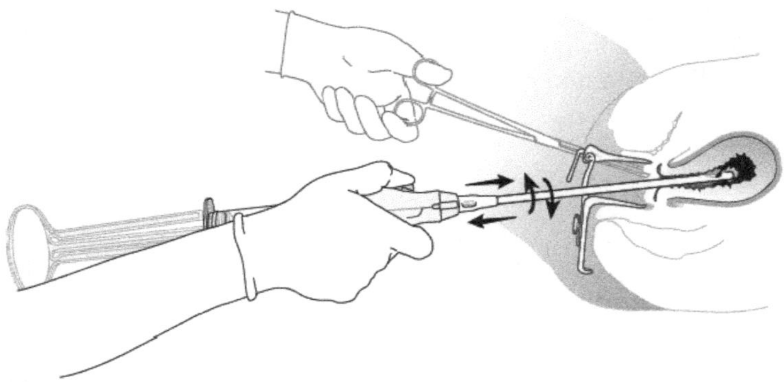

While applying traction to the tenaculum, insert the cannula through the cervix and into the upper uterine cavity. Attach the prepared aspirator to the cannula, release the vacuum by pressing the buttons, and evacuate the contents of the uterus using a combination of rotary and back-and-forth motions. Signs of complete evacuation include contraction of the uterus and detection of a gritty sensation as the cannula moves across the endometrial surface, with no further tissue passing through the cannula.

Figure 25-7C Evacuating the contents of the uterus

events such as a missed ectopic pregnancy. If ectopic pregnancy is suspected, strongly consider sending the tissue for an urgent microscopic exam and obtaining a serum quantitative hCG, to be repeated in 48 to 72 hours unless the pathologist sees chorionic villi.

Second-Trimester Dilation and Evacuation

After the first trimester, the most common method for abortion in the United States is dilation and evacuation (D&E), a procedure that combines aspiration with the use of extracting forceps.[23] In the United States, most women prefer D&E to medical induction methods that typically entail hospitalization, higher cost, and a prolonged period of labor.[108] Although D&E requires surgical expertise, it is safer than older *instillation methods* of induction that involved infusion or injection of prostaglandins, hypertonic saline, or urea into the amniotic cavity. Data on the comparative safety of D&E and modern induction methods are limited. One study reported a higher adverse event rate with misoprostol induction compared with D&E—based solely on the greater need for curettage to remove retained placenta[109]—while another found overall fewer adverse events with D&E. However, serious events were rare with both approaches.[110]

Using preoperative sonography to obtain an accurate estimation of gestational age enhances the safety of D&E abortion, and intraoperative sonography may be helpful as well. To permit evacuation of the larger products of conception, the cervix requires more dilation for a second-trimester D&E than for a first-trimester aspiration. Thus, preoperative cervical preparation using osmotic dilating devices, mifepristone, misoprostol, or a combination is recommended (see Adjunctive Techniques). After administering anesthesia, the clinician removes the osmotic dilators and empties the uterus using appropriate instruments. In the United States, the federal Partial Birth Abortion Ban Act of 2003 [18 U.S.C. 1531 (2003)] effectively prohibits *intentionally* extracting an intact fetus past certain anatomic landmarks[111] unless fetal demise has occurred before extraction (which may be accomplished with medication such as digoxin or potassium chloride).

Second-Trimester Induction Abortion

Second-trimester induction abortion involves administration of medications that cause the uterus to contract and eventually expel the fetus and placenta. Although induction is used commonly in many European countries, it accounts for only a small proportion of abortions after the first trimester in the United States.[23] Modern induction agents have largely replaced older instillation methods, conferring a considerable safety advantage.

Mifepristone and misoprostol, or misoprostol alone, may be used for labor induction abortion in the second trimester. Based on current evidence, the most effective approach is mifepristone followed in 24 to 48 hours by repeated doses of misoprostol.[112] A commonly used regimen is 200 mg of mifepristone orally, followed in 36 to 48 hours by 800 mcg of misoprostol vaginally, and an additional 400 mcg orally or vaginally every 3 hours for up to 5 doses. If used as a single agent, the optimal dosing for misoprostol is 400 mcg vaginally or sublingually every 3 hours, and initiating induction with a loading dose of 600 to 800 mcg may be more effective.[112] With misoprostol-alone regimens, the median time to abortion is 10 to 19 hours, and 70% to 90% of women will abort within 24 hours.[112,113] Pretreatment with mifepristone enhances efficacy and shortens the time required to induce abortion by about 50%.[113] The Royal College of Obstetricians and Gynaecologists (RCOG) in the United Kingdom has endorsed the mifepristone-misoprostol combination for abortion at 14 weeks' gestation or more when providers with specialized skills for D&E are not available.[6] Other less favorable and less frequently used methods include vaginal administration of dinoprostone, an E_2 prostaglandin approved by the FDA for second-trimester abortion, and intravenous administration of high-dose oxytocin.[112]

All second-trimester induction methods have side effects specific to the medications used. Although retained placenta requiring curettage was common with older induction methods, its frequency has decreased to less than 10% with use of mifepristone or misoprostol induction regimens.[113,114]

ADJUNCTIVE TECHNIQUES

Clinicians use several adjunctive techniques to facilitate abortion procedures, including pretreatment with osmotic dilators, administration of perioperative uterotonic agents, and different techniques for analgesia and anesthesia. Use of osmotic dilators decreases the risk of cervical laceration or perforation,[115,116] although the minimal risk of uterine injury in first-trimester abortion may not justify their routine use. The Society of Family Planning recommends cervical preparation routinely before second-trimester D&E abortion and advises that clinicians consider cervical preparation in the first trimester when they anticipate challenges dilating the cervix (e.g., for adolescents or for women undergoing later-first trimester procedures).[117,118]

Osmotic dilating devices. Two types of osmotic dilators currently are available in the United States: *Laminaria japonica* or *digitata* consist of sterile stalks of dried seaweed, and Dilapan-S is a synthetic polyacrylonitrile (plastic) rod. The clinician places osmotic dilators so they extend through the endocervical canal and dilate both the internal and external os.

The devices absorb fluid and expand. The major effect of laminaria is mechanical (exerting radial pressure on the cervix), while the predominant effect of Dilapan-S is likely chemical (inducing prostaglandin release). Thus, using a combination of these two types of dilating tents is reasonable. Laminaria tents reach maximum dilation in 12 to 24 hours, so they are most commonly inserted the day before the D&E procedure. In contrast, Dilapan-S devices dilate quickly, achieving most of their effect within 4 to 6 hours, so their use often allows clinicians to complete second-trimester D&E abortions in a shorter time frame than in the past. Many clinicians use a combination of osmotic dilators, and serial insertions may be necessary for procedures later in pregnancy.[117]

Misoprostol. Treatment with misoprostol prior to D&E causes cervical softening, effacement, and dilation (called ripening) that can reduce the need for additional mechanical dilation or make it easier. Vaginal insertion of misoprostol has greater efficacy and fewer side effects than oral administration.[119,120] Numerous studies suggest that an optimal regimen for first-trimester cervical preparation is 400 mcg administered vaginally 3 hours prior to the procedure.[118,121] This regimen is as effective as overnight laminaria for first-trimester cervical preparation.[119] The same dose of misoprostol administered sublingually 2 to 4 hours before aspiration abortion primes the cervix as well as vaginal misoprostol, but with a higher incidence of side effects.[120–122] Although less well-studied, buccal misoprostol has pharmacokinetics similar to vaginal misoprostol[123] and may represent an effective alternative route of administration.[118,124]

Experienced providers may use misoprostol safely in lieu of osmotic dilators before early second-trimester abortions or in combination with osmotic dilators for later D&E procedures.[117] Optimal regimens for these uses are not well defined.[117] When misoprostol is used with dilating tents, procedure times are shorter but patients are likely to experience more pain.[125] Misoprostol also has the potential problem of inducing contractions, so its use entails a greater risk of unscheduled delivery when used at home after the first trimester. Side effects include nausea, vomiting, diarrhea, cramping, and fever or shivering. Although uterine rupture has been reported following misoprostol use in the second trimester, primarily in a uterus with a scar from prior uterine surgery, these cases are rare and do not contraindicate its use, as demonstrated by several large case series.[117]

Mifepristone. Mifepristone also is an excellent cervical ripening agent, but longer preparation times (24 to 48 hours) result in better effects. It is used off-label for cervical ripening at later gestational ages. Cervical preparation with mifepristone as a single ripening agent given 24 hours prior to D&E at 14 to 16 weeks' gestation did not increase procedure time when compared with osmotic dilators.[126] In another study, individuals undergoing D&E from 16 weeks' through 23 weeks' gestation were randomized to cervical preparation with osmotic dilators alone, or in conjunction with mifepristone or misoprostol.[127] There was no difference in operative time between the groups. Providers found the procedure subjectively easier with mifepristone plus dilating tents compared with tents alone, and mifepristone was better tolerated than misoprostol.[127] Mifepristone also may allow for fewer visits for cervical preparation and fewer osmotic dilators when used for D&E procedures between 19 weeks and 23 weeks and 6 days.[128]

Uterotonic agents. Agents such as vasopressin, oxytocin, prostaglandins, and ergotamines (e.g., methylergonovine maleate or Methergine) strengthen uterine contractility, and they may constrict blood vessels as well. Since all four types of uterotonic agents operate at different gene sites, their use in combination is not redundant. Prophylactic use of uterotonic agents in second-trimester abortions may help reduce blood loss.[129] Adding vasopressin or oxytocin to the cervical anesthetic solution provides a simple means of administration, as does direct injection of methylergonovine, dilute vasopressin, or oxytocin into the cervix at the end of the procedure. For severe bleeding, undiluted oxytocin may be safely given as an intravenous push. Many providers give patients oral methylergonovine to use at home for a few days, particularly following second-trimester abortions, although the efficacy of this practice is not established.[130]

Pain control options. Many options are available for pain control during abortion, and the choice of agent often depends upon the clinical setting. Local analgesia and oral pain control options are widely used, whereas intravenous sedation and general anesthesia require specialized equipment and trained providers. Clinicians should discuss available options for pain control when obtaining informed consent for an abortion, as many patients feel that such decisions should be individualized.[131]

Medication abortion. For patients undergoing medication abortion, oral analgesia is usually given. Pain control regimens are not well studied,[132,133] but NSAIDs are a mainstay. Their mechanism of action is to inhibit enzymes that produce endogenous prostaglandins, and they do not appear to affect the efficacy of misoprostol in inducing uterine contractions. Patients taking mifepristone and misoprostol have similar duration and intensity of pain whether NSAIDs are taken at regular intervals or as needed. They tend to ingest more pills when taken at regular intervals.[134] Clinicians may also prescribe medications containing a narcotic such as acetaminophen/codeine or oxycodone, with instructions to use as needed.

First-trimester aspiration procedures. First-trimester aspiration procedures may be performed with cervical anesthesia and oral or IV options for analgesia or sedation. Practice patterns vary, and researchers have studied different approaches. Cervical anesthesia commonly is accomplished using 0.5 or 1% lidocaine given paracervically or intracervically at 2 or 4 injection sites in addition to the tenaculum site. Cervical anesthesia reduces pain regardless of gestational age in the first trimester; the earlier the gestation, the greater the benefit with dilation pain.[135] Evidence shows that deeper injections are superior to shallow injections. A 3-minute wait time does not improve pain scores.[136] A randomized controlled trial found that individuals who received paracervical anesthesia with a combined ketorolac and lidocaine solution reported less pain with cervical dilation compared with those who received oral ibuprofen and lidocaine alone.[137]

The effect of anxiolytics, oral and intravenous pain medications or sedatives, and non-pharmacologic interventions on pain also has been studied.[138] Midazolam reduces pre-procedure anxiety, but it does not affect pain or anxiety during the aspiration procedure.[139] Intramuscular ketorolac given 30 to 60 minutes prior to uterine aspiration appears to be similar to oral ibuprofen given 60 to 90 minutes pre-procedure for pain control during dilation, aspiration, and post-procedure.[140] Patients report higher intraoperative pain scores and less satisfaction with oral oxycodone and lorazepam compared with IV fentanyl and midazolam (intravenous sedation).[141] Inhaled nitrous oxide is an alternative to oral sedation.[142] While ketorolac reduces pain with cervical dilation when included with a paracervical block,[137] a 30 mg dose given intravenously prior to anesthesia induction with lidocaine and propofol has the same effect on postoperative pain as placebo and does not change blood loss.[143] When compared with placebo hydrocodone/acetaminophen used in conjunction with oral lorazepam, ibuprofen, and paracervical anesthesia does not decrease pain and may increase postoperative nausea.[144]

Induction abortion. Most patients undergoing induction abortion require analgesia. Options include oral medications (NSAIDs or opiates)[145] or patient-controlled IV or epidural analgesia,[146] all of which are effective and acceptable to patients. Paracervical block for induction abortion has no effect on pain intensity, amount of morphine used, or duration of induction.[147]

D&E. For patients undergoing D&E, a paracervical block reduces pain associated with osmotic dilator placement,[148] though the infusion of liquid lidocaine into the uterus at the time of cervical preparation with dilator tents does not have a significant effect.[149] IV sedation is the most common pain control modality used for D&E in the U.S. A one-time direct venous injection of 50 to 100 mcg of fentanyl with or without midazolam (moderate sedation) has been studied in women undergoing D&E up to 18 weeks' gestation in an outpatient setting, and is safe and effective.[150] A few studies have examined the safety of deep IV sedation without tracheal intubation for patients undergoing first and second-trimester surgical abortion, and found that anesthesia-related complications, such as intubation and hypoxemia, are extremely rare.[150–152]

MANAGING POSTABORTION ADVERSE EVENTS AND MORBIDITY

Take seriously any complaint or problem after an abortion procedure. Advise all abortion patients to watch for warning signs (see Table 25-3), and tell them how to contact you in case they have questions or problems.

Prompt recognition and management can be critical in preventing the rare serious outcome.

THE SAFETY OF ABORTION

Modern methods of abortion are remarkably safe. Since the nationwide legalization of abortion in the United States, abortion-related mortality has decreased by 90%, with most of the decline occurring from 1973 to 1976. The risk of dying from a modern legal abortion is less than 1 in 100,000 procedures, which represents the lowest mortality risk of all pregnancy outcomes. Pregnancy-related death rates are twice as high for spontaneous abortion and 8 times higher for continuing pregnancy and childbirth.[153] The single greatest factor influencing the safety of abortion is gestational age. Abortions are safer when performed early in pregnancy, which emphasizes the importance of access for individuals seeking abortion.[154]

Medication abortion using mifepristone regimens has proven safe and effective. A review of reports from the 202 Planned Parenthood sites that provided early medication abortions using mifepristone and vaginal misoprostol during 2001 to early 2004 found an overall success rate of 99.7%. Only 206 morbidity events were reported among 95,163 patients—a rate of 2 events per 1,000 abortions.[154,155] Heavy bleeding was the most common morbidity, occurring in 2 per 1,000 treatments, though few patients required blood transfusions (0.5 transfusions per 1,000 abortions). Infections requiring parenteral antibiotics occurred at a rate of 0.2 per 1,000 mifepristone abortions.

In the decade following FDA approval of mifepristone, more than a million individuals in North America have used mifepristone in combination with misoprostol for early abortion; 10 fatalities were reported in this cohort, for a mortality rate of less than 1 per 100,000 abortions.[43,156] One woman died from hemorrhage resulting from a ruptured ectopic pregnancy,[157] and 9 women died of pelvic infection complicated by septic shock. The causative agent in 8 cases of infection was *Clostridium sordellii*, a toxin-producing bacterium that has been associated with rare, serious infections following childbirth, spontaneous abortion (miscarriage), gynecological procedures, and other clinical events.[68,158,159] The CDC identified *Clostridium perfringens* as the pathogen in one case of infection, and the last *Clostridium*-related death occurred in 2009.[160] The clinical manifestations of *Clostridium sordellii* toxic shock infections differ from those typically seen in women with endometritis[68](see below). Intensive investigations by health authorities have not established a causal relationship between the medications used for early abortion and these adverse events, and contamination of mifepristone and misoprostol tablets has been ruled out. Updated labeling for mifepristone reminds providers to remain aware of the possibility of unrecognized ectopic pregnancy or infection throughout the treatment period.

Immediate and Short-Term Adverse Events and Morbidity

Adverse events and morbidity following abortion, while not common,[161,162] include the following immediate and short-term problems:

Bleeding. Regardless of whether they have undergone medication or aspiration methods, almost all patients have at least some bleeding during and after an abortion. Typically, bleeding persists for at least several days, with light bleeding or spotting continuing for as long as 2 to 4 weeks. In medication abortion patients, the absence of bleeding after misoprostol administration may indicate unsuccessful abortion.

Promptly evaluate any bleeding that is excessive or prolonged. The most common causes of hemorrhage after aspiration or D&E abortion are uterine atony and retained placental or fetal tissue. Atony, which typically occurs immediately after the procedure, almost always responds to uterotonic agents and uterine massage. Individuals with retained tissue may present with heavy bleeding several days to a few weeks following the abortion (see Incomplete Abortion, below). After a medication abortion, less than 1 in 100 patients require aspiration or curettage to stop bleeding, and less than 1 in 1,000 require transfusion.[7] Bleeding that requires treatment is often not due to immediate hemorrhage but to persistent or delayed bleeding that occurs 3 to 5 weeks following mifepristone administration.[85] Medication abortion patients and providers, therefore, need to remain vigilant for bleeding even if findings appear normal on the follow-up examination.

Incomplete abortion. When part of the pregnancy tissue remains in the uterus, the abortion procedure is *incomplete*. This problem occurs in less than 3% of aspiration procedures.[161,162] Retained pregnancy tissue is likely to cause continued bleeding and cramping that prompt women to seek care. Treatment with misoprostol, oral methylergonovine maleate, or vacuum aspiration is appropriate. Medication abortion regimens take a longer time to empty the uterus than does aspiration, and an ultrasound examination may show residual tissue after the pregnancy sac has passed. This normal finding does not require intervention unless the patient is bleeding excessively or has symptoms or signs of an infection.[94]

Continuing pregnancy. In less than 1% of cases, an attempt to terminate pregnancy fails altogether.[7,163] A patient with a continuing pregnancy may have ongoing symptoms of pregnancy and a soft or enlarged uterus. Ultrasound or hCG testing may help to identify this problem. (See Chapter 24, Pregnancy Testing and Management of Early Pregnancy.) Providing or referring the patient for an effective means to terminate the pregnancy is appropriate treatment.

Meticulous tissue examination after an aspiration abortion minimizes the risk of a continuing pregnancy. Failure to visualize products of conception (gestational sac plus placental tissue / chorionic villi) in the aspirate warrants further investigation for a continuing intrauterine or ectopic pregnancy. Failed aspiration abortion occurs more often in patients with uterine abnormalities, such as a bicornuate uterus or a cavity distorted by fibroids. Treatment options include medication abortion (if the patient is still within an eligible gestational age limit) or re-aspiration using ultrasound visualization for guidance as needed. Ongoing pregnancy due to failed medication abortion potentially involves an increased risk for fetal malformation, so encourage the patient to consider carefully before deciding to continue the pregnancy to term.[7]

Intrauterine blood clots (hematometra). Intrauterine blood clots can occur immediately or as long as a few days after an aspiration abortion; their presence may cause severe cramping and pain. Sometimes called the *postabortal* or *redo syndrome*, this problem occurs after approximately 0.14% of first-trimester vacuum aspiration abortion procedures.[163] Typical findings on the pelvic examination include a large, tense, and tender uterus with little or no bleeding from the cervix. A simple vacuum aspiration remedies the problem; pain and cramping resolve within a few minutes.

Cervical, uterine, or abdominal organ trauma. External cervical tears can occur if the tenaculum detaches from the cervix. Management options include applying pressure and observing, applying ferric subsulfate (Monsel's) solution, or, rarely, placing suture. A small midline uterine perforation in the first trimester can be managed safely with careful observation for 2 to 4 hours, and hospitalization is not necessary unless evidence arises of internal bleeding, abdominal pain, or rebound tenderness. More severe cervical or uterine trauma, including perforation with damage to nearby abdominal organs or vessels, is rare.[163] Depending on their severity, these adverse events may require exploratory surgery to identify and repair the uterus or abdominal organ injury, or even hysterectomy. To decrease the risk of such injuries, providers typically prepare the cervix with osmotic dilators or pharmacologic agents before second-trimester abortion.[115,117] Avoiding routine use of a uterine sound or sharp curette during aspiration abortion also may reduce the risk.

Uterine rupture has been reported with use of misoprostol for induction of labor at term and rarely in conjunction with mifepristone or other uterotonic agents in second-trimester medication abortion. Most cases occur in women with a previous uterine scar.[164]

Infection. Most U.S. studies report an infection rate of less than 2% following procedural abortion.[162,165] Infection rates are low following medication-induced abortion in the first and second trimesters.[166]

Measures to minimize the risk of infection after aspiration abortion or D&E include screening for pre-existing reproductive tract infections (with treatment before or at the time of the abortion) or administering prophylactic antibiotics at the time of the abortion, using a no-touch technique, and emptying the uterus completely during aspiration or D&E. Short course regimens of routine peri-abortal antibiotics for infection prevention are effective.[167] Many providers use doxycycline or azithromycin; nitroimidazoles (metronidazole or tinidazole) and other tetracyclines are appropriate alternatives.[167] A short course of azithromycin or metronidazole may be less expensive than tetracyclines, including doxycycline. Although some providers use additional antibiotic prophylaxis for individuals who may be at increased risk for subacute bacterial endocarditis, the American Heart Association does not recommend prophylaxis for genitourinary procedures.[168]

Common symptoms of postabortal pelvic infection include some combination of persistent cramping, abdominal pain, fever, discharge, and malaise. Treatment of uncomplicated pelvic infection includes broad-spectrum antibiotics and aspiration of retained tissue, if present. Metronidazole is equally effective orally and parenterally, thereby permitting the option of outpatient treatment in appropriately selected patients. Hospitalization for intravenous antibiotic therapy is warranted in patients with severe illness or suspected pelvic abscess and in those who are immunocompromised, are unable to tolerate oral medications, or who fail to respond to outpatient therapy.

The few patients who developed toxic shock from *Clostridium sordellii* infection presented with atypical findings, including flu-like symptoms, and absence of fever.[68] Suspect an atypical infection if a patient manifests the following symptoms or signs in the days following misoprostol use for medication abortion:

- Nausea, vomiting, diarrhea, weakness with or without abdominal pain
- Tachycardia or hypotension
- Lack of fever with little tenderness on pelvic examination
- High hemoglobin or hematocrit value
- Marked leukocytosis (unusually high white blood cell count)

If you suspect an atypical infection, refer the patient immediately to the emergency room with a copy of the mifepristone Medication Guide. Call the emergency room to explain why you are making the referral. Hospital personnel may know little about medication abortion or *Clostridium sordellii* or *perfringens*, particularly since the last reported case of clostridial infection associated with induced abortion occurred in 2009.

Long-Term Health Outcomes

Individuals who seek abortion services may ask about possible long-term health effects. Public debate about long-term effects has been used inappropriately as a rationale for limiting access to legal abortion services.

Reassuring expert reviews of this topic have been published.[169] The study of long-term health outcomes is methodologically challenging; as new research findings are published, pay attention to the quality of study design and the criteria for determining causality. Conclusions in three key areas are briefly summarized below.

Future Reproductive Health and Fertility

Research to date has found no association between mifepristone-misoprostol abortion and the risk of subsequent ectopic pregnancy, preterm birth, or low birthweight infants.[170,171] Some registry-based observational studies and systematic reviews have suggested a modest increase in the risk of preterm birth in pregnancies subsequent to a first-trimester vacuum aspiration.[172–175] Increased risks for spontaneous abortion or preterm delivery and low birthweight infants have been reported in pregnancies subsequent to a second-trimester D&E abortion, but adequate preparation of the cervix before the procedure may mitigate these risks.[176–178]

Psychological Health

The contention that induced abortion causes lasting psychological harm is misleading and unsubstantiated. No causal association is evident between induced abortion and mental health problems.[179,180] If abortion caused incapacitating emotional responses frequently, this association would be evident because abortion is such a common procedure. Temporary feelings of loss or sadness may follow what is sometimes a difficult decision to terminate a pregnancy, but these normal reactions do not constitute mental health problems. Psychiatric problems following abortion are rare,[181] and they are more likely to occur among individuals with preexisting mental health conditions.[182] Relief is a predominant emotion after abortion, and long-term follow-up studies confirm that most individuals remain satisfied with their decision to have had an abortion.[183]

Breast Cancer

The question of whether induced abortion has any effect on the risk of subsequent breast cancer has received intense scrutiny. Epidemiologic research on this topic is complex, as study design methods can lead to spurious associations. For example, recall bias may explain some of the positive associations found in case-control studies that compare abortion histories of healthy women with those of women who have breast cancer, because healthy women are less likely than women with cancer to report sensitive events such as prior abortion. Prospective studies have found no association between induced abortion and breast cancer.[184–186] Numerous authoritative organizations, including the National Cancer Institute and the American College of Obstetricians and Gynecologists (ACOG), have concluded that no evidence supports a true association between induced abortion and subsequent risk of breast cancer.[187,188]

POSTABORTION CONTRACEPTION

Fertility returns quickly following abortion. Ovulation, and with it the possibility of another pregnancy, may occur as soon as 8 days after abortion.[189] However, many patients may not be interested in discussing contraception at the time of a visit for an abortion.[190] Providers should offer contraceptive counseling that respects the individual's autonomy.

Many factors influence a patient's choice of contraception. Individuals who are experiencing intimate partner violence may choose injectables, as they are private and cannot be tampered with.[191] Lack of insurance coverage and availability may prevent individuals from choosing the method they desire.[192–194] Should a patient desire contraception on the same day of the abortion, providers can help identify any personal, situational, or method-related factors that may contribute to the patients' satisfaction and success with their chosen method. If the patient is receptive to counseling, the provider may explain the availability of emergency contraception and, if possible, provide a supply to have on hand in case of future need. With the exception of the copper IUD, back-up contraception is needed for a week if the patient initiates a method more than 5 to 7 days from the time of abortion.

Providers may place intrauterine contraception safely at the time pregnancy expulsion is confirmed following mifepristone and misoprostol for first-trimester abortion. Individuals who delay placement beyond this time are less likely to return for intrauterine contraception. Studies have demonstrated expulsion rates of 4% to 12% for copper IUDs and the levonorgestrel intrauterine system when placed 1 to 4 weeks after early medication abortion.[195–197]

When intrauterine contraception is placed immediately after a first-trimester aspiration or D&E, continuation at 6 months post-procedure is more common compared with delayed insertion, but expulsion rates may be higher.[198,199] Reported expulsion rates when devices are placed immediately following first- and second-trimester procedures range from 3.1 to 6.8%, versus 0 to 5% when placement is delayed by 2 to 6 weeks. However, the proportion of participants in the delayed placement groups who did not return for intrauterine contraception placement ranged from 45% to 71%; hence, when viewed at 6 months or later, many more in the immediate insertion group are protected by IUDs.[200–202] Intrauterine contraception placement is not recommended if uterine perforation or post-procedure hemorrhage occur.[203]

Progestin-only methods such as the etonogestrel subdermal contraceptive implant and depot medroxyprogesterone acetate (DMPA) may be initiated on the same day that a patient takes mifepristone for a medication abortion.[204–206] Available evidence demonstrates that the implant does not affect mifepristone's efficacy.[207,208] One study found that participants who received DMPA on the same day as mifepristone had a greater frequency of ongoing pregnancies compared with those who received it after the abortion (3.6% vs. 0.9%).[209] Although patients in the same-day mifepristone and DMPA group reported greater satisfaction with their assignment, clinicians should thoroughly counsel individuals considering this approach about the increased risk of ongoing pregnancy and need for close monitoring and possible further treatment.

The patient may start a combined estrogen/progestin method of contraception immediately after an aspiration or D&E. Many providers initiate the hormonal method on the same day as the abortion. If initiated within 5 days, a back-up contraceptive method is not needed.[204,210]

Author Disclosures—Nippita: none. Paul: none.

References

1. Finer LB, Frohwirth LF, Dauphinee LA, Singh S, Moore AM. Reasons U.S. women have abortions: quantitative and qualitative perspectives. Perspect Sex Reprod Health 2005;37:110–118. doi:10.1363/3711005.
2. Biggs MA, Gould H, Foster DG. Understanding why women seek abortions in the US. BMC Womens Health 2013;13:29. doi:10.1186/1472-6874-13-29.
3. Janiak E, Kawachi I, Goldberg A, Gottlieb B. Abortion barriers and perceptions of gestational age among women seeking abortion care in the latter half of the second trimester. Contraception 2014;89:322–327. doi:10.1016/j.contraception.2013.11.009.
4. Drey EA, Foster DG, Jackson RA, Lee SJ, Cardenas LH, Darney PD. Risk factors associated with presenting for abortion in the second trimester. Obstet Gynecol 2006;107: 128–135. doi:10.1097/01.AOG.0000189095.32382.d0.
5. Kiley JW, Yee LM, Niemi CM, Feinglass JM, Simon MA. Delays in request for pregnancy termination: comparison of patients in the first and second trimesters. Contraception 2010;81:446–451. doi:10.1016/j.contraception.2009.12.021.
6. Royal College of Obstetricians and Gynaecologists. The care of women requesting induced abortion, 2 2011. At https://www.rcog.org.uk/globalassets/documents/guidelines/abortion-guideline_web_1.pdf. Accessed June 10, 2017.
7. American College of Obstetricians and Gynecologists. Medical management of first-trimester abortion. Obstet Gynecol 2014;123:676–692. doi:10.1097/01.AOG.0000444454.67279.7d.
8. Jones B, Dalven J. Abortion law and policy in the USA. In: Paul M, Lichtenberg ES, Borgatta L, Grimes DA, Stubblefield PG, Creinin MD, eds. Management of unintended and abnormal pregnancy: comprehensive abortion care. Oxford: Blackwell-Wiley; 2009:36–47.
9. Fried MG. The economics of abortion access in the US: restrictions on government funding for abortion is the post-Roe battleground. Conscience 26:11–15. At http://www.ncbi.nlm.nih.gov/pubmed/16619422. Accessed June 11, 2017.

10. Henshaw SK, Joyce TJ, Dennis A, Finer LB, Blanchard K. Restrictions on Medicaid funding for abortions: a literature review, 2009. At https://www.guttmacher.org/sites/default/files/report_pdf/medicaidlitreview.pdf. Accessed June 11, 2017.
11. Stewart FH, Shields WC, Hwang AC. The federal abortion ban: a clinical and moral dilemma, and international policy setback. Contraception 2004;69:433–435. doi:10.1016/j.contraception.2004.03.001.
12. Weitz TA, Yanow S. Implications of the federal abortion ban for women's health in the United States. Reprod Health Matters 2008;16:99–107. doi:10.1016/S0968-8080(08)31374-3.
13. Barot S, Cohen S. The Global Gag Rule and fights over funding UNFPA: The issues that won't go away. Guttmacher Policy Rev 2015;18:27–33. At http://www.guttmacher.org/pubs/gpr/18/2/gpr1802715.pdf.
14. Nash E, Gold RB, Mohammed L, Cappello O, Ansari-Thomas Z. Laws affecting reproductive health and rights: state policy trends at midyear, 2017 | Guttmacher Institute.; 2017. At https://www.guttmacher.org/article/2017/07/laws-affecting-reproductive-health-and-rights-state-policy-trends-midyear-2017. Accessed August 6, 2017.
15. Benson Gold R, Nash E. Flouting the facts: state abortion restrictions flying in the face of science. Guttmacher Policy Rev 2017;20(2017). At https://www.guttmacher.org/gpr/2017/05/flouting-facts-state-abortion-restrictions-flying-face-science. Accessed July 4, 2017.
16. Joffe CE. Dispatches from the Abortion Wars: The costs of fanaticism to doctors, patients, and the rest of us. Beacon Press; 2009.
17. Grossman D. The use of public health evidence in Whole Woman's Health v Hellerstedt. JAMA Intern Med 2017;177:155–156. doi:10.1001/jamainternmed.2016.6839.
18. Finer LB, Zolna MR. Declines in Unintended Pregnancy in the United States, 2008–2011. N Engl J Med 2016;374:843–852. doi:10.1056/NEJMsa1506575.
19. Daniels K, Daugherty J, Jones J. Current contraceptive status among women aged 15–44: United States, 2011–2013. NCHS Data Brief 2014;(173):1–8. At http://www.ncbi.nlm.nih.gov/pubmed/25500343. Accessed June 30, 2017.
20. Cates W, Grimes DA, Schulz KF. The public health impact of legal abortion: 30 Years later. Perspect Sex Reprod Health 2003;35:25–28. doi:10.1111/j.1931–2393.2003.tb00081.x.
21. Jones RK, Jerman J. Abortion incidence and service availability in the United States, 2014. Perspect Sex Reprod Health 2017;49:17–27. doi:10.1363/psrh.12015.
22. Guttmacher Institute. U.S. abortion rate continues to decline, hits historic low. https://www.guttmacher.org/news-release/2017/us-abortion-rate-continues-decline-hits-historic-low.
23. Jatlaoui TC, Ewing A, Mandel MG, et al. Abortion surveillance - United States, 2013. MMWR Surveill Summ 2016;65:1–44. doi:10.15585/mmwr.ss6512a1.
24. Advancing New Standards in Reproductive Health. Turnaway Study. At https://www.ansirh.org/research/turnaway-study. Accessed August 12, 2017.
25. Greene Foster D, Dobkin LM, Upadhyay UD. Denial of abortion care due to gestational age limits. Contraception 2013;87:3–5. doi:10.1016/j.contraception.2012.09.020.
26. Biggs MA, Upadhyay UD, McCulloch CE, Foster DG. Women's mental health and well-being 5 years after receiving or being denied an abortion. JAMA Psychiatry 2017;74:169. doi:10.1001/jamapsychiatry.2016.3478.
27. American College of Obstetricians and Gynecologists. Abortion training and education. Committee Opinion No. 612. Obstet Gynecol 2014;124:1055–1059. doi:10.1002/14651858.CD003677.pub4.not.
28. O'Connell K, Jones HE, Simon M, et al. First-trimester surgical abortion practices: a survey of National Abortion Federation members. Contraception 2009;79:385–392. doi:10.1016/j.contraception 2008.11.005.
29. Jones RK, Jerman J. Abortion incidence and service availability in the United States, 2014. Perspect Sex Reprod Health 2017;49:17–27. doi:10.1363/psrh.12015.
30. Jerman J, Frohwirth L, Kavanaugh ML, Blades N. Barriers to abortion care and their consequences for patients traveling for services: qualitative findings from two states. Perspect Sex Reprod Health 2017;49:95–102. doi:10.1363/psrh.12024.

31. Johns NE, Foster DG, Upadhyay UD. Distance traveled for Medicaid-covered abortion care in California. BMC Health Serv Res 2017;17:287. doi:10.1186/s12913-017-2241-0.

32. White K, Turan JM, Grossman D. Travel for abortion services in Alabama and delays obtaining care. Women's Heal Issues. May 2017. doi:10.1016/j.whi.2017.04.002.

33. Jerman J, Jones RK and Onda T. Characteristics of U.S. abortion patients in 2014 and changes since 2008. New York: Guttmacher Institute, 2016. At https://www.guttmacher.org/report/characteristics- us-abortion-patients-2014. Accessed July 3, 2017.

34. Sonfield A, Hasstedt K and Gold RB. Moving forward: family planning in the era of health reform, New York: Guttmacher Institute, 2014. At https://www.guttmacher.org/sites/default/files/report_pdf/family-planning-and-health-reform.pdf. Accessed July 3, 2017.

35. Jones RK, Frohwirth L, Moore AM. More than poverty: disruptive events among women having abortions in the USA. J Fam Plan Reprod Heal care 2013;39:36–43. doi:10.1136/jfprhc-2012-100311.

36. Cockrill K, Upadhyay UD, Turan J, Greene Foster D. The stigma of having an abortion: development of a scale and characteristics of women experiencing abortion stigma. Perspect Sex Reprod Health 2013;45:79–88. doi:10.1363/4507913.

37. Perrucci AC. Decision assessment and counseling in abortion care: philosophy and practice. Lanham, MD: Rowman & Littlefield, 2012.

38. National Abortion Federation. Clinical policy guidelines for abortion care 2018. At https://prochoice.org/resources/clinical-policy-guidelines/. Accessed March 2, 2018.

39. Clark W, Panton T, Hann L, Gold M. Medication abortion employing routine sequential measurements of serum hCG and sonography only when indicated. Contraception 2007;75:131–135. doi:10.1016/j.contraception.2006.08.001.

40. Guttmacher Institute. Medication abortion. At https://www.guttmacher.org/state-policy/explore/medication-abortion. Accessed August 12, 2017.

41. Winikoff B. Acceptability of medical abortion in early pregnancy. Fam Plann Perspect 2013;27:142–148, 185. doi:10.2307/2136257.

42. Yarnall J, Swica Y, Winikoff B. Non-physician clinicians can safely provide first trimester medical abortion. Reprod Health Matters 2009;17(33):61–69. doi:10.1016/S0968-8080(09)33445-X.

43. United States Food and Drug Administration. Postmarket Drug Safety Information for Patients and Providers - Mifeprex (mifepristone) Information. At https://www.fda.gov/Drugs/DrugSafety/PostmarketDrugSafetyInformationforPatientsandProviders/ucm111323.htm. Accessed July 5, 2017.

44. Jain JK, Dutton C, Harwood B, Meckstroth KR, Mishell DR. A prospective randomized, double-blinded, placebo-controlled trial comparing mifepristone and vaginal misoprostol to vaginal misoprostol alone for elective termination of early pregnancy. Hum Reprod 2002;17:1477–1482. doi:10.1093/humrep/17.6.1477.

45. Tang OS, Gemzell-Danielsson K, Ho PC. Misoprostol: pharmacokinetic profiles, effects on the uterus and side-effects. Int J Gynaecol Obstet 2007;99 Suppl 2:S160-7. doi:10.1016/j.ijgo.2007.09.004.

46. da Silva Dal Pizzol T, Knop FP, Mengue SS. Prenatal exposure to misoprostol and congenital anomalies: Systematic review and meta-analysis. Reprod Toxicol 2006;22: 666–671. doi:10.1016/j.reprotox.2006.03.015.

47. Creinin MD, Vittinghoff E, Keder L, Darney PD, Tiller G. Methotrexate and misoprostol for early abortion: a multicenter trial. I. Safety and efficacy. Contraception 1996;53: 321–327. At http://www.ncbi.nlm.nih.gov/pubmed/8773418. Accessed July 5, 2017.

48. Wiebe E, Dunn S, Guilbert E, Jacot F, Lugtig L. Comparison of abortions induced by methotrexate or mifepristone followed by misoprostol. Obstet Gynecol 2002;99: 813–819. At http://www.ncbi.nlm.nih.gov/pubmed/11978292. Accessed July 5, 2017.

49. Aiken ARA, Digol I, Trussell J, Gomperts R. Self reported outcomes and adverse events after medical abortion through online telemedicine: population based study in the Republic of Ireland and Northern Ireland. BMJ 2017;357:j2011. doi:10.1136/bmj.j2011.

50. Peyron R, Aubeny E, Targosz V, et al. Early termination of pregnancy with mifepristone (RU 486) and the orally active prostaglandin misoprostol. N Engl J Med 1993;328:1509–1513. doi:10.1056/NEJM199305273282101.
51. Spitz IM, Bardin CW, Benton L, Robbins A. Early pregnancy termination with mifepristone and misoprostol in the United States. N Engl J Med 1998;338:1241–1247. doi:10.1056/NEJM199804303381801.
52. World Health Organisation Task Force on Post-Ovulatory Methods of Fertility. Comparison of two doses of mifepristone in combination with misoprostol for early medical abortion: a randomised trial. BJOG 2000;107:524–530. doi:10.1111/j.1471-0528.2000.tb13273.x.
53. Shannon CS, Winikoff B, Hausknecht R, et al. Multicenter trial of a simplified mifepristone medical abortion regimen. Obstet Gynecol 2005;105:345–351. doi:10.1097/01.AOG.0000152003.94320.59.
54. Schaff EA, Stadalius LS, Eisinger SH, Franks P. Vaginal misoprostol administered at home after mifepristone (RU486) for abortion. J Fam Pract 1997;44:353–360. At http://www.ncbi.nlm.nih.gov/pubmed/9108832. Accessed July 6, 2017.
55. Fielding SL, Edmunds E, Schaff EA. Having an abortion using mifepristone and home misoprostol: a qualitative analysis of women's experiences. Perspect Sex Reprod Health 2002;34:34–40. At http://www.ncbi.nlm.nih.gov/pubmed/11990637. Accessed July 5, 2017.
56. Kopp Kallner H, Fiala C, Gemzell-Danielsson K. Assessment of significant factors affecting acceptability of home administration of misoprostol for medical abortion. Contraception 2012;85:394–397. doi:10.1016/j.contraception.2011.08.009.
57. Løkeland M, Iversen OE, Engeland A, Økland I, Bjørge L. Medical abortion with mifepristone and home administration of misoprostol up to 63 days' gestation. Acta Obstet Gynecol Scand 2014;93:647–653. doi:10.1111/aogs.12398.
58. Raymond EG, Shannon C, Weaver MA, Winikoff B. First-trimester medical abortion with mifepristone 200 mg and misoprostol: a systematic review. Contraception 2013;87:26–37. doi:10.1016/j.contraception.2012.06.011.
59. Winikoff B, Dzuba IG, Chong E, et al. Extending outpatient medical abortion services through 70 days of gestational age. Obstet Gynecol 2012;120:1070–1076. doi:http://10.1097/AOG.0b013e31826c315f.
60. Abbas D, Chong E, Raymond EG. Outpatient medical abortion is safe and effective through 70 days gestation. Contraception 2015;92:197–199. doi:10.1016/j.contraception.2015.06.018.
61. Winikoff B, Dzuba IG, Creinin MD, et al. Two distinct oral routes of misoprostol in mifepristone medical abortion. Obstet Gynecol 2008;112:1303–1310. doi:10.1097/AOG.0b013e31818d8eb4.
62. Hamoda H, Ashok PW, Flett GMM, Templeton A. A randomised controlled trial of mifepristone in combination with misoprostol administered sublingually or vaginally for medical abortion up to 13 weeks of gestation. BJOG An Int J Obstet Gynaecol 2005;112:1102–1108. doi:10.1111/j.1471-0528.2005.00638.x.
63. Tang OS, Chan CCW, Ng EHY, Lee SWH, Ho PC. A prospective, randomized, placebo-controlled trial on the use of mifepristone with sublingual or vaginal misoprostol for medical abortions of less than 9 weeks gestation. Hum Reprod 2003;18:2315–2318. At http://www.ncbi.nlm.nih.gov/pubmed/14585880. Accessed July 6, 2017.
64. Bracken H, Dabash R, Tsertsvadze G, et al. A two-pill sublingual misoprostol outpatient regimen following mifepristone for medical abortion through 70 days' LMP: a prospective comparative open-label trial. Contraception 2014;89:181–186. doi:10.1016/j.contraception.2013.10.018.
65. Raghavan S, Comendant R, Digol I, et al. Two-pill regimens of misoprostol after mifepristone medical abortion through 63 days' gestational age: a randomized controlled trial of sublingual and oral misoprostol. Contraception 2009;79:84–90. doi:10.1016/jcontraception.2008.09.001.

66. Creinin MD, Fox MC, Teal S, et al. A randomized comparison of misoprostol 6 to 8 hours versus 24 hours after mifepristone for abortion. Obstet Gynecol 2004;103: 851–859. doi:10.1097/01.AOG.0000124271.23499.84.
67. Creinin MD, Schreiber CA, Bednarek P, et al. Mifepristone and misoprostol administered simultaneously versus 24 hours apart for abortion: a randomized controlled trial. Obstet Gynecol 2007;109:885–894. doi:10.1097/01.AOG.0000258298.35143.d2.
68. Fischer M, Bhatnagar J, Guarner J, et al. Fatal toxic shock syndrome associated with clostridium sordellii after medical abortion. N Engl J Med 2005;353:2352–2360. doi:10.1056/NEJMoa051620.
69. Chen MJ, Creinin MD. Mifepristone With Buccal Misoprostol for Medical Abortion. Obstet Gynecol 2015;126:12–21. doi:10.1097/AOG.0000000000000897.
70. von Hertzen H, Huong N, Piaggio G, et al. Misoprostol dose and route after mifepristone for early medical abortion: a randomised controlled noninferiority trial. BJOG 2010;117:1186–1196. doi:10.1111/j.1471-0528.2010.02636.x.
71. Ashok PW, Penney GC, Flett GM, Templeton A. An effective regimen for early medical abortion: a report of 2000 consecutive cases. Hum Reprod 1998;13:2962–2965. At http://www.ncbi.nlm.nih.gov/pubmed/9804263. Accessed September 15, 2017.
72. Schaff EA, Fielding SL, Eisinger SH, Stadalius LS, Fuller L. Low-dose mifepristone followed by vaginal misoprostol at 48 hours for abortion up to 63 days. Contraception 2000;61:41–46. At http://www.ncbi.nlm.nih.gov/pubmed/10745068. Accessed September 15, 2017.
73. Blum J, Raghavan S, Dabash R, et al. Comparison of misoprostol-only and combined mifepristone-misoprostol regimens for home-based early medical abortion in Tunisia and Vietnam. Int J Gynaecol Obstet 2012;118:166–171. doi:10.1016/j.ijgo.2012.03.039.
74. Miller S, Lehman T, Campbell M, et al. Misoprostol and declining abortion-related morbidity in Santo Domingo, Dominican Republic: a temporal association. BJOG 2005;112:1291–1296. doi:10.1111/j.1471-0528.2005.00704.x.
75. Ngoc NTN, Blum J, Raghavan S, et al. Comparing two early medical abortion regimens: mifepristone+misoprostol vs. misoprostol alone. Contraception 2011;83:410–417. doi:10.1016/j.contraception.2010.09.002.
76. Morris JL, Winikoff B, Dabash R, et al. FIGO's updated recommendations for misoprostol used alone in gynecology and obstetrics. Int J Gynecol Obstet 2017;138:363–366. doi:10.1002/ijgo.12181.
77. Jones RK. How commonly do US abortion patients report attempts to self-induce? Am J Obstet Gynecol 2011;204:23.e1-4. doi:10.1016/j.ajog.2010.08.019.
78. Kahn JG, Becker BJ, MacIsaac L, et al. The efficacy of medical abortion: A meta-analysis. Contraception 2000;61:29–40. doi:10.1016/S0010-7824(99)00115-8.
79. Creinin MD, Vittinghoff E, Schaff E, Klaisle C, Darney PD, Dean C. Medical abortion with oral methotrexate and vaginal misoprostol. Obstet Gynecol 1997;90:611–616. At http://www.ncbi.nlm.nih.gov/pubmed/9380325. Accessed July 6, 2017.
80. Wiebe ER. Oral methotrexate compared with injected methotrexate when used with misoprostol for abortion. Am J Obstet Gynecol 1999;181:149–152. doi:10.1016/S0002-9378(99)70451-5.
81. Creinin MD, Shulman T. Effect of nonsteroidal anti-inflammatory drugs on the action of misoprostol in a regimen for early abortion. Contraception 1997;56:165–168. doi:10.1016/S0010-7824(97)00120-0.
82. Tang OS, Lee SWH, Ho PC. A prospective randomized study on the measured blood loss in medical termination of early pregnancy by three different misoprostol regimens after pretreatment with mifepristone. Hum Reprod 2002;17:2865–2868. At http://www.ncbi.nlm.nih.gov/pubmed/12407040. Accessed July 6, 2017.
83. Davis A, Westhoff C, De Nonno L. Bleeding patterns after early abortion with mifepristone and misoprostol or manual vacuum aspiration. J Am Med Womens Assoc 2000; 55:141–144. At http://www.ncbi.nlm.nih.gov/pubmed/10846324. Accessed July 6, 2017.
84. Tang OS, Gao PP, Cheng L, Lee SW, Ho PC. A randomized double-blind placebo-controlled study to assess the effect of oral contraceptive pills on the outcome of medical

abortion with mifepristone and misoprostol. Hum Reprod 1999;14:722–725. At http://www.ncbi.nlm.nih.gov/pubmed/10221703. Accessed July 6, 2017.

85. Allen RH, Westhoff C, De Nonno L, Fielding SL, Schaff EA. Curettage after mifepristone-induced abortion: Frequency, timing, and indications. Obstet Gynecol 2001;98: 101–106. doi:10.1016/S0029-7844(01)01375-8.
86. Cleland K, Creinin MD, Nucatola D, Nshom M, Trussell J. Significant adverse events and outcomes after medical abortion. Obstet Gynecol 2013;121:166–171. doi:http://10.1097/AOG.0b013e3182755763.
87. Dayananda I, Maurer R, Fortin J, Goldberg AB. Medical abortion follow-up with serum human chorionic gonadotropin compared with ultrasonography. Obstet Gynecol 2013;121:607–613. doi:10.1097/AOG.0b013e3182839fda.
88. Ngoc NTN, Bracken H, Blum J, et al. Acceptability and feasibility of phone follow-up after early medical abortion in Vietnam. Obstet Gynecol 2014;123:88–95. doi:10.1097/AOG.0000000000000050.
89. Bracken H, Lohr PA, Taylor J, Morroni C, Winikoff B. RU OK? The acceptability and feasibility of remote technologies for follow-up after early medical abortion. Contraception 2014;90:29–35. doi:10.1016/j.contraception.2014.03.016.
90. Platais I, Tsereteli T, Comendant R, Kurbanbekova D, Winikoff B. Acceptability and feasibility of phone follow-up with a semiquantitative urine pregnancy test after medical abortion in Moldova and Uzbekistan. Contraception 2015;91:178–183. doi:10.1016/j.contraception.2014.11.004.
91. Chen MJ, Rounds KM, Creinin MD, Cansino C, Hou MY. Comparing office and telephone follow-up after medical abortion. Contraception 2016;94:122–126. doi:10.1016/j.contraception.2016.04.007.
92. Clark W, Bracken H, Tanenhaus J, Schweikert S, Lichtenberg ES, Winikoff B. Alternatives to a routine follow-up visit for early medical abortion. Obstet Gynecol 2010; 115(2, Part 1):264–272. doi:10.1097/AOG.0b013e3181c996f3.
93. Rossi B, Creinin MD, Meyn LA. Ability of the clinician and patient to predict the outcome of mifepristone and misoprostol medical abortion. Contraception 2004;70: 313–317. doi:10.1016/j.contraception.2004.04.005.
94. Cowett AA, Cohen LS, Lichtenberg ES, Stika CS. Ultrasound evaluation of the endometrium after medical termination of pregnancy. Obstet Gynecol 2004;103(5, Part 1): 871–875. doi:10.1097/01.AOG.0000124782.69622.48.
95. Pocius KD, Bartz D, Maurer R, Stenquist A, Fortin J Goldberg AB. Serum human chorionic gonadotropin (hCG) trend within the first few days after medical abortion: a prospective study. Contraception 2017;95:263–8.
96. Creinin MD. Change in serum β-human chorionic gonadotropin after abortion with methotrexate and misoprostol. Am J Obstet Gynecol 1996;174:776–778. doi:10.1016/S0002-9378(96)70463-5.
97. Barnhart KT. Ectopic pregnancy. N Engl J Med 2009;361:379–387. doi:10.1056/NEJMcp0810384.
98. Godfrey EM, Anderson A, Fielding SL, Meyn L, Creinin MD. Clinical utility of urine pregnancy assays to determine medical abortion outcome is limited. Contraception 2007;75:378–382. doi:10.1016/j.contraception.2007.01.021.
99. Weitz T, Anderson P, Taylor D. Advancing scope of practice for advanced practice clinicians: more than a matter of access. Contraception 2009;80:105–107. doi:10.1016/j.contraception.2009.04.013.
100. Goldberg AB, Dean G, Kang M-S, Youssof S, Darney PD. Manual versus electric vacuum aspiration for early first-trimester abortion: a controlled study of complication rates. Obstet Gynecol 2004;103:101–107. doi:10.1097/01.AOG.0000109147.23082.25.
101. Wen J, Cai QY, Deng F, Li YP. Manual versus electric vacuum aspiration for first-trimester abortion: A systematic review. BJOG An Int J Obstet Gynaecol 2008;115: 5–13. doi:10.1111/j.1471-0528.2007.01572.x.
102. Bird ST, Harvey SM, Beckman LJ, Nichols MD, Rogers K, Blumenthal PD. Similarities in women's perceptions and acceptability of manual vacuum aspiration and electric

vacuum aspiration for first trimester abortion. Contraception 2003;67:207–212. At http://www.ncbi.nlm.nih.gov/pubmed/12618255. Accessed July 11, 2017.

103. Dean G, Cardenas L, Darney P, Goldberg A. Acceptability of manual versus electric aspiration for first trimester abortion: A randomized trial. Contraception 2003;67:201–206. doi:10.1016/S0010-7824(02)00485-7.

104. Dean G, Colarossi L, Porsch L, Betancourt G, Jacobs A, Paul ME. Manual compared with electric vacuum aspiration for abortion at less than 6 weeks of gestation: a randomized controlled trial. Obstet Gynecol 2015;125:1121–1129. doi:10.1097/aog.0000000000000787.

105. Varli IH, Lindelius A, Bergström M. Is preoperative vaginal cleansing necessary for control of infection after first trimester vacuum curettage? Acta Obstet Gynecol Scand 2005;84:650–653. doi:10.1111/j.0001-6349.2005.00689.x.

106. Meckstroth KR, Paul ME. First trimester aspiration abortion. In: Paul ME, Lichtenberg ES, Borgatta L, Grimes DA, Stubblefield PG, Creinin MD, eds. Management of unintended and abnormal pregnancy: comprehensive abortion care. Oxford: Wiley-Blackwell; 2009:135–156.

107. Renner RM, Jensen JT, Nichols MD, Edelman AB. Pain control in first-trimester surgical abortion: a systematic review of randomized controlled trials. Contraception 2010;81:372–388. doi:10.1016/j.contraception.2009.12.008.

108. Grimes DA, Smith MS, Witham AD. Mifepristone and misoprostol versus dilation and evacuation for midtrimester abortion: A pilot randomised controlled trial. BJOG An Int J Obstet Gynaecol 2004;111:148–153. doi:10.1046/j.1471-0528.2003.00034.x.

109. Autry AM, Hayes EC, Jacobson GF, Kirby RS. A comparison of medical induction and dilation and evacuation for second-trimester abortion. Am J Obstet Gynecol 2002;187:393–397. doi:10.1067/mob.2002.123887.

110. Sonalkar S, Ogden SN, Tran LK, Chen AY. Comparison of complications associated with induction by misoprostol versus dilation and evacuation for second-trimester abortion. Int J Gynecol Obstet. June 2017. doi:10.1002/ijgo.12229.

111. Partial-Birth Abortion Ban Act of 2003. At https://www.congress.gov/bill/108th-congress/senate-bill/3/text. Accessed June 11, 2017.

112. Borgatta L, Kapp N, Society of Family Planning. Labor induction abortion in the second trimester: SFP Guideline 20111. Contraception 2011;84:4–18. doi:10.1016/j.contraception.2011.02.005.

113. Kapp N, von Hertzen H. Medical methods to induce abortion in the second trimester. In: Paul ME, Lichtenberg ES, Borgatta L, Grimes DA, Stubblefield PG, Creinin MD, eds. Management of unintended and abnormal pregnancy: comprehensive abortion care. Oxford: Wiley-Blackwell; 2009:178–192.

114. Kapp N, Borgatta L, Stubblefield P, Vragovic O, Moreno N. Mifepristone in second-trimester medical abortion: a randomized controlled trial. Obstet Gynecol 2007;110: 1304–1310. doi:10.1097/01.AOG.0000289577.32274.a5.

115. Grimes DA, Schulz KF, Cates WJ. Prevention of uterine perforation during curettage abortion. JAMA 1984;251:2108–2111. At http://www.ncbi.nlm.nih.gov/pubmed/6708260. Accessed July 20, 2017.

116. Schulz K, Grimes D, Cates W. Measures to prevent cervical injury during suction curettage abortion. Lancet 1983;321:1182–1185. doi:10.1016/S0140-6736(83)92464-9.

117. Fox MC, Krajewski CM. Cervical preparation for second-trimester surgical abortion prior to 20 weeks' gestation: SFP Guideline #2013-4. Contraception 2014;89:75–84. doi:10.1016/j.contraception.2013.11.001.

118. Allen RH, Goldberg AB. Cervical dilation before first-trimester surgical abortion (< 14 weeks' gestation). Contraception 2016;93:277–291. doi:10.1016/j.contraception.2015.12.001.

119. MacIsaac L, Grossman D, Balistreri E, Darney P. A randomized controlled trial of laminaria, oral misoprostol, and vaginal misoprostol before abortion. Obstet Gynecol 1999;93:766–770. doi:10.1016/S0029-7844(98)00493-1.

120. Carbonell Esteve JL, Mari JM, Valero F, et al. Sublingual versus vaginal misoprostol (400 mcg) for cervical priming in first-trimester abortion: a randomized trial. Contraception 2006;74:328–333. doi:10.1016/j.contraception.2006.03.031.

121. Kapp N, Lohr PA, Ngo TD, Hayes JL. Cervical preparation for first trimester surgical abortion. In: Cochrane Database of Systematic Reviews. Chichester, UK: John Wiley & Sons, Ltd; 2010. www.ncbi.nlm.nih.gov/pubmed/20166091.

122. Tang OS, Mok KH, Ho PC. A randomized study comparing the use of sublingual to vaginal misoprostol for pre-operative cervical priming prior to surgical termination of pregnancy in the first trimester. Hum Reprod 2004;19:1101–1104. doi:10.1093/humrep/deh143.

123. Meckstroth KR, Whitaker AK, Bertisch S, Goldberg AB, Darney PD. Misoprostol administered by epithelial routes. Obstet Gynecol 2006;108:582–590. doi:10.1097/01.AOG.0000230398.32794.9d.

124. Panchal HB, Godfrey EM, Patel A. Buccal misoprostol for cervical ripening prior to first trimester abortion. Contraception 2010;81:161–164. doi:10.1016/j.contraception.2009.10.002.

125. Drey EA, Benson LS, Sokoloff A, Steinauer JE, Roy G, Jackson RA. Buccal misoprostol plus laminaria for cervical preparation before dilation and evacuation at 21–23 weeks of gestation: a randomized controlled trial. Contraception 2014;89:307–313. doi:10.1016/j.contraception.2013.10.013.

126. Borgatta L, Roncari D, Sonalkar S, et al. Mifepristone vs. osmotic dilator insertion for cervical preparation prior to surgical abortion at 14–16 weeks: A randomized trial. Contraception 2012;86:567–571. doi:10.1016/j.contraception.2012.05.002.

127. Goldberg AB, Fortin JA, Drey EA, et al. Cervical preparation before dilation and evacuation using adjunctive misoprostol or mifepristone compared with overnight osmotic dilators alone. Obstet Gynecol 2015;126:599–609. doi:10.1097/AOG.0000000000000977.

128. Shaw KA, Shaw JG, Hugin M, Velasquez G, Hopkins FW, Blumenthal PD. Adjunct mifepristone for cervical preparation prior to dilation and evacuation: a randomized trial. Contraception 2015;91:313–319. doi:10.1016/j.contraception.2014.11.014.

129. Schulz KF, Grimes DA, Christensen DD. Vasopressin reduces blood loss from second-trimester dilatation and evacuation abortion. Lancet 1985;326:353–356. doi:10.1016/S0140-6736(85)92496-1.

130. O'Connell K, Jones HE, Lichtenberg ES, Paul M. Second-trimester surgical abortion practices: a survey of National Abortion Federation members. Contraception 2008;78:492–499. doi:10.1016/j.contraception.2008.07.011.

131. Allen RH, Fortin J, Bartz D, Goldberg AB, Clark MA. Women's preferences for pain control during first-trimester surgical abortion: a qualitative study. Contraception 2012;85:413–418. doi:10.1016/j.contraception.2011.08.019.

132. Fiala C, Cameron S, Bombas T, Parachini M, Saya L, Gemzell-Danielsson K. Pain during medical abortion, the impact of the regimen: A neglected issue? A review. Eur J Contracept Reprod Heal Care 2014;19:404–419. doi:10.3109/13625187.2014.950730.

133. Jackson E, Kapp N. Pain control in first-trimester and second-trimester medical termination of pregnancy: a systematic review. Contraception 2011;83:116–126. doi:10.1016/j.contraception.2010.07.014.

134. Raymond EG, Weaver MA, Louie KS, et al. Prophylactic compared with therapeutic ibuprofen analgesia in first-trimester medical abortion: a randomized controlled trial. Obstet Gynecol 2013;122:558–564. doi:10.1097/AOG.0b013e31829d5a33.

135. Renner R-M, Nichols MD, Jensen JT, Li H, Edelman AB. Paracervical block for pain control in first-trimester surgical abortion. Obstet Gynecol 2012;119:1030–1037. doi:10.1097/AOG.0b013e318250b13e.

136. Allen RH, Singh R. Society of Family Planning Clinical Guidelines Pain control in surgical abortion Part 1-Local anesthesia and minimal sedation. Contraception 2018. doi: 10.1016/j.contraception.2018.01.014

137. Cansino C, Edelman A, Burke A, Jamshidi R. Paracervical block with combined ketorolac and lidocaine in first-trimester surgical abortion: a randomized controlled trial. Obstet Gynecol 2009;114:1220–1226. doi:10.1097/AOG.0b013e3181c1a55b.

138. Renner RM, Jensen JT, Nichols MD, Edelman AB. Pain control in first-trimester surgical abortion: a systematic review of randomized controlled trials. Contraception 2010;81:372–388. doi:10.1016/j.contraception.2009.12.008.
139. Bayer LL, Edelman AB, Fu R, et al. An evaluation of oral midazolam for anxiety and pain in first-trimester surgical abortion. Obstet Gynecol 2015;126:37–46. doi:10.1097/AOG.0000000000000913.
140. Braaten KP, Hurwitz S, Fortin J, Goldberg AB. Intramuscular ketorolac versus oral ibuprofen for pain relief in first-trimester surgical abortion: a randomized clinical trial. Contraception 2014;89:116–121. doi:10.1016/j.contraception.2013.10.009.
141. Allen RH, Fitzmaurice G, Lifford KL, Lasic M, Goldberg AB. Oral compared with intravenous sedation for first-trimester surgical abortion. Obstet Gynecol 2009;113:276–283. doi:10.1097/AOG.0b013e3181938758.
142. Singh RH, Montoya M, Espey E, Leeman L. Nitrous oxide versus oral sedation for pain management of first-trimester surgical abortion—a randomized study. Contraception 2017;96:118–123. doi:10.1016/j.contraception.2017.06.003.
143. Roche NE, Li D, James D, Fechner A, Tilak V. The effect of perioperative ketorolac on pain control in pregnancy termination. Contraception 2012;85:299–303. doi:10.1016/j.contraception.2011.10.001.
144. Micks EA, Edelman AB, Renner R-M, et al. Hydrocodone-acetaminophen for pain control in first-trimester surgical abortion: a randomized controlled trial. Obstet Gynecol 2012;120:1060–1069. doi:http://10.1097/AOG.0b013e31826c32f0.
145. Hamoda H, Ashok PW, Flett GMM, Templeton A. Analgesia requirements and predictors of analgesia use for women undergoing medical abortion up to 22 weeks of gestation. BJOG An Int J Obstet Gynaecol 2004;111:996–1000. doi:10.1111/j.1471-0528.2004.00235.x.
146. Smith R-L, Siddiqui N, Henderson T, Teresi J, Downey K, Carvalho JCA. Analgesia for medically induced second trimester termination of pregnancy: a randomized trial. J Obstet Gynaecol Canada 2016;38:147–153. doi:10.1016/j.jogc.2015.12.015.
147. Andersson I-M, Benson L, Christensson K, Gemzell-Danielsson K. Paracervical block as pain treatment during second-trimester medical termination of pregnancy: an RCT with bupivacaine versus sodium chloride. Hum Reprod 2016;31:67–74. doi:10.1093/humrep/dev286.
148. Soon R, Tschann M, Salcedo J, Stevens K, Ahn HJ, Kaneshiro B. Paracervical block for laminaria insertion before second-trimester abortion. Obstet Gynecol July 2017:1. doi:10.1097/AOG.0000000000002149.
149. Mercier RJ, Liberty A. Intrauterine lidocaine for pain control during laminaria insertion: a randomized controlled trial. Contraception 2014;90:594–600. doi:10.1016/j.contraception.2014.07.008.
150. Wilson LC, Chen BA, Creinin MD. Low-dose fentanyl and midazolam in outpatient surgical abortion up to 18 weeks of gestation. Contraception 2009;79:122–128. doi:10.1016/j.contraception.2008.08.005.
151. Mancuso AC, Lee K, Zhang R, Hoover EA, Stockdale C, Hardy-Fairbanks AJ. Deep sedation without intubation during second trimester surgical termination in an inpatient hospital setting. Contraception 2017;95:288–291. doi:10.1016/j.contraception.2016.09.012.
152. Dean G, Jacobs AR, Goldstein RC, Gevirtz CM, Paul ME. The safety of deep sedation without intubation for abortion in the outpatient setting. J Clin Anesth 2011;23:437–442. doi:10.1016/j.jclinane.2011.05.001.
153. Raymond EG, Grimes DA. The comparative safety of legal induced abortion and childbirth in the United States. Obstet Gynecol 2012;119:215–219. doi:10.1097/AOG.0b013e31823fe923.
154. Zane S, Creanga AA, Berg CJ, et al. Abortion-related mortality in the United States. Obstet Gynecol 2015;126:258–265. doi:10.1097/AOG.0000000000000945.
155. Henderson JT, Hwang AC, Harper CC, Stewart FH. Safety of mifepristone abortions in clinical use. Contraception 2005;72:175–178. doi:10.1016/j.contraception.2005.03.011.

156. Sinave C, Le Templier G, Blouin D, Léveillé F, Deland E. Toxic shock syndrome due to Clostridium sordellii: a dramatic postpartum and postabortion disease. Clin Infect Dis 2002;35:1441–1443. doi:10.1086/344464.

157. Shannon C, Brothers LP, Philip NM, Winikoff B. Ectopic pregnancy and medical abortion. Obstet Gynecol 2004;104:161–167. doi:10.1097/01.AOG.0000130839.61098.12.

158. Cohen AL, Bhatnagar J, Reagan S, et al. Toxic shock associated with Clostridium sordellii and Clostridium perfringens after medical and spontaneous abortion. Obstet Gynecol 2007;110:1027–1033. doi:10.1097/01.AOG.0000287291.19230.ba.

159. Ho CS, Bhatnagar J, Cohen AL, et al. Undiagnosed cases of fatal Clostridium-associated toxic shock in Californian women of childbearing age. Am J Obstet Gynecol 2009;201:459.e1-7. doi:10.1016/j.ajog.2009.05.023.

160. Meites E, Zane S, Gould C. Fatal Clostridium sordellii infections after medical abortions. N Engl J Med 2010;363:1382–1383. doi:10.1056/NEJMc1001014.

161. Upadhyay UD, Desai S, Zlidar V, et al. Incidence of emergency department visits and complications after abortion. Obstet Gynecol 2015;125:175–183. doi:10.1097/AOG.0000000000000603.

162. White K, Carroll E, Grossman D. Complications from first-trimester aspiration abortion: a systematic review of the literature. Contraception 2015;92:422–438. doi:10.1016/j.contraception.2015.07.013.

163. Taylor D, Upadhyay UD, Fjerstad M, Battistelli MF, Weitz TA, Paul ME. Standardizing the classification of abortion incidents: the Procedural Abortion Incident Reporting and Surveillance (PAIRS) Framework. Contraception 2017;96:1–13. doi:10.1016/j.contraception.2017.05.004.

164. Goyal V. Uterine rupture in second-trimester misoprostol-induced abortion after cesarean delivery. Obstet Gynecol 2009;113:1117–1123. doi:10.1097/AOG.0b013e31819dbfe2.

165. Lichtenberg ES, Grimes DA. Surgical complications: prevention and management. In: Paul ME, Lichtenberg ES, Borgatta L, Grimes DA, Stubblefield PG, Creinin MD, eds. Management of Unintended and Abnormal Pregnancy: Comprehensive Abortion Care. Blackwell-Wiley; 2009.

166. Shannon C, Brothers LP, Philip NM, Winikoff B. Infection after medical abortion: A review of the literature. Contraception 2004;70:183–190. doi:10.1016/j.contraception.2004.04.009.

167. Achilles SL, Reeves MF, Society of Family Planning. Prevention of infection after induced abortion. Contraception 2011;83:295–309. doi:10.1016/j.contraception.2010.11.006.

168. Wilson W, Taubert KA, Gewitz M, et al. Prevention of infective endocarditis: a guideline from the American Heart Association Rheumatic Fever, Endocarditis, and Kawasaki Disease Committee, Council on Cardiovascular Disease in the Young, and the Council on Clinical Cardiology, Council on Cardiovascular Surgery and Anesthesia, and the Quality of Care and Outcomes Research Interdisciplinary Working Group. Circulation 2007;116:1736–1754. doi:10.1161/CIRCULATIONAHA.106.183095.

169. Hogue C, Boardman L. Answering questions about long-term outcomes. In: Paul ME, Lichtenberg ES, Borgatta L, Grimes DA, Stubblefield PG, Creinin MD, eds. Management of Unintended and Abnormal Pregnancy: Comprehensive Abortion Care. Oxford: Blackwell-Wiley; 2009:252–263.

170. Virk J, Zhang J, Olsen J. Medical abortion and the risk of subsequent adverse pregnancy outcomes. N Engl J Med 2007;357:648–653. doi:10.1056/NEJMoa070445.

171. Liao H, Wei Q, Duan L, Ge J, Zhou Y, Zeng W. Repeated medical abortions and the risk of preterm birth in the subsequent pregnancy. Arch Gynecol Obstet 2011;284:579–586. doi:10.1007/s00404-010-1723-7.

172. Klemetti R, Gissler M, Niinimaki M, Hemminki E. Birth outcomes after induced abortion: a nationwide register-based study of first births in Finland. Hum Reprod 2012;27:3315–3320. doi:10.1093/humrep/des294.

173. Bhattacharya S, Lowit A, Bhattacharya S, et al. Reproductive outcomes following induced abortion: a national register-based cohort study in Scotland. BMJ Open 2012;2:e000911. doi:10.1136/bmjopen-2012-000911.

174. Saccone G, Perriera L, Berghella V. Prior uterine evacuation of pregnancy as independent risk factor for preterm birth: a systematic review and metaanalysis. Am J Obstet Gynecol 2016;214:572–591. doi:10.1016/j.ajog.2015.12.044.
175. Scholten BL, Page-Christiaens GCML, Franx A, Hukkelhoven CWPM, Koster MPH. The influence of pregnancy termination on the outcome of subsequent pregnancies: a retrospective cohort study. BMJ Open 2013;3:e002803. doi:10.1136/bmjopen-2013-002803.
176. Kalish RB, Chasen ST, Rosenzweig LB, Rashbaum WK, Chervenak FA. Impact of midtrimester dilation and evacuation on subsequent pregnancy outcome. Am J Obstet Gynecol 2002;187:882–885. doi:10.1067/mob.2002.127139.
177. Chasen ST, Kalish RB, Gupta M, Kaufman J, Chervenak FA. Obstetric outcomes after surgical abortion at ≥20 weeks' gestation. Am J Obstet Gynecol 2005;193:1161–1164. doi:10.1016/j.ajog.2005.05.078.
178. Oliver-Williams C, Fleming M, Monteath K, Wood AM, Smith GCS. Changes in association between previous therapeutic abortion and preterm birth in Scotland, 1980 to 2008: a historical cohort study. PLoS Med 2013;10:e1001481. doi:10.1371/journal.pmed.1001481.
179. Herd P, Higgins J, Sicinski K, Merkurieva I. The implications of unintended pregnancies for mental health in later life. Am J Public Health 2016;106:421–429. doi:10.2105/AJPH.2015.302973.
180. Steinberg JR, Rubin LR. Psychological aspects of contraception, unintended pregnancy, and abortion. Policy Insights from Behav Brain Sci 2014;1:239–247. doi:10.1177/2372732214549328.
181. Munk-Olsen T, Laursen TM, Pedersen CB, Lidegaard Ø, Mortensen PB. Induced first-trimester abortion and risk of mental disorder. N Engl J Med 2011;364:332–339. doi:10.1056/NEJMoa0905882.
182. Steinberg JR, McCulloch CE, Adler NE. Abortion and mental health. Obstet Gynecol 2014;123:263–270. doi:10.1097/AOG.0000000000000092.
183. Rocca CH, Kimport K, Roberts SCM, Gould H, Neuhaus J, Foster DG. Decision rightness and emotional responses to abortion in the United States: a longitudinal study. PLoS One 2015;10:e0128832. doi:10.1371/journal.pone.0128832.
184. Guo J, Huang Y, Yang L, et al. Association between abortion and breast cancer: an updated systematic review and meta-analysis based on prospective studies. Cancer Causes Control 2015;26:811–819. doi:10.1007/s10552-015-0536-1.
185. Braüner CM, Overvad K, Tjønneland A, Attermann J. Induced abortion and breast cancer among parous women: A Danish cohort study. Acta Obstet Gynecol Scand 2013;92:700–705. doi:10.1111/aogs.12107.
186. Melbye M, Wohlfahrt J, Olsen JH, et al. Induced abortion and the risk of breast cancer. N Engl J Med 1997;336:81–85. doi:10.1056/NEJM199701093360201.
187. National Cancer Institute. Abortion, Miscarriage, and Breast Cancer Risk.; 2003. At https://www.cancer.gov/types/breast/abortion-miscarriage-risk#summary-report.
188. Committee on Gynecologic Practice. ACOG Committee Opinion No. 434: Induced Abortion and Breast Cancer Risk. Obstet Gynecol 2009;113:1417–1418. doi:10.1097/AOG.0b013e3181ac067d.
189. Schreiber CA, Sober S, Ratcliffe S, Creinin MD. Ovulation resumption after medical abortion with mifepristone and misoprostol. Contraception 2011;84:230–233. doi:10.1016/j.contraception.2011.01.013.
190. Matulich M, Cansino C, Culwell KR, Creinin MD. Understanding women's desires for contraceptive counseling at the time of first-trimester surgical abortion. Contraception 2014;89:36–41. doi:10.1016/j.contraception.2013.09.013.
191. Steinauer JE, Upadhyay UD, Sokoloff A, Harper CC, Diedrich JT, Drey EA. Choice of the levonorgestrel intrauterine device, etonogestrel implant or depot medroxyprogesterone acetate for contraception after aspiration abortion. Contraception 2015;92: 553–559. doi:10.1016/j.contraception.2015.06.013.
192. Krashin JW, Stuart GS, Garrett J, et al. Contraception insurance coverage and receipt of long-acting reversible contraception or depot medroxyprogesterone

acetate on the day of abortion. Obstet Gynecol 2017;130:109–117. doi:10.1097/AOG.0000000000002070.

193. Goyal V, Canfield C, Aiken ARA, Dermish A, Potter JE. Postabortion contraceptive use and continuation when long-acting reversible contraception is free. Obstet Gynecol 2017;129:655–662. doi:10.1097/AOG.0000000000001926.

194. Thompson KMJ, Speidel JJ, Saporta V, Waxman NJ, Harper CC. Contraceptive policies affect post-abortion provision of long-acting reversible contraception. Contraception 2011;83:41–47. doi:10.1016/j.contraception.2010.06.008.

195. Shimoni N, Davis A, Ramos ME, Rosario L, Westhoff C. Timing of copper intrauterine device insertion after medical abortion. Obstet Gynecol 2011;118:623–628. doi:10.1097/AOG.0b013e31822ade67.

196. Betstadt SJ, Turok DK, Kapp N, Feng K-T, Borgatta L. Intrauterine device insertion after medical abortion. Contraception 2011;83:517–521. doi:10.1016/j.contraception.2010.10.006.

197. Pohjoranta E, Suhonen S, Mentula M, Heikinheimo O. Intrauterine contraception after medical abortion: factors affecting success of early insertion. Contraception 2017;95:257–262. doi:10.1016/j.contraception.2016.10.012.

198. Okusanya BO, Oduwole O, Effa EE. Immediate postabortal insertion of intrauterine devices. Cochrane Database Syst Rev 2014;28. doi:10.1002/14651858.CD001777.pub4.

199. Steenland MW, Tepper NK, Curtis KM, Kapp N. Intrauterine contraceptive insertion postabortion: a systematic review. Contraception 2011;84:447–464. doi:10.1016/j.contraception.2011.03.007.

200. Cremer M, Bullard KA, Mosley RM, et al. Immediate vs. delayed post-abortal copper T 380A IUD insertion in cases over 12 weeks of gestation. Contraception 2011;83:522–527. doi:10.1016/j.contraception.2010.10.005.

201. Bednarek PH, Creinin MD, Reeves MF, et al. Immediate versus delayed IUD insertion after uterine aspiration. N Engl J Med 2011;364:2208–2217. doi:10.1056/NEJMoa1011600.

202. Hohmann HL, Reeves MF, Chen BA, Perriera LK, Hayes JL, Creinin MD. Immediate versus delayed insertion of the levonorgestrel-releasing intrauterine device following dilation and evacuation: a randomized controlled trial. Contraception 2012;85:240–245. doi:10.1016/j.contraception.2011.08.002.

203. Patil E, Bednarek PH. Immediate intrauterine device insertion following surgical abortion. Obstet Gynecol Clin North Am 2015;42:583–591. doi:10.1016/j.ogc.2015.08.002.

204. Gemzell-Danielsson K, Kallner HK. Post abortion contraception. Women's Heal 2015;11:779–784. doi:10.2217/whe.15.72.

205. Barros Pereira I, Carvalho RM, Graça LM. Intra-abortion contraception with etonogestrel subdermal implant. Eur J Obstet Gynecol Reprod Biol 2015;185:33–35. doi:10.1016/j.ejogrb.2014.11.025.

206. Douthwaite M, Candelas JA, Reichwein B, Eckhardt C, Ngo TD, Domínguez A. Efficacy of early induced medical abortion with mifepristone when beginning progestin-only contraception on the same day. Int J Gynecol Obstet 2016;133:329–333. doi:10.1016/j.ijgo.2015.11.009.

207. Hognert H, Kopp Kallner H, Cameron S, et al. Immediate versus delayed insertion of an etonogestrel releasing implant at medical abortion—a randomized controlled equivalence trial. Hum Reprod 2016;31:2484–2490. doi:10.1093/humrep/dew238.

208. Raymond EG, Weaver MA, Tan Y-L, et al. Effect of immediate compared with delayed insertion of etonogestrel implants on medical abortion efficacy and repeat pregnancy. Obstet Gynecol 2016;127:306–312. doi:10.1097/AOG.0000000000001274.

209. Raymond EG, Weaver MA, Louie KS, et al. Effects of depot medroxyprogesterone acetate injection timing on medical abortion efficacy and repeat pregnancy. Obstet Gynecol 2016;128:739–745. doi:10.1097/AOG.0000000000001627.

210. Fine PM, Tryggestad J, Meyers NJ, Sangi-Haghpeykar H. Safety and acceptability with the use of a contraceptive vaginal ring after surgical or medical abortion. Contraception 2007;75:367–371. doi:10.1016/j.contraception.2007.01.009.

Contraceptive Efficacy

26

James Trussell, PhD
Abigail R.A. Aiken, MD, MPH, PhD

- Pregnancy rates during *perfect use* reflect how effective methods can be in preventing pregnancy when used *consistently and correctly* according to instructions.
- Pregnancy rates during *typical use* reflect how effective methods are for the average person who does not always use methods correctly or consistently.
- For methods that require substantial user effort to sustain adherence, typical use pregnancy rates generally vary widely across different groups, primarily due to differences in the propensity to use the method perfectly.
- There are few empirically based estimates of pregnancy rates during perfect use. For some methods there are none, and for most others there is only one; more are needed.

In the current chapter, we explain the derivation of the estimates of the first-year probabilities of pregnancy during *typical* use (column 2) and *perfect* use (column 3) in Table 26-1.[1–4] We also provide tables summarizing the literature on contraceptive efficacy for each method. These are arranged in the order in which they appear in summary Table 26-1. The studies cited in these tables were all conducted in the United States unless otherwise noted. In the epidemiology literature, the term *efficacy* refers to how well an intervention (in this case a contraceptive method) works in clinical trials, and the term *effectiveness* refers to how well it works in the "real world" (*i.e.*, a non-trial-based setting). We use both trial- and non-trial-based evidence in this chapter. Throughout the book, we use the terms "efficacy" and "effectiveness" interchangeably to mean generally how well a method works. Finally, this chapter explains the derivation of the estimated proportion of women continuing use of each method for 1 year; this is the complement of the proportion discontinuing use within the first year for method-related reasons, including contraceptive failure, side effects, and method switch. A general explanation of the sources of evidence and the logic underlying the summary table on contraceptive efficacy (Table 3-2, identical to Table 26-1) is provided in Chapter 3 on Efficacy, Safety, and Personal Considerations; we suggest reading the effectiveness section of that chapter first. Both typical- and perfect-use pregnancy rates can be measured in clinical trials, but experts generally rely on typical-use rates calculated with population-based survey data in order to reflect the actual experience across a range of contraceptive users with differing demographic characteristics. While one drawback of this approach is reliance upon women's recall of key information, there are also important drawbacks to calculating typical-use contraceptive failure rates in clinical trials. Populations in clinical trials are more highly selected (and thus less generalizable to the wider population), and their behaviors may be affected by frequent contact with investigators and study staff (particularly for methods that are highly user-dependent). We would prefer using survey data to base typical-use estimates for all methods requiring adherence, but we can do so for only five methods since the others are used too infrequently to allow population-based estimation. We therefore base the estimates for these remaining methods on clinical studies because there is no alternative.

NO METHOD

Our estimate of the percentage of women becoming pregnant among those not using contraception is based on populations not using contraception (Hutterites), and on couples in clinical studies who stopped using contraceptives because they wanted to conceive. Table 26-2 summarizes the studies of the 12-month probability of pregnancy among these women. None of these is ideal for our needs, since all but one were studies of couples planning a pregnancy after stopping contraceptive use. What we want is an estimate of the fraction of women now using contraception who would become pregnant if contraception simply vanished and women did not alter their sexual behavior. Perhaps the most relevant is the study among Hutterites, an Anabaptist sect that does not use contraception, where the estimate is 88.8%.[5] However, this is an estimate of pregnancies leading to the first live birth among married women who reported no fetal losses. The proportion would be higher if women with fetal losses were included. However, this group of women was young, with a median age at marriage of 21, so presumably having a higher than average rate of fertility. Therefore, we arbitrarily lowered our estimate to 85%. This estimate is certainly on the high end of the range of plausible estimates: 80%, 75%, and 70% are also plausible.

Available evidence in the United States suggests that only 40% to 46% of women who do not use contraception (but who still wish to avoid pregnancy) become pregnant within 1 year.[6,7] However, such women are almost certainly self-selected for low fecundity or low frequency of intercourse. They may not use contraception because, in part, they are aware that they are unlikely to conceive based on prior experiences of not getting pregnant despite not using contraception. The probability of pregnancy of 85%, therefore, is our best guess of the fraction of women currently using reversible methods of contraception who would become pregnant within 1 year if they were to discontinue contraception but not otherwise change their behavior. Couples who have regular unprotected intercourse for a year without achieving pregnancy are clinically defined as infertile (but by no means are they necessarily sterile).

TYPICAL USE OF WITHDRAWAL, MALE CONDOM, ORAL CONTRACEPTIVE PILLS, AND DEPO-PROVERA

Our estimates of the probability of pregnancy during the first year of typical use for withdrawal (20%), the male condom (13%), the pill (7%), and Depo-Provera (4%) are derived from the 2006-10 National Surveys of Family Growth (NSFG) corrected for under-reporting of abortion.[8] These current estimates are generally lower than the previous estimates derived from the 2002 NSFG (also corrected for abortion under-reporting), except withdrawal (19.9% versus 18.4%). The most notable decrease in the estimated probability of pregnancy is for the male condom (12.6% versus 17.4%).[7]

The correction for under-reporting of abortion may produce estimates that are too high because women in abortion clinics (surveys of whom provided the information for the correction) tend to over-report use of a contraceptive method at the time they became pregnant. Moreover, women in personal interviews for the NSFG also might over-report use of a contraceptive method at the time of an unintended pregnancy that led to a live birth. Evidence for this suspicion is provided by uncorrected first-year probabilities of pregnancy of 3.7% for the IUD and 2.3% for Norplant (methods with little or no scope for user error) in the 1995 NSFG; these probabilities are much higher than rates observed in clinical trials of these methods.[9] Such over-reporting of contraceptive use is unsurprising; women may feel less stigmatized in acknowledging an unintended pregnancy if reported as stemming from contraceptive failure versus from contraceptive non-use. Thus, biases in opposite directions affect these estimates. Pregnancy rates based on the NSFG alone would tend to be too low because induced abortions (and contraceptive failures leading to induced abortions) are under-reported, but they would tend to be too high because contraceptive failures leading to live births are over-reported. We reason that the former bias is the more important one.

The NSFG does not ask for brand of pill; thus combined and progestin-only pills cannot be distinguished. However, since use of the combined pill is far more common than use of the progestin-only pill, the results from the NSFG overwhelmingly reflect typical use of combined pills.[10] The efficacy of progestin-only pills may be lower than that for combined pills since progestin-only pills are probably less forgiving of nonadherence to the dosing schedule (see Chapter 9).

TYPICAL AND PERFECT USE OF THE SPONGE

Our estimates of the probabilities of pregnancy during the first year of typical and perfect use of the sponge correspond with results of a reanalysis of data from a clinical trial in which women were randomly assigned to use the diaphragm or sponge.[11] The probability of failure during typical use was 17%. The probability of failure among parous users (27.4%) was twice as high as that among nulliparous users (14.0%). The results indicate that within the first year of perfect use, the range of sponge failure will be 11.4% to 12.0% among all women, 19.4% to 20.5% among parous women, and 9.0% to 9.5% among nulliparous women. We take as our estimate the midpoints of these ranges: 12%, 20%, and 9%, respectively.[11]

TYPICAL AND PERFECT USE OF THE DIAPHRAGM

Results are based on the only clinical trial of the SILCS diaphragm (now called the Caya diaphragm, used with contraceptive gel.[12] That study estimated a 6-month probability of failure during typical use of 10.4%; from this, we extrapolated a 12-month probability of 17.4% under the assumption that the probability of failure during the second 6 months is 75% of that in the first 6 months (the median of the four estimates for the sponge, cap, and diaphragm);[13] during perfect use we extrapolated the 6-cycle probability of 7.9% to a 13-cycle probability of 16.3% under the assumption that the per-cycle probability remains constant under perfect use. Thus, we conclude that the first-year probability of failure for this diaphragm used with contraceptive gel is similar for typical and perfect use, 17.4% and 16.3% respectively.

The only other diaphragms currently available in the United States are Milex: Arcing and Omniflex. These have been made of silicone since the late 1970s; before that time they were made of latex.[14] There are no published efficacy studies. The latest estimate of the probability of pregnancy during typical use of the Ortho (now discontinued) and Milex diaphragms is based on the 1995 NSFG; use of the diaphragm has virtually disappeared, and would not reflect the experience of current users of Milex.[15]

TYPICAL AND PERFECT USE OF THE FEMALE CONDOM

The typical-use estimate for the female condom is based on the results of a 6-month clinical trial of the Reality female condom (later called the FC female condom); 12.4% of women in the United States experienced a pregnancy during the first 6 months of use.[13] We extrapolated the 12-month probability of pregnancy for users of Reality in the United States (21%) under the assumption that the probability of failure during the second 6 months is 75% of that in the first 6 months.[13] The probability of pregnancy during 6 months of perfect use of Reality by U.S. women who met the adherence criteria stipulated in the study protocol was 2.6%. Those who reported fewer than 4 acts of intercourse during the month prior to any follow-up visit, who did not use Reality at every act of intercourse, who at any time reported not following the Reality instructions, or who used another method of contraception were censored at the beginning of the first interval where nonadherence was noted.[16] Under the assumption that the probability of pregnancy in the second 6 months of perfect use would be the same, the probability of pregnancy during a year of perfect use would be 5.1%. There have been no efficacy trials of the second version of the female condom, the FC2 female condom.

PERFECT USE OF WITHDRAWAL

Our estimate of the proportion becoming pregnant during a year of perfect use of withdrawal (4%) is simply a guess based on the reasoning that the risk of pregnancy resulting from pre-ejaculatory fluid is modest. Although three studies found no motile sperm in the pre-ejaculate,[17–19] the most recent study did not replicate this result, perhaps because the samples were examined within 2 minutes of production.[20] In that study, 37% of subjects produced pre-ejaculatory samples that contained motile sperm, and the sperm concentration and the percentage of motile sperm were similar in an individual's pre-ejaculatory and ejaculatory specimens. However, the actual number of sperm in the pre-ejaculate was low.

TYPICAL AND PERFECT USE OF SPERMICIDES

Our estimate of the proportion of users becoming pregnant during a year of typical use of spermicides (21%) is based on a recent randomized NIH trial of 5 spermicides.[21] We extrapolated a 1-year probability from the 6-month probability reported for each method by assuming the probability of failure in the second 6 months would be 75% of that in the first 6 months,[13] and took as our estimate the mean of the 4 estimates of products still marketed (excluding the 52.5 mg gel).

Our estimate of the proportion becoming pregnant during 1 year of perfect use of spermicides (16%) is based on the same NIH trial of 5 spermicides.[21] We assumed that the pregnancy rate per cycle during perfect use would be constant, extrapolated a 1-year probability from the 6-cycle probability reported for each method, and took as our estimate the mean of the 4 estimates of products still marketed (excluding the 52.5 mg gel). Our estimate is considerably higher than would be expected from the extensive literature on the contraceptive efficacy of spermicides.

Six studies outside the United States,[22–27] in addition to several U.S. studies reviewed earlier,[1] have yielded very low probabilities of pregnancy during the first year of typical use of spermicides, much lower than any estimates for barriers with spermicides. The efficacy literature on spermicides is dominated by studies of suppositories, foams, and film; high spermicide efficacy is documented only in these studies. There are few studies of creams and gels used alone, and those with the lowest pregnancy rates are more than 30 years old (Table 26-3). We consider it likely that the spermicide studies suffer from flaws in analysis or design that are not apparent in the brief published descriptions. For example, an FDA advisory committee was openly skeptical of one German study:[22] "the way in which the survey was designed and the manner in which the various incentives were offered" (physicians reportedly received a fee for completing survey data forms) "would clearly make the data resulting from the survey unacceptable to any scientific group or regulatory agency."[28,29]

The first clinical trial of Emko vaginal foam is also one of the few studies to compute separate pregnancy rates for cycles in which the product was used at every act of intercourse and for cycles in which unprotected intercourse occurred.[30] The design of that trial was also quite sophisticated. Women were randomly assigned to six groups. Each group used three different spermicidal products for three cycles each. The six groups represented all possible permutations of orders of use of the three products. If the pregnancy rate for three cycles of consistent use (not perfect use, which requires both consistent *and* correct use) of Emko vaginal foam is extrapolated, then the implied proportion becoming pregnant in the first year of consistent use is 8.9%.

A recent randomized clinical trial comparing the efficacy of a film and a foaming tablet—the first trial of spermicides conducted according to modern standards of design, execution, and analysis—supports the conclusion that the contraceptive efficacy of spermicides is considerably lower than was previously thought.[31] In that trial, 6-month probabilities of pregnancy during consistent use were 28% for the tablet and 24% for the film, probabilities that were nearly identical to those during typical use in that trial and about the same as the 12-month probability of pregnancy during typical use of spermicides in the 1995 NSFG (the most recent estimate).[32]

TYPICAL AND PERFECT USE OF FERTILITY AWARENESS-BASED METHODS

The typical- and perfect-use effectiveness of fertility awareness based methods (FABM) is challenging to estimate in national surveys in the United States given low use of these methods, and because several clinical trials have used inappropriate methodological approaches.[1] The probability of pregnancy during typical use of FABM in Table 26-1 (15%) is an unpublished estimate based on the 2006-2010 NSFG adjusted for under-reporting of abortion.[33] The estimate was not published because the 257 observations did not meet the pre-specified minimum of 50 observations at each month for the first 12 months. Of FABM observations that could be analyzed, 80% were calendar rhythm. The 15% typical-use failure rate for FABM overall is substantially lower than the previous estimate (24%);[7] it is unclear if this change relates to instability in the estimates given small sample sizes, to better use of these methods over time in the intervening period, or to other factors. Probabilities of failure during typical use for individual FABM—including the Ovulation Method (23%), the TwoDay method (14%), the Standard Days method (12%), Natural Cycles (8%), and the symptothermal method (2%)—are taken from the only clinical studies of these five methods that also contain correctly computed perfect-use estimates.[34–38] None of these studies was conducted in the United States. We find the results for the symptothermal method (study conducted in Germany) unbelievable, although we cannot identify any errors in study design or analysis.

The perfect-use estimates for fertility awareness-based methods are based on the only empirical estimates for these methods: 3.2% for the ovulation method, 3.5% for the TwoDay method, 4.8% for the Standard Days method, 1.0% for Natural Cycles, and 0.4 per 100 woman years for the symptothermal method.[34–38]

PERFECT USE OF THE MALE CONDOM

Our estimate of the probability of pregnancy during a year of perfect use of the male condom is based on results from the only three studies of the male condom meeting modern standards of design, execution, and analysis.[39–41] In each study, couples were randomly assigned to use either a latex condom or a polyurethane condom. All three studies reported efficacy during consistent use but only one reported efficacy during perfect use;[40] in that study the 6-cycle probability of pregnancy during perfect use (0.7%) was 70% of that (1%) during typical use. We assumed that in the other two studies the 6-cycle probability of pregnancy during perfect use would also be 70% of the 6-cycle probability during typical use, assumed that the pregnancy rate per cycle during perfect use would be constant, extrapolated a 1-year probability from the 6-cycle probability reported for the latex condom in each trial, and took as our estimate the median (2%, also the mean) of those 3 estimates. This estimate is consistent with an estimate based on studies of condom breakage and slippage.[42] Under the assumption that 1.5% of condoms break or slip off the penis and that women have intercourse twice a week, then about 1.5% of women would experience condom breaks during the half-week that they are at risk of pregnancy during each cycle. The per-cycle probability of conception would be reduced by 98.5%, from 0.1358 to only 0.0020, if a condom failure results in no protection whatsoever against pregnancy, so that about 2.6% of women would become pregnant each year.[43] Unfortunately, breakage and slippage rates did not accurately predict pregnancy rates during consistent use in one clinical trial of the latex and polyurethane male condom,[39] and estimates of condom breakage and slippage during intercourse or withdrawal vary substantially across studies in developed countries,[42] from a low of 0.6% among commercial sex workers in Nevada's legal brothels[42] to a high of 7.2% among monogamous couples in North Carolina.[44]

PERFECT USE OF ORAL CONTRACEPTIVE PILLS, DEPO-PROVERA, AND NEXPLANON, AND TYPICAL USE OF NEXPLANON

Although the lowest reported pregnancy rate for the combined pill during typical use is 0% (Table 26-12), recent studies indicate that pregnancies do occur, albeit rarely, during perfect use.[45,46] Hence, we set the perfect-use estimate for the pill at the very low level of 0.3%. The lowest reported pregnancy rate for the progestin-only pill exceeds 1% (see Table 26-11). Whether the progestin-only pill is less effective than the combined pill during perfect use is unknown.

The perfect-use estimate for Depo-Provera (0.2%) is the weighted average of the results from the seven trials of the 150 mg intramuscular dose (90-day or 3-month) and the two trials of the 104 mg subcutaneous dose shown in Table 26-13.[47–54] These trials yield an estimate of efficacy during perfect rather than typical use either because women late for an injection were discontinued or because all pregnancies reported occurred during actual use (after one injection but before the next was scheduled). In the two trials of DMPA-SC, there were no reported pregnancies during perfect use in either study.[53,54]

Information about Nexplanon is taken from studies of Implanon, because the dose of etonogestrel is the same and no new efficacy studies were required for approval. Implanon failures are rare.[55] We took the pregnancy rate during typical use of Implanon (0.1%) from a recent multi-center study,[56] and we set the probability during perfect use equal to that during typical use.

TYPICAL AND PERFECT USE OF EVRA AND NUVARING

The typical- (7%) and perfect-use (0.3%) estimates for the Evra patch and NuvaRing were set equal to those for the pill. It is possible that the patch and ring will prove to have better efficacy than the pill during typical use, because of better adherence with the dosing schedule. However, such superior efficacy has not been demonstrated in randomized trials. While in one trial the failure rate was lower among women randomly assigned to use the Evra patch (1.2%) than among those assigned to use the pill (2.2%), the difference was not statistically significant ($p = 0.6$).[57] In a subsequent paper that argues that better adherence to the dosing schedule leads to better contraceptive efficacy of the patch than the pill during typical use, the authors acknowledge that it would require a trial with 24,143 subjects to demonstrate such superiority and conclude that "studies of this size to compare effectiveness may not be practical."[58] Women were randomly assigned to the NuvaRing or the pill in two studies. In one, the pregnancy rates were identical (1.2 per 100 women-years of exposure).[59] In the second, the pregnancy rates did not differ significantly (0.25 versus 0.99 per 100 women-years of exposure).[60]

TYPICAL AND PERFECT USE OF INTRAUTERINE DEVICES (IUDs)

The estimate for typical use of the ParaGard IUD (0.8%) is taken directly from the largest study for that method.[61] The typical-use estimate for Mirena (52 mg LNG) (0.07%) is taken from the largest study of this method.[62] The typical-use estimates for Sklya (13.5 mg LNG) (0.4%), Kyleena (19.5 mg LNG) (0.2%), and Liletta (52 mg LNG) (0.1%) are taken from the only studies of these methods.[63,64] All of the estimates are below 1%; they suggest that effectiveness is higher with LNG than with copper and that effectiveness increases with LNG dose. The estimate for perfect use of the

ParaGard (0.6%) was obtained by removing the pregnancies that resulted when the device was not known to be in situ,[65] on the perhaps-questionable assumption that these pregnancies should be classified as user failures and the empirically-based assumption that expulsions are so uncommon that the denominator of the perfect-use pregnancy rate is virtually the same as the denominator for the typical-use rate (Table 26-14). The perfect-use estimates for Mirena (0.05%), Skyla (0.3%), and Kyleena (0.2%) were derived under the assumption that the same proportions were user failures as for ParaGard (25%). No differences in the typical-use and perfect-use estimates for Kyleena and Mirena are apparently due to the fact that only one significant digit is shown. The perfect-use rate for Liletta (0.1%) was obtained by removing the 1 pregnancy that occurred after an expulsion.

TYPICAL AND PERFECT USE OF PERMANENT CONTRACEPTION

The weighted average of the results from the nine vasectomy studies in Table 26-17 analyzed with life-table procedures is 0.02% becoming pregnant in the year following the procedure.[66–74] In eight of these studies, pregnancies occurred after the ejaculate had been declared to be sperm-free. This perfect-use estimate of 0.02% is undoubtedly too low, because clinicians are understandably loath to publish articles describing their surgical failures and journals would be reluctant to publish an article documenting poor surgical technique. The difference between typical-use and perfect-use pregnancy rates for vasectomy would depend on the frequency of unprotected intercourse after the procedure had been performed but before the ejaculate had been certified to be sperm-free. We arbitrarily set the typical- and perfect-use estimates to 0.15% and 0.10%, respectively. For tubal occlusion (except for the Essure implant), there is no scope for user error. The typical- and perfect-use estimates (both 0.5%) are the pooled results from the U.S. Collaborative Review of Sterilization, a prospective study of 10,685 women undergoing tubal occlusion.[75] We are less concerned about publication bias with female than with male permanent contraception because the largest studies of tubal occlusion are based on prospective, multicenter clinical trials, not retrospective reports from one investigator.

CONTRACEPTIVE CONTINUATION

Contraceptives will be effective at preventing unintended pregnancy only if individuals or couples continue to use them once they have initiated use. The proportions of users continuing use at the end of the first year for withdrawal, fertility awareness-based methods, the male condom, the pill, and Depo-Provera were obtained from the 2002 NSFG. For spermicides, the sponge, and the diaphragm, the proportions were obtained from the 1995 NSFG; the most recent years for which these estimates are available.[7,9] Only method-related reasons for discontinuation (contraceptive failure, changing methods, or termination of contraceptive use while still at risk for unintended pregnancy) were counted. Other reasons for discontinuing use of a method (such as attempting to get pregnant or not having intercourse) are not counted in the discontinuation rate because these reasons are unrelated to the method and do not apply to women seeking to avoid pregnancy and at risk of becoming pregnant. For the female condom, we adjusted the continuation rate for the male condom to reflect a higher pregnancy rate.

We set the continuation rates for the Evra patch and NuvaRing equal to that for the pill. We took the continuation rate for Nexplanon from a multicenter trial of Implanon.[56]

Discontinuation rates of two IUDs (for reasons related to the contraceptive) are based on clinical trials. The estimate for the Copper T 380A IUD was taken directly from the large study for that method.[61] The estimate for the Mirena LNG IUD is the weighted average from three studies of that method.[76–78]

EMERGENCY CONTRACEPTION

See Chapter 10.

THE LACTATIONAL AMENORRHEA METHOD (LAM)

LAM is a highly effective, temporary method of contraception. If the woman feeds the infant from only her breast (or gives supplemental non-breast-milk feeds to a minor extent only) and if the woman has not experienced her first postpartum menses, then breastfeeding provides more than 98% protection from pregnancy in the first 6 months following a birth.[79,80] Four prospective clinical studies of the contraceptive effect of LAM demonstrated cumulative 6-month life-table perfect-use pregnancy rates of 0.5%, 0.6%, 1.0%, and 1.5% among women who relied solely on LAM.[81–84]

Author Disclosure—Trussell: Agile, Evofem, Merck. Aiken: Agile.

References

1. Trussell J, Kost K. Contraceptive failure in the United States: a critical review of the literature. Stud Fam Plann 1987;18:237–83.
2. Trussell J, Hatcher RA, Cates W, Stewart FH, Kost K. Contraceptive failure in the United States: an update. Stud Fam Plann 1990;21:51–4.
3. Trussell J. Contraceptive failure in the United States. Contraception 2004;70:89–96.
4. Trussell J. Contraceptive failure in the United States. Contraception 2011;83:397–404.
5. Sheps MC. An analysis of reproductive patterns in an American isolate. Popul Stud 1965;19:65–80.
6. Grady WR, Hayward MD, Yagi J. Contraceptive failure in the United States: estimates from the 1982 National Survey of Family Growth. Fam Plann Perspect 1986;18: 200–9.
7. Vaughan B, Trussell J, Kost K, Singh S, Jones R. Discontinuation and resumption of contraceptive use: results from the 2002 National Survey of Family Growth. Contraception 2008;78:271–83.
8. Sundaram A, Vaughan B, Kost K, Bankole A, Finer L, Singh S, Trussell J. Contraceptive failure in the United States: Estimates from the 2006–2010 National Survey of Family Growth. Perspect Sexual Reprod Health 2017;49:7–16.
9. Trussell J, Vaughan B. Contraceptive failure, method-related discontinuation and resumption of use: results from the 1995 National Survey of Family Growth. Fam Plann Perspect 1999;31:64–72, 93.
10. Hall KS, Trussell J. Types of combined oral contraceptives used by US women. Contraception 2012;86:659–65.
11. Trussell J, Strickler J, Vaughan B. Contraceptive efficacy of the diaphragm, the sponge and the cervical cap. Fam Plann Perspect 1993;25:100–5, 135.
12. Schwartz JL, Weiner DH, Lai JJ, et al. Contraceptive efficacy, safety, fit, and acceptability of a single-size diaphragm developed with end-user input. Obstet Gynecol 2015;125: 895–903.
13. Trussell J, Sturgen K, Strickler J, Dominik R. Comparative contraceptive efficacy of the female condom and other barrier methods. Fam Plann Perspect 1994;26:66–72.
14. Personal communication from Robert Shaw dated February 9, 2017.
15. Trussell J. Estimates of contraceptive failure from the 1995 National Survey of Family Growth. Contraception 2008 Jul;78:85.
16. Farr G, Gabelnick H, Sturgen K, Dorflinger L. Contraceptive efficacy and acceptability of the female condom. Am J Public Health 1994;84:1960–4.
17. Ilaria G, Jacobs JL, Polsky B, et al. Detection of HIV-1 DNA sequences in pre-ejaculatory fluid. Lancet 1992;340:1469.
18. Pudney J, Oneta M, Mayer K, Seage G, Anderson D. Pre-ejaculatory fluid as potential vector for sexual transmission of HIV-1. Lancet 1992;340:1470.
19. Zukerman Z, Weiss DB, Orvieto R. Does preejaculatory penile secretion originating from Cowper's gland contain sperm? J Assist Reprod Genet 2003;20:157–9.
20. Killick SR, Leary C, Trussell J, Guthrie KA. Sperm content of pre-ejaculatory fluid. Hum Fertil 2011;14:48–52.
21. Raymond EG, Chen PL, Luoto J. Contraceptive effectiveness and safety of five nonoxynol-9 spermicides: a randomized trial. Obstet Gynecol 2004;103:430–9.
22. Brehm H, Haase W. Die alternative zur hormonalen kontrazeption? Med Welt 1975;26:1610–7. German.
23. Dimpfl J, Salomon W, Schicketanz KH. Die spermizide barriere. Sexualmedizin 1984;13:95–8. German.
24. Florence N. Das kontrazeptive vaginal-suppositorium: ergebnisse einer klinischen fünfjahresstudie. Sexualmedizin 1977;6:385–6. German.
25. Godts P. Klinische prüfung eines vaginalem antikonzipiens. Ars Medici 1973;2:589–93. German.

26. Iizuka R, Kobayashi T, Kawakami S, et al. Clinical experience with the Vaginal Contraceptive Film containing the spermicide polyoxyethylene nonylphenyl ether (C-Film study group). Jpn J Fertil Steril 1980;25:64–8. (In Japanese; translation supplied by Apothecus Inc.)
27. Salomon W, Haase W. Intravaginale kontrazeption. Sexualmedizin 1977;6:198–202. German.
28. Over-the-Counter Contraceptives and Other Vaginal Drug Products Review Panel (Elizabeth B. Connell, Chairman). Encare Oval. Memorandum to Food and Drug Administration Commissioner Donald Kennedy, February 9, 1978.
29. Stewart FH, Stewart G, Guest FJ, Hatcher RA. My body, my health: the concerned woman's guide to gynecology. New York: John Wiley & Sons; 1979.
30. Mears E. Chemical contraceptive trial: II. J Reprod Fertil 1962;4:337–43.
31. Raymond E, Dominik R, The Spermicide Trial Group. Contraceptive effectiveness of two spermicides: a randomized trial. Obstet Gynecol 1999;93:896–903.
32. Trussell J. Estimates of contraceptive failure from the 1995 National Survey of Family Growth. Contraception 2008;78:85.
33. Personal communication from Aparna Sundaram and Barbara Vaughan, October 6, 2016.
34. Trussell J, Grummer-Strawn L. Further analysis of contraceptive failure of the ovulation method. Am J Obstet Gynecol 1991;165:2054–9.
35. Arévalo M, Jennings V, Nikula M, Sinai I.Efficacy of the new TwoDay Method of family planning. Fertil Steril 2004;82:885–92.
36. Arévalo M, Jennings V, Sinai I. Efficacy of a new method of family planning: the Standard Days method. Contraception 2002;65:333–8.
37. Berglund Scherwitzl E, Lundberg O, Kopp-Kalner H, Gemzell Danielsson K, Trussell J, Scherwitzl R. Perfect-use and typical-use Pearl Index of a contraceptive modible app. Contraception 2017;96:420–5.
38. Frank-Herrmann P, Heil J, Gnoth C, et al. The effectiveness of a fertility awareness based method to avoid pregnancy in relation to a couple's sexual behaviour during the fertile time: a prospective longitudinal study. Hum Reprod 2007;22:1310–9.
39. Frezieres RG, Walsh TL, Nelson AL, Clark VA, Coulson AH. Evaluation of the efficacy of a polyurethane condom: results from a randomized controlled clinical trial. Fam Plann Perspect 1999;31:81–7.
40. Walsh TL, Frezieres RG, Peacock K, Nelson AL, Clark VA, Bernstein L. Evaluation of the efficacy of a nonlatex condom: results from a randomized, controlled clinical trial. Perspect Sex Reprod Health 2003;35:79–86.
41. Steiner MJ, Dominik R, Rountree RW, Nanda K, Dorflinger LJ. Contraceptive effectiveness of a polyurethane condom and a latex condom: a randomized controlled trial. Obstet Gynecol 2003;101:539–47.
42. Albert AE, Warner DL, Hatcher RA, Trussell J, Bennett C. Condom use among female commercial sex workers in Nevada's legal brothels. Am J Public Health 1995;85:1514–20.
43. Kestelman P, Trussell J. Efficacy of the simultaneous use of condoms and spermicides. Fam Plann Perspect 1991;23:226–7, 232.
44. Steiner M, Piedrahita C, Glover L, Joanis C. Can condom users likely to experience condom failure be identified? Fam Plann Perspect 1993;25:220–3, 226.
45. Hernádi L, Marr J, Trummer D, De Leo V, Petraglia F. Efficacy and safety of a low-dose combined oral contraceptive containing drospirenone 3 mg and ethinylestradiol 20 mcg in a 24/4-day regimen. Contraception 2009;80:18–24.
46. Kroll R, Reape KZ, Margolis M. The efficacy and safety of a low-dose, 91-day, extended-regimen oral contraceptive with continuous ethinyl estradiol. Contraception 2010;81:41–8.
47. Mishell DR, El-Habashy MA, Good RG, Moyer DL. Contraception with an injectable progestin. Am J Obstet Gynecol 1968;101:1046–53.

48. World Health Organization. Multinational comparative clinical trial of long-acting injectable contraceptives: norethisterone enanthate given in two dosage regimens and depot-medroxyprogesterone acetate. Final report. Contraception 1983;28:1–20.
49. Schwallie PC, Assenzo JR. Contraceptive use-efficacy study utilizing medroxyprogesterone acetate administered as an intramuscular injection once every 90 days. Fertil Steril 1973;24:331–9.
50. Scutchfield FD, Long WN, Corey B, Tyler CW. Medroxyprogesterone acetate as an injectable female contraceptive. Contraception 1971;3:21–35.
51. Sangi-Haghpeykar H, Poindexter AN, Bateman L, Ditmore JR. Experiences of injectable contraceptive users in an urban setting. Obstet Gynecol 1996;88:227–33
52. World Health Organization. A multicentered Phase III comparative clinical trial of depot-medroxyprogesterone acetate given three-monthly at doses of 100 mg or 150 mg: I. Contraceptive efficacy and side effects. Contraception 1986;34:223–35.
53. Jain J, Jakimiuk AJ, Bode FR, Ross D, Kaunitz AM.Contraceptive efficacy and safety of DMPA-SC. Contraception 2004;70:269–75.
54. Kaunitz AM, Darney PD, Ross D, Wolter KD, Speroff L. Subcutaneous DMPA vs. intramuscular DMPA: a 2-year randomized study of contraceptive efficacy and bone mineral denisty. Contraception 2009;80:7–17.
55. Graesslin O, Korver T. The contraceptive efficacy of Implanon: a review of clinical trials and marketing experience. Eur J Contracept Reprod Health Care 2008;13 Suppl 1:S4–12.
56. Bahamondes L, Brache V, Meirik O, Ali M, Habib N, Landoulsi S; WHO Study Group on Contraceptive Implants for Women. A 3-year multicentre randomized controlled trial of etonogestrel- and levonorgestrel-releasing contraceptive implants, with non-randomized matched copper-intrauterine device controls. Hum Reprod 2015;30:2527–38.
57. Audet MC, Moreau M, Koltun WD, Waldbaum AS, Shangold G, Fisher AC, Creasy GW. Evaluation of contraceptive efficacy and cycle control of a transdermal contraceptive patch vs. an oral contraceptive. JAMA 2001;285:2347–54.
58. Archer DF, Cullins V, Creasy GW, Fisher AC. The impact of improved compliance with a weekly contraceptive transdermal system (Ortho Evra®) on contraceptive efficacy. Contraception 2004;69:189–95.
59. Oddsson K, Leifels-Fischer B, de Melo NR, Wiel-Masson D, Benedetto C, Verhoeven CH, Dieben TO. Efficacy and safety of a contraceptive vaginal ring (NuvaRing) compared with a combined oral contraceptive: a 1-year randomized trial. Contraception 2005;71:176–82.
60. Ahrendt HJ, Nisand I, Bastianelli C, et al. Efficacy, acceptability and tolerability of the combined contraceptive ring, NuvaRing, compared with an oral contraceptive containing 30 microg of ethinyl estradiol and 3 mg of drospirenone. Contraception 2006;74: 451–7.
61. Sivin I, Shaaban M, Odlind V, et al. A randomized trial of the Gyne T 380 and Gyne T 380 Slimline intrauterine copper devices. Contraception 1990;42:379–89
62. Heinemann K, Reed S, Moehner S, Minh TD. Comparative contraceptive effectiveness of levonorgestrel-releasing and copper intrauterine devices: the European Active Surveillance Study for Intrauterine Devices. Contraception 2015;91:280–3.
63. Nelson A, Apter D, Hauck B, et al. Two low-dose levonorgestrel intrauterine contraceptive systems: a randomized controlled trial. Obstet Gynecol 2013;122;1205–13.
64. Eisenberg DL, Schreiber CA, Turok DK, Teal SB, Westhoff CL, Creinin MD; ACCESS IUS Investigators. Three-year efficacy and safety of a new 52-mg levonorgestrel-releasing intrauterine system. Contraception 2015;92:10–6.
65. Sivin, I. (Center for Biomedical Research, Population Council). Email to: James Trussell (Office of Population Research, Princeton University) 1992.
66. Alderman PM. The lurking sperm: a review of failures in 8879 vasectomies performed by one physician. JAMA 1988;259:3142–4.
67. Moss WM. A comparison of open-end versus closed-end vasectomies: a report on 6220 cases. Contraception 1992;46:521–5.

68. Philp T, Guillebaud J, Budd D. Complications of vasectomy: review of 16,000 patients. Br J Urol 1984;56;745–8.
69. Margaret Pyke Centre. One thousand vasectomies. Br Med J 1973;4:216–21.
70. Kase S, Goldfarb M. Office vasectomy review of 500 cases. Urology 1973;1:60–2.
71. Klapproth HJ, Young IS. Vasectomy, vas ligation and vas occlusion. Urology 1973;1: 292–300.
72. Schmidt SS. Vasectomy. JAMA 1988;259:3176.
73. Marshall S, Lyon RP. Variability of sperm disappearance from the ejaculate after vasectomy. J Urol 1972;107:815–7.
74. Jamieson DJ, Costello C, Trussell J, Hillis SD, Marchbanks PA, Peterson HB; US Collaborative Review of Sterilization Working Group. The risk of pregnancy after vasectomy. Obstet Gynecol 2004;103:848–50. Erratum in: Obstet Gynecol 2004;104:200.
75. Peterson HB, Xia Z, Hughes JM, Wilcox LS, Tylor LR, Trussell J. The risk of pregnancy after tubal sterilization: findings from the U.S. Collaborative Review of Sterilization. Am J Obstet Gynecol 1996;174:1161–70.
76. Luukkainen T, Allonen H, Haukkamaa M, et al. Effective contraception with the levonorgestrel-releasing intrauterine device: 12-month report of a European multicenter study. Contraception 1987;36:169–79.
77. Sivin I, El Mahgoub S, McCarthy T, et al. Long-term contraception with the Levonorgestrel 20 mcg/day (LNG-IUS) and the Copper T 380Ag intrauterine devices: a five-year randomized study. Contraception 1990;42:361–78.
78. Cox M, Blacksell S. Clinical performance of the levonorgestrel intra-uterine system in routine use by the UK Family Planning and Reproductive Health Research Network: 12-month report. Br J Fam Plann 2000;26:143–7.
79. Kennedy KI, Rivera R, McNeilly AS. Consensus statement on the use of breastfeeding as a family planning method. Contraception 1989;39:477–96.
80. Kennedy KI, Labbok MH, Van Look PFA. Lactational amenorrhea method for family planning. Int J Gynaecol Obstet 1996;54:55–7.
81. Kazi A, Kennedy KI, Visness CM, Khan T. Effectiveness of the lactational amenorrhea method in Pakistan. Fertil Steril 1995;64:717–23.
82. Labbok MH, Hight-Laukaran V, Peterson AE, Fletcher V, von Hertzen H, Van Look PFA. Multicenter study of the Lactational Amenorrhea Method (LAM): I. Efficacy, duration, and implications for clinical application. Contraception 1997;55:327–36.
83. Pérez A, Labbok MH, Queenan JT. Clinical study of the lactational amenorrhoea method for family planning. Lancet 1992;339:968–70.
84. Ramos R, Kennedy KI, Visness CM. Effectiveness of lactational amenorrhea in prevention of pregnancy in Manila, the Philippines: non-comparative prospective trial. BMJ 1996;313:909–12.

Table 26-1 Percentage of women experiencing an unintended pregnancy during the first year of typical use and the first year of perfect use of contraception and the percentage continuing use at the end of the first year. United States.

Method	% of Women Experiencing an Unintended Pregnancy within the First Year of Use		% of Women Continuing Use at One Year[3]
	Typical Use[1]	Perfect Use[2]	
No method[4]	85	85	
Spermicides[5]	21	16	42
Female condom[6]	21	5	41
Withdrawal	20	4	46
Diaphragm[7]	17	16	57
Sponge	17	12	36
Parous Women	27	20	
Nulliparous Women	14	9	
Fertility awareness-based methods[8]	15		47
Ovulation method[8]	23	3	
TwoDay method[8]	14	4	
Standard Days method[8]	12	5	
Natural Cycles[8]	8	1	
Symptothermal method[8]	2	0.4	
Male condom[6]	13	2	43
Combined and progestin-only pills	7	0.3	67
Evra patch	7	0.3	67
NuvaRing	7	0.3	67
Depo-Provera	4	0.2	56
Intrauterine contraceptives			
ParaGard (copper T)	0.8	0.6	78
Skyla (13.5 mg LNG)	0.4	0.3	
Kyleena (19.5 mg LNG)	0.2	0.2	
Liletta (52 mg LNG)	0.1	0.1	
Mirena (52 mg LNG)	0.1	0.1	80
Nexplanon	0.1	0.1	89
Tubal occlusion	0.5	0.5	100
Vasectomy	0.15	0.1	100

Emergency Contraceptives: Use of emergency contraceptive pills or placement of a copper intrauterine contraceptive after unprotected intercourse substantially reduces the risk of pregnancy. (See Chapter 10.)

Lactational Amenorrhea Method: LAM is a highly effective, *temporary* method of contraception.[9] (See Chapter 17.)

Source: See text.

(continued)

Table 26-1 Percentage of women experiencing an unintended pregnancy during the first year of typical use and the first year of perfect use of contraception and the percentage continuing use at the end of the first year. United States.—*(continued)*

[1]Among *typical* couples who initiate use of a method (not necessarily for the first time), the percentage who experience an accidental pregnancy during the first year if they do not stop use for any reason other than pregnancy. Estimates of the probability of pregnancy during the first year of typical use for fertility awareness-based methods, withdrawal, the male condom, the pill, and Depo-Provera are taken from the 2006–2010 National Survey of Family Growth (NSFG) corrected for under-reporting of abortion. See the text for the derivation of estimates for the other methods.

[2]Among couples who initiate use of a method (not necessarily for the first time) and who use it *perfectly* (both consistently and correctly), the percentage who experience an accidental pregnancy during the first year if they do not stop use for any other reason. See the text for the derivation of the estimate for each method.

[3]Among couples attempting to avoid pregnancy, the percentage who continue to use a method for 1 year.

[4]This estimate represents the percentage who would become pregnant within 1 year among women now relying on reversible methods of contraception if they abandoned contraception altogether. See text.

[5]150 mg gel, 100 mg gel, 100 mg suppository, 100 mg film.

[6]Without spermicides.

[7]With spermicidal cream or jelly.

[8]About 80% of segments of FABM use in the 2006-2010 NSFG were reported as calendar rhythm. Specific FABM methods are too uncommonly used in the U.S. to permit calculation of typical use failure rates for each using NSFG data; rates provided for individual methods are derived from clinical studies. The Ovulation and TwoDay methods are based on evaluation of cervical mucus. The Standard Days method avoids intercourse on cycle days 8 through 19. Natural Cycles is a fertility app that requires user input of basal body temperature (BBT) recordings and dates of menstruation and optional LH urinary test results. The Symptothermal method is a double-check method based on evaluation of cervical mucus to determine the first fertile day and evaluation of cervical mucus and temperature to determine the last fertile day.

[9]However, to maintain effective protection against pregnancy, another method of contraception must be used as soon as menstruation resumes, the frequency or duration of breastfeeds is reduced, bottle feeds are introduced, or the baby reaches 6 months of age.

Table 26-2 Summary of studies of pregnancy rates among women neither contracepting nor breastfeeding[a]

Reference	N for Analysis	Life-Table 12-Month % Pregnant	Characteristics of the Sample	LFU (%)[g]	Comments
Sivin and Stern, 1979	420	78.1	48% nulliparous	?	Following removal of copper–medicated IUD for planned pregnancy
Tatum, 1975	553	84.6		17.2	Following removal of copper–medicated IUD for planned pregnancy
Sivin, 1987	96	87	All parous	?	Chile, Dominican Republic, Finland, Sweden, United States; following removal of Norplant for planned pregnancy
Tietze and Lewit, 1970	378	88.2	89% aged 15–29	19.0	Following removal of nonmedicated IUD for planned pregnancy
Sheps, 1965	397	88.8	All married Hutterites	?	Conceptions leading to the first live birth following marriage among women reporting no fetal losses before the first conception
Gnoth et al.,2003	346	92 (12 c.y.)	Mean age = 29	1.7[c]	Germany; women using Symptothermal method to conceive.
Belhadj et al., 1986	110	94.0[c]	All parous; aged 18–36	9.1	Brazil, Chile, Dominican Republic, Singapore, United States; following removal of medicated IUD for planned pregnancy
Wiegratz et al., 2006	1,180	94.0	Mean age = 27	44.7[c]	Germany; following discontinuation of an OC containing 30 µg EE and 2 mg of dienogest

Notes:

[a]Updated from Trussell and Kost (1987), Table 1.

[c]Calculated by James Trussell from data in the article.

[g]Most of these studies incorrectly report the loss to follow-up probability as the number of women lost at any time during the study divided by the total number of women entering the study. Thus, these are the probabilities presented in the table. However, the correct measure of LFU would be a gross life-table probability. When available, gross 12-month probabilities are denoted by the letter "g."

[f]Nonresponse rate for entire survey.

For table references, see reference section.

Table 26-3 Summary of studies of contraceptive failure: spermicides[a]

			Risk of Pregnancy						
			Life-Table	Pearl Index Pregnancy Rate					
Reference	Method Brand	N for Analysis	12-Month % Pregnant	Index	Total Exposure	Maximum Exposure	Characteristics of the Sample	LFU (%)[g]	Comments
Edelman, 1980	S'positive	200		0.0	2,682 Mo.	?		?	Study conducted by Jordan-Simner, Inc., as reported by Edelman
Squire et al., 1979	Semicid Suppository	326	0.3				69% aged 20–34; 55% married; "well educated"; "highly motivated"; 24% prior use of oral contraceptives	0.0[c]	89% reported exclusive use of foam
Soloman and Haase, 1977	Patentex (Encare) Oval	1,652		0.3[c]	34,506 Cy.	54 Mo.	13% aged 15–20, 48% aged 21–30, 33% aged 31–40, 6% aged 41–45, 42% nulliparous	?	Subjects who used for less than one year excluded? Germany
Iizuka et al., 1980	Vaginal Contraceptive Film (C-Film)	168		0.6	2,161 Mo.	?	All women had been pregnant before; 20% aged <25, 64% aged 25–34,17% aged 35+	?	Japan
Brehm and Haase, 1975	Patentex (Encare) Oval	10,017		0.9[c]	63,759 Cy.	?	18% aged <21, 20% aged >35; 46% parity 0	?	Germany; FDA rejected this study because of flawed design (see text)
Florence, 1977	a-gen 53	103		1.2[c]	2,255 Cy.	61 Mo.	17% aged 17–20, 51% aged 21–30, 20% aged 31–40,12% aged 41+	?	Belgium

(continued)

Table 26-3 Summary of studies of contraceptive failure: spermicides[a]—(continued)

			Risk of Pregnancy						
			Life-Table	Pearl Index Pregnancy Rate					
Reference	Method Brand	N for Analysis	12-Month % Pregnant	Index	Total Exposure	Maximum Exposure	Characteristics of the Sample	LFU (%)[g]	Comments
Dimpfl et al., 1974	Pantentex (Encare) Oval	482	1.5				22% aged <21, 25% aged >31; 44% parity 0; 60% married	?	Denmark, Germany, Poland, Switzerland
Bushnell, 1965	Emko Vaginal Foam	130		1.8	2,737 Mo.	57 Mo.	Aged 17–51; 76% aged 20–35	?	
Godts, 1973	a-gen 53	56		1.9[c]	1,344 Cy.	32 Mo.	21% aged 18–20, 46% aged 21–30, 18% aged 31–40, 14% aged 41+; all gravid	?	
Carpenter and Martin, 1970	Emko Pre-fil Vaginal Foam	1,778		3.4[c]	17,200 Cy.	18 Cy.	69% aged 21–35; 24% ≥12 years education; 44% no previous contraceptive experience	14.2[c]	All women agreed to exclusive use of foam
Brigato et al., 1982	Vaginal Contraceptive Film (C-Film)	37		3.9[c]	924 Mo.	?		?	Italy
Wolf et al., 1957	Preceptin Vaginal Gel	112		4.2[c]	1,145 Mo.	?	All aged 13–40; mean age = 25[i]; all married	6.9[c]	
Bernstein, 1971	Emko Pre-fil Vaginal Foam	2,932		4.3[c]	28,332 Cy.	20 Cy.	70% aged 21–35; 39% ≥12 years education	16.1[c]	All women agreed to exclusive use of foam
Tyler, 1965	Delfen Vaginal Foam	672		6.0	9,486 Cy.	≥16 Mo.	Rates for full applicator doses and half doses combined	?	

(continued)

Table 26-3 Summary of studies of contraceptive failure: spermicides[a]—*(continued)*

			Risk of Pregnancy						
			Life-Table	Pearl Index Pregnancy Rate					
Reference	Method Brand	N for Analysis	12-Month % Pregnant	Index	Total Exposure	Maximum Exposure	Characteristics of the Sample	LFU (%)[g]	Comments
Apothecus, 1992	Vaginal Contraceptive Film (C-Film)	761		6.5	6,501 Mo.	?			Belgium, Netherlands, Britain, Germany, Switzerland, Denmark, Sweden, Israel, Egypt; results never published; quality of study unknown
Kleppinger, 1965	Delfen Vaginal Foam	138		7.5	1,116 Mo.	19 Mo.	53% aged 21–30; 27% postpartum	0.0[c,g]	
Dubrow and Kuder, 1958	Delfen Vaginal Cream	338		7.6	633 Mo.	12 Mo.	Mean age = 25; 93% ≤12 years education; 39% black; 45% Puerto Rican[t]	59.5[c]	
Dubrow and Kuder, 1958	Preceptin Vaginal Gel	835		8.1	3,728 Mo.	23 Mo.	Mean age = 25; 93% ≤12 years education; 39% black; 45% Puerto Rican[t]	45.1[c]	
Wolf et al., 1957	Delfen Vaginal Cream	875		8.9[c]	5,232 Mo.	30 Mo.	All aged 13–40; mean age = 25[t]; all married	13.0[c]	
Frankman et al., 1975	Vaginal Contraceptive Film (C-Film)	237		9.0	1,866 Mo.	23 Mo.		?	Sweden; data included in Apothecus (1992)

(continued)

Table 26-3 Summary of studies of contraceptive failure: spermicides[a]—(continued)

Reference	Method Brand	N for Analysis	Risk of Pregnancy: Life-Table 12-Month % Pregnant	Pearl Index Pregnancy Rate: Index	Pearl Index Pregnancy Rate: Total Exposure	Pearl Index Pregnancy Rate: Maximum Exposure	Characteristics of the Sample	LFU (%)[g]	Comments
Rovinsky, 1964	Delfen Vaginal Cream	251		9.1	2,915 Mo.	67 Mo.	70% aged 20–34; 55% Puerto Rican; 10% ≥13 years education	28.0[c]	
Raymond et al., 2004	100 mg suppository (Encare)	299	10.0[d]				44% aged 18–25	22	Random assignment to 100 mg suppository, 52.5 mg gel, 100 mg gel, 150 mg gel or 100 mg film
Raymond et al., 2004	100 mg film (Ortho Options Contraceptive Film)	295	11.9[d]				43% aged 18–25	24	Random assignment to 100 mg film, 52.5 mg gel, 100 mg gel, 150 mg gel or 100 mg suppository
Vessey et al., 1982		?		11.9	303 Yr.	?	All white; at recruitment aged 25–39 and married; at enrollment, all women had been using the diaphragm, IUD, or pill successfully for at least 5 months	0.3[t,v]	Britain; Oxford/FPA study

(continued)

Table 26-3 Summary of studies of contraceptive failure: spermicides[a]—*(continued)*

Reference	Method Brand	N for Analysis	Risk of Pregnancy: Life-Table 12-Month % Pregnant	Pearl Index Pregnancy Rate: Index	Pearl Index Pregnancy Rate: Total Exposure	Pearl Index Pregnancy Rate: Maximum Exposure	Characteristics of the Sample	LFU (%)[g]	Comments
Jones and Forrest, 1992		267	13.4				Aged 15–44[t]	21[r]	NSFG 1988; probability when standardized and corrected for estimated underreporting of abortion = 30.2[s]
Raymond et al., 2004	150 mg gel (Ortho Options Conceptrol)	300	14.0[d]		43% aged 18–25	21	Random assignment to 150 mg gel, 52.5 mg gel, 100 mg gel, 100 mg film or 100 mg suppository		
Vaughan et al., 1977		596	14.9[s]				Aged 15–44; all married[t]	19.0[r]	NSFG 1973
Trussell and Vaughan, 1999		164	15.3				Aged 15–44[t]	21[r]	NSFG 1995
Raymond et al., 2004	100 mg gel (Ortho Options Conceptrol)	295	15.5[d]				46% aged 18–25	25	Random assignment to 100 mg gel, 52.5 mg gel, 150 mg gel, 100 mg film or 100 mg suppository
Trussell, 2008		272	16.4				Aged 15–44[t]	21[r]	NSFG 1995; probability when corrected for estimated underreporting of absorption = 28.2

(continued)

Table 26-3 Summary of studies of contraceptive failure: spermicides[a]—(continued)

Reference	Method Brand	N for Analysis	Risk of Pregnancy: Life-Table 12-Month % Pregnant	Pearl Index Pregnancy Rate: Index	Total Exposure	Maximum Exposure	Characteristics of the Sample	LFU (%)[g]	Comments
Fu et al., 1999		?	16.6					21[r]	NSFG 1995; probability when standardized and corrected for estimated underreporting of abortion = 29.0[s]
Grady et al., 1983		1,106	17.5[s,c]				Aged 15–44; all married[t]	18.2[r]	NSFG 1973 and 1976
Schirm et al., 1982		1,106	17.9[s]				Aged 15–44; all married[t]	18.2[r]	NSFG 1973 and 1976
Mears, 1962	Emko Aerosol Foam (nonoxynol 10–11)	425		18.0[c]	722 Cy.	3 Cy.	Pearl index of 9.3 among consistent and 48.4 among inconsistent users	>20[c,t]	Britain; postal trial; random assignment to foam, foaming tablet, or pessary with crossover design
Kasabach, 1962	Koromex A Jelly	242		21.0[c]	2,058 Mo.	24 Mo.	36% aged 25–35; all married; 68% "had a high school education"; all parous	19.3[c]	
Bracher and Santow, 1992		89	21.5				27% aged <20, 56% aged 20–29, 17% aged 30+; 49% parity 0; 87% married or cohabiting	25[r]	Australian Family Survey; first use of method

(continued)

Table 26-3 **Summary of studies of contraceptive failure: spermicides[a]**—*(continued)*

Reference	Method Brand	N for Analysis	Risk of Pregnancy: Life-Table 12-Month % Pregnant	Pearl Index Pregnancy Rate: Index	Total Exposure	Maximum Exposure	Characteristics of the Sample	LFU (%)[g]	Comments
Grady et al., 1986		284	21.8[s]				Aged 15–44; all married[t]	20.6[r]	NSFG 1982
Raymond et al., 2004	52.5 mg gel (Advantage S)	296	22.2[d]				43% aged 18–25	20	Random assignment to 52.5 mg gel, 100 mg gel, 150 mg gel, 100 mg film or 100 mg suppository
Dingle and Tietze, 1963	Lactikol	170		23.5	1,789 Mo.	36 Mo.	Median age = 24.5	3.2[t]	
Frank, 1962	Koromex A Jelly	824		24.8[c]	5,767 Mo.	12 Mo.	72% aged 21–35	17.0[c]	
Raymond et al., 1999	Vaginal Contraceptive Film	369	24.9[d]				Aged 18–35; 17% nulligravid	5.8	Mexico, Ecuador, Guatemala, Ghana, United States; random assignment to Vaginal Contraceptive Film or Conceptrol foaming tablets

(continued)

Table 26-3 Summary of studies of contraceptive failure: spermicides[a]—(continued)

			Risk of Pregnancy						
			Life-Table	Pearl Index Pregnancy Rate					
Reference	Method Brand	N for Analysis	12-Month % Pregnant	Index	Total Exposure	Maximum Exposure	Characteristics of the Sample	LFU (%)[g]	Comments
Raymond et al., 1999	Conceptrol foaming tablets	365	28.0[d]				Aged 18–35; 16% nulligravid	7.3	Mexico, Ecuador, Guatemala, Ghana, United States; random assignment to Conceptrol foaming tablets or Vaginal Contraceptive Film
Tietze and Lewit, 1967	Emko Vaginal Foam	779	28.3				86% < age 30; all married; 47% ≥ high school completion; 75% nonwhite	6.9[g]	
Dingle and Tietze, 1963	Durafoam	421		28.5	2,985 Mo.	36 Mo.	Median age = 26.1	3.2[t]	
Mears, 1962	Genexol Pessary (nonoxynol 10–11)	425		30.3	730 Cy.	3 Cy.		>20[c,t]	Britain; postal trial; random assignment to foam, foaming tablets, or pessary with crossover design

(continued)

Table 26-3 **Summary of studies of contraceptive failure: spermicides[a]**—*(continued)*

Reference	Method Brand	N for Analysis	Risk of Pregnancy: Life-Table 12-Month % Pregnant	Pearl Index Pregnancy Rate: Index	Pearl Index Pregnancy Rate: Total Exposure	Pearl Index Pregnancy Rate: Maximum Exposure	Characteristics of the Sample	LFU (%)[g]	Comments
Tietze and Lewit, 1967	Cooper Creme and Creme Jel, Koromex A, Lactikol Creme and Jelly, Lanesta Gel	806	36.8				79% < age 30; all married; 53% ≥ high school completion; 75% nonwhite	3.4[g]	
Mears, 1962	Volpar Foaming Tablets (phenyl mercuric acetate)	425		48.2[c]	728 Cy.	3 Cy.	Pearl index of 44.4 among consistent and 64.1 among inconsistent users	>20[c,t]	Britain; postal trial; random assignment to foam, foaming tablet, or pessary with crossover design
Mears and Please, 1962	Staycept Cream (hexyl resorcinol)	678		49.6[c]	707 Cy.	3 Cy.	Pearl index of 31.4 among consistent and 132.0 among inconsistent users	>41[c,t]	Britain; postal trial; random assignment to cream, foaming tablet, or pessary with crossover design
Mears and Please, 1962	Genexol Pessary (quinine)	678		52.2	647 Cy.	3 Cy.		>41[c,t]	Britain; postal trial; random assignment to cream, foaming tablet, or pessary with crossover design

(continued)

Table 26-3 Summary of studies of contraceptive failure: spermicides[a]—(continued)

			Risk of Pregnancy						
				Pearl Index Pregnancy Rate					
Reference	Method Brand	N for Analysis	Life-Table 12-Month % Pregnant	Index	Total Exposure	Maximum Exposure	Characteristics of the Sample	LFU (%)[g]	Comments
Smith et al., 1974	Vaginal Contraceptive Film (C-Film)	63[c]		55.7[c]	194[c] Mo.	<15[c]	Aged 16–35	9.5[c]	Britain; trial terminated for ethical reasons
Mears and Please, 1962	Volpar Foaming Tablets (phenyl mercuric acetate)	678		59.0[c]	705 Cy.	3 Cy.	Pearl index of 47.8 among consistent and 106.7 among inconsistent users	>41[c,t]	Britain; postal trial; random assignment to cream, foaming tablet, or pessary with crossover design

Notes:

[a]Updated from Trussell and Kost (1987), Table 2.

[c]Calculated by James Trussell from data in the article.

[d]6-month probability; 12-month probability not available.

[g]Most of these studies incorrectly report the loss to follow-up probability (LFU) as the number of women lost at any time during the study divided by the total number of women entering the study. Thus, these are the probabilities presented in the table. However, the correct measure of LFU would be a gross life-table probability. When available, gross 12-month probabilities are denoted by the letter "g."

[r]Nonresponse rate for entire survey.

[s]Standardized: Vaughan et al., (1977) (1973 NSFG)—intention (the average of probabilities for preventers and delayers); Grady et al., (1983) (1973 and 1976 NSFG)—intention. Our calculation (the average of probabilities for preventers and delayers); Schirm et al., (1982) (1973 and 1976 NSFG)—intention, age, and income; Grady et al., (1986) (1982 NSFG)—intention, age, poverty status, and parity; Jones and Forrest, (1992) (1988 NSFG)—age, marital status, and poverty status; Fu et al., (1999) (1995 NSFG)—age, union status, poverty status.

[t]Total for all methods in the study.

[v]The authors report that LFU for "relevant reasons (withdrawal of cooperation or loss of contact)" was 0.3% per year in the 1982 study. In the 1982 study, women had been followed for 9.5 years on average; if 0.3% are LFU per year, then 2.8% would be LFU in 9.5 years. LFU including death and emigration is about twice as high as LFU for "relevant reasons."

For table references, see reference section.

Table 26-4 Summary of studies of contraceptive failure: Female condom

			Risk of Pregnancy						
			Life-Table 6-Month % Pregnant	Pearl Index Pregnancy Rate					
Reference	Method Brand	N for Analysis		Index	Total Exposure	Maximum Exposure	Characteristics of the Sample	LFU (%)	Comments
Farr et al., 1994	Reality Female Condom	221	12.4				40% nulliparous	2.3	U.S. participants only

Table 26-5 Summary of studies of contraceptive failure: withdrawal

Reference	N for Analysis	Risk of Pregnancy: Life-Table 12-Month % Pregnant	Pearl Index Pregnancy Rate: Index	Pearl Index Pregnancy Rate: Total Exposure	Pearl Index Pregnancy Rate: Maximum Exposure	Characteristics of the Sample[w]	LFU (%)[g]	Comments
Vessey et al., 1982	?		6.7	674 Yr.	?	All white; at recruitment aged 25–39 and married; at enrollment, all women had been using the diaphragm, IUD, or pill successfully for at least 5 months	0.3[t,v]	Britain; Oxford/FPA study
Bracher and Santow, 1992	94	14.2				25% aged <20, 66% aged 20–29, 9% aged 30+; 57% parity 0; 92% married or cohabiting	25[r]	Australian Family Survey; first use of method
Westoff et al., 1961	~74		16.7	1,287 Mo.	?	All married; all white	5.7[r]	FGMA study
Cliquet et al., 1977	2,316	17.3				All aged 30–34 living in Belgium; 93% living as married[t]	22[r]	Belgium; 1971 National Survey on Family Development (NEGO II)
Trussell, 2008	438	18.7				Aged 15–44[t]	21[r]	NSFG 1995; probability when corrected for underreporting of abortion = 28.4
Kost et al., 2008	848	18.8				Aged 15–44[t]	27.5[r]	NSFG 2002; probability when corrected for underreporting of abortion = 18.4

(continued)

Table 26-5 Summary of studies of contraceptive failure: withdrawal—*(continued)*

Reference	N for Analysis	Risk of Pregnancy: Life-Table 12-Month % Pregnant	Pearl Index Pregnancy Rate: Index	Pearl Index Pregnancy Rate: Total Exposure	Pearl Index Pregnancy Rate: Maximum Exposure	Characteristics of the Sample[w]	LFU (%)[g]	Comments
Trussell and Vaughan, 1999	440	18.8				Aged 15–44[t]	21[r]	NSFG 1995
Sundaram et al., 2016	1,808	19.9						2006–2010 NSFG adjusted for under-reporting of abortion
Fu et al., 1999	?	20.1					21[r]	NSFG 1995; probability when standardized and corrected for estimated underreporting of abortion = 27.1[s]
Debusschere, 1980	3,561	20.8				Aged 16–44 living in Flanders; 85% married[t]	40[r]	Belgium; 1975–1976 National Survey on Family Development (NEGO III)
Peel, 1972	62		21.9	1,640 Mo.	60 Mo.	All married	2.9[t]	Britain; Hull Family Survey

Notes:

[a]Updated from Trussell and Kost (1987), Table 1.

[c]Calculated by James Trussell from data in the article.

[g]Most of these studies incorrectly report the loss to follow-up probability (LFU) as the number of women lost at any time during the study divided by the total number of women entering the study. Thus, these are the probabilities presented in the table. However, the correct measure of LFU would be a gross life-table probability. When available, gross 12-month probabilities are denoted by the letter "g."

[r]Nonresponse rate for entire survey.

[s]Fu et al., (1999) (1995 NSFG)—age, union status, poverty status.

[t]Total for all methods in the study.

[v]The authors report that LFU for "relevant reasons (withdrawal of cooperation or loss of contact)" was 0.3% per year in the 1982 study. In the 1982 study, women had been followed for 9.5 years on average; if 0.3% are LFU per year, then 2.8% would be LFU in 9.5 years. LFU including death and emigration is about twice as high as LFU for "relevant reasons."

[w]Unless otherwise noted, characteristics refer to females.

For table references, see reference section.

Table 26-6 Summary of studies of contraceptive failure: diaphragm with spermicide[a]

Reference	N for Analysis	Risk of Pregnancy				Characteristics of the Sample	LFU (%)[g]	Comments
		Life-Table 12-Month % Pregnant	Pearl Index Pregnancy Rate					
			Index	Total Exposure	Maximum Exposure			
Stim, 1980	1,238		1.1[c]	911 Yr.	4 Yr.	Median age = 24	19.5	Fit-free diaphragm without spermicides; continuous wearing with brief daily removal for cleaning but not within 6 hours after intercourse; 1,238 women given device, with follow-up of 997
Lane et al., 1976	2,168	2.1[c]				61% aged 21–34; 71% unmarried; 92% white	1.2[c,g]	Probability downward biased due to improper exposure allocated to women LFU
Vessey and Wiggins, 1974	4,052		2.4	5,909 Mo.	>60 Mo.	All white; at recruitment aged 25–39 and married; all had been using the diaphragm for at least 5 months at enrollment; no previous pill use	1.0[v]	Britain; Oxford/FPA study
Vessey et al., 1982	?		5.5	2,582 Yr.	24 Mo.	All white and aged 25–34; all married at recruitment; at enrollment, all women had been using the diaphragm, IUD, or pill successfully for at least 5 months	0.3[t,v]	Britain; Oxford/FPA study

(continued)

Table 26-6 Summary of studies of contraceptive failure: diaphragm with spermicide[a]—*(continued)*

		Risk of Pregnancy						
			Pearl Index Pregnancy Rate					
Reference	N for Analysis	Life-Table 12-Month % Pregnant	Index	Total Exposure	Maximum Exposure	Characteristics of the Sample	LFU (%)[g]	Comments
Mauck et al., 1999	403	7.9[d]				Mean age = 28.8; 25% nulligravid	4.2[c]	Ortho All-Flex diaphragm; random assignment to Ortho All-Flex diaphragm or FemCap
Trussell, 2008	165	8.0				Aged 15–44[t]	21[r]	NSFG 1995; probability when corrected for estimated under-reporting of abortion = 11.5
Trussell and Vaughan, 1999	166	8.1				Aged 15–44[t]	21[r]	NSFG 1995
Loudon et al., 1991	269		8.7	2,350 Mo.	12 Mo.	Mean age = 28.6; 57% gravidity 0; 68% married or cohabiting; 54% already using the diaphragm at start of trial	>3.7	Britain; random assignment of spermicide: either C-Film or jelly
Fu et al., 1999	?	9.2					21[r]	NSFG 1995; probability when standardized and corrected for estimated underreporting of abortion = 15.9s
Dubrow and Kuder, 1958	873		9.3	5,814 Mo.	48 Mo.	Mean age = 25; 39% black; 45% Puerto Rican; 93% ≤12 years education[t]	38.0[c]	

(continued)

Table 26-6 Summary of studies of contraceptive failure: diaphragm with spermicide[a]—*(continued)*

Reference	N for Analysis	Risk of Pregnancy: Life-Table 12-Month % Pregnant	Pearl Index Pregnancy Rate: Index	Pearl Index Pregnancy Rate: Total Exposure	Pearl Index Pregnancy Rate: Maximum Exposure	Characteristics of the Sample	LFU (%)[g]	Comments
Jones and Forrest, 1992	472	10.4				Aged 15–44[t]	21[r]	NSFG 1988; probability when standardized and corrected for estimated underreporting of abortion = 22.0s
Hall, 1973	347	10.6				Approximately 75% aged 20–24; 47% black; 38% Hispanic; all postpartum	16.0	
Bounds and Guillebaud, 1984	123	10.9				90% aged 20–34; all married/consensual union; "most" ≥13 years education; 96% white	0.0	Britain; random assignment to the diaphragm or sponge
Edelman et al., 1984	717	12.5				88% aged 20–34; 55% never married; 76% ≥13 years education; 94% white; 39% used oral contraceptives prior to entering study	37.8[c,g]	Random assignment to the diaphragm or sponge
McIntyre and Higgins, 1986	717	12.9				88% aged 20–34; 55% never married; 76% ≥13 years education; 94% white; 39% used oral contraceptives prior to entering study	37.8[c,g]	A reanalysis of data used by Edelman et al. (1984); random assignment to the diaphragm or sponge

(continued)

Table 26-6 **Summary of studies of contraceptive failure: diaphragm with spermicide[a]**—*(continued)*

		Risk of Pregnancy						
			Pearl Index Pregnancy Rate					
Reference	N for Analysis	Life-Table 12-Month % Pregnant	Index	Total Exposure	Maximum Exposure	Characteristics of the Sample	LFU (%)[g]	Comments
Vaughan et al., 1977	166	13.1[s]				Aged 15–44; all married[t]	19.0[r]	NSFG 1973
Dingle and Tietze, 1963	189		14.3	2,012 Mo.	36 Mo.	Median age = 22.8	3.2[t]	
Grady et al., 1983	349	14.3[c,s]				Aged 15–44; all married[t]	18.2[r]	NSFG 1973 and 1976
Bernstein et al., 1986	707[c]	16.7				96% aged ≤35; 17% married; 97% ≥ high school completion	33.5[c,g]	Random assignment to the diaphragm or cervical cap
Barnhart et al., 2007	297	17.0				Mean age = 28.4	15.5[c]	
Grady et al., 1986	257	17.0[s]				Aged 15–44; all married[t]	20.6[r]	NSFG 1982
Schwartz et al., 2015	397	17.8				Mean age = 29, 29% nulliparous		SILCS (Caya) diaphragm. 12-month LT extrapolated from 6-month LT probability. 12-month extrapolated LT probability = 14.0 during perfect use

(continued)

Table 26-6 Summary of studies of contraceptive failure: diaphragm with spermicide[a]—*(continued)*

Reference	N for Analysis	Risk of Pregnancy: Life-Table 12-Month % Pregnant	Pearl Index Pregnancy Rate: Index	Pearl Index Pregnancy Rate: Total Exposure	Pearl Index Pregnancy Rate: Maximum Exposure	Characteristics of the Sample	LFU (%)[g]	Comments
Tietze and Lewit, 1967	1,197	17.9				86% aged <30; all married; 60% ≥ high school completion; 50% white	7.2[g]	
Schirm et al., 1982	349	18.6[s]				Aged 15–44; all married[t]	18.2[r]	NSFG 1973 and 1976
Kovacs et al., 1986	324	20.9[t]				28% aged 24–26	52.2	Australia
Bracher and Santow, 1992	219	21.0				12% aged <20; 77% aged 20–29, 11% aged 30+; 56% parity 0; 87% married or cohabiting	25[r]	Australian Family Survey; first use of method
Bounds et al., 1995	80	21.2				Mean age = 29.6; 60% nulliparous	1.3	Britain; probability during consistent use = 12.3; random assignment to diaphragm with spermicide or diaphragm only
Smith et al., 1995	110	24.1				Mean age = 28.8	26.0	Britain; fit-free diaphragm without spermicide; continuous wearing with brief daily removal for cleaning but not within 6 hours after intercourse

(continued)

Table 26-6 **Summary of studies of contraceptive failure: diaphragm with spermicide[a]**—*(continued)*

Reference	N for Analysis	Risk of Pregnancy: Life-Table 12-Month % Pregnant	Pearl Index Pregnancy Rate: Index	Pearl Index Pregnancy Rate: Total Exposure	Pearl Index Pregnancy Rate: Maximum Exposure	Characteristics of the Sample	LFU (%)[g]	Comments
Bounds et al., 1995	84	28.6				Mean age = 29.5; 55% nulliparous	0.0[g]	Britain; diaphragm without spermicide; probability during consistent use = 19.3; random assignment to diaphragm only or diaphragm with spermicide

Notes:

[a]Updated from Trussell and Kost (1987), Table 5.

[c]Calculated by James Trussell from data in the article.

[d]6-month probability; 12-month probability not available.

[g]Most of these studies incorrectly report the loss to follow-up (LFU) probability as the number of women lost at any time during the study divided by the total number of women entering the study. Thus, these are the probabilities presented in the table. However, the correct measure of LFU would be a gross life-table probability. When available, gross 12-month probabilities are denoted by the letter "g."

[r]Nonresponse rate for entire survey.

[s]Standardized: Vaughan et al., (1977) (1973 NSFG)—intention (the average of probabilities for preventers and delayers); Grady et al., (1983) (1973 and 1976 NSFG)—intention. Our calculation (the average of probabilities for preventers and delayers); Schirm et al., (1982) (1973 and 1976 NSFG)—intention, age, and income; Grady et al., (1986) (1982 NSFG)—intention, age, poverty status, and parity; Jones and Forrest, (1992) (1988 NSFG)—age, marital status, and poverty status; Fu et al., (1999) (1995 NSFG)—age, union status, poverty status.

[t]Total for all methods in the study.

[v]The authors report that LFU for "relevant reasons (withdrawal of cooperation or loss of contact)" was 0.3% per year in the 1982 study and "about 10 per 1,000" per year in the 1974 study. In the 1982 study, women had been followed for 9.5 years on average; if 0.3% are LFU per year, then 2.8% would be LFU in 9.5 years. LFU including death and emigration is about twice as high as LFU for "relevant reasons."

For table references, see reference section.

Table 26-7 Summary of studies of contraceptive failure: sponge[a]

Reference	N for Analysis	Life-Table 12-Month % Pregnant	Characteristics of the Sample	LFU (%)[g]	Comments
Jones and Forrest, 1992	227	14.5	Aged 15–44[t]	21[r]	NSFG 1988
Edelman et al., 1984	722	17.0	89% aged 20–34, 28% married; 77% ≥13 years education; 94% white, 49% never-married; 38% used oral contraceptives prior to entering study	33.2[c,g]	Random assignment to the diaphragm or sponge
McIntyre and Higgins, 1986	723	17.4	89% aged 20–34, 28% married; 77% ≥13 years education; 94% white, 49% never-married; 38% used oral contraceptives prior to entering the study	33.2[c,g]	A reanalysis of data used by Edelman et al. (1984); random assignment to the diaphragm or sponge; much higher probability for parous women
Trussell and Vaughan, 1999	111	18.4	Aged 15–44[t]	21[r]	NSFG 1995
Bounds and Guillebaud, 1984	126	24.5	92% aged 20–34; all married/consensual union; "most" ≥13 years education; 99% white	1.7[g]	Britain; random assignment to the diaphragm or sponge

Notes:

[a]Updated from Trussell and Kost (1987), Table 4.

[c]Calculated by James Trussell from data in the article.

[g]Most of these studies incorrectly report the loss to follow-up (LFU) probability as the number of women lost at any time during the study divided by the total number of women entering the study. Thus, these are the probabilities presented in the table. However, the correct measure of LFU would be a gross life-table probability. When available, gross 12-month probabilities are denoted by the letter "g."

[r]Nonresponse rate for entire survey.

[t]Total for all methods in the study.

For table references, see reference section.

Table 26-8 Summary of studies of contraceptive failure: cervical cap and other female barrier methods with spermicide[a]

			Risk of Pregnancy						
			Life-Table	Pearl Index Pregnancy Rate					
Reference	Method Brand	N for Analysis	12-Month % Pregnant	Index	Total Exposure	Maximum Exposure	Characteristics of the Sample	LFU (%)[g]	Comments
Shihata and Trussell, 1991	FemCap	106	4.8					0.0[g]	Probability based on 13 cycles
Denniston and Putney, 1981	Prentif Cavity-rim	110	8.0[b,n]				98% aged 20–35; 70% nulliparous	20.9[c]	
Cagen, 1986	Prentif Cavity-rim	620	8.1[n]				87% aged 20–34; 80% always used spermicide and 14% never did	38.5[c]	LFU = "no response"
Koch, 1982	Prentif Cavity-rim	372	8.4				76% aged 20–29; 65% college graduates	8.0[c]	Women advised also to use condom for the first several cap uses
Mauck et al., 1996	Lea's Shield	79	8.7[b]				Mean age = 29.6; mean education = 14.2 years; 19% nulliparous	6.4[b,g]	
Richwald et al., 1989	Prentif Cavity-rim	3,433	11.3				Mean age 29.0; 91% white non-Hispanic; 80% unmarried; almost 60% college graduates; 64% one or more previous pregnancies; 6.1% failure rate among perfect users, 11.9% among imperfect users	18[g]	Women advised to use extra spermicide or use condoms during first 2 months of use; 15 sites; 14 in Los Angeles, 1 in Santa Fe

(continued)

Table 26-8 Summary of studies of contraceptive failure: cervical cap and other female barrier methods with spermicide[a]—*(continued)*

			Risk of Pregnancy						
			Life-Table	Pearl Index Pregnancy Rate					
Reference	Method Brand	N for Analysis	12-Month % Pregnant	Index	Total Exposure	Maximum Exposure	Characteristics of the Sample	LFU (%)[g]	Comments
Mauck et al., 1999	FemCap	355	13.5[d]				Mean age = 29.1; 23% nulligravid	3.7[c]	Random assignment to FemCap or Ortho All-Flex diaphragm
Powell et al., 1986	Prentif Cavity-rim and Vimule	477	16.6				67% aged 25–34 "about half" unmarried; 97% high school graduates; 17% using the pill when fitted for cap	43.8[c]	Canada; back-up methods encouraged (including the emergency contraceptive pills used by 23 women in cases of cap dislodgement)
Bernstein et al., 1986	Prentif Cavity-rim	687[c]	17.4				95% aged ≤35, 16% married, 96% ≥ high school completion	26.3[c,g]	Random assignment to the diaphragm or cervical cap
Kassell and McElroy, 1981	Prentif Cavity-rim	90		18.1[c]	731 Mo.	12 Mo.	Mean age = 23.6; mean education = 14.7 years	10.0[c]	
Boehm, 1983	Prentif Cavity-rim	47		18.1[c]	397 Mo.	12 Mo.		31.6	All women reported exclusive use of cap
Lehfeldt and Sivin, 1984	Prentif Cavity-rim	130	19.1				37% aged 16–25; 72% college graduates; 91% nulliparous	7.2[c]	All women agreed to exclusive use of cap

(continued)

Table 26-8 Summary of studies of contraceptive failure: cervical cap and other female barrier methods with spermicide[a]—*(continued)*

			Risk of Pregnancy						
			Life-Table	Pearl Index Pregnancy Rate					
Reference	Method Brand	N for Analysis	12-Month % Pregnant	Index	Total Exposure	Maximum Exposure	Characteristics of the Sample	LFU (%)[g]	Comments
Smith and Lee, 1984	Prentif Cavity-rim and Vimule	33	27.0				80% aged 20–29; clients at university student health service	1.5–4.6[c]	Regular users for whom the cap (with spermicide) was the sole method used "during the fertile portion of the cycle"

Notes:

[a]Updated from Trussell and Kost (1987), Table 4.

[b]6-month net probability; 12-month probability not available.

[c]Calculated by James Trussell from data in the article.

[g]Most of these studies incorrectly report the loss to follow-up (LFU) probability as the number of women lost at any time during the study divided by the total number of women entering the study. Thus, these are the probabilities presented in the table. However, the correct measure of LFU would be a gross life-table probability. When available, gross 12-month probabilities are denoted by the letter "g."

[n]Only net probabilities available for this study.

For table references, see reference section.

Table 26-9 Summary of studies of contraceptive failure: fertility awareness methods[a]

Reference	Method	N for Analysis	Risk of Pregnancy: Life-Table 12-Month % Pregnant	Risk of Pregnancy: Pearl Index Pregnancy Rate: Index	Total Exposure	Maximum Exposure	Characteristics of the Sample	LFU (%)[g]	Comments
Frank-Hermann et al., 2007	Symptothermal method	900	1.6				88% aged < 35	?	Germany
Trussell and Grummer Strawn, 1990	Ovulation	725	3.2				Mean age = 30; proven fertility; agreed to use OM alone; cohabiting; 765 of 869 learned OM to satisfaction of teachers; 725 entered effectiveness study	?	Reanalysis of W.H.O. (1981) trial; probability based on 13 cycles of *perfect* use
Arévalo, et al., 2004	TwoDay	450	3.5				23% aged 18–24; 29% aged 25–29; 26% aged 30–34; 22% aged 35–39; all parous	4.4	Guatemala, Peru, and the Philippines
Berglund Scherwitzl et al., 2016	Natural Cycles	4,054	6.4				79% nulliparous	1.5	Mostly Sweden
Rice et al., 1981	Calendar + BBT	723	8.2				Aged 19–44; 9% aged 19–24, 54% aged 25–34, 37% aged 35–44; all parity 1+	3.4[c]	United States, France, Colombia, Canada, Mauritius
Berglund Scherwitzl et al., 2017	Natural Cycles	22,785	8.3				Mean age = 29	1.8	Mostly Sweden (79%)

(continued)

Table 26-9 Summary of studies of contraceptive failure: fertility awareness methods[a]—*(continued)*

			Risk of Pregnancy						
			Life-Table	Pearl Index Pregnancy Rate					
Reference	Method	N for Analysis	12-Month % Pregnant	Index	Total Exposure	Maximum Exposure	Characteristics of the Sample	LFU (%)[g]	Comments
Dolack, 1978	Ovulation	329		10.5[c]	3,354 Cy.	?	Aged 19–48; mean age = 28; 40% had used oral contraceptives prior to study	18.0[c]	
Arévalo et al., 2002	Standard Days	478	12.0					7.1	Bolivia, Peru, Philippines
Johnston et al., 1978	CervicalMucus + BBT + Other Signs	268	13.3[c]				73% aged 22–32; all married or de facto married; 48% ≥12 years education (n = 460)	33.9[c,t]	Australia; probability based on 13 cycles
Wade et al., 1981	Cervical Mucus + BBT + Calendar	239	13.9[c]				Aged 20–39; 78% married	11.4[c,g]	Random assignment to OM or CM + BBT + Cal
Johnston et al., 1978	Calendar + BBT + Other Signs	192	14.3				73% aged 22–32; all married or de facto married; 48% ≥12 years education (n = 460)	33.9[c,t]	Australia; probability based on 13 cycles
Tietze et al., 1951	Calendar	409		14.4	7,267 Mo.	>60 Mo.	57% aged 25–34	13.4[c,t]	
Vessey et al., 1982	Rhythm	?		15.5	161 Yr.	?	All white; at recruitment aged 25–39 and married; at enrollment, all women had been using the diaphragm, IUD, or pill successfully for at least 5 months	0.3[t,v]	Britain; Oxford/FPA study

(continued)

Table 26-9 Summary of studies of contraceptive failure: fertility awareness methods[a]—(continued)

			Risk of Pregnancy						
				Pearl Index Pregnancy Rate					
Reference	Method	N for Analysis	Life-Table 12-Month % Pregnant	Index	Total Exposure	Maximum Exposure	Characteristics of the Sample	LFU (%)[g]	Comments
Klaus et al., 1979	Ovulation	?	15.8[n]				67% aged 18–34; 52% ≥13 years education; some use of concurrent methods	2.9[n]	Probability based on only 12 cycles
Johnston et al.,1978	Cervical Mucus + BBT + Other Signs + Other Methods	94	16.0				78% aged 22–32; all married or de facto married; 53% ≥12 years education ("other" not limited to rhythm)	33.9[c,t]	Australia; probability based on 13 cycles
Grady et al., 1986	Rhythm	167	16.1[s]				Aged 15–44; all married[t]	20.6[r]	NSFG 1982
Ball, 1976	Ovulation	124		16.8[c]	1,626 Cy.	22 Cy.	Aged 20–39	1.6[c]	Australia
Bracher and Santow, 1992	Rhythm	137	17.9				14% aged <20, 75% aged 20–29, 11% aged 30+; 46% parity 0; 92% married or cohabiting	25[r]	Australian Family Survey; first use of method
Kambic et al., 1981, 1982	Ovulation or Cervical Mucus + BBT	235	18.2[n]				81% aged 20–34; 83% married; approx. 30% used barrier methods concurrently[t]	6.5[n]	
Grady et al., 1983	Rhythm	412	18.3[s,c]				Aged 15–44; all married[t]	18.2[r]	NSFG 1973 and 1976

(continued)

Table 26-9 Summary of studies of contraceptive failure: fertility awareness methods[a]—*(continued)*

Reference	Method	N for Analysis	Risk of Pregnancy: Life-Table 12-Month % Pregnant	Pearl Index Pregnancy Rate: Index	Pearl Index Pregnancy Rate: Total Exposure	Pearl Index Pregnancy Rate: Maximum Exposure	Characteristics of the Sample	LFU (%)[g]	Comments
Johnston et al., 1978	Ovulation + Other Methods	71	18.8				80% aged 22–32; all married or de facto married; 49% ≥12 years education ("other" not limited to rhythm)	33.9[c,t]	Australia; probability based on 13 cycles
Vaughan et al., 1977	Rhythm	220	19.1[s]				Aged 15–44; all married[t]	19.0[r]	NSFG 1973
Trussell, 2008		249	19.6				Aged 15–44[t]	21[r]	NSFG 1995; probability when corrected for estimated underreporting of abortion = 22.6
W.H.O., 1981	Ovulation	725	19.6				Mean age about 30; proven fertility; agreed to use OM alone; 54% desired no more children; 765 of 869 learned OM to satisfaction of teachers; 725 entered effectiveness study	?	New Zealand, India, Ireland, Philippines, El Salvador; probability based on 13 cycles
Trussell and Vaughan, 1999		250	19.8				Aged 15–44[t]	21[r]	NSFG 1995

(continued)

Table 26-9 Summary of studies of contraceptive failure: fertility awareness methods[a]—(continued)

			Risk of Pregnancy						
			Life-Table	Pearl Index Pregnancy Rate					
Reference	Method	N for Analysis	12-Month % Pregnant	Index	Total Exposure	Maximum Exposure	Characteristics of the Sample	LFU (%)[g]	Comments
Fu et al., 1999		?	20.2					21[r]	NSFG 1995; probability when standardized and corrected for estimated underreporting of abortion = 25.3[s]
Jones and Forrest, 1992	Rhythm	289	20.9				Aged 15–44[t]	21[r]	NSFG 1988; probability when standardized and corrected for estimated underreporting of abortion = 31.4[s]
Bartzen, 1967	BBT	335		21.3[c]	4,824 Cy.	58 Mo.	Aged 19–45; mean age = 28	11.6[c]	
Kost et al., 2008		236	23.0				Aged 15–44[t]	27.5[r]	NSFG 2002; probability when corrected for estimated underreporting of abortion = 25.3
Schirm et al., 1982	Rhythm	412	23.7[s]				Aged 15–44; all married[t]	18.2[r]	NSFG 1973 and 1976

(continued)

Table 26-9 Summary of studies of contraceptive failure: fertility awareness methods[a]—*(continued)*

			Risk of Pregnancy						
			Life-Table	Pearl Index Pregnancy Rate					
Reference	Method	N for Analysis	12-Month % Pregnant	Index	Total Exposure	Maximum Exposure	Characteristics of the Sample	LFU (%)[g]	Comments
Marshall, 1976	Ovulation + BBT	84		23.9[c]	1,195 Cy.	32 Mo.	67% aged 20–34	1.2[c]	Britain
Johnston et al., 1978	Ovulation	586	26.4				69% aged 22–32; all married or de facto married; 44% ≥12 years education	33.9[c,t]	Australia; probability based on 13 cycles
Wade et al., 1981	Ovulation	191	37.2[c]				Aged 20–39; 74% married	13.8[c,g]	Random assignment to OM or CM + BBT + Cal

Notes:

[a]Updated from Trussell and Kost (1987), Table 3.

[c]Calculated by James Trussell from data in the article.

[g]Most of these studies incorrectly report the loss to follow-up probability (LFU) as the number of women lost at any time during the study divided by the total number of women entering the study. Thus, these are the probabilities presented in the table. However, the correct measure of LFU would be a gross life-table probability. When available, gross 12-month probabilities are denoted by the letter "g."

[n]Only net probabilities for this study.

[r]Nonresponse rate for entire survey.

[s]Standardized: Vaughan et al., (1977) (1973 NSFG)—intention (the average of probabilities for preventers and delayers); Grady et al., (1983) (1973 and 1976 NSFG)—intention. Our calculation (the average of probabilities for preventers and delayers); Schirm et al., (1982) (1973 and 1976 NSFG)—intention, age, and income; Grady et al., (1986) (1982 NSFG)—intention, age, poverty status, and parity; Jones and Forrest, (1992) (1988 NSFG)—age, marital status, and poverty status; Fu et al., (1999) (1995 NSFG)—age, union status, poverty status.

[t]Total for all methods in the study.

[v]The authors report that LFU for "relevant reasons (withdrawal of cooperation or loss of contact)" was 0.3% per year in the 1982 study. In the 1982 study, women had been followed for 9.5 years on average; if 0.3% are LFU per year, then 2.8% would be LFU in 9.5 years. LFU including death and emigration is about twice as high as LFU for "relevant reasons."

For table references, see reference section.

Table 2-10 Summary of studies of contraceptive failure: condom[a]

		Risk of Pregnancy						
		Life-Table	Pearl Index Pregnancy Rate					
Reference	N for Analysis	12-Month % Pregnant	Index	Total Exposure	Maximum Exposure	Characteristics of the Sample[w]	LFU (%)[g]	Comments
Potts and McDevitt, 1975	397	2.1[b]				77% males ≥age 40; all married	4.8[c]	Britain; postal trial of spermicidally lubricated condom
Steiner et al., 2003	436	3.3[d]				72% living with partner	5.8	Kimono Select latex condom; random assignment to Kimono Select latex or eZ-on plastic condom
Peel, 1972	96		3.9	3,689 Mo.	60 Mo.	All married	2.9[t]	Britain; Hull Family Survey
Frezieres et al., 1999	383	4.1[d]				Mean age of male and female subjects = 27	3.9[c]	Avanti plastic condom; random assignment to Avanti plastic or Ramses latex condom
Glass et al., 1974	2,057	4.2				All white; at recruitment aged 25–39 and married; at enrollment, all women had been using the diaphragm, IUD, or pill successfully for at least 5 months	<1.0[v]	Britain; Oxford/FPA study
Vessey et al., 1988	?		4.4	10,000c Yr.	24 Mo.	All white; at recruitment aged 25–39 and married; at enrollment, all women had been using the diaphragm, IUD, or pill successfully for at least 5 months	?	Britain; Oxford/FPA study

(continued)

Table 2-10 Summary of studies of contraceptive failure: condom[a]—*(continued)*

Reference	N for Analysis	Risk of Pregnancy: Life-Table 12-Month % Pregnant	Pearl Index Pregnancy Rate: Index	Total Exposure	Maximum Exposure	Characteristics of the Sample	LFU (%)[g]	Comments
John, 1973	85		5.7[c]	261 Yr.	>7 Yr.	?	?	Britain; retrospective study
Vessey et al., 1982	?		6.0	4,317 Yr.	24 Mo.	All white and aged 25–34; all married at recruitment; at enrollment all women were using the diaphragm, IUD, or pill successfully for at least 5 months	0.3[t,v]	Britain; Oxford/FPA study
Frezieres et al., 1999	384	6.2[d]				Mean age of male and female subjects = 27	2.9[c]	Ramses latex condom; random assignment to Ramses latex or Avanti plastic condom
Jones and Forrest, 1992	1,728	7.2				Aged 15–44[t]	21[r]	NSFG 1988; probability when standardized and corrected for estimated underreporting of abortion = 15.8s
Walsh et al., 2003	415	7.9[d]				74% > high school education[t]	0.7	Trojan-Enz or LifeStyles latex condom; random assignment to Trojan-Enz latex or LifeStyles latex condom or Tactylon plastic condom
Bracher and Santow, 1992	262	8.1				16% aged <20, 65% aged 20–29, 19% aged 30+; 48% parity 0; 83% married or cohabiting	25[r]	Australian Family Survey; first use of method

(continued)

Table 2-10 Summary of studies of contraceptive failure: condom[a]—*(continued)*

Reference	N for Analysis	Risk of Pregnancy: Life-Table 12-Month % Pregnant	Pearl Index Pregnancy Rate: Index	Pearl Index Pregnancy Rate: Total Exposure	Pearl Index Pregnancy Rate: Maximum Exposure	Characteristics of the Sample	LFU (%)[g]	Comments
Trussell, 2008	2,909	8.6				Aged 15–44[t]	21[r]	NSFG 1995; probability when corrected for estimated underreporting of abortion = 17.8
Trussell and Vaughan, 1999	2,925	8.7				Aged 15–44[t]	21[r]	NSFG 1995
Steiner et al., 2003	442	9.2[d]				73% living with partner	5.1	eZ-on plastic condom; random assignment to eZ-on plastic or Kimono Select latex condom
Schirm et al., 1982	1,223	9.6[s]				Aged 15–44; all married[t]	18.2[r]	NSFG 1973 and 1976
Grady et al., 1983	1,223	9.7[s,c]				Aged 15–44; all married[t]	18.2[r]	NSFG 1973 and 1976
Fu et al., 1999	?	9.7					21[r]	NSFG 1995; probability when standardized and corrected for estimated underreporting of abortion = 14.[s]
Vaughan et al., 1977	696	10.1[s]				Aged 15–44; all married[t]	19.0[r]	NSFG 1973
Walsh et al., 2003	415	10.8[d]				74% > high school education[t]	0.7	Tactylon plastic condom; random assignment to Tactylon plastic or Trojan-Enz latex or LifeStyles latex condom

(continued)

Table 2-10 Summary of studies of contraceptive failure: condom[a]—*(continued)*

Reference	N for Analysis	Risk of Pregnancy: Life-Table 12-Month % Pregnant	Pearl Index Pregnancy Rate: Index	Pearl Index Pregnancy Rate: Total Exposure	Pearl Index Pregnancy Rate: Maximum Exposure	Characteristics of the Sample	LFU (%)[g]	Comments
Sundaram et al., 2016	6,819	12.6						2006-2010 NSFG adjusted for under-reporting of abortion
Grady et al., 1986	526	13.8[s]				Aged 15–44; all married[t]	20.6[r]	NSFG 1982
Westoff et al., 1961	~212		13.8[c]	10,062 Mo.	?	All married	5.7[r]	FGMA study
Kost et al., 2008	3,845	13.9				Aged 15–44[t]	27.5[r]	NSFG 2002; probability when corrected for estimated underreporting of abortion = 17.4

Notes:

[a]Updated from Trussell and Kost (1987), Table 6.

[b]24-month probability; 12-month probability not published.

[c]Calculated by James Trussell from data in the article.

[d]6-month probability; 12-month probability not available.

[g]Most of these studies incorrectly report the loss to follow-up probability (LFU) as the number of women lost at any time during the study divided by the total number of women entering the study. Thus, these are the probabilities presented in the table. However, the correct measure of LFU would be a gross life-table probability. When available, gross 12-month probabilities are denoted by the letter "g."

[r]Nonresponse rate for entire survey.

[s]Standardized: Vaughan et al., (1977) (1973 NSFG)—intention (the average of probabilities for preventers and delayers); Grady et al., (1983) (1973 and 1976 NSFG)—intention. Our calculation (the average of probabilities for preventers and delayers); Schirm et al., (1982) (1973 and 1976 NSFG)—intention, age, and income; Grady et al., (1986) (1982 NSFG)—intention, age, poverty status, and parity; Jones and Forrest, (1992) (1988 NSFG)—age, marital status, and poverty status; Fu et al., (1999) (1995 NSFG)—age, union status, poverty status.

[t]Total for all methods in the study.

[v]The authors report that LFU for "relevant reasons (withdrawal of cooperation or loss of contact)" was 0.3% per year in 1982 study. In the 1982 study, women had been followed for 9.5 years on average; if 0.3% are LFU per year, then 2.8% would be LFU in 9.5 years. LFU including death and emigration is about twice as high as LFU for "relevant reasons."

[w]Unless otherwise noted, characteristics refer to females.

For table references, see reference section.

Table 26-11 Summary of studies of contraceptive failure: progestin-only pill[a]

			Risk of Pregnancy						
				Pearl Index Pregnancy Rate					
Reference	Method Brand	N for Analysis	Life-Table 12-Month % Pregnant	Index	Total Exposure	Maximum Exposure	Characteristics of the Sample	LFU (%)[g]	Comments
Broome and Fetherby, 1990	Femulen, Micronor, Microval, Neogest	358		0.2	18,125 Mo.	150 Mo.		?	At a minimum, 14,103 months (78% of the total exposure) capture use beyond the first year; 46% of women used for >4 years and 13% used for >8 years. Retrospective chart review; England
Collaborative Study Group, 1998	Desogestrel 75 mcg (Cerazette)	979		0.41	728 Yr.	13 Cy.	Mean age = 29.6 years. ~ 1/3 breast feeding		Finland, Germany, Netherlands, Norway, Sweden, United Kingdom; random assignment to desogestrel 75 mcg or levonorgestrel 30 mcg
Bisset et al., 1990	Femulen, Micronor, Neogest, Microval	1,042		1.01	24,942 Mo.	?			United Kingdom. Retrospective chart review; cases with no followup excluded
Postlethwaite, 1979	Femulen (Ethynodiol diacetate 0.5 mg)	309	1.1[c]				Aged 17–48	21.0[c]	Britain

(continued)

Table 26-11 **Summary of studies of contraceptive failure: progestin-only pill[a]**—*(continued)*

Reference	Method Brand	N for Analysis	Risk of Pregnancy: Life-Table 12-Month % Pregnant	Risk of Pregnancy: Pearl Index Pregnancy Rate: Index	Risk of Pregnancy: Pearl Index Pregnancy Rate: Total Exposure	Risk of Pregnancy: Pearl Index Pregnancy Rate: Maximum Exposure	Characteristics of the Sample	LFU (%)[g]	Comments
Shroff et al., 1987	Femulen (Ethynodiol diacetate 0.5 mg)	425	1.1[n]				72% aged 16–34; 25% nulligravid	12.7[c]	Britain; authors employed by manufacturer
Board, 1971	Micronor (Norethindrone 0.35 mg)	154		1.3	1,882 Mo.	19 Mo.		?	
Collaborative Study Group, 1998	Levonorgestrel 30 mcg (Microval)	327		1.55	258 Yr.	13 Cy.	Mean age = 29.6 years. ~ 1/3 breast feeding	?	Finland, Germany, Netherlands, Norway, Sweden, United Kingdom; random assignment to levonorgestrel 30 mcg or desogestrel 75 mcg
Keifer, 1973	Micronor (Norethindrone 0.35 mg)	151		1.68	2,141 Mo.	26 Mo.	Aged 18–45; 84% aged 21–35; 74% previous oral contraceptive users; at least 32% current users at start	4.6[c]	

(continued)

Table 26-11 Summary of studies of contraceptive failure: progestin-only pill[a]—*(continued)*

			Risk of Pregnancy						
				Pearl Index Pregnancy Rate					
Reference	Method Brand	N for Analysis	Life-Table 12-Month % Pregnant	Index	Total Exposure	Maximum Exposure	Characteristics of the Sample	LFU (%)[g]	Comments
Vessey et al., 1985		?		1.98[c]	404 Yr.	12 Mo.	All white and aged 25–34; all married at recruitment; at enrollment, all women had been using the diaphragm, IUD, or pill successfully for at least 5 months	0.3[t,v]	Britain; Oxford/FPA study
Korba and Paulson, 1974	Ovrette (Norgestrel 0.075 mg)	2,202		2.19[c]	29,006 Mo.	67 Mo.		?	Authors employed by manufacturer
McQuarrie et al., 1972	Micronor (Norethindrone 0.35 mg)	318		2.64[c]	3,453 Cy.	27 Mo.	Aged 16–42; mean age = 26; all white	2.2[c]	
Nelson, 1973	Megestrol acetate (0.5 mg)	342		2.7	3,552 Mo.	41 Mo.		14.6[c]	

(continued)

Table 26-11 **Summary of studies of contraceptive failure: progestin-only pill**[a]—*(continued)*

Reference	Method Brand	N for Analysis	Risk of Pregnancy: Life-Table 12-Month % Pregnant	Pearl Index Pregnancy Rate: Index	Pearl Index Pregnancy Rate: Total Exposure	Pearl Index Pregnancy Rate: Maximum Exposure	Characteristics of the Sample	LFU (%)[g]	Comments
Jubhari et al., 1974	Quingestanol acetate (0.3 mg)	382	2.9[n]				Mean age = 23; "predominantly white, single and nulliparous"	14.0	
Hawkins and Benster, 1977	Norethisterone (0.35 mg)	200	6.8				Mean age = 25; postpartum women, 71% within 3 months of delivery[t]	5.2[c]	Britain
Hawkins and Benster, 1977	Megestrol acetate (0.5 mg)	174	8.7				Mean age = 25; postpartum women, 71% within 3 months of delivery[t]	8.4[c]	Britain
Sheth et al., 1982	Levonorgestrel (0.30 mg)	128	9.5[n]				Mean age = 25.7	2.1[t]	Yugoslavia, India

(continued)

Table 26-11 Summary of studies of contraceptive failure: progestin-only pill[a]—*(continued)*

			Risk of Pregnancy						
				Pearl Index Pregnancy Rate					
Reference	Method Brand	N for Analysis	Life-Table 12-Month % Pregnant	Index	Total Exposure	Maximum Exposure	Characteristics of the Sample	LFU (%)[g]	Comments
Hawkins and Benster, 1977	Chlormadinone acetate (0.5 mg)	182	9.6				Mean age = 26; postpartum women, 71% within 3 months of delivery[t]	3.3[c]	Britain
Sheth et al., 1982	Norethisterone (0.35 mg)	130	13.2[n]				Mean age = 25.6	2.1[t]	Yugoslavia, India

Notes:

[a]Updated from Trussell and Kost (1987), Table 8.

[c]Calculated by James Trussell from data in the article.

[g]Most of these studies incorrectly report the loss to follow-up (LFU) probability as the number of women lost at any time during the study divided by the total number of women entering the study. Thus, these are the probabilities presented in the table. However, the correct measure of LFU would be a gross life-table probability. When available, gross 12-month probabilities are denoted by the letter "g."

[n]Only net probabilities available for this study.

[t]Total for all methods in the study.

[v]The authors report that LFU for "relevant reasons (withdrawal of cooperation or loss of contact)" was 0.3% per year in the 1982 study. In the 1985 study, women had probably been followed for 12.5 years on average; if 0.3% are LFU per year, then 3.7% would be LFU in 12.5 years. LFU including death and emigration is about twice as high as LFU for "relevant reasons."

For table references, see reference section.

Table 26-12 Summary of studies of contraceptive failure: combined oral contraceptives, vaginal rings, and patches[a]

			Risk of Pregnancy						
				Pearl Index Pregnancy Rate					
Reference	Method Brand	N for Analysis	Life-Table 12-Month % Pregnant	Index	Total Exposure	Maximum Exposure	Characteristics of the Sample	LFU (%)[g]	Comments
Teichmann et al., 2009	Lybrel	323		0.0	3,072 Cy.		Aged 18–49; mean age = 27.6	<2.8[c]	Random assignment to Lybrel or Alesse
Preston, 1972	Norlestrin 2.5 (80% dose)	378	0.0[c]				Aged 15–46; 46% aged 25–34; 36% white; 64% on pill at start	9.5	Author employed by manufacturer; pill not marketed
Ledger, 1970	Ortho-Novum 1/80	144	0.0[c]				All aged 14–43; mean age = 24; mostly graduate students or wives of students	14.0[c]	
Woutersz, 1981	Lo/Ovral	1,700		0.12	22,489 Cy.	53 Cy.	65% aged 20–29; 55% on pill at start	23.8	Author employed by manufacturer
Korba and Heil, 1975	Ovral	6,806		0.19	127,872 Cy.	110 Cy.	Mean age = 25; 26% white; approximately 80% had not used other oral contraceptives within 3 months	?	Mexico, Puerto Rico, United States; author employed by manufacturer

(continued)

Table 26-12 Summary of studies of contraceptive failure: combined oral contraceptives, vaginal rings, and patches[a]—(continued)

			Risk of Pregnancy						
				Pearl Index Pregnancy Rate					
Reference	Method Brand	N for Analysis	Life-Table 12-Month % Pregnant	Index	Total Exposure	Maximum Exposure	Characteristics of the Sample	LFU (%)[g]	Comments
Lammers andoOp ten Berg, 1991	Mercilon	1,684		0.20	25,970 Cy.	36 Cy.	23% aged <20, 51% aged 20–29, 14% aged 30–34; 12% aged 35+	?	Authors employed by manufacturer; Belgium, Denmark, Finland, France, Hungary, Netherlands, Norway, Poland, Sweden, Switzerland, West Germany, Yugoslavia
Ellis, 1987	Ortho-Novum 7/7/7	619		0.22	909[c] Yr.	?	Mean age = 24.5; 40.5% nulligravid	?	United States, Canada, France
Ahrendt et al., 2006	NuvaRing			0.24	408.8 Yr.			2.2[e]	Austria, Belgium, Denmark, France, Germany, Italy, Norway, Spain, Sweden, Switzerland; random assignment to Yasmin or NuvaRing
Morigi and Pasquale, 1978	Modicon	1,168		0.24[c]	16,345 Cy.	53 Cy.	Aged 13–54; 85% aged 19–36; 61% previous use of oral contraceptives	?	Mexico, Puerto Rico, Canada, United States; author employed by manufacturer

(continued)

Table 26-12 **Summary of studies of contraceptive failure: combined oral contraceptives, vaginal rings, and patches[a]**—*(continued)*

			Risk of Pregnancy						
			Life-Table	Pearl Index Pregnancy Rate					
Reference	Method Brand	N for Analysis	12-Month % Pregnant	Index	Total Exposure	Maximum Exposure	Characteristics of the Sample	LFU (%)[g]	Comments
Hughes, 1978	Ovamin	453		0.24[c]			Aged 16–40; % new users not stated	11.9[c]	Britain
Vessey et al., 1982	50 µg estrogen	?		0.25	10,400 Yr.	24 Mo.	All white and aged 25–34; all married at recruitment; at enrollment, all women had been using the diaphragm, IUD, or pill successfully for at least 5 months	0.3[t,v]	Britain; Oxford/FPA study
Runnebaum et al., 1992	Ortho-Cyclen	59,701		0.27[c]	342,348 Cy.	6 Cy.	Mean age = 24.0; 32% parous	?	Germany
Kaunitz et al., 1999	Ortho-Novum 7/7/7	321	0.30				Mean age = 27.8; 65% used hormonal contraception in prior month	6.9[c]	Trial design discontinued subjects who did not adhere to dosing schedule
Bannemerschult et al., 1997	Alesse	805		0.30	4,400 Cy.	6 Cy.	Mean age = 25.6	0.6[c]	Germany; some women who did not return for follow-up visits were excluded
Royal College, 1974		23,611		0.34	?	48 Mo.	75% aged 20–34; all married/living as married; 62% on pill at start (20% new users)	32.0[c]	Britain

(continued)

Table 26-12 Summary of studies of contraceptive failure: combined oral contraceptives, vaginal rings, and patches[a]—(continued)

			Risk of Pregnancy						
				Pearl Index Pregnancy Rate					
Reference	Method Brand	N for Analysis	Life-Table 12-Month % Pregnant	Index	Total Exposure	Maximum Exposure	Characteristics of the Sample	LFU (%)[g]	Comments
Woutersz, 1983	Nordette	1,130		0.35	11,064 Cy.	31 Cy.	71% aged 20–30; 48% no use of hormones and not pregnant within 60 days of start	8.1[c]	Author employed by manufacturer
Merki-Feld et al., 2007	NuvaRing	2,667		0.35	15,900	?	Mean age = 28 years	0.9%[c]	Switzerland
Vessey et al., 1982	<50 μg estrogen	?		0.38	3,158 Yr.	24 Mo.	All white and aged 25–34; all married at recruitment; at enrollment, all women had been using the diaphragm, IUD, or pill successfully for at least 5 months	0.3[t,v]	Britain; Oxford/FPA study
Kaunitz, 2000	Ortho-Novum 7/7/7	2,675	0.39[d]				Mean age = 28.5[t]	6.0[c]	Random assignment to Ortho-Novum 7/7/7 or Cyclessa; 2.5% of subjects discontinued for noncompliance
Parsey and Pong, 2000	Yasmin	326		0.41	3,201 Cy.	13 Cy.	Mean age = 26.4	?	

(continued)

Table 26-12 Summary of studies of contraceptive failure: combined oral contraceptives, vaginal rings, and patches[a]—*(continued)*

			Risk of Pregnancy						
			Life-Table	Pearl Index Pregnancy Rate					
Reference	Method Brand	N for Analysis	12-Month % Pregnant	Index	Total Exposure	Maximum Exposure	Characteristics of the Sample	LFU (%)[g]	Comments
Hernádi et al., 2009	Yaz	1,101	0.5				Aged 18–35 at recruitment; mean age = 24.7	1.9[c]	Czech Republic, Italy, Hungary, Slovak Republic, Latvia, Belgium
Kaunitz, 2000	Cyclessa	2,643	0.51[d]				Mean age = 28.5[t]	5.8[c]	Random assignment to Cyclessa or Ortho-Novum 7/7/7; 2.4% of subjects discontinued for non-compliance
Anderson et al., 2003	Seasonale	456	0.55					8.6	Random assignment to Seasonale or Nordette; noncompliant patients excluded
Gauthier et al., 1992	Ortho Tri-Cyclen	661	0.57[b]				Mean age = 27.9; 24% nulligravid	?	France; 2 authors employed by manufacturer

(continued)

Table 26-12 **Summary of studies of contraceptive failure: combined oral contraceptives, vaginal rings, and patches[a]**—*(continued)*

Reference	Method Brand	N for Analysis	Risk of Pregnancy: Life-Table 12-Month % Pregnant	Pearl Index Pregnancy Rate: Index	Pearl Index Pregnancy Rate: Total Exposure	Pearl Index Pregnancy Rate: Maximum Exposure	Characteristics of the Sample	LFU (%)[g]	Comments
Åkerlund et al., 1993	Mercilon	485		0.57[c]	4,543 Cy.	12 Mo.	Mean age = 23.8	?	Denmark, Norway, Sweden; random assignment to Mercilon or Marvelon; cycles excluded if the pill-taking period was less than 18 or more than 33 days or if the pill-free period was less than 5 or more than 9 days
Anderson et al., 2006	Seasonique	1,006	0.6				Mean age = 27.4	14.8	
Preston, 1974 and 1972	Norlestrin 2.5 (60% dose)	1,192		0.63[c]	14,536 Cy.	>18 Cy.	Aged 14–47; 35% aged 25–34; 47% white; 56% on pill at start	13.7	Author employed by manufacturer; pill not marketed
Roumen et al., 2001	NuvaRing	1,145		0.64[c]	12,109 Cy.	13 Cy.	Mean age = 28.2	?	Austria, Belgium, Denmark, Finland, France, Germany, Israel, Netherlands, Norway, Spain, Sweden, United Kingdom

(continued)

Table 26-12 Summary of studies of contraceptive failure: combined oral contraceptives, vaginal rings, and patches[a]—*(continued)*

			Risk of Pregnancy						
				Pearl Index Pregnancy Rate					
Reference	Method Brand	N for Analysis	Life-Table 12-Month % Pregnant	Index	Total Exposure	Maximum Exposure	Characteristics of the Sample	LFU (%)[g]	Comments
Archer et al., 1999	Alesse	1,708	0.69[b]				Mean age = 27.2	12.1	Cycles in which 3 or more consecutive active pills were missed and all subsequent cycles from that subject were excluded from the analysis
Smallwood et al., 2001	Evra patch	1,664	0.7				Mean age = 28.7	?	Australia, Austria, Belgium, France, Israel, Netherlands, Sweden, Switzerland, United Kingdom, United States
Palacios et al., 2010	Natazio	1,377		0.73	23,368 Cy.	20 Cy.	Mean age = 30	0.002[c]	Austria, Germany, Spain
London et al., 1992	Triphasil (Tri-Levlen)	2,124		0.80	11,306 Cy.	6 Cy.	Mean age = 25.5	?	Random assignment to Triphasil or Ortho Tri-Cyclen

(continued)

Table 26-12 Summary of studies of contraceptive failure: combined oral contraceptives, vaginal rings, and patches[a]—*(continued)*

			Risk of Pregnancy						
			Life-Table	Pearl Index Pregnancy Rate					
Reference	Method Brand	N for Analysis	12-Month % Pregnant	Index	Total Exposure	Maximum Exposure	Characteristics of the Sample	LFU (%)[g]	Comments
Åkerlund et al., 1993	Marvelon (Ortho-Cept, Desogen)	497		0.83[c]	4,688 Cy.	12 Mo.	Mean age = 23.1	?	Denmark, Norway, Sweden; random assignment to Marvelon or Mercilon; cycles excluded if the pill-taking period was less than 18 or more than 33 days or if the pill-free period was less than 5 or more than 9 days
Corson, 1990	Lo/Ovral	737		0.94[c]	9,727 Cy.	24 Cy.	Mean age = 24.3	?	Random assignment to Lo/Ovral or Ortho-Cyclen
London et al., 1992	Ortho Tri-Cyclen	2,110		0.94	11,006 Cy.	6 Cy.	Mean age = 25.6	?	Random assignment to Ortho Tri-Cyclen or Triphasil
Preston, 1974 and 1972	Norlestrin 2.5 (40% dose)	1,393		0.94[c]	15,265 Cy.	>18 Cy.	Aged 13–42; 27% aged 25–34; 39% white; 49% on pill at start	16.3	Author employed by manufacturer; pill not marketed

(continued)

Table 26-12 Summary of studies of contraceptive failure: combined oral contraceptives, vaginal rings, and patches[a]—*(continued)*

			Risk of Pregnancy						
			Life-Table	Pearl Index Pregnancy Rate					
Reference	Method Brand	N for Analysis	12-Month % Pregnant	Index	Total Exposure	Maximum Exposure	Characteristics of the Sample	LFU (%)[g]	Comments
Ahrendt et al., 2006	Yasmin	484		0.99	404.8 Yr.	13 Cy.		3.3[c]	Austria, Belgium, Denmark, France, Germany, Italy, Norway, Spain, Sweden, Switzerland; random assignment to Yasmin or NuvaRing
The Mircette Study Group, 1998	Mircette	1,226		1.02	14,050 Cy.	13 Cy.	Mean age = 28.3	6.8[c]	
Endrikat et al., 1995	Mercilon	219		1.04[c]	2,496 Cy.	12 Cy.	Mean age = 25.0	?	Austria, France; random assignment to Mercilon or Meliane; cycles excluded if more than two pills were missed or pill-taking was irregular
Oddsson et al., 2005	Microgynon	518	1.07				Mean age = 27.2; 53% nulligravid	6.4[c]	Random assignment to Microgynon or NuvaRing; Belgium, Brazil, Chile, Denmark, Finland, France, Germany, Italy, Norway, Spain, Sweden

(continued)

Table 26-12 Summary of studies of contraceptive failure: combined oral contraceptives, vaginal rings, and patches[a]—*(continued)*

			Risk of Pregnancy						
				Pearl Index Pregnancy Rate					
Reference	Method Brand	N for Analysis	Life-Table 12-Month % Pregnant	Index	Total Exposure	Maximum Exposure	Characteristics of the Sample	LFU (%)[g]	Comments
Ellsworth, 1986	Triphasil	1,264		1.09	8,349 Cy.	34 Cy.	All < age 38	?	17 U.S. centers
Corson, 1990	Ortho-Cyclen	736		1.11[c]	9,351 Cy.	24 Cy.	Mean age = 24.6	?	Random assignment to Ortho-Cyclen or Lo/Ovral
Dieben et al., 2002	NuvaRing	2,322	1.18				Mean age = 28.2	?	United States, Canada, Europe; Pearl index for United States = 1.75; European results published separately by Roumen et al. (2001)
Teichmann et al., 2009	Alesse	318		1.19	3,270 Cy.	12 Cy.	Aged 18–48; mean age = 27.2	<2.2[c]	Random assignment to Alesse or Lybrel
Oddsson et al., 2005	NuvaRing	512	1.2				Mean age = 27.0; 57% nulligravid	6.4[c]	Random assignment to NuvaRing or Microgynon; Belgium, Brazil, Chile, Denmark, Finland, France, Germany, Italy, Norway, Spain, Sweden

(continued)

Table 26-12 Summary of studies of contraceptive failure: combined oral contraceptives, vaginal rings, and patches[a]—*(continued)*

			Risk of Pregnancy						
			Life-Table	Pearl Index Pregnancy Rate					
Reference	Method Brand	N for Analysis	12-Month % Pregnant	Index	Total Exposure	Maximum Exposure	Characteristics of the Sample	LFU (%)[g]	Comments
Bachmann et al., 2004	Yaz	1,018	1.26				Mean age = 24.7	4.6	Argentina, Austria, Brazil, Poland, United States
Audet et al., 2001	Evra patch	811	1.3				Mean age = 28.0	3.9[c]	Random assignment to Evra patch or Triphasil
Anderson et al., 2003	Nordette	226	1.45					9.3	Random assignment to Nordette or Seasonale; noncompliant patients excluded
Preston, 1974 and 1972	Norlestrin 1.0 (60% dose)	1,872		1.47[c]	20,341 Cy.	>18 Cy.	Aged 14–44; 30% aged 25–34; 42% white; 55% on pill at start	13.1	Author employed by manufacturer; pill not marketed
Preston, 1974	Norlestrin 1.0 (20% dose)	276		1.59[c]	2,449 Cy.	?		?	Author employed by manufacturer; pill not marketed
Archer et al., 2006	Lybrel	2,134		1.6	?	13 Cy.	Mean age = 28.8	10.5[c]	Subjects discontinued if they missed ≥ 3 consecutive pills or ≥ 5 pills in any pill pack

(continued)

Table 26-12 Summary of studies of contraceptive failure: combined oral contraceptives, vaginal rings, and patches[a]—*(continued)*

			Risk of Pregnancy						
			Life-Table	Pearl Index Pregnancy Rate					
Reference	Method Brand	N for Analysis	12-Month % Pregnant	Index	Total Exposure	Maximum Exposure	Characteristics of the Sample	LFU (%)[g]	Comments
Audet et al., 2001	Triphasil	605	1.8				Mean age = 27.8	7.9[c]	Random assignment to Triphasil or Evra patch
Nakajima et al., 2007	Loestrin 24 Fe	705		1.82	?	6 Cy.	Aged 18–45; mean age = 28.9	8.4	Random assignment to Loestrin 24 Fe or Loestrin Fe
Vaughan et al., 1977		2,434		2.0[s]			Aged 15–44; all married[t]	19.0[r]	NSFG 1973
Bracher and Santow, 1992		1,830	2.2				42% aged <20, 49% aged 20–29, 9% aged 30+; 67% parity 0; 45% married or cohabiting	25[r]	Australian Family Survey, first use of method
Schirm et al., 1982		4,487	2.4[s]				Aged 15–44; all married[t]	18.2[r]	NSFG 1973 and 1976
Grady et al., 1983		4,487	2.5[c,s]				Aged 15–44; all married[t]	18.2[r]	NSFG 1973 and 1976
Bounds et al., 1979	Microgynon-30	55	2.6[c]				Aged 16–39; mean age = 26; 62% used oral contraceptives as last contraceptive before study	5.5[c]	Britain; probability based on only 12 cycles

(continued)

Table 26-12 Summary of studies of contraceptive failure: combined oral contraceptives, vaginal rings, and patches[a]—*(continued)*

			Risk of Pregnancy						
				Pearl Index Pregnancy Rate					
Reference	Method Brand	N for Analysis	Life-Table 12-Month % Pregnant	Index	Total Exposure	Maximum Exposure	Characteristics of the Sample	LFU (%)[g]	Comments
Kroll et al., 2010	LoSeasonique	2,185		2.74	20,937 Cy.	4 91-day Cy.	Mean age = 26.7	13.9	
Grady et al., 1986		856	2.9[s]				Aged 15–44; all married[t]	20.6[r]	NSFG 1982
Nakajima et al., 2007	Loestrin Fe	181		2.98	?	6 Cy.	Aged 18–45; mean age = 28.5	8.6	Random assignment to Loestrin Fe or Loestrin 24 Fe
Jones and Forrest, 1992		3,041	5.1				Aged 15–44; all married[t]	21[r]	NSFG 1988; probability when standardized and corrected for estimated under-reporting of abortion = 7.3s
Preston, 1974	Norlestrin 1.0 (40% dose)	313		5.80[c]	1,570 Cy.	?		?	Author employed by manufacturer; pill not marketed
Bounds et al., 1979	Loestrin-20	55	5.9[c]				Aged 16–39; mean age = 26; 65% used oral contraceptives as last contraceptive before study	5.5[c]	Britain; probability based on only 12 cycles

(continued)

Table 26-12 Summary of studies of contraceptive failure: combined oral contraceptives, vaginal rings, and patches[a]—*(continued)*

			Risk of Pregnancy						
			Life-Table	Pearl Index Pregnancy Rate					
Reference	Method Brand	N for Analysis	12-Month % Pregnant	Index	Total Exposure	Maximum Exposure	Characteristics of the Sample	LFU (%)[g]	Comments
Trussell, 2008		2,127	6.7				Aged 15–44[c]	21[r]	NSFG 1995; probablility when corrected for estimated underreporting of abortion = 8.8
Trussell and Vaughan, 1999		2,130	6.9				Aged 15–44[t]	21[r]	NSFG 1995
Sundaram et al., 2016		3,307	7.2						2006–2010 NSFG adjusted for underreporting of abortion
Fu et al., 1999		?	7.3					21[r]	NSFG 1995; probability when standardized and corrected for estimated underreporting of abortion = 8.1[s]
Kost et al., 2008		2,451	7.7				Aged 15–44[t]	27.5[r]	NSFG 2002; probablility when corrected for estimated underreporting of abortion = 8.7

(continued)

Table 26-12 Summary of studies of contraceptive failure: combined oral contraceptives, vaginal rings, and patches[a]—*(continued)*

			Risk of Pregnancy						
				Pearl Index Pregnancy Rate					
Reference	Method Brand	N for Analysis	Life-Table 12-Month % Pregnant	Index	Total Exposure	Maximum Exposure	Characteristics of the Sample	LFU (%)[g]	Comments
Preston, 1974	Norlestrin 2.5 (20% dose)	178		10.45[c]	871 Cy.	?		?	Author employed by manufacturer; pill not marketed

Notes:

[a]Updated from Trussell and Kost (1987), Table 8.

[b]12-cycle probability; 12-month probability not available.

[c]Calculated by James Trussell from data in the article.

[d]6-cycle probability.

[g]Most of these studies incorrectly report the loss to follow-up (LFU) probability as the number of women lost at any time during the study divided by the total number of women entering the study. Thus, these are the probabilities presented in the table. However, the correct measure of LFU would be a gross life-table probability. When available, gross 12-month probabilities are denoted by the letter "g."

[r]Nonresponse rate for entire survey.

[s]Standardized: Vaughan et al., (1977) (1973 NSFG)—intention (the average of probabilities for preventers and delayers); Grady et al., (1983) (1973 and 1976 NSFG)—intention. Our calculation (the average of probabilities for preventers and delayers); Schirm et al., (1982) (1973 and 1976 NSFG)—intention, age, and income; Grady et al., (1986) (1982 NSFG)—intention, age, poverty status, and parity; Jones and Forrest, (1992) (1988 NSFG)—age, marital status, and poverty status; Fu et al., (1999) (1995 NSFG)—age, union status, poverty status.

[t]Total for all methods in the study.

[v]The authors report that LFU for "relevant reasons (withdrawal of cooperation or loss of contact)" was 0.3% per year in the 1982 study. In the 1982 study, women had probably been followed for 9.5 years on average; if 0.3% are LFU per year, then 2.8% would be LFU in 9.5 years. LFU including death and emigration is about twice as high as LFU for "relevant reasons."

For table references, see reference section.

Table 26-13 Summary of studies of contraceptive failure: injectables[a]

Reference	Method Brand	N for Analysis	Life-Table 12-Month % Pregnant	Characteristics of the Sample	LFU (%)[g]	Comments
Kaunitz et al., 2009	Depo-Provera SC 104 mg (90-Day)	266	0.0[c]	Mean age = 25.9	?	Random assignment to Depo-Provera SC or Depo-Provera IM
Kaunitz et al., 2009	Depo-Provera 150 mg (90-Day)	268	0.0[c]	Mean age = 25.8	?	Random assignment to Depo-Provera IM or Depo-Provera SC
Jain et al., 2004	Depo-Provera SC 104 mg (90-Day)	1,779	0.0	Mean age = 30.6		Brazil, Bulgaria, Canada, Chile, Estonia, Indonesia, Latvia, Lithuania, Mexico, Norway, Pakistan, Peru, Poland, Romania, Russia, United Kingdom, United States
W.H.O., 1988	Depo-Provera 25 mg + Estradiol Cypionate 5 mg (30-Day)	1,168	0.0	Aged 18–35; mean age = 26; proven fertility	11.4[g]	Egypt, Thailand, Mexico, Guatemala, Cuba, Indonesia, Pakistan, U.S.S.R., Philippines, Italy, Hungary, Chile
W.H.O., 1986	Depo-Provera 150 mg (90-Day)	607	0.0	Mean age = 27.7[t]	8.6[g]	7 developing countries
Mishell et al., 1968	Depo-Provera 150 mg (90-Day)	100	0.0[c]	59% aged 21–30	24.0[c]	Injection immediately postpartum
Howard et al., 1982	Norigest 200 mg (56-Day)	383	0.0[c]		6.5[n]	Britain
Kaunitz et al., 1999	Lunelle	782	0.0	Mean age = 27.3; 44% used hormonal contraception in prior month	8.6[c]	Trial design discontinued subjects who did not adhere to dosing schedule

(continued)

Table 26-13 Summary of studies of contraceptive failure: injectables[a]—*(continued)*

Reference	Method Brand	N for Analysis	Life-Table 12-Month % Pregnant	Characteristics of the Sample	LFU (%)[g]	Comments
Hall et al., 1997	Cyclofem (Lunelle)	3,183	0.0		12.9[c]	Brazil, Chile, Colombia, Peru. Perfect use analysis since trial design discontinued women who were late for injections
W.H.O., 1983	Depo-Provera 150 mg (90-Day)	1,587	0.1	Mean age = 27.4[t]	8.1	87% of women from 9 developing countries
W.H.O., 1988	Norigest 50 mg + Estradiol Valerate 5 mg (30-Day)	1,152	0.18	Aged 18–35; mean age = 26.7; proven fertility	10.5[g]	Egypt, Thailand, Mexico, Guatemala, Cuba, Indonesia, Pakistan, U.S.S.R., Philippines, Italy, Hungary, Chile
Sangi-Haghpeykar et al., 1996	Depo-Provera 150 mg (3-Month)	536	0.2	25% nulligravid; mean age = 24.4; primarily low income	5.4[c]	
Scutchfield et al., 1971	Depo-Provera 150 mg (90-Day)	650	0.2[c]	66% aged 20–34; 50% married	6.8[n]	
Schwallie and Assenzo, 1973	Depo-Provera 150 mg (90-Day)	3,857	0.3	86% aged 20–39	18.6	Primarily United States; also Chile, Jamaica, Mexico; authors employed by manufacturer
W.H.O., 1983	Norigest 200 mg (60-Day)	789	0.4	Mean age = 27.4[t]	7.1	87% of women from 9 developing countries
W.H.O., 1986	Depo-Provera 100 mg (90-Day)	609	0.4	Mean age = 27.7[t]	8.2[g]	7 developing countries
W.H.O., 1983	Norigest 200 mg (84-Day)	796	0.6	Mean age = 27.4[t]	7.4	87% of women from 9 developing countries

(continued)

Table 26-13 Summary of studies of contraceptive failure: injectables[a]—*(continued)*

Reference	Method Brand	N for Analysis	Life-Table 12-Month % Pregnant	Characteristics of the Sample	LFU (%)[g]	Comments
W.H.O., 1977	Depo-Provera 150 mg (84-Day)	846	0.7	87% aged 20–34	6.2	10 developing countries
Schwallie and Assenzo, 1972	Depo-Provera 300 mg (180-Day)	991	2.3[n]	88% aged 20–39	28.9	United States, Chile; authors employed by manufacturer
Fu et al., 1999	Depo-Provera 150 mg	?	2.8		21[r]	NSFG 1995; probability when standardized and corrected for estimated underreporting of abortion = 2.6[s]
Trussell, 2008	Depo-Provera 150 mg (90-Day)	209	2.9	Aged 15–44[t]	21[r]	NSFG 1995; probability when corrected for estimated underreporting of abortion = 5.4
Trussell and Vaughan, 1999	Depo-Provera 150 mg (90-Day)	209	3.2	Aged 15–44[t]	21[r]	NSFG 1995
W.H.O., 1977	Norigest 200 mg (84-Day)	832	3.6	84% aged 20–34	5.8	10 developing countries
Sundaram et al., 2016	Depo Provera	893	4.0			2006–2010 NSFG adjusted for under-reporting of abortion
Kost et al., 2008	Depo-Provera 150 mg (90-Day)	715	7.5	Aged 15–44[t]	27.5[r]	NSFG 2002; probability when corrected for estimated underreporting of abortion = 6.7

Notes:

[a]Updated from Trussell and Kost (1987), Table 9.

[c]Calculated by James Trussell from data in the article.

[g]Most of these studies incorrectly report the loss to follow-up (LFU) probability as the number of women lost at any time during the study divided by the total number of women entering the study. Thus, these are the probabilities presented in the table. However, the correct measure of LFU would be a gross life-table probability. When available, gross 12-month probabilities are denoted by the letter "g."

[n]Only net probabilities available for this study.

[r]Nonresponse rate for entire survey.

[s]Fu et al., (1995 NSFG)—age, union status, poverty status.

[t]Total for all methods in the study.

For table references, see reference section.

Table 26-14 Summary of studies of contraceptive failure: intrauterine contraceptives[a]

Reference	Method Brand	N for Analysis	Life-Table 12-Month % Pregnant	Characteristics of the Sample	LFU (%)[g]	Comments
Luukkainen et al., 1987	Mirena	1,821	0.1	15% aged 17–25, 60% aged 26–35, 25% aged 36–40; 7% parity 0, 27% parity 1, 50% parity 2, 16% parity 3+	5.7[c]	Denmark, Finland, Hungary, Norway, Sweden
Sivin et al., 1990	Mirena	1,124	0.2	Mean age = 26.6; mean parity = 2.4	5.7[g,x]	Brazil, Chile, Dominican Republic, Egypt, Singapore, United States
Eisenberg et al., 2015	Liletta	1,568	0.1	Mean age = 26 years, 62% nulliparous	?	
Nelson et al., 2013	Kyleena	1,452	0.2	Mean age = 27 years, 40% nulliparous	?	Argentina, Canada, Chile, Finland, France, Hungary, Mexico, Netherlands, Norway, Sweden, United States
Sivin et al., 1990	TCu380A Slimline	698	0.3	Mean age = 28.5; mean parity = 2.7; 47.4% prior IUD use	6.0	Randomized trial of TCu380A and TCu380A Slimline. Egypt, Chile, Sweden, Dominican Republic, Brazil
Sivin et al., 1990	TCu380A	298	0.4	Mean age = 28.1; mean parity = 2.6; 49.0% prior IUD use	9.7	Randomized trial of TCu380A and TCu380A Slimline. Egypt, Chile, Sweden, Dominican Republic, Brazil
Nelson et al., 2013	Skyla	1,432	0.4	Mean age = 27 years, 39% nulliparous	?	Argentina, Canada, Chile, Finland, France, Hungary, Mexico, Netherlands, Norway, Sweden, United States
Cox and Blacksell, 2000	Mirena	692	0.6	All parous	?	United Kingdom
Heinemann et al., 2015	Mirena	41,001	0.7	Mean age = 37.4 years	1.7%	European Active Surveillance Study for Intrauterine Devices

(continued)

Table 26-14 Summary of studies of contraceptive failure: intrauterine contraceptives[a]—*(continued)*

Reference	Method Brand	N for Analysis	Life-Table 12-Month % Pregnant	Characteristics of the Sample	LFU (%)[g]	Comments
Sivin and Stern, 1979	TCu380A	3,536	0.8	72% aged 20–29; 64% nulliparous	18.3[n]	
Gibor and Mitchell, 1980	Progestasert	6,261	2.0[n]		?	Authors employed by manufacturer; United States (51%), Canada (5%), and at least 11 other countries
Trussell and Vaughan, 1999		59	3.7	Aged 15–44[t]	21[r]	NSFG 1995
Bracher and Santow, 1992		408	3.9	10% aged <20, 68% aged 20–29, 22% aged 30+; 25% parity 0; 87% married or cohabiting	25[r]	Australian Family Survey, first use of method
Vaughan et al., 1977		576	4.2[s]	Aged 15–44; all married[t]	19.0[r]	NSFG 1973
Schirm et al., 1982		1,070	4.6[s]	Aged 15–44; all married[t]	18.2[r]	NSFG 1973 and 1976
Grady et al., 1983		1,070	4.8[c,s]	Aged 15–44; all married[t]	18.2[r]	NSFG 1973 and 1976
Grady et al., 1986		235	5.9[s]	Aged 15–44; all married[t]	20.6[r]	NSFG 1982

Notes:

[a]Updated from Trussell and Kost (1987), Table 7.

[c]Calculated by James Trussell from data in the article.

[g]Most of these studies incorrectly report the loss to follow-up (LFU) probability as the number of women lost at any time during the study divided by the total number of women entering the study. Thus, these are the probabilities presented in the table. However, the correct measure of LFU would be a gross life-table probability. When available, gross 12-month probabilities are denoted by the letter "g."

[n]Only net probabilities available for this study.

[r]Nonresponse rate for entire survey.

[s]Standardized: Vaughan et al., (1977) (1973 NSFG)—intention (the average of probabilities for preventers and delayers); Grady et al., (1983) (1973 and 1976 NSFG)—intention. Our calculation (the average of probabilities for preventers and delayers); Schirm et al., (1982) (1973 and 1976 NSFG)—intention, age, and income; Grady et al., (1986) (1982 NSFG)—intention, age, poverty status, and parity.

[t]Total for all methods in the study.

[x]Irving Sivin, personal communication to James Trussell, August 13, 1992.

For table references, see reference section.

Table 26-15 Summary of studies of contraceptive failure: implants[a]

Reference	Method Brand	N for Analysis	Risk of Pregnancy				Characteristics of the Sample	LFU (%)[g]	Comments
			Life-Table 12-Month % Pregnant	Pearl Index Pregnancy Rate					
				Index	Total Exposure	Maximum Exposure			
Harvey, et al., 2009	Implanon	976		0	1,196.9 Yr.	3 Yr.	43% nulligravid	21.4[c]	Australia; retrospective chart review
Graesslin and Korver 2008; Darney et al., 2009	Implanon	923		0	24,100 Cy.	4 Yr.	Aged 18–40	2.2	Asia, Chile, Europe, United States
Lipetz et al., 2009	Implanon	493		0	808.4 Yr.	3 Yr.		3.2[c]	Wales; review of case notes for cost study
Flores	Implanon	417		0	958.5 Yr.	3 Yr.	Mean age = 25.8	18.9	Mexico City
Arribas-Mir, et al., 2009	Implanon	372		0	893.4 Yr.	3 Yr.	Mean age = 27.2; 42.7% nulliparous	4.3	Grenada, Spain
Lakha and Glasier, 2006	Implanon	324		0	?	4 Yr.	Mean age = 26	14.5[c]	Edinburgh; 33 women did not return for implant removal until at least 1 month after 3 years of use; the longest duration of use was 4 years and 8 days
Zheng et al., 1999a	Implanon	200		0	644.6 Yr.	4 Yr.		1.0[c]	

(continued)

Table 26-15 Summary of studies of contraceptive failure: implants[a]—*(continued)*

			Risk of Pregnancy						
			Life-Table	Pearl Index Pregnancy Rate					
Reference	Method Brand	N for Analysis	12-Month % Pregnant	Index	Total Exposure	Maximum Exposure	Characteristics of the Sample	LFU (%)[g]	Comments
Smith and Reuter, 2002	Implanon	190		0	?	?		≥ 37.4	England; audit and postal survey
Thamkhantho, et al., 2008	Implanon	163		0	88.7 Yr.	1 Yr.		45.4	Bangkok; of the 89 women who returned for the 1-year follow-up none was LFU thereafter
Rai et al., 2004	Implanon	147		0	?	30 Mo.		30.6	London; retrospective chart review
Agarwal and Robinsom, 2005	Implanon	106		0	?	3 Yr.	Aged 15–43; 37% nulliparous	19[c]	Luton, England; 2 clients retained device for 3 and 8 months after its expiration date, respectively but neither became pregnant
Zheng et al., 1999b	Implanon	100		0	341.6 Yr.	4 Yr.		3.0[c]	China
Gezginc et al., 2007	Implanon	80		0	?	?	Mean age = 33	?	Turkey
Booranabunyat and Taneepanichskul, 2004	Implanon	53		0	306 Mo.	6 Mo.	Aged 35–48	0.0	Bangkok

(continued)

Table 26-15 Summary of studies of contraceptive failure: implants[a]—*(continued)*

Reference	Method Brand	N for Analysis	Risk of Pregnancy: Life-Table 12-Month % Pregnant	Pearl Index Pregnancy Rate: Index	Pearl Index Pregnancy Rate: Total Exposure	Pearl Index Pregnancy Rate: Maximum Exposure	Characteristics of the Sample	LFU (%)[g]	Comments
Yildizbas et al., 2007	Implanon	41		0	20.5 Yr.	6 Mo.	Aged 18–40	0.0	Turkey
Bahamondes et al., 2015	Implanon	995	0.1					2.5	Multi-center study in Brazil, Chile, Dominican Republic, Hungary, Thailand, Turkey, Zimbabwe

Notes:

[a]Updated from Trussell and Kost (1987), Table 9.

[c]Calculated by James Trussell from data provided by Sivin (1992).

[g]Proportion LFU in the first year (number of women LFU in the first year divided by the number entering the study); gross 12-month life-table probabilities denoted by the letter "g."

[f]Nonresponse rate for entire survey.

[s]Fu et al., (1999) (1995 NSFG)—age, union status, poverty status.

[t]Total for all methods in the study.

For table references, see reference section.

Table 26-16 Summary of studies of contraceptive failure: tubal occlusion[a]

			Risk of Pregnancy						
			Life-Table	Pearl Index Pregnancy Rate					
Reference	Procedure	N for Analysis	12-Month % Pregnant	Index	Total Exposure	Maximum Exposure	Characteristics of the Sample	LFU (%)[g]	Comments
Engel, 1978	Laparoscopy	182	0.0[c]				"No failures" presumably some women followed for at least 12 months	?	
Valle and Battifora, 1978	Laparoscopy	165	0.0[c]				"Failure rate after 2 years follow-up is zero" all aged 22–38; 80% had at least 12 months follow-up	?	
Vessey et al., 1983	Procedures other than laparotomy and laparoscopy	345		0.0	331 Yr.	12 Mo.	All white; at recruitment aged 25–39 and married; at enrollment, all women had been using the diaphragm, IUD, or pill successfully for at least 5 months	0.3[v]	Britain; Oxford/FPA study
Chi et al., 1980	Culdoscopy: Pomeroy	392	0.0				Mean age = 32[t]	?	IFRP (19 countries)
Loffer and Pent, 1977	Laparoscopy	1,717		0.0[c]		>6 Mo.	Duration of follow-up not reported	?	

(continued)

Table 26-16 Summary of studies of contraceptive failure: tubal occlusion[a]—*(continued)*

			Risk of Pregnancy						
			Life-Table	Pearl Index Pregnancy Rate					
Reference	Procedure	N for Analysis	12-Month % Pregnant	Index	Total Exposure	Maximum Exposure	Characteristics of the Sample	LFU (%)[g]	Comments
Chi et al., 1987	Minilaparotomy: Pomeroy	445	0.0[c]				Median age = 32	31.6	IFRP (19 countries)
Cooper et al., 2003	Essure implant	449	0.0[c]				Mean age = 31.9	2.2[c]	United States, Australia
Kerin et al., 2003	Essure implant	198	0.0				Mean age = 35	?	United States, Australia, Belgium, Spain
Arjona et al., 2008	Essure implant	1,612	0.0[c]				Mean age = 36.6	?	Spain; 3 women became pregnant before the 3-month followup
Vleugals and Voersema, 2005	Essure implant	161	0.0[c]				Mean age = 37.4	?	The Netherlands
Peterson et al., 1996	Postpartum partial salpingectomy	1,637	0.06				43% aged 18–27, 38% aged 28–33, 18% aged 34+	8.8	U.S. Collaborative Review of Sterilization
Peterson et al., 1996	Unipolar coagulation	1,432	0.07				20% aged 18–27, 39% aged 28–33, 42% aged 34+	5.0	U.S. Collaborative Review of Sterilization

(continued)

Table 26-16 Summary of studies of contraceptive failure: tubal occlusion[a]—*(continued)*

			Risk of Pregnancy						
				Pearl Index Pregnancy Rate					
Reference	Procedure	N for Analysis	Life-Table 12-Month % Pregnant	Index	Total Exposure	Maximum Exposure	Characteristics of the Sample	LFU (%)[g]	Comments
Dominik et al., 2000	Filshie Clip	1,063	0.11					31.3[c]	Dominican Republic, Guatemala, Haiti, Malaysia, Mexico, Panama, Venezuela
Sokal et al., 2000	Filshie Clip	1,378	0.17				Mean age = 31	18.1[c]	Brazil, Dominican Republic, Indonesia, Kenya, Mexico, Panama, Peru, Thailand
Sokal et al., 2000	Tubal Ring	1,355	0.17				Mean age = 31	17.6[c]	Brazil, Dominican Republic, Indonesia, Kenya, Mexico, Panama, Peru, Thailand
Bhiwandiwala et al., 1982	Rocket Clip	630	0.18[u]					42.1[c,t]	IFRP (27 countries)
Peterson et al., 1996	Bipolar coagulation	2,267	0.23				31% aged 18–27, 35% aged 28–33, 35% aged 34+	10.5	U.S. Collaborative Review of Sterilization
Chi et al., 1980	Minilaparotomy	3,988	0.24				Mean age = 32[t]	?	IFRP (19 countries)

(continued)

Table 26-16 Summary of studies of contraceptive failure: tubal occlusion[a]—*(continued)*

			Risk of Pregnancy						
			Life-Table	Pearl Index Pregnancy Rate					
Reference	Procedure	N for Analysis	12-Month % Pregnant	Index	Total Exposure	Maximum Exposure	Characteristics of the Sample	LFU (%)[g]	Comments
Bhiwandiwala et al., 1982	Electro-coagulation	6,542	0.26[u]					42.1[c,t]	IFRP (27 countries)
Vessey et al., 1983	Laparotomy: all procedures	743		0.28	716 Yr.	12 Mo.	All white; at recruitment aged 25–39 and married; at enrollment, all women had been using the diaphragm, IUD, or pill successfully for at least 5 months	0.3[t,v]	Britain; Oxford/FPA study
Mumford et al., 1980	Minilaparoscopy: Pomeroy	2,022	0.3[u]					?	IFRP (23 countries)
Chi et al., 1980	Electro-coagulation	3,594	0.32[c]					?	IFRP (19 countries)
Bhiwandiwala et al., 1982	Tubal Ring	5,046	0.47[u]					42.1[c,t]	IFRP (27 countries)
Mumford et al., 1980	Minilaparoscopy: Ring	1,324	0.51[u]					?	IFRP (23 countries)

(continued)

Table 26-16 Summary of studies of contraceptive failure: tubal occlusion[a]—*(continued)*

			Risk of Pregnancy						
			Life-Table	Pearl Index Pregnancy Rate					
Reference	Procedure	N for Analysis	12-Month % Pregnant	Index	Total Exposure	Maximum Exposure	Characteristics of the Sample	LFU (%)[g]	Comments
Vessey et al., 1983	Laparoscopy: Tubal Diathermy	776		0.53	755 Yr.	12 Mo.	All white; at recruitment aged 25–39 and married; at enrollment, all women had been using the diaphragm, IUD, or pill successfully for at least 5 months	.3[t,v]	Britain: Oxford/FPA study
Chi et al., 1981	Tubal Ring	4,106	0.54[c]					?	IFRP (19 countries)
Peterson et al., 1996	All methods combined	10,685	0.55				33% aged 18–27, 35% aged 28–33, 32% aged 34+	10.8	U.S. Collaborative Review of Sterilization
Chi et al., 1980	Laparoscopy: Rocket Clip	457	0.59				Mean age = 32[t]	?	IFRP (19 countries)
Peterson et al., 1996	Rubber band	3,329	0.59				30% aged 18–27, 36% aged 28–33, 34% aged 34+	12.1	U.S. Collaborative Review of Sterilization
Mumford et al., 1980	Laparoscopy: Rings	4,262	0.60[u]					?	IFRP (23 countries)

(continued)

Table 26-16 Summary of studies of contraceptive failure: tubal occlusion[a]—(continued)

Reference	Procedure	N for Analysis	Risk of Pregnancy: Life-Table 12-Month % Pregnant	Pearl Index Pregnancy Rate: Index	Pearl Index Pregnancy Rate: Total Exposure	Pearl Index Pregnancy Rate: Maximum Exposure	Characteristics of the Sample	LFU (%)[g]	Comments
Vessey et al., 1983	Laparoscopy: Rings, Clips, etc.	379		0.60	334 Yr.	12 Mo.	All white; at recruitment aged 25–39 and married; at enrollment, all women had been using the diaphragm, IUD, or pill successfully for at least 5 months	0.3[t,v]	Britain; Oxford/FPA study
Dominik et al., 2000	Hulka Clip	1,062	0.69					33.1[c]	Dominican Republic, Guatemala, Haiti, Malaysia, Mexico, Panama, Venezuela
Peterson et al., 1996	Interval partial salpingectomy	425	0.73				28% aged 18–27, 32% aged 28–33, 40% aged 34+	7.3	U.S. Collaborative Review of Sterilization
Chi et al., 1987	Minilaparotomy: Rings and Clips	1,146		0.79	1,143 Yr.	12 Mo.	Median age = 32 years	13.5	IFRP (19 countries)
Vancaillie et al., 2008	Adiana implant	570	1.07				Median age = 31	3.0[c]	United States, Mexico, Australia; 3 women became pregnant before bilateral occlusion was confirmed

(continued)

Table 26-16 Summary of studies of contraceptive failure: tubal occlusion[a]—*(continued)*

			Risk of Pregnancy						
				Pearl Index Pregnancy Rate					
Reference	**Procedure**	**N for Analysis**	**Life-Table 12-Month % Pregnant**	**Index**	**Total Exposure**	**Maximum Exposure**	**Characteristics of the Sample**	**LFU (%)[g]**	**Comments**
Yoon et al., 1977	Falope Ring	902		1.33[c]	3,617[c] Mo.	12 Mo.		21.0[c]	
Peterson et al., 1996	Spring Clip	1,595	1.82				44% aged 18–27, 30% aged 28–33, 26% aged 34+	16.4	U.S. Collaborative Review of Sterilization
Hulka et al., 1976	Spring Clip	1,079	2.3[2]					9.5[c]	United States, UK, Jamaica, Thailand, Singapore, El Salvador (defective clips)
Chi et al., 1981	Spring Clip	1,699	4.19[c]					?	IFRP (19 countries) (defective clips)
Chi et al., 1980	Culdoscopy: Tantalum Clip	498	8.19				Mean age = 32[t]	?	IFRP (19 countries)

Notes:

[a] Updated from Trussell and Kost (1987), Table 10.

[c] Calculated by James Trussell from data in the article.

[g] Most of these studies incorrectly report the loss to follow-up (LFU) probability as the number of women lost at any time during the study divided by the total number of women entering the study. Thus, these are the probabilities presented in the table. However, the correct measure of LFU would be a gross life-table probability. When available, gross 12-month probabilities are denoted by the letter "g."

[t] Total for all methods in the study.

[u] Study did not report whether the cumulative life-table probability was net or gross.

[v] The authors report that LFU for "relevant reasons (withdrawal of cooperation or loss of contact)" was 0.3% per year in the 1983 study. In the 1983 study, women had probably been followed for 10 years on average; if 0.3% are LFU per year, then 3.0% would be LFU in 10 years. LFU including death and emigration is about twice as high as LFU for "relevant reasons."

For table references, see reference section.

Table 26-17 Summary of studies of contraceptive failure: vasectomy[a]

Reference	N for Analysis	Risk of Pregnancy: Life-Table 12-Month % Pregnant	Pearl Index Pregnancy Rate: Index	Total Exposure	Maximum Exposure	Characteristics of the Sample	LFU (%)[g]	Comments
Moss, 1992	6,220	0.0[c]					?	1 pregnancy 10 years after vasectomy
Schmidt, 1988	5,000	0.0[c]					?	Presumably 0 pregnancies
Alderman, 1988	5,331	0.0[c]				5,331 of 8,879 had at least 2 post-op semen tests	?	Canada; 4 pregnancies, 4.5–8.6 years after vasectomy
Philip et al., 1984	16,039	0.0[c]				16,039 of 16,796 provided requested post-op semen samples	?	Britain; 6 pregnancies, 1.3–3 years after vasectomy; 3 pregnancies in first year among 757 men who did not supply post-op semen samples
Kase and Goldfarb, 1973	500	0.0[c]				2% ≥aged 41	?	1 pregnancy 15 months after vasectomy
Vessey et al., 1982	?		0.08	2,500 Yr.	24 Mo.	Females all white; females at recruitment aged 25–39 and married; at enrollment, all women had been using the diaphragm, IUD, or pill successfully for at least 5 months	0.3[t,v]	Britain; Oxford/FPA study
Margaret Pyke Center, 1973	1,000	0.1[c]				24% ≥age 41	?	Britain; 1 pregnancy in first year

(continued)

Table 26-17 Summary of studies of contraceptive failure: vasectomy[a]—*(continued)*

Reference	N for Analysis	Risk of Pregnancy: Life-Table 12-Month % Pregnant	Pearl Index Pregnancy Rate: Index	Pearl Index Pregnancy Rate: Total Exposure	Pearl Index Pregnancy Rate: Maximum Exposure	Characteristics of the Sample	LFU (%)[g]	Comments
Klapproth and Young, 1973	1,000	0.2[c]				35% ≥age 41	10.0?	2 pregnancies, 3 and 4 months after vasectomy
Marshall and Lyon, 1972	200	0.5[c]				Age 25–60; "majority" aged 35–39	?	1 pregnancy 3 months after vasectomy
Jamieson et al., 2004	544	0.74					6.1	U.S. Collaborative Review of Sterilization; women interviewed after husbands' vasectomy

Notes:

[a]Updated from Trussell and Kost (1987), Table 10.

[c]Calculated by James Trussell from data in the article.

[g]Most of these studies incorrectly report the loss to follow-up (LFU) probability as the number of women lost at any time during the study divided by the total number of women entering the study. Thus, these are the probabilities presented in the table. However, the correct measure of LFU would be a gross life-table probability. When available, gross 12-month probabilities are denoted by the letter "g."

[t]Total for all methods in the study.

[v]The authors report that LFU for "relevant reasons (withdrawal of cooperation or loss of contact)" was 0.3% per year in the 1982 study. In the 1982 study, women had probably been followed for 9.5 years on average; if 0.3% are LFU per year, then 2.8% would be LFU in 9.5 years. LFU including death and emigration is about twice as high as LFU for "relevant reasons."

For table references, see reference section.

Table References

Aérvalo M, Jennings V, Nikula M, Sinai I. Efficacy of the new TwoDay Method of family planning. Fertil Steril 2004;82:885–92.

Agrawal A, Robinson C. An assessment of the first 3 years' use of Implanon in Luton. J Fam Plann Reprod Health Care 2005;31:310–2.

Ahrendt HJ, Nisand I, Bastianelli C, et al. Efficacy, acceptability and tolerability of the combined contraceptive ring, NuvaRing, compared with an oral contraceptive containing 30 microg of ethinyl estradiol and 3 mg of drospirenone. Contraception 2006;74:451–7.

Åkerlund M, Røde A, Westergaard J. Comparative profiles of reliability, cycle control and side effects of two oral contraceptive formulations containing 150 μg desogestrel and either 30 μg or 20 μg ethinyl oestradiol. Brit J Obstet Gynaecol 1993;100:832–8.

Alderman PM. The lurking sperm: a review of failures in 8879 vasectomies performed by one physician. JAMA 1988;259:3142–4.

Anderson FD, Hait H, the Seasonale-301 Study Group. A multicenter, randomized study of an extended cycle oral contraceptive. Contraception 2003;68:89–96.

Anderson FD, Gibbons W, Portman D, the Seasonique™ Study Group. Safety and efficacy of an extended-regimen oral contraceptive utilizing continuous low-dose ethinyl estradiol. Contraception 2006;73:229–34.

Apothecus Pharmaceutical Corporation. VCF®: Vaginal Contraceptive Film™. East Norwich NY: Apothecus Inc, 1992.

Archer DF, Jensen JT, Johnson JV, Borisute H, Grubb GS, Constantine GD. Evaluation of a continuous regimen of levonorgestrel/ethinyl estradiol: phase 3 study results. Contraception 2006;74:439–45.

Archer DF, Maheux R, DelConte A, O'Brien FB. North American levonorgestrel study group (NALSG). Efficacy and safety of a low-dose monophasic combination oral contraceptive containing 100 μg levonorgestrel and 20 μg ethinyl estradiol (Alesse). Am J Obstet Gynecol 1999;181 Suppl 1:S39–44.

Arévalo M, Jennings V, Sinai I. Efficacy of a new method of family planning: the Standard Days Method. Contraception 2002;65:333–8.

Arjona JE, Miño M, Cordón J, Povedano B, Pelegrin B, Castelo-Branco C. Satisfaction and tolerance with office hysteroscopic tubal sterilization. Fertil Steril 2008;90:1182–6.

Arribas-Mir L, Rueda-Lozano D, Agrela-Cardona M, et al. Insertion and 3-year follow-up experience of 372 etonogestrel subdermal contraceptive implants by family physicians in Granada, Spain. Contraception 2009;80:457–62.

Audet MC, Moreau M, Koltun WD, Waldbaum AS, Shangold G, Fisher AC, Creasy GW. Evaluation of contraceptive efficacy and cycle control of a transdermal contraceptive patch vs an oral contraceptive. JAMA 2001;285:2347–54.

Bachmann G, Sulak PJ, Sampson-Landers C, Benda N, Marr J. Efficacy and safety of a low-dose 24-day combined oral contraceptive containing 20 micrograms ethinylestradiol and 3 mg drospirenone. Contraception 2004;70:191–8.

Bahamondes L, Brache V, Meirik O, Ali M, Habib N, Landoulsi S; WHO Study Group on Contraceptive Implants for Women. A 3-year multicentre randomized controlled trial of etonogestrel- and levonorgestrel-releasing contraceptive implants, with non-randomized matched copper-intrauterine device controls. Hum Reprod 2015;30:2527–38.

Ball M. A prospective field trial of the ovulation method of avoiding conception. Eur J Obstet Gynecol Reprod Biol 1976;6:63–6.

Bannemerschult R, Hanker JP, Wunsch C, Fox P, Albring M, Brill K. A multicenter, uncontrolled clinical investigation of the contraceptive efficacy, cycle control, and safety of a new low dose oral contraceptive containing 20 μg ethinyl estradiol and 100 μg levonorgestrel over six treatment cycles. Contraception 1997;56:285–90.

Barnhart KT, Rosenberg MJ, MacKay HT, et al. Contraceptive efficacy of a novel spermicidal microbicide used with a diaphragm: a randomized controlled trial. Obstet Gynecol 2007;110:577–86.

Bartzen PJ. Effectiveness of the temperature rhythm system of contraception. Fertil Steril 1967;18:694–706.

Belhadj H, Sivin I, Diaz S, et al. Recovery of fertility after use of the levonorgestrel 20 mcg/d or copper T 380 Ag intrauterine device. Contraception 1986;34:261–7.

Berglund Scherwitzl E, Gemzell Danielsson K, Sellberg JA, Scherwitzl R. Fertility awareness-based mobile application for contraception. Eur J Contracept Reprod Health Care 2016;21:234–41.

Berglund Scherwitzl E, Lundberg O, Kopp-Kalner H, Gemzell Danielsson K, Trussell J, Scherwitzl R. Perfect-use and typical-use Pearl Index of a contraceptive modible app. Contraception 2017;96:420–425.

Bernstein GS. Clinical effectiveness of an aerosol contraceptive foam. Contraception 1971;3:37–43.

Bernstein GS, Clark V, Coulson AH, et al. Use effectiveness study of cervical caps. Final report. Washington (DC): National Institute of Child Health and Human Development, 1986 July Contract No.: 1-HD-1-2804.

Bhiwandiwala PP, Mumford SD, Feldblum PJ. A comparison of different laparoscopic sterilization occlusion techniques in 24,439 procedures. Am J Obstet Gynecol 1982;144:319–31.

Bisset AM, Dingwall-Fordyce I, Hamilton MIK. The efficacy of the progestogen-only pill as a contraceptive method. Br J Family Plann 1990;16:84–7.

Board JA. Continuous norethindrone, 0.35 mg, as an oral contraceptive agent. Am J Obstet Gynecol 1971;109:531–5.

Boehm D. The cervical cap: effectiveness as a contraceptive. J Nurse Midwifery 1983;28:3–6.

Booranabunyat S, Taneepanichskul S. Implanon use in Thai women above the age of 35 years. Contraception 2004;69:489–91.

Bounds W, Guillebaud J. Randomised comparison of the use-effectiveness and patient acceptability of the Collatex (Today) contraceptive sponge and the diaphragm. Br J Fam Plann 1984;10:69–75.

Bounds W, Guillebaud J, Dominik R, Dalberth BT. The diaphragm with and without spermicide: a randomized, comparative efficacy trial. J Reprod Med.1995;40:764–74.

Bounds W, Vessey M, Wiggins P. A randomized double-blind trial of two low dose combined oral contraceptives. Brit J Obstet Gynaecol 1979;86:325–9.

Bracher M, Santow G. Premature discontinuation of contraception in Australia. Fam Plann Perspect 1992;24:58–65.

Brehm H, Haase W. Die alternative zur hormonalen kontrazeption? Med Welt 1975;26:1610–7. German.

Brigato G, Pisano G, Bergamasco A, Pasqualini M, Cutugno G, Luppari T. Vaginal topical chemical contraception with C-Film. Ginecol Clinica 1982;3:77–80. (In Italian; translation supplied by Apothecus Inc.)

Broome M, Fotherby K. Clinical experience with the progestogen-only pill. Contraception 1990;42:489–95.

Bushnell LF. Aerosol foam: a practical and effective method of contraception. Pac Med Surg 1965;73:353–5.

Cagen R. The cervical cap as a barrier contraceptive. Contraception 1986;33:487–96.

Carpenter G, Martin JB. Clinical evaluation of a vaginal contraceptive foam. Adv Plann Parent 1970;5:170–5.

Chi IC, Laufe LE, Gardner SD, Tolbert MA. An epidemiologic study of risk factors associated with pregnancy following female sterilization. Am J Obstet Gynecol 1980;136:768–73.

Chi IC, Mumford SD, Gardner SD. Pregnancy risks following laparoscopic sterilization in nongravid and gravid women. J Reprod Med 1981;26:289–94.

Chi IC, Siemens AJ, Champion CB, Gates D, Cilenti D. Pregnancy following minilaparotomy tubal sterilization: an update of an international data set. Contraception 1987;35:171–8.

Cliquet RL, Schoenmaeckers R, Klinkenborg L. Effectiveness of contraception in Belgium: results of the second national fertility survey, 1971 (NEGO II). J Biosoc Sci 1977;9:403–16.

Collaborative Study Group on the Desogestrel-containing Progestogen-only Pill. A double-blind study comparing the contraceptive efficacy, acceptability and safety of two progestogen-only pills containing desogestrel 75 micrograms / day or levonorgestrel 30 micrograms / day. Eur J Contracept Reprod Health Care 1998;3:169–178.

Cooper JM, Carignan CS, Cher D, Kerin JF. Microinsert nonincisional hysteroscopic sterilization. Obstet Gynecol 2003;102:59–67.

Cox M, Blacksell S. Clinical performance of the levonorgestrel intra-uterine system in routine use by the UK Family Planning and Reproductive Health Research Network: 12-month report. Br J Fam Plann 2000;26:143–7.

Darney P, Patel A, Rosen K, Shapiro LS, Kaunitz AM. Safety and efficacy of a single-rod etonogestrel implant (Implanon): results from 11 international clinical trials. Fertil Steril 2009;91:1646–53.

Debusschere R. Effectiviteit van de anticonceptie in Vlaanderen: resultaten van het NEGO-III-onderzoek 1975–1976. Bevolking en Gezin 1980;1:5–28. German.

Denniston GC, Putney D. The cavity rim cervical cap. Adv Plann Parent 1981;16:77–80.

Dieben TOM, Roumen JME, Apter D. Efficacy, cycle control and user acceptability of a novel combined contraceptive vaginal ring. Obstet Gynecol 2002;100:585–93.

Dimpfl J, Salomon W, Schicketanz KH. Die spermizide barriere. Sexualmedizin 1984;13:95–8. German.

Dingle JT, Tietze C. Comparative study of three contraceptive methods: vaginal foam tablets, jelly alone, and diaphragm with jelly or cream. Am J Obstet Gynecol 1963;85:1012–22.

Dolack L. Study confirms values of ovulation method. Hospital Progress 1978;59: 64–6,72–3.

Dominik R, Gates D, Sokal D, et al. Two randomized controlled trials comparing the Hulka and Filshie Clips for tubal sterilization. Contraception 2000;62:169–75.

Dubrow H, Kuder K. Combined postpartum and family-planning clinic. Obstet Gynecol 1958;11:586–90.

Edelman DA. Nonprescription vaginal contraception. Int J Gynecol Obstet 1980;18:340–4.

Edelman DA, McIntyre SL, Harper J. A comparative trial of the Today contraceptive sponge and diaphragm. Am J Obstet Gynecol 1984;150:869–76.

Eisenberg DL, Schreiber CA, Turok DK, Teal SB, Westhoff CL, Creinin MD; ACCESS IUS Investigators. Three-year efficacy and safety of a new 52-mg levonorgestrel-releasing intrauterine system. Contraception. 2015;92:10–6.

Ellis JW. Multiphasic oral contraceptives: efficacy and metabolic impact. J Reprod Med 1987;32:28–36.

Ellsworth HS. Focus on triphasil. J Reprod Med 1986;31:559–64.

Endrikat J, Jaques MA, Mayerhofer M, Pelissier C, Müller U, Düsterberg B. A twelve-month comparative clinical investigation of two low-dose oral contraceptives containing 20 μg ethinylestradiol/75 μg gestodene and 20 μg ethinylestradiol/150 μg desogestrel, with respect to efficacy, cycle control and tolerance. Contraception 1995;52:229–35.

Engel T. Laparoscopic sterilization: electrosurgery or clip application? J Reprod Med 1978;21:107–10.

Farr G, Gabelnick H, Sturgen K, Dorflinger L. Contraceptive efficacy and acceptability of the female condom. Am J Public Health 1994;84:1960–4.

Flores JB, Balderas ML, Bonilla MC, Vazquez-Estrada L. Clinical experience and acceptability of the etonogestrel subdermal contraceptive implant. Int J Gynaecol Obstet 2005;90:228–33.

Florence N. Das kontrazeptive vaginal-suppositorium: ergebnisse einer klinischen fünfjahresstudie. Sexualmedizin 1977;6:385–6. German.

Frank R. Clinical evaluation of a simple jelly-alone method of contraception. Fertil Steril 1962;13:458–64.

Frank-Herrmann P, Heil J, Gnoth C, et al. The effectiveness of a fertility awareness based method to avoid pregnancy in relation to a couple's sexual behaviour during the fertile time: a prospective longitudinal study. Hum Reprod 2007;22:1310–9.

Frankman O, Raabe N, Ingemansson CA. Clinical evaluation of C-Film, a vaginal contraceptive. J Int Med Res 1975;3:292–6.

Frezieres RG, Walsh TL, Nelson AL, Clark VA, Coulson AH. Evaluation of the efficacy of a polyurethane condom: results from a randomized controlled clinical trial. Fam Plann Perspect 1999;31:81–7.

Fu H, Darroch JE, Haas T, Ranjit N. Contraceptive failure rates: new estimates from the 1995 National Survey of Family Growth. Fam Plann Perspect 1999;31:56–63.

Gezginc K, Balci O, Karatayli R, Colakoglu MC. Contraceptive efficacy and side effects of Implanon. Eur J Contracept Reprod Health Care 2007;12:362–5.

Gibor Y, Mitchell C. Selected events following insertion of the Progestasert system. Contraception 1980;21:491–503.

Glass R, Vessey M, Wiggins P. Use-effectiveness of the condom in a selected family planning clinic population in the United Kingdom. Contraception 1974;10:591–8.

Gnoth C, Godehardt D, Godehardt E, Frank-Herrmann P, Freundl G. Time to pregnancy: results of the German prospective study and impact on the anagement of infertility. Hum Reprod 2003;18:1959–66.

Godts P. Klinische prüfung eines vaginalem antikonzipiens. Ars Medici 1973;28:584–93. German.

Grady WR, Hayward MD, Yagi J. Contraceptive failure in the United States: estimates from the 1982 National Survey of Family Growth. Fam Plann Perspect 1986;18:200–9.

Grady WR, Hirsch MB, Keen N, Vaughan B. Contraceptive failure and continuation among married women in the United States, 1970–75. Stud Fam Plann 1983;14:9–19.

Graesslin O, Korver T. The contraceptive efficacy of Implanon: a review of clinical trials and marketing experience. Eur J Contracept Reprod Health Care 2008;13 Suppl 1:S4–12.

Hall P, Bahamondes L, Diaz J, Petta C. Introductory study of the once-a-month, injectable contraceptive Cyclofem in Brazil, Chile, Colombia, and Peru. Contraception 1997;56:353–9.

Hall RE. Continuation and pregnancy rates with four contraceptive methods. Am J Obstet Gynecol 1973;116:671–81.

Harvey C, Seib C, Lucke J. Continuation rates and reasons for removal among Implanon users accessing two family planning clinics in Queensland, Australia. Contraception 2009;80:527–32.

Hawkins DF, Benster B. A comparative study of three low dose progestogens, chlormadinone acetate, megestrol acetate and norethisterone, as oral contraceptives. Br J Obstet Gynaecol 1977;84:708–13.

Hernádi L, Marr J, Trummer D, De Leo V, Petraglia F. Efficacy and safety of a low-dose combined oral contraceptive containing drospirenone 3 mg and ethinylestradiol 20 mcg in a 24/4-day regimen. Contraception 2009;80:18–24.

Howard G, Blair M, Chen JK, Fotherby K, Muggeridge J, Elder MG, Bye PG. A clinical trial of norethisterone oenanthate (Norigest) injected every two months. Contraception 1982;25:333–43.

Hughes I. An open assessment of a new low dose estrogen combined oral contraceptive. J Int Med Res 1978;6:41–5.

Hulka JF, Mercer JP, Fishburne JI, et al. Spring clip sterilization: one-year follow-up of 1,079 cases. Am J Obstet Gynecol 1976;125:1039–43.

Iizuka R, Kobayashi T, Kawakami S, et al. Clinical experience with the Vaginal Contraceptive Film containing the spermicide polyoxyethylene nonylphenyl ether (C-Film study group). Jpn J Fertil Steril 1980;25:64–8. (In Japanese; translation supplied by Apothecus Inc.)

Jain J, Jakimiuk AJ, Bode FR, Ross D, Kaunitz AM. Contraceptive efficacy and safety of DMPA-SC. Contraception 2004;70:269–75.

Jamieson DJ, Costello C, Trussell J, Hillis SD, Marchbanks PA, Peterson HB; for the US Collaborative Review of Sterilization Working Group. The risk of pregnancy after vasectomy. Obstet Gynecol. 2004;103(5 Pt 1):848–50. Erratum in: Obstet Gynecol 2004;104:200.

John APK. Contraception in a practice community. J R Coll Gen Pract 1973;23:665–75.

Johnston JA, Roberts DB, Spencer RB. A survey evaluation of the efficacy and efficiency of natural family planning services and methods in Australia: report of a research project. Sydney: St. Vincent's Hospital; 1978.

Jones EF, Forrest JD. Contraceptive failure rates based on the 1988 NSFG. Fam Plann Perspect 1992;24:12–9.

Jubhari S, Lane ME, Sobrero AJ. Continuous microdose (0.3 mg) quingestanol acetate as an oral contraceptive agent. Contraception 1974;9:213–9.

Kambic R, Kambic M, Brixius AM, Miller S. A thirty-month clinical experience in natural family planning. Am J Public Health 1981;71:1255–8. Erratum in: Am J Public Health 1982;72:538.

Kasabach HY. Clinical evaluation of vaginal jelly alone in the management of fertility. Clin Med 1962;69:894–7.

Kase S, Goldfarb M. Office vasectomy review of 500 cases. Urology 1973;1:60–2.

Kassell NC, McElroy MP. Emma Goldman Clinic for Women study. In: King L, (ed). The cervical cap handbook for users and fitters. Iowa City: Emma Goldman Clinic for Women; 1981. p. 11–9.

Kaunitz AM. Efficacy, cycle control, and safety of two triphasic oral contraceptives: Cyclessa (desogestrel/ethinyl estradiol) and Ortho-Novum 7/7/7 (norethindrone/ethinyl estradiol): a randomized clinical trial. Contraception 2000;61:295–302.

Kaunitz AM, Darney PD, Ross D, Wolter KD, Speroff L. Subcutaneous DMPA vs. Intramuscular DMPA: a 2-year randomized study of contraceptive efficacy and bone mineral denisty. Contraception 2009;80:7–17.

Kaunitz AM, Garceau RJ, Cromie MA, Lunelle Study Group. Comparative safety, efficacy, and cycle control of Lunelle monthly contraceptive injection (medroxyprogesterone acetate and estradiol cypionate injectable suspension) and Ortho-Novum 7/7/7 oral contraceptive (norethindrone/eithinyl estradiol triphasic). Contraception 1999;60:179–87.

Keifer W. A clinical evaluation of continuous Norethindrone (0.35 mg). In: Ortho Pharmaceutical Corporation. A clinical symposium on 0.35 mg. Norethindrone: continuous regimen low-dose oral contraceptive. Proceedings of a symposium, New York City, February 22, 1971. Raritan: Ortho Pharmaceutical Corporation, 1973;9–14.

Kerin JF, Cooper JM, Price T, Herendael BJ, Cayuela-Font E, Cher D, Carignan CS. Hysteroscopic sterilization using a micro-insert device: results of a multicentre Phase II study. Hum Reprod 2003;18:1223–30.

Klapproth HJ, Young IS. Vasectomy, vas ligation and vas occlusion. Urology 1973;1: 292–300.

Klaus H, Goebel JM, Muraski B. Use-effectiveness and client satisfaction in six centers teaching the Billings ovulation method. Contraception 1979;19:613–29.

Kleppinger RK. A vaginal contraceptive foam. Penn Med J 1965;68:31–4.

Koch JP. The Prentif contraceptive cervical cap: a contemporary study of its clinical safety and effectiveness. Contraception 1982;25:135–59.

Korba VD, Heil CG. Eight years of fertility control with norgestrel-ethinyl estradiol (Ovral): an updated clinical review. Fertil Steril 1975;26:973–81.

Korba VD, Paulson SR. Five years of fertility control with microdose norgestrel: an updated clinical review. J Reprod Med 1974;13:71–5.

Kost K, Singh S, Vaughan B, Trussell J, Bankole A. Estimates of contraceptive failure from the 2002 National Survey of Family Growth. Contraception 2008;77:10–21.

Kovacs GT, Jarman H, Dunn K, Westcott M, Baker HWG. The contraceptive diaphragm: is it an acceptable method in the 1980s? Aust NZ J Obstet Gynaecol 1986;26:76–9.

Kroll R, Reape KZ, Margolis M. The efficacy and safety of a low-dose, 91-day, extended-regimen oral contraceptive with continuous ethinyl estradiol. Contraception 2010;81:41–8.

Lakha F, Glasier AF. Continuation rates of Implanon in the UK: data from an observational study in a clinical setting. Contraception 2006;74:287–9.

Lampe L, Andersson K, Atterfeldt P, et al. Effective contraception with the levonorgestrel-releasing intrauterine device: 12-month report of a European multicenter study. Contraception 1987;36:169–79.

Lane ME, Arceo R, Sobrero AJ. Successful use of the diaphragm and jelly by a young population: report of a clinical study. Fam Plann Perspect 1976;8:81–6.

Ledger WJ. Ortho 1557-O: a new oral contraceptive. Int J Fertil 1970;15:88–92.

Lehfeldt H, Sivin I. Use effectiveness of the Prentif cervical cap in private practice: a prospective study. Contraception 1984;30:331–8.

Lipetz C, Phillips C, Fleming C. Actual cost of providing long-acting reversible contraception: a study of Implanon cost. J Fam Plann Reprod Health Care 2009;35:75–9.

Loffer FD, Pent D. Risks of laparoscopic fulguration and transection of the fallopian tube. Obstet Gynecol 1977;49:218–22.

Loudon NB, Barden ME, Hepburn WB, Prescott RJ. A comparative study of the effectiveness and acceptability of the diaphragm used with spermicide in the form of C-film or a cream or jelly. Br J Fam Plann 1991;17:41–4.

Luukkainen T, Allonen H, Haukkamaa M, et al. Effective contraception with the levonorgestrel-releasing intrauterine device: 12-month report of a European multicenter study. Contraception 1987;36:169–79.

Margaret Pyke Centre. One thousand vasectomies. Br Med J 1973;4:216–21.

Marshall J. Cervical-mucus and basal body-temperature method of regulating births: field trial. Lancet 1976;2:282–3.

Marshall S, Lyon RP. Variability of sperm disappearance from the ejaculate after vasectomy. J Urol 1972;107:815–7.

Mauck C, Callahan M, Weiner DH, Dominik R, FemCap investigators' group. A comparative study of the safety and efficacy of FemCap, a new vaginal barrier contraceptive, and the Ortho All-Flex diaphragm. Contraception 1999;60:71–80.

Mauck C, Glover LH, Miller E, et al. Lea's Shield®: a study of the safety and efficacy of a new vaginal barrier contraceptive used with and without spermicide. Contraception 1996;53:329–35.

McIntyre SL, Higgins JE. Parity and use-effectiveness with the contraceptive sponge. Am J Obstet Gynecol 1986;155:796–801.

McQuarrie HG, Harris JW, Ellsworth HS, Stone RA, Anderson AE. The clinical evaluation of norethindrone in cyclic and continuous regimens. Adv Plann Parent 1972;7:124–30.

Mears E. Chemical contraceptive trial: II. J Reprod Fertil 1962;4:337–43.

Mears E, Please NW. Chemical contraceptive trial. J Reprod Fertil 1962;3:138–47.

Merki-Feld GS, Hund M. Clinical experience with NuvaRing in daily practice in Switzerland: cycle control and acceptability among women of all reproductive ages. Eur J Contracept Reprod Health Care 2007;12:240–7.

The Mircette Study Group. An open-label, multicenter, noncomparative safety and efficacy study of Mircette, a low-dose estrogen-progestin oral contraceptive. Am J Obstet Gynecol 1998;179 Suppl:S2–8.

Mishell DR, El-Habashy MA, Good RG, Moyer DL. Contraception with an injectable progestin. Am J Obstet Gynecol 1968;101:1046–53.

Morigi EM, Pasquale SA. Clinical experience with a low dose oral contraceptive containing norethisterone and ethinyl oestradiol. Curr Med Res Opin 1978;5:655–62.

Moss WM. A comparison of open-end versus closed-end vasectomies: a report on 6220 cases. Contraception 1992;46:521–5.

Mumford SD, Bhiwandiwala PP, Chi IC. Laparoscopic and minilaparotomy female sterilisation compared in 15,167 cases. Lancet 1980;2:1066–70.

Nakajima ST, Archer DF, Ellman H. Efficacy and safety of a new 24-day oral contraceptive regimen of norethindroneacetate 1 mg/ethinyl estradiol 20 μ (Loestrin® 24 Fe). Contraception 2007;75:16–22.

Nelson JH. The use of the mini pill in private practice. J Reprod Med 1973;10:139–43.

Nelson A, Apter D, Hauck B, Schmelter T, Rybowski S, Rosen K, Gemzell-Danielsson K. Two low-dose levonorgestrel intrauterine contraceptive systems: a randomized controlled trial. Obstet Gynecol 2013;122;1205–13.

Oddsson K, Leifels-Fischer B, de Melo NR, et al. Efficacy and safety of a contraceptive vaginal ring (NuvaRing) compared with a combined oral contraceptive: a 1-year randomized trial. Contraception 2005;71:176–82.

Palacios S, Wildt L, Parke S, Machlitt A, Römer T, Bitzer J. Efficacy and safety of a novel oral contraceptive based on oestradiol (oestradiol valerate/dienogest): a Phase III trial. Eur J Obstet Gynecol Reprod Biol 2010;149:57–62.

Parsey KS, Pong A. An open-label, multicenter study to evaluate Yasmin, a low-dose combination oral contraceptive containing drospirenone, a new progestogen. Contraception 2000;61:105–11.

Peel J. The Hull family survey: II. Family planning in the first five years of marriage. J Biosoc Sci 1972;4:333–46.

Peterson HB, Xia Z, Hughes JM, Wilcox LS, Tylor LR, Trussell J. The risk of pregnancy after tubal sterilization: findings from the U.S. Collaborative Review of Sterilization. Am J Obstet Gynecol 1996;174:1161–70.

Philp T, Guillebaud J, Budd D. Complications of vasectomy: review of 16,000 patients. Br J Urol 1984;56;745–8.

Postlethwaite DL. Pregnancy rate of a progestogen oral contraceptive. Practitioner 1979;222:272–5.

Potts M, McDevitt J. A use-effectiveness trial of spermicidally lubricated condoms. Contraception 1975;11:701–10.

Powell MG, Mears BJ, Deber RB, Ferguson D. Contraception with the cervical cap: effectiveness, safety, continuity of use, and user satisfaction. Contraception 1986;33:215–32.

Preston SN. A report of a collaborative dose-response clinical study using decreasing doses of combination oral contraceptives. Contraception 1972;6:17–35.

Preston SN. A report of the correlation between the pregnancy rates of low estrogen formulations and pill-taking habits of females studied. J Reprod Med 1974;13:75–7.

Rai K, Gupta S, Cotter S. Experience with Implanon in a northeast London family planning clinic. Eur J Contracept Reprod Health Care 2004;9:39–46.

Raymond EG, Chen PL, Luoto J. Contraceptive effectiveness and safety of five nonoxynol-9 spermicides: a randomized trial. Obstet Gynecol 2004;103:430–9.

Raymond E, Dominik R, the spermicide trial group. Contraceptive effectiveness of two spermicides: a randomized trial. Obstet Gynecol 1999;93:896–903.

Rice FJ, Lanctôt CA, Garcia-Devesa C. Effectiveness of the sympto-thermal method of natural family planning: an international study. Int J Fertil 1981;26:222–30.

Richwald GA, Greenland S, Gerber MM, Potik R, Kersey L, Comas MA. Effectiveness of the cavity-rim cervical cap: results of a large clinical study. Obstet Gynecol 1989;74:143–8.

Roumen FJME, Apter D, Mulders TMT, Dieben TOM. Efficacy, tolerability and acceptability of a novel contraceptive vaginal ring releasing etonogestrel and ethinyl oestradiol. Hum Reprod 2001;16:469–75.

Rovinsky JJ. Clinical effectiveness of a contraceptive cream. Obstet Gynecol 1964;23:125–31.

Royal College of General Practitioners. Oral contraceptives and health. New York: Pitman Publishing Corporation; 1974.

Salomon W, Haase W. Intravaginale kontrazeption. Sexualmedizin 1977;6:198–202. German.

Sangi-Haghpeykar H, Poindexter AN, Bateman L, Ditmore JR. Experiences of injectable contraceptive users in an urban setting. Obstet Gynecol 1996;88:227–33.

Schirm AL, Trussell J, Menken J, Grady WR. Contraceptive failure in the United States: the impact of social, economic, and demographic factors. Fam Plann Perspect 1982;14:68–75.

Schmidt SS. Vasectomy. JAMA 1988;259:3176.

Schwallie PC, Assenzo JR. Contraceptive use-efficacy study utilizing Depo-Provera administered as an injection once every six months. Contraception 1972;6:315–27.

Schwallie PC, Assenzo JR. Contraceptive use-efficacy study utilizing medroxyprogesterone acetate administered as an intramuscular injection once every 90 days. Fertil Steril 1973;24:331–9.

Schwartz JL, Weiner DH, Lai JJ, et al. Contraceptive efficacy, safety, fit, and acceptability of a single-size diaphragm developed with end-user input. Obstet Gynecol 2015;125:895–903.

Scutchfield FD, Long WN, Corey B, Tyler CW. Medroxyprogesterone acetate as an injectable female contraceptive. Contraception 1971;3:21–35.

Sheps MC. An analysis of reproductive patterns in an American isolate. Popul Stud 1965;19:65–80.

Sheth A, Jain U, Sharma S, et al. A randomized, double-blind study of two combined and two progestogen-only oral contraceptives. Contraception 1982;25:243–52.

Shihata AA, Trussell J. New female intravaginal barrier contraceptive device: preliminary clinical trial. Contraception 1991;44:11–9.

Shroff NE, Pearce MY, Stratford ME, Wilkinson PD. Clinical experience with ethynodiol diacetate 0.5 mg daily as an oral contraceptive. Contraception 1987;35:121–34.

Sivin I, El Mahgoub S, McCarthy T, et al. Long-term contraception with the Levonorgestrel 20 mcg/day (LNG-IUS) and the Copper T 380Ag intrauterine devices: a five-year randomized study. Contraception 1990;42:361–78.

Sivin I, Shaaban M, Odlind V, et al. A randomized trial of the Gyne T 380 and Gyne T 380 Slimline intrauterine copper devices. Contraception 1990;42:379–89.

Sivin I, Stern J. Long-acting, more effective copper T IUDs: a summary of U.S. experience, 1970–1975. Stud Fam Plann 1979;10:263–81.

Smallwood GH, Meador ML, Lenihan JP, Shangold GA, Fisher AC, Creasy GW, and the ORTHO EVRA/EVRA 002 Study Group. Efficacy and safety of a transdermal contraceptive system. Obstet Gynecol 2001;98:799–805.

Smith A, Reuter S. An assessment of the use of Implanon in three community services. J Fam Plann Reprod Health Care 2002;28:193–6.

Smith C, Farr G, Feldblum PJ, Spence A. Effectiveness of the non-spermicidal fit-free diaphragm. Contraception 1995;51:289–91.

Smith GG, Lee RJ. The use of cervical caps at the University of California, Berkeley: a survey. Contraception 1984;30:115–23.

Smith M, Vessey MP, Bounds W, Warren J. C-Film as a contraceptive. Br Med J 1974;4:291.

Sokal D, Gates D, Amatya R, Dominik R, and the Clinical investigator team. Two randomized controlled trials comparing the tubal ring and Filshie Clip for tubal sterilization. Fertil Steril 2000;74:525–33.

Steiner MJ, Dominik R, Rountree RW, Nanda K, Dorflinger LJ. Contraceptive effectiveness of a polyurethane condom and a latex condom: a randomized controlled trial. Obstet Gynecol 2003;101:539–47.

Stim EM. The nonspermicidal fit-free diaphragm: a new contraceptive method. Adv Plan Parent 1980;15:88–98.

Squire JJ, Berger GS, Keith L. A retrospective clinical study of a vaginal contraceptive suppository. J Reprod Med 1979;22:319–23.

Sundaram A, Vaughan B, Kost K, Bankole A, Finer L, Singh S, Trussell J. Contraceptive failure in the United States: Estimates from the 2006–2010 National Survey of Family Growth. Perspect Sexual Reprod Health 2017;49:7–16.

Tatum HJ. Comparative experience with newer models of the copper T in the United States. In: Hefnawi F, Segal SJ, (eds). Analysis of intrauterine contraception. Amsterdam (Netherlands): North Holland, 1975. p. 155–63.

Teichmann A, Apter D, Emerich J, et al. Continuous daily levonorgestrel/ethinyl estradiol vs. 21-day, cyclic levonorgestrel/ethinyl estradiol: efficacy, safety and bleeding in a randomized, open-label trial. Contraception 2009;20:504–11.

Thamkhantho M, Jivasak-Apimas S, Angsuwathana S, Chiravacharadej G, Intawong J. One-year assessment of women receiving sub-dermal contraceptive implant at Siriraj Family Planning Clinic. J Med Assoc Thai 2008;91:775–80.

Tietze C, Lewit S. Comparison of three contraceptive methods: diaphragm with jelly or cream, vaginal foam, and jelly/cream alone. J Sex Res 1967;3:295–311.

Tietze C, Lewit S. Evaluation of intrauterine devices: ninth progress report of the cooperative statistical program. Stud Fam Plann 1970;1:1–40.

Tietze C, Poliakoff SR, Rock J. The clinical effectiveness of the rhythm method of contraception. Fertil Steril 1951;2:444–50.

Trussell J. Estimates of contraceptive failure from the 2002 National Survey of Family Growth. Contraception 2008;78:85.

Trussell J, Grummer-Strawn L. Contraceptive failure of the ovulation method of periodic abstinence. Fam Plann Perspect 1990;22:65–75.

Trussell J, Hatcher RA, Cates W, Stewart FH, Kost K. Contraceptive failure in the United States: an update. Stud Fam Plann 1990;21:51–4.

Trussell J, Kost K. Contraceptive failure in the United States: a critical review of the literature. Stud Fam Plann 1987;18:237–83.

Trussell J, Vaughan B. Contraceptive failure, method-related discontinuation and resumption of use: results from the 1995 National Survey of Family Growth. Fam Plann Perspect 1999;31:64–72, 93.

Tyler ET. Current developments in systemic contraception. Pac Med Surg 1965;93:79–85.

Valle RF, Battifora HA. A new approach to tubal sterilization by laparoscopy. Fertil Steril 1978;30:415–22.

Vancaillie TG, Anderson TL, Johns DA. A 12-month prospective evaluation of transcervical sterilization using implantable polymer matrices. Obstet Gynecol 2008;112:1270–7.

Vaughan B, Trussell J, Menken J, Jones EF. Contraceptive failure among married women in the United States, 1970–1973. Fam Plann Perspect 1977;9:251–8.

Vessey M, Huggins G, Lawless M, McPherson K, Yeates D. Tubal sterilization: findings in a large prospective study. Br J Obstet Gynaecol 1983;90:203–9.

Vessey M, Lawless M, Yeates D. Efficacy of different contraceptive methods. Lancet 1982;1:841–2.

Vessey MP, Lawless M, Yeates D, McPherson K. Progestogen-only oral contraception. Findings in a large prospective study with special reference to effectiveness. Br J Fam Plann 1985;10:117–21.

Vessey MP, Villard-Mackintosh L, McPherson K, Yeates D. Factors influencing use-effectiveness of the condom. Br J Fam Plann 1988;14:40–3.

Vessey M, Wiggins P. Use-effectiveness of the diaphragm in a selected family planning clinic population in the United Kingdom. Contraception 1974;9:15–21.

Vleugels MPH, Veersema S. Hysteroscopic sterilization in the outpatient department without anasthesis. Gynecol Surg 2005;2:155–8.

Wade ME, McCarthy P, Braunstein GD, et al. A randomized prospective study of the use-effectiveness of two methods of natural family planning. Am J Obstet Gynecol 1981;141:368–76.

Walsh TL, Frezieres RG, Peacock K, Nelson AL, Clark VA, Bernstein L. Evaluation of the efficacy of a nonlatex condom: results from a randomized, controlled clinical trial. Perspect Sex Reprod Health 2003;35:79–86.

Wiegratz I, Mittman K, Dietrich H, Zimmermann T, Kuhl H. Fertility after discontinuation of treatment with an oral contraceptive containing 30 mg of ethinyl estradiol and 2 mg of dienogest. Fertil Steril 2006;85:1812–9.

Westoff CF, Potter RG, Sagi PC, Mishler EG. Family growth in metropolitan America. Princeton: Princeton University Press; 1961.

Wolf L, Olson HJ, Tyler ET. Observations on the clinical use of cream-alone and gel-alone methods of contraception. Obstet Gynecol 1957;10:316–21.

World Health Organization. A multicentered phase III comparative clinical trial of depot-medroxyprogesterone acetate given three-monthly at doses of 100 mg or 150 mg: I. Contraceptive efficacy and side effects. Contraception 1986;34:223–35.

World Health Organization. A multicentered phase III comparative study of two hormonal contraceptive preparations given once-a-month by intramuscular injection: I. Contraceptive efficacy and side effects. Contraception 1988;37:1–20.

World Health Organization. A prospective multicentre trial of the ovulation method of natural family planning. II. The effectiveness phase. Fertil Steril 1981;36:591–8.

World Health Organization. Multinational comparative clinical evaluation of two long-acting injectable contraceptive steroids: norethisterone oenanthate and medroxyprogesterone acetate. Contraception 1977;15:513–33.

World Health Organization. Multinational comparative clinical trial of long-acting injectable contraceptives: norethisterone enanthate given in two dosage regimens and depot-medroxyprogesterone acetate. Final report. Contraception 1983;28:1–20.

Woutersz TB. A low-dose combination oral contraceptive: experience with 1,700 women treated for 22,489 cycles. J Reprod Med 1981;26:615–20.

Woutersz TB. A new ultra-low-dose combination oral contraceptive. J Reprod Med 1983;28:81–4.

Wyeth Laboratories. NORPLANT® SYSTEM Prescribing Information. Philadelphia (PA): Wyeth Laboratories; 1990 Dec 10.

Yildizbas B, Sahin HG, Kolusari A, Zeteroglu S, Kamaci M. Side effects and acceptability of Implanon: a pilot study conducted in eastern Turkey. Eur J Contracept Reprod Health Care 2007;12:248–52.

Yoon IB, King TM, Parmley TH. A two-year experience with the Falope ring sterilization procedure. Am J Obstet Gynecol 1977;127:109–12.

Zheng SR, Zheng HM, Qian SZ, Sang GW, Kaper RF. A long-term study of the efficacy and acceptability of a single-rod hormonal contraceptive implant (Implanon) in healthy women in China. Eur J Contracept Reprod Health Care 1999a;4:85–93.

Zheng SR, Zheng HM, Qian SZ, Sang GW, Kaper RF. A randomized multicenter study comparing the efficacy and bleeding pattern of a single-rod (Implanon) and a six-capsule (Norplant) hormonal contraceptive implant. Contraception 1999b;60:1–8.

Appendix 1

Digital Resources for Health & Medical Information*

Brian Nguyen, MD, MSCP
Leo Han, MD, MPH

- Advances in information and communication technology have produced a vast universe of digital health and medical resources for both healthcare providers and patients.
- While digital resources are easily accessible and constantly being updated, their quality can be variable or sources not reputable. Consumers of reproductive health information may be more vulnerable to misinformation given the lack of a consistent sex education in the United States and the young age at which this information becomes relevant.
- The Centers for Disease Control and Prevention's Medical Eligibility Criteria and Selected Practice Recommendations website and mobile app should be a key resource for *Contraceptive Technology* readers. These digital resources will have answers to

*Contraceptive Technology does not endorse, approve, or affiliate with any organization, entity, website or mobile application identified or mentioned in this Appendix. Likewise, Contraceptive Technology has not received any remuneration or other compensation for listing or identifying any organization, entity, website or mobile application in this Appendix. The views expressed in this Appendix are solely those of Contraceptive Technology and the authors, and are provided for informational and educational purposes.

most contraceptive questions healthcare providers might have when initiating contraceptives with their patients. These resources are also maintained regularly.

- **Top three family planning websites:**

The Center for Disease Control and Prevention: www.cdc.gov	Essential resource for healthcare providers. Reliable and regularly-updated home to the • U.S. Medical Eligibility Criteria (MEC) • Selected Practice Recommendations (SPR) • Sexually Transmitted Disease [STD] Treatment Guidelines • Updates on infectious disease outbreaks (e.g., Zika, drug resistant-gonorrhea)
Bedsider: www.bedsider.org	Essential resource recommendation for patients. Designed with the patient's interests and health literacy in mind, the website delivers accurate information with tools to help patients obtain access to and decide on an ideal method of contraception.
The Emergency Contraception Website: http://not-2-late.com http://ec.princeton.edu	Resource for all research, policy, and clinically related information about emergency contraception (EC), including the appropriate Yuzpe dose by pill-type, as well as where to direct patients to obtain EC.

- **Top three "must-have" family planning apps (*available on Apple iOS and Android platforms*)[§]:**

Contraceptive Guidance for Health Care Providers from the CDC	Easy-to-use, easily searchable mobile app version of the U.S. Medical Eligibility Criteria and Selected Practice Recommendations (MEC/SPR).
STD Treatment Guidelines from the CDC	Easy-to use mobile app with the most evidence-based screening and treatment regimens from the CDC.
Agency for Healthcare Research & Quality's Electronic Preventative Services Selector (AHRQ ePSS)	Interactive, patient characteristic-specific mobile app that compiles and simplifies preventative health recommendations from the U.S. Preventative Services Task Force (USPSTF) for the primary care clinician.

- *Contraceptive Technology* authors have a website (www.contraceptive technology.com) and a twitter feed (@ContraceptTech).

[§]Contraceptive Technology is an independent publication and has not been authorized, sponsored, or otherwise approved by Apple Inc. or Google Inc. The Android robot is reproduced or modified from work created and shared by Google and used according to terms described in the Creative Commons 3.0 Attribution License.

1 INTRODUCTION

The following section provides general background information regarding the rise and importance of digital health resources as well as a curated guide to digital resources relevant to family planning in the form of websites, mobile applications, and social media.

1.1 The Rise of Digital Resources

Prior to the rise of the internet, the volume of digital resources was limited to digital transcriptions of written media and audio and visual recordings from large academic institutions and publishers. Access to digital resources with the most up-to-date information was limited to affiliated parties, libraries, and individuals who could privately afford to purchase them. Consequently, access to digital health and medical information was primarily limited to trained healthcare providers (HCPs). Prior to the internet, patients were reliant on their HCPs to be their primary source of guidance for health and medical information and decision-making. However, rapid developments in the internet and communication technology in the last two decades have made information freely accessible and transformed the provider-patient relationship such that HCPs are today not only responsible for providing information but also for guiding their patients' search for and use of digital information.

Estimates from the United Nations and World Bank as of 2016 indicate that approximately half of the world population is using the internet, constituting nearly 3.5 billion users. As fewer than 5% of the world's population was using the internet two decades ago, this development represents unprecedented growth.[1] As both a freely accessible repository for information and a forum for the continuous discussion and development of new information in the form of websites, the internet is a vast universe of digital resources. In the United States, more than 80% of adults use the internet, nearly 75% of whom have used it to find health information in the past year; women are more likely than men to do so (79% vs. 65%).[2] With recent developments in mobile technology, the availability of digital health and medical information has never been greater. According to U.S. survey data from 2013, 85% of U.S. adults own a mobile phone and nearly one third of them have used their mobile phones to access digital health and medical information.[3] As of 2017, the majority of U.S. internet use was accessed via mobile technology and fueled by mobile-platform software applications, known as "apps."[4] These are transforming the landscape of digital resources to include not only a wider breadth of available information but also user-specific tools that directly influence patient health or help patients access healthcare.

1.2 The Impact of Digital Resources

Digital resources are convenient, portable, and economical. Computers are in almost every clinic room today and in almost every home. Smartphones contain web apps that are usually built as focused resources or as tools to help patients directly by reminding them to engage in specific health maintenance behaviors, tracking symptoms, or directing them to specific services. Nearly 1 in 5 smartphone users has at least one health-related app on her or his phone.[5]

The availability of these digital resources has the potential to empower the patient by increasing individual awareness of and access to health-related knowledge and services, which may contribute to the sense of autonomy needed to achieve true patient-centered care.[6] Given the quantity of information found on the internet and patients' ability to access this information both conveniently and anonymously (particularly with respect to sensitive topics such as reproductive and sexual health), patients commonly resort to digital resources first and prior to meeting with HCPs such that they are better able to have effective exchanges and make informed decisions.[7] Digital resources have transformed how healthcare is provided, moving towards a model of improved quality through informed choices and shared decision-making.[8,9] Additionally, digital resources serve as a tremendous tool for patients to continue to expand their knowledge after time-limited clinical encounters.

The amount of clinical research being published continues to grow at an increasing rate.[10] Healthcare providers are thus responsible for more information than ever and expected to constantly maintain up-to-date knowledge of medical evidence, healthcare policy, and professional guidelines. Fortunately, digital resources help HCPs maintain their expertise. Online digital resources provide clinicians with mobile, easily accessible, up-to-date, immediate answers to their patients' clinical questions. In developing countries, expanding access to digital resources has enabled academic physicians to train other HCPs, helping to address the global shortage of medical personnel and protecting the human right to health.

1.3 The Perils of Digital Resources

While the expansion of information technology has created a digital universe of medical resources, finding the most reliable resource with the right information can be a challenge. Increases in the volume of digital information may have the opposite effect of decreasing the chances of finding the most appropriate source of information in the least amount of time.[11] As there exists no restriction on the content that can be uploaded to the internet or on the types of apps that are developed for mobile phones, digital resources do not necessarily receive oversight from experts and can vary widely in their quality.[12] Unlike traditional print sources that have publishers and editors to ensure the quality of content, digital resources do not have the same controls. In a systematic review of 79 studies that examined the accuracy and utility of digital health resources found on the internet, nearly 75% of the studies expressed concerns regarding the quality of digital content.[13] While there are many high-quality digital resources available to consumers, there are arguably many more "resources" that represent anecdotal evidence, specific opinion, or commercial interest.

Furthermore, in a study examining how lay users searched for answers to specific health-related queries on the internet, users endorsed the importance of the credibility of their sources of information; however, in observations of their browsing practices, these users never examined the "About Us" sections of websites to verify credibility and, when interviewed, could not recall the sources from where they derived their health information.[14] Inexperienced or unguided users of digital resources may likely be met with frustration, misinformation, or incomplete information. Finally, social media platforms also increase the person-to-person passage of information. The interconnectedness of people through the internet means even more ways health information can be found, amplified, and distorted.[15]

While lay consumers of digital information and resources are at the greatest risk of encountering these issues, early learners in the medical field are also at risk, given reports that medical students frequently rely on digital resources for their learning.[16] Senior medical faculty have raised concerns about the ability of early learners to discern reputable from non-reputable sources,[17] which may ultimately have an impact on how students counsel and practice when they become HCPs.

While digital resources for health and medical information can be more comprehensive than those that can be provided by a HCP during a clinical encounter, these resources do not always relay how the information should be used or how it may fit into the context of a patient's condition or concern. For this reason, helping patients navigate the digital landscape plays a new but increasingly important role in the overall counseling that HCPs provide.

1.4 The Range of Digital Resources

The distinctions between websites and mobile apps are becoming increasingly blurred. Many professional organizations now offer the user the ability to subscribe and receive content updates via e-mail, as well as view content that is tailored to their specific interests. Additionally, several organizations have optimized their websites to be viewed on mobile phones, with others developing their own mobile health apps. Consequently, rather than divide the following resource guide by website and mobile health app, we will provide a directory of relevant resources linked to a professional organization, followed by a general description of the types of commercial resources currently available. The goal of including commercial resources is not to endorse any particular one but rather to ensure that readers are aware of the landscape of resources being accessed by their patients.

1.5 Digital Resources within Contraceptive Technology

As *Contraceptive Technology* is primarily a print publication, its content will remain static until the next edition. This section was thus written to address this problem and direct the reader to additional, credible digital resources (websites and mobile apps) and consensus organizations that are well accepted by healthcare professionals.

In this section, we also provide a list with guidance specific to the HCP audience of *Contraceptive Technology* and their patients in how to better navigate and use the expanse of digital health and medical resources. As more than 75% of patients will begin their search for health information by using popular search engines such as Google, Bing, or Yahoo, they may face difficulty in parsing out the most appropriate sources for their queries[2]. HCPs today should thus have a repository of useful digital resources. HCPs can then direct patients to these trusted sites or applications for further information.

Our list is neither exhaustive nor does it guarantee that listed sites will be regularly maintained or updated. While we strived to choose digital resources without commercial interests or undertones, some of these still may contain endorsement of specific branded products or services. This list does not mean to make any endorsements of anything other than the digital resources themselves. The information in this section is accurate only up to the time of this edition's publication.

2 DIGITAL RESOURCES FROM PROFESSIONAL GROUPS AND SOCIETIES**

2.1 Contraceptive Guidance for Health Care Providers from the CDC *iOS* (C) (www.cdc.gov/reproductivehealth/contraception/contraception_guidance.htm)

Digital resources listed with indication of intended audience as follows: **(C) clinicians, **(P)** patients, **(C, P)** for both clinicians and patients. Mobile app available on the following platforms: Android *iOS* Apple

The Centers for Disease Control and Prevention (CDC) is an essential resource for issues related to reproductive, maternal, and infant health. True to its name, CDC is also the first resource for clinical concerns regarding epidemics or outbreaks such as the Zika virus (www.cdc.gov/zika/index.html) and changes to clinical recommendations based upon changes in disease prevalence and antibiotic resistance, particularly in the case of sexually transmitted infections (www.cdc.gov/std/default.htm). Most pertinent to contraception, the CDC website has made digitally available in many formats their indispensable 2016 U.S. Medical Eligibility Criteria for Contraceptive Use (U.S. MEC) and 2016 U.S. Selected Practice Recommendations for Contraceptive Use (U.S. SPR). Full versions of the MEC and SPR, complete with clarification, comments, and evidence are available from this portal. In addition, the popular color-coded MEC charts and patient-centered effectiveness charts are downloadable from the website. The CDC has also released a user-friendly phone app (CDC Contraception) that is available for both iPhone and Android platforms. The MEC can be searched by condition or method with the app, while the SPR is organized by topic. This app is free to download and use.

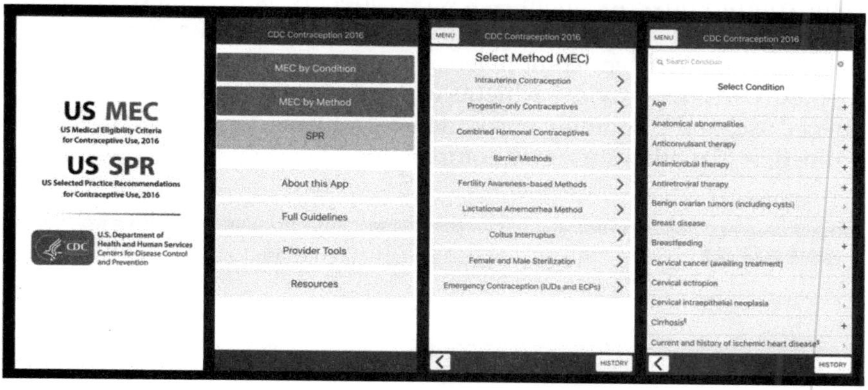

Of note, for patients who decline contraception, the CDC also offers a valuable online resource for preconception and reproductive life planning (www.cdc.gov/preconception/hcp/index.html). The website includes evidence-based recommendations for preconception counseling as well as reproductive life planning tools (www.cdc.gov/preconception/RLPtool.html) and informational resources that providers can print and offer directly to their patients.

2.2 STD Treatment Guidelines from the CDC *iOS* (C)

(www.cdc.gov/std/treatment) Clinicians providing reproductive health care will need the most up-to-date STI/STD treatment guidelines. While many HCPs may be familiar with the website, they may not always be at a computer on which to browse the site, or they may find the site too cumbersome for the procurement of quick algorithms for treatment. Fortunately, the CDC has also developed a free mobile app (CDC STD Tx Guide) for download as well. It has a very simple interface and is easy to use.

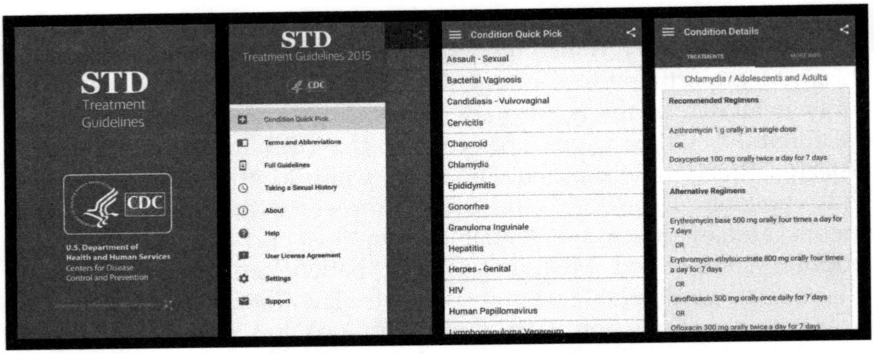

2.3 Bedsider (www.bedsider.org) (C,P)

If you have a patient who wants information about choosing the right contraceptive for them, www.bedsider.org is a visually engaging, patient-centered website full of interactive, informative features that provide simplified yet comprehensive answers. For each contraceptive method, Bedsider provides patients with information on efficacy, cost, side effects, use, and commonly encountered problems. Unique to Bedsider is a function that allows users to compare methods side-by-side, stratifying

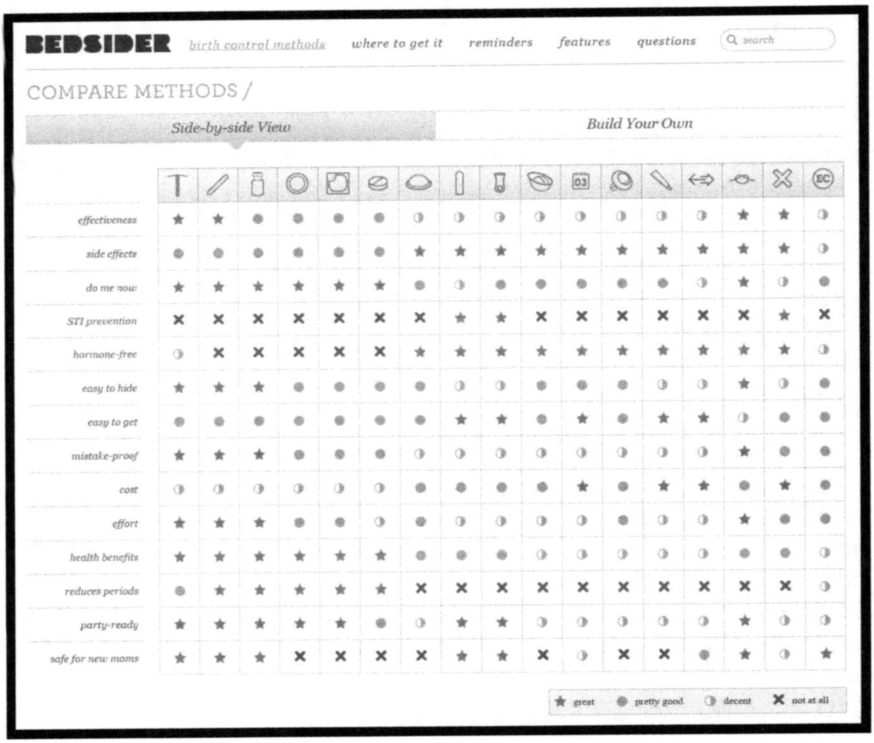

											03						EC
effectiveness	★	★	●	●	●	●	◑	◑	◑	◑	◑	◑	◑	◑	★	★	◑
side effects	●	●	●	●	●	●	★	★	★	★	★	★	★	★	★	★	◑
do me now	★	★	★	★	★	★	●	◑	●	●	●	●	●	◑	★	◑	●
STI prevention	✕	✕	✕	✕	✕	✕	✕	★	★	✕	✕	✕	✕	✕	✕	★	✕
hormone-free	◑	✕	✕	✕	✕	✕	★	★	★	★	★	★	★	★	★	★	◑
easy to hide	★	★	★	●	●	●	●	◑	◑	●	●	●	◑	◑	★	◑	●
easy to get	●	●	●	●	●	●	●	★	★	●	★	●	★	★	◑	●	●
mistake-proof	★	★	★	●	●	●	◑	◑	◑	◑	◑	◑	◑	◑	★	●	●
cost	◑	◑	◑	◑	◑	◑	●	●	●	●	★	●	★	★	●	★	●
effort	★	★	★	●	●	◑	●	◑	◑	◑	◑	●	◑	◑	★	●	●
health benefits	★	★	★	★	★	★	●	●	●	◑	◑	◑	◑	◑	●	●	◑
reduces periods	●	★	★	★	★	★	✕	✕	✕	✕	✕	✕	✕	✕	✕	✕	◑
party-ready	★	★	★	★	★	●	◑	★	★	◑	◑	◑	◑	◑	★	◑	◑
safe for new moms	★	★	★	✕	✕	✕	✕	★	★	✕	◑	✕	✕	●	★	◑	★

★ great ● pretty good ◑ decent ✕ not at all

for multiple characteristics that may be important to a potential user. Beyond information about contraceptives, Bedsider also includes articles about contraceptive behavior pertinent to both men and women. The site includes multimedia video "stories" from real users of the method describing their experiences, as well as blog posts, articles, and humorous, informational videos. While Bedsider does not have a mobile app, it offers users the opportunity to create a user account and connect to other followers of Bedsider on social media outlets such as Facebook and Twitter. Bedsider is a digital resource developed by the National Campaign to Prevent Teen and Unplanned Pregnancy (now called Power to Decide), a private non-profit organization. Bedsider content is approved by the Medical Advisory Committee of the National Campaign to Prevent Teen and Unplanned Pregnancy and receives no funding from pharmaceutical companies or the government.

2.4 The Agency for Healthcare Research & Quality (www.ahrq.gov/) *iOS* (C)

As family planning is considered to be an essential component of preventative healthcare, its provision is often paired with the provision of other preventive health services. The most up-to-date guidelines are located on the Agency for Healthcare Research and Quality's (AHRQ) website. The AHRQ works within the U.S. Department of Health and Human Services and links to the U.S. Preventative Services Task Force (USPSTF) guidelines. Additionally, the site is connected to the National Guidelines Clearinghouse, a centralized repository of guidelines from national and international health organizations. While the website is a comprehensive repository, users may find it difficult to find a streamlined set of practice guidelines. In such an event, users may be recommended their mobile health app, the Electronic Preventative Services Selector (ePPS). This app is available for both Apple and Android platforms and allows HCPs

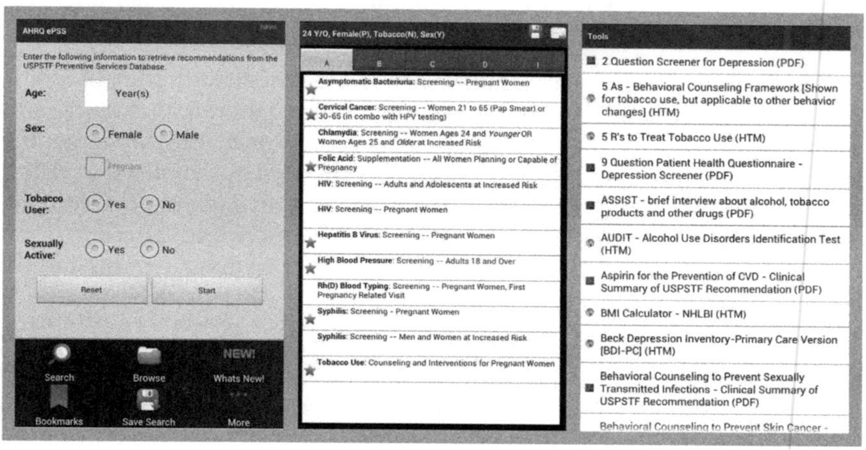

to search and browse recommendations multiple ways. Additionally, the guidelines can be accessed offline once downloaded, making it a valuable resource for rural primary care providers.

2.5 Family Planning National Training Center (www.fpntc.org & www.ctcfp.org) iOS (C)

The Family Planning National Training Center (FPNTC) and Clinical Training Center for Family Planning (CTCFP) are separate websites that have similar, but not identical, resources. They are clinical training resources in family planning supported by the Office of Population Affairs (OPA). The sites are a treasure trove of resources for HCPs and clinic administrators regarding provision of high quality, efficient, family planning services. In addition to the sites, they have a counseling app (Quality Family Planning, QFP) for HCPs with categorized counseling tools for both women and men seeking reproductive, preventative health services.

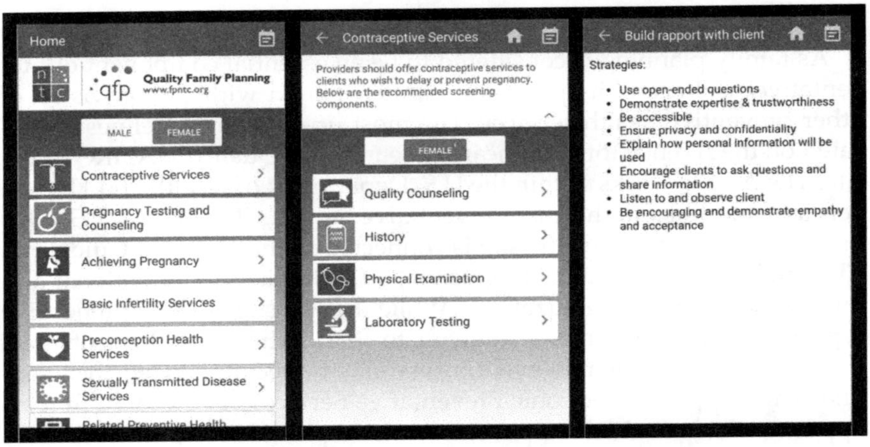

2.6 American Society for Colposcopy and Cervical Pathology iOS (C) (www.asccp.org)

The American Society for Colposcopy and Cervical Pathology (ASCCP) is a non-profit specialty society dedicated to education and training surrounding the treatment of cervical-related cancers and other lower genital tract disorders. Its website offers invaluable practice guidelines that reflect the rapidly changing guidelines surrounding the screening, treatment, and expectant management of patients due to recent advances in HPV testing and vaccination. The website is also a portal for one of the largest sources of training in colposcopy.

Of greatest value, however, is the mobile app developed by the ASCCP, which is available for both Apple and Android platforms. The mobile app is indispensable to any women's healthcare primary provider, as it distills unwieldly guidelines into a specific management plan based upon the patient's risk factors and screening/pathologic findings, including recommendations for follow up. As of this section's publication date, users had to pay $9.99 in order to download the app.

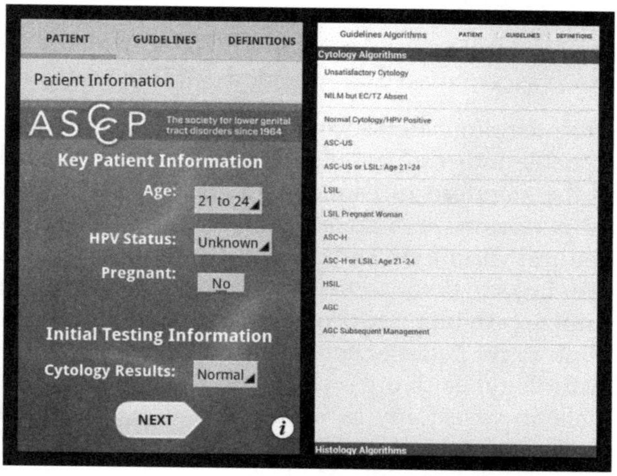

2.7 The Emergency Contraception Website (C, P) (ec.princeton.edu/emergency-contraception.html or http://not-2-late.com)

Once a static digital resource for determining an appropriate *Yuzpe* dose for use as emergency contraception, this non-profit site started by Dr. James Trussell now serves as an excellent resource for EC-related info for both providers and patients. The site still provides the recommended Yuzpe dose by pill brand, but in addition, now also has a thorough FAQ section, information on how to procure EC for patients (as well as links to bedsider.org for finding prescribing HCPs), and even an "ask the expert" section where patients who still have unanswered questions may submit them by email to be answered by an EC expert.

2.8 The American College of Obstetricians and Gynecologists (ACOG) website (www.acog.org) *iOS* (C, P)

The American College of Obstetricians and Gynecologists is known for putting out the guidelines that serve as the standard of care for general Obstetrician-Gynecologists. In addition to the well-known, periodically released and updated *Practice Guidelines* and *Committee Opinions*, ACOG offers a number of Patient Education FAQs on topics including postpartum sterilization, sterilization for men and women, emergency contraception, hysteroscopic sterilization, LARC, and many others (www.acog.org/Patients). Extensive advice regarding coding can be found there as well. Many of the materials do not require membership, but some sections of the ACOG website require membership login for access, such as the practice bulletins which guide the practice of many Obstetrician-Gynecologists. ACOG provides a free app on both Android and Apple mobile platforms.

The app allows users to receive up-to-date information valuable for clinical practice, as well as information on national and local meetings. The app also includes an Estimated Due Date Calculator for pregnancy, based on guidance from ACOG.

2.9 The American Urological Association (AUA) website (www.auanet.org/guidelines/vasectomy-(2012-amended-2015) *iOS* (C, P)

The American Urological Association (AUA) website offers a freely accessible, searchable index of frequently updated professional guidelines that serve as the standard of care for urological practice, including the provision and performance of male sterilization or vasectomy. Given significant procedural variations in vasectomy among providers, the posted guidelines offer links to detailed to discussions on best practices and techniques to optimize provider performance. The AUA website also provides a direct weblink to its patient-centered foundation, Urology Care Foundation (www.urologyhealth.org), which provides printable patient education materials on vasectomy as well as a podcast that interviews men choosing to undergo vasectomy. The AUA offers providers a free app on both Android and Apple mobile platforms, which may be useful for accessing and browsing practice guidelines.

2.10 The World Health Organization (WHO): Programme in Sexual and Reproductive Health (www.who.int/reproductivehealth/publications/family_planning/en) (C)

For those who are have more internationally focused practice questions, the WHO puts out their version of the MEC and SPR online in their contraceptive portal. While they do not have the visually intuitive charts that the CDC makes, they do have resources in both Spanish and French. More important, the latest WHO statements and guidelines are found online in multiple languages and updated frequently.

2.11 GirlsHealth.Gov (girlshealth.gov/know-the-facts-first/index.html) (P)

Developed by the Office on Women's Health under the U.S. Department of Health and Human Services, GirlsHealth.gov is a website offering guidance to teenage girls, providing information about their bodies, facts on sex and STDs, ways to protect oneself from risky sexual behaviors, and how to negotiate relationships. Many of these topics are presented in colorful, interactive activities; however, the site itself is difficult to navigate, as one of its most valuable functionalities, the STD testing site locator, is located at the bottom of the page.

2.12 Planned Parenthood Federation of America *iOS* (P) (www.plannedparenthood.org/)

Planned Parenthood is one of the nation's leading providers of family planning services. Its webpage serves as a place where patients can connect to clinical services and chat and text with live experts until almost midnight, Eastern Standard Time. Planned Parenthood invites users to ask questions about issues ranging from missed pills and unprotected intercourse to sexually transmitted infections. Live experts are trained to provide factual answers but not provide diagnoses. Planned Parenthood also offers a mobile app on both Apple and Android platforms, which goes beyond providing information to allowing users to order birth control from their phone for users in some states. Additionally, functions are being developed to allow the treatment of UTIs and for the procurement of at-home STD testing kits. Users can obtain face-to-face, online consultations with HCPs. While the app is free to download, actual medical services obtained via the app are paid for upon linkage with and verification of the user's health insurance plan.

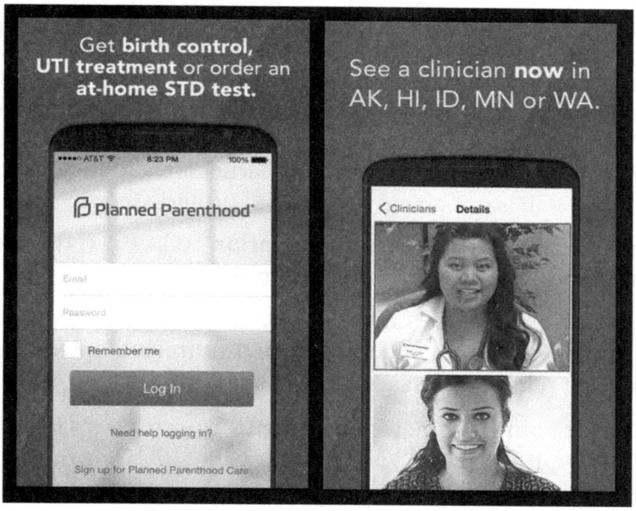

(www.plannedparenthood.org/teens)

Providing up-to-date, clear, and medically accurate information, the Planned Parenthood for Teens website helps young people of all gender identities to better understand their sexual health. It has nice crisp webpage and delves into adolescent topics such as sexting, bullying, and LGBTQ issues.

(www.plannedparenthood.org/learn/birth-control/birth-control-pill)

Given concerns about misinformation and the complexity of information found online surrounding correct use of the birth control pill, Planned Parenthood has developed a website with video instruction and answers to frequently asked questions and concerns regarding pill use.

2.13 National Domestic Violence Hotline (www.ndvh.org) (P)

The preponderance of intimate partner violence and reproductive coercion among women being seen in a family planning clinic setting has been well-established; HCPs should be routinely screening patients for the possibility of their partner being a source of abuse whether it be physical, sexual, psychological, or financial. Additionally, HCPs should screen for reproductively coercive behaviors such as tampering with contraceptive pills or unwillingness to consistently use condoms. HCPs should be prepared to offer resources such as the website for the National Domestic Violence Hotline, which offers information on how to contact them by phone or via a discreet online chat interface. Advocates are available for callers 24 hours a day, 7 days per week.

2.14 The Office of Population Affairs (C) (www.hhs.gov/opa)

The Office of Population Affairs (OPA) administers the Title X program, the federal program dedicated to the provision of family planning and other reproductive health services. While the site has basic information and links to information on family planning, it also has a search bar for finding the closest Title X clinic, which may be useful for HCPs looking for a place where their patients may obtain contraception, particularly long-acting reversible methods if the HCP is not already trained to provide them.

2.15 American Sexual Health Association (C, P) (www.ashasexualhealth.org/sexual-health/teens-and-young-adults)

This association provides a wealth of resources on sexual health for both men and women, and specific resources directed at teens and young adults. This is a relatively basic site with static content.

2.16 Center for Young Women's Health and Young Men's Health (Boston Children's Hospital) (http://youngwomenshealth.org and http://youngmenshealthsite.org) (P)

These websites provide information for adolescents, including guides on a variety of sexual health topics such as contraception, STIs, LGBT health, and puberty.

2.17 Go Ask Alice! (www.goaskalice.columbia.edu) (C)

Geared at young adults, this question-and-answer website contains a large database of questions about a variety of reproductive and sexual health concerns.

2.18 The Guttmacher Institute (C) (www.guttmacher.org/united-states/contraception)

For those seeking more epidemiological or policy-focused information on contraception and abortion, the Guttmacher institute produces continuously updated fact sheets and articles on contraceptive usage, contraceptive coverage, and regulations surrounding contraceptive provision in the US.

3 DIGITAL RESOURCES FROM COMMERCIAL GROUPS

The market for digital health apps is enormous and continually expanding. A 2015 survey conducted by the Institute for Healthcare Informatics found over 165,000 healthcare-related apps across both Apple and Android platforms. Of nearly 100,000 health apps available through Apple, 7% were relevant to women's health and pregnancy.[19] The potential for mobile apps to improve patient education and care is well-recognized by HCPs who desire to promote the use of apps. However, there is currently a lack of expertise and resources with which to make evidence-based, unbiased, commercial-free referrals to apps that may be clinically useful to patients and healthcare providers. While the Apple platform requires a certification process for content and functionality, the Android platform does no quality screening. Consequently, some apps exist in the online stores that claim to be able to determine when a woman ovulated, independent of her cycle, and others claim to be able to determine the gender of a woman's pregnancy as influenced by her date of conception.[20] Additionally, many of the apps on both platforms are developed by groups with profit interests. These groups may not be advised by a professional committee from the healthcare field, and their apps may not have been validated by such a committee. These apps often cost the user money to download; those that are free are commonly subject the user to advertisements. For these reasons, we will not be discussing apps individually but instead describing the landscape of apps according to categories relevant to contraceptive technology to make HCPs aware of resources that are accessible to patients. Examples of apps listed do not serve as any endorsement of the app.

3.1 Menstrual cycle and fertility tracking

Menstrual tracking apps tend to be marketed by their ability to inform the user about one of two conditions that are based upon the same physiological premise: (1) fertility tracking apps to notify users when intercourse is optimal for conception and (2) contraceptive apps to notify users of the days when intercourse is less likely to lead to pregnancy. According to one survey, more than half of women initiating contraception report tracking their menses.[21] Menstrual cycle tracking apps are the fourth most popular health app among adults and the second most popular health app among adolescent females.[22] While many are free, most charge a small fee ($0.99 to $9.99). Some of these apps (e.g., Clue) market themselves as a form of "nonhormonal" contraception and have substantial commercial financial backing. Given the uptake of these apps, one group conducted a survey of available menstrual tracking apps in 2016, finding more than 225 apps. Fewer than 20 of these apps were accurate, and only 5% of them had ever involved a professional health care consultant or cited any medical literature. Most available apps simply did not function as advertised or contained misleading information or misinformation. To provide an accurate assessment, menstrual tracking apps should require the user to collect data over multiple cycles and account for several other factors that may have an impact on a user's cycling. As a result, the authors of the survey concluded that apps could not be a primary tool for assisting with conception or contraception without the oversight of a HCP.[23,24] To date only one app appears to have a validation study of any kind (Natural Cycles),[25] and another is currently under way.[26]

Despite their shortcomings, tracking apps are more than fancy, pixelated alternatives to traditional cycle beads. A few theoretical advantages include the following features:

3.1.1 Sophisticated tracking mechanisms

While traditional fertility predicting methods rely on a cycle length within a fairly normal range, some apps use proprietary algorithms to provide unique fertility predictions based on user-provided data. Some use additional inputs such as data from a thermometer (e.g., Natural Cycles, Kindara) and user reports of cervical mucus (e.g., Ovia). Others integrate data from multiple user inputs (e.g., Glow) as well as provide fertility recommendations for women using birth control (e.g., Clue). Nevertheless, almost none of the technological claims has a validating study and all of these apps ultimately come from a place of commercial interest (Glow for example has an IVF function that facilitates consultation with a reproductive endocrinologist and claims that IVF cycles are cheaper through Glow).

3.1.2 Push alerts

Unlike Cycle Beads (see Chapter 12 on Fertility Awareness-Based Methods), apps not only automatically advance daily, but they can send notifications to patients of "at risk days." What apps cannot do is prevent women from having intercourse on "fertile" days, and in fact, in the single validation study that is available, 51% of women logged unprotected intercourse during a day she was at risk for pregnancy.[25]

3.2 Symptom tracking

For practitioners working with patients who experience menstrual-cycle-related health conditions, apps provide an opportunity for patients to keep a digital diary. Many fertility tracking apps also allow patients to record their bleeding pattern over time (e.g., Kindara, Clue, SpotOn). This feature can help patients track symptoms to help distinguish between heavy menstrual bleeding and intercycle bleeding for diagnostic purposes, assess the quantity of bleeding the patient is experiencing, and assess the effectiveness of treatments. Some apps are also available to track additional symptoms such as painful periods, mood-related symptoms, headaches, and pelvic pain. From these apps, HCPs can evaluate the cyclicity of symptoms prior to contraception as well as the frequency of symptoms after contraceptive initiation, whether for treatment or for monitoring side effects. Variants of these apps are marketed toward specific conditions such as menopause (e.g., Menopause View) and endometriosis (e.g., Futter).

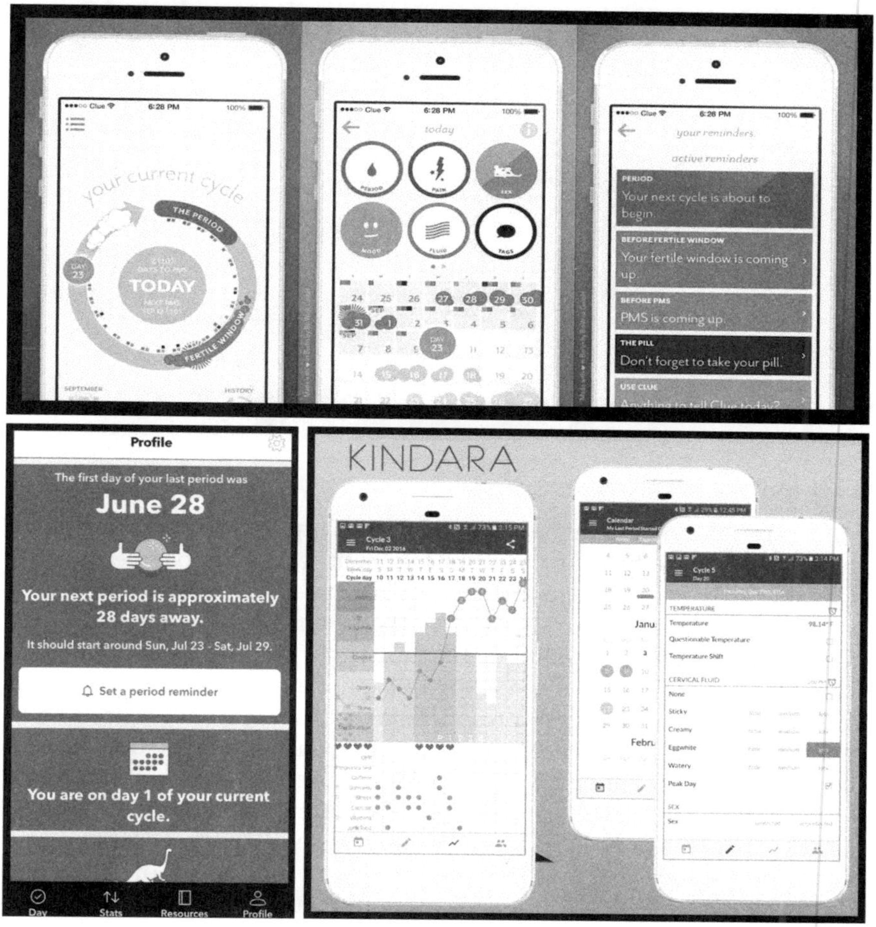
your current cycle
THE PERIOD
TODAY
FERTILE WINDOW
today
your reminders
active reminders
PERIOD
Your next cycle is about to begin.
BEFORE FERTILE WINDOW
Your fertile window is coming up.
BEFORE PMS
PMS is coming up.
THE PILL
Don't forget to take your pill.
USE CLUE
Profile
The first day of your last period was
June 28
Your next period is approximately 28 days away.
It should start around Sun, Jul 23 - Sat, Jul 29.
Set a period reminder
You are on day 1 of your current cycle.
Day
Stats
Resources
Profile
KINDARA

3.3 Birth control/Pill reminders

After fertility tracking, this is the second most prevalent app type available.[27] There are some dedicated reminder apps (e.g., Bedsider Birth Control Reminders), which are essentially glorified calendar alarms. However, they do allow the user to input which short-acting method (e.g., pills, patches, shots, or rings) is used and then tailor the reminder to the recommended dosing schedule. For the most part, this is also a functionality built into many of the fertility trackers apps (e.g., Spot On, Planned Parenthood).

No validation studies of reminder apps have been done to date. However, a well-conducted RCT of a daily text-message reminder did not improve pill adherence.[28] It remains unclear if adherence would be improved with a better designed app that provides back-up alarms and task management software to establish routines and confirm task completion.[29]

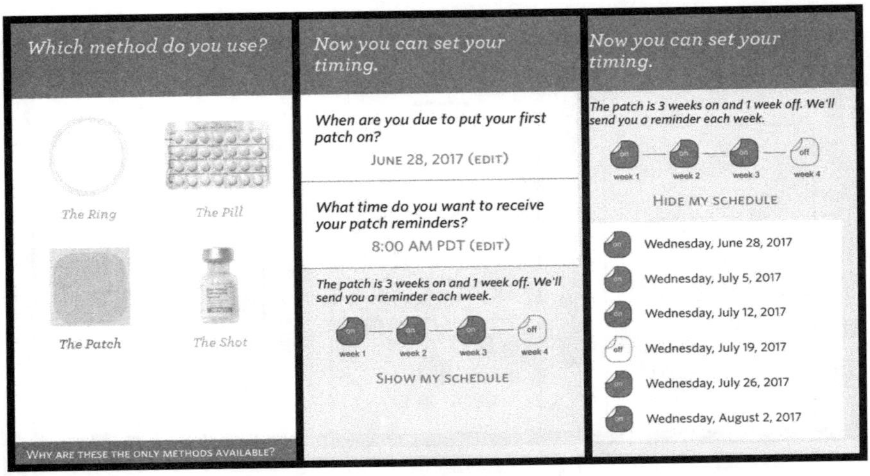

3.4 Contraception Delivery Apps

Contraception on demand has taken on a whole new definition in the digital age. At the time of this publication, at least 10 apps/websites are available (e.g., Nurx, Lemonaid, Pandia) that offer contraceptive prescriptions without having users leave their home. Via the apps, patients go through a health screening either through a tele-visit (e.g., Skype) or through answering a brief screening questionnaire. Then, for a small fee, patients receive an electronic prescription that they can have sent to a designated pharmacy for pickup. Some services will even provide the medication directly to patients via the postal service. There are some useful variations on this theme. For example, the Planned Parenthood Care app allows patients to order tests for STI testing, Nurx allows patients to obtain both contraceptive pills and HIV pre-exposure prophylaxis (or PrEP), and Maven allows patients to book a tele-appointment for other kinds of counseling related to women's health issues. Some accept the patient's insurance for billing purposes, while others do not but will provide the patient with a low-cost, generic alternative where possible. One drawback is the state-by-state availability of such services. At the time of writing, no site covered more than 20 states although all claimed "more states coming" on their respective websites. As states update their tele-medicine laws related to consent, licensure, prescribing, and reimbursement (as of 2017, only two states lacked tele-medicine reimbursement policies: Connecticut and Rhode Island), this particular type of digital resource will likely expand.

While these apps offer a convenient way to obtain a specific reproductive health services, they do not supplant encounters with reproductive specialists or the patient's primary HCP who may better contextualize all of a patient's medical issues and needs through counseling and who can place a contraceptive implant or an intrauterine device.

3.5 Pregnancy Test Apps

Multiple apps on the market currently claim to function as pregnancy tests. While most have a disclaimer that there is no medical basis for the app or that it is to be used only as a joke or prank, not all of them are labeled clearly. To date, there is no known app for any platform that can determine if a woman is pregnant.

4 CONCLUSION AND FUTURE DIRECTIONS

The amount of digital information available to HCPs today is unprecedented and is expected to continue to grow. Nevertheless, continued increases in the number of available resources may not translate into effective knowledge if the sources do not control for quality. Many of the resources listed in *Contraceptive Technology* represent sources that we believe will continue to be maintained by professional organizations and thus be updated to reflect the most current knowledge. However, it is impossible to overemphasize the turnover speed of the web. In writing this Appendix, the authors saw numerous examples of news articles profiling "hot" websites, apps or digital services that no longer existed at the time of writing. With respect to mobile health applications, we discussed many of the shortcomings of currently available technology; however, we do so to point out a gap in having medical professionals and HCPs involved in the guidance of using these resources. It is our hope that this resource becomes a springboard for HCPs to collaborate with patients in the digital space.

Author Disclosures—Nguyen: none. Han: none.

References

1. Internet Live Stats. Number of Internet users (2016). www.internetlivestats.com/internet-users/. Accessed Sep 20, 2017.
2. Fox S, Duggan M. Health online 2013. Washington, DC: Pew Internet & American Life Project. www.pewinternet.org/2013/01/15/health-online-2013/#. Accessed Sep 20, 2017.
3. Fox S, Duggan M. Information triage. Pew Research Center. Pew Research Internet Project. www.pewinternet.org/2013/01/15/information-triage/. Accessed Sep 20, 2017.
4. Lella A, Lipsman A. The 2017 US mobile app report. comScore. www.comscore.com/Insights/Presentations-and-Whitepapers/2017/The-2017-US-Mobile-App-Report. Accessed Sep 20, 2017.

5. Fox S, Duggan M. Mobile health 2012. Pew internet and American life project. www.pewinternet.org/2012/11/08/mobile-health-2012/. Accessed Sep 20, 2017
6. Clarke MA, Moore JL, Steege LM, et al. Health information needs, sources, and barriers of primary care patients to achieve patient-centered care: A literature review. Health Inform J 2016;22:992–1016.
7. Rupert DJ, Gard Read J, Amoozegar JB, et al. Peer-Generated Health Information: The role of online communities in patient and caregiver health decisions. J Health Commun 2016;21:1187–1197.
8. Ziebland S, Powell J, Briggs P, et al. Examining the role of patients' experiences as a resource for choice and decision-making in health care: a creative, interdisciplinary mixed-method study in digital health. Programme Grants for Applied Research 2016;4:1–214.
9. McMullan M. Patients using the Internet to obtain health information: how this affects the patient–health professional relationship. Patient Educ Couns 2006;63:24–8.
10. Larsen PO, Von Ins M. The rate of growth in scientific publication and the decline in coverage provided by Science Citation Index. Scientometrics 2010;84:575–603.
11. Damman OC, Hendriks M, Rademakers J, Delnoij DM, and Groenewegen PP. How do healthcare consumers process and evaluate comparative healthcare information? A qualitative study using cognitive interviews. BMC Pub Health 2009;9:423.
12. Hirsch M, Aggarwal S, Barker C, Davis CJ, and Duffy JM. Googling endometriosis: a systematic review of information available on the Internet. Am J Obstet Gynecol 2016;216:451–458.
13. Eysenbach G, Powell J, Kuss O, and Sa ER. Empirical studies assessing the quality of health information for consumers on the world wide web: a systematic review. JAMA 2002;287:2691–700.
14. Eysenbach G, Kohler C. How do consumers search for and appraise health information on the world wide web? Qualitative study using focus groups, usability tests, and in-depth interviews. BMJ 2002;324:573–7.
15. Wilson K, Keelan J. Social media and the empowering of opponents of medical technologies: the case of anti-vaccinationism. J Med Internet Res 2013;15:e103.
16. Prasannan L, Gabbur N, Haughton M. Use of web resources among medical students at a large urban medical center. Obstet Gynecol 2014;123:118S.
17. Implementing digital resources for clinicians' and patients' varying needs. Med Inform Internet Med 2005;30:107–22.
18. Kazmerski T, McCauley HL, Jones K, Borrero S, Silverman JG, Decker MR, et al. Use of reproductive and sexual health services among female family planning clinic clients exposed to partner violence and reproductive coercion. Matern Child Hlth J 2015;19:1490–6.
19. Quintiles IMS. Patient Adoption of mHealth. Report by the IMS Institute for Healthcare Informatics, 2015. www.imshealth.com/files/web/IMSH%20Institute/Reports/Patient%20Adoption%20of%20mHealth/IIHI-Patient-Adoption-mhealth-Exhibits-Full.pdf. Accessed Sep 20, 2017.
20. Boulos MNK, Brewer AC, Karimkhani C, Buller DB, Dellavalle RP. Mobile medical and health apps: state of the art, concerns, regulatory control and certification. OJPHI 2014;5:229.
21. Nippita S, Oviedo JD, Velasco MG, Westhoff CL, Davis AR, Castaño PM. A randomized controlled trial of daily text messages versus monthly paper diaries to collect bleeding data after intrauterine device insertion. Contraception 2015;92:578–584.
22. Wartella E, Rideout V, Montague H, Beaudoin-Ryan L, Lauricella A. Teens, health and technology: A national survey. Media and Communication 2016;4:13–23.
23. Moglia ML, Nguyen HV, Chyjek K, Chen KT, Castaño PM. Evaluation of smartphone menstrual cycle tracking applications using an adapted APPLICATIONS scoring system. Obstet Gynecol 2016;127:1153–1160.
24. Duane M, Contreras A, Jensen ET, White A. The performance of fertility awareness-based method apps marketed to avoid pregnancy. J Am Board Fam Med 2016;29:508–511.

25. Berglund Scherwitzl E, Gemzell Danielsson K, Sellberg JA, and Scherwitzl R. Fertility awareness-based mobile application for contraception. Eur J Contracep Repr Health Care 2016;21:234–241.
26. Simmons RG, Shattuck DC, Jennings VH. Assessing the efficacy of an app-based method of family planning: the Dot Study Protocol. JMIR research protocols 2017;6:e5.
27. Mangone ER, Lebrun V, and Muessig KE. Mobile phone apps for the prevention of unintended pregnancy: a systematic review and content analysis. JMIR mHealth uHealth 2016;4:e6.
28. Hou MY, Hurwitz S, Kavanagh E, Fortin J, and Goldberg AB. Using daily text-message reminders to improve adherence with oral contraceptives: a randomized controlled trial. Obstet Gynecol 2010;116:633–640.
29. Stawarz K, Cox AL, Blandford A. Don't forget your pill!: designing effective medication reminder apps that support users' daily routines. In Proceedings of the 32nd annual ACM conference on Human factors in computing systems, 2014.

Index

A

B

C

D

E

F

G

H

I

J

K

L

M

N

O

P

Q

R

S

T

U

V

W

X

Y

Z

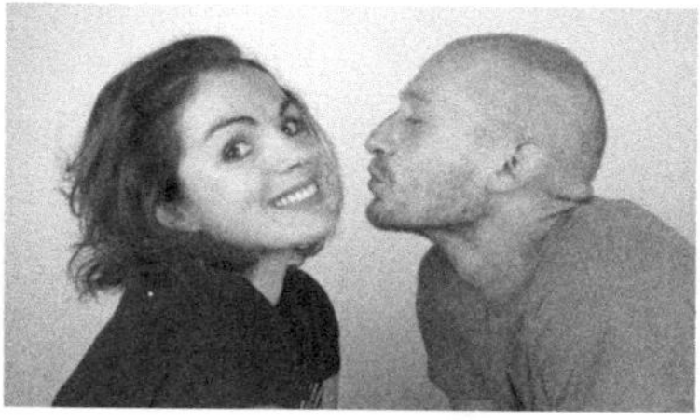

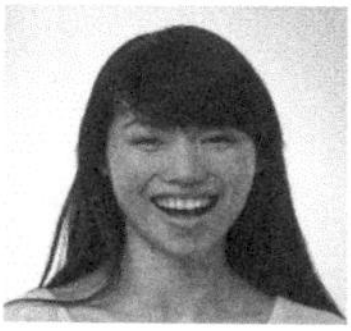

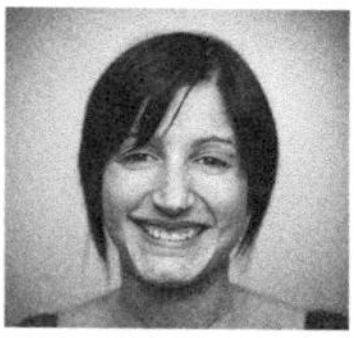

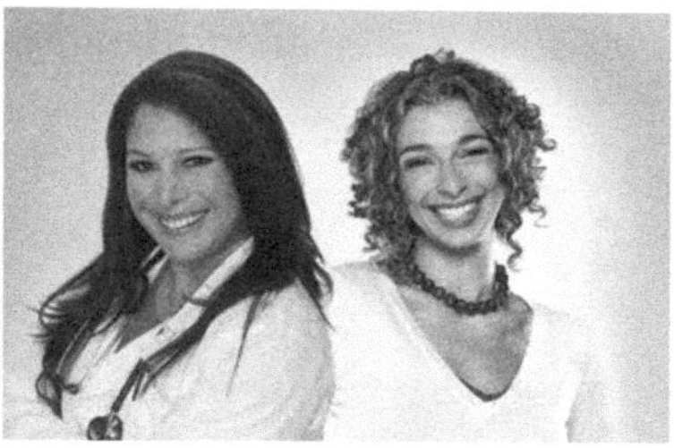

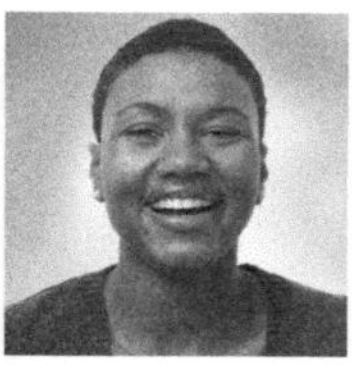

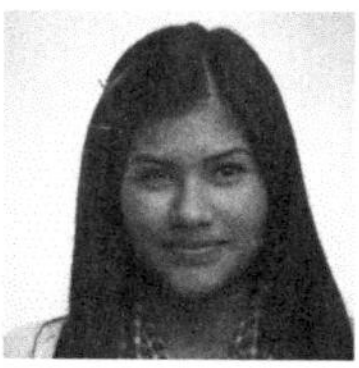

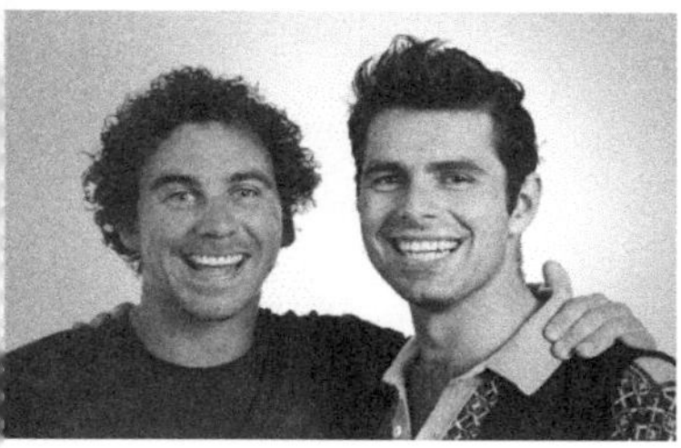

Contraception Options Chart

Front

Back

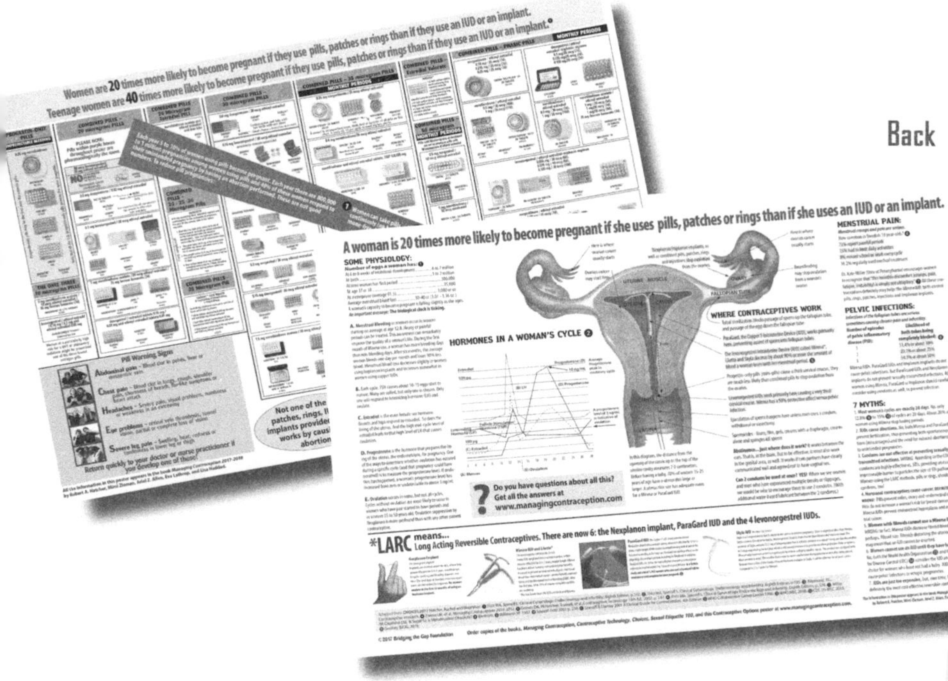

This large 24"X36" chart is printed and laminated both sides.

One side shows all the birth control pills from the lowest to the highest dosages. Great for the clinician determining which pill to prescribe and also very helpful for the patient that can't remember the name of the pill she is taking but can identify the package.

The other side shows **ALL** the contraceptive methods with emphasis on the LARC METHODS (Long Acting Reversible Contraceptives). It has an illustration of the uterus showing where and how contraceptives work. There is also an illustration of an IUD placement and MUCH MUCH MORE!!!

GREAT TEACHING TOOL!!!

To order copies go to
managingcontraception.com
email info@managingcontraception.com call 404 875 5001
Or use **order form** in back of this book

ORDER FORM

For quick and easy online ordering, visit
ContraceptiveTechnology21st.com

BY MAIL:
Managing Contraception, LLC
PO Box 79299
Atlanta, GA 30357

BY FAX:
(404) 875-5030

BY PHONE:
(404) 875-5001

ORDERED BY

Name ____________________ Title ____________________
Organization ____________________
Address ____________________
City ____________________ State ____________ Zip ____________
E-mail Address ____________________
Phone ____________________ Fax ____________________

SHIP TO (Only if different from Ordered By)

Name ____________________ Title ____________________
Organization ____________________
Address ____________________
City ____________________ State ____________ Zip ____________
Phone ____________________ E-mail Address ____________________

Item Code #	Description	Qty.	Price Ea.	Item Total
4004	New Sexual Ettiquette 101 & More			
3007	Managing Contraception 14th Edition			
5100	Choices English			
5000	Choices Spanish			
6405	Contraceptive Option Chart (24"x 36")			
6410	Mini Contraceptive Option Charts (25 per pack)			
9019	Contraceptive Technology 20th Edition			
9040	Contraceptive Technology 21st Ed. (Paperback)			
9042	Contraceptive Technology 21st Edition (Hardback)			
9045	Contraceptive Technology 21st Edition (EBook)			

Payment Method:

☐ MasterCard ☐ VISA ☐ Discover
☐ American Express ☐ Check
☐ Purchase Order #____________________
(For Organizations Only)

* Credit Card Number:
____
* Expiration Date ____________________
* Security Code ____________________
* Signature ____________________
* Name on Card ____________________
* Billing Address on Card ____________________
____
* Phone ________ ____________________

***REQUIRED**

Merchandise Subtotal: ____________

GA Sales Tax (7%)
(For GA Shipments only) ____________

Subtotal ____________

*Shipping (Add 18%)
or ask for quote ____________

TOTAL $____________

*International Shipping: Alaska, Hawaii, Puerto Rico, Canada and all others not in the 48 contiguous United States, call for shipping prices.
Prices valid until superceded by subsequent publication.

Thank You for Your Order!

www.ManagingContraception.com

Summer 201